The Risk Assessment of Environmental and Human Health Hazards: A Textbook of Case Studies

The Risk Assessment of Environmental and Human Health Hazards: A Textbook of Case Studies

Edited by

DENNIS J. PAUSTENBACH
ChemRisk™ Division, McLaren Environmental Engineering, Alameda, California

WILEY

A WILEY-INTERSCIENCE PUBLICATION
JOHN WILEY & SONS
New York · Chichester · Brisbane · Toronto · Singapore

Library of Congress Cataloging in Publication Data:

The Risk assessment of environmental hazards/edited by Dennis J.
    Paustenbach.
        p.   cm.
    "A Wiley-Interscience publication."
    Includes index.
    ISBN 0-471-84998-7
    1. Health risk assessment. 2. Environmental health.
3. Pollution.   I. Paustenbach, Dennis J.

RA427.3.R57 1989
363. 1 –dc 19   87-35056
                                                                      CIP
Printed in the United States of America

10 9 8 7 6 5 4 3 2

Contributors

CARL L. ALDEN, The Proctor & Gamble Company, Miami Valley Laboratories, Cincinnati, Ohio

BRUCE N. AMES, Department of Biochemistry, University of California, Berkeley, California

MELVIN E. ANDERSEN, Biochemical Toxicology Branch, Armstrong Aerospace Medical Research Laboratories, Wright–Patterson Air Force Base, Ohio

ROBERT L. ANDERSON, The Proctor & Gamble Company, Miami Valley Laboratories, Cincinnati, Ohio

ANGELA D. ARMS, Health and Safety Research Divison Oak Ridge National Laboratory, Oak Ridge, Tennessee

WILLIAM E. BISHOP, The Proctor & Gamble Company, Environmental Safety Department, Ivorydale Technical Center, Cincinnati, Ohio

SCOTT BOUTWELL, Dames and Moore, San Jose, California

SUSAN M. BRETT, Environ Corporation, Washington, DC

JAMES L. BYARD, James L. Byard and Associates, Toxicology Consultant, Inc., E1 Macero, California

HARVEY J. CLEWELL III, Biochemical Toxicology Branch, Armstrong Aerospace Medical Research Laboratories, Wright–Patterson Air Force Base, Ohio

BERNARD L. COHEN, Department of Physics, University of Pittsburgh, Pittsburgh, Pennsylvania

LOUIS ANTHONY COX, Jr., U.S. West Advanced Technologies, Englewood, Colorado

DAVID W. CRAWFORD, Envirologic Data Corporation, Portland, Maine

MELISSA DUBINSKY, International Technology Corporation, Oak Ridge, Tennessee

R. C. GAMMAGE, Health and Safety Research Division, Oak Ridge National Laboratory, Oak Ridge, Tennessee

LISA C. GANDY, National Hazardous Materials Training Center, Division of Interdisciplinary Toxicology, University of Arkansas for Medical Sciences, Little Rock, Arkansas

MICHAEL L. GARGAS, Biochemical Toxicology Branch, Armstrong Aerospace Medical Research Laboratories, Wright–Patterson Air Force Base, Ohio

LOIS SWIRSKY GOLD, Biology and Medicine Division, Lawrence Berkeley Laboratory, Berkeley, California

ROBERT J. GOLDEN, Karch & Associates, Inc., Washington, DC

NAOMI H. HARLEY, Department of Environmental Medicine, New York University, New York, New York

YUTAKA IWATA, Stauffer Chemical Company, Richmond, California

E. MARSHALL JOHNSON, Thomas Jefferson Medical College, Philadelphia, Pennsylvania

NATHAN J. KARCH, Karch & Associates, Inc., Washington, DC

RUSSELL E. KEENAN, Envirologic Data Corporation, Portland, Maine

JAMES B. KNAAK, California Department of Health Services, Sacramento, California

DANIEL KREWSKI, Health Protection Branch, Health & Welfare Canada, Ottawa, Ontario, Canada

PETER K. LAGOY, ICF Clement Associates, Washington, DC

LESTER B. LAVE, Graduate School of Industrial Administration, Carnegie–Mellon University, Pittsburgh, Pennsylvania

F. H. LAWRENCE, Envirologic Data Corporation, Portland, Maine

MAXWELL W. LAYARD, Failure Analysis Associates, Palo Alto, California

BETH A. LEONARD, McKinsey & Company, Pittsburgh, Pennsylvania

HON-WING LEUNG, Syntex Corporation, Palo Alto, California

DAVID LIPSKY, Environmental Division, Dynamic Corporation, Fort Lee, New Jersey

RANJIT J. MACHADO, Environ Corporation, Washington, DC

KEITH T. MADDY, California Department of Food and Agriculture, Sacramento, California

RENAE MAGAW, Biology and Medicine Division, Lawrence Berkeley Laboratory, Berkeley, California

THOMAS C. MARSHALL, International Technology Corporation, Oak Ridge, Tennessee

L. DANIEL MAXIM, Everest Consulting Associates, Cranbury, N.J.

IAN C. T. NISBET, ICF Clement Associates, Washington, DC

A. OXMAN, Department of Clinical Epidemiology and Biostatistics, McMaster University Hamilton, Ontario, Canada

DENNIS J. PAUSTENBACH, McLaren Environmental Engineering, ChemRisk Division, Alameda, California

GARY RAND, Florida Power & Light, Juno Beach, Florida

RICHARD H. REITZ, Toxicology Research Laboratory, The Dow Chemical Company, Midland, Michigan

PAOLO F. RICCI, Lawrence Berkeley Laboratory and University of California, Berkeley, California

JOSEPH V. RODRICKS, Environ Corporation, Washington, DC

MARY M. SAUER, Envirologic Data Corporation, Portland, Maine

JOYCE S. SCHLESINGER, Environ Corporation, Washington, DC

CARL O. SCHULZ, COSAR, Inc., Columbia, South Carolina

ROBERT L. SIELKEN, Jr., Sielken, Inc., Bryan, Texas

ABRAHAM SILVERS, Electric Power Research Institute, Palo Alto, California

F. A. SMITH, Toxicology Research Laboratory, The Dow Chemical Company, Midland, Michigan

LINDA TOLLEFSON, Epidemiology and Clinical Toxicology Unit, Center for Food Safety and Applied Nutrition, U.S. Food and Drug Administration, Washington, DC

G. W. TORRANCE, Department of Clinical Epidemiology and Biostatistics, McMaster University, Hamilton, Ontario, Canada

CURTIS C. TRAVIS, Health and Safety Research Division, Oak Ridge National Laboratory, Oak Ridge, Tennessee

DUNCAN TURNBULL, Environ Corporation, Washington, DC

CHRIS WHIPPLE, Electric Power Research Institute, Palo Alto, California

ROBIN K. WHITE, Health and Safety Research Division, Oak Ridge National Laboratory, Oak Ridge, Tennessee

D. M. WOLTERING, The Proctor & Gamble Company, Environmental Safety Department, Ivorydale Technical Center, Cincinnati, Ohio

CRAIG ZAMUDA, Office of Emergency and Remedial Response, U.S. Environmental Protection Agency, Washington, DC

Foreword

Having twice served as Administrator of the Environmental Protection Agency, first in the early 1970s and, most recently, in the mid-1980s, I am convinced that significant differences exist between those two periods of time. In the early 1970s our overriding concern was the gross pollution of our air and our water; this was pollution that we could smell, see, and feel, and that had a significant effect on the environment in which we lived or played. In the mid- to late-1970s, our focus changed and we became more concerned about toxic pollutants—those that affect our health. Cancer and its causes became significant factors in how we feel about environmental contaminants. The concern over cancer coupled with our ability to detect vanishingly small amounts of contaminants dramatically increased the reach and costs of present-day environmental regulations.

The difference in our perception of environmental threats has led us to different approaches in dealing with those threats. It seemed to me in the early 1970s that money alone would solve most of our pollution problems. It soon became obvious that there would never be enough money and that there would always be new environmental problems to solve. The challenge was how to make intelligent judgments about the health risks posed by the myriad of pollutants of concern and which to address first.

When I went back to EPA in 1983, one of my primary goals was to introduce into the EPA decision-making process the concepts of risk assessment and risk management, and to ensure that everybody understood that there was a clear and necessary distinction between the two concepts.

Risk assessment is the scientific evaluation of the human health impacts posed by a particular substance or mixture of substances. Risk management involves a whole host of factors, such as technological feasibility, cost, and public reaction; factors that must be purged from the risk assessment process to the extent possible.

We also tried at the EPA in the mid-1980s to bring some commonality to the risk assessment process for substances that were dealt with by other agencies of the federal government such as the Occupational Safety and Health Administration, the Food and Drug Administration, and the Consumer Product Safety Commission. Our effort in this regard has been modestly successful. It is fair to say that, as a result of the dedication and determination of many in the federal government in recent years, the quantitative approach to analyzing environmental problems, which is the essence of risk assessment, has become generally accepted.

As is clearly demonstrated in this text, many of the ideas which we proposed in 1983 have been implemented in recent assessments. Unlike earlier attempts, scientists have become more comfortable with describing the uncertainties in the assessment process.

They also feel more comfortable about stating that sufficient scientific data are not available to reach a firm conclusion.

It is also apparent from the assessments presented in this text that we are more skilled at estimating human exposure and more willing to acknowledge the uncertainties in our estimates of the possible risks associated with exposure to carcinogens and developmental toxicants. Perhaps the most important breakthrough is that the final decision, the risk management judgment, is no longer confused with the scientific evaluation of the data. This change is important and hopefully permanent.

An area where I felt scientists and risk assessors, in particular, could do a better job was in the communication of risk. We need to describe the hazards posed by suspect substances as clearly as possible, tell people what the known or suspected health problems are, admit our uncertainties, and help the public understand the risk in a larger context. There are a number of examples in this text which do a good job of showing how to present these issues in a comprehensible form.

Scientists should be willing to take a larger role in explaining risks and the risk assessment process to the public. Unfortunately, due to the great pressures on regulatory agencies, the regulated community, and the consultants who serve each of them, scientists have rarely had the opportunity to reduce these often voluminous assessments into papers suitable for publication. Indeed, only a handful of risk assessments addressing specific contaminated sites or chemicals have been published.

For many reasons, Dr. Paustenbach's text is an important and timely contribution to the fields of environmental and occupational health. The breadth of our environmental concerns is clearly illustrated by the diversity of issues discussed here.

He and his colleagues are to be congratulated for having prepared a reference text which presents a large number of rather complex evaluations. This text can serve as an important reference point against which risk assessments of the coming years can be compared. It is my hope that future evaluations will be much improved as a result of the information presented here.

WILLIAM D. RUCKELSHAUS

Former Administrator
United States Environmental Protection Agency
June 1, 1988

Preface

By the 1970s it had become clear that humans had unknowingly contaminated much of their drinking water and their air. Scientists throughout the world recognized that dramatically different approaches had to be developed regarding the management of hazards which might affect our health. In response, industry and government began to invest unprecedented sums of money into the identification, evaluation, and control of industrial chemicals and wastes.

During the years 1970–1985 nearly 25 major pieces of legislation were passed which attempted to regulate the manufacture, transportation, and use of hazardous materials. Our knowledge of toxicology, industrial hygiene, environmental control, analytical chemistry, and the basic sciences related to environmental issues increased at a rate that was nothing short of remarkable.

With this increased awareness came the need to direct our economic and technological resources to solve the environmental and occupational problems. Our first challenge was to prioritize the various hazards. Not unexpectedly, regulators and legislators sought methods to describe these hazards quantitatively. Out of this need to prioritize in an objective manner arose the field of health risk assessment. Risk assessment was soon recognized as a process through which all pertinent scientific data describing a particular problem were brought together so that a comprehensive evaluation could be conducted.

A necessary and logical consequence of these assessments was the evaluation of the cost–benefit relation of various clean-up or control options. The presentation of the cost–risk–benefit relation appealed to risk managers since it helped them to evaluate accurately the wisdom of spending various sums of money.

By 1984 it was clear that the government had identified risk assessment as a critical and integral part of regulatory decision-making. Soon thereafter, risk assessments were required as part of remedial investigation and feasibility studies for the clean-up of hazardous waste sites, to obtain permits for discharging chemicals into waterways or into the atmosphere, for evaluating the reasonableness of proposed regulations, and were used to help determine causation in toxic tort litigation cases.

The early years of risk assessment were not without their shortcomings. Risk assessments conducted during the late 1970s and throughout the 1980s suffered from numerous inadequacies. Improvements were needed in assessments conducted by regulatory agencies, as well as those by consultants and corporations. Like any other new scientific undertaking, risk assessment suffered the pains of maturing from its infancy, which some trace back to the investigative work of the early toxicologists who practiced during the 1940s.

Because of the youth of this field there has been a lack of uniform agreement on the meaning of the term risk assessment. As recently as five years ago, a report evaluating the probability that an earthquake would occur in Northern California within the next decade and a 300-page document that attempted to refute allegations that disposable diapers containing trace levels of dioxin posed a cancer hazard were each called risk assessments. However, it now seems reasonably clear that as we enter the 1990s virtually all regulatory and legislative decisions regarding the environmental problems that will be attacked and the funds that will allocated will be based on information derived from risk assessments. In light of their importance, it seemed that a text which contained much of the basic information for conducting such assessments was long overdue.

This book was written with the objective of helping to bring to the scientific community the most thorough and current approaches to quantitative evaluate the health risks of occupational and environmental hazards. We now have within our grasp, unlike in the past, the capacity to conduct risk assessments with much greater accuracy. The introduction and widespread use of computers, as well as the focusing of some of America's best talent on environmental issues, has reaped significant rewards in the 1980s. Although it is true that there is still a great deal we do not know about the mechanisms of carcinogenicity or developmental toxicity, or exactly how to predict the behavior of chemicals in the atmosphere or in complex geological formations, we can make decisions about environmental problems that are infinitely better than the arbitrary ones of the 1950s, 1960s, and early 1970s.

Risk assessments offer an opportunity for the public to develop an understanding of the critical issues. It is my belief that if emotionalism and subjective claims carry more weight than a thorough and objective analysis, mankind will almost surely compromise its ability to achieve all the goals of which it is capable. If we wish to maintain a standard of living close to that to which we have become accustomed in the developed countries, we need to evaluate the various controllable risks in a uniform and scientifically defensible manner. Such evaluations should help ensure that significant hazards are controlled while insignificant ones are dismissed.

In short, I remain confident that if uniform, reasonable, objective, and defensible risk assessments are used to address environmental and occupational health problems, America will have a much better chance of reaching its objectives and yet maintain a safe and healthy environment.

In spite of the importance of risk assessments, the scientist who wishes to learn how to develop an analysis of a potential or alleged health hazard is hard pressed to know where to begin. Very few environmental assessments describing the likelihood of an adverse effect following repeated low level exposure to a chemical have been published in the scientific literature; perhaps fewer than a dozen. Generally, these few attempts lack thoroughness or a high quality scientific peer review. The purpose of this text is to help advance the art of risk assessment by sharing high quality examples prepared by the foremost authorities within the scientific community. Emphasis has been placed on those assessments that evaluate the potential health hazards associated with exposure to chemical and physical agents in our environment.

The contributors to this text are the premier persons in the field. Approximately 50 contributors were drawn from more than a dozen scientific disciplines. They have been responsible for conducting a large fraction of the important assessments in the United States. Luminaries from the fields of biochemistry, toxicology, chemistry, medicine, health physics, radiation biology, nuclear and environmental engineering, avian and aquatic toxicology, statistics, economics, and risk assessment have participated.

The book contains 12 chapters that address the fundamental components of a health risk assessment and issues related to risk characterization and management. With these examples, in hand, scientists should be well armed to tackle nearly any hazard requiring evaluation. The hope was that in the coming years even better evaluations would be conducted and, accordingly, more scientifically based decisions would be reached. Over the two years during which this text was written, I read and edited every chapter. As the contributors will attest, each received a review equal to that associated with the better peer reviewed scientific journals.

Even though most chapters were originally developed to satisfy a regulatory requirement, a litigation challenge, or a social concern, most of them required significant additional work to be suitable for publication. Although I reviewed and critiqued each chapter I am unable to endorse uniformly each of the methods used by the various contributors or the conclusions which they reached. In light of the consensus view that these authors represent the best scientists in their fields, it would be presumptuous to have insisted that all of them approach their analysis in the same manner that I might have chosen.

It was an honor to have the opportunity to assemble this group of scientists and to serve as editor. Their qualifications are impeccable and these are validated by the quality of each chapter. I thank each scientist who participated in this project and I appreciate their commitment to meet an ambitious timetable.

Undertakings of this type are often at the expense of a number of personal relationships. My wife, Louise, and my son, Mark, exhibited extraordinary patience during the months of preparation. Projects like these, by their very nature, are rather selfish since they are pursued because of a personal and/or professional goal. Further, as is nearly always the case, the spouse must assume an even more disproportionately heavy role in the family with little hope of appreciation or acknowledgment by the outside world. I appreciated Louise's and Mark's support during the journey.

My administrative assistant, Dale Zwirn, deserves special acknowledgment, since she never once complained about the additional work load or the peculiar personalities of some of the contributors and the editor. The outstanding typing support provided by Rosie Helmer and others at Syntex Corporation's word processing group was invaluable.

I am optimistic that those who study the various case studies will find them enlightening as well as thought provoking. The text has been organized in such a way that it could be used in an undergraduate or graduate level course in environmental toxicology, public health, industrial hygiene, environmental engineering, or health risk assessment. Ideally, it will serve to encourage health professionals and scientists from related fields to pursue the art of risk assessment.

It is my hope that you will learn as much from reading this text as I did in assembling it.

Dennis J. Paustenbach

Palo Alto, California
October 1988

Contents

Section H
RISK MANAGEMENT

**The Risk Assessment of
Environmental and Human Health Hazards:
A Textbook of Case Studies**

Introduction: A Primer for Conducting Human or Environmental Health Risk Assessments

Dennis J. Paustenbach

McLaren Environmental Engineering, ChemRisk Division, Alameda, California

INTRODUCTION

In recent years, a number of handbooks and guidelines which describe general approaches to preparing health risk assessments have been developed. For example, the U.S. Environmental Protection Agency (EPA) has published generic risk assessment guidelines for carcinogens (EPA, 1986a), developmental toxicants (1986b), exposure assessment (1986c), mixtures (1986d), municipal waste combustors (1986e), systemic toxicants (1988a) as well as female (1988b) and male reproductive (1988c) toxicants. The EPA has also issued a handbook for conducting endangerment assessments (EPA, 1986f) and risk assessments of Superfund sites (EPA, 1986g). In addition, the State of California has published a handbook for conducting assessments of carcinogenic substances (California Department of Health Services, 1985) and guidelines for safe use determinations for compliance with California's Proposition 65 (California Department of Health Services, 1988).

As discussed by a special National Academy of Sciences committee convened in 1983, most human or environmental health hazards can be evaluated by dissecting the analysis into four parts. These are hazard identification, dose–response assessment, exposure assessment, and risk characterization. Each is clearly defined in the committee's report *Risk Assessment in the Federal Government* (NAS, 1983).

Perhaps the most important recommendation of the committee was to encourage the separation of risk assessment from risk management. One result of this separation is that the risk assessor is faced with the challenge to communicate all the information needed by the risk manager in such a manner that its implications will be readily understood. The following sections recommend that numerous scientific papers, including the chapters from this book, be consulted when preparing health risk assessments. The papers cited are not intended to represent a compilation of all the important papers but rather to illustrate that a wealth of information is available to scientists responsible for conducting these assessments.

HAZARD IDENTIFICATION

The hazard identification step in risk assessment contains a description of a particular chemical or physical agent's capacity to adversely affect, at some dose, the health of biota,

1

fish, wildlife, or humans. It is defined as the process of determining whether exposure to an agent can cause an increased incidence of a health condition (cancer, birth defect, etc.). It involves characterizing the nature and strength of the evidence of causation. Numerous reference texts which describe the toxic effects of as many as 2,000 of the most commonly used chemicals are currently available. Fewer texts describing the potential adverse effects of xenobiotics on cattle, sheep, fish, birds, and various types of wildlife have been written because of the smaller number of toxicity studies which have been conducted on these nontraditional species.

Compilations of toxicity test results can be found in the following texts:

- *Patty's Industrial Hygiene and Toxicology*, Volumes 2a, 2b, and 2c (1982) by Clayton and Clayton.
- *Casarett and Doull's Toxicology: The Basic Science of Poisons*, 3rd edn. (1986) by Klaassen et al.
- *Dangerous Properties of Industrial Materials* (1984) by Sax.
- *Toxic and Hazardous Industrial Chemicals Safety Manual* (1976) by the International Technical Information Institute.
- *Effects and Dose–Response Relationships of Metals* (1976) by Nordberg.
- *Clinical Toxicology of Commercial Products* (1984) by Gosselin et al.
- *Hamilton and Hardy's Industrial Toxicology* (1984) by Finkel et al.
- *Clinical Toxicology* (1972) by Thiennes and Haley.
- *Registry of Toxic Effects of Chemical Substances* (1986h) by the Environmental Protection Agency (EPA).
- *Handbook of Toxic and Hazardous Chemicals and Carcinogens* (1985) by Sitnig.
- *Occupational Diseases: A Guide to Their Recognition* (1976) by the National Institute for Occupational Safety and Health.
- *Encyclopedia of Occupational Health and Safety* (1983) by the World Health Organization (see Parmeggiai, 1983).
- *Chemical Hazards of the Workplace* (1988) by Proctor et al.
- *Chemical Hazards to Human Reproduction* (1983) by Nisbet and Karch.
- *Catalog of Teratogenic Agents* (1980) by Shepard.

Each year, new information on the potential adverse effects of xenobiotics on fishes becomes available. A few texts have reviewed the overall approach to hazard identification and catalogued some of the adverse effects on fish and other wildlife. The following are good resources:

- Chapter 9 in this text, "Evaluating the environmental safety of detergent chemicals: Including a case study of cationic surfactants" (1989) by Woltering and Bishop.
- Chapter 10 in this text, "Risk assessment for nitrilotriacetic acid (NTA)" by Anderson and Alden.
- *Handbook of Adverse Effects on the Fathead Minnow* (1984) by Brooke et al.
- *Fundamentals of Aquatic Toxicology* (1985) by Rand and Petrocelli.
- *Environmental Hazard Assessment of Effluents* (1986) by Bergmann et al.
- *Aquatic Toxicology and Hazard Assessment: Sixth Symposium.* (1983) by Bishop et al.
- *Analyzing the Hazard Evaluation Process* (1979) by Dickson et al.

- *Biotransformation and Fate of Chemicals in the Aquatic Environment* (1980) by Maki et al.

Except for the intentional toxic effects posed by pesticides, no general reference text appears to have been written which reviews the adverse effects of industrial chemicals on the health or reproductive capacity of birds, large and small wildlife, etc. General discussions of the hazard identification process for avian species include:

- Chapter 27 in this text, "An environmental risk assessment of a pesticide" (1989) by Rand.
- Chapter 29 in this text, "Endangerment assessment for the bald eagle population near the Sand Springs petrochemical complex Superfund site" (1989) by Gandy.
- Chapter 28 in this text, "Examination of potential risks from exposure to dioxin in sludge used to reclaim abandoned strip mines" (1989) by Keenan et al.
- *Fate and Effects of Kepone in the James River* (1984) by Bender and Huggett.
- *Principles for Evaluating Chemicals in the Environment* (1975) by the National Academy of Sciences.
- Environmental risk assessment of surfactants: Fate and environmental effects in Lake Biwa Basin (1988) by Sueishi et al.
- Soil–food-chain–pesticide–wildlife relationships in aldrin-treated fields (1973) by Korschgen.
- "The risk of chemicals to aquatic environment" (1982) by Southworth et al.
- *Toxicology of Pesticides* (1975) by Hayes.
- *Pesticides Studied in Man* (1982) by Hayes.

Sampling and Statistical Aspects

An important aspect of hazard identification is a description of the pervasiveness of the hazard. For example, most environmental assessments require knowledge of the concentration of the material in the environment, weighted in some way to account for the geographical magnitude of the contamination; that is, a 1-acre or 300-acre site, a 1,000-gal/min or 1,000,000 gal/min stream. All too often environmental incidents have been described by statements like "concentrations as high as 150 ppm" of a chemical were measured at a 1,000-acre waste site. However, following closer examination, we may find that only 1 of 200 samples collected on a 20-acre portion of a 1,000-acre site showed this concentration and that 2 ppm was the geometric mean level of contamination in the 200 samples.

An appropriate sampling program is critical in the conduct of a health risk assessment. This topic could arguably be part of the exposure assessment but it has been placed within hazard identification because, if the degree of contamination is small, no further work may be necessary. Accurate sampling strategies are also important in occupational risk assessment where time-weighted average samples collected over the entire work day, rather than those collected over shorter periods, are known to be the best way to assess the chronic inhalation hazard. When evaluating the potential hazard to wildlife, a thorough sampling plan is no less important since a representative number of fish, birds, rattlesnakes, mice, worms, or other species needs to be collected before the seriousness of the hazard can be described.

Schemes or approaches for collecting representative samples of soil, water, air, and other media are perhaps better defined than those used for the collection of birds, fish, mice, or food stuffs. Regrettably, the wealth of information on sampling theory and the importance of random sampling which has been developed within the statistics community has not been incorporated into the practice of environmental risk assessment. Scientists involved in these activities should find the following texts to be useful in designing sampling plans:

- *Sampling Techniques* (1977) by Cochran.
- *Statistical Theory* (1980) by Lindgreen.
- *Statistical Methods for Environmental Pollution Monitoring* (1987) by Gilbert.

Not only is it important that samples be collected in a random or representative manner, but the number of samples must be sufficient to conduct a statistically valid analysis. The number needed to insure statistical validity will be dictated by the variability between the results. The larger the variance, the greater the number of samples needed to define the problem.

Since environmental data are almost always log–normally distributed, perhaps the most useful piece of information in conducting an evaluation is the geometric mean (GM) concentration and the geometric standard deviation (GSD). For these analyses to be valid, one must know that the samples were collected in a random and representative manner. An accurate description of the severity of the hazard will not be possible if the samples are not obtained in a manner which is representative and one which rules out the possibility of bias. In addition, the integrity of the samples, their transport, and their analysis must be insured. The following references or texts should be useful for those attempting to evaluate environmental data:

- Statistical design and data analysis requirements (1985) by Leidel and Busch.
- A method for evaluating the mean exposure from a log-normal distribution (1987) by Rappaport and Selvin.
- *Handbook for Interpreting Soil Data* (1984) by Environmental Protection Agency.
- Statistical evaluation reflecting the skewness in the distribution of TCDD levels in human adipose tissue (1987b) by Sielken.

Environmental Fate

When assessing the potential environmental hazard of a chemical in drinking water, air, fly ash, soil, or groundwater, it is important to understand the behavior of the toxicant in that particular media. For example, the potential groundwater contamination posed by dioxin in soil is dramatically different from the hazard posed by the contamination of soil by perchloroethylene (PERC) or other more water soluble chemicals. Even though dioxin may be orders of magnitude more toxic than PERC, it poses a much lesser hazard to groundwater since it is virtually insoluble in water (less than 2 parts per trillion) and because it binds tenaciously to soils and virtually all other solids. A consideration of these types of phenomena is important to the hazard characterization process and has been addressed in the following publications:

- Chapter 7 in this text, "Comprehensive methodology for assessing the risks to humans and wildlife posed by contaminated soils" (1989) by Paustenbach.

- Chapter 8 in this text, "Hazard assessment of 1, 1, 1-trichloroethane in groundwater" (1989) by Byard.
- Water and soil pollutants (1986) by Menzer and Nelson.
- *Dynamics, Exposure, and Hazard Assessment of Toxic Chemicals* (1980) by Haque.
- *Environmental Risk Analysis for Chemicals* (1982) by Conway.
- *Chemodynamics, Environmental Movement of Chemicals in Air, Water, and Soil* (1979) by Thibodeaux.
- *Soils Contaminated by Petroleum: Environmental and Public Health Effects* (1988) by Calabrese and Kostecki.
- Behavior assessment model for trace organics in soil. Part IV (1984) by Jury et al.
- Photolysis of chemicals (1984) by Wong et al.

Chemical and Physical Properties

A thorough understanding of the chemical and physical properties of the toxicant is very useful when attempting to understand the severity of the hazard. For example, when chemicals such as the heavy metals, PCB, DDT, or the dioxins are not heated, the inhalation hazard is low because of their low volatility. On the other hand, because their persistence or long biologic half-life, these chemicals may pose a significant hazard if they enter the food chain and accumulate in fish and/or the adipose tissue, meat, or milk of cows. In addition, the chemical and physical properties of a chemical will influence its bioavailability when it enters living organisms. The following references should provide insight into understanding the importance of chemical and physical properties in the hazard identification step and, indeed, the entire risk assessment process:

- *Environmental Assessment Technical Handbook* (1984) by the U.S. Food and Drug Administration.
- *The Handbook of Chemistry and Physics* (1988) by Weast.
- Outline and criteria for evaluating the safety of new chemicals (1981) by Beck et al.
- *Handbook of Organic Industrial Solvents* (1988) by American Mutual Insurance Alliance.
- *Understanding Chemicals in the Environment* (1979) by Maki et al.
- *A Review and Analysis of Parameters for Assessing Transport of Environmentally Released Radionuclides in Agriculture* (1984) by Baes et al.
- Correlation of bioconcentration factors of chemicals in aquatic and terrestrial organisms with their physical and chemical properties (1980) by Kenaga.
- Some physical factors in toxicology assessment tests (1979) by Freed et al.
- Bioavailability of soil-bound TCDD: Dermal bioavailability in the rat (1988) by Shu et al.
- Bioavailability of soil-bound TCDD in the rat: Oral bioavailability in the rat (1987) by Shu et al.
- Influence of solvents and absorbents on dermal and intestinal absorption of TCDD (1980) by Poiger and Schlatter.
- Uptake and selective retention in rats of orally administered chlorinated dioxins and dibenzofurans from fly-ash and fly-ash extract (1984) by Van den Berg et al.

DOSE–RESPONSE ASSESSMENT

The process of characterizing the relationship between the dose of a substance and the likelihood of an adverse health effect in the exposed population is called the dose–response assessment. This step should take into account such factors as sex, lifestyle, and other modifying factors, as well as the low-dose extrapolation. For purposes of most risk assessments, the greatest degree of uncertainty will be associated with the extrapolation from the high doses tested in animals to human exposure at the concentrations found in the environment. Typically, environmental exposure is 100- to 100,000-fold below the lowest dose tested in the animal study. It is important in the dose–response assessment that the method used to extrapolate and the justification for selecting that method be described in detail.

Classic Toxicants

Over the past two decades, toxicologists have tended to focus their discussion of approaches to dose–response extrapolation of data obtained in cancer bioassays. However, the need to evaluate the risk associated with doses much lower than those tested in experimental animals is equally important when assessing chemicals whose primary adverse effects include reproductive or developmental toxicity, or where the adverse effect occurs in the liver, kidney, nervous system, respiratory tract, central and peripheral nervous system, the immune system, or other organs. In the numerous scientific papers which have reviewed the various approaches to extrapolating animal data to identify safe levels of exposure for humans, virtually all have focused on the use of the safety factor or uncertainty factor approach, since all adverse effects other than cancer and mutation-based developmental effects are believed to have a threshold—a dose below which no adverse effect should occur.

The following are excellent references which discuss approaches to setting exposure limits for chemicals which are thought to have thresholds:

- Statistics versus safety factors and scientific judgment in the evaluation of safety for man (1972) by Weil.
- 100-fold margin of safety (1954) by Lehmann and Fitzhugh.
- Regulatory history and experimental support of uncertainty (safety factors) (1983) by Dourson and Stara.
- *Methodological Approaches to Deriving Environmental and Occupational Health Standards* (1978) by Calabrese.
- A new method for determining allowable daily intakes (1985) by Crump.
- New approaches in the derivation of acceptable daily intakes (ADI) (1986) by Dourson.
- Safety assessments of chemicals with threshold effects (1985) by Lu.
- Occupational exposure limits, pharmacokinetics, and unusual work schedules (1985) by Paustenbach.
- *Drinking Water and Health—Volumes I–VIII* (1977–1987) by the National Academy of Sciences.
- Neurobehavioral toxicity as a basis for risk assessment (1988) by Weiss.
- Acceptable daily intake: Inception, evaluation and application (1988) by Lu.

Developmental and Reproductive Toxicants

Since 1980 a number of researchers have discussed various approaches to setting acceptable daily intakes or exposure limits for developmental toxicants, as well as reproductive toxicants. At one point it was suggested that cancer models used for extrapolating cancer bioassay data might be a plausible approach to setting acceptable limits of exposure to these compounds. However, since a threshold is generally believed to exist for developmental and reproductive toxicants, cancer models are currently considered inappropriate.

The following papers either present or review the various approaches to setting limits for these categories of toxicants:

- Chapter 21 in this text, "A case study of developmental toxicity risk estimation based on animal data" (1989) by Johnson.
- Chapter 22 in this text, "Risk assessment methodologies for developmental and reproductive toxicants: A study of the glycol ethers" (1989) by Paustenbach.
- The relative teratogenic index and teratogenic potency: Proposed components of developmental toxicity risk assessment (1982) by Fabro et al.
- *Risk Assessment Guidelines for Developmental Toxicants* (1986b) by Environmental Protection Agency.
- A tier system for developmental toxicity evaluations based on considerations of exposure and effect relationships (1987) by Johnson.
- Entire issue of *Carcinogenesis, Mutagenesis and Teratogenesis* (June, 1987).
- Evaluation of developmental toxicity data: A discussion of some pertinent factors, and a proposal (1987) by Hart et al.
- A scheme for prioritizing developmental toxins (1987b) by Wang and Schwetz.
- Cross species extrapolations and the biologic basis for safety factor determinations in developmental toxicology (1988) by Johnson.
- Issues in qualitative and quantitative risk analysis for developmental toxicology (1988) by Kimmel and Gaylor.
- Estimation of human reproductive risk from animal studies: Determination of interspecies extrapolation factors for steroid hormone effects on the male (1988) by Meistrich.
- Quantification of the genetic risk of environmental mutagens (1988) by Ehling.
- *Proposed Guidelines for Assessing Female Reproductive Risk* (1988b) by Environmental Protection Agency.
- *Proposed Guidelines for Assessing Male Reproductive Risk* (1988c) by Environmental Protection Agency.

Carcinogens

Lastly, the area within which the dose–response evaluation has received the most thorough discussion involves extrapolation for chemical carcinogens. A good deal of the basis for the modeling of chemical carcinogens comes from our experience with human exposure to radiation. Even though experience with gamma radiation may give us some insight into the validity of the extrapolation models for some initiators, it remains premature to assume that these models are appropriate for estimating the low-dose response for all chemical carcinogens. In fact, there are many in the scientific community who believe that at least three major categories of carcinogens are likely: cytotoxicants, initiators, and promoters (Andersen, 1988). Each type would require a different approach to assessing the low-dose response (Williams and Weisburger, 1981).

Some of the differences between chemical- and radiation-induced carcinogenesis are that gamma, beta, and alpha radiation are all known to be genotoxic, whereas not all chemical carcinogens act through a genotoxic mechanism. This is an important point, since the ability of a chemical to interact directly with DNA is the primary rationale for assuming a linear response at very low doses. Low-dose linearity for radiation may be appropriate because it is an initiator and because the dose to which people are exposed is linearly related to the internal dose received at the target organ. However, the internal or delivered dose of a chemical carcinogen to which humans may be exposed will often not be linear at the target organ. For example, carcinogens ingested in food must first be diluted in the stomach, transferred into the bloodstream, and transported to other organs, including the liver, where they will be either redistributed as the parent compound or metabolized. Since most environmental chemicals must be metabolized to become reactive and because the conversion to the metabolite and the likelihood that it will interact with DNA will often be dose-dependent, this process will frequently be nonlinear. The parent chemical or metabolite must then be transported through the cell membrane and then through the cytoplasm of the cell before possible interaction with DNA. Pharmacokinetic analyses can be very helpful in estimating the likely target-tissue dose based on the administered dose level.

The potential strengths and weaknesses of the most commonly accepted approaches to estimating the low-dose response go far beyond the scope of this discussion and the reader is encouraged to study the following publications, which address this topic:

- Chapter 4 in this text, "A time-to-response perspective on ethylene oxide carcinogenicity" (1989) by Sielken.
- Chapter 5 in this text, "Use of physiological pharmacokinetics in cancer risk assessments: A study of methylene chloride" (1989) by Andersen et al.
- Chapter 23 in this text, "A physiologically based pharmacokinetic approach for assessing the cancer risk of tetrachloroethylene" (1989) by Travis et al.
- "Safety" testing of carcinogenic agents (1961) by Mantel and Bryan.
- Fundamental carcinogenic processes and their implications for low dose risk assessment (1976) by Crump et al.
- Statistical aspects of dichotomous dose response data (1978) by Brown.
- *Carcinogenic Risk Assessment* (1977) by Cornfield.
- A general scheme for the incorporation of pharmacokinetics in low dose risk estimation for chemical carcinogenesis (1980) by Anderson et al.
- Risk assessment and regulatory decision making (1981) by Munro and Krewski.
- Determining safe levels of exposure: Safety factors or mathematical models (1984) by Krewski et al.
- An improved procedure for low-dose carcinogenic risk assessment from animal data (1981) by Crump.
- Carcinogenic risk assessment for chloroform: An alternative to EPA's procedures (1981) by Reitz et al.
- Linear interpolation algorithm for low dose risk assessment of toxic substances (1980) by Gaylor and Kodell.
- The multistage model with time-dependent dose pattern: Applications of carcinogenic risk assessment (1984) by Crump and Howe.

- Quantitative risk assessment: State of the art for carcinogenesis (1983) by Park and Snee.
- The role of pharmacokinetics in risk assessment (1986) by Reitz et al.
- Pharmacokinetics in low-dose extrapolation using animal cancer data (1988) by Whittemore et al.
- Some issues in the quantitative modeling portion of cancer risk assessment (1985) by Sielken.
- Quantitative cancer risk assessments for 2, 3, 7, 8-TCDD (1987a) by Sielken.
- A response to Crump's evaluation of Sielken's dose–response assessment for TCDD (1987d) by Sielken.

Biologically Based Disposition and Cancer Models

Perhaps one of the most important breakthroughs, which should allow us to conduct much more accurate carcinogenic risk assessments, was a mathematical approach used by Bischoff and Brown (1966) and later further refined by Fiserova-Bergerova (1975) and by Ramsey and Andersen (1984). This procedure, known as physiologically based pharmacokinetics (PB-PK), allows scientists to extrapolate the biologically important dose delivered to target organs more accurately than other approaches (Menzel, 1987). Physiologically based toxicokinetic models differ from the conventional compartmental models in that they are based to a large extent on the actual physiology of the organism. Instead of compartments defined by the experimental data themselves, actual organ and tissue groups are used with weights and blood flows from the literature (Bischoff and Brown, 1966; Himmelstein and Lutz, 1979). Instead of composite rate constants determined by fitting the data, actual physicochemical and biochemical constants of the compound are used. The result is a model that predicts the qualitative behavior of the experimental time course *without being based on it*. Refinement of the model to incorporate additional insights gained from comparison with experimental data yields a model that can be used for quantitative extrapolation well beyond the range of experimental conditions (Clewell and Andersen, 1985). Such approaches may also give insight on the reasonableness of low-dose linearity on a chemical-by-chemical basis. These analyses, coupled with pharmacodynamic models, are likely to allow us to make dramatic improvements in the way we assess risks associated with low level exposures. Additional improvements will almost certainly be realized when approaches which account for such biological process as cell proliferation, the multistage cancer process, and time-to-tumor are used.

The following references are important for understanding physiologically based pharmacokinetic (PB-PK) models or the more newly termed biologically based disposition models, as well as the biologically based low-dose extrapolation models:

- A physiologically based description of the inhalation pharmacokinetics of styrene in rats and humans (1984) by Ramsey and Andersen.
- Physiological pharmacokinetic modeling (1987) by Menzel.
- Physiologically-based pharmacokinetics and the risk assessment process for methylene chloride (1987) by Andersen et al.
- A physiologically-based pharmacokinetic model for carbon tetrachloride (1988) by Paustenbach et al.
- Risk assessment extrapolations and physiological modeling (1985) by Clewell and Andersen.
- Biologically motivated cancer risk models (1987) by Thorslund, et al.

- Biologically structured models and computer simulation: Application to chemical carcinogenesis (1988) by Conolly et al.
- Mutation and cancer: A model for human carcinogenesis (1981) by Moolgavkar and Knudson.
- A stochastic two-stage model for cancer risk assessment (1988) by Moolgavkar et al.

EXPOSURE ASSESSMENT

Over the past five years, a good deal of attention has been directed to the exposure assessment part of risk assessment. This is logical, since many of the risk assessments performed during the 1970s tended to make too many conservative assumptions which, as a result, frequently overestimated the actual exposure.

The exposure assessment is the process wherein the intensity, frequency, and duration of human exposure to an agent are estimated. The process may also address the exposure of wildlife to chemical agents. An exposure assessment should quantitatively estimate the magnitude (size) of the exposed population, the routes of entry, and the uncertainties in the exposure estimates. In this process, three routes of entry generally need to be considered: inhalation, dermal absorption, and ingestion.

The following references are useful for conducting exposure assessments and for calculating the uptake of xenobiotics by humans and wildlife:

Inhalation

- Chapter 19 in this text, "Assessment of potential health hazards associated with PCDD and PCDF emissions from a municipal waste combustor" (1989) by Lipsky.
- Chapter 12 in this text, "A risk assessment of a former pesticide production facility" (1989) by Marshall et al.
- Chapter 22 in this text, "Risk assessment methodologies for developmental and reproductive toxicants: A study of the glycol ethers" (1989) by Paustenbach.
- Chapter 14 in this text, "Problems associated with the use of conservative assumptions in exposure and risk analysis" (1989) by Maxim.
- Chapter 17 in this text, "Formaldehyde exposure and risk in mobile homes" (1989) by Gammage and Travis.
- Chapter 18 in this text, "Environmental lung cancer risk from radon daughter exposure" (1989) by Harley.
- Report of the Task Group on Reference Man (1975) by Snyder.
- Guidelines for exposure assessment (1986c) by the Environmental Protection Agency.
- Methodology for the Assessment of Health Risks Associated with Multiple Pathway Exposure to Multiple Waste Combustors (1986e) by the Environmental Protection Agency.

Dermal Absorption

- Chapter 24 in this text, "The worker hazard posed by re-entry into pesticide-treated foliage" (1989) by Knaak et al.

- Chapter 8 in this text, "Hazard assessment of 1,1,1-trichloroethane in groundwater" (1989) by Byard.
- Assessment of health risks from exposure to contaminated soil (1985) by Hawley.
- *The Handbook of Dermaltoxicology* (1975) by Maibach.
- *Exposure Tests for Organic Compounds in Industry* (1973) by Piotrowski.
- Absorption of some glycol ethers through human skin in vitro (1984) by Dugard et al.
- Bioavailability of soil-bound TCDD: Oral bioavailability in the rat (1987) by Shu et al.
- Health risk assessment of human exposure to soil amended with sewage sludge contaminated with polychlorinated dibenzodioxins and dibenzofurans (1986) by Eschenroeder et al.

Ingestion

- Chapter 26 in this text, "A comprehensive risk assessment of DEHP as a component of baby pacifiers, teethers, and toys" (1989) by Turnbull and Rodricks.
- Chapter 6 in this text, "Superfund risk assessments: The process and past experience at uncontrolled hazardous waste sites" (1989) by Zamuda.
- Chapter 25 in this text, "Methylmercury in fish: Assessment of risk for U.S. consumers" (1989) by Tollefson.
- Chapter 13 in this text, "The endangerment assessment for the Smuggler Mountain site, Pitkin County, Colorado: A case study" (1989) by LaGoy et al.
- Health implications of 2,3,7,8-tetrachlorodibenzo-*p*-dioxin (TCDD) contamination of residential soil (1984) by Kimbrough et al.
- Bioavailability of soil-borne PLB's ingested by farm animals (1985) by Fries.
- A method for estimating soil ingestion by children (1987) by Clausing et al.
- Bioavailability of soil-bound TCDD: Oral bioavailability in the rat (1987) by Shu et al.
- Infant exposure assessment for breast milk dioxins and furans derives from waste incineration emissions (1987) by Smith.
- Chapter 15 in this text, "Risk analyses of buried waste from electricity generation" (1989) by Cohen.
- Chapter 16 in this text, "Assessment of a waste site contaminated with chromium" (1989) by Golden and Karch.
- Dioxin in soil: Bioavailability after ingestion by rats and guinea pigs (1984) by McConnell et al.

RISK CHARACTERIZATION

The quantitative estimate of the risk is the topic of principal interest to the regulatory agency or risk manager in arriving at decisions. The risk manager must consider the results of the risk characterization when evaluating the economics, societal aspects, and various benefits of the risk assessment. In general, efforts to improve the risk characterization process has received the least amount of study to date. One needs only to review some of the decisions which have been reached in toxic tort cases by federal agencies and by industry to understand that improvements are needed.

Certainly, factors such as societal pressure, technical uncertainties, and severity of the potential hazard influence how decision makers respond to the risk assessment. However, better risk characterizations could be developed in risk assessments than has typically been the case. The following texts and publications are useful sources of information which should be helpful in improving the way risks are characterized.

- Chapter 30 in this text, "Legal and philosophical aspects of risk analysis" (1989) by Anthony et al.
- Chapter 31 in this text, "A decision-oriented framework for evaluating environmental risk management strategies: A case study of lead in gasoline" (1989) by Krewski et al.
- *Risk Assessment in the Federal Government: Managing the Process* (1983) by the National Academy of Sciences.
- *Societal Risk Assessment: How Safe is Safe Enough* (1980) by Schwing and Albers.
- *Risk Evaluation and Management: Contemporary Issues in Risk Analysis* (1986) by Covello et al.
- Risk analysis and risk management: An historical perspective (1985) by Covello and Mumpower.
- *Of Acceptable Risk* (1976) by Lowrance.
- *Modern Science and Human Values* (1984) by Lowrance.
- *Risk Watch: The Odds of Life* (1984) by Urquhart and Heilmann.
- *The Good News is the Bad News is Wrong* (1984) by Wattenberg.
- Chapter 32 in this text, "Regulating coke oven emissions" (1989) by Lave and Leonard.
- Chapter 33 in this text, "Ranking possible carcinogens: One approach to risk management" (1989) by Ames et al.

Environmental Risks

The process by which the risks to wildlife and ecosystems are characterized is slightly different than that used for humans. In order to describe the hazard posed by fairly widespread dissemination of xenobiotics, one needs to understand the physical properties of the compounds, their environmental fate, and their toxic effects, not only to humans, but also to aquatic species and other wildlife. Perhaps no other industry has so thoroughly evaluated the potential adverse effects of widespread distribution of xenobiotics in the environment as the detergent industry. This insight is not unexpected, since each day literally millions of pounds of detergents are released into our waterways with potential uptake by a diverse number of organisms, including humans. Some of the more important issues in the evaluation of these hazards have been addressed in the following publications:

- Chapter 27 in this text, "An environmental risk assessment of a pesticide" (1989) by Rand.
- Chapter 9 in this text, "Detergent chemicals: A case study of a cationic surfactant" (1989) by Woltering and Bishop.
- Chapter 10 in this text, "Risk assessment of NTA in drinking water" (1989) by Anderson and Alden.
- Chapter 29 in this text, "Endangerment assessment for the bald eagle population near the Sand Springs petrochemical complex Superfund site" (1989) by Gandy.
- Soil ingestion as a pathway of metal uptake into grazing livestock (1981) by Thornon and Abrahams.

- Chapter 28 in this text, "Examination of potential risks from exposure to dioxin in sludge used to reclaim abandoned strip mines" (1989) by Keenan et al.
- Evaluation of residual PCB contamination present on Michigan farms in 1978 (1986) by Fries and Jacobs.
- *Environmental Hazard Assessment of Effluents* (1986) by Bergmann et al.
- *Fundamentals of Aquatic Toxicology* (1985) by Rand and Petrocelli.
- Chemosphere pesticide reserves in birds and mammals (1973) by Stickel.
- Environmental risk assessment of surfactants: Fate and environmental effects on Lake Biwa Basin (1988) by Sueishi et al.

PITFALLS IN ENVIRONMENTAL HEALTH RISK ASSESSMENT

Each of the four parts of a risk assessment offers an opportunity for scientists to fall into traps that can dramatically influence the results of the evaluation. During the past fifteen years many of the important pitfalls have been identified. The following publications have focused on some of the shortcomings which have crept into risk assessment:

- Conservatism in regulatory analysis (1985) by Nichols and Zeckbauser.
- Chapter 14 in this text, "Problems associated with the use of conservative assumptions in exposure and risk analysis" (1989) by Maxim.
- A review of the Food and Drug Administration analysis for polychlorinated biphenyls (1984) by Maxim and Harrington.
- A critical analysis of risk assessment of TCDD contaminated soils (1986) by Paustenbach et al.
- The marigold syndrome (1985) by Havender.
- Some issues in the quantitative modeling portion of cancer risk assessment (1985) by Sielken.
- *Cancer Risk Assessment Guidelines* (1985) by Office of Science and Technology Policy.
- *A Proposed System for Food Safety* (1980) by the Food Safety Council.
- De Minimus Risk (1988) by Whipple.
- The perils of prudence: How conservative risk assessments distort regulation (1988) by Nichols and Zeckhauser.
- Evaluating the benefits of uncertainty reduction in environmental health risk management (1987) by Finkel and Evans.

SUMMARY

This brief chapter reviewed the key issues which need to be addressed in developing a risk assessment. It is hoped that this text will assist those who need to evaluate the risks posed by environmental and occupational hazards. The art of risk assessment has made significant progress since the early 1980s. Through the sharing of the experiences and knowledge of the authors who have contributed to this effort, it can be expected that the overall quality of risk assessment will increase significantly in the coming years.

REFERENCES

American Mutual Insurance Alliance (1988). *Handbook of Organic Industrial Solvents*, AMIA, Chicago, II.

Ames, B. N., Magaw, R., and Gold, L. S. (1987). Ranking possible carcinogenic hazard. *Science* **236**, 271–273.

Andersen, M. E. (1981). A physiologically-based toxicokinetic description of the metabolism of inhaled gases and vapors: Analysis at steady-state. *Toxicol. Appl. Pharmacol.* **60**, 509–526.

Andersen, M. E., Clewell, H. J., Gargas, M. L., Smith, F. A., and Reitz, R. H. (1987). Physiologically-based pharmacokinetics and the risk assessment process for methylene chloride. *Toxicol Appl. Pharmacol.* **87**, 185–205.

Anderson, M. W. et al. (1980). A general scheme for the incorporation of pharmacokinetics in low dose risk estimation for chemical carcinogenesis. .*Toxicol. Appl. Pharm.* **55**, 154–161.

Angle, C. R., and McIntire, M. S. (1974). Lead in air, dustfall, soil, housedust, milk and water: Correlation with blood lead of urban and suburban school children. *Trace Substances Environ. Health* **8**, 23–28.

Armitage, P., and Doll, R. (1954). The age distribution of cancer and a multistage theory of carcinogensis. *Br. J. Cancer* **8**, 1–12.

Baes, C. F., II, Sharp, R. D., Sjoreen, A., and Shor, R. (1984). *A Review and Analysis of Parameters for Assessing Transport of Environmental Released Radionuclides in Agriculture*, ORNL-5786. U.S. Department of Energy, Oak Ridge National Laboratory, Oak Ridge, TN.

Barnard, R. C. (1984). Science, policy and the law: A developing partnership in reducing the risk of cancer. In P. F. Diesler, Jr., Ed., *Reducing the Carcinogenic Risks in Industry*. Dekker, New York.

Bartek, M. J., and LaBudde, J. A. (1975). Percutaneous absorption, in vitro. In H. Maibach, Ed., *Animal Models in Dermatology*. Churchill-Livingstone, Edinburgh and London, p. 103.

Beck, L. W., Maki, A. W., Artman, N. R., and Wilson, E. R. (1981). Outline and criteria for evaluating the safety of new chemicals. *Regul. Toxicol. Pharmacol.* **1**, 19–58.

Bender, M. E., and Huggett, R. J. (1984). Fate and effects of kepone in the James River. *Rev. Environ. Toxicol.* **1**, 5–50.

Bentkover, J. D., Covello, V. T., and Mumpower, J. (1986). *Benefits Assessment: The State of the Art*. Riedel Publ. Boston, MA.

Bergmann, H. L., Kimerle, R. A., and Maki, A. W. (1986). *Environmental Hazard Assessment of Effluents*. Pergamon, New York.

Binder, S., Sokal, D., and Maughan, D. (1986). Estimating the amount of soil ingested by young children through tracer elements. *Arch. Environ. Health* **41**, 341–345.

Bischoff, K. B., and Brown, R. G. (1966). Drug distribution in mammals. *Chem. Eng. Prog., Symp. Ser.* **62**, 33–45.

Bishop, W. E., Cardwell, R. D., and Heidolph, B. B. (1983). *Aquatic Toxicology and Hazard Assessment: Sixth Symposium*, STP 737. Am. Soc. Test. Mater., Philadelphia, PA.

Branson, D. R., and Dickson, K. L. (1981). *Aquatic Toxicology and Hazard and Assessment: Fourth Symposium*, STP 737. Am. Soc. Test. Mater., Philadelphia, PA.

Briggs, G. G., Bromilow, R. H., and Evans, A. A. (1982). Relationships between lipophilicity and root uptake and translocation of non-ionized chemicals by barley. *Toxicol. Environ. Chem.* **7**, 173–189.

Brooke, L. T., Call, D. J., Geiger, D. L., and Northcott, C. E. (1984). Acute toxicities of organic chemicals to fathead minnows. Center for Lake Superior Environmental Studies, University of Wisconsin, Superior, WI.

Browman, M. G., and Chester, S. (1977). The solid-water interface: Transfer of organic pollutants across the solid-water interface. In I. H. Suffet, Ed., *Fate of Pollutants in the Air and Water Environment*, Part I. Wiley, New York.

Brown, C. (1978). Statistical aspects of extrapolation of dichotomous dose response data. *J. Natl. Cancer Inst.* **60**, 101–108.

Brown, H. S., Guble, R., and Tatelbaum, S. (1988). Methodology for assessing hazards of contaminants to seafood. *Regul. Toxicol. Pharmacol.* **8**, 76–100.

Brown, K. G., and Hoel, D. G. (1986). Statistical modeling of animal bioassay data with variable dosing regimens: Example—Vinyl chloride. *Risk Anal.* **6**, 155–166.

Bus, J. S., and Gibson, J. E. (1985). Body defense mechanisms to toxicant exposure. In L. J. Cralley and L. V. Cralley, Eds., *Patty's Industrial Hygiene and Toxicology*, 2nd ed., Vol. 3B. Wiley, New York, pp. 143–174.

Cairns, J., Jr., Dickson, K. L., and Maki, A. W. (Eds.) (1978). *Estimating the Hazards of Chemical Substances to Aquatic Life*, STP 657. Am. Soc. Test. Mater., Philadelphia, PA.

Calabrese, E. J. (1978). *Methodological Approaches to Deriving Environmental and Occupational Health Standards.* Wiley, New York.

Calabrese, E. J., and Kostecki, P. T. (1988). *Soils Contaminated by Petroleum: Environment and Public Health Effects.* Wiley, New York.

Calabrese, E. J., Gilbert, C. E., Kostecki, P. T., Barnes, R., Stanek, E., Veneman, P., Pastides, H., and Edwards, C. (1988). *Epidemiological Study to Estimate How Much Soil Children Eat.* Division of Public Health, University of Massachusetts, Amherst.

California Department of Health Services (1985). *Guidelines for Chemical Carcinogens: Risk Assessments and Their Scientific Rationale* CDHS, Sacramento, CA.

California Department of Health Services (1988). *Guidelines and Safe Use Determination Procedures for the Safe Drinking Water and Toxic Enforcement Act of 1986.* CDHS, Sacramento, CA.

Castanho, M. (1987). Methods of soil sampling. *Comments Toxicol.* **1**, 221–227.

Chemical Manufacturers Association (1984). *Risk Mangagement of Existing Chemicals.* CMA, Washington, DC.

Chiou, C. T. (1981). Partition coefficient and water solubility in environmental chemistry. In J. Saxena and F. Fisher, Eds., *Hazard Assessment of Chemicals.* Academic Press, New York, pp. 117–153.

Chiou, C. T., V. H., Schmedding, D. W., and Kohnert, R. L. (1977). Partitions coefficient and bioconcentration of selected organic solvents. *Environ. Sci. Technol.* **11**, 475–479.

Christian, M. S. (1983). Assessment of reproductive toxicology: State-of-the-art. In M. S. Christian, W. M. Galbraith, P. Voytek, and M. A. Mehlmann, Eds., *Assessment of Reproductive and Teratogenic Hazards.* Princeton Univ. Press, Princeton, NJ.

Clausing, O., Brunekreef, A. B., and van Wijnen, J. H. (1987). A method for estimating soil ingestion by children. *Int. Arch. Occup. Environ. Health* **59**, 73–82.

Clayson, D. B., Krewski, D., and Munro, I. (Eds.) (1985). *Toxicological Risk Assessment*, Vols. 1 and 2. CRC Press, Boca Raton, FL.

Clayton, G. D., and Clayton, F. E. (1982). *Patty's Industrial Hygiene and Toxicology*, 3rd rev. ed., Vols. 2A, 2B, and 2C. Wiley, New York.

Clewell, H. J., and Andersen, M. E. (1985). Risk assessment extrapolations and physiological modeling. *Toxicol. Ind. Health* **1**, 111–132.

Cochran, W. G. (1977). *Sampling Techniques*, 3rd ed. Wiley, New York.

Conolly, R. B., Reitz, R. H., Clewell, H. J., and Andersen, M. E. (1988). Biologically structured models and computer simulation: Application to chemical carcinogenesis. *Toxicol. Appl. Pharmacol.* (in press).

Conway, R. A. (1982). *Environmental Risk Analysis for Chemicals.* Van Nostrand-Reinhold, New York.

Cooper, M. (1957). *Pica*. Thomas, Springfield, IL.

Cornfield, J. (1977). Carcinogenic risk assessment. *Science* **198**, 693–699.

Covello, V. T., and Mumpower, J. (1985). Risk analysis and risk management: An historical perspective. *Risk Anal.* **5**, 103–120.

Covello, V. T., Menkes, J., and Mumpower, J. (Eds.) (1986). *Risk Evaluation and Management. Contemporary Issues in Risk Analysis*, Vol. 1. Plenum Press, New York.

Covello, V. T. et al. (1987). *Uncertainty in Risk Assessment, Risk Management, and Decision Making*, Adv. Risk Anal., Vol. 4. Plenum Press, New York.

Crandall, R. W., and Lave, B. L. (Eds.) (1981). *The Scientific Basis of Risk Assessment*. Brookings Institution, Washington, DC.

Crosby, D., and Wong, Z. (1976). Photodegradation of TCDD. *Science.*

Crouch, E. A. C., and Wilson, R. (1982). *Risk/Benefit Analysis*. Ballinger Press, Cambridge, MA.

Crouch, E. A. C., Wilson, R., and Zeise, L. (1983). The risks of drinking water. *Water Resour. Res.* **19**, 1359–1375.

Crump, K. S. (1981). An improved procedure for low-dose carcinogenic risk assessment from animal data. *J. Environ. Toxicol.* **5**, 339–346.

Crump, K. S. (1985). A new method for determining allowable daily intakes.

Crump, K. S., and Howe, R. B. (1984). The multistage model with time-dependent dose pattern: Applications of carcinogenic risk assessment. *Risk Anal.* **4**, 163–176.

Crump, K. S., Hoel, D. G., Langley, C. H., and Peto, R. (1976). Fundamental carcinogenic processes and their implications for low dose risk assessment. *Cancer Res.* **36**, 2973–2979.

Dedrick, R. L. (1973). Animal scale-up. *J. Pharmacokinet. Biopharm.* **1**, 435–461.

De Weese, L. R., McEwen, L. C., Hensler, G. L., and Petersen, B. E. Organochlorine contaminants in passeriformes and other avian prey of the peregrine falcon in the western United States. *Environ. Toxicol Chem.* **5**, 675–693.

Dickson, K. L., Maki, A. W., and Cairns, J., Jr., (Eds.) (1979). *Analyzing the Hazard Evaluation Process*. Am. Fish. Soc., Washington, DC.

di Domencio, A., Silano, V., Viviano, G., and Zapponi, G. (1980). Accidental release of 2, 3, 7, 8-tetrachlorodibenzo-p-dioxin. Part II. TCDD distribution in the soil surface layer. *Ecotoxicol. Environ. Saf.* **4**, 298–320.

Dourson, M. (1986). New approaches in the derivation of acceptable daily intakes (ADI). *Comments Toxicol.* **1**, 35–48.

Dourson, M. L., and Stara, J. F. (1983). Regulatory history and experimental support of uncertainty (safety factors). *Regul. Toxicol. Pharmacol.* **3**, 224–238.

Dugard, P. H., Walker, M., Mawdsley, S. J., and Scott, R. C. (1984). Absorption of some glycol ethers through human skin in vitro. *Environ. Health Perspect.* **57**, 193–198.

Ehling, U. H. (1988). Quantification of the genetic risk of environmental mutagens. *Risk Anal.* **8**, 45–58.

El Sayed, E. I., Graves, J. B., and Bonner, F. L. (1967). Chlorinated Hydrocarbon insecticide residues in selected insects and birds found in association with cotton fields. *J. Agric. Food Chem.* **15**(6), 1014–1017.

Environmental Protection Agency (EPA) (1979). *Water Related Fate of 129 Priority Pollutants*, Vols. 1 and 2, PB80-204381. USEPA, Washington, DC.

Environmental Protection Agency (EPA) (1982). *Air Quality Criteria for Particulate Matter and Sulfur Oxides*, Vol. 2, EPA-600-8-82-029bF. Office of Environmental Criteria and Assessment, USEPA, Research Triangle Park, NC, pp. 5-106–5-112.

Environmental Protection Agency (EPA) (1984). *Handbook for Interpreting Soil Data*. USEPA, Research Triangle Park, NC.

Environmental Protection Agency (EPA) (1986a). Guidelines for carcinogen risk assessment. *Fed. Regist.* **51**, CFR 2984, No. 185, 33,992–34,003.

Environmental Protection Agency (EPA) (1986b). Guidelines for developmental toxicity risk assessment. *Fed. Regist.* **51**, CFR 2984, No. 185, 34,028–34,040.

Environmetal Protection Agency (EPA) (1986c). Guidelines for exposure assessment. *Fed. Regist.* **51**, CFR 2984, No. 185, 34,041–34,054.

Environmental Protection Agency (EPA) (1986d). Guidelines for the health assessment of chemical mixtures. *Fed. Regist.* **51**, CFR 2984, No. 185, 34,014–34,025.

Environmental Protection Agency (EPA) (1986e). *Methodology for the Assessment of Health Risks Associated with Multiple Pathway Exposure to Municipal Waste Combustors*. Office of Air Quality Planning and Standards, USEPA, Research Triangle Park, NC.

Environmental Protection Agency (EPA) (1986f). *Superfund Health Assessment Manual*, EPA 540/1-86/060. Office of Emergency and Remedial Response, USEPA, Research Triangle Park, NC.

Environmental Protection Agency (EPA) (1986g). *Draft Superfund Exposure Assessment Manual*, OSWFR Directive 9285.5-1. USEPA, Research Triangle Park, NC.

Environmental Protection Agency (EPA) (1986h). *Registry of Toxic Effects of Chemical Substances*. USEPA, Research Triangle Park, NC.

Environmental Protection Agency (EPA) (1987a). *Handbook for Conducting Endangerment Assessments*. USEPA, Research Triangle Park, NC.

Environmental Protection Agency (EPA) (1987b). *An Approach to Estimating Exposure to 2,3,7,8-TCDD* (Draft). EPA Exposure Assessment Group, Washington, DC.

Environmental Protection Agency (EPA) (1988a). Guidelines for health assessment of systemic toxicants. *Fed. Regist.* (in draft).

Environmental Protection Agency (EPA) (1988b). Proposed guidelines for assessing female reproductive risk. *Fed. Regist.* **53**, No. 126, 24834–24847 (June 30).

Environmental Protection Agency (EPA) (1988c). Proposed guidelines for assessing male reproductive risk. *Fed. Regist.* **53**, No. 126, 24850–2486 (June 30).

Ernst, W. (1977). Determination of the bioconcentration potential of marine organisms—A steady-state approach. *Chemosphere* **11**, 731–740.

Eschenroeder, A., Jaeger, R. J., Ospital, J. J., and Doyle, C. (1986). Health risk assessment of human exposure to soil amended with sewage sludge contaminated with polycholorinated dibenzodioxins and dibenzofurans. *Vet. Hum. Toxicol.* **28**, 356–442.

Fabro, S., Schull, G., and Brown, N. A. (1982). The relative teratogenic index and teratogenic potency: Proposed components of developmental toxicity risk assessment. *Teratogen., Carcinogen. Mutagen.* **2**, 61–76.

Finkel, A. M., and Evans, J. S. (1987). Evaluating the benefits of uncertainty reduction in environmental health risk management. *J. Air Pollut. Control Assoc.* **37**, 1164–1171.

Fiserova-Bergerova, V. (1975). Mathematical modeling of inhalation exposure. *J. Combust. Toxicol.* **3**, 201–210.

Food Safety Council (1980). *A Proposed System for Food Safety Assessment: Final Report of the Scientific Committee*. Nutrition Foundation, Washington, DC.

Freed, V. H., Chiou, C. T., Schmeddling, D., and Kohnert, R. (1979). Some physical factors in toxicological assessment tests. *Environ. Health Perspect.* **30**, 75–80.

Fries, G. F. (1982). Potential polychlorinated biphenyl residues inanimal products from application of contaminated sewage sludge to land. *J. Environ. Qual.* **11**, 14–20.

Fries, G. F. (1985). Bioavailability of soil-borne polybrominated biphenyls ingested by farm animals. *J. Toxicol. Environ. Health* **16**, 565–579.

Fries, G. F., and Jacobs, L. W. (1986). Evaluation of residual polybrominated biphenyl contamination present on Michigan farms in 1978. *Mich., Agric. Exp. Stn., Res. Rep.* **477**.

Fries, G. F., and Paustenbach, D. J. (1987). A critical evaluation of the factors used in assessing incinerator emissions as a potential source of TCDD in foods of animal origin. *Int. Dioxin Symp., 7th*, Abstr. RC-05.

Friess, S. (1987). History of risk assessment. In *Pharmacokinetics in Risk Assessment: Drinking Water and Health,* Vol. 8. National Academy of Science, Washington, DC, pp. 3–7.

Gaylor, D. W., and Kodell, R. L. (1980). Linear interpolation algorithm for low dose risk assessment of toxic substances. *J. Environ. Pathol. Toxicol.* **4,** 305–312.

Gilbert, R. O. (1987). *Statistical Methods for Environmental Pollution Monitoring.* Van Nostrand-Reinhold, New York.

Gosselin, R. E., Gleason, M. N., Hodge, H. C., and Smith, R. P. (1984). *Clinical Toxicology of Commercial Products,* 5th ed. Williams & Wilkins, Baltimore, MD.

Hallenbeck, W. H., and Cunningham, K. M. (1986). *Quantitative Risk Assessment for Environmental and Occupational Health.* Lewis Publishers, Chelsea, MA.

Hamaker, J. W. (1975). The interpretation of soil leaching experiments. In R. Haque and V. H. Freed, Eds., *Environmental Dynamics of Pesticides.* Plenum Press, New York, pp. 115–133.

Hamaker, J. W., and Kerlinger, W. O. (1969). Vapor pressure of pesticides. *Adv. Chem. Ser.* **86,** 39–54.

Hamaker, J. W., and Thompson, J. M. (1972). Adsorption. In C. A. I. Goring and J. M. Haymaker, Eds., *Organic Chemicals in the Soil Environment,* Vol. 1. Dekker, New York, pp. 51–122.

Haque, R. (Ed.) (1980). *Dynamics, Exposure and Hazard Assessment of Toxic Chemicals.* Ann Arbor Science, Ann Arbor, MI.

Hart, W. L., Reynolds, R. C., Krasavage, W. J., Kly, T. S., Bell, R. H., and Raleigh, R. L. (1987). Evaluation of developmental toxicity data: A discussion of some pertinent factors, and a proposal. *Risk Anal.* **8,** 59–69.

Hartley, H. O., and Sielken, R. L. (1977). Estimation of "safe doses" in carcinogenic experiments. *J. Environ. Pathol.* **1,** 241–252.

Havender, W. R. (1984). EDB and the marigold option. *Regulation.* (Jan/Feb), 13–17.

Hawley, J. (1985). Assessment of health risks from exposure to contaminated soil. *Risk Anal.* **5,** 289–302.

Hayes, W. J., Jr. (1975). *Toxicology of Pesticides.* Waverly Press, Baltimore, MD.

Hayes, W. J., Jr. (1982). *Pesticides Studied in Man.* Williams & Wilkins, Baltimore, MD.

Healy, W. B., and Drew, K. R. (1970). Ingestion of soil by hoggets grazing Swedes. *N.A.A. Agric. Res.* **13,** 940–944.

Himmelstein, K. J., and Lutz, R. J. (1979). A review of the application of physiologically based pharmacokinetic modeling. *J. Pharmacokinet. Biopharm.* **7,** 127–137.

Hohenemser, C., and Kasperson, J. X. (Eds.) (1982). *Risk in the Technological Society.* Westview Press, Denver, CO.

Hutt, P. (1984). Legal considerations in risk assessment under federal regulatory statues. In J. Rodricks and R. Tardiff, Eds., *Assessment and Management of Chemical Risks.* Am. Chem. Soc., Washington, DC, pp. 84–95.

International Technical Information Institute (1976). *Toxic and Hazardous Industrial Chemicals Safety Manual.* ITII, Toranomon-Tachikawa Bldg., 6-5, 1 Chome, Nishi-Shimbashi, Minato-ku, Tokyo, Japan.

Jarvinen, A. W., and Tyo, R. M. (1979). Toxicity to minnows of endrin in food and water. *Arch. Environ. Chem. Toxicol.*

Johnson, E. M. (1987). A tier system for developmental toxicity evaluations based on considerations of exposure and effect relationships. *Teratology* **35,** 405–427.

Johnson, E. M. (1988). Cross-species extrapolations and the biologic basis for safety factor determinations in developmental toxicology. *Regul. Toxicol Pharmacol.* **8,** 22–36.

Johnson, P. (1980). The perils of risk avoidance. *Regulation* (May/June), 15–19.

Jury, W. A., Farmer, W. J., and Spencer, W. F. (1983). Behavior assessment model for trace organics in soil. Part I. Description of the model. *J. Environ. Qual.* **12,** 558–564.

Jury, W. A., Farmer, W. J., and Spencer, W. F. (1984). Behavior assessment model for trace organics in soil. Part IV. Review of experimental evidence. *J. Environ. Qual.* **13**, 580–586.

Kenaga, E. (1980). Correlation of bioconcentration factors of chemicals inaquatic and terrestrial organisms with their physical and chemical properties. *Ecotoxicol. Environ. Saf.* **4**, 26–38.

Kimbrough, R. (1986). Estimation of amount of soil ingested, inhaled or available for dermal contact. *Comments Toxicol.* **1**, 217–221.

Kimbrough, R., Falk, H. Stehr, P., and Fries G. (1984). Health implications of 2, 3, 7, 8-tetrachlorodibenzo-p-dioxin (TCDD) contamination of residential soil. *J. Toxicol. Environ. Health* **14**, 47–93.

Kimmel, C. A., and Gaylor, D. W. (1988). Issues in qualitative and quantitative risk analysis for developmental toxicology. *Risk Anal.* **8**, 15–20.

Klaassen, C. D., Amdur, M. O., and Doull, J. (Eds.) (1986). *Casarett and Doull's Toxicology: The Basic Science of Poisons*, 3rd ed. Macmillan, New York.

Korschgen, L. J. (1973). Soil–Food-chain–pesticide–wildlife relationships in aldrin-treated fields. *J. Wildl. Manage.* **34**(1), 186–199.

Krewski, D., Brown, C., and Murdoch, D. (1984). Determining safe levels of exposure: Safety factors or mathematical models. *Fundam. Appl. Toxil.* **4**, S383–S394.

Krewski, D. and Brown, C. (1981). Carcinogenic risk assessment: A guide to the literature. *Biometrics* **37**, 353–366.

Krzeminski, S. F., Gilbert, J. T., and Ritts, J. A. (1977). A pharmacokinetic model for predicting pesticide residues in fish. *Arch. Environ. Contam. Toxicol.* **5**, 157–165.

LaGoy, P. (1987). Estimated soil ingestion rates for use in risk assessment. *Risk Anal.* **7**, 355–359.

Lave, L. B. (Ed.) (1983). *Quantitative Risk Assessment in Regulation.* Brookings Institution, Washington, DC.

Lehmann, A., and Fitzhugh, O. G. (1954). 100-fold margin of safety. *Q. Bull.—Assoc. Food Drug Off. U.S.* **18**, 33–35.

Leidel, N., and Busch, K. A. (1985). Statistical design and data analysis requirements. In L. J. Cralley and L. V. Cralley, Eds., *Pattys Industrial Hygiene Toxicology*, 2nd ed., Vol. 3A, Wiley, New York.

Lepow, M. L., Bruckman, L., Robino, R. A., Markowitz, S., Gillette, M., and Kapish, J. (1974). Role of airborne lead in increased body burden of lead in Hartford children. *Environ. Health Perspect.* **6**, 99–101.

Lindgreen, B. W. (1980). *Statistical Theory*, 2nd ed. Macmillan, New York.

Lowrance, W. (1976). *Of Acceptable Risk.* Wm. Kaufmann, Inc., Los Altos, CA.

Lowrance, W. (1984). *Modern Science and Human Values.* Oxford Univ. Press, London and New York.

Lu, F. C. (1985). Safety assessments of chemicals with threshold effects. *Regul. Toxicol. Pharmacol.* **5**, 121–132.

Lu, F. C. (1988). Acceptable daily intake: Inception, evolution, and application. *Regul. Toxicol. Pharmacol.* **8**, 45–60.

Mackay, D., and Paterson, S. (1982). Calculating fugacity. *Environ. Sci. Technol.* **15**(9), 1006–1014.

Marzulli, F. N. and Maibach, H. I. (1983). *Dermatotoxicology.* 2nd ed. Hemisphene Pub. Washington, DC.

Maki, A. (1979). An analysis of decision criteria in environmental hazard evaluation programs. In K. L. Dickson, A. W. Maki, and J. Cairns, Jr., Eds., *Analyzing the Hazard Evaluation Process.* Am. Fish. Soc., Washington, DC, pp. 83–100.

Maki, A., Dickson, K. L., and Cairns, J., Jr. (Eds.) (1979). *Understanding Chemicals in the Environment.*

Maki, A., Dickson, K. L., and Cairns, J., Jr. (Eds.) (1980). *Biotransformation and Fate of Chemicals in the Aquatic Environment.*

Mantel, N., and Bryan, W. R. (1961). "Safety" testing of carcinogenic agents. *J. Natl. Cancer Inst. (U.S.)* **27**, 455–460.

Martin, W. E. (1964). Loss of Sr-90, Sr-89 and I-131 from fallout of contaminated plants. *Radiat. Bot.* **4**, 275–281.

Maxim, L. D., and Harrington, L. (1984). A review of the Food and Drug Administration risk analysis for polychlorinated biphenyls. *Regul. Toxicol. Pharmacol.* **4**, 192–199.

McColl, R. S. (1987). *Environmental Health Risks: Assessment and Management.* Institute for Risk Research, Waterloo, Ontario.

McConnell, E., Lucier, G., Rumbaugh, R., Albro, P., Harvan, D., Hass, J., and Harris M. (1984). Dioxin in soil: Bioavailability after ingestion by rats and guinea pigs. *Science* **223**, 1077–1079.

Meistrich, M. L. (1988). Estimation of human reproductive risk from animal studies: Determination of interspecies extrapolation factors for steriod hormone effects on the male. *Risk Anal.* **8**, 27–34.

Menzel, D. (1987). Physiological pharmacokinetic modeling. *Environ. Sci. Technol.* **21**, 944–950.

Menzer, R. E., and Nelson, J. O. (1986). Water and soil pollutants. In C. D. Klaassen, M. O. Amdur, and J. Doull, Eds., *Casarett and Doull's Toxicology*, 3rd ed. Macmillan, New York, pp. 825–853.

Moolgavkar, S. H. (1978). The multistage theory of carcinogenesis and the age distribution of cancer in man. *JNCI, J. Natl. Cancer Inst.* **61**, 49–52.

Moolgavkar, S. H. (1986). Carcinogenesis modeling: From molecular biology to epidemiology. *Annu. Rev. Public Health* **7**, 151–169.

Moolgavkar, S. H., and Knudson, A. G. (1981). Mutation and cancer: A model for human carcinogenesis. *JNCI, J. Natl. Cancer Inst.* **66**, 1037–1052.

Moolgavkar, S. H., and Venzon, D. J. (1979). Two event models for carcinogenesis: Incidence curves for childhood and adult tumors. *Math. Biosci.* **47**, 55–77.

Moolgavkar, S. H., Day, N. E., and Stevens, R. G. (1980). Two-stage model for carcinogenisis: Epidemiology of breast cancer in females. *JNCI, J. Natl. Cancer Inst.* **65**, 559–569.

Moolgavkar, S. H., Dewanji, A., and Venzon, D. J. (1988). A stochastic two-stage model for cancer risk assessment. I. The hazard function and probability of tumor. *Risk Anal.* (in press).

Motto, H. L., Daines, R. H., Chilko, D. M., and Motto, C. K. (1970). *Environ. Sci. Technol.* **4**, 231–237.

Munro, I. C., and Krewski, D. R. (1981). Risk assessment and regulatory decision making. *Food Cosmet. Toxicol.* **19**, 549–560.

National Academy of Sciences (NAS) (1975). *Principles for Evaluating Chemicals in the Environment.* NAS, Washington, DC.

National Academy of Sciences (NAS) (1977–1987). *Drinking Water and Health*, Vols. 1–8. NAS, Washington, DC.

National Academy of Sciences (NAS) (1983). *Risk Assessment in the Federal Government: Managing the Process.* National Academy Press, Washington, DC.

National Institute for Occupational Safety and Health (1976). *Occupational Diseases: A Guide to Their Recognition.* NIOSH, Cincinnati, OH.

National Research Council (1980). *Lead in the Human Environment.* NRC, Washington, DC.

National Research Council (1987). *Pharmacokinetics in Risk Assessment: Drinking Water and Health*, Vol. 8. National Academy of Science, Washington, DC.

Neely, W. G., Branson, D. R., and Blau, G. E. (1974). The use of the partition coefficient to measure the bioconcentration potential of organic chemicals in fish. *Environ. Sci. Technol.* **8**, 1113–1115.

Nichols, A. L., and Zeckhauser, R. J. (1985). Conservatism in regulatory analysis. *Science.*

Nichols, A. L., and Zeckhauser, R. J. (1988). The perils of prudence: How conservative risk assessments distort regulation. *Regul. Toxicol. Pharmacol.* **8**, 61–75.

Nisbet, I. C. T., and Karch, N. J. (1983). *Chemical Hazards to Human Reproduction.* Noyes Data Corp., Park Ridge, NJ.

Nordberg (1976). *Effects and Dose-Response Relationsships of Metals.* Elsevier; Amsterdam, Netherlands.

Office of Science and Technology Policy (1985). *Cancer Risk Assessment Guidelines.* OSTP, Washington, DC.

Office of Technology Assessment (1981). *Assessment of Technologies for Determining Cancer Risks from the Environment.* OTA, Washington, DC.

Park, C. N., and Snee, R. D. (1983). Quantitative risk assessment: State of the art for carcinogenesis. *Am. Stat.* **37**(4), 427–441.

Parmeggiai, L. (Ed.) (1983). *Encyclopaedia of Occupational Health and Safety*, 3rd ed., Vols. 1 and 2. International Labor Office, World Health Organ., Geneva.

Paustenbach, D. J. (1985). Occupational exposure limits, pharmacokinetics, and unusual work schedules. In L. J. Cralley and L. V. Cralley (Eds.), *Patty's Industrial Hygiene Toxicology*, 2nd ed., Vol. 3A. Wiley, New York, Chapter 5.

Paustenbach, D. J., Shu, H. P., and Murray, F. J. (1986). A critical analysis of risk assessment of TCDD contaminated soils. *Regul. Toxicol. Pharmacol.* **6**, 284–307.

Paustenbach, D. J., Clewell, H. J. III, Gargas, M. L., and Andersen, M. E. (1988). A physiologically-based pharmacokinetic model for inhaled carbon tetrachloride. *Toxicol. Appl. Pharm.* (in press).

Piotrowski, J. L. (1973). *Exposure Tests for Organic Compounds in Industry.* National Institute of Occupational Safety and Health, Cincinnati, OH.

Poiger, H., and Schlatter, C. (1980). Influence of solvents and absorbents on dermal and intestinal adsorption of TCDD. *Food Cosmet. Toxicol.* **18**, 477–481.

Proctor, N. H., Hughes, J. P., and Fischman, M. (1988). *Chemical Hazards of the Workplace*, 2nd ed. Lippincott, Philadelphia, PA.

Ramsey, J. R., and Andersen, M. E. (1984). A physiologically-based description of the inhalation pharmacokinetics of styrene in rats and humans. *Toxicol. Appl. Pharmacol.* **73**, 159–175.

Rand, G. M., and Petrocelli, S. R. (1985). *Fundamentals of Aquatic Toxicology.* McGraw-Hill, New York.

Rappaport, S. M., and Selvin, J. (1987). A method for evaluating the mean exposure from a log-normal distribution. *Am. Ind. Hyg. Assoc. J.* **48**, 374–379.

Reinecke, A. J., and Nash, R. G. (1984). Toxicology of TCDD and bioavailability by earthworms. *Soil Biol. Biochem.* **16**, 45–49.

Reitz, R. H., Quast, J. F., Stott, W. T., Watanabe, P. G., and Gehring, P. J. (1980). Pharmacokinetics and macromolecular effects of chloroform in rats and mice: Implications for carcinogenic risk estimation. In *Water Chlorination.* Ann Arbor Science Press, Michigan, Chapter 85, pp. 983–993.

Reitz, R. H., Fox, T. R., and Watanabe, P. G. (1986). The role of pharmacokinetics in risk assessment. *Basic Life Sci.* **38**, 499–507.

Rodricks, J. V. (1988). Origins of risk assessment in food-safety decisionmaking. *J. Am. Coll. Toxicol* (in press).

Rodricks, J. V., Brett, S. N., and Wrenn, G. C. (1987). Risk decisions in federal regulatory agencies. *Regul. Toxicol. Pharmacol.* **7**, 307–320.

Roels, H., Buchet, J. P., and Lauwerys, R. R. (1980). Exposure to lead by the oral and pulmonary routes of children living in the vicinity of a primary lead smelter. *Environment* **22**, 81–94.

Romney, E. M., Lindberg, N. G., Hawthorne, H. A., Bystrom, B. B., and Larson, K. H. (1963). Contamination of plant foliage with radioactive nuclides. *Annu. Rev. Plant Physiol.* **14**, 271–279.

Rowe, W. D. (1977). *An Anatomy of Risk.* Wiley, New York.

Russell, R. S. (1966). Entry of radioactive materials into plants. In R. S. Russell, Ed. *Radioactivity and Human Diet*, Pergamon Press, New York, Chapter 5.

Sax, N. I. (1984). *Dangerous Properties of Industrial Materials*, 6th ed. Van Nostrand, New York.

Sayre, J. W., Charney, E., Vostal, J., and Pless, B. (1974). House and hand dust as a potential source of childhood lead exposure. *Am. J. Dis. Child.* **127**, 167–170.

Schaeffer, D. J. (1981). Is "No-threshold" a "Non-concept". *Environ. Manage.* **5**, 475–481.

Schardein, J. L. (1983). Teratogenic risk assessment. *Issues Rev. Toxicol.* **1**, 181–214.

Schardein, J. L., Schwetz, B. A., and Kepel, M. E. (1985). Species sensitivities and prediction of teratogenic potential. *Environ. Health Perspect.* **61**, 55–67.

Schaum, J. (1983). *Risk Analysis of TCDD Contaminated Soil*. Office of Health and Environmental Assessment, U.S. Environ. Prot. Agency, Washington, DC.

Schwing, R. C., and Albers, W. A., Jr. (Eds.) (1980). *Societal Risk Assessment: How Safe is Safe Enough*. Plenum Press, New York.

Shepard, T. H. (1980). *Catalog of Teratogenic Agents*, 3rd ed. John Hopkins Univ. Press, Baltimore, MD.

Shu, H., Paustenbach, D., Murray, J., Marple, L., Brunck, B., Dei Rossi, D., Webb, A. S., and Tietelbaum, T. (1987). Bioavailability of soil-bound TCDD: Oral bioavailability in the rat. *Fundam. Appl. Toxicol.* **10**, 648–654.

Shu, H., Tietelbaum, P., Webb, A. S., Marple, L., Brunck, B., Dei Rossi, D., Murray, J., and Paustenbach, D. (1988). Bioavailability of soil-bound TCDD: Dermal bioavailability in the rat. *Fundam. Appl. Toxicol.* **10**, 335–343.

Sielken, R. L. (1985). Some issues in the quantitative modeling portion of cancer risk assessment. *Regul. Toxicol. Pharmacol.* **5**, 175–181.

Sielken, R. L. (1987a). Quantitative cancer risk assessment for 2,3,7,8-TCDD. *Food Chem. Toxicol.* **25**, 257–267.

Sielken, R. L. (1987b). Statistical evaluation reflecting the skewness in the distribution of TCDD levels in human adipose tissue. *Chemosphere* **16**(8–9), 2135–2140.

Sielken, R. L. (1987c). The capabilities, sensitivity, pitfalls, and future of quantitative risk assessment. In R. Stephen McColl, Ed., *Environmental Health Risks: Assessment and Management*. Univ. of Waterloo Press, Waterloo, Ontario, pp. 95–131.

Sielken, R. L. (1987d). A response to Crump's evaluation of Sielken's dose-response assessment for TCDD.

Silkworth, J., McMartin, D., DeCaprio, A., Rej, R., O'Keefe, P., and Kaminsky, L. (1982). Acute toxicity in guinea pigs and rabbits of soot from a polychlorinated biphenyl-containing transformer fire. *Toxicol. Appl. Pharmacol.* **65**, 425–429.

Sitnig, M. (1985). *Handbook of Toxic and Hazardous Chemicals and Carcinogens*. Noyes Data Corp., Park Ridge, NJ.

Smith, A. H. (1987). Infant exposure assessment for breast milk dioxins and furans derived from waste incineration emissions. *Risk Anal.* **7**, 347–353.

Smith, J. H., Bomberger, D. C., and Haynes, D. L. (1981). Volatilization rates of intermediate and low volatility chemicals from water. *Chemosphere* **10**, 281–289.

Snyder, W. S. (1975). *Report of the Task Group on Reference Man*, ICRP No. 23. Pergamon Press, New York.

Southworth, G. R., Parkhust, B. R., Herbes, S. E., and Tsai, S. C. (1982). The risk of chemicals to aquatic environment. In R. A. Conway, Ed., *Environmental Risk Analysis for Chemicals*. Van Nostrand, New York.

Spacie, A., and Hamelink, J. (1985). Bioaccumulation. In G. M. Rand and S. R. Petrocelli, Eds., *Fundamentals of Aquatic Toxicology*. McGraw-Hill, New York.

Spencer, W. F., and Farmer, W. J. (1980). Assessment of the vapor behavior of toxic organic chemicals. In R. Haque, Ed., *Dynamics, Exposure and Hazard Assessment of Toxic Chemicals.* Ann Arbor Science, Ann Arbor, MI, pp. 143–161.

Sprague, J. B. (1973). The ABCs of pollutant bioassay using fish. In J. Cairns, Jr. and K. L. Dickson, Eds., *Biological Methods for the Assessment of Water Quality.* Am. Soc. Test. Mater., Philadelphia, PA, pp. 6–30.

Stickel, L. F. (1973). Chemosphere pesticide reserves in birds and mammals. In C. A. Edwards, Ed., *Environmental Pollution by Pesticides.* Plenum Press, New York.

Stickel, W. H., Hayne, D. W., and Stickel, L. F. (1965). Effects of heptachlorocontaminated earthworms on woodcocks. *J. Wildl. Manage.* **29**(1), 132–146.

Stokinger, H. E. (1981). Threshold limit values. Part I. In *Dangerous Properties of Industrial Materials Report.* Van Nostrand-Reinhold, New York, pp. 8–13.

Sueishi, T., Morioka, T., Kaneko, H., Kvsaka, M., Yagi, S., and Chikami, S. (1988). Environmental risk assessment of surfactants: Fate and environmental effects in Lake Biwa Basin. *Regul. Toxicol. Pharmacol.* **8**, 5–21.

Thibodeaux, L. J. (1979). *Chemodynamics: Environmental Movement of Chemicals in Air, Water and Soil.* Wiley, New York.

Thiennes, C. H., and Haley, T. J. (1972). *Clinical Toxicology,* 5th ed. Lea & Febinger, Philadelphia, PA.

Thornton, I., and Abrahams, P. (1981). Soil ingestion as a pathway of metal intake into grazing livestock. In *Proceedings of the International Conference on Heavy Metals in the Environment.* CEP Consultants, Edinburgh, pp. 167–122.

Thorslund, T. W., Brown, C. C., and Charnley, G. (1987). Biologically motivated cancer risk models. *Risk Anal.* **7**, 109–119.

Travis, C. C., Richter, S. A., Crouch, C. E., Wilson, R., and Klema, E. D. (1987). Cancer risk management. *Environ. Sci. Technol.* **21**, 415 420.

Tucker, R. K., and Crabtree, D. G. (1970). *Handbook of Toxicity of Pesticides to Wildlife,* Fish Wildl. Serv. USDI, Resour. Publ. No. 84. Denver Wildlife Research Center, Denver, CO.

Turnbull, D., and Rodricks, J. (1985). Assessment of possible carcinogenic risk to humans resulting from exposure to di(2-ethylhexyl)phthalate(DEHP). *J. Am. Coll. Toxicol.* **4**, 111–145.

Urquhart, J., and Heilmann, K. (1984). *Risk Watch: The Odds of Life.* Facts on File Publ., New York.

U.S. Food and Drug Administration (1984). *Environmental Assessment Technical Handbook.* Center for Food Safety and Applied Nutrition and Center for Veterinary Medicine, USFDA, Washington, DC.

Van den Berg, M., Olie, K., and Hutzinger, O. (1984). Uptake and selective retention in rats of orally administered chlorinated dioxins and dibenzofurans from fly-ash and fly-ash extract. *Chemosphere* **12**, 537–544.

Wang, G. M., and Schwetz, B. A. (1987). An evaluation system for ranking chemicals with tetratogenic, potential. *Teratogen. Carcinogen. Mutagen.* **7**, 133–139.

Wattenberg, B. J. (1984). *The Good News is the Bad News is Wrong.* Simon & Schuster, New York.

Weast, R. C. (1988). *Handbook of Chemistry and Physics.* CRC Press, Inc. Cleveland, Ohio.

Weil, C. S. (1970). Selection of number of the valid sampling units and a consideration of their combination in toxicological studies involving reproduction, teratogenesis or carcinogenesis. *Food Cosmet. Toxicol.* **8**, 177–182.

Weil, C. S. (1972). Statistics versus safety factors and scientific judgment in the evaluation of safety for man. *Toxicol. Appl. Pharmacol.* **21**, 454–463.

Weiss, B. (1988). Neurobehavioral toxicity as a basis for risk assessment. *Trends Pharmacol. Sci.* **9**(2), 59–62.

Wester, R. C., and Noonan, P. K. (1980). Relevance of animal models for percutaneous absorption. *Int. J. Pharm.* **7**, 99–110.

Whipple, C. (1988). *De Minimus Risk.* Macmillan, New York.

Whittemore, A. S., Grosser, S. L., and Silvers, A. (1986). Pharmacokinetics in low-dose extrapolation using animal cancer data. *Fundam. Appl. Toxicol.* **7**, 183–190.

Williams, G. M., and Weisburger, J. H. (1981). Systematic carcinogen testing through a decision point approval. *Annu. Rev. Pharmacol. Toxicol.* **21**, 393–416.

Wilson, J. G. (1973). *Environment and Birth Defects.* Academic Press, New York.

Wilson, J. G. (1983). In M. S. Christian, W. M. Galbraith, P. Voytek, and M. A. Mehlmann, Eds., *Assessment of Reproductive and Teratogenic Hazards.* Princeton Univ. Press, Princeton, NJ.

Wipf, H. K., Homberger, E., Neimer, N., Ranalder, U. B., Vetter W., and Vuilleumeir, J. P. (1982). TCDD-levels in soil and plant samples from the Seveso area. In O. Hutzinger et al., Eds., *Chlorinated Dioxins and Related Compounds: Impact on the Environment.* Pergamon Press, New York, pp. 115–126.

World Health Organization (WHO) (1987). *Occupational Exposure Limits for Airborne Toxic Substances,* 3rd ed., Occup. Saf. Health Ser., No. 37. International Labor Office, WHO, Geneva.

Zielhuis, R. L., and van der Kreek, F. W. (1979a). The use of a safety factor in setting health based permissible levels for occupational exposure. Part I. A proposal. *Int. Arch. Occup. Environ. Health* **42**, 191–201.

Zielhuis, R. L., and van der Kreek, F. W. (1979b). Calculation of a safety factor in setting health based permissible levels for occupational exposure. Part II. Comparison of extrapolated and published permissible levels. *Int. Arch. Occup. Environ. Health* **42**, 203–215.

A

BASIC PRINCIPLES

1

A Survey of Health Risk Assessment

Dennis J. Paustenbach

McLaren Environmental Engineering, ChemRisk Division, Alameda, California

1 INTRODUCTION

Since 1970 the field of risk assessment has received widespread attention within both the scientific and regulatory communities [Starr, 1969; National Academy of Sciences (NAS) 1983; Ruckelshaus, 1984b; National Academy of Engineering (NAE), 1986]. It has also attracted the attention of the public (Wall Street Journal, 1987) and the legal system (Barnard, 1984). Beginning in the 1980s, the public began to develop an expectation that risk analysis would help bring order to what appeared to be an unmanageable quantity of scientific and medical data regarding the potential health hazards posed by physical and chemical agents in our environment. It was hoped that risk assessment methodologies would help regulators make better decisions. Such analyses represented a logical progression from the 1950s when scientists tended to give decisionmakers only the "black and white," "yes it is," or "no it isn't" insight obtained from toxicity testing. Another reason that risk assessments have become important to risk managers, policymakers, and the public is that they often offer a range of options, each having a specific cost and benefit.

Properly conducted risk assessments have received fairly broad acceptance, in part because they put into perspective the terms *toxic*, *hazard*, and *risk*. Regrettably, the terms have not always been used correctly by either the lay press or those within the scientific community. Toxicity, as noted by Paracelsus in the 1500s, is an inherent property of all substances. All chemical and physical agents can produce adverse health effects, that is, toxicity, at some dose or under specific exposure conditions (concentration plus duration). In short, the dose makes the poison. In contrast, exposure to a chemical e.g., benzene, that has the *capacity* to produce a particular type of adverse effect, for example, leukemia, represents a hazard. Risk, however, is the *probability* or likelihood that an adverse outcome will occur in a person or a group that is exposed to a particular concentration or dose of the hazardous agent. Therefore, risk is generally a function of exposure or dose. In this text, the process or procedure used to estimate the likelihood that humans or ecological systems will be affected adversely by a chemical or physical agent under a specific set of conditions is called *health risk assessment*.

The term *risk assessment*, however, is not used exclusively to describe the likelihood of an adverse response to a chemical or physical agent. In fact, risk assessment has been used to describe the likelihood of a diverse number of unwanted events. These include industrial explosions, workplace injuries, failure of machine parts, a wide variety of natural catastrophes (e.g., earthquakes, tidal waves, hurricanes, volcanic eruptions, tornadoes, blizzards), injury or death due to an array of voluntary activities (e.g., skiing, football, sky diving, flying, hunting), diseases (e.g., cancer, leukemia, developmental toxicity caused by chemical exposure), death due to natural causes (e.g., heart attack, cancer, diabetes), death due to lifestyle (e.g., smoking, alcoholism, diet), and a number of other endpoints (Schwing and Albers, 1980).

The purpose of risk assessments is to provide complete information to risk managers, specifically, policymakers and regulators, so that the best possible decision can be made. As discussed by numerous researchers, factors other than those addressed in a risk assessment can influence decisions about risk (Lowrance, 1976, 1985). In light of the dramatic increase in the number of pieces of legislation that have been passed during the past 30 years (Fig. 1), it is clear that society has been uncomfortable about the regulatory agencies ability to "manage" the risks posed by chemical and physical hazards. Starr (1969), in his groundbreaking article on risk assessment—"Social benefits versus technological risk"—as well as in his 1985 lecture "Risk management, assessment, and acceptability," discussed some of the conflicts that face those who conduct risk assessments. For example, he noted that "public acceptance of any risk is more dependent on public confidence in risk management than on the quantitative estimates of risk consequences, probabilities, and magnitudes." He was one of the first scientists to draw the distinction between voluntary and involuntary risks—an issue that continues to be a difficult one for risk managers who must often regulate involuntary risks, which would

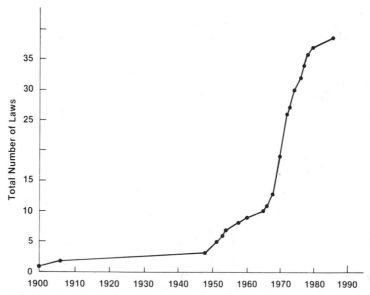

Figure 1. Federal legislation dealing with the manufacture, use, transportation, sale, or disposal of hazardous materials. From Paustenbach (1984).

clearly be considered inconsequential when compared with voluntary risks generally accepted by the public (Crouch and Wilson, 1987).

1.1   Risk Assessment versus Risk Management

A health risk assessment is a written document wherein all the pertinent scientific information, regarding toxicology, human experience, environmental fate, and exposure are assembled, critiqued, and interpreted. The goal of the assessment is to estimate the likelihood of an adverse effect on humans, wildlife, or ecological systems posed by a specific level of exposure to a chemical or physical hazard. Risk assessments of environmental hazards, in contrast to the analyses of the likelihood of the occurrence of any undesirable event, for example, earthquakes and machine failure, are thoroughly dependent on the degree of exposure. As a result, assessments of health hazards posed by workplaces, hazardous waste sites, ambient air pollutants, water pollutants, soil contaminants, and food contaminants are dependent on both the potency of the agent and the level of exposure. The same principles apply to assessments of plants, fish, birds, insects, large and small mammals, reptiles, and other wildlife.

The term risk assessment has been misused by dozens of scientists whose papers have appeared in the scientific literature during the past 10 years. All too often, risk assessment has incorrectly been characterized as the process used to estimate the low-dose response following exposure to carcinogenic chemicals. Perhaps the best and most widely cited definition of risk assessment is the one suggested by the National Academy of Science (NAS, 1983). In its report, the NAS committee recommended.

> risk assessment to mean the characterization of the potential adverse health effects of human exposures to environmental hazards. Risk assessments include several elements: description of the potential adverse health effects based on an evaluation of results of epidemiologic, clinical, toxicologic, and environmental research; extrapolation from those results to predict the type and estimate the extent of health effects in humans under given conditions of exposure; judgments as to the number and characteristics of persons exposed at various intensities and durations; and summary judgments on the existence and overall magnitude of the public-health problem. Risk assessment also includes characterization of the uncertainties inherent in the process of inferring risk.

The NAS committee emphasized that the processes of risk assessment and risk management were to be separate activities. They offered the following definition for risk management (NAS, 1983):

> The Committee uses the term risk management to describe the process of evaluating alternative regulatory actions and selecting among them. Risk management, which is carried out by regulatory agencies under various legislative mandates, is an agency decision-making process that entails consideration of political, social, economic, and engineering information with risk-related information to develop, analyze, and compare regulatory options and to select the appropriate regulatory response to a potential chronic health hazard. The selection process necessarily requires the use of value judgments on such issues as the acceptability of risk and the reasonableness of the costs of control.

One goal of the committee was to encourage scientists, policymakers, and the public to separate clearly the risk assessment from the risk management process. Until this time, many assessments were so laden with value judgments and the subjective views of the risk assessors that the risk manager was unable to separate the scientific data from the wishes of the risk scientist. Perhaps the most significant accomplishment of the NAS committee was the identification of this problem.

1.2 The Assessment Process

Risk assessment can be divided into four major steps: hazard identification, dose–response assessment, exposure assessment, and risk characterization (NAS, 1983). For some perceived hazards, the risk assessment might stop with the first step, hazard identification, if no adverse effect is identified or if an agency elects to take regulatory action without further analysis. The NAS committee suggested the following definitions of the four steps:

> *Hazard identification* is the most easily recognized of the actions of regulatory agencies. It is defined here as the process of determining whether human exposure to an agent could cause an increase in the incidence of a health condition (cancer, birth defect, etc.) or whether exposure by a nonhuman receptor, for example, fish, birds, or other wildlife, might adversely be affected. It involves characterizing the nature and strength of the evidence of causation. Although the question of whether a substance causes cancer or other adverse health effects in humans is theoretically a yes–no question, there are few chemicals or physical agents on which the human data are definitive [National Research Council (NRC), 1983]. Therefore, the question is often restated in terms of effects in laboratory animals or other test systems: "Does the agent induce cancer in test animals?" Positive answers to such questions are typically taken as evidence that an agent may pose a cancer risk for any exposed human. Information from short-term in vitro tests and structural similarity to known chemical hazards may, in certain circumstances, also be considered as adequate information of identifying a hazard.

> *Dose–response assessment* is the process of characterizing the relation between the dose of an agent administered or received and the incidence of an adverse health effect in exposed populations and estimating the incidence of the effect as a function of exposure to the agent. This process considers such important factors as intensity of exposure, age pattern of exposure, and possibly other variables that might affect response, such as sex, lifestyle, and other modifying factors. A dose–response assessment usually requires extrapolation from high to low doses and extrapolation from animals to humans, or one laboratory animal species to a species of wildlife. A dose–response assessment should describe and justify the methods of extrapolation used to predict incidence and it should characterize the statistical and biologic uncertainties in these methods. When possible, the uncertainties should be described numerically rather than qualitatively.

> *Exposure assessment* is the process of measuring or estimating the intensity, frequency, and duration of human or animal exposure to an agent currently present in the environment or of estimating hypothetical exposures that might arise from the release of new chemicals into the environment. In its most complete form, an exposure assessment should describe the magnitude, duration, schedule, and route of exposure; the size, nature, and classes of the human, animal, aquatic, or wildlife populations exposed; and the uncertainties in all estimates. The exposure assessment can often be used to identify feasible prospective control options and to predict the effects of available control technologies for controlling or limiting exposure.

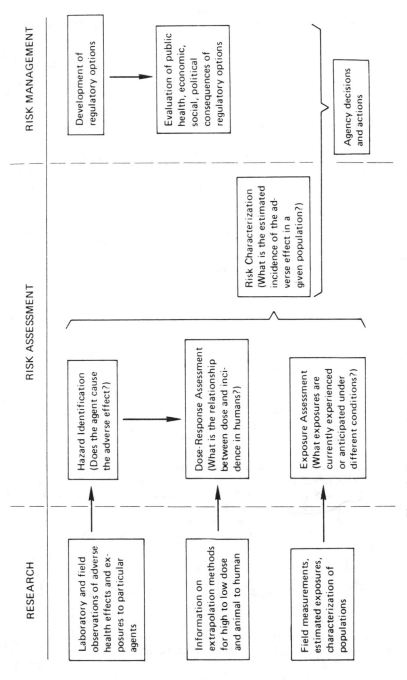

Figure 2. Elements of the risk assessment and risk management processes. From NAS (1983).

31

Risk characterization is the process of estimating the incidence of a health effect under the various conditions of human or animal exposure described in the exposure assessment. It is performed by combining the exposure and dose–response assessments. The summary effects of the uncertainties in the preceding steps should be described in this step.

The relation between the four steps of the risk assessment process and risk management are depicted in Fig. 2. The information needed to perform each step is also shown.

2   HEALTH RISK ASSESSMENTS: A BRIEF HISTORY

The origin of risk assessment, in its most basic form, can be traced back to that of early humans. Certainly, after humans recognized that the meat of animals represented a source of food when edible plants were not available, they had to weigh the hazard of being mauled by a wild animal, which they hoped to kill and eat, versus the benefit of thwarting starvation. The historical record does not permit us to know how well early humans balanced this risk–benefit relationship; however, it is safe to assume that those who first conducted these assessments fared less well than those who later conducted similar analyses. Almost certainly, the scientists of the 21st century, when studying the risk analyses conducted in the 1980s, will draw a similar analogy to those conducted by primitive humans.

2.1   The Earliest Years (ca. 3200 B.C. to A.D. 500)

A thoughtful review of the history of risk analysis has been developed by Covello and Mumpower (1985) and much of the subsequent discussion draws on their work. With respect to the early years, they noted the following:

In the Tigris–Euphrates valley about 3200 B.C. there lived a group called the Asipu. One of their primary functions was to serve as consultants for risky, uncertain, or difficult decisions. If a decision needed to be made concerning a forthcoming risky venture, a proposed marriage arrangement, or a suitable building site, one could consult with a member of the Asipu. The Asipu would identify the important dimensions of the problem, identify alternative actions, and collect data on the likely outcomes (e.g., profit or loss, success or failure) of each alternative. The best available data from their perspective were signs from the gods, which the priest-like Asipu were especially qualified to interpret. The Asipu would then create a ledger with a space for each alternative. If the signs were favorable, they would enter a plus in the space; if not, they would enter a minus. After the analysis was completed, the Asipu would recommend the most favorable alternative. The last step was to issue a final report to the client, etched upon a clay tablet. [Oppenheim, 1977].

According to Grier, the practices of the Asipu mark the first recorded instance of a simplified form of risk analysis. The similarities between the practices and procedures of modern risk analysts and those of their Babylonian forebears underscore the point that people have been dealing with problems of risk for a long time, often in a sophisticated and quantitative way.

Covello and Mumpower (1985) implied that religious beliefs played a significant role in the evolution of probability theory and risk analysis.

An important thread leading to modern quantitative risk analysis can be traced to early religious ideas concerning the probability of an afterlife. This should hardly be surprising, considering the salience and seriousness of the risks involved (at least for true believers). Beginning with Plato's *Phaedo* in the 4th century B.C., numerous treatises have been written discussing the risk to one's soul in the afterlife based on how one conducts oneself in the here and now.

One of the most sophisticated analyses of this issue was carried out by Arnobius the Elder, who lived in the 4th century A.D. in North Africa. Arnobius was a major figure in a pagan church that was competing at the time with the fledgling Christian church. Members of Arnobius' church, who maintained a temple to Venus complete with virgin sacrifices and temple prostitution, led a decadent life in comparison to the austere Christians. Arnobius taunted the Christians for their lives of pointless self abnegation; but, after a revelatory vision, renounced his previous beliefs and attempted to convert to Christianity. The bishop of the Christian church, suspicious of Arnobius' motives and the sincerity of his conversion, refused him the rite of baptism. In an effort to demonstrate the authenticity of his conversion, Arnobius authorized an eight-volume monograph entitled *Against the Pagans*. In this work, Arnobius made a number of arguments for Christianity, one of which is particularly relevant to the history of probabilistic risk analysis. After thoroughly discussing the risks and uncertainties associated with decisions affecting one's soul, Arnobius proposed a 2×2 matrix. There are, he argued, two alternatives: "accept Christianity" or "remain a pagan." There are also, he argued, two possible, but uncertain, states of affairs: "God exists" or "God does not exist." If God does not exist, there is no difference between the two alternatives (with the minor exception that Christians may unnecessarily forgo some of the pleasures of the flesh enjoyed by pagans). If God exists, however, being a Christian is far better for one's soul then being a pagan.

2.2 Environmental Risks (ca. A.D. 500–1300)

Contamination of the air, water, and land has long been recognized as a potential health problem, but the need to control pollution was not recognized for a rather long period. Covello and Mumpower (1985), in reviewing this topic observed:

> Air pollution (due to dust and smoke from wood and coal fires) has been a ubiquitous problem in congested urban areas since ancient times [Hughes, 1975]. The first act of government intervention did not occur until 1285, however, when King Edward I of England responded to a petition from members of the nobility and others concerning the offensive coal smoke in London. Smoke arising from the burning of soft coal had long been a problem in London [White, 1967; Brake, 1975]. Edward's response to the petition was one that is now commonly practiced by government risk managers—he established a commission in 1285 to study the problem. In response to the commission's report, several private sector actions were taken, including a voluntary decision by a group of London smiths in 1298 not to "... work at night on account of the unhealthiness of coal and damage to their neighbors." [Hughes, 1975] These voluntary efforts were not sufficient, however, and in 1307 Edward issued a royal proclamation prohibiting the use of soft coal in kilns. Shortly after this, Edward was forced to establish a second commission, the main function of which was to determine why the royal proclamation was not being observed.

Apparently, relatively few advances in the area of health risk assessment, as we would think of it today, were made for nearly 2100 years after the initial observation that the environment could affect human health. The association between malaria and swamps, for example, was established in the 5th century B.C. even though the precise reason for the association remained obscure. Covello and Mumpower (1985) noted that in *Airs, Water, and Places*, thought to have been written by Hippocrates in the 4th or 5th century B.C., an attempt was made to set forth a causal relation between disease and the environment. As early as the 1st century B.C., the Greeks and Romans had observed the adverse effects of exposure to lead (Gilfillan, 1965; Nriagu, 1983). Specifically, the Roman Vitruvious (cited in Hughes, 1975), wrote:

> We can take example by the workers in lead who have complexions affected by pallor. For when, in casting, the lead receives the current of air, the fumes from it occupy the members of the body, and burning them thereon, rob the limbs of the virtues of the blood. Therefore it seems that water should not be brought in lead pipes if we desire to have it wholesome.

2.3   Occupational Hazard Assessment (ca. 1300–1900)

During the 16th to 18th centuries, the basis for our current approach to health risk assessment, including a sensitivity to the importance of dose–response, became well established. The following advancements were identified by Covello and Mumpower (1985):

- A study by Agricola [1556] linking adverse health effects to various mining and metallurgical practices.
- A study by Evelyn [1661] linking smoke in London to various types of acute and chronic respiratory problems.
- A study by Ramazzini [1700, 1713] indicating that nuns living in Apennine monasteries appeared to have higher frequencies of breast cancer (Ramazzini suggested that this might be due to their celibacy, an observation that is in accord with recent observations that nulliparous women may develop breast cancer more frequently than woman who have had children) [Macmahon and Cole, 1969; Sherman and Korenman, 1974].
- A study by Hill [1781] linking the use of tobacco snuff with cancer of the nasal passage.
- A study by Sir Percival Pott [1775] indicating that juvenile chimney sweeps in England were especially susceptible to scrotal cancer at puberty.
- A study by Ayrton-Paris [1822] as well as by Hutchinson [1887] indicating that occupational and medicinal exposures to arsenic can lead to cancer.
- A study by Chadwick [1842] linking nutrition and sanitary conditions in English slums to various types of ailments.
- A study by Snow [1855] linking cholera outbreaks to contaminated water pumps.
- Studies by Unna [1894] and Dubreuilh [1896] linking sunlight exposure with skin cancer.
- A study by Rehn [1895] linking aromatic amines with bladder cancer.

Covello and Mumpower (1985) observed that

> despite these studies, progress toward establishing causal links between adverse health effects and different types of hazardous activities was exceedingly slow. It appears that at least two major obstacles impeded progress. The first was the paucity of scientific models of biological, chemical, and physical processes, especially prior to the 17th and 18th centuries. Related to this was the lack of instrumentation and the lack of rigorous observational and experimental techniques for collecting data and testing hypotheses.

2.4   Occupational Disease Recognition (1900–1930)

During the early years of the 20th century, it became clear that the industrial revolution had been responsible for introducing health hazards that were adversely affecting a large number of workers (McCord, 1937; Lanier, 1985). Dozens of scientific papers appeared in the literature which discussed various unique diseases observed in numerous workplaces.

Some of the best accounts were chronicled by Alice Hamilton (Sicherman, 1984). Because of the relatively large numbers of diseases recognized to be associated with exposure to toxicants in the workplace, Harvard University established its industrial hygiene program in 1937. During the ensuing years, numerous other graduate programs in occupational hygiene were established in an effort to train professionals who could recognize, evaluate, and control the causative agents.

2.5   Toxicology Studies and Risk Assessment (1930–1940)

According to Friess (1987), beginning in the 1930s the need to protect humans from the adverse effects of chemicals in the workplace, the marketplace, and the environment became a commonly recognized goal in the United States and Europe. The general approach to risk assessment evolved over time, but it was characterized by acceptance of the premise that human health was related to the degree of exposure and the toxicity of the chemical. The setting of permissible exposure limits for the workplace introduced the concept of acceptable levels of exposure to toxic agents (Paustenbach and Langner, 1986).

Friess (1987) has suggested that what we currently call risk assessment began roughly in the 1930s. He noted that assessments took the form of an initial review of the epidemiological data of the worker/user populations for a specific chemical, and the dose–response data collected in tests involving animals. Following the deliberations of a committee of specialists in the health sciences or by an individual, the epidemiologic and animal toxicologic data for the chemical were assessed, and then the dosage–response relation for each serious health effect in the human was estimated (Stokinger, 1981; Lanier, 1985). The relation could be displayed either as a curve of dosage versus anticipated response or, in an attempt to linearize the relation, as a curve of log dosage versus percentage response. Friess noted that:

> whatever the display mode, however, the predicted human dose/response curve was then used for two purposes. It could be used to predict human response amplitudes under a specified exposure scenario. Secondly, accepting a 5 percent response amplitude as being essentially a no-effect level within the limits of biological variability in populations, the curve could be used to establish the human No Observable Effect Level (NOEL). This procedure was, and is, a primitive quantitative risk assessment methodology.

2.6   Concern over Low-Level Health Risks (1940–1950)

During the 600 years between 1348 and 1948, society's concern for health risks usually focused on those factors that could increase the risk of infectious disease. This was appropriate since these were the greatest hazard. For example, the 1348–1349 epidemic of the Black Death (bubonic plague) killed over one-quarter of the population of Europe— approximately 25 million people (Winslow, 1923; Helleiner, 1967; Ziegler, 1969). However, beginning in the late 1940s, after having eliminated many of the truly serious threats to health (often achieved through better understanding, control, and the use of medicinal drugs), our attention began to be diverted to the more subtle and insidious, yet much lower risk, hazards (Eisenbud, 1978). Specifically, society began to focus on the hazards posed by agents found in our environment.

The tremendous increase in the synthesis and manufacture of organic chemicals (Fig. 3), coupled with the potential problems described in Carson's *Silent Spring* (1962), suggested that pollution of our environment might very well be the next "Black Death" if

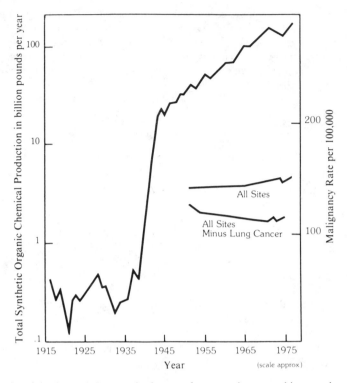

Figure 3. In spite of the dramatic increase in the manufacture and presumed increased exposure to synthesized organic chemicals, there has been no apparent increased risk in the cancer rate, even after correction for smoking and other lifestyle factors [American Industrial Health Council (AIHC), 1983].

attention were not directed to this threat. Interestingly, concurrent with the increased manufacture of industrial chemicals was the introduction and widespread use of pesticides, including herbicides. Furthermore, at about the same time the U.S. Food and Drug Administration (FDA) began to study and identify those chemicals that could safely be added to foods and drugs.

2.7   Setting Acceptable Daily Intakes (1950–1970)

The 20 years between 1950 and 1970 were important ones in toxicology and risk assessment (Friess, 1987). At least two key review papers in the 1950s serve as milestones: that of Barnes and Denz in 1954 and that by Lehmann and his colleagues at the U.S. Food and Drug Administration in 1959 (Friess, 1987). The rationale for and size of the safety factor to be used in the animal–human NOEL extrapolation evolved from these publications. For a chemical with a well-defined toxic action at a target tissue, which appears to display a dose threshold and is at least moderately reversible, a safety factor (later called an uncertainty factor) of 100 was proposed. The first factor of 10 was used to extrapolate the NOEL from animals to humans and the second factor of 10 was to account for the variability in sensitivities within human populations. For more serious irreversible types of effects, even including carcinogenesis, additional safety factors (range 2–10 and higher) were added to the fundamental 100. For example, at times during the 1960s and 1970s, safety factors of 1000 were applied to the apparent NOEL for tumorigenesis observed in chronic animal bioassays in an effort to estimate the NOEL in human populations (Weil, 1972).

2.8   The Cancer Hazard (1970–1985)

Progress toward the assessment of environmental stressors (e.g., chemical and physical agents) remained at the level of "the dose makes the poison" until about 1974. Some observers, including the author, believe that the vinyl chloride experience may very well have been a critical turning point in the evolution of modern risk assessment. Vinyl chloride (VC) was a chemical that had long been thought so harmless as to be considered sufficiently safe for use as an anesthetic agent for surgery. However, following an epidemiological study of workers involved in its manufacture, it was determined that VC could cause cancer at levels that were tasteless, odorless, and produced no detectable adverse effects! The vinyl chloride experience sensitized risk scientists and health professionals to the fact that it was quite possible that the background incidence of cancer (believed primarily to be due to diet, smoking, and other lifestyle factors) was so high as to mask the adverse effect of a large number of carcinogenic agents present in our air, water, and food. As a result, new approaches to setting acceptable levels of exposure to carcinogens began to be investigated.

The concept of a threshold dose at which no adverse effects would be expected for carcinogens was first challenged in the early 1960s. The classic paper by Mantel and Bryan (1961), which described an approach to estimating virtually safe doses (VSDs), appealed to regulatory agencies who believed that a NOEL for carcinogens might not exist. Soon thereafter, for regulatory purposes, most human exposure to carcinogens was assumed to present a finite incremental cancer risk, irrespective of whether repair processes were operable after the chemical interacted with DNA (Crump et al., 1976). From this regulatory philosophy evolved the widespread use of mathematical models; those which estimate the excess lifetime cancer risk for humans based on the dose–response curve obtained in animal bioassays.

The acceptance of models that predict the potential upper-bound excess cancer risk represented an important turning point in the history of environmental regulation, and risk management. Through the use of reasonably standard statistical approaches, the risk estimation approach introduced by Mantel and Bryan in 1961 offered an alternative to the "safety" standard demanded by the Delaney Amendment of 1958. This was later refined by Crump and co-workers (1976) in a very influential paper entitled "Fundamental carcinogenic processes and their implications for low dose risk assessment." The approach described by Crump and co-workers became the standard one used by U.S. regulatory agencies during the 1970s and 1980s for estimating the plausible upper bound of the cancer risk.

2.9   Recent Concerns Regarding Risk Assessment (1980s)

Friess (1987) has suggested that the years between 1980 and 1990 will be considered a time when public health officials, toxicologists, statisticians, and risk assessors began to question the appropriateness of using so-called cancer models (which are more correctly called dose response models) to estimate the incidence of tumors in exposed human populations. During this time period, valid scientific arguments were put forth that these models relied on too many assumptions that might apply to initiators of tumorigenesis but that they were probably not appropriate for the nongenotoxic chemicals, including promoters (Weisburger and Williams, 1981; Shu et al., 1987) and carcinogens which produce tumors through repeated cytotoxic events (Andersen, 1988).

During the 1980s, the public had also become uneasy about the appropriateness of such models in making risk management decisions. The questioning of such approaches was clearly illustrated by two pieces that appeared in the *Wall Street Journal*—one in 1984 and the other in 1987. The first addressed the reasonableness of EPA's decision to ban ethylene dibromide (EDB) as a grain fumigant and the second discussed formaldehyde. Havender (1983) reviewed the ethylene dibromide experience.

Recently, we went through yet another in the parade of hysterias over a carcinogen in the nation's food supply that began with the great cranberry scare of 1959. This time the threat was a grain fumigant, ethylene dibromide, or EDB....

Does EDB cause cancer in laboratory animals? No knowledgeable person denies this, since all 10 long-term, high dose tests involving male and female rats and mice were unequivocally positive, as was a skin-painting test on mice. Clearly, EDB must be handled with care. But does this mean that the traces now being found in supermarket food pose a significant hazard to the public and warrant a ban?

According to EPA's estimates, the average person consumes 5 to 10 micrograms of EDB a day—a quantity far too small to be seen with the unaided eye. (By comparison, we typically ingest 140,000 micrograms of pepper—a known carcinogen—each day.) That quantity is less than a quarter-millionth of what, on a body weight basis, the rats were given.

In other words, one would have to eat at least 250,000 times as much food every day as we normally do, or some 400 tons daily over a lifetime, to equal the dose that produced cancer in laboratory animals. This huge difference, dwarfing even the 1,000-bottles-of-diet-pop-a-day equivalent human dose that made the saccharin rat tests look ridiculous, is itself enough to justify skepticism about the hazard faced by consumers.

The other reason for not going into a panic over EDB-contaminated foods is that its risk vanishes into insignificance against the background of risks from other, natural carcinogens in food.

Aflatoxin, a mold present in many of the same grain-based foods as EDB (as well as in peanut butter, milk and apple juice) is some 1,000 times more potent than EDB as a carcinogen. Its allowed level in solid food is 20 ppb, which means that consumers are exposed to as much as 20,000 times the carcinogenic hazard from aflatoxin than they would get from EDB present in food at 1 ppb (the "emergency" action level of Florida and some other states).

Against this natural background of dietary carcinogens the risk from 10 micrograms of EDB a day is trivial. Indeed a muffin baked from the most contaminated mix found in California would have, because most of the EDB bakes off, only a fraction of the hazard of a peanut butter-and-jelly sandwich. If one can eat that sandwich with equanimity, then one should be at least as tranquil about eating corn muffins.

The second commentary, by the editor of the *Wall Street Journal*, described his impression of the wisdom of EPA's position on formaldehyde (Wall Street Journal, 1987):

Just presenting the 95% upper-confidence limit not only grossly distorts the perception of risk, but also unduly alarms the public.

Staffers at the Environmental Protection Agency are calling this widely used medical and industrial chemical [formaldehyde] a "probable human carcinogen," supposedly endangering the health of thousands of Americans. Some EPA officials are therefore urging strict federal regulations on formaldehyde.

To support this claim, the EPA recently produced some seemingly shocking—and highly publicized—statistics on the alleged cancer risks from formaldehyde exposure. The agency purports that three out of every 10,000 garment workers exposed to formaldehyde fumes risk getting cancer. For mobile-home dwellers exposed to formaldehyde-treated pressed wood, the cancer risk over 10 years is said to be two in 10,000. And for residents of conventional homes, the perceived risk is one in 10,000. Given the current widespread fear of cancer, these numbers were certain to scare many people....

EPA's "likely estimate" for cancer risks from formaldehyde exposure among garment workers is actually 4 in 1 *billion*. Similarly, for mobile-home dwellers the "likely" estimate is 2 in 10 billion, and for conventional-home residents 6 in 100 billion....

A recent Harvard School of Public Health analysis criticized harshly the federal government's handling of formaldehyde risk assessment. It said that "the true extent of uncertainty about the magnitude of estimated cancer risk is not conveyed to policy makers." As a result, it concluded, "policy guidelines are substituted for scientific judgment in the government risk-assessment process."

The experiences with saccharin, EDB, dioxin, formaldehyde, and methylene chloride suggest that the 1980s were difficult years for regulatory agencies that had been mandated to protect the public health—in part, because the human hazard posed by typical levels of exposure in the environment was probably much lower than that predicted by exposure assessments and low-dose extrapolation models.

2.10 Biologically Based Disposition Models (1980–1990)

A potentially major advancement in health risk assessment may well have occurred in 1984 with the publication of a paper by Ramsey and Andersen. This manuscript described a procedure known as physiologically based pharmacokinetic modeling wherein actual organs and tissue groups were used with weights and blood flows to predict the qualitative time course and distribution of a chemical in the test species. Although their research was an extension of the earlier work of Kety (1951), Mapleson (1963), Riggs (1963), Bischoff (1967), Fiserova-Bergerova (1975), and Davis and Mapleson (1981), and all this was an extension of the seminal work of Haggard (1924), they applied these procedures in a form that was understandable and readily applicable. Moreover, Clewell and Andersen (1985; 1986) showed that with the advent of personal computers, these approaches were within the grasp of virtually all scientists.

The significance of the Ramsey–Andersen work was more widely recognized when the approach was applied to the risk assessment of the bioassay data on methylene chloride (Andersen et al., 1987). Soon after its critical review by several U.S. regulatory agencies, a symposium was jointly sponsored by the National Academy of Science, EPA, FDA, and others, wherein the merit and applications of the PB-PK methodology were discussed. The significance of PB-PK modeling was made evident by the publication of the proceedings of this meeting in Volume VIII of the National Academy of Science's series on *Drinking Water and Health* (1987). At the present time, these approaches are the ones considered likely to move quantitative risk assessment (and low-dose extrapolation models) to the next level of refinement. The importance of this approach is characterized by attempts to incorporate all the available biologic data and our understanding of the mechanisms of cancer into a quantitative estimate of delivered dose and response (Clewell and Andersen, 1985; Menzel,

1987). More recently, the term physiologically based pharmacokinetic model has been replaced by the more descriptive "biologically based disposition model" (Andersen, 1988).

2.11 Biologically based Cancer Models (1980–1995)

Although the development and use of biologically based disposition models represented a significant improvement in our approach to estimating the low-dose response, perhaps an even more important contribution was the development of biologically based cancer models (Moolgavkar, 1986). The first and perhaps most promising of these models was developed by Moolgavkar and Knudson (1981). Despite the diversity of the disease processes categorized under the heading of cancer, their model is very compelling even though it is quite simple. It is a form of the two-stage model initially described by Armitage and Doll in the 1950s (1954; 1960). In this model, cancer is explained as the end result of two mutagenic events (u1 and u2), corresponding to mutations at a critical gene locus which in the human is duplicated within the genetic material of the cell. As discussed by Andersen (1988), the first event produces an intermediate cell type that may have different growth characteristics than the normal cell but one that is not aggressively malignant. A second irreversible event is necessary to complete the cell transformation process, alter the second locus of the critical gene, and obtain the cancer cell which grows into a tumor by clonal expansion.

Using this model, one can explain how genotoxicants alter mutation rates, how cytotoxicants alter cell death and birth rates of the normal and intermediate cells, and how promoters convey growth advantages on the intermediate cell populations. It can be anticipated that this approach, which has already been applied by Thorslund et al. (1987) and Conolly et al. (1988), and improved upon by Moolgavkar (1986) and Moolgavkar et al. (1988), will be the foundation upon which future cancer risk estimates will be based. Most importantly, the use of biologically based disposition models coupled with the biologically based cancer models should produce estimates of risks at low doses which are more realistic and believable than current approaches. It is plausible that such approaches could be used in regulatory decision making as early at 1990 if sufficient attention is directed to these efforts by scientists within government, academia, and industry.

3 HAZARD IDENTIFICATION (CHEMICAL, PHYSICAL, AND TOXICOLOGICAL PROPERTIES)

About 10 years ago it was recognized that the physical and chemical properties of a substance play a large role in predicting its fate in the environment—an essential part of hazard identification (Cairns et al., 1978; Dickson et al., 1979; Maki et al., 1980; Veith et al., 1980). Tests to understand these properties began to be conducted on new products (Tables 1 and 1A). Together, the toxicity data and the information on fate describe the environmental hazard (Table 2). Some of the early work involved the study of the relation of physicochemical properties of the organophosphates to their persistence and transport in either biological or environmental systems. It was shown, for example, that the octanol–water partition coefficient gives an indication of the possibility for biological magnification (Kenaga, 1975; Metcalf et al., 1975). Similarly, it was shown that the stability of the compound, as evidenced by its resistance to hydrolysis and other degradative reactions, will often account for its persistence—thus allowing the possibility of transport in water or air (Fig. 4 and Table 3). Although it could be argued that physical property

TABLE 1. Candidate Tests for Screening Ecological Impact of New Products

I. Chemical fate (transport, persistence)
- A. Transport
    1. Adsorption isotherm (soil)
    2. Partition coefficient (water–octanol)
    3. Water solubility
    4. Vapor pressure
- B. Other physicochemical properties
    1. Boiling/melting/sublimation points
    2. Density
    3. Dissociation constant
    4. Flammability/explodability
    5. Particle size
    6. pH
    7. Chemical incompatibility
    8. Vapor-phase UV spectrum for halocarbons
    9. UV and visible absorption spectra in aqueous solution
- C. Persistence
    1. Biodegradation
        a. Shake flask procedure following carbon loss
        b. Respirometric method following oxygen (BOD) and/or carbon dioxide
        c. Activated sludge test (simulation of treatment plant)
        d. Methane and CO_2 productions in anaerobic digestion
    2. Chemical degradation
        a. Oxidation (free-radical)
        b. Hydrolysis (25°C, pH 5.0 and 9.0)
    3. Photochemical transformation in water

II. Ecological effects
- A. Microbial effects
    1. Cellulose decomposition
    2. Ammonification of urea
    3. Sulfate reduction
- B. Plant effects
    1. Algae inhibition (fresh and seawater, growth, nitrogen fixation)
    2. Duck weed inhibition (increase in fronds or dry weight)
    3. Seed germination and early growth
- C. Animal effects testing
    1. Aquatic invertebrates (*Daphnia*) acute toxicity (first instar)
    2. Fish acute toxicity (96 hr)
    3. Quail dietary LC_{50}
    4. Terrestial mammal test
    5. *Daphnia* life cycle test
    6. *Mysidopsis bahia* life cycle
    7. Fish embryo–juvenile test
    8. Fish bioconcentration test

Source: Toxic substances control; discussion of premanufacture testing policy and technical issues; request for comment, *Federal Register*, **44**, 53, Part IV, pp. 1639–16292, March 16, 1979.

TABLE 1A. Summary of the Environmental Fate Testing Programs[a] to Evaluate Three Different Chemicals to be Sold by a Manufacturer

Test Type	NTA	Type A Zeolite	LAS
Screening Tests			
CO_2 evolution	>95% (TCO_2)	N.A. (inorganic)	>95% (TCO_2)
Octanol–water partition coefficient	N.A.[b] (ionic salt)	N.A. (insoluble in octanol)	125
Microbial inhibition	N.A. (CO_2 evolution tests demonstrate no inhibition)	N.A. (insoluble, unreactive)	N.A. (CO_2 evolution test demonstrate no inhibition)
Semicontinuous activated sludge	92% removal efficiency	80–90% removal	>91% removal efficiency
Settling test	N.A. (water soluble)	40–60% removal	N.A. (water soluble)
Confirmatory Tests			
Adsorption isotherms	<30% on organic and inorganic solids	N.A.	Some affinity for organics and inorganics; effective in removal from water
Hydrolysis rate	N.A. (stable in acids and bases)	Half-life approx 55 days	N.A. ($TCO_2 \sim 90\%$)
Metal complexation	Readily complexes metals	Readily complexes metals	N.A.
Ozonation	N.A. ($TCO_2 \sim 90\%$)	N.A.	N.A. ($TCO_2 \sim 90\%$)
Chlorination	N.A. ($TCO_2 \sim 90\%$)	N.A.	N.A. ($TCO_2 \sim 90\%$)
Photolysis	N.A. ($TCO_2 \sim 90\%$)	N.A.	N.A. ($TCO_2 \sim 90\%$)
Biodegradation rates	N.A. ($TCO_2 \sim 90\%$)	N.A. (inorganic)	N.A. ($TCO_2 \sim 90\%$)
Continuous activated sludge	>90% removal efficiency	90% removal efficiency	>90% removal efficiency
Biological inhibition of wastewater treatment process	N.A. (CO_2 tests demonstrate no inhibition)	N.A.	N.A. (CO_2 tests demonstrate no inhibition)
Sludge properties	N.A. (water soluble)	No effects on settleability	N.A. (water soluble)

[a]These are programs that the Procter and Gamble's guidelines suggested for the sodium salt of nitrilotriacetic acid (NTA), sodium aluminosilicate (Type A zeolite), and linear alkylbenzenesulfonate (LAS).
[b]N.A., Guidelines indicate test is not needed or applicable.
Source: Beck et al. (1981).

TABLE 2. Environmental Processes and Properties which Influence the Degree of Hazard

Process	Key Environmental Property[a]
	Physical Transport
Meteorological transport	Wind velocity
Biouptake	Biomass
Sorption	Organic content of soil or sediments, mass loading of aquatic systems
Volatilization	Turbulence, evaporation rate, reaeration coefficients, soil organic content
Runoff	Precipitation rate
Leaching	Adsorption coefficient
Fallout	Particulate concentration, wind velocity
	Chemical Processes
Photolysis	Solar irradiance, transmissivity of water or air
Oxidation	Concentrations of oxidants and retarders
Hydrolysis	pH, sediment or soil basicity or acidity
Reduction	Oxygen concentration, ferrous ion concentration, and complexation state
	Biological Processes
Biotransformation	Microorganism population and acclimation level

[a]At constant temperature.
Source: Mill, T., "Data Needed to Predict the Environmental Fate of Organic Chemicals," presented at Symposium on Environmental Fate and Effects, American Chemical Society, Miami, Florida, September, 1978. Proceedings published by Ann Arbor Science.

data are part of the exposure assessment, this information (like toxicity data) is placed within the domain of hazard identification since these properties often dictate the presence of an environmental hazard.

3.1 Water Solubility

Water solubility is an important parameter in understanding environmental fate, which in turn influences the outcome of environmental risk assessments. Together with other physicochemical properties, it can be a useful predictor of the tendency of a chemical to move and distribute between the various environmental compartments [Food and Drug Administration, (USFDA), 1984]. In general, highly water-soluble chemicals are more likely to be transported and distributed by the hydrologic cycle than relatively water-insoluble chemicals. However, many of those chemicals that are known to be significant environmental contaminants, for example, DDT and polychlorinated biphenyls, are those that have very low water solubilities (Tinsley, 1979). Their wide distribution seems to be due to their high stability in soil and water and, to a much lesser degree, their vapor transport following evaporation from water. The solubilities of various halogenated hydrocarbons are shown in Table 4 and of some pesticides in Table 5.

The degree of water solubility, or insolubility, also influences the extent to which a chemical may sorb to particulate matter, such as soil or sediment, or cross a lipid–water

TABLE 3. Mechanisms Affecting Environmental Fate of Chemicals

I. Original input to environment during manufacturing, distribution, use, and disposal
   A. To water
      1. Treatment plant effluents at manufacturing and/or formulating plants
      2. Spills during manufacturing (original and formulating) and distribution
      3. Disposal after use
   B. To soil
      1. Direct applications as an agricultural chemical or for vegetation control
      2. Land disposal, e.g., landfill or land cultivation operations
      3. Spills
   C. To atmosphere
      1. Stack emission during manufacture
      2. Fugitive volatilization losses, e.g., from leaks, storage tank vents, and wastewater treatment
      3. Losses during use and subsequent disposal

II. Mechanisms for transformation and transport within and between environmental compartments
   A. Water
      1. Transport from water to atmosphere, sediments, or organisms
         a. Volatilization
         b. Adsorption onto sediments; desorption
         c. Absorption into cells (protista, plants, animals); desorption
      2. Transformations
         a. Biodegradation (affected by living organisms)
         b. Photochemical degradation (nonmetabolic degradation requiring light energy), direct or via a sensitizer
         c. Chemical degradation (effected by chemical agents), e.g., hydrolysis, free-radical oxidation
   B. Soil
      1. Transport to water, sediments, atmosphere, or cells
         a. Dissolution in rain water
         b. Adsorption on particles carried by runoff
         c. Volatilization from leaf or soil surfaces
         d. Uptake by protista, plants, and animals
      2. Transformation
         a. Biodegradation
         b. Photodegradation on plant and soil surfaces
   C. Atmosphere
      1. Transport from atmosphere to land or water
         a. Adsorption to particulate matter followed by gravitational settling or rain washout
         b. Washout by being dissolved in rain
         c. Dry deposition (direct absorption in water bodies)
      2. Transport within atmosphere
         a. Turbulent mixing and diffusion within troposphere
         b. Diffusion to stratosphere
      3. Atmospheric transformations
         a. Photochemical degradation by direct absorption of light, or by accepting energy from an excited donor molecule (sensitizer), or by reacting with another chemical that has reached an excited state
         b. Oxidation by ozone
         c. Reaction with free radicals
         d. Reactions with other chemical contaminants

Source: R. A. Conway (1982). Introduction to environmental risk analysis, in *Environmental Risk Analysis for Chemicals*, R. A. Conway, Ed., Van Nostrand Reinhold. Based in part on P. H. Howard, J. Saxena, and H. Sikka, Determining the fate of chemicals, *Environmental Science and Technology*, **12**(4) 3989–407 (1978).

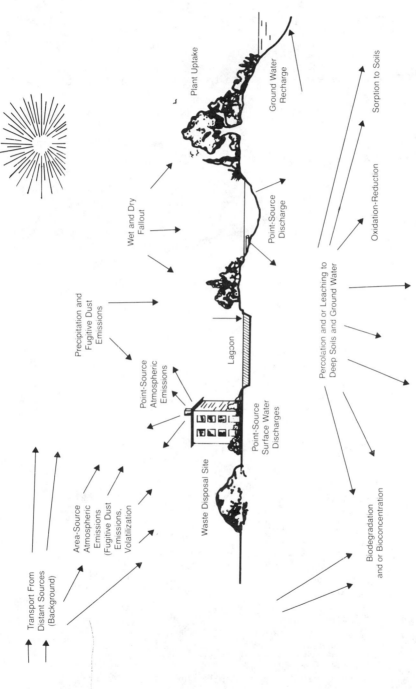

Figure 4. Schematic illustrating the transport and fate of atmospheric emissions into various parts of the environment.

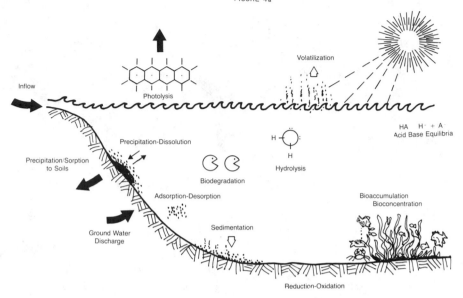

Figure 5. Schematic illustrating the various avenues for degradation and movement of xenobiotics in the environment.

TABLE 4. Water Solubilities of Various Halogenated Aliphatic Hydrocarbons[a]

Halogenated Aliphatic Hydrocarbon	Solubility (mg/L)
Chloromethane	6,450–7,250 at 20°C
Dichloromethane	13,000–20,000 at 25°C
Trichlormethane (chloroform)	8,200 at 20°C
Tetrachloromethane (carbon tetrachloride)	785 at 20°C
Chloroethane	5,740 at 20°C
1,1-Dichloroethane	5,470 at 20°C
1,2-Dichloroethane	5,500 at 20°C
1,1,1-Trichloroethane	8,690 at 20°C
1,1,2-Trichloroethane	440–4,400 at 20°C
1,1,2-Trichloroethane	4,500 at 20°C
1,1,2,2-Tetrachloroethane	2,900 at 20°C
Hexachloroethane	50 at 22°C
Chloroethane (vinyl chloride)	60 at 10°C
1,1-Dichloroethane	400 at 20°C
1,2-trans-Dichloroethane	600 at 20°C
Trichloroethane	1,100 at 20°C

[a]Modified from lecture materials from Tetra Tech, Inc.; distributed at EPA Water Quality Assessment Workshop, June 1981.

TABLE 5. Water Solubilities of Various Pesticides[a]

Pesticide	Solubility
Acrolein	20.8% at 20°C
Aldrin	17–180 ppb at 25°C
DDD	20–100 ppb at 25°C
DDE	1.2–140 ppb at 20°C
Dieldrin	186–200 ppb at 25°C
Endosulfan	100–260 ppb at 20°C
Endrin	220 ppb at 25°C
Heptachlor	56–180 ppb at 25°C
Heptachlor epoxide	200–350 ppb at 25°C
Hexachlorocyclohexane	0.70–21.3 ppm at 25°C
Lindane	5–12 ppm at 25°C

[a]Modified from lecture materials from Tetra Tech, Inc.; distributed at EPA Water Quality Assessment Workshop, June 1981.

interface. Many of the environmental fate processes, such as hydrolysis, chemical reduction and oxidation, biodegradation, and photodegradation (Figure 5), are influenced by a chemical's water solubility (Tables 4 and 5). A chemical's water solubility, along with its vapor pressure, can be used to predict the extent to which a chemical will volatilize from water into air. Knowledge of a chemical's water solubility can also be used to determine appropriate experimental designs in tests of ecological effects and in tests for other physicochemical and fate parameters (by allowing preliminary approximation of those parameters).

3.2   Photodegradation (Direct)

Direct photodegradation involves the absorption of light in the ultraviolet–visible (UV–Vis) region by a molecule with a resultant increase in the molecular energy level; the increased energy then chemically transforms the molecule. Determination of the UV absorption spectrum of a substance is a prerequisite to direct photodegradation studies since compounds that do not absorb light in this specturm will not decompose by direct photodegradation. A molecule that absorbs light in the ultraviolet–visible region, however, does not necessarily undergo chemical transformation since the energy of the molecule may be dissipated in some other manner and the molecule returned to its initial state (USFDA, 1984).

Hydrolysis and biodegradation are generally considered to be the most important degradation pathways for organic chemicals in the aqueous environment, while photodegradation is more important for chemicals in the vapor or gaseous phase (Figure 5). Biodegradation is generally considered the predominant pathway in the soil environment, although screening tests for determining the degradation of chemicals in soil have not always distinguished between biological, chemical, or photochemical degradation. Photodegradation is a less significant degradation mechanism in soil and water systems because of the limited opportunity for exposure of the substance to sunlight. Therefore, for most chemicals found primarily in water or soil, hydrolysis and biodegradation studies should be performed before other tests. The results from these studies can then be used to decide if additional degradation studies are required. If no degradation pathways have been identified in the environment and if the chemical absorbs in the UV spectrum, then the direct photodegradability of the substance should be evaluated to determine if the chemical is likely to bioaccumulate in the environment if not well controlled.

3.3 Photodegradation (Indirect)

Atmospheric photodegradation involves primarily indirect mechanisms. Indirect photo-degradation is the process whereby chemicals react with intermediates that are formed as a result of direct photodegradation. Most frequently in the atmosphere, the indirect process involves free radical formation resulting from the interaction of sunlight with natural constituents, followed by reaction of the free radical with the chemical. This free radical reaction can result in the propagation of more reactive species and continued free radical reactions (USFDA, 1984).

Hydroxyl radicals have been implicated as the most important reactive species in the photooxidation of organic compounds (Doyle et al., 1975). A reactivity scale of hydrocarbons based on reactions with hydroxyl radicals has been formulated by Glasson and Tuesday (1970), Environmental Protection Agency (EPA) (1974), and Darnall et al. (1976). In general, chemicals containing C–H or C–C bonds will be susceptible to hydroxyl radical attack in the troposphere and will be indirectly photodegraded. Some of the volatile fully halogenated compounds have been alleged to pose a significant hazard to the stratospheric ozone layer. A preliminary estimate of the transfer of halogen from the troposphere to the stratosphere can be determined using models proposed by Crutzen et al. (1978) and Neely (1977).

Significant volatility of a chemical should be demonstrated before indirect photodegradation tests of a chemical in its vapor phase are considered. The design of such studies should be based on the reactivity of the substance with hydroxyl radicals. As noted above, biodegradation or hydrolysis (or both) are considered more important degradation processes in soil and water than direct photodegradation. Furthermore, Crosby and Li (1969) have observed that it is both reasonable and probable that in many instances photodegradation will provide the same products as metabolism by plants and microorganisms. They noted that photodegradation is a process that can "open up" a chemical structure ordinarily resistant to metabolism and thus result in an accelerated disappearance of the chemical from the environment. It can also induce chemical transformations entirely separate from those possible by living organisms (USFDA, 1984).

3.4 Biodegradation in Soil

Biodegradation of an organic chemical refers to the reduction in molecular complexity owing to the metabolic activity of living organisms, usually microorganisms and particularly bacteria and fungi. When an organic chemical is totally biodegraded in the presence of oxygen (aerobic biodegradation), the end products are inorganic carbon dioxide and water and may also include organic compounds involved in the normal metabolic processes of aerobic microorganisms. Depending on the structure of the chemical, end products may also include other inorganic salts (e.g., nitrates, sulfates). In contrast, when an organic chemical is totally biodegraded in the absence of oxygen (anaerobic biodegradation), the end products theoretically are methane, carbon monoxide, and carbon dioxide and some of the various organic compounds involved in the normal metabolic processes of anaerobic microorganisms (USFDA, 1984).

The carbon dioxide evolution test methods for the biodegradation of xenobiotics usually evaluate the potential biodegradation of an organic chemical to carbon dioxide and water in natural systems, both soil and water. The test is applicable to all chemicals irrespective of water solubility or vapor pressure. The amount of carbon dioxide produced over a given period compared to the amount theoretically possible is used as a measure of biodegradation. Results from this test are considered positive if the actual amount of carbon dioxide produced during the test period in all soils tested is 50% or greater than the amount of carbon dioxide that theoretically could be produced from the test chemical. Positive test results indicate that the test chemical will persist indefinitely in soil systems, but reliable biodegradation in the environment may not be assumed (USFDA, 1984).

In contrast, negative test results (less than 50% theoretical carbon dioxide production from the test chemical in all soils treated) do not allow distinction among the following: the test chemical may be completely resistant to biodegradation, resistant to biodegradation because of sorption or complexing, biodegraded at a very slow rate, only partially biodegraded (i.e., the identity of the test compound is changed but the compound is not completely changed to carbon dioxide and water), or biodegraded under different biodegradation test conditions (e.g., with lower concentrations of test chemical). In short, this is a screening test. If negative test results are obtained, it may be necessary to rerun the test to analyze for partial biodegradation of the test chemical or to test for biodegradation of the chemical under different conditions. When a negative test result occurs in only one or two of the soils tested, further analysis or testing may also be necessary to determine if the test chemical is actually resistant to biodegradation, degraded at a very slow rate, or only partially degraded in some soil systems (USFDA, 1984).

Environmentally realistic biodegradation results are difficult to obtain in the laboratory because of the many variables that affect the rate and extent of biodegradation, for example, temperature, pH, oxygen level, concentration of test chemical and viable microorganisms, and type of microbial species (EPA, 1979). Importantly, in nature most chemicals are at far lower concentrations than are used in laboratory tests. At these lower concentrations, the rates and even the occurrence of biodegradation can differ markedly. Chemicals are also more likely to be more toxic or inhibitory to microorganisms at concentrations used in laboratory tests than at environmental concentrations. Use of a radiolabeled (carbon-14) test chemical or of an analytical technique specific for the test chemical allows the use of lower test concentrations (and would also allow determination of partial biodegradation), thus allowing laboratory results to be more reflective of the actual environment.

Biodegradation is the main process by which organic chemicals, following introduction into the environment, are reduced in complexity. Although an organic chemical may be transformed by abiotic mechanisms (e.g., chemical oxidation, hydrolysis, photodegradation) that depend only on light and/or thermal energy, these abiotic mechanisms rarely lead to appreciable changes in chemical structure. Photochemical reactions are much less important for chemicals below the soil surface since the UV light cannot penetrate past about the top $\frac{1}{10}$–1 cm (Paustenbach, 1987). In contrast, the enzyme-catalyzed metabolic processes of biological systems have the energy, as well as the specificity, to bring about major changes in structure and stability (USFDA, 1984).

3.5 Vapor Pressure and Density

Vapor pressure is an important property governing the tendency of a chemical substance to be transported in air and is thus an important parameter in predicting the distribution of chemicals into environmental compartments. For example, vapor pressure data can be used to estimate the losses due to volatilization. This estimate can be used in conjunction with values for other parameters of environmental fate (e.g., sorption–desorption and degradation) in deciding whether additional tests are necessary for a more complete description of the test chemical's instability and degradation pathways.

Equilibrium vapor pressure can be thought of as the solubility of a chemical substance in air and is dependent on the nature of the chemical and temperature. The vapor pressure of any chemical increases with an increase in temperature. This is because as temperature increases, the kinetic energy or movement of molecules increases, and more high-energy molecules are available to escape into the gaseous state. Vapor pressure values are therefore, meaningful only if accompanied by the temperature at which they were measured. Vapor pressures of many organic chemicals of environmental interest increase three- to fourfold for each 10°C increase in temperature (USFDA, 1984).

Volatility is the evaporative loss of a substance to the air from the surface of a liquid or solid. Although potential volatility of a chemical is related to its inherent vapor pressure,

TABLE 6. Vapor Pressure and Volatilization Half-Life of Various Halogenated Aliphatic Hydrocarbons[a]

Halogenated Aliphatic Hydrocarbon	Vapor Pressure (torr) at 20°C	Volatilization Half-Life[b] (min^2)
Chloromethane	3700	27
Dichloromethane	362	21
Trichloromethane (chloroform)	150	21
Tetrachloromethane (carbon tetrachloride)	90	29
Chloroethane	1000	21
1,1-Dichloroethane	180	22
1,2-Dichloroethane	61	29
1,1,1-Trichloroethane	96	20
1,1,2-Trichloroethane	19	21
1,1,2,2-Tetrachloroethane	5	56
Hexachloroethane	0.4	45
Chloroethene (vinyl chloride)	2660	26
1,1-Dichloroethene	591	22
1,2-trans-Dichloroethene	200	22
Trichloroethene	57.9	21
Tetrachloroethene	14	26
1,2-Dichloropropane	42	<50
1,3-Dichloropropene	25	31
Hexachlorobutadiene	0.15	
Hexachlorocyclopentadiene	0081 at 25°C	
Bromomethane	1420	
Bromodichloromethane	50	
Dibromochloromethane	15	
Tribromomethane	10	
Dichlorodifluoromethane	4306	
Trichlorofluoromethane	667	

[a] Modified from lecture materials from Tetra Tech, Inc.; distributed at EPA Water Quality Assessment Workshop, June 1981.
[b] From Dilling (1977). Values were obtained by stirring 1 ppm solutions in an open container at 200 rpm at 25°C; average solution depth was 6.5 cm.

TABLE 7. Equilibrium Vapor Pressure and Vapor Density at 30°C

Compound	Vapor Pressure (torr)	Molecular Weight	Vapor Density (g/L)
Lindane	1.28×10^{-4}	291	1.97×10^{-6}
Dieldrin	1.0×10^{-5}	399	2.1×10^{-7}
$p,p,$-DDT	7.16×10^{-7}	354	1.36×10^{-8}
$o,p,$-DDT	5.5×10^{-6}	354	1.03×10^{-7}

Source: Tinsley (1979).

actual volatilization (or vaporization) rates will depend on environmental conditions and on factors that can lessen or enhance the effective vapor pressure or behavior of a chemical at a solid–air or liquid–air interface. For example, some chemicals with very low vapor pressures and low water solubility, such as DDT and polychlorinated biphenyls, because of their low concentrations in the environment, may still be mobilized to a significant extent through volatilization. The volatilization half-lives of various aliphatic hydrocarbons are shown in Table 6 and the vapor pressures of select pesticides are presented in Table 7.

3.6 Dissociation Content

An understanding of the dissociation constant or pK can be useful in the experimental design of tests to measure the environmental fate parameters and ecological effects of a particular chemical. For example, the potential hydrolysis of a chemical known to dissociate should be tested at pH values above and below its pK. Knowledge of the pK may be useful in the selection of soils to test for sorption–desorption of a chemical, as only soils with certain pH values might potentially bind it.

The dissociation constant is an equilibrium constant. An equilibrium constant is a measure of the degree to which ionizable chemicals break up into charged constituents owing to the effect of the solvent on the dissolved chemical. By definition, pK is equal in value to the pH at which 50% ionization occurs. Some chemicals have one pK and some chemicals have several.

The distribution of a chemical in the environment is partly a function of the pK of the chemical and the pH of the environment in which the chemical is found. Together, these factors determine the extent to which a substance will exist in the ionized or nonionized form. The extent of ionization of molecules of a chemical will affect the availability of the chemical to enter into physical, chemical, and biological reactions (USFDA, 1984).

Ionic charge can affect a chemical's solubility in water. The ionic charge of a chemical also affects its potential to bind to certain soils and sediments. Anion and cation exchange processes in soils depend on the nature of the soil, pK of the chemical, and pH of the surrounding medium. Most soils are negatively charged. In general, positively charged ions (cations) have a greater potential to bind to negatively charged soil particles than do negatively charged ions (anions) or nonionized species. The ionic charge of a chemical will also affect its potential to partition between lipid or octanol and water, and thus its ability to pass through membranes and its availability to be metabolized (Hayes, 1975). In general, only the nonionized form of an organic substance is capable of entering and passing through lipid membranes (USFDA, 1984).

3.7 Ultraviolet–Visible (UV–Vis) Absorption Spectrum

Absorption spectra give some indication of the wavelengths at which a chemical may be susceptible to direct photodegradation. Before a chemical can undergo a direct photochemical reaction, it must have the ability to absorb energy from wavelengths in the UV–Vis range of the electromagnetic spectrum. Whether photodegradation of a chemical will occur depends on the total energy absorbed in the specific wavelength regions. As an aside, energy absorption is characterized by both the molar extinction coefficient (absorptivity) and the bandwidth. It is worth noting that the absence of measurable absorption does not preclude the possibility of photodegradation through other means, for example, indirect photodegradation of gases [Organization for Economic Cooperation and Development (OECD), 1981].

The UV–Vis absorption spectrum is a quantitative measure of the ability of a substance to absorb radiation in the electromagnetic spectral region between 200 and 750 nm. It is generally measured with a spectrophotometer and presented as a function of wavelength or wave number. Because of the low cost of this test, it is usually a worthwhile one when first evaluating a chemical that might enter the environment.

3.8 Sorption and Desorption

One of the most important factors governing the behavior of chemicals in soil and sediment is the sorption–desorption process. Sorption is a general expression for a process in which a chemical moves from one phase to be accumulated in another, particularly in cases in which the second phase is solid (Weber, 1927b). Sorption of a chemical by soil and sediment can result from adsorption or partitioning. Adsorption is the adhesion of molecules to surfaces of solid bodies with which they are in contact. Ionic species and metal ions exhibit this surface condensation phenomenon. Desorption is the reverse process of sorption. The major forces acting to sorb molecules to the soil include hydrophobic bonding, van der Waals forces, cation exchange, anion exchange, and coordination bonding (Hamaker and Thompson, 1972; Hamaker, 1975; Haque and Schmedding, 1975; Browman and Chesters, 1977; Chiou et al., 1979).

Some of the factors influencing the relative distribution of a test chemical between sorbed and solution phases include physical and chemical parameters of the molecule (e.g., size, shape, water solubility, pK, and polarity), properties of the soil or sediment (e.g., amount and type of clay and organic matter, cation exchange capacity, particle size, and pH, as well as temperature, water content, and salt concentration), and properties of the water in which the test chemical is dissolved (e.g., ionic strength and pH). The organic matter content is probably the most important soil or sediment property determining the sorption of nonionic chemicals (Weed and Weber, 1974; Hamaker, 1975; Stern and Walker, 1978; Chiou et al., 1979; Karickhoff et al., 1979). Figure 6 demonstrates how the percentages of sand, silt, and clay characterize the type of soil, which in turn dictates how it interacts with xenobiotics. The role of specific soil and sediment properties in dictating the sorption of ionic chemicals varies with the type and extent of the charge of the chemical and with the type and extent of the charge of the soil or sediment (USFDA, 1984). Table 8 illustrates the relation between water solubility and the soil adsorption coefficient.

3.9 Partition Coefficient

The n-octanol–water partition coefficient has often been used to predict the bioaccumulation potential in aquatic and terrestrial organisms and to estimate the amount of sorption

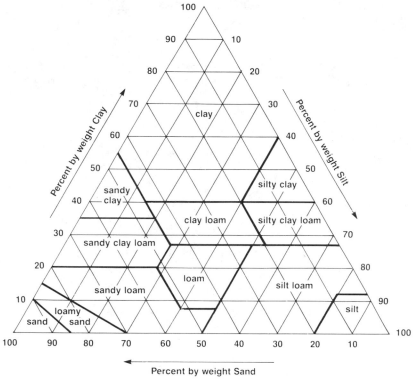

Figure 6. Triangle diagram illustrating the various classifications of soil and the criteria by which it is classified.

to soil and sediment. It is a very useful test to the risk assessor. The processes governed by the partition coefficient are major factors in determining the movement of chemicals in the biosphere. The n-octanol–water partition coefficient (K_{ow}) describes the tendency of a nonionized organic chemical to accumulate in lipid (fatty) tissue and to sorb onto soil particles or onto the surface of organisms or other particulate matter coated with organic material. Although a powerful tool for understanding organic chemicals, it is not as good a predictor for inorganic chemicals, for metal organic complexes, or for dissociating and ionic organic compounds (USFDA, 1984).

Although numerous systems have been used to measure partition coefficients, such as hexane–water or benzene–water, it has become customary in environmental fate assessment to use the n-octanol–water system. n-Octanol is considered a good medium for simulating natural fatty substances. Also, the n-octanol–water system is widely used as a reference system, and many data using this system have been reported in the literature (Leo et al., 1971; Sato and Nakajima, 1979; Tulp and Hutzinger, 1978; Gargas and Andersen, 1987). The n-octanol–water partition coefficients and partition coefficients for a variety of chemicals are presented in Tables 9 and 10, respectively.

If the molecular structure of a relatively simple chemical is known, it is often possible to estimate the n-octanol–water partition coefficient. This is because the partition pheno-menon exhibits a reasonable additive–constitutive property for these molecules. That is,

TABLE 8. Water Solubility, Soil Adsorption Coefficient, and Bioconcentration Factor Data: Experimental and Calculated

Chemical (Use)	Water Solubility[a] (ppm)	Soil Adsorption Coefficient		Bioconcentration Factor Predicted from[b]		Bioconcentration Factor[a]
		K_{oc}[a]	K_{oc}[b]	WS	K_{oc}	
Acephate (I)[c]	650,000		3	0.3		
Alachlor (H)	242	190	210	28	9	
Aldicarb (I)	7,800		32	4		
Aldrin (I)	0.013	410	47,600	7,160	22	
Ametryn (H)	185	392	250	33	21	
Aniline	36,600		13	2		
Anthracene	0.073	26,000	18,400	2,700	2,300	
Asulam (H)	5,000	300	40	5	16	
Atrazine (H)	33	149	640	86	7	
Benefin (H)	<1	10,700	>4,400	>620	850	
Bentazon (H)	500	0	140	19	0	
Benzene	1,780	83	71	9	3	
Bifenox (H)	0.35		7,800	1,120		
Biphenyl	7.5		1,400	198		340
Bromacil (H)	8.5	72	1,350	185	3	
Bromobenzene	446	150	150	20		
Butralin (H)	1	8,200	4,400	618	630	
x-sec-Butyl-4-chloro diphenyloxide	0.14		13,000	1,870		298
Captan (F)	<0.5		>6,400	>910		
Carbaryl (I)	40	230	570	77	12	
Carbofuran (I)	415		160	21		
Carbon tetrachloride (IF)	800		110	14		18
Carbophenothion (I)	0.34	45,400	7,900	1,140	4,300	
Chloramben (H)	700	21	120	15	0.8	
Chloramben, methyl ester (H)	120	507	310	41	28	
Chlorbromuron (H)	50	460	510	68	25	
Chlordane (I)	0.056		21,300	3,140		11,400
Chlorobenzene	448		150	20		12
4-Chlorobiphenyl	1.65		3,300	465		590
4-Chlorodiphenyloxide	3		2,400	330		736
Chloroneb (F)	8	1,200	1,400	190	71	
6-Chloropicolinic acid	3,400	9	50	6.3	0.3	
Chloroxuron (H)	2.7	3,200	2,500	350	220	
Chlorpropham (H)	88	590	370	50	33	
Chlorpyrifos (I)	0.3	13,600	8,500	1,220	1,100	450
Chlorpyrifos methyl (I)	4.0	3,300	2,000	280	230	
Chlorthiamid (H)	950	107	100	13	5	
Crotoxyphos (I)	1,000	170	100	13	8	
Crufomate (I)	200		240	31		
Cyanazine (H)	171	200	260	34	10	
Cycloate (H)	85	345	380	50	18	
2,4-D acid (H)	900	20	100	13	0.8	

Source: Kenaga (1980).

54

TABLE 9. Solubilities and Partition Coefficients of Various Compounds

Compound	Solubility in Water (ppm)	Log (n-Octanol–Water Partition Coefficient)
Benzene	1,710 (20°C)	2.13
Toluene	470 (16°C)	2.69
Fluorobenzene	1,540 (30°C)	4.27
Chlorobenzene	448 (30°C)	2.84
Bromobenzene	446 (30°C)	2.99
Iodobenzene	340 (30°C)	3.25
p-Dichlorobenzene	79 (25°C)	3.38
Naphthalene	30	3.37
Diphenyl ether	21 (25°C)	4.20
Tetrachloroethylene	400 (25°C)	2.60
Chloroform	7,950 (25°C)	1.97
Carbon tetrachloride	800	2.64
p,p'-DDT	0.0031–0.0034 (25°C)	6.19
p,p'-DDE	0.040 (20°C)	5.69
Benzoic acid	2,700 (18°C)	1.87
Salicylic acid	1,800 (20°C)	2.26
Phenylacetic acid	16,000 (20°C)	1.41
Phenoxyacetic acid	12,000 (10°C)	1.26
2,4-D	890 (25°C)	2.81
2,4,5,2′,5′-PCB	0.010 (24°C)	6.11
2,4,5,2′,4′,5′-PCB	0.00095 (24°C)	6.72
4,4′-PCB	0.062 (20°C)	5.58

Source: Freed et al. (1979).

TABLE 10. Partition Coefficients (K_{ow}) of Various Chemicals

Chemical	Log K_{ow} (room temperature)
Benzoic acid	1.87
Chloroform	1.97
Benzene	2.13
Salicyclic acid	2.26
Fluorobenzene	2.27
Tetrachloroethylene	2.60
Carbon tetrachloride	2.64
Toluene	2.69
Chlorobenzene	2.84
Malathion	2.89
p-Dichlorobenzene	3.81
Dichlorfenthion	5.14
4,4′-PCB	5.58
p,p-DDE	5.69
2,4,5,2′,5′-PCB	6.11
p,p-DDT	6.19
2,4,5,2′,4′,5′-PCB	6.72

Source: Chiou et al. (1977).

the partition coefficient of a simple molecule can be considered as an additive function of the partition coefficients of component parts of the molecule (Leo et al., 1971), particularly if the components are nonpolar.

3.10 Bioconcentration Factor (BCF)

During the early 1960s, it was hoped that the octanol–water partition coefficient (K_{ow}) would offer environmental toxicologists and risk assessors a simple technique for identifying those chemicals that were likely to accumulate in the environment (Table 11). The experience with DDT seemed to confirm that the octanol–water partition could identify those chemicals that could bioaccumulate in fish as well as biomagnify in the food chain (microbe to fly to fish to bird). In the late 1970s, it was shown that bioconcentration in the environment could only be partly explained by the octanol–water partition.

The experience with DDT was an important one (see Table 12). Mortalities and reproductive failure in fish and fish-eating birds were linked to unusually high concentrations of DDT or its metabolites in the fat of these animals. Since the top-level carnivores, especially birds, had higher residue concentrations of these chemicals than the food they consumed, it was logical to postulate that accumulation occurred primarily by transfer through the food chain (Spacie and Hamelink, 1985). This idea was supported indirectly by the observation that DDT residues increased in a stepwise fashion from one trophic level to the next (Woodwell et al., 1967). The net efficiency of energy transfer between trophic levels is only about 10%. If the transfer efficiency for a chemical contaminant from food to consumer were greater, say 50–100%, and if there were no significant losses from the organism, then residues would continue to accumulate throughout the life of the consumer. The higher the trophic level, the greater would be the body burden of residues. Although the actual mechanism for such a process was not clear, the concept of *biomagnification* or *transfer up the food chain* became popular (Spacie and Hamelink, 1985).

By the early 1980s it was shown that any one of several simple formulas based primarily on physical properties and especially the octanol–water partition could not predict the

---

TABLE 11. Methods for Estimating the Bioconcentration Factor (BCF) Using Physical Property Data

Octanol–Water Partition Coefficient (K_{ow})

$$K_{ow} = \frac{\text{concentration of chemical in octanol phase}}{\text{concentration of chemical in aqueous phase}}$$

For example, $\log \mathrm{BCF} = 0.76 \log K_{ow} - 23$

Water Solubility (S)

For example, $\log \mathrm{BCF} = 2.791 - 0.564 \log S$

Adsorption Coefficients for Soil and Sediments (K_{oc})

$$K_{oc} = \frac{\text{g adsorbed/g organic carbon}}{\text{g/mL solution}}$$

For example, $\log \mathrm{BCF} = 1.119 \log K_{oc} - 1.579$

TABLE 12. Log BCF and Bioconcentration Potential (DDE = 100) for 30 Organic Chemicals as Determined with the Fathead Minnow in 32-day Exposures

Chemical	Mean Exposure C_w (μg/L)	Log BCF	BCF	Bioconcentration Potential[a]
Tris-(2, 3-Dibromopropyl phosphate)	47.7	0.44	2.7	<0.1
5-Bromoindole	4.3	1.15	14	<0.1
Hexachlorocyclopentadiene	20.9	1.47	29	<0.1
Diphenylamine	43.7	1.48	30	<0.1
Chlorinated paraffin	49.2	1.69	49	<0.1
Toluene diamine	1.0	1.96	91	0.2
N-Phenyl-2-naphylamine	52.1	2.17	147	0.3
Tricresyl phosphate	31.6	2.22	165	0.3
Lindane	3.4	2.26	180	0.4
Pentachlorophenol	11.1	2.89	770	1.5
2, 4, 6-Tribromoanisole	4.8	2.94	865	1.7
1, 2, 4-Trichlorobenzene	1.6	3.32	2,800	5.5
Hexachloronorbornadiene	[b]	3.81	6,400	13
Methoxychlor	3.5	3.92	8,300	16
Heptachlor	3.1	3.98	9,500	19
Heptachloronorbornene	—[b]	4.05	11,100	22
Heptachlorepoxide	1.3	4.16	14,400	28
Mirex	1.2	4.26[c]	18,100	35
Hexabromocyclododecane	6.2	4.26	18,100	35
Hexabromobiphenyl	5.3	4.26	18,100	35
Hexachlorobenzene	2.6	4.27	18,500	36
p, p'-DDT	6.5	4.47[c]	29,400	58
Octachlorostyrene	7.1	4.52	33,000	65
o, p'-DDT	5.1	4.57[c]	37,000	72
Chlordane	5.9	4.58	37,800	74
Aroclor® 1016	8.7	4.63[d]	42,500	83
p, p'-DDE	7.3	4.71[e]	51,000	100
Aroclor® 1248	4.0	4.85	70,500	138
Aroclor® 1254	4.3	5.00[c]	100,000	196
Aroclor® 1260	1.0	5.28	194,000	300

[a]Bioconcentration potential calculated relative to p, p'-DDE = 100.
[b]Calculated from bioassay with these chemicals.
[c]Geometric mean of two tests.
[d]Geometric mean of five tests.
[e]Geometric mean of three tests.
Source: Veith et al. (1979).

concentration of a chemical in various media in the environment. As might have been expected, the processes of biomagnification and bioaccumulation were found to be rather complex and therefore not describable by a simple formula or set of formulas. Instead, detailed dynamic models were found to be necessary to distinguish the various routes of uptake by fish and other aquatic species. It is now fairly clear that the degree of accumulation in aquatic organisms depends on the type of food chain, on the availability and persistence of the contaminant in water, metabolism, and especially on the physicochemical properties of the contaminant.

TABLE 13. Terminology Useful in Understanding Behavior of Chemicals in Aquatic Systems[a]

Term	Definition
Uptake	Transfer of a chemical into or onto an aquatic organism. The uptake phase of an accumulation test is the period during which test organisms are exposed to the chemical.
Depuration	Elimination of a chemical from an organism by desorption, diffusion, excretion, egestion, biotransformation, or another route. The depuration phase of a test is the period during which previously exposed organisms are held in uncontaminated water.
Half-life or half-time	Time required for an organism held in clean water to eliminate 50% of the total body burden of tissue concentration of a chemical.
Bioavailability	Term used for the fraction of the total chemical in the surrounding environment which is available for uptake by organisms. The environment may include water, sediment, suspended particles, and food items.
Partitioning	Distribution of a chemical between two immiscible solvents. The partition coefficient (P or K_{ow}) is the ratio of the chemical concentrations in the two solvents at equilibrium. Partition coefficients are commonly measured between n-octanol and water.
Steady-state or dynamic equilibrium	The state at which the competing rates of uptake and elimination of a chemical within an organism or tissue are equal. An apparent steady state is reached when the concentration of a chemical in tissue remains essentially constant during a continuous exposure. Bioconcentration factors are usually measured at steady state.
Compartment	Quantity of chemical that displays uniform rates of uptake and elimination in a biological system and whose kinetics can be distinguished from those of other compartments.
Bioconcentration	The tendency of a chemical to accumulate in a living organism to levels in excess of the concentration in its surrounding environment; e.g., concentration of kepone in fish is hundreds of times higher than the kepone concentration in the water and the concentration of 2, 3, 7, 8-TCDD in a beach mouse can be several hundred times higher than that of the soil in which it lives.
Biomagnification	The process by which the concentration of a chemical in an organism is much greater than in its surrounding environment due not only to bioconcentration but also the uptake of food which has progressively bioconcentrated that chemical in its environment; e.g. flies that bioconcentrate DDT are eaten by frogs, which in turn are eaten by small fish, which are eaten by larger fish, which are eaten by birds.

[a] Based, in part, on Spacie and Hamelink (1985).

58

Spacie and Hamelink (1985) have reviewed the various factors that must be considered to assess the fate of chemicals in the environment and especially in aquatic systems. They noted that the distribution of a chemical in aquatic organisms is not quite as simple to model or measure as it is in in vitro tests using organic solvents, for example, the partition coefficient. Since animals move about, feed, grow, and actively transport and transform chemicals within their tissues, it is difficult to describe all the factors that can affect chemical uptake and distribution. Mass balance or kinetic models are usually required to describe all the various steps in the accumulation, distribution, and elimination of residues. Models similar to those used by pharmacologists to describe the time course of drugs in the human body are transferable to aquatic systems. Some terms important to understanding the behavior of chemicals are defined in Table 13.

As discussed by Hamelink (1977), the primary assumption underlying bioconcentration measurements is that compounds can be taken up directly from the water. This process may or may not be reversible, and it can be influenced by metabolism of the

TABLE 14. Comparison of Estimated Values with Laboratory Measurements of BCF

	Estimated BCF			Laboratory
Compound	From K_{ow}	From S	From K_{oc}	Measure BCF
Nitrobenzene	99	9.1	—	15.1
Carbon tetrachloride	17	14	—	30
p-Dichlorobenzene	220	53	—	215[a]
1, 2, 4-Trichlorobenzene	970	91	—	2,800
Hexachlorobenzene	5,600	4,100	280	18,500
DDT	14,000	23,000	27,000	29,400
Aroclor 1254 (PCB)	49,000	8,300	4,000	100,000
Chlordane	21,000	120	—	37,800

[a]Muscle only.
Source: Pfeifer (1984).

TABLE 15. Bioconcentration of Kepone from Water by Estuarine Organisms

Species	Concentrations in water (μg/L)	Duration of Exposure (days)	Body Burden (μg/kg)[a]	BCF[b]
Crassostrea virginica	0.03	30	210	× 7,000
(oysters)	0.39	30	2,200	× 5,641
M. bahia	0.03	21	120	× 4,000
(mysids)	0.41	21	4,800	× 11,700
P. pugio	0.02	28	90	× 4,500
(grass shrimp)	0.40	28	4,570	× 11,425
C. variegatus	0.05	28	370	× 7,400
(sheepshead minnow)				
L. xanthurus	0.03	30	90	× 3,000
(spot)	0.04	30	940	× 2,350

[a]Whole-body residue concentrations at the end of exposure.
[b]Ratio of the mean whole-body burden at the end of exposure to the mean measured concentration of kepone in water during the exposure.
Source: Macek et al. (1979).

compound within the animal. Regardless of the factors involved, there exists a theoretical equilibrium level where the amount of compound entering an animal is equal to the amount being "lost" when the concentration in the water is held constant. In actuality, the animal may lose some chemicals very slowly, yet the net rate of accumulation may be balanced by their growth rate, which yields a stable concentration over time (see Table 14). The condition under which the concentration in the animal stays constant is defined as the steady state, often recognized as a plateau in the uptake rate.

The establishment of a bioconcentration factor (BCF) does not mean that aquatic animals in natural environments acquire residues solely from the water. They may take up chemicals both directly from the water and in their food. Kepone uptake by estuarine organisms is a good case in point (Table 15). The relative contribution from each source depends on the substance, the concentration in the water, length of exposure, nature and degree of contamination in their food, the growth rate of the animal, and metabolism by the animal, but the theoretical limits to an accumulation process are presumed to lie at a value roughly equivalent to the BCF. Thus, by knowing the true BCF for a given chemical, it is possible to make comparisons between different chemicals regarding their accumulation potential.

3.11   Hydrolysis

Hydrolysis is one of the most common reactions occurring in the environment, and therefore represents one of the most potentially important pathways for a chemical. Rates of hydrolysis are independent of many rapidly changing factors that normally affect other degradative processes, such as the amount of sunlight, presence or absence of microbial populations, and extent of oxygen supply. Hydrolysis rates are typically influenced by pH, temperature, and concentration of the chemical, but these properties change seasonally, and slowly, in the aquatic environment (Mabey and Mill, 1978).

Hydrolysis refers to the reaction of an organic chemical (RX) with water, with the resultant net exchange of a group X from the organic chemical for the OH group from the water at the reaction center:

$$RX + HOH \rightleftarrows ROH + HX.$$

In aqueous systems, rates of hydrolysis usually show first-order kinetics; that is, the rate of the reaction depends only on the concentration of the organic chemical. This is because

TABLE 16. Hydrolysis Rates (Half-Life) at pH 7.4

Compound	Half-Life at Temperatures		ΔH (kcal/mole)
	37.5°C	20°C	
Phosmet	1.1 h	7.1 h	19.3
Dialifor	41.8 h	14.0 h	21.2
Malathion	1.3 d	10.5 d	21.6
Methyl chlorpyrifos	2.6 d	12.5 d	16.2
Dicapthon	5.5 d	29.0 d	17.2
Chlorpyrifos	13.4 d	53.0 d	14.2
Parathion	26.8 d	130.0 d	16.3

Source: Freed et al. (1979).

water is present in such excess that its concentration does not change during the reaction and thus does not affect reaction rate (USFDA, 1984).

The pH of water has a significant effect on the rate of hydrolysis reactions. The pH of natural waters may vary from 5 to 9; the pH of acid precipitation and leachate from mine waste may be as low as 3–4. Hydrolysis data are important in the design and interpretation of other environmental fate and effects tests. If a substance is extremely susceptible to hydrolysis, the loss of the compound via hydrolysis must be taken into account, for example, in aquatic toxicity tests and photodegradation tests. Some examples of rates of hydrolysis are shown in Table 16.

3.12   Algae Assay

Algae are simple photosynthetic organisms found in many terrestrial and aquatic habitats. These range from moist soils and surfaces exposed to air, to freshwater ponds, lakes, reservoirs, streams, estuaries, and oceans (Palmer, 1977). In fact, algae may be present wherever there is sufficient moisture and sunlight. Algae are important because they occur symbiotically with fungi in lichens and because they may be associated with, or found in, the cells and tissues of various animal groups (e.g., sponges, *Hydra*, corals). Algae probably carry out a significant percentage of all photosynthesis that occurs on earth, and they constitute the major component of aquatic ecosystems responsible for the fixation of energy from sunlight (USFDA, 1984). The oxygen generated as a result of this photosynthetic activity is utilized by aquatic animals and contributes in large part to the total reservoir of atmospheric oxygen. Algae are also important because they aid in transforming organic wastes to stable effluents (Palmer, 1977). Because they serve as the foundation of most aquatic food chains and are utilized by many herbivores as a major food source, algae are extremely important in the functioning of aquatic ecosystems (EPA, 1971; Miller and Zepp, 1979). For example, changes in algal growth rate, species composition, maximal standing crop, and photosynthetic rate can have profound effects on other parts of aquatic food chains and other pathways in food webs of aquatic ecosystems.

Many of the problems associated with eutrophication or nutrient enrichment of aquatic ecosystem are due to nutrient uptake and stimulation of algal biomass. Massive algal growths may occur, causing taste, odor, and oxygen-depletion problems. The latter may in turn cause fish kills and adversely affect commercial sport fisheries. Some algae release extracellular products, which are toxic to fish, birds, and mammals. Therefore, obtaining an estimate in the laboratory of effects on this significant group is an important part of assessing the potential effects of chemicals on aquatic ecosystems. This is true even though it is acknowledged that it is difficult to extrapolate from data derived in laboratory assay tests to natural aquatic ecosystems (USFDA, 1984).

3.13   Cellulose Decomposition

Cellulose is a highly water-insoluble unbranched polysaccharide (complex carbohydrate) and is one of the most abundant organic materials in plants, where it serves as a major supporting material. Dead plant matter, consisting largely of cellulose, is degraded by a number of species of bacteria and fungi, referred to as decomposers in the carbon cycle. This degradation is accomplished in a stepwise manner going from cellulose to cellobiose to glucose to organic acids and CO_2. Respiratory activity in the producers, herbivores, and carnivores accounts for the return of a considerable amount of biologically fixed carbon as gaseous CO_2 to the atmosphere; however, the most substantial return is accomplished by the respiratory activity of decomposers in their processing of waste materials and dead remains of other trophic (food-web) levels (Kormondy, 1969).

The degradation of cellulose is of particular interest to farmers since the fertility of farmland depends in part on the presence of organisms that degrade dead plant matter. The organisms that decompose the various types of cellulose are some of the most important microorganisms contributing to the humification processes in soils. The inhibition of, or interference with, cellulose degradation by toxic chemicals adversely affects the recycling of carbon and soil fertility by retarding the breakdown of the vast amounts of cellulose that enter the soil.

3.14   Nitrogen Transformation

Although gaseous nitrogen (N_2) makes up the greatest part of the atmosphere, green plants obtain their nitrogen from the soil solution in the form of ammonia (NH_3) and/or nitrates (NO_3). The main aspects of the biogeochemical cycle for nitrogen are the fixation of gaseous nitrogen, the ammonification of organically found nitrogen, and the processes of nitrification and denitrification. Ammonification is a key initial step in the reintroduction of nitrogen from protein wastes into the soil and is one of the more readily measured reactions of the nitrogen cycle (USFDA, 1984).

The breakdown of proteins and other nitrogen-containing organics in soil and the production of ammonia are the work of widespread and varied microflora. The amino groups are split off to form ammonia in a series of reactions collectively called ammonification. Urea, a waste product found in urine, is also decomposed by numerous microorganisms, resulting in the formation of ammonia. This reaction can serve as a convenient assay method for ammonification activity. There is a strong correlation between an organism's ability to degrade urea and its capacity to degrade protein.

The ammonification test is potentially applicable to all test chemicals except water-insoluble gases. Information from such testing would be used to assess the likelihood that the test chemical interferes with the normal conversion of organically bound nitrogen into ammonia, a critical step in the cycle, which supplies the combined nitrogen required by almost all microorganisms, high plants, and animals (USFDA, 1984).

3.15   Seed Germination

Seeds germinate and grow into plants that are able to utilize and convert radiant energy (sunlight) directly, through the process of photosynthesis, into chemical energy that is stored in the form of sugars, starches, and other organic chemicals. These chemicals are in turn used by humans or by other organisms as energy sources. Plants also synthesize other compounds essential to many animals and humans and furnish atmospheric oxygen through photosynthesis. Thus, the maintenance of the biosphere depends on the normal functioning of the plant throughout its life cycle. Angiosperms (dicotyledon and monocotyledon flowering plants) are of particular importance and concern since they are ecologically significant organisms in many ecosystems. They comprise the dominant vegetation in most parts of the United States and are also the source of all major food crops.

Many plant species are especially sensitive to chemicals in the seed germination stage. Certain vital cellular and subcellular processes associated with germination, such as cell elongation, cell differentiation, mitosis, and protein and enzyme synthesis, may be affected by xenobiotics (USFDA, 1984). Tests to evaluate seed germination have been developed and these should be used to evaluate chemicals that can be expected to be widely used in the environment, for example, pesticides.

3.16 Sulfur Transformation

Sulfur is essential to all living organisms as a part of sulfur-containing amino acids. The sulfur cycle is one of the major biogeochemical cycles and involves the release of sulfur as hydrogen sulfide (H_2S) from organic compounds (plant and animal wastes) by anaerobic microbial degradation, enabling the sulfur to be recycled again through living organisms.

Anaerobic microbial degradation of organic wastes is carried out by bacteria, which are able to use sulfate rather than oxygen as the acceptor of electrons that are gained upon oxidation of the organic material. These heterotrophic sulfate-reducing bacteria are widely distributed in nature where anoxic conditions exist—as in sewage, sediments, muds, and bovine rumina. Two groups of bacteria are able to reduce sulfate to H_2S (Frobisher et al., 1974). The best known of these are the *Desulfovibrio* organisms. These organisms have been thoroughly studied because they are responsible for serious odor and corrosion problems associated with sulfate reduction. However, these problems tend to obscure the necessary and beneficial role played by *Desulfovibrio* in the sulfur cycle (USFDA, 1984).

3.17 Microbial Growth Inhibition

The main objective of this test is to determine the lowest concentration of test chemical that will inhibit the growth of tested microbial strains or species. Widespread microbial growth inhibition may result in ecosystem-level effects, which may include, depending on the organisms inhibited, reduction in plant growth or quality through nutritional disturbances (i.e., interruption of nutrient cycling) and interference with the natural degradative functions of microorganisms that play a dominant role in transformations of biotic and xenobiotic wastes. Microorganisms serve many important functions associated with the major biogeochemical cycles, for example, carbon, nitrogen, and sulfur. An introduction to and discussion of microbial ecology may be found in Brock (1966).

4 TOXICOLOGY TESTING

The purpose of toxicological testing is to characterize the potential adverse effects of a chemical on humans through the use of laboratory animals or in vitro systems. The ultimate objective is to identify those substances that might injure humans who might come into contact with them and thus to prevent injury. The most fundamental concept in toxicology is that a relation exists between the dose of an agent and the response that is produced in a mammalian system. Three tenants are basic to toxicology. First, the magnitude of the biologic response is a function of the concentration of the agent and the site of action. Second, the concentration at the site of action is related in some predictable and describable manner with the administered dose. Third, the dose and response are causally related.

4.1   Mammalian Toxicist Tests

4.1.1   Acute Test (Mammalian). The objectives of acute toxicity testing are to define the intrinsic toxicity of the chemical, to assess the susceptible species, to identify target organs, to provide information for risk assessment after acute exposure to the chemical, and to provide information for the design and selection of dose levels for prolonged studies (Chan et al., 1982). A battery of tests under different conditions and exposure routes should be conducted on chemicals that are likely to be made in large quantity or where human exposure cannot be prevented. In general, a basic acute test battery should be conducted on nearly every chemical to which humans may be routinely or occasionally exposed. This battery usually includes oral, dermal, and inhalation toxicity tests and skin and eye irritation studies. Other tests such as acute preneonatal and neonatal exposure, dermal contact sensitization, and phototoxicity should be considered, depending on the likely degree of human exposure.

An acute test to estimate the oral LD_{50} may require as many as 50 animals. Often, three or more doses are used and five or more animals of each sex are treated. The number of animals used in the dermal and inhalation tests is usually less, while skin and eye irritation tests often require even fewer animals. Standard protocols have been developed and these should be used if the test results are to be submitted to help support justification of a registration or to meet some other regulatory criteria.

4.1.2   Subchronic Tests (Mammalian). Subchronic studies are designed to examine the adverse effects resulting from repeated exposure over a portion of the average life span of an experimental animal. For rodents, these tests are usually 30–90 days in duration. Properly designed subchronic studies give valuable information on the cumulative toxicity of a substance, target organs, physiological effects, and metabolic tolerance of a compound following repeated low-dose (relative to acute toxicity testing dose levels) exposure. By monitoring many different parameters of toxicity, including histopathologic evaluation, a wide variety of adverse effects can be detected. The results from such studies can also provide information that will aid in selecting dose levels for chronic, reproductive, and carcinogenicity studies. Subchronic studies are also valuable for establishing dose levels at which no toxicological effects are evident—a critical figure in risk assessment. For chemicals where chronic human exposure to low doses is likely, the conduct of subchronic animal studies should be given serious consideration.

The exposure period in subchronic studies may vary, depending on the objective of the study, the species selected for the study, and the route of administration. A generalization that is often made is that subchronic studies do not exceed 10% of the animal's life span. Like most generalizations, this is not always the case. Oral and inhalation subchronic studies are generally carried out for 3 months in shorter-lived animals (rodents) and about 1 year in longer-lived animals (dogs, monkeys). Subchronic dermal studies are usually performed in 1 month or less. The most common routes of administration used in subchronic toxicity studies are oral, dermal, and respiratory. Wherever feasible, subchronic toxicity studies should expose the animals by the route through which humans are most likely to be exposed (Hayes, 1982).

4.1.3   Chronic Tests (Mammalian). Long-term toxicity tests are usually defined as studies of longer than 3 months duration, that is, greater than 10% of the life span in the laboratory rat. These types of study are conducted in all species of laboratory animals and in some economically important animals. This class of tests encompasses the lifetime toxicity studies, multigeneration reproduction studies, and carcinogenicity studies.

There are two basic reasons for conducting chronic toxicity tests: to produce a toxic effect and to define a safe level of exposure (Stevens and Gallo, 1982). The chronic study is defined so as to identify any of the myriad of potential toxic effects of a xenobiotic on structural and functional entities. In contrast to the carcinogenicity studies, which are designed to measure tumor induction, the chronic toxicity study uses a holistic approach to define the etiology of an adverse response to identify the appropriate margin of safety between any proposed use (exposure) levels and those that might produce toxicity (Stevens and Gallo, 1982).

Fairly large numbers of rodents are used in these tests. The classic chronic toxicity study in rats usually consists of three treatment groups and a control group, all of equal number at the outset, in which the xenobiotic is administered 7 days per week for at least 2 years. Because of the shorter life span of mice, the compound need be given for only 18 months. A second nonrodent species is often required to assure safety and the choice is usually the purebred beagle. The choice of a larger animal permits more extensive clinical analyses since more blood can be collected from each animal with greater frequency than is possible with rodents. There are several schools of thought on the use of the second species but the dog should be used with caution since it is a carnivore and often metabolizes compounds differently than an omnivore or herbivore (Stevens and Gallo, 1982).

The most intellectually challenging task for the toxicologist responsible for directing a chronic toxicity study is the selection of the dose levels to be tested. There are several suggested approaches. One of these is the approach of the National Cancer Institute's Bioassay Program, which is to conduct a 3-month range-finding study with enough doses to find a level that suppresses body weight gain slightly, that is, 10%. This dose is defined as the maximum tolerated dose (MTD) and is selected as the highest dose. Generally $\frac{1}{4}$ MTD and $\frac{1}{8}$ MTD are selected as the other two test doses.

4.1.4 Developmental Toxicity (Mammalian).

Once known as teratology tests, these toxicological studies have been defined more appropriately as tests for developmental toxicity (Nisbet and Karch, 1983; EPA, 1986c). There are four ways in which altered in utero development can be demonstrated: (i) death of the conceptus, (ii) gross structural abnormality, (iii) in utero growth retardation, or (iv) decrement of anticipated postnatal functional capabilities. These can arise from a variety of causes (Wilson, 1973).

Three terms are often used to describe the results of developmental toxicity tests. For the sake of risk assessment, *teratogenic* should be used to describe those chemicals that have been shown to produce gross structural abnormalities. *Embryotoxic* and *fetotoxic* appear to be the most ill-defined terms. Several papers have used embryotoxic as the sum of all possible toxic actions affecting the embryo, including teratogenic, embryolethal, and other effects. Black and Marks (1986) have proposed that embryotoxicity should describe the loss of an embryo and the term fetotoxicity should be used for less severe effects. Fetotoxicity has also been used to describe the toxic or degenerative effect on fetal tissues and organs after organogenesis (Rao et al., 1981; EPA, 1986c). Some authors have suggested that fetotoxicity should be equated with transient effects such that bones and organs would be expected to continue to develop to their normal appearance and function. The EPA guidelines for developmental toxicants (1986c), in contrast, have suggested that embryotoxic and fetotoxic be used to describe a very wide range of adverse effects and that these terms only differentiate the time when the effects are apparent.

4.1.5 Reproductive Toxicity (Mammalian).

In contrast to tests that evaluate developmental toxicity, reproductive tests evaluate chemicals for their ability to affect adversely the fertility of either parent. A number of functional, morphological, and biochemical parameters are available to assess toxic effects on both male and female reproductive function. The functional parameters include reproductive efficiency, cogenesis, and fertilization. Morphological parameters are gross pathology and histopathology. The biochemical parameters include molecular aspects (normal synthesis and metabolism), accessory cell function, and hormonal status. Species survival requires the production and eventual union of the male and female gametes, each with its complement of healthy genes. Of these events and processes, oogenesis, spermatogenesis, and fertilization, are studied to evaluate the reproductive process (Dixon and Hall, 1982).

These tests typically are conducted for three generations of the test species. Depending on the protocol, the parent may be exposed continuously throughout the key periods prior to and following conception. Thus far, the three-generation protocol has been successful for identifying chemicals that might adversely affect reproduction.

4.2 Aquatic Toxicology

Aquatic toxicology has been defined as the study of the effects of chemicals and other foreign agents on aquatic organisms with special emphasis on adverse or harmful effects (Rand and Petrocelli, 1985). Aquatic toxicity tests are used to evaluate the concentrations of the chemical and the duration of exposure required to produce the criterion effect. The effects of a chemical may be of such minor significance that the aquatic organism is able to carry on its functions in a normal manner and that only under conditions of additional stress (e.g., changes in pH, dissolved oxygen, and temperature) can a chemically induced effect be detected. On the other hand, at sufficiently high concentrations, some chemicals many have the capacity to cause illness and death in some or all aquatic life. A number of species are typically used in these tests (Table 17).

Two general approaches may be used to conduct these tests, and each has advantages and limitations. (i) Effects can be studied in controlled laboratory experiments with a limited number of variables. (ii) Effects can be studied in a natural ecosystem (in situ). Until

TABLE 17. Standard Test Species Used in Aquatic Toxicology Testing

Fresh Water	Salt Water
Acute	
Fathead minnow	Mummichog
Bluegill sunfish	Sheepshead minnow
Channel catfish	Silverside
Trout/salmon	Flounder
Daphnia magna	Stickleback
Daphnia pulex	Grass shrimp
Ceriodaphnia sp.	Oysters
Chronic	
Fathead minnow	Silverside
Daphnia sp.	Sheepshead minnow
Ceriodaphnia sp.	Mysid shrimp

now, the laboratory setting has been favored because of ease and decreased cost compared to that associated with field studies.

4.2.1 Acute Effects (Aquatic). Acute effects are those that occur rapidly as a result of short-term exposure to a chemical. In fish and other aquatic organisms, effects that occur within a few hours, days, or weeks are considered acute. Generally, acute effects are relatively severe. The most common adverse effect measured in aquatic organisms is lethality or mortality. A chemical is considered acutely toxic if by its direct action it kills 50% or more of the exposed population of test organisms in a relatively short period of time, such as 96 hours to 14 days (Rand and Petrocelli, 1985).

4.2.2 Subacute Effects (Aquatic). Subchronic and chronic toxic effects may occur when a chemical produces deleterious effects as a result of a single exposure, but more often they are a consequence of repeated or long-term exposures. There may be a relatively long latency (time to occurrence) period for the expression of these effects, particularly if the exposure concentration is very low. To evaluate these effects, subchronic tests are often 10–90 days in duration. Tests to evaluate the removal of a chemical from fish, so-called depuration studies, require several days but are informative in helping to assess the possible subacute and chronic effects of a water contaminant (Table 18).

4.2.3 Chronic (Aquatic). Chronic effects may also be lethal or sublethal. A typical lethal effect is failure of the chronically exposed organisms to produce viable offspring. The most common sublethal effects in aquatic species are behavioral changes (e.g., swimming, attraction–avoidance, and prepredator relation), physiological changes (e.g., growth, reproduction, and development), biochemical changes (e.g., blood enzyme and ion levels), and histological changes. Some sublethal effects may indirectly result in lethalities. For example, certain behavioral changes (e.g., swimming or olfactory) may diminish the ability of aquatic organisms to find food or to escape from predators and ultimately lead to death.

TABLE 18. **Time Required by Fish to Eliminate 50% of Residue Burden ($t_{1/2}$) during Depuration in Uncontaminated Flowing Water**

Chemical	Species	$t_{1/2}$ (days)
DEHP	Bluegill	<3
TCB	Bluegill	<7
Leptophos	Bluegill	<10
Cadmium	Shrimp	<10 [22]
Endrin	Catfish	<10 [13]
Kepone	Sheepshead minnow	<28 [19]
Kepone	Oysters	<4 [19]
Aroclor 1254	Grass shrimp	<14 [27]
Aroclor 1254	Spot	<42 [28]
Aroclor 1254	Fathead minnow	<42[a]
DDT	Rainbow trout	>160 [12]
	Lake trout	>125 [29]

[a]Unpublished data, Dr. Gil Veith, National Environmental Research Laboratory, U.S. Environmental Protection Agency, Duluth, Minnesota.
Source: Macek et al. (1979).

Chronic aquatic testing will often be necessary to understand the full range of possible adverse effects of repeated long-term exposure on aquatic species. For example, some sublethal effects may have little or no effect on the organism because they are rapidly reversible or diminish or cease with time (e.g., growth may be reduced at high concentrations early in a toxicity study but may not be significantly different from that in controls by the end of the study). In laboratory studies, sublethal effects can go unnoticed in acute tests. The only way to study sublethal toxicity in the laboratory is by using long-term exposures. Numerous types of aquatic tests have been developed for evaluating each of these adverse effects of chronic exposure. These have been described by several authors (Mayer and Hamelink, 1977; Rand and Petrocelli, 1985).

4.3 Domestic Animal Toxicology

The effects of low-level exposure to xenobiotics unintentionally present in the environment have been studied infrequently in domestic animals, especially cows, goats, and sheep. In general, their exposure to chemical contaminants, which have been of widespread concern to humans or aquatic life, has been negligible. More recently, especially because of broadscale environmental contamination that has been reported at times with PCB, PBB, DDT, and heptachlor, a greater number of studies have been conducted (Fries, 1982, 1985; Jones et al., 1986). Standardized tests for evaluating the effects of xenobiotics on domestic animals have been established for intentional feed additives but not for toxicity testing of unintentional additives. Because of an increased concern for hazards such as the airborne release of metals and TCDD by incinerators, the evaluation of domestic animals used for food will almost certainly increase in the coming years (Fries and Paustenbach, 1987).

4.4 Earthworms and Other Wildlife

One of the most interesting and challenging areas in environmental assessment is the characterization of the potential hazard to lower wildlife and insects. Heretofore, this area has received little attention, although it could arguably be an important dimension in the evaluation of hazardous waste sites and other hazards. Only a handful of industrial chemicals have been studied thoroughly for their potential adverse effect on lower forms of wildlife such as earthworms, field mice, snakes, ants, or turtles with the exception perhaps of some pesticides (Oliver, 1984; Reineke and Nash, 1984; Young, 1983; Young and Cockerham, 1985).

When a fairly significant area of land or the environment could be contaminated by a chemical, it is prudent to have a thorough understanding of the physical and chemical properties of that chemical in order to appreciate the overall exposure potential. If it is determined that a potentially significant degree of exposure to wildlife might occur, various levels of testing should be considered. For the pesticides, the EPA has established numerous requirements and has been testing to evaluate the potential adverse affects on aquatic species, large and small animals, lower species, and some plants. These are an excellent source of information for developing tests to evaluate the industrial chemicals or physical agents. Several thoughtful approaches for establishing batteries of tests for new chemicals—including the tier approach—have been proposed, and these should be considered (Beck et al., 1981; Dickson et al., 1982). One of the debated areas is whether to conduct laboratory or field studies to evaluate the hazard to wildlife. In general, laboratory studies are deemed more appropriate as a screening test since the data are easier to collect and interpret, thus making the studies more cost effective (Young and Cockerham, 1985).

4.5   Avian Toxicology

With the development of literally hundreds of pesticides during the past 40 years, the need to evaluate their potential adverse effect on wildlife, and especially birds, became very clear. By 1979, the EPA under the Federal Insecticide, Fungicide, and Rodenticide Act (FIFRA) established guidelines for assessing the potential effects of pesticides on avian species.

4.5.1   *Avian Dietary LC_{50}.*

The toxicity testing of birds is not unlike that of mammals or fish. Under FIFRA, testing is required on two avian species, one species of wild waterfowl (preferably the mallard) and one species of upland game bird (preferable the bobwhite or other native quail or the ring-necked pheasant). Birds used in these tests should be 10–17 days of age at the beginning of the test period and the test animals should be observed over at least an 8-day period. During the first 5 days, birds are on a treated diet followed by at least 3 days of observation on clean diets. The results of this test are useful for setting acceptable application levels and for identifying doses for further testing.

4.5.2   *Avian Reproduction.*

One of the primary concerns about the presence of xenobiotics in the environment with respect to the avian hazard is the potential adverse effect on reproduction. Since this can be a rather insidious effect if it were to occur in the field—for example, the population could be markedly diminished before observation begins, it is of critical importance. Testing used to evaluate reproductive toxicity is usually performed on the bobwhite and the mallard. Avian reproduction testing is often required by FIFRA if any of the following conditions apply:

1. Pesticide residues resulting from the proposed use are persistent in the environment to the extent that toxic amounts are expected on avian feed.
2. Pesticide residues are stored or accumulated in plant or animal tissues.
3. Pesticide is proposed for use under conditions where birds may be subjected to repeated or continued exposure to the pesticide, especially preceding or during the breeding season.

To satisfy this last requirement, birds are exposed to treated diets beginning not less than 10 weeks before egg laying and extending throughout the laying season. At least two treatment level groups are used. Concentrations for the test substance should be based on residues expected under the proposed use and a multiple, such as 5. Some scientists have suggested that it may be cost effective to consider multiple-level testing, at least three exposure levels, to determine effect and no-effect levels. This may be especially useful for new pesticides that show promise on several crops and where avian exposure may vary or where levels of environmental exposure are not established, or both.

4.5.3   *Pen Field Studies.*

Simulated testing and actual field testing for mammals and birds are sometimes the best approaches to evaluating safety. These have become more commonplace since 1980 and are likely to become routine for those chemicals that have significant toxicity or where there is persistence. The decision to conduct field tests is usually based on consideration of the physicochemical properties of the pesticide, the proposed use pattern, the likelihood of wildlife exposure to the pesticide under field conditions and at levels expected to be toxic to wildlife, and on review of laboratory data. The major problems with field studies are that they are cumbersome, difficult to analyze, troubled by the unpredictable nature of the wild, and very expensive.

4.5.4   Full-Scale Field Studies.   Full-scale field tests are often productive if use of the pesticide, or another chemical, is anticipated to have some likelihood of adversely affecting wildlife. Universally acceptable standards for conducting full-scale field tests are not possible because of the variety of ways a pesticide may enter the environment and impact wildlife. In the full-scale field test, the objective is to determine the impact on wildlife populations. Such tests are applicable to use patterns associated with a major wildlife habitat. These would include forests, rangeland, and croplands such as cotton, corn, sorghum, soybeans, rice, and alfalfa. A limited number of full-scale field studies had been conducted through 1985.

4.5.5   Rules of Thumb for Risk Assessment of Avian Hazards.   The following guidelines, which can be used in risk assessment calculations, have been offered by Kenaga (1972). Although perhaps dated, these are helpful for conducting assessments where the risk to avian species is a concern:

1. Body weights of birds can be estimated reasonably to within $\pm 20\%$ of the actual weight when not known exactly, by use of available literature values.

2. The quantity of food eaten per day by birds can be reasonably estimated when not known exactly. In general, species weighing over 100 grams eat less than 20% of the body weight in food per day, and those under 10 grams may eat as much as 60% in dry weight food per day. Based on a linear relationship of body weight to food intake, percent of body weight eaten per day can be estimated within a 2-fold factor.

3. The upper limits of the amount of residues of a pesticide on various species, shapes, and sizes of plant food and insects immediately after application can be reasonably estimated. In general, the highest residues may be expected on treated food particles which have the highest surface area to weight–volume ratios and greatest exposure to the pesticide application. The upper limits of pesticide residues on plants and their decline with time on various types of crops, as correlated from data on many pesticides, are known.

4. Based upon the information developed in this report on a unit basis, a 1 pound per acre dosage of a non-cumulative pesticide could result in a 35-fold difference (7–240 ppm) between maximum pesticide residues in different sized natural bird food particles. Also a 20-gram bird of nearly any species will likely eat 5 times as much food in mg per kg of body weight per day as a 1,000-gram bird of nearly any species. Thus, it is possible that a 20-gram bird could eat 100 times or more pesticide than a 1,000-gram bird, in terms of mg/kg/day. Variations in concentrations and dosages of pesticides and variations in good consumption rates of different weights of birds can be estimated to obtain specified mg/kg/day. As has been shown, the maximum residues estimated here rarely occur in nature and therefore mitigating circumstances of stability of the residues, food habits of the birds, etc. would result in corresponding reduction of this estimate.

5. The estimated or calculated mg/kg/day of intake of pesticides from residues on bird food should be matches with toxicological responses from similar dosages in laboratory or field test results with birds, preferably by use of ad lib dietary feeding tests, rather than acute oral, injection or other less correlatable tests, not as suitable for environmental interpretation. Subacute and chronic laboratory toxicity tests are often conducted with diets containing a constant concentration rate of pesticides over a period of days, weeks, or months. Interpretation of such laboratory tests should take into consideration the frequently large and quick rate of decline in pesticide residues which occur on natural bird food, or the dietary intake of birds in such tests should be adjusted accordingly. In addition, the test methods should provide for the study of metabolites of the pesticide or other derived molecules if any occur. Food acceptance of the pesticide in the diet of birds and the relative toxicity of the pesticide to representative species of birds must also be taken into account.

5   EXPOSURE ASSESSMENT

As discussed in the NAS guidelines (1983), the exposure assessment is as important as the hazard identification portion of a risk assessment. In fact, it is quite likely that the major improvements in risk assessment that will be achieved in the near future will be due to improvements in our ability to estimate the uptake of chemicals caused by specific exposure scenarios.

5.1   Environmental Exposure Estimation

When conducting an environmental risk assessment, one of the most difficult aspects is the estimation of the likely degree of exposure to the chemical. Often, this question can be answered through direct measurement or modeling. The latter approach is needed for those settings where exposure is imminent if corrective action is not taken, for example landfills, waste sites, or lagoons above drinking water aquifers. Often, the future contamination of ambient air or drinking water predicted by these models is less than that which could be measured; thus, a modeling approach is needed to help prevent the future contamination of important exposure pathways. As illustrated in Fig. 4 the distribution of a chemical in the environment can be widespread, so it is important to characterize its physical properties in order to predict its behavior.

The environmental fate of a chemical can be predicted through both physical and mathematical simulation approaches (Metcalf et al., 1975; Baughman and Lassiter, 1978; Branson, 1978). In general, equations can be used to describe the dominant modes of transport and the metabolism of the chemical substance, if any, as well as any potentially significant sources of the substance. Often, a deterministic mathematical model is used, for example, differential equations can be used to describe both the individual rates of transformation and the transport processes, thus permitting a description of the environmental chemistry and fate of the chemical. Typical chemical and biological properties that are important in the prediction of environmental concentrations, and the tests for measuring them, were discussed in Section 3 (hazard identification) of this chapter.

5.2   Human Exposure Estimation

The primary routes of exposure to chemicals in the environment are inhalation of dusts and vapors, dermal contact with contaminated soils or dusts, and ingestion of contaminated foods, water, or soil/dust (Kimbrough et al., 1984; Schaum, 1984; Hawley, 1985; Eschenroeder et al., 1986; EPA, 1986e; Paustenbach et al., 1986; Paustenbach, 1987). Initial efforts to quantitatively estimate the uptake of environmental contaminants by humans were first conducted by scientists in the field of radiological health (Romney et al., 1963; Martin, 1964; Russell, 1966; Land, 1980; Moghissi et al., 1980; Bresson et al., 1981; Baes et al., 1984) and their work can be a source of valuable information when conducting assessments of chemical contaminants. General methodologies for estimating the human uptake of contaminants have been proposed (Bresson et al., 1981; Schaum, 1984; Eschenroeder et al., 1986; Paustenbach, 1987).

5.2.1   Uptake via Inhalation. To estimate the amount of a chemical absorbed by humans through inhalation, the following parameters must be measured or estimated:

1. Contaminant concentration in air (gas, vapors, or particulates).
2. Particle size distribution (for chemicals adsorbed onto particles).
3. Contaminant concentration in dust (may vary with particle size).
4. Respiration rate.
5. Degree of pulmonary absorption (e.g., bioavailability).
6. Duration of exposure.

The most direct method for determining a contaminant's concentration in air is by actual measurement. Unfortunately, field data are not always available and estimates must be made. However, the range over which values could reasonably span is relatively narrow. This characteristic, for example, the limited distribution of possible contaminant levels, can give us confidence that post hoc estimates of inhalation exposure will be acceptable for most uses of risk assessment.

If the source of the airborne chemical is the soil and the contaminant is relatively volatile, for example, chlorinated solvents, the vapor concentration at ground level can be estimated. This is dependent on its concentration in the soil, its vaporization rate, the distance above the soil where exposure is likely to occur, and the degree of atmospheric mixing. Computer models have been developed to solve the appropriate equations. If the soil contaminant is relatively nonvolatile, for example, metals or dioxins, the inhaled dose is primarily driven by the concentration of airborne particulates to which the contaminant is adsorbed. Often, the smaller particles contain a higher concentration of the toxicant than the large particles so this must be considered in the calculation.

In many locations around the United States, the airborne concentration of total suspended particulates (TSPs) can be estimated from published data. Generally, measures of TSPs are collected by high-volume air samplers and represent the weight of all particles having an aerodynamic diameter of less than 20 μm. In many geographic locations, the EPA has conducted exhaustive studies of airborne dust levels and has considered such

TABLE 19. Respiratory Rates for Various Ages and Sexes

	Adult Man	Adult Woman	Child (10 y)	Infant (1 y)	Newborn
Minute Volume for Reference Man					
Resting (L/min)	7.5	6.0	4.8	1.5	0.5
Light activity (L/min)	20.0	19.0	13.0	4.2	1.5
Liters of air Breathed for Reference Man					
8 h working "light activity"	9,600[†]	9,100[‡]	6,240[§]	2,500[‖] (10 h)	90[¶] (1 h)
8 h nonoccupational activity	9,600[†]	9,100[‡]	6,240[§]		
8 h resting	3,600[†]	2,900[‡]	2,300[§]	1,300[‖] (14 h)	690[¶] (23 h)
Total	2.3×10^4	2.1×10^4	1.5×10^4	0.38×10^4	0.08×10^4
% of total air breathed at work	42	43			

Source: Report of the Task Group on Reference man. (Snyder, 1975).

TABLE 20. "Rule of Nines" for Estimating Surface Area of Certain Regions of Total Body

Head and neck	9%
Upper limbs (each 9%)	18%
Lower limbs (each 18%)	36%
Front of trunk	18%
Back of trunk	18%
Perineum	1%
Outstretched palm and fingers	1%

Source: Report of the Task Group on Reference man (Snyder, 1975).

variables as meteorological conditions, geographic terrain, and traffic patterns. These studies provide good to excellent estimates of ambient particulate concentrations for nearly all locations in the United States (Schaum, 1984).

Not all TSPs present a respiratory hazard to humans, since only some of the particles are inhalable, that is, are taken into the nose or mouth during breathing. Inhalable particulates are generally defined as those less than 20 μm in aerodynamic diameter (Schaum, 1984). To provide an accurate estimate of uptake, only the values for the inhalable and respirable fractions of TSPs need be considered. If the inhalation hazard is due to contaminated soil, it must be remembered that not all inhalable particulates will orginate from the contaminated site. In fact, probably no more than 50% of the TSPs in the area around a site will have originated from crustal material, that is, soil (Trijonis et al., 1980). Also, differences in the indoor and outdoor airborne particulate concentrations must be considered.

The amount of contaminated particulates or vapor available for systemic uptake is dependent on the person's respiration rate. The indoor respiration rate can be estimated as similar to the resting rate, whereas the outdoor respiration rate should be based on the occupational respiration rate, that is, one that is based on moderate activity (Table 19). Typically, it has been assumed that the resting ventilation rate is about $5 \, m^3$ every 8 hours for a 70 kg person and about $10 \, m^3$ every 8 hours for a physical laborer (Kimbrough et al., 1984; Paustenbach et al., 1986).

The pulmonary absorption coefficient, or bioavailability, can markedly influence the degree of uptake, especially for the nonrespirable fraction. Since relatively low concentrations of volatilized solvents are present at most environmentally contaminated sites, the pulmonary absorption coefficient for vapors can be considered 100% for these purposes. For inhaled particulates, bioavailability depends on the physicochemical properties of the contaminant, as well as the physicochemical properties of the particulates themselves, and the site of particulate deposition within the pulmonary system.

5.2.2 Dermal Uptake.

To estimate dermal exposure to contaminated soil, dusts, or liquids, and the subsequent absorption of the chemical contaminant, the following parameters need to be known or estimated:

1. Contaminant concentration in soil or dust.
2. Soil/dust deposition rate from air and from direct soil contact.
3. Area of exposed skin.

4. Dermal absorption coefficient (i.e., bioavailability).

5. Duration of exposure.

The deposition rate of dust from air has been estimated by Eschenroeder et al. (1986) and Hawley (1985), while direct soil contamination can be inferred from Sayre et al. (1974) or Roels et al., 1980. Other parameters can be estimated on a case-by-case basis.

Volatilized solvents, such as vapors, can be inhaled and/or absorbed through the skin (Piotrowski, 1972). Generally, the dermal uptake of vapors is very small, often less than 1% of the amount taken up by inhalation. In general, dermal uptake of vapors is so small that this route of entry can be neglected. The surface area of various portions of the skin are presented in Table 20.

For chemical contaminants adsorbed onto soil particles, one of the most important parameters that influences uptake is bioavailability. The bioavailability of chemicals on soil can depend on the physicochemical properties of the contaminant and the soil, the length of time the contaminant has been in contact with soil (e.g., aging), and the length of time the contaminated soil is in contact with the skin (Poiger and Schlatter, 1980; Paustenbach et al., 1986; Shu et al., 1988b). Although often overlooked, soil can be characterized by three factors: percent organics, sand, and silt. Furthermore, these factors influence the number and types of binding sites.

5.2.3   Uptake Due to Ingestion.
The risks associated with the ingestion of chemical contaminants are dictated by the following parameters:

1. Amount of contaminated medium ingested per day (i.e., soil, food, and liquids).

2. Contaminant concentration in each medium.

3. Gastrointestinal absorption coefficient (i.e., bioavailability).

Ingested contaminated media can include foods, fluids, and soil. The average daily intake of various foods has been compiled by the U.S. Food and Drug Administration (U.S. FDA) and these can be used if no site-specific information on the food ingestion of the exposed population is available (Pennington, 1983).

If there is no information when estimating water consumption, one can rely on the value for average water intake used by the EPA of 1 L/day for children (10 kg) and 2 L/day for adults (70 kg). Although these figures have been used in assessments for a number of years, they appear to represent an overestimate of the actual amount ingested by most persons. A more extensive description of age-specific water intake has been developed by Pennington (1983). When estimating uptake, the amount of contaminant present in each medium should be assessed using a valid, randomized sampling program. The statistical analysis of the data should employ a log–normal, rather than the more typical Gaussian distribution (Rappaport and Selvin, 1987).

For many risk assessments involving hazardous waste sites, it has been suggested that the major source of oral uptake of xenobiotics is from the direct ingestion of contaminated soil (Kimbrough et al., 1984). The amount of soil ingested by children has been estimated by numerous investigators (Lepow et al., 1974; Duggan and Williams, 1977; Schaum, 1984; Paustenbach et al., 1986; Clausing et al., 1987; LaGoy, 1987). There is general agreement that soil ingestion is greatest in preschool-aged children and that the amount decreases with age. More recently, a systematic approach involving the analysis of fecal samples has been proposed to estimate the amount of soil ingested by children (Binder et al., 1987;

Calabrese et al., 1988). A comprehensive review of the available data has been conducted by Paustenbach (1987). The value of soil uptake by the typical child is best estimated as either 50 or 100 mg/day (ages 2–6).

Finally, to calculate absorbed dose via ingestion, the gastrointestinal absorption coefficient (e.g., bioavailability) for the chemical contaminant must be known or estimated (Poiger and Schlatter, 1980). The medium in which the chemical contaminant is found, for example, dirt, meat, and fly ash, clearly influences bioavailability (Shu et al., 1988). Studies thus far suggest that bioavailability on soil can vary from 0.55 to 95% for certain chemicals on various kinds of soil. The bioavailability of xenobiotics in liquids is generally in the 75–100% range.

5.2.4 *Estimating Daily Dose.*

To compare an individual's uptake of contaminants from the environment with doses that have been shown to cause adverse effects in humans or animals, risk assessors often estimate the maximum daily dose (MDD) and lifetime average daily dose (LADD) resulting from environmental exposure. These are usually expressed in units of weight of contaminant absorbed per unit body weight per day (mg/kg·day). For chemicals with acute effects, the MDD is compared with the no observed effect level (NOEL) observed in short-term animal studies, and for chemicals possessing carcinogenic potential in long-term bioassays, the LADD is generally compared with the NOEL identified in these tests.

The ratio of the dose that caused no adverse effect in animal or human studies (NOEL) and the exposure dose is known as the *margin of safety*. The MDD is usually based on a feasible "worst-case" uptake scenario for a given day of exposure and the ADD is based on the "average" daily dose (ADD), or lifetime average daily dose (LADD) computed over 70 years. If exposure is not for a lifetime, the LADD is calculated by multiplying the ADD by the fraction of the lifetime over which that exposure occurred. To calculate MDD, ADD, and LADD, the pattern and duration of an individual's exposure must be estimated, as well as the uptake parameters described earlier.

5.2.5 *Physiological Parameters for Humans.*

The response of a person exposed to a pollutant depends not only on the nature and the concentration of the toxicant but also on a variety of other factors including age, food habits, lifestyle, and many physiological parameters. In many cases these parameters are known, and these can be used in risk assessment calculations (Moghissi et al., 1980). Recognizing that many factors must be estimated, the International Committee for Radiological Protection (ICRP) has assembled data describing "reference men," "reference women," and "reference children" (Snyder, 1975). Although ICRP specifies that caution should be used in the application of these data for areas other than radiation protection, a great deal of the information gathered by ICRP is applicable for estimating the uptake of environmental contaminants by humans. For example, Tables 19 through 21 contain data on some physiologic parameters for various ages and sexes.

5.2.6 *Breathing Rate.*

In general, the breathing rates of animals and humans have been well documented (Guyton, 1947; Altman and Ditmer, 1964; Snyder, 1975). See Table 19. For laboratory animals, uptake can usually be estimated by a general equation. Studies with rats and hamsters enclosed in a chamber are consistent with a ventilation rate (QP) calculated according to the equation

$$QP = (15 \, \text{L/h})(\text{BW})^{0.74}.$$

The use of 0.74 as the exponent for body weight (BW) was proposed by Guyton (1947) based on studies with anesthetized animals. This equation predicts an alveolar ventilation rate of 348 L/h in a 70-kg human (total ventilation rate = 1.5 times alveolar ventilation rate or 522 L/h). This rate of ventilation is intermediate between the value reported by the ICRP (Snyder, 1975) for a resting human (300 L/h) and the value utilized by EPA for its risk calculations (20 m^3/24 h or 833 L/h), which corresponds to humans performing mild exercise.

5.2.7   Surface Area.   The surface area of the entire human body as well as the anatomical parts have been measured. This information has been presented in several papers and texts (Snyder, 1975) and is useful when estimating the uptake of various chemicals because of skin contact with liquids or contaminated soil. Some of this information is presented in Table 20.

5.2.8   Body Weight.   The changes in body weight of virtually all important laboratory species and humans have been collected and tabulated from the time of birth until maturity. The best reference for animals is the *Biology Data Book* (Altman and Ditmer, 1964) and ICRP's reference man (Snyder, 1975) contains the best information for humans. It is important to correct for weight changes over time when conducting a risk assessment. There are at least two factors why this improves the assessment process: first, the uptake of foods per unit body weight is much greater during the early years and second, the body burden may decrease over time if the bulk of the exposure is during the early years, for example, intentional soil ingestion by toddlers but not adults.

5.2.9   Cardiac Output.   This parameter is useful in some calculations of uptake, especially those involving airborne toxicants. The following equation has been found fairly accurate for estimating cardiac output (QC) for both animals and humans:

$$QC = (15 \, \text{L/h})(\text{BW})^{0.74}.$$

It gives values consistent with those reported in the medical literature (Snyder, 1975; Davis and Mapleson, 1981).

5.2.10   Water Consumption.   The water consumption of humans and animals seems to be very similar on a body weight basis. The following equation has been used to estimate water consumption:

$$\text{water consumption} = 0.102(\text{BW})^{0.7}.$$

Estimates of the typical water consumption of 2.0 L/day for 70-kg humans and 9.7 mL/day for 34.5-g mice are not inconsistent with this equation and these appear to be consistent with the upper values of field data for various animal species.

5.2.11   Characteristics of Skin.   The capacity of human skin to absorb liquid and solid xenobiotics has been evaluated by a number of researchers over the past 20 years. In addition, increasing numbers of in vitro tests using either animal or human skin have been developed and conducted in recent years in an attempt to provide a better estimate of the human situation. However, for obvious reasons, most tests for estimating uptake by humans have been conducted in animals. Some tests conducted on humans have been reviewed (Piotrowski, 1972; Maibach and Gellen, 1982). Various approaches used to estimate uptake based on various types of data can be found in Shu et al. (1988b) and Dugard et al. (1984).

Scientists attempting to use animal test data to estimate dermal uptake by humans must remember that these data are very likely to overestimate the actual human uptake via the skin since there is general agreement among researchers that rat skin and rabbit skin are more permeable to many chemicals than is human skin. A number of investigators have compared the dermal penetration of a variety of drugs and pesticides among rabbit, rat, pig, and human skin (Bartek et al., 1972; Bartek and La Budde, 1975; Wester and Noonan, 1980). Based on a review of studies conducted in various species, Wester and Noonan (1980) concluded: "Clearly, percutaneous absorption in the rabbit and rat would not be predictive of that in man." In short, it is important that scientists attempting to estimate dermal uptake in humans understand the known relationship between humans and animals for chemicals similar to those of interest.

5.2.12   Adipose Tissue.
Although it is possible to estimate, after the fact, the degree of exposure to a chemical through use of assumptions, this is an approach that could underestimate or overestimate the true exposure by a factor of 10-fold or more depending on the specific conditions of exposure (Hattemer-Frey and Travis, 1987; Paustenbach, 1987). A better approach to estimate the actual absorbed dose is to measure the parent chemical or metabolite in urine, blood, breath, air, faces, hair, or the adipose tissue of previously exposed persons. For the volatile or extensively metabolized chemicals, it is usually only possible to estimate the absorbed dose (exposure) within hours or a few days after exposure has ceased. For those chemicals with a longer biologic half-life, for example, greater than 30 days, it may be possible to estimate the average daily uptake from adipose tissue levels.

The following example calculation illustrates how prior exposure to stable or long-lived chemicals can be estimated post hoc based on adipose tissue levels. This approach has been used to estimate the daily uptake of numerous pesticides whose biologic half-life is in excess of several months (Williams et al., 1984; Leung et al., 1988).

Example Calculation (Estimating TCDD Exposure from Fat Levels)

Background. Since TCDD is highly lipophilic and has a long biologic half-life in humans, it is expected to accumulate in adipose tissue with repeated daily exposure. TCDD levels in the adipose tissue of nonoccupationally exposed persons in the United States is about 7 ppt (MMR, 1987; Sielken, 1987b). Using a basic pharmacokinetic approach (Gehring, 1984), one can estimate the daily uptake needed to reach the steady-state adipose tissue level in the general population. Estimation of the amounts of TCDD absorbed is based on the following assumptions:

- TCDD concentration in human adipose tissue is 7 ppt (Sielken, 1987b).
- The TCDD concentration in the liver is 0.7 ppt (Poiger and Schlatter, 1980).
- TCDD concentration in other tissues is estimated to be 0.84 ppt based on their fat content.
- The average human weighs 70 kg and has 15% body fat and a 1.75-kg liver (Snyder, 1975).
- The assumed half-life for excretion in humans is 7 years (2600 days) (Leung et al., 1988).

The total body burden for the general population may be estimated as follows:

$$(10.5 \text{ kg fat})(7 \text{ ng/kg}) = \quad 73.50$$
$$(1.75 \text{ kg liver})(0.7 \text{ ng/kg}) = \quad 1.23$$
$$(57.75 \text{ kg other tissue})(0.84 \text{ ng/kg}) = \underline{\quad 48.51}$$
$$\text{Total body burden} = 123.24 \text{ ng}$$

It is reasonable to assume that this total body burden represents a steady-state (SS) level acquired from repetitive exposure to background levels. Assuming exposure occurs daily, the total dose absorbed daily (D_t) can be calculated from the equation (Gehring, 1984)

$$D_t = SS/(1.44)(t_{1/2}),$$

where for 7 ppt, $SS = 410$ ng. For a 7-year half-life, the daily uptake would need to be 0.048 ng/day or 0.68 pg/kg·day to reach 7 ppt.

Similarly, the steady-state level of TCDD in adipose tissue resulting from ingestion of foods that results in a daily dose of 1 pg/kg·day (the estimated uptake in the diet of western man) can be estimated:

$$D_t = SS/1.44(1800 \text{ days})$$

$$\text{daily dose} = (70 \text{ kg}) (1.0 \text{ pg/kg·day}) = 70.0 \text{ pg/day}$$

then,

$$0.07 \text{ ng/day} = SS/(1.44)1800$$

$$\text{steady-state body burden} = SS = 181.4 \text{ ng}.$$

From the steady-state body burden, the concentration in adipose can be calculated:

$$(10.5 \text{ kg fat})(X) + (1.75 \text{ kg liver})(X)(0.7/7) + (57.75 \text{ kg})(X)(0.84/7) = 181 \text{ ng},$$

$$X = 181/17.6 = 10.3 \text{ ppt},$$

where X = steady-state TCDD concentration in adipose tissue.

5.2.13   Mother's Milk.

In the 1970s and 1980s, it was recognized that chemicals with a long biologic half-life, for example, those that are lipophilic, were not only stored in the adipose tissue of humans but were also released in the lipids of moher's milk during breast-feeding. Each of the more than 20 chemicals currently found in human adipose tissue will, to some degree, be present in mother's milk. The potential health effects of these chemicals on the newborn has been questioned since 1985 but the available data indicate that for the majority of persons, the benefits of breast-feeding significantly outweigh the potential or theoretical increased risk of cancer due to the presence of chemical carcinogens (Smith, 1987).

For sake of risk assessment calculations, it is probably acceptable to assume that babies ingest about 100 mL/day of milk fat per kg of body weight during the first 3–6 months of life. It is important to note that the fat content of mother's milk during the early stages is 4.2 g/kg·day and only 2.0 g/kg·day during the later stages (Smith, 1987). Other figures have been suggested (Snyder, 1975) and these should be considered by scientists responsible for such assessments (Table 21).

TABLE 21. **Typical Milk Consumption According to Age (mL/d)**

Age (y)	Male	Female
0.25	750	600
0.50	1000	800
0.75	850	650
1	580	500
2	500	440
3	490	440
4	490	430
5	490	430

Source: Report of the task group on reference man.

6 DOSE–RESPONSE ASSESSMENT (EXTRAPOLATION MODELS)

Perhaps the most misunderstood area in risk assessment is the unfounded belief that the results of low-dose extrapolation models are synonymous with quantitative risk assessment. As shown in Fig. 7, the results of these models should be but one part of the assessment process. Regrettably, the fact that regulatory agencies have placed such emphasis on the point estimates from the most popular model has helped fuel the misunderstanding about their role in the whole process (Park and Snee, 1983).

The dose–response evaluation, at least when assessing the cancer risk, defines the relation between the dose of an agent and the probability of induction of a carcinogenic effect in the animal species tested. This component usually entails an extrapolation from the generally high doses administered to experimental animals or exposures noted in epidemiologic studies to the exposure levels expected from human contact with the agent in the environment. This portion of the assessment should also include a discussion of the likely validity of these extrapolations. The ultimate purpose of the dose–response evaluation is to identify the dose of a substance which is not likely to have an adverse impact on the exposed species, generally humans. Two approaches are available for estimating that acceptable level of exposure: safety factors or uncertainty factors and mathematical modeling.

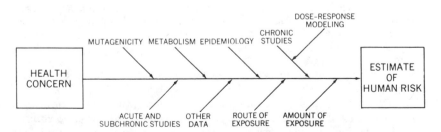

Figure 7. Data that go into the risk assessment process. As shown, the dose–response models are only one part of the analysis. Many of the other factors have not been given serious consideration when estimating the human risk. From Park and Snee (1983).

6.1   Safety Factors and Thresholds

For much of the past 40 years, the safety factor approach has been used to identify the dose (based usually on animal data) at which humans would not be expected to be adversely affected (Barnes and Denz, 1954; Dourson and Stara, 1983; Paustenbach and Langer, 1986). Until recently, the approach was also used for carcinogens, developmental toxins, and all systemic toxicants. Although much less complex than the mathematical models that were later developed for estimating the risk of exposure to carcinogenic agents, limits based on safety factors have generally been effective at preventing disease among exposed persons (Stokinger, 1970; Dourson and Stara, 1983; Flamm and Winbush, 1984; Friess, 1987).

Traditional toxicological procedures define a safe level of exposure for humans as some arbitrary fraction of that dose level at which no effects were observed, that is, the no observed effect level (NOEL), in a group of test animals. For food additives and pesticides where toxic effects other than cancer are a concern, an acceptable daily intake has often been established through the application of a 100-fold safety factor to the chronic NOEL. The purpose of the uncertainty factor is to account for the possibility that humans may be up to 10 times more sensitive than the animals species tested and that a 10-fold variation in sensitivity within the human population may exist (Lehman and Fitzhugh, 1954). The magnitude of the safety factor may be modified depending on the chemical and kinetic properties of the test compounds and the effect induced, as well as on the quality of the available toxicological data.

The use of safety factors to derive acceptable human exposure levels rests at least tacitly on the assumption of the existence of a threshold dose below which no adverse effects will occur (Munro and Krewski, 1981; Krewski et al., 1984). However, because the threshold concept may not be universally applicable to carcinogens, the regulation of carcinogens in our food, air, and water has come to be influenced by mathematical modeling to estimate acceptable doses. The uncertainty as to the low-dose effects of carcinogenic agents has resulted in the proposed use of safety factors as high as 5000-fold (Weil, 1972; Truhaut, 1979).

As discussed by Munro and Krewski (1981),

> in mathematical terms, the absence of a threshold precludes the possibility that a sufficiently low level of exposure will be free of any attendant degree of hazard. Biological arguments in favor of the no-threshold concept for carcinogenesis are generally based on the fact that irreversible self-replicating lesions may result from a mutation in a single somatic cell, often following the administration of only a single dose. Arguments against this position draw on the existence of metabolic detoxification: DNA repair, immunological surveillance and other mechanisms that may operate to nullify effects at low doses. Even admitting their existence, thresholds are likely to vary among individuals. The determination of a population threshold thus presents the difficult statistical program of determining the minimum of the individual thresholds, a minimum which may well be effectively zero in some cases (Brown, 1976).

The safety factor approach has been criticized on the grounds that the observed no-effect level will depend on the sample size, with response rates of 0/10 and 0/1000 obviously having different toxicological and statistical significance (Munro and Krewski, 1981; Crump, 1984). In addition, there is always the possibility of observing no effects even though the test compound may affect an appreciable proportion of very large populations. For example, with 50 animals per test group there is a better than even chance of observing no effects with a compound for which the population risk is actually as high as 1% (Cornfield et al., 1978). For this reason some scientists have suggested using the probit

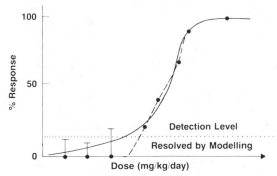

Figure 8. The rationale for using low-dose extrapolation models is that it is not possible to conduct animal studies at doses as low as those typically encountered in the environment. Using statistical principles, it is possible to estimate the likely range of results for those data collected at low doses and from this estimate the response at much lower doses. This figure illustrates how the models can describe the data in the high-dose region but at low doses the presumption of linearity and the need to account for the uncertainty introduced by studying only 100 animals per dose forces the models to predict risks that almost certainly are greater than those that exist.

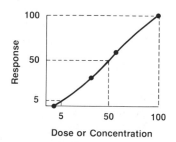

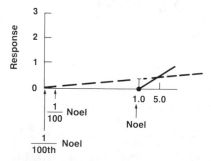

Figure 9. Illustration of the region in which mathematical models are used to estimate the likely carcinogenic response at doses 1/100th and 1/1000th the no observed effect level (NOEL).

model plus a safety factor (Gaylor and Kodell, 1980). For carcinogens which act through a nongenotoxic mechanism, that is, repeated cytotoxicity and promoters this approach may be reasonable (Andersen, 1988). One shortcoming of the uncertainty factor approach is that it does not account for the slope of the dose–response curve. For example, a moderate safety factor may provide an adequate margin of safety if the dose–response relation is relatively steep but may not be sufficiently conservative if the dose–response curve is relatively shallow.

6.2   Mathematical Models and Virtual Safe Doses

It is important to recognize that since direct estimates of risk at low levels of exposure would require the testing of prohibitively large numbers of animals, models must be used to help account for this shortcoming. The purpose of so-called cancer models is to estimate a virtually safe dose (VSD) more recently termed "a risk specific dose," based on the extrapolation of experimental results well outside the dose range used in animal tests; usually 3–4 orders of magnitude below the NOEL. Statistical procedures for estimating the low-dose response involve a mathematical model relating the probability of a specific response at very low doses. In these approaches, the uncertainty that the NOEL would be observed if, for example, 1000 animals were tested, is estimated using bounding procedures. As shown in Fig. 8, the upper bound of the NOEL is used to identify the slope of linear extrapolation.

Because of the statistical and biological problems inherent in the identification of a true no-effect level, most mathematical models for carcinogens have eliminated the concept of threshold or dose where no response would be expected (Fig. 9). Cornfield (1977) and Schaffer (1977) have discussed kinetic models that lead to the existence of thresholds under steady-state conditions, but these have not been used in important regulatory decisions. As noted by Brown and co-workers (1978), the basis for assuming no threshold is that one cannot dismiss the possibility of a response being induced, for example, if a reactive metabolite were produced during the approach to steady state, some degree of risk would be present no matter how small the dose. In the 1970s and 1980s, it was widely held that absolute safety could not be guaranteed unless a threshold could be demonstrated on theoretical grounds. In response, a virtually safe level of exposure associated with some very low level of risk, a VSD could be estimated, began to be discussed and accepted. In the 1980s, the term VSD began to be displaced by the term de minimis level of risk.

A number of cancer models have been discussed in the literature (Krewski and Brown, 1981). Statistical models are based on the notion that each individual in the population has his or her own tolerance to the test compound. Any level of exposure below this tolerance will have no effect on the individual, while any level of exposure exceeding the tolerance will result in a positive response. These tolerances are presumed to vary among individuals in the population with the lack of a population threshold reflected in the fact that the minimum tolerance is allowed to be zero. Specification of a functional form of the distribution of tolerances determines the shape of the dose–response curve and thus defines a particular statistical model.

Munro and Krewski (1981) have summarized the characteristics of some of the low-dose extrapolation models:

Stochastic models are based on the premise that a positive response is the result of the random occurrence of one or more biological events. The one-hit model (Hoel et al., 1975) is based on the concept that a response will occur after the target site has been hit by a single biologically effective unit of dose. The multi-hit model (Rai & Van Ryzin, 1981) is a direct extension of one-hit model, assuming that more than one hit is required in order to induce a response. [This model may also be viewed as a tolerance distribution model, where the tolerance distribution is gamma. This formulation allows the "hit" parameter k to assume non-integral values.] The multi-state model, on the other hand, is based on the assumption that the induction of irreversible self-replicating toxic effects such as carcinogenesis is the result of the occurrence of a number of different random biological events, the time rate of occurrence of each event being in strict linear proportion to the dose rate (Crump, 1979; Crump, Hoel, Langley & Peto, 1976). Despite their biological rationale, these stochastic models must also be considered somewhat arbitrary until the mechanisms of carcinogenesis are more fully understood.

The shape of the dose–response curves for the above models in the low-dose region will have considerable impact on estimates of risk associated with low levels of exposure. For example, the one-hit model is linear at low doses and will thus generally provide relatively high estimates of risk at low dose levels. The logit, Weibull and multi-hit models are linear at low doses only when the shape parameters β, m and k in these models are equal to unity. When these parameters are greater than unity, the dose–response curves for these models approach zero at a slower than linear, or sublinear rate. The multi-stage model is linear at low doses only when the linear coefficient in the model (β_1) is positive and is sublinear otherwise. The probit model is inherently sublinear at low doses and generally leads to relatively low estimates of risk at low dose levels. [Mathematically, the probit model is extremely flat in the low-dose region, with the dose–response curve approaching zero more rapidly than any power of dose.]

As noted by Munro and Krewski (1981), the dose–response curve for the logit, Weibull, and multihit models can approach zero at a faster than linear, or supralinear, rate although the biological plausibility of this behavior seems questionable.

Crump and Masterman (1979) have pointed out that low-dose linearity in the logit, Weibull, and multihit models is compatible only with dose–response curves that are linear at low and moderate doses and exhibit downward curvature at high doses. Thus, those frequently encountered data sets exhibiting a strong degree of upward curvature at moderate- or high-dose levels would preclude the existence of low-dose linearity according to these models. The multistage model, however, does provide for data that are linear at low doses and exhibit upward curvature at higher doses. This characteristic, along with others, has been the reason that the multistage model developed by Crump has been the one most widely used by U.S. regulatory agencies during the period from 1977 to the present (EPA, 1986a).

Some persons have suggested that a less conservative approach than that implicit in the multistage model should be considered. One simple extrapolation procedure (Gaylor and Kodell, 1980; Van Ryzin, 1980) that can provide for the possibility of low-dose linearity involves fitting a suitable model to the experimental data and then extrapolating linearly from some point on the fitted curve where the excess risk is still within the observable range. This procedure not only accommodates low-dose linearity but provides a conservative upper limit on risk at low levels of exposure whenever the true dose–response curve is sublinear in the low-dose region (Park and Snee, 1983). An alternative linear extrapolation procedure that exploits the linearity property of the upper confidence limits on risk based on the multistage model has been discussed by Crump (1981).

6.2.1 Shortcomings of Low-Dose Models.
As discussed by Munro and Krewski (1981), because most of the low-dose extrapolation models fit the data more or less equally well in the observable range, it is not possible to select an appropriate model or range of risks using statistical goodness-of-fit criteria alone (Food Safety Council, 1980; Sielken, 1987a, 1988). Theoretical results by Crump (1981) have shown that statistical discrimin-

ation between two plausible models is difficult even with an experiment designed specifically for this purpose. Even more important than the mathematical shortcomings is the inability of the models to account for the all-important biological factors that modify response to chemical exposure at low levels. Among these are the role of the immune system to recognize and destroy aberrant cells, repair of DNA, pharmacokinetics, and enzyme induction and inhibition (Bus and Gibson, 1985).

Another criticism of placing an emphasis on the results of models is that equally reasonable models can yield markedly different results in the region of concern (Fig. 10 and 11). Here it is shown that five different classes of dose–response models can yield results of five to eight orders of magnitude. Sometimes, the model selection is not as much a problem as the decision as to "what endpoint to model." As shown in Fig. 10, depending on whether total tumors or hepatocellular tumors are evaluated, the various models can yield markedly different results. Here again, it is difficult to distinguish policy from science in such decisions. The procedure used to bound the risk has also been questioned as unnecessarily conservative and this is illustrated in Fig. 12 (Young, 1987). This figure illustrates that the application of a bounding procedure encompasses a wide range of possible outcomes.

An evaluation of the human carcinogenic risk associated with low-level exposure to a xenobiotic is a complex process that requires analysis of a variety of data. This evaluation

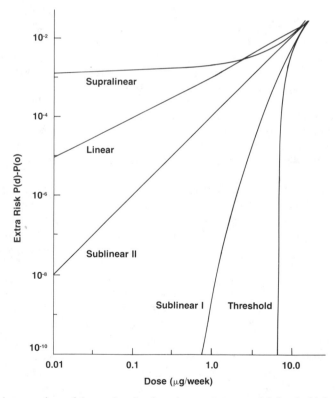

Figure 10. A comparison of the results of various dose–response models for the high- and low-dose regions. From NAS (1983).

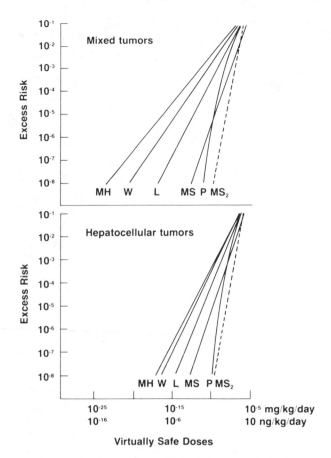

Figure 11. A comparison of the risk estimates obtained for a chemical using the most common dose–response models where both mixed tumors and hepatocellular tumors are considered separately. When total tumors are considered the best surrogate for predicting the human risk, the virtually safe dose (VSD) is much lower than when only liver tumors are considered. The plot also demonstrates the differences in the best estimates of predicted risks for the most frequently used models. For example, the multihit model (MH) is more conservative than the Weibull (W), which is more conservative than the logit (L), multistage (MS), probit (P), and multistage with two stages (MS-2) (From Munro and Krewski, 1981).

should include data from studies of acute, subchronic, and chronic effects on animals, metabolism in several species, mutagenicity, route of exposure, mechanism of action, epidemiology, and pharmacokinetics. The major failing of the widespread use of low-dose extrapolation models is that they often reduce a decision process that requires thoughtful and critical analysis of complex and often conflicting data to one driven by a computer analysis of four or more data points on a dose–response curve. Although every regulatory agency that deals with carcinogens [NAS, 1983; Office of Science and Technology Policy (OSTP), 1985; EPA, 1986a] advocates the necessity for careful evaluation of all available data, most regulatory decisions have been overly responsive to the results of these models at the expense of the biologic information. The very existence of the weight-of-evidence

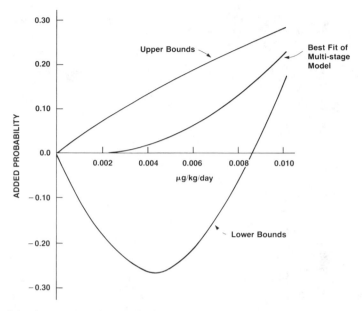

Figure 12. It has been suggested that both the upper and lower bounds on the added probability of developing a tumor be presented with each risk assessment. This plot illustrates the marked difference between the upper and lower bounds and the best fit of the multistage model for carcinomas observed in the female rat in the study by Kociba and co-workers using 2,3,7,8-TCDD. From Sielken (1987a).

approach, which incorporates an assessment of the uncertainty in the animal data, acknowledges the importance of dealing rationally with all data (OSTP, 1985; EPA, 1986a). The one problem in relying heavily on modeling rodent bioassay data is that it gives decision makers the mistaken impression that not only is the analysis routine but that a degree of certainty is awarded the analysis which in fact does not exist.

The Food Safety Council (1980) summarized its views regarding the best use of low-dose extrapolation models in risk management decisions as follows:

> Human risk assessment is a very inexact exercise, based largely upon theoretical assumptions concerning interspecies extrapolations. The uncertainties involved should be fully recognized by the scientific community and society. The methods used by all the mathematical models attempt to predict how many test animals will respond at low exposure levels, based upon observed responses at high dose levels. The models tell us little about predicted human responses at any exposure level. This requires judgmental decisions based upon broad biological assumption, or comparative metabolic data, when they are available. Quantitative risk assessment can, at best, provide a range for the incidence of potential toxic effects in humans.

The Office of Science and Technology Policy (OSTP, 1985) recently developed guidelines for using low-dose models which are very useful for assessing the risk of environmental exposure to chemical carcinogens:

> No single mathematical procedure is recognized as the most appropriate for low-dose extrapolation in carcinogenesis. When relevant biological evidence on mechanism of action exists (e.g., pharmacokinetics, target organ dose), the models or procedures employed should be

consistent with the evidence. When data and information are limited, however, and when much uncertainty exists regarding the mechanism of carcinogenic action, models or procedures which incorporate low-dose linearity are preferred when compatible with the limited information.

At present, mechanisms of the carcinogenesis process are largely unknown and data are generally limited. If a carcinogenic agent acts by accelerating the same carcinogenic process that leads to the background occurrence of cancer, the added effect of the carcinogen at low doses is expected to be virtually linear (Crump et al., 1976).

The Agency will review each assessment as to the evidence on carcinogenesis mechanisms and other biological or statistical evidence that indicates the suitability of a particular extrapolation model. Goodness-of-fit to the experimental observations is not an effective means of discriminating among models (OSTP, 1985). A rationale will be included to justify the use of the chosen model. In the absence of adequate information to the contrary, the linearized multistage procedure will be employed. Where appropriate, the results of using various extrapolation models may be useful for comparison with the linearized multistage procedure. When longitudinal data on tumor development are available, time-to-tumor models may be used.

It should be emphasized that the linearized multistage procedure leads to a plausible upper limit to the risk that is consistent with some proposed mechanisms of carcinogenesis. Such an estimate, however, does not necessarily give a realistic prediction of the risk. The true value of the risk is unknown, and may be as low as zero. The range of risks, defined by the upper limit given by the chosen model and the lower limit which may be as low as zero, should be explicitly stated. An established procedure does not yet exist for making "most likely" or "best" estimates of risk within the range of uncertainty defined by the upper and lower limit estimates. If data and procedures become available, the Agency will also provide "most likely" or "best" estimates of risk. This will be most feasible when human data are available and when exposures are in the dose range of the data.

In certain cases, the linearized multistage procedure cannot be used with the observed data, for example, when the data are nonmonotonic or flatten out at high doses. In these cases, it may be necessary to make adjustments to achieve low-dose linearity.

Dr. Robert Sielken, an authority in cancer risk assessment, has posed a series of questions that can serve as criteria for the validity of the low-dose extrapolation. This list is useful in that satisfaction of some or most of these criteria can give increased confidence in the risk estimates from cancer models (Sielken, 1985).

All quantitative models for cancer risk are *not* equal. Nor are they all equally relevant or equally reflective of the available scientific information. There are several questions which the government regulator, industrial executive, or a staff member should ask in order to better ascertain the value of a particular quantitative cancer risk assessment. Several of these questions are stated here. A *negative* answer to almost any one of these questions can seriously diminish the relevance and value of the risk assessment [emphasis supplied].

1. Were all the events which are called a "carcinogenic response" of equal severity or consequence?
2. Does the quantitative model reflect the time the carcinogenic response occurs?
3. If a time-to-response model has been used, is the stated probability of a carcinogenic response inflated by ignoring competing routes?
4. Does the family of curves represented by the dose response model contain enough curves of differing shapes to reflect the observed curvature in the experimental data?
5. Has the dose level been expressed on a biologically relevant scale?
6. Are the experimental data at the high doses relevant to the low dose behavior?

7. Are the animals used for experimentation and the carcinogenic responses observed in these animals relevant to humans?

8. Are the experimental data consistent across the animals which are considered relevant to humans?

9. If animal to human extrapolation is to be used for cancer risk assessment, then have the relevant biological differences in the species been identified and incorporated into the risk assessment?

10. Have any differences between the route of the experimental exposure and the route of human exposure been accounted for?

11. Are the exposure durations and patterns (once in a lifetime, intermittent, continuous, etc.) the same in the experimental data as they are in the human population at risk?

12. Are the inferences made from short-term tests consistent with the inferences made from long-term studies?

13. Are the inferences drawn from animal-based models consistent with those from human epidemiological data?

14. Have the human exposures been carefully identified with respect to routes, durations, dose levels, and patterns (continuous, intermittent, etc.)?

15. Has the statistical variability in the quantitative risk assessment, caused by the variability in the experiment, been characterized?

16. Have the assumptions, policy decisions, and value judgments incorporated into the quantitative risk assessment been clearly stated and the impact on the quantitative risk assessment been evaluated and recorded?

17. Are the risks characterized in understandable and appropriate terms?

18. Are the stated risks actually estimates of the risks as opposed to upper bounds or lower bounds of the risks?

19. If the uncertainty of the risk estimate is described in terms of bounds on the risk, then have both upper and lower bounds been recorded as well as their method of determination, including the assumptions made in that determination and their impact?

20. Have the quantitative risk assessments been based on outdated guidelines or procedures?

Because of the uncertainties involved in estimating the risks of low levels of exposure, some regulatory authorities have advocated the use of conservative risk assessment procedures (Interagency Regulatory Liaison Group, 1979; EPA, 1986a,b). While linear extrapolation may be appropriate for potent electrophilic carcinogens, the use of such conservative procedures for less potent substances, which may induce tumors through perturbation of normal physiology, may not be warranted (Weisberger and Williams, 1981; 1986). The most suitable model for estimating the low dose response for promotors and other chemicals that do no act through genotoxic mechanisms is not clear. In general, estimates of risk based on the probit model will be liberal because of extreme steepness in the low-dose region (Hartley and Sielken, 1977). This may also be true to a lesser degree with the multihit and logit models (Haseman et al., 1981), both of which are generally in close agreement. The biologically-based models appear to be most relevant.

There has been a good deal of debate about the alleged shortcomings of allowing agencies to rely heavily on the results of any cancer model and, in particular, the multistage model. The following comments submitted to EPA by the American Industrial Health Council (AIHC) summarize many of the criticisms to date (AIHC, 1983).

Three agencies (EPA, OSHA and CSC) are using a computer program for the multistage model usually referred to as Global 79 or, in slightly modified form, as Global 82 developed by Dr. Kenneth Crump. The mathematics in the model have been disclosed, but AIHC believes that assumptions and characteristics of the model should be set forth so the values generated can be fully evaluated in the multidisciplinary risk characterization step.

Three characteristics of the computer programs of the multistage model are worth noting:

(i) the program has a procedure for calculating a linearized 95% upper confidence limit on added risk, but does not apply that procedure to calculate the 95% lower limit on added risk.

(ii) the model does not calculate confidence limits in a statistical fashion, independent of the linearized constraint.

(iii) the calculation of the most likely value is constrained by rejection of negative parameter values so that all points on the projected dose response curve are positive.

Generation of lower confidence limits on added risk and an unconstrained most probable value would provide data that assist in judging the biological relevance of the model and the values it generates. This additional information will assist in the exercise of scientific judgment in interpreting the results.

Confidence limits are usually calculated to reflect the uncertainty due to the limited number of animals in the experiment and ability of the model to fit the curvature of the data. It should be noted that the linearized upper confidence limit procedure in Global 79 and 82 determines upper confidence limits in a different manner. Global 79 and 82 impose an additional constraint of low dose linearity.

There are sound scientific reasons for displaying all six values if the current linearized multistage model is used:

Constrained maximum likelihood

Unrestricted maximum likelihood

95% upper confidence limit and 95% lower confidence limit, with and without the linear constraint.

Normally upper and lower confidence limits are essentially error bands and serve the same purpose as standard error band calculations in statistical analyses. Thus both maximum likelihood values and 95% confidence limit should be reported separately with and without the constraints. However, when an additional linear constraint is imposed and confidence limits reflect deviation from the usual calculation of confidence limits.

Just as there would be severe criticism if experimental data were selectively reported for whatever reason good or bad, AIHC believes that the results of statistical modeling should not be selectively reported.

Scientific evaluation is based on a consideration of all the data, weighing relevance, validity and quality of the data. That evaluation assumes all data are available and unbiased evaluation of those data, not pre-selected data and pre-selected evaluation procedures.

As in most legitimate debates, the arguments raised in support of using the results of the low-dose extrapolation models for regulatory purposes cannot be rebutted out-of-hand. The position of the California Department of Health Services (1986) represents a good survey of the rationale for accepting the results of the multi-stage or other similar models:

It is apparent [from this discussion] that the choice of mathematical models to represent dose–response relationships involves a substantial element of scientific judgement. Although several models are available, all are subject to criticism. Empirically, several different models can be fitted to most data sets, and it is unlikely that further experimentation, even with large groups of animals, will decisively discriminate between possible models. On theoretical grounds, each model has certain desirable features and limitations. The multistage model has good flexibility to fit a wide range of empirical data and has a reasonable biological basis. However, it, too, may not be optimal in all circumstances.

Within this background of scientific uncertainty, the following conclusions appear to be reasonable guidelines for dose–response assessment in the light of the foregoing survey of scientific knowledge:

- It is not appropriate to apply the concept of "thresholds" to carcinogenesis unless dose–response data are available that are inconsistent with a nonthreshold model.

- The effect of a carcinogen can generally be assumed to be additive to that of ongoing processes or other agents that give rise to "background" incidence of cancer. Exceptions to this general assumption are appropriate when the carcinogen under discussion can be shown to operate by a mechanism that is distinct from those leading to background incidence or to act synergistically with other carcinogenic exposures.

- The current knowledge of the mechanisms of carcinogenic action provides little guidance as to the appropriate choice of dose–response models. Although the assumption of low-dose linearity is most generally accepted for carcinogens that interact directly with DNA (first-stage carcinogens, or "initiators"), dose additivity (with the assumptions discussed previously) will lead to low-dose linearity for carcinogens that act at any stage.

Until the biologically–based disposition and biologically–based cancer models achieve widespread acceptance in the scientific and regulatory communities, it is unlikely that the aforementioned regulatory position will change markedly.

7   RISK CHARACTERIZATION

Although we have come a long way in understanding how we might do a better job in the hazard identification, dose–response assessment, and exposure assessment portions of risk assessment, we have only scratched the surface in our understanding of how to best characterize the risks and how to present them most appropriately to decisionmakers. If there is any doubt about this claim, one need only read newspaper accounts of the scientific positions of regulatory agencies attempting to characterize the severity of a hazard:

> Excess deaths from lung cancer due to workplace arsenic are down 98%, says the Occupational Safety and Health Administration, based on risk assessment studies. The arsenic standard of OSHA requires engineering controls and other measures to reduce worker exposure from 500 to $10 \mu g/m^3$. Three risk assessments performed under federal court order on the standard's efficacy indicate that excess deaths (relative to the general population) dropped 8–10 per 1000 workers from the 375 to 465 per 1000 that would have occurred under the previous $500 \mu g/m^3$ standard (Chemical Engineering, 1983).

Among the numerous shortcomings of this news clipping is that the reader is likely to infer that under the "old" OSHA standard, as many as 46.5% of the worker population was likely to die prematurely due exclusively to occupational exposure to arsenic. In actuality, there was a good deal of discussion within the scientific community whether any increased cancer risk had been observed in epidemiology studies of workers who had been exposed to levels in the vicinity of $500 \mu g/m^3$. In addition, in an attempt to demonstrate the potential benefits of regulation, much more certainty was attached to the possible results of the regulation than was present in the low-dose extrapolation process. Since the hallmark of a good risk characterization is a thorough description of the range of plausible outcomes, this report would have been more fair had it stated that the old regulation may have posed a risk as great as about 400 in 1,000 and as low as 1 in 1,000,000. As shown here and in most press releases of the past decade, the degree of uncertainty is rarely developed within the risk assessment nor is the significance of the risk communicated in a thorough, easily understood, and objective manner.

7.1 Fundamentals

The risk characterization step is a discussion which sums up all the information that has been gathered and presents it in a useful and understandable manner. To do this, the risk characterization should contain not only a risk estimate for a given exposure scenario but also a summary of the relevant biological information, the assumptions used and their limitations, and a discussion of uncertainties in the risk assessment, both qualitative and quantitative (Preuss and Ehrlich, 1987).

When characterizing the risks associated with exposure to a carcinogen, developmental or reproductive toxicant, a mutagen, or a mixture of different chemicals, emphasis needs to be placed on the dose–response relationship. Since issuance of the OSTP and EPA risk assessment guidelines of 1984 and 1986, much importance has been placed on adding a discussion to the risk characterization, which addresses the weight of evidence for selecting certain parameters or assumptions in the assessment. The weight-of-evidence thought process has grown out of a concern that often only one piece of "negative data" seemed to dominate a risk assessment, even when a more scientifically solid "positive data" set was available. In all likelihood, assessments conducted in the coming years will place a much greater emphasis on comparing the quality of both negative and positive data before allowing spurious data from either category to dominate a regulatory action. A number of good papers which illustrate the importance of the weight-of-evidence approach have been published since 1985 (Rodricks and Turnbull, 1985; Paustenbach et al., 1986; Shu et al., 1987; Paynter et al., 1988).

Another key component of the risk characterization is a complete discussion and analysis of the uncertainties. The portions of the assessment which benefit most from an uncertainties and sensitivity analysis are the dose–response and exposure segments. A good deal of work has been conducted in the area of the low-dose extrapolation models and it has been shown how simulations can illustrate some of the shortcomings in placing too much emphasis on point estimates of risk.

Recently, specific mathematical techniques have been developed for assessing both uncertainty and parameter sensitivity when attempting to estimate dose, especially for multipathway exposures; that is, inhalation and dermal uptake of vapors and particles, ingestion of contaminants via the food chain and incidental soil ingestion, and so on. Specifically, probability distributions are estimated to describe the uncertainty around each of the components in the exposure calculations. From this, the probability distribution of the results of the exposure assessment can be estimated (Bogan and Spears, 1987). Such approaches offer the hope that rather than having to state that "it is plausible that someone might absorb as much as 100 fg/kg·day of a given chemical which is released by automobiles and can be taken up both by direct contact and the food chain," we might be able to say that "the data indicate that perhaps 0.5% of the population might absorb as much as 100 fg/kg·day, 76% might absorb 5 fg/kg·day, and 23.5% is likely to absorb less than 1 fg/kg·day."

8   RISK MANAGEMENT

While the scientific community has placed much attention on the best methods for developing a comprehensive and objective risk assessment, these assessments will not serve the intended purpose if a poor decision is ultimately reached by the risk manager. During the 1980s, our attention focused on the technical intricacies of hazard identification, low-dose extrapolation, and risk characterization. However, as was dramatically illustrated by California Proposition 65 (Abelson, 1987), the public must be assured that high-quality and responsive management decisions are being reached or they may choose to take matters into their own hands.

The goal of risk management is to select the option that balances the benefits of an action against the real or perceived risks. Such choices are the central role of a regulatory agency. Consequently, the National Academy of Science work group on risk assessment insisted that the risk assessment and risk management functions be clearly separated. Up until the time of their report (NAS, 1983), many assessments interwove such risk management issues as cost, feasibility, and reasonableness into the scientific justification of acceptable levels of exposure—two different issues that must be kept separate in the risk assessment. As shown in Fig. 12, risk managers need to weigh the cost of an action such as setting a clean-up level, with the change in risk. The relationship between cost and risk reduction shown here is typical; risk reduction is not linearly related to cost.

Risk managers have a number of choices available to them when presented with the need to make a decision regarding human or environmental exposure to an agent. This process may be systematized to the extent that the following factors are balanced against the perceived risk (Munro and Krewski, 1981):

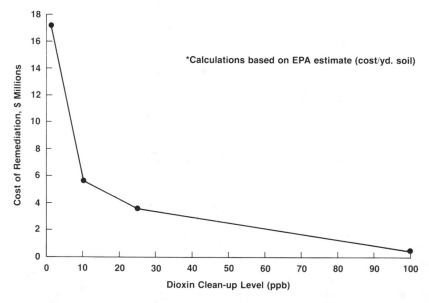

Figure 13. Estimated cost of soil removal and destruction (clean-up) for various target soil clean-up levels at the Castlewood site in Missouri. The plot is based on EPA estimates of the number of yards of soil contaminated at various concentration of dioxin and their estimated cost for incinerating. From: Paustenbach et al. (1986). Copyright 1986, Academic Press.

- Consumer expectations.
- Education to permit informed choice by consumers.
- Cost to industry and ultimately to consumers.
- Ability to control exposure—consumption monitoring programs.
- Impact on trade.
- Availability of less hazardous substitutes.
- Ability to enforce regulations.
- Impact on future regulatory policy.

Numerous options are available to the risk manager but the basic ones are banning, limiting use, and no restrictions.

Recognition of the many uncertainties in the exposure analysis and low-dose extrapolation has encouraged some skeptics to subscribe to the view that risk assessment is a dubious enterprise and too uncertain to be relied on for risk management decisions. Although low-level risks are inherently uncertain regardless of the approach used to evaluate them, current approaches to assessing health risks are much better than the guesses of prior years. At the very least, a most valuable use of risk assessment is to identify those activities that are worthy of further study or regulation due to their importance versus those activities that pose a trivial hazard. Using this approach, scientists and administrators can direct their efforts to the areas where regulations will give the best payback.

As noted above, an important aspect of risk management is to be sure that the significant risks are receiving proper attention and that decisionmakers are not getting bogged down in the trivial ones. The term de minimus became a common one within risk management circles during the 1980's. De minimis risks are those judged to be too small to be of social concern, or too small to justify the use of risk management resources for control. Properly applied, a de minimis risk concept can help set priorities for bringing regulatory attention to risk in a socially beneficial way. Although the de minimis approach ignores risks below some low limit, it too is in the long-standing tradition of risk management methods that are intended to err on the side of safety in matters of uncertainty (Whipple, 1986).

8.1   Risk Criteria

Beginning in the late 1970s and early 1980s, regulatory agencies frequently adopted a risk criteria of 1 in 1,000,000 as one that represented a de minimis risk when fairly large populations could be exposed to a suspect carcinogen. The so-called risk estimates, which were based on the results of dose–response models applied to bioassay data, as discussed by the current commissioner of the USFDA, need to be put into perspective if they are to be properly used by risk managers. Specifically, the commissioner made the following observations (Young, 1987):

> In applying the de minimis concept and in setting other safety standards, FDA has been guided by the figure of "one in a million." Other Federal agencies have also used a one in a million level such as the Occupational Safety and Health Administration and the Environmental Protection Agency. Both agencies rely on the one in one million increased risk over a lifetime as a reasonable criterion for separating high-risk problems warranting agency attention from negligible risk problems that do not.

The risk level of one in one million is often misunderstood by the public and the media. It is not an actual risk—i.e., we do not expect one out of every million people to get cancer if they drink decaffeinated coffee. Rather, it is a mathematical risk based on scientific assumptions used in risk assessment.

FDA uses a conservative estimate to risk to ensure that the risk is not understated. We interpret animal test results conservatively and we are extremely careful when we extrapolate risks to humans. When FDA uses the risk level of one in one million, it is confident that the risk to humans is virtually nonexistent.

The widely held fallacy that all occupational and environmental regulations have as their goal a theoretical increased risk of cancer of 1 in 1,000,000 was recently addressed by Travis et al. (1987). They conducted a retrospective examination of the level of risk which triggered regulatory action in 132 decisions. Three variables were considered: (1) individual risk (an upper-limit estimate of the probability that the most highly exposed individual in a population will develop cancer as a result of a lifetime exposure), (2) population risk (an upper-limit estimate of the number of additional incidences of cancer in the exposed population), and (3) population size. The findings of Travis et al. (1987) can be summarized as follows:

1. Every chemical with an individual lifetime risk above 4×10^{-3} received regulation. Those with values below 1×10^{-6} remained unregulated.
2. For small populations, regulatory action never resulted for individual risks below 1×10^{-4}.
3. For effects resulting from exposures to the entire U.S. population, a risk level below 1×10^{-6} never triggered action; above 3×10^{-4} it always triggered action.

In short, regulatory agencies have found risk in excess of 1 in 1,000,000 acceptable if experienced by small populations. Travis et al. (1987) made the following observation:

> Perhaps the most surprising aspect of our study is the consistency found among federal agencies' methods in the use of cancer risk estimates for regulatory decisions. With the possible exception of USFDA decisions concerning de minimis risks, the history of federal decision making indicates that all agencies are fairly consistent in their implicit definitions of de miminis and de minimis levels of risk. If the above three guidelines were adopted explicitly, consistency with past decisions would be maintained and the process of regulatory decision making would be simplified considerably.

Not only have regulatory agencies taken exception to the unilateral application of 1 in 1,000,000 risk, but many common human activities entail risks greatly in excess of 1 in 1,000,000. Rodricks et al. (1987) have discussed these:

> Examination of the risks of common human activities demonstrates... a lifetime risk of 1 in 100,000 or more is within the realm of, or orders of magnitude below, everyday risks that generally do not cause undue concern. These are risks that people, while they are aware of them and may have *some* concern or fear over them, do not in general alter their behavior to avoid. As Table 1 illustrated, the risks from many activities greatly exceed the level of one in 100,000. In comparison to these background risks of "everyday activities," a lifetime risk of 1 in 100,000 is relatively small. Accordingly, regulatory action will not generally be justifiable unless risks are substantially higher than this 1 in 100,000 "benchmark."

Finally, it is interesting to note that the incidence of cancer for the American population and for people in highly industrialized countries is about 1 in 4. Smoking and lifestyle factors such as diet account for this background rate. If regulatory action were taken to limit further risk to 1 in 1,000,000, this would be equivalent to lowering the cancer incidence in a million people from 250,001 to 250,000. It is for this reason and the economic strain on the regulated party that upper-bound theoretical risks greater than 1 in 1,000,000 are frequently deemed acceptable by regulatory agencies. Often, theoretical risks in the vicintiy of 1 in 50,000 to 1 in 100,000 are acceptable in environmental standards. When the population potentially exposed to a chemical is much less than 1,000,000, for example, manufacturing workers or pesticide applicators, then risk criteria on the order of 1 in 1,000 have often been deemed reasonable (Rodricks et al., 1987).

Although scientists within the regulated community will frequently agree with the various positions put forth by scientists within the various regulating agencies, there remains a genuine concern that conservative or "health protective" assumptions or models will be mishandled or misunderstood (through excessive simplification) by the press or the public. For example, in an effort to illustrate the potential severity of a hazard, reporters often cite only the highest measured or highest predicted level of exposure and the associated risk for the "worst case" person (who may not exist under any scenario). Regrettably, our society has encouraged the media to dwell on sensational reporting rather than a careful, balanced, and objective scientific presentation of the pertinent data.

A major problem faced by scientists and policymakers is how best to present the results of analyses in a fair and thorough manner, yet in a manner that is understandable. Dr. Fred Hoerger, a scientist who has been involved in regulatory affairs and environmental policy for 20 years, has illustrated one potential problem with the way some risk assessments have been conducted using the following story (Hoerger, 1985):

> One of the major problems with risk assessment today is the extreme over-simplification resulting from the use of quantitative mathematical models for extrapolating from high doses to low doses.... As indicated earlier, mathematical models give a range of risk estimates. The upper bound estimate is the worst case estimate of risk. By its derivation, it is very, very, unlikely that the number represents the true risk. For example, an extrapolation showing an upper bound risk of 10 in a million may have an associated lower bound or risk of zero—the extrapolation only tells us that either number is equally plausible, and our communication seldom mentions the lower bound estimate.

> I will illustrate upper bound estimates by departing from health concerns and turning to another environmental concern: the weather.

> It can be said that the upper bound estimate of rainfall for the United States is 15,000 inches per year. Most of us are accustomed to thinking of yearly rainfall averaging a few inches to perhaps 50 or 60 inches per year in Miami, Florida. As a result, my estimate of 15,000 inches per year sounds outlandish. For a moment, let me justify my estimate on the basis of "prudent" predicting principles. Historical records show that the highest single day rainfall was 43 inches in Alvin, Texas in 1979. Simply multiplying this number by the number of days in a year and extending it to the United States gives my estimate of 15,000 inches.

> Yes, there are faults in my logic. The 43 inch rainfall is certainly an extreme case. Again, we know that there are climatic differences between Alvin, Texas and Phoenix, Arizona or Sacramento, California. And again, we know that conditions for such extreme rain occur only rarely anywhere in the United States. In risk assessment terminology, I used a worst case assumption, a linearized extrapolation, and ignored the mechanisms of rain formation.

The popular print and electronic news media often find it necessary to make very fast interpretations of a risk assessment brought to its attention. Without understanding the complex nature of the data base on which the assessment is made, it is very easy for the media to reach the same kind of conclusions that led to my 15,000 inch rainfall data base. The consequences of such reporting are enormous in promoting irrational public concern and for political solutions to highly complex technical problems.

8.2   Some Basics in Risk Management

The problems with which risk managers must grapple have received a good deal of attention since 1985 and these have been discussed in a number of texts (Kates et al., 1985; Covello et al., 1986, 1987; Merkhofer, 1986; Sjöberg, 1986; Colby et al., 1987; Johnson and Covello, 1987; Lave and Upton, 1987; McColl, 1987). Because of the significant number of considerations and subjective evaluations that go into risk management decisions, and because the focus of this text is on the objective aspects of risk assessment, only some fundamental aspects are discussed here.

During William Ruckelshaus' tenure as administrator of the U.S. EPA, he frequently talked about risk management. He noted that although there is an objective way to assess risk, there is no purely objective way to manage it. Furthermore, he noted that we cannot ignore the subjective perception of risk in the ultimate management of a particular substance and that "no amount of data is a substitute for good judgment." The following views by Ruckelshaus (1984) are a reasonable summary of some of the challenges faced by risk managers:

> We must search for ways to describe risk in terms that the average citizen can comprehend. Telling a family that lives close to a manufacturing facility that no further controls on the plant's emissions are needed because, according to our linear model, their risk is only 10^{-6}, is not very reassuring. We need to describe the suspect substances as clearly as possible, tell people what the known or suspected health problems are, and help them compare that risk to those with which they are more familiar.

> To effectively manage the risk, we must seek new ways to involve the public in the decision-making process. Whether we believe in participatory democracy or not, it is a part of our social regulatory fabric. Rather than praise or lament it, we should seek more imaginative ways to involve the various segments of the public affected by the substance at issue. They need to become involved early, and they need to be informed if their participation is to be meaningful....

> For this to happen, scientists must be willing to take a larger role in explaining the risks to the public—including the uncertainties inherent in any risk assessment. Shouldering this burden is the responsibility of all scientists, not just those with a particular policy end in mind. In fact, all scientists should make clear when they are speaking as scientists, ex cathedra, and when they are recommending policy they believe should flow from scientific information....

> Lest anyone misunderstand, I am not suggesting that all the elements of managing risk can be reduced to a neat mathematical formula. Going through a discipline approach can help to organize our thoughts so that we include all the elements that should be weighed. We will build up a set of precedents that will be useful for later decision-making and will provide more predictable outcomes for any social regulatory programs we adopt.

> In a society in which democratic principles dominate, the perceptions of the public must be weighed. Instead of objective and subjective risks, the experts sometimes refer to "real" and "imaginary" risk. There is a certain arrogance in this—an elitism that has ill served us in the past. Rather than decry the ignorance of the public and seek to ignore their concerns, our

governmental processes must accommodate the will of the people and recognize its occasional wisdom. As Thomas Jefferson observed. "If we think [the people] are not enlightened enough to exercise their control with a wholesome descretion, the remedy is not to take it from them, but to inform their descretion."

8.3   Acceptable Levels of Risk: One Approach to Risk Management

One of the most important and difficult tasks facing the risk manager is that involving the identification of a level of acceptable risk. Even though it has been well acknowledged for thousands of years that all activities in which humans participate involve some level of risk, in recent years Western society has wanted to reduce involuntary risks to levels once considered trivial. This rather abrupt change in societal expectations has driven the risk manager into unfamiliar waters since it is no longer sufficient to say that a chemical is bad or good, carcinogenic or noncarcinogenic, teratogenic or nonteratogenic. Rather, the risk manager must decide if a chemical, at a particular dose, poses a risk that outweighs its benefits. More often, the risk manager must answer the question: Does the economic and societal cost of reducing or eliminating the risk outweigh the benefit? Whipple (1986) has addressed this issue:

> The concept of de minimis risk level appears to be an important tool which the risk manager can use to help resolve some of the challenges which face him. The term de minimis is used in law to describe trivial issues not deserving of a court's time and attention. When applied to health and safety risks and their regulation, the term refers to a risk that avoids regulatory attention by virtue of its small size. This concept has several potential regulatory applications. A de minimis rationale can be used either to determine the regulatory standard or to decide that no standard is required. In the latter case, whole classes of small risks may be excluded from regulatory consideration.

The concept of de minimis risk has been offered in recent years as a way to help identify the insignificant risks that do not deserve our attention so that we can focus on the truly important ones. Whipple (1986) believes that the de minimis concept as applied to health risks has grown in its importance over the past 5–10 years.

> The impetus to establish a consistent de minimis approach to risk regulation has increased in recent years for several reasons. First, technologies for identifying risks have improved in several ways. Improvements in analytical chemistry permit the detection of hazardous substances at the part-per-billion or even part-per-trillion level; only a decade ago such exposures would have been ignored simply because they would have been undetectable. (Radiation is an exception to this rule, since it has been detectable at low levels for decades. This helps to explain why many de minimis proposals have arisen from the radiation protection area.)

> Second, our view of the nature of low-level risks has shifted somewhat over the past decade. An initial concern that we face rare but potent carcinogens seems to have given way to the view that carcinogens are fairly commonplace and significantly varied in their potency. Recent studies that reveal widespread exposures to natural carcinogens in food (Ames, 1983a) have troubling implications for a risk-management policy based on elimination of carcinogens (Ames, 1983b; Epstein et al., 1984), and strengthens the argument for adopting a carcinogen-management policy that bases regulatory action on both carcinogenic potency and exposure.

Interestingly, even though the logic of such an approach may appear compelling, a number of questions have been raised about the legal acceptability of a de minimis interpretation of some regulations and these may preclude its use in a number of settings.

Recently, Dr. Joe Rodricks (Rodricks, 1988), who was formerly a senior Scientific Advisor at the U.S. FDA, reviewed the early history about how U.S. regulatory agencies matured from the ban or no ban policy dictated by the Delaney Amendment to the current philosophy regarding "acceptable levels of risk." The following excerpts summarize his recollection of how this occurred (Rodricks, 1988):

> I believe we can locate the origins of risk assessment as a regulatory tool in FDA's attempt, during the 1960s and 1970s, to deal with the various uses of diethylstibesterol (DES). DES is a synthetic estrogen which is a human and animal carcinogen. The part of the story I want to relate concerns the use of DES as a growth promotant in animals used for human food. There is, of course, another important DES story, associated with its use as a human drug; but risk assessment begins with FDA's attempts to deal with the problems created by residues of DES in food.
>
> Why do I believe that DES is so important in the history of the regulatory uses of risk assessment? The Delaney Clause of the food additive amendments was introduced in 1958 and the Clause prohibited the direct addition of carcinogens to foods. This prohibition was based on the notion, put forward by many scientists at the time, that no safe level of exposure to a carcinogen could be established, as it could for other classes of toxic agents.
>
> Until at least 1962, this Clause applied to carcinogenic animal drugs such as DES; even though such drugs were not directly added to food, there was a potential that they might enter food through their use in animals we use for food.
>
> For several reasons, some of which I shall touch upon later, Congress amended the food laws in 1962 to allow the use of carcinogenic drugs such as DES in food animals, but only under certain highly restrictive conditions. Those restrictions stated that, under its intended conditions of use, there should be *no residue* of the drug in edible animal products when those products were examined by a method of analysis found acceptable by the FDA. This statement is a paraphrase of the law, but the phrase "no residue" does appear in this so-called "Des-proviso."
>
> This modification of the Delaney Clause for carcinogenic animal drugs permitted the use of DES as a growth promotant. In 1963, FDA issued regulations approving the use of DES as a feed additive for cattle, later approved its use in sheep, and established an official method of analysis that could be used to search for residues in edible animal products. It is important to describe that official method of analysis. It wasn't a chemical assay; it was called the "mouse uterine bioassay." Because DES has estrogenic properties, one can use a biological assay system to detect its presence. One would take tissue, specifically liver, from DES-treated animals, and feed the tissue to immature female mice. After 21-days of feeding the weight of the mouse uterus was measured to determine whether there was a uterotrophic response. The assay was relatively crude, difficult to perform, and was characterized by a low degree of accuracy and precision. The assay had none of the characteristics of a regulatory enforcement assay, especially speed, but FDA did approve it for detecting DES residues.
>
> The mouse uterine assay could detect an estrogenic response equivalent to DES liver levels of about two parts-per-billion or greater. The assay could not detect residue levels below two parts-per-billion. This approval by FDA thus carried with it the implicit assumption that residues of DES present at concentrations below two parts per billion, which were almost certainly going to be present, were not unsafe—i.e., that there was no significant risk to humans associated with DES liver levels below two parts-per-billion. Part of the reasoning behind this assumption was that, as some FDA scientists believed at the time, DES produced its carcinogenic response only at dose levels that were estrogenically active (i.e., cancer was thought to be secondary to the estrogenic response and if one could not measure an estrogenic response, then one should be below a threshold for carcinogenicity). Later it became clear that there wasn't much proof for that assumption, but it carried a lot of weight in FDA in the early to late 1960s.
>
> This view, which allowed some drug residues below a specified detection limit, would seem to

contradict the earlier view of the Agency that it could not establish safe levels for carcinogens. I surmise that some Agency scientists then believed that there were exceptions to that view, exemplified by the estrogen-mediated carcinogenicity hypothesis for DES. I also believe that it was this view of DES that led Congress to modify the Delaney Clause, because it was led to believe that there was no significant cancer risk associated with DES levels below two parts-per-billion. It is also possible, of course, that Congress believed that "no residue" was equivalent to *zero* residue, when in fact it can only mean "no residue above the detection limit" of whatever assay one happens to apply. But whatever it was Congress believed (assuming it makes any sense at all to talk about "Congressional beliefs"), the effect of the animal drug amendment was to allow some finite level of carcinogen to be present in meat, milk, or eggs, and to require FDA to specify the allowable upper limit on this level.

If FDA were to take the position that the only allowable level was absolute zero, then there was no need for the amendment. No drug could ever be approved, because no method of analysis could ever ensure the absolute absence of residues.

As you might have guessed, USDA scientists began examining all edible tissues from DES-treated animals using chemical methods—no one ever used the mouse uterine assay for enforcement—and they began to find DES residues below two parts-per-billion. And every time they lowered the sensitivity of the analytical method, they found a higher frequency of residues. FDA kept modifying the conditions of use of DES to try to find those under which no residues might appear (for example, by changing drug withdrawal times), but USDA continued to detect residues. FDA finally decided to act against the use of DES. To complete its action against the animal drug uses of DES took nearly a decade of work on the part of the Agency.

During that time FDA rejected the estrogen-mediated carcinogenicity hypothesis as unsubstantiated, performed some risk assessments on DES, decided the risks were too high, and acted against DES. In 1979, Commissioner Donald Kennedy ordered revocation of the approvals for the animal drug uses of DES.

The issues surrounding DES created within the FDA a dilemma about other carcinogens that were used in the same way. Specifically, the question arose as to how FDA should decide what method detection limits ought to be required for residues of other carcinogens. To answer the question on detection limits required an answer to the question of what maximum intake level of a carcinogen FDA could ignore without jeopardizing the public health.

In 1973, FDA proposed to use a procedure for specifying maximum acceptable carcinogen intake levels that was first set forth in the scientific literature by Professor Nathan Mantel. Mantel's proposed procedure was based on the results from risk assessment, coupled with a definition of insignificant risk. This combination resulted in what Professor Mantel labeled a "virtually safe dose" for carcinogens, and which FDA later called a "safe" dose. (At FDA we did not allow "virtually safe" intakes, only "safe" intakes.) With this proposal was established the notion that some very low level of cancer risk would not pose a significant public health threat.

FDA looked at a whole series of other methods for defining "no residue" and rejected them all, because none allowed the Agency to take into account the cancer bioassay data in a systematic way in making decisions about what the maximum carcinogen exposure level ought to be. The Mantel procedure, and later risk assessment procedures adopted at FDA, allowed the chemical-specific bioassay potency information to be used in setting limits on exposure—the more potent the carcinogen, the lower the maximum level of acceptable intake. FDA still operates on the principle of "insignificant carcinogenic risk." In 1977 and 1985 there are Federal Register notices in which FDA sets forth the reasons for its belief that the lifetime risk level chosen—one-in-one million estimated using a linear extrapolation model—poses no significant carcinogenic risk to people.

I also need to add that, during this whole period, there were other forces at work that caused FDA and other regulatory agencies to search for some systematic and quantitative way to take into account carcinogenicity data when setting limits on carcinogen exposures. I find four trends that led to reinforcement of the position that FDA was taking with respect to the carcinogenic animal drugs.

First, the number of animal tests for carcinogenicity that were being conducted was increasing quickly and, with that, the number of animal carcinogens. There were thus many more carcinogens to deal with and most were commercially important substances. (Many of the carcinogens that NCI identified in the early years of its testing program were not particularly important commercially.) In addition, the chemists were at work finding more and more carcinogens in more and more places: trace constituents of food additives and color additives, natural contaminants such as the aflatoxins, and industrial pollutants such as PCB's. These findings created the need for a method to establish maximum allowable intake levels for carcinogens.

Another force that led to the incorporation of risk assessment into regulatory proceedings was that new methods for risk assessment began appearing in the scientific literature; indeed, there was substantial growth in this whole area of scientific inquiry during the 1970s.

Finally, there were many new federal laws enacted during the early 1970s, and they also helped create conditions for the growth of risk assessment in regulation. Risk assessment became firmly lodged in the regulatory programs of the federal government in 1979 with the publication of the Interagency Regulatory Liaison Group document on the subject. More recent documents published by the National Research Council (1983) and the Office of Science and Technology Policy (1985) have reaffirmed the basis of and need for risk assessment procedures in regulation of environmental and occupational carcinogens and carcinogens in consumer products. Even considering all the uncertainties in risk assessment, it remains as the only useful and systematic means available to give us some sense of the relative public health importance of low risk agents.

I have gone through this little history to make the following essential point: that once FDA came to accept that there were levels of carcinogenic risk too low to require regulation, and that risk assessment could be used to help identify those levels, then there was no *logical* basis for rejecting the use of this same approach for setting non-zero limits on human intakes of classes of carcinogens other than the animal drugs. FDA did, in fact, extend that methodology to other classes of regulated agents, and those extensions bring us to the present, in which we find FDA proposing to apply this same approach to directly added food ingredients—i.e., substances clearly falling under the requirements of the Delaney Clause.

8.4   Worst Case Assumptions

One serious problem that has slowly crept into risk assessment is the tendency of some assessors, especially those in regulatory agencies and/or consultants to these agencies, is the repeated adoption of conservative assumptions in their calculations. The stated rationale is to ensure that the true risk to which anyone will be exposed will be less than that predicted by the assessment procedure. Although this might appear to be an admirable goal, such approaches to "protect" everyone from potential harm have a number of shortcomings. One problem with the repeated use of exceedingly unlikely exposure scenarios is that it is extremely difficult to compare various assessments since different scientists can incorporate differing levels of conservatism in their assumptions. Many exposure scenarios have been called "worst case," as if to imply that they are feasible or plausible, but frequently, the scenarios described are only remotely possible for only a handful of persons.

Assessments based on assumptions generally thought to be conservative are routinely used by agencies when evaluating the public risk associated with exposure to potential carcinogens. For example, conservative risk assessment assumptions are used by EPA's Carcinogen Assessment Group to estimate a plausible upper bound for risk; the plausible lower bound is taken to be zero risk except where direct human evidence indicates otherwise. These upper-bound risk estimates are based on data from the most sensitive sex, strain, and species of test aminal and for the cancer tumor type (often including benign tumors) and tissue that maximize the estimated potency. Extrapolation of animal results to humans are calculated from the ratio of surface areas, an approach more conservative than scaling by weight, and extrapolation from high- to low-dose response is based on a dose–response model that exhibits linearity at low doses (Whipple, 1986). The selection of the most sensitive sex, strain, and species is usually justified on the grounds that humans are genetically diverse, differ widely in health status, and are exposed to many other potentially harmful agents (Anderson, 1983). Frequently, humans will not be more sensitive. Further, the assumption of low-dose linearity will generally add sufficient conservatism to protect virtually all persons especially if risks of one in 100,000, or less, are adopted.

As discussed by Whipple (1986), worst case assumptions have become rather routine in many risk assessments. However, serious risk management problems can arise from the repeated use of such conservative approaches:

> Certainly the perception of many risk analysis is that conservative risk-assessment assumptions are protective. High-risk estimates are associated with stringent standards. An analyst's own sense of responsibility encourages conservatism. Although the social costs of false alarms are acknowledged, to give a incorrect assurance of safety is believed to be far worse. The relative social cost of risk underestimation is taken to outweigh that of overestimation....

> But to find that analytical conservatism is generally protective requires three assumptions: (1) that the disparity in social costs between false negatives and false positives is great, (2) that risk-management decisions are insensitive to resource restraints and do not incur significant opportunity costs, and (3) that activities or agents identified as hazardous (whether true positives or false positives) can be eliminated without creation of significant new risks. The potential protectiveness of conservatism also depends on whether risk managers compensate for conservatism in standard setting....

> An additional factor encouraging conservatism is how a regulatory agency's decisions might be judged in hindsight. An overcontrolled risk will probably drop from sight once a decision is implemented and control investments made, despite continuing social costs. But an undercontrolled risk, possibly discovered through the identification of victims, is far more disturbing for a regulatory agency.

> If risk reductions are limited by resource scarcity, however, the logical regulatory objective is to allocate the scarce resource in a way that maximizes social benefits. Opportunity costs, the value of benefits forgone from possible alternative uses of the scarce resource, become important under these circumstances. Money or regulatory attention spent on one risk is not available for another, so it is important not to waste resources on trivial risks. Here, conservatism is counterproductive, and risks are increased if resources are shifted from significant risks to small, exaggerated risks. Under this fixed-allocation or zero-sum case, risk reductions are maximized when the cheapest and easiest risk reductions are given highest priority. Here, conservatism estimates shift resources to uncertain risks, increasing expected health consequences.

> Often a regulatory action that reduces one risk will increase another (Whipple, 1985). This is especially true when the particular benefit obtained is considered essential but the method for achieving the benefit carries risks. The important issue here is the recognition that the appropriate measure for analysis of a risk-reducing action is the net risk reduction. In that event, uneven conservatism in risk assessment can have a perverse effect by leading to the substitution of a large

risk for a small one. The cyclamate ban, leading to greater use of saccharine, may be one such instance. (Risks from both substances are significantly uncertain.) Electricity production is also a good example, because utilities are obligated to provide service. A restriction on coal use can lead to greater oil use. If regulatory considerations make nuclear power unattractive, then perhaps a utility will choose coal instead; the net change in public risk would need to be evaluated.

In some cases—for example, those involving carcinogens—it may be possible to compare risks that have common conservative assumptions and arrive at a reasonable relative ranking. But for dissimilar technologies—for example, coal and nuclear electricity—the comparison of conservative risk estimates does not include conservative assumptions common to both estimates. In these cases conservatism is less useful and less protective than are mean estimates of risk.

Considering the many ways in which a conservative analysis can fail to protect, intentional use of conservative risk estimates is not beneficial to public health. In addition to misallocating scarce resources, conservatism can lead to unwise risk transfer and encourage risk regulators to compensate for perceived conservatism. When this happens, risk regulation becomes less predictable and more arbitrary.

Certainly a society can manage risk to the population as a whole by limiting individual risks. This is, in fact, the approach taken by the Nuclear Regulatory Commission (1983) in its proposed safety goals for nuclear power plants. Individual risk limits are appropriate in cases where individuals face relatively high risks. But when individual risks are neither high nor inequitably distributed and the need for management arises because a large number of people face a low-to-moderate risk, the individual risk approaches can lead to misallocation of resources. To take a hypothetical example, a 10^{-6}/year risk of death to 1,000 people produces a 10^{-3} expected fatalities per year, which is equivalent to an expectation of one fatality per thousand years. This same risk of 10^{-6}/yr applied to the entire U.S. population of 230 million produces an expectation of 230 fatalities per year. If judgment of whether either situation represents de minimis risk is based solely on the degree of individual risk involved, the regulatory response (or nonresponse) to the two situations is likely to be comparable. Yet common sense tells us that greater effort and expenditure are justified to save 230 lives than 0.001 life.

In all likelihood, as society grows more comfortable with the thought that all activities involve some level of risk, the uniform approaches for identifying de minimis levels of risk will be established. Until then, it is clear that the label "de minimis" will be divided on a case-by-case basis.

Several authors have specifically addressed the problems of repetitively using conservative assumptions in risk assessments (Nichols and Zeekhauser, 1988; Maxim, 1989).

8.5   Federal Guidelines on Risk Assessment

Shortly after risk assessments became rather commonplace, and expected, in regulatory proceedings, various policies were proposed to ensure that risk assessments met certain criteria. These have been discussed by Bentkover et al. (1986):

> Early requirements for developing economic and environmental impact assessments were defined in Section 102 of the National Environmental Policy Act of 1969, in Executive Order (E.O.) 11949 (and the preceding E.O. 11821), and in the Office of Management of Budget (OMB) Directive A107 for inflationary impact statements. These regulations required that economic and environmental impact statements be developed and included in all recommendations or reports on proposals for legislation and other Federal actions.

> On March 23, 1978, E.O. 12044 was issued, directing each Executive Branch agency to undertake several specific steps aimed at the improvement of existing and future regulations. This E.O. required:

1. Simplification of regulations to minimize cost and paperwork burdens on the public.
2. Reform of the regulatory development process to include publishing, at least semiannually, an agenda of significant regulations under development or review.
3. Agency-head approval.
4. Regulatory analysis exploring alternatives and their economic consequences, along with a detailed explanation of the basis for selection among alternatives.
5. Periodic review of existing regulations.

The key portion of Executive Order 12044 to risk assessors lies in the need to discuss the various alternatives and cost–benefit relation associated with each alternative. Executive Order 12291, issued on February 17, 1981, called for a detailed regulatory analysis on all new major rules. These rules, which resulted in an annual effect on the economy of $100 million or more, were considered major. Bentkover has summarized the importance of his order (Bentkover et al., 1986):

> The effect of this order was threefold. First, it expanded the definition of "major rule" and so incorporated a greater number of regulations within its purview. Second, it granted the OMB authority to order that a rule not designated major by an agency head may be so designated. Third, it required that any set of related rules be considered together as a major rule. Executive Order 12291 established the following analysis requirements for major rules:

> 1. Administrative decisions shall be based on adequate information concerning the need for and consequences of proposed government actions.
> 2. Regulatory action shall not be undertaken unless the potential benefits to society from the regulation outweigh the potential costs to society.
> 3. Regulatory objectives shall be chosen to maximize the net benefits to society.
> 3. Among alternative approaches to any given regulatory objective, the alternative involving the least net cost to society shall be chosen.
> 5. Agencies are to set regulatory priorities with the aim of maximizing the aggregate net benefits to society, taking into account the condition of the particular industries affected by regulations, the condition of the national economy, and other regulatory actions contemplated for the future [Section 2(a)–(e)].

In addition, a new process for conducting regulatory impact analysis (RIA) was required. It specified that an RIA must contain the following (Bentkover et al., 1986):

> 1. A description of the potential benefits of the rule, including any beneficial effects that cannot be quantified in monetary terms, and the identification of those likely to receive the benefits;
> 2. A description of the potential costs of the rule, including any adverse effects that cannot be quantified in monetary terms, and the identification of those likely to bear the costs;
> 3. A determination of the potential net benefits of the rule, including an evaluation of effects that cannot be quantified in monetary terms;
> 4. A description of alternative approaches that could substantially achieve the same regulatory goal at lower cost, together with an analysis of this potential benefit and costs and a brief explanation of the legal reasons why such alternatives, if proposed, could not be adopted; and
> 5. Unless covered by the description required under paragraph (4) of this subsection, an explanation of any legal reasons why this rule cannot be based on the requirements set forth in Section 2 of this Order.

8.6 The Court's View on Risk Assessment

In the early 1980's, the Supreme Court had an opportunity to give an opinion on the use of risk assessment in regulations. In one instance, the Fifth Circuit's Court of Appeals set aside the Consumer Product Safety Commission's ban of urea formaldehyde foam insulation and it required changes in the future risk assessment methodologies to be used by CPSC and other agencies (AIHC, 1983).

The court concluded that CPSC's finding of unreasonable risk of cancer was unsupported. It rejected the risk assessment methodology followed by CPSC, which at the time was the same methodology used by the Cancer Assessment Group (CAG) at EPA and by OSHA. Specifically, CPSC calculated the risk of cancer from exposure to formaldehyde emissions from the foam insulation using the multistage model with a linearized 95% upper confidence level. CPSC applied this model to extrapolate from whatever experimental data base resulted in the highest estimate of risk. In CPSC's case, the data base was the CIIT rat study. Another rat study and a CIIT mouse study were not used.

The court held that the CPSC methodology did not provide substantial evidence to support a finding of unreasonable cancer risk. It was unreasonable, the court concluded, to base a risk assessment on a single study and to disregard other studies:

> While the Commission correctly notes that the epidemiologic evidence is not conclusive, its exclusive reliance on the Chemical Institute study in its Global 79 risk assessment is equally unsupportable....

> As Dr. Higginson aptly stated, it is not good science to rely on a single experiment, particularly one involving only 240 subjects, to make precise estimates of cancer risk. [Slip op. at 3641, 3641 (AIHC, 1983)]

The court also felt that it was not appropriate to base decisions only on upper confidence limit results of a model to generate "up-to" estimates since it would not provide substantial evidence to support a finding of unreasonable risk.

The exposure assumptions and data used by CPSC were considered unrepresentative and imprecise and it was felt they could not be used as the basis of an "exacting, precise, and extremely complicated risk assessment model."

> The predictions made by the risk assessment model are no better than the data base. We have concluded that this base was inadequate.

Some analysts have claimed that the formaldehyde decision required that basic changes be made in the methodology used by CPSC and other U.S. regulatory agencies (AIHC, 1983; Barnard, 1984):

- The *formaldehyde* decision makes clear that extrapolation should be made using the available data sets, not just one data set. A scientific explanation of the differences in the results may be called for, but these factors do not justify preselection of a single data set for risk estimation.
- Exposure data must be valid and precise in order to form the basis of a quantitative risk assessment.
- One extrapolation model should not be used exclusively. As the EPA Science Advisory Board recommended in reviewing air emission criteria documents prepared by EPA, other models should also be fitted.
- Finally, and very important, the results reported should be "most likely" or "most

probably" results. Upper confidence limits, which provide only "up-to" estimates, are not substantial evidence to support a finding of human risk (AIHC, 1983).

It is interesting to note that the court's recommendations were not unlike those put forth in the National Academy of Science position document (NAS, 1983), or in the later state-of-the-art documents by the Office of Science and Technology Policy (OSTP, 1985) and the EPA cancer risk assessment guidelines (EPA, 1986a).

9   OVERVIEW

Because of the number of environmental concerns, it is clear that there will continue to be a need to conduct comprehensive analyses of the potential of chemical(s) to affect adversely human health or the environment, that is, risk assessment. The field of health risk assessment, as applied to environmental hazards, has been raised to a level of importance which necessitates that uniform and scientifically valid methodologies be used in these assessments. The increased number of published assessments and government reports have been helpful in advancing the art.

It is important that scientists involved in risk assessment be attentive to all the scientific data needed to describe the degree of risk associated with a given hazard. It is also important that assessors maintain a clear conceptual distinction between the scientific assessment of risks and the objectives of risk management. Risk assessment and risk management have different goals, and although assessors may wish to influence the managers, it is in everyone's best interest that scientists provide the most accurate and fair description of the risk so that the risk manager can have the most objective information on which he/she will base their decision. If risk management considerations are seen to affect either the scientific interpretations or the choice of inference options in a risk assessment, the credibility of the assessment will be compromised. Each of us must make every effort to maintain a separation of the two processes.

In short, risk assessments will continue to be needed as long as they provide an objective and balanced interpretation of all the pertinent scientific information regarding toxicity and the degree of human or environmental exposure. If risk assessors fail to remove their own biases from their assessments, it is likely that risk managers will eventually be forced to make their decisions much like they did in the past—actions heavily influenced by the perceptions of special interest groups, political pressure, and fears held by the public rather than fact. If this occurs, society will almost surely expend its resources on projects that will not yield the optimum return on its investment while truly important hazards could remain unaddressed.

REFERENCES

Abelson, P. H. (1987). California's Proposition 65 (editorial). *Science* **237**, 1553.

Adolph, E. F. (1949). Quantitative relations in the physiological constitutions of mammals. *Science* **109**, 579–585.

Agricola, G. (1556). *De re metallica* (1st ed. reprint, translated by H. C. Hoover and L. C. Hoover. Dover, New York, 1950).

Altman, P. L., and Dittmer, D. S. (1964). *Biology Data Book*, Biological Handbooks. Fed. Am. Soc. Exp. Biol., Washington, DC, p. 101.

American Industrial Health Council (1983). *Significant Developments Regarding Government Cancer Risk Assessment Methodology*. AIHC, Washington, DC.

American Society for Testing and Materials (1980). Conducting acute toxicity tests with fishes, macroinvertebrates, and amphibians. In *Annual Book of ASTM Standards*, E729–780. ASTM, Philadelphia, PA.

Ames, B. N. (1983). Dietary carcinogens and anticarcinogens. *Science* **221**, 1256–1263.

Ames, B. N., Magaw, R., and Gold, L. S. (1987). Ranking possible carcinogenic hazards. *Science* **236**, 271–280.

Ames, B. N. (1987). Six common errors relating to environmental pollution. *Regul. Toxicol. Pharm.* **7**, 379–383.

Anderson, E. L. (1983). Quantitative approaches in use to assess cancer risks. *Risk Anal.* **3**, 277–295.

Andersen, M. E. (1988). Quantitative risk assessment and industrial hygiene. *Amer. Ind. Hyg. Assn. J.* (in press).

Andersen, M. E., Clewell, H. J., Gargas, M. L., Smith, F. A., and Reitz, R. A. (1987). Physiologically based pharmacokinetics and the risk assessment process for methylene chloride. *Toxicol. Appl. Pharm.* **87**, 185–205.

Angle, C. R., and McIntire, M. S. (1974). Lead in air, dustfall, soil, housedust, milk and water: Correlation with blood lead of urban and suburban school children. *Trace Substances Environ. Health* **8**, 23–28.

Armitage, P. and Doll, R. (1954). The age distribution of cancer and a multistage theory of carcinogenesis. *Brit. J. Cancer* **8**, 1–12.

Armitage, P. and Doll, R. (1961). Stochastic models for carcinogenesis. In J. Newman, Ed., *Proceedings of the Fourth Berkeley Symposium on Mathematical Statistics and Probability*, Vol. 4. University of California Press, Berkeley, CA. pp. 19–38.

Ayrton–Paris, J. A. (1822). *Pharmaecologia.*

Baes, C. F., III (1982). Predictions of radionuclide K_d values from soil–plant concentration ratios. *Trans. Am. Nucl. Soc.* **41**, 53–54.

Baes, C. F., III, Sharp, R. D., Sjoreen, A., and Shor, R. (1984). *A Review and Analysis of Parameters for Assessing Transport of Environmentally Released Radionuclides through Agriculture*, ORNL-5786. U.S. Department of Energy, Oak Ridge National Laboratory, Oak Ridge, TN.

Barltrop, D. (1973). Sources and significance of environmental lead for children. In *Environmental Health Aspects of Lead*. Commission of European Communities, Center for Information and Documentation, Luxembourg, pp. 675–681.

Barnard, R. C. (1984). Science, policy and the law: A developing partnership in reducing the risk of cancer. In P. F. Diesler, Jr., Ed., *Reducing the Carcinogenic Risks In Industry*. Dekker, New York.

Barnes, J. M., and Denz, F.A. (1954). Experimental methods used in determining chronic toxicity. *Pharmacol. Rev.* **6**, 191–242.

Bartek, M. J., and LaBudde, J. A. (1975). Percutaneous absorption. In H. Maibach, Ed., *Animal Models in Dermatology*. Churchill–Livingstone, New York, pp. 103–120.

Beck, L. W., Maki, A. W., Artman N. R., and Wilson, E. R. (1981). Outline and criteria for evaluating the safety of new chemicals. *Regul. Toxicol. Pharmacol.* **1**, 19–58.

Bentkover, J. D., Covello, V. T., and Mumpower, J. (1986). *Benefits Assessment: The State of the Art*. Reidel Publ., Boston, MA.

Bergmann, H. L., Kimerle, R. A., and Maki, A. W. (1986). *Environmental Hazard Assessment of Effluents*. Pergamon, New York.

Binder, S., Sokal, D., and Maughan, D. (1987). Estimating the amount of soil ingested by young children through tracer elements. *Arch. Environ. Health* **41**, 341–345.

Bischoff, K. B. (1967). Applications of a mathematical model for drug distribution in mammals. In D. Hershey, Ed., *Chemical Engineering in Medicine and Biology*. Plenum, New York.

Bishop, W. E., Cardwell, R. D., and Heidolph, B. B. (1983). *Aquatic Toxicology and Hazard*

Assessment: Sixth Symposium, STP 737. American Society Testing and Materials, Philadelphia, PA.

Black, D. L., and Marks, T. A. (1986). Inconsistent use of terminology in animal developmental toxicology studies: A discussion. *Teratology* **33**, 333–338.

Bogan, K. T., and Spear, R. C. (1987). Integrating uncertainty and interindividual variation in environmental risk assessment. *Risk Anal.* **7**, 427–436.

Branson, D. R., and Dickson, K. L. (1981). *Aquatic Toxicology and Hazard Assessment: Fourth Symposium*, STP 737. American Society Testing and Materials, Philadelphia, PA.

Breidenstein, B. C. (1984). *Contribution of Red Meat to the U.S. Diet*. National Livestock and Meat Board, Chicago, IL.

Bresson, G., Pages, P., Lombard, J., and Fagnani, F. (1981). Occupational radiological risks in uranium mining. In *Interconference on Radiation Hazards in Mining*. Society of Mining Engineers, New York, pp. 111–114.

Briggs, G. G., Bromilow, R. H., and Evans, A. A. (1982). Relationships between lipophilicity and root uptake and translocation of non-ionized chemicals by barley. *Toxicol. Environ. Chem.* **7**, 173–189.

Brooke, L. T., Call, D. J., Geiger, D. L., and Northcott, C. E. (Eds.) (1984). *Acute Toxicities of Organic Chemicals to Fathead Minnows*. Center for Lake Superior Environ. Stud., University of Wisconsin-Superior, Superior.

Browman, M. G., and Chesters, G. (1977). The solid-water interface: Transfer of organic pollutants across the solid-water interface. In I. H. Suffet, Ed., *Fate of Pollutants in the Air and Water Environment*, Part I. Wiley, New York, pp. 49–101.

Brown, C. (1978). Statistical aspects of extrapolation of dichotomous dose-response data. *J. Natl. Cancer Inst.* **60**, 101–108.

Brown, H. S. (1986). A critical review of current approaches to determining "How clean is clean" at hazardous waste sites. *Hazard. Waste Hazard. Mater.* **3**, 233–260.

Brown, M. S. (1983). Regulatory reform: Alternatives to regulation for managing risks to health, safety and environment. In F. Homburger, Ed., *Safety Evaluation and Regulation of Chemicals*. Karger, New York, pp. 121–125.

Brunekreef, B., Noy, D., Biersteker, K., and Boleij, J. (1983). Blood lead levels of dutch city children and their relationship to lead in the environment. *J. Air Pollut. Control Assoc.* **33**, 872–876.

Buchet, J., Roels, H., Lauwerys, R. et al. (1980). Repeated surveillance of exposure to cadmium, manganese, and arsenic in school-age children living in rural, urban and nonferrous smelter areas in Belgium. *Environ. Res.* **22**, 95–108.

Bus, J. S., and Gibson, J. E. (1985). Body defense mechanisms to toxicant exposure. In L. J. Cralley and L. V. Cralley, Eds., *Patty's Industrial Hygiene and Toxicology*, Vol. 3B. Wiley, New York, pp. 143–174.

Butte, N. F., Garza, C., Stuff, J. E., Smith, E. O., and Nichols, B. L. (1984). Effect of maternal diet and body composition on lactational performance. *Am. J. Clin. Nutr.* **39**, 296–306.

Cairns, J., Jr., Dickson, K. L., and Maki, A. W. (1978). *Estimating the Hazards of Chemical Substances to Aquatic Life*, STP 657. American Society for Testing and Materials Philadelphia, PA.

Calabrese, E. J., Gilbert, C. E., et al. (1988). Epidemiology study to estimate how much soil children eat. A report by the division of public health, Univ. of Mass., Amherst.

Calabrese, E. J. (1978). *Methodological Approaches to Deriving Environmental and Occupational Health Standards*. Wiley, New York.

California Department of Health Services (1986). *Guidelines for the assessment of carcinogenic substances*. CDHS, Sacramento, CA.

Carson, R. (1962). *Silent Spring*. Houghton Mifflin, Boston, MA.

Chadwick, E. (1842). *Report of the Sanitary Condition of the Labouring Population of Gt. Britain* (ed with introduction by M. W. Flinn) Edinburgh Univ. Press, Edinburgh, 1965).

Chan, P. K., O'Hara, G. P., and Hayes, A. W. (1982). Principles and methods for acute and subchronic toxicity. In A. W. Hayes, Ed., *Principles and Methods in Toxicology*. Raven Press, New York.

Chanlett, E. (1979). *Environmental Protection*. McGraw–Hill, New York, pp. 66–148.

Chemical Manufactures Association (1984). *Risk Management of Existing Chemicals*. CMA, Washington, DC.

Chemical Engineering (1983). Excess deaths from lung cancer due to workplace arsenic are down 98%. *Chemical Engineering*, Sept 28th.

Chiou, C. T. (1981). Partition coefficient and water solubility in environmental chemistry. In J. Saxena and F. Fisher, Eds., *Hazard Assessment of Chemicals*. Academic Press, New York, pp. 117–153.

Chiou, C. T., Freed, V. H., Schmedding, D. W., and Kohnert, R. L. (1977). Partitions coefficient and bioconcentration of selected organic solvents. *Environ. Sci. Technol.* **11**, 475–479.

Chiou, C. T., Peters, L. J., and Freed, V. J. (1979). A physical concept of soil-water equilibria for nonionic organic compounds. *Science* **206**, 831–832.

Chou, C. C., Milstein, R. J., Smith, W. S., Ruiz, H. V., Molina, M. J., and Rowland, F. S. (1978). Stratospheric photodissociation of several saturated perhalo chlorofluorocarbon compounds in current technological use (Fluorocarbons -13, -113, -114, and -115). *J. Phys. Chem.* **82**, 1–6.

Clausing, O., Brunekreef, A. B., and van Wijnen, J. H. (1987). A method for estimating soil ingestion by children. *Inter. Arca. Occup. Environ. Hth.* **59**, 73–82.

Clayson, D. B., Krewski, D., and Munro, I. (Eds.) (1985). *Toxicological Risk Assessment*, Vol. 1 and 2. CRC Press, Boca Raton, FL.

Clewell, H. J., and Andersen, M. E. (1985). Risk assessment extrapolations and physiological modeling. *Toxicol. Ind. Health* **1**, 111–132.

Clewell, H. J., III, and Andersen, M. E. (1986). A multiple dose-route physiological model for volatile chemicals using acslipl. *In Languages for Continuous System Simulation*, F. D. Collier, Ed. Society for Computer Simulation Publication. San Diego, CA, pp. 95–101.

Colby, A., Kohlberg, L. et al. (1987). *The Measurement of Moral Judgment*, Vols. 1 and 2. Cambridge Univ. Press, London and New York.

Conolly, R. B., Reitz, R. H., Clewell, H. J., and Andersen, M. E. (1988a). Computer Simulation of Chemical Carcinogenesis. *Toxicology Letters* (in press).

Conolly, R. B., Reitz, R. H., Clewell, H. J. and Andersen, M. E. (1988b). Biologically-structured models and computer simulation: Application to chemical carcinogenesis *Comments Toxicol* (in press).

Consultancy, J. C. (1986). *Risk Assessment for Hazardous Installations*. Commission of the European Communities, Pergamon, Oxford.

Cornfield, J. (1977). Carcinogenic risk assessment. *Science* **198**, 693–699.

Cornfield, J., Carlborg, F. W., and van Ryzin, J. (1978). Setting tolerances on the basis of mathematical treatment of dose-response data extrapolated to low doses. In G. L. Plaa and W. A. M. Duncan, Eds., *Proceedings of the First International Congress on Toxicology*. Academic Press, NY. pp. 143–164.

Covello, V. T., and Mumpower, J. (1985). Risk analysis and risk management: An historical perspective. *Risk Anal.* **5**, 103–120.

Covello, V. T., Menkes, J., and Mumpower, J. (Eds.) (1986). *Risk Evaluation and Management: Contemporary Issues in Risk Analysis*, Vol. 1. Plenum Press, New York.

Covello, V. T. et al. (1987). Uncertainty in risk assessment, risk management, and decision making. *Adv. Risk Anal.* **4**.

Cowherd, C., Muleski, G., Englehart, P., and Gillette, G. (1968). *Rapid Assessment of Exposure to Particulate Emissions from Surface Contamination Sites*, EPA Control No. 68–01–6861.

Crosby, D. G., and Li, M. (1969). Herbicide photodecomposition. In P. C. Kearney and D. D. Kaufmann, Eds., *Degradation of Herbicides*. Dekker, New York, pp. 321–363.

Crouch, E. A. C., and Wilson, R. (1982). *Risk/Benefit Analysis*. Ballinger, Cambridge, MA.

Crouch, E. A. C., and Wilson, R. (1981). Regulation of carcinogens. *Risk Anal.* **1**, 47–57.

Crouch, E. A. C., Wilson, R., and Zeise, L. (1983). The risks of drinking water. *Water Resour. Res.* **19**, 1359–1375.

Crump, K. S. (1979). Dose-response problems in carcinogenesis. *Biometrics* **35**, 157–167.

Crump, K. S. (1981). An improved procedure for low-dose carcinogenic risk assessment from animal data. *J. Environ. Toxicol.* **5**, 339–346.

Crump, K. S. (1984). A new method for determining allowable daily intakes. *Foundam. Appl. Toxicol.* **4**, 854–877.

Crump, K. S., and Masterman, D. (1979). Review and evaluation of methods of determining risk for chronic low-level carcinogenic insult. In *Environmental Contaminants in Food*. Office of Technology Assessment, U.S. Congress, Washington, DC, p. 154.

Crump, K. S., Hoel, D. G., Langley, C. H., and Peto, R. (1976). Fundamental carcinogenic processes and their implications for low dose risk assessment. *Cancer Res.* **36**, 2973–2979.

Crump, K. S., Guess, A., and Peto, R. (1977). Uncertainty estimates for low-dose extrapolations of animal carcinogenicity data. *Cancer Res* **37**, 3475–3483.

Crutzen, P. J., Isaksen, I. A. S., and McAfee, J. R. (1978). The impact of the chlorocarbon industry on the ozone layer. *JGR, J. Geophys. Res.* **83**, 345–363.

Daniels, S. L., Hoerger, F. D., and Moolenaar, R. J. (1985). Environmental exposure assessment: Experience under the toxic substances control act. *Environ. Toxicol. Chem.* **4**(1), 107–118.

Darnall, K. R., Lloyd, A. C., Winer, A. M., and Pitts, J. N., Jr. (1976). Reactivity scale for atmospheric hydrocarbons based on reaction with hydroxyl radicals. *Environ. Sci. Technol.* **10**, 692–696.

Davis, N. R., and Mapleson, W. W. (1981). Structure and quantification of a physiological model of the distribution of injected agents and inhaled anaesthetics. *Br. J. Anaesth.* **53**, 399–404.

Dedrick, R. L. (1973). Animal scale-up. *J. Pharmacokin Biopharm.* **1**, 435–461.

Dickson, K. L., Maki, A. W., and Cairns, J., Jr. (Eds.) (1979). *Analyzing the Hazard Evaluation Process*. American Fisheries Society, Washington, DC.

Dickson, K. L., Maki, A. W. and Cairns, J., Jr. (Eds.) (1982). *Modeling the Fate of Chemicals in the Aquatic Environment*. Ann Arbor Science, Ann Arbor, MI.

Dixon, R. L., and Hall, J. L. (1982). Reproductive toxicology. In A. W. Hayes, Ed., *Principles and Methods of Toxicology*, Chap. 4. Raven, New York.

Dourson, M. L., and Stara, J. F. (1983). Regulatory history and experimental support of uncertainty (safety factors). *Regul. Toxicol. Pharmacol.* **3**, 224–238.

Doyle, G. J., Lloyd, A. C., Darnall, K. R., Winer, A. M., and Pitts, J. N., Jr. (1975). Gas phase kinetic study of relative rates of reaction of selected aromatic compounds with hydroxyl radicals in an environmental chamber. *Environ. Sci. Technol.* **9**, 237–241.

Dubreuilh. W. (1896). Des Hyperkeratoses Circonscrites *Ann. Dermatol. Syphilig Ser.*, 3, pp. 1158–1204.

Dugard, P. H., Walker, M., Mawdsley, S. J., and Slott, R. C. (1984). Absorpsion of some glycol ethers through human skin. *Environ. Health. Perspect.* **57**, 193–198.

Duggan, M. J., and Williams, S. (1977). Lead-in-dust in city streets. *Sci. Total Environ.* **7**, 91–97.

Earle, V. M., III (1978). The fantasy of life without risk. *Fortune*, Feb. 16, pp. 113–116.

Eisenbud, M. (1978). *Environment, Technology, and Health: Human Ecology in Historial Perspective*. New York Univ. Press, New York.

El Beit, I. O. D. (1981). Factors affecting soil residues of dieldrin, Endosulfan, Y-HCH, Dimethoate, and Pyrolan. *Ecotoxicol. Environ. Safety* **5**, 135–160.

Environmental Protection Agency (EPA) (1986a). Guidelines for carcinogen risk assessment. *Fed. Regist.* **51** CFR 2984, No. 185, 33, 992–34, 003.

Environmental Protection Agency (EPA) (1986b). Guidelines for exposure assessment. *Fed. Regist.* **51**, CFR 2984, No. 185, 34, 042–34, 054.

Environmental Protection Agency (EPA) (1986c). Guidelines for health assessment of suspect developmental toxicants. *Fed. Regist.* **51** CFR 2984, No. 185, 34, 028–34, 041.

Environmental Protection Agency (EPA) (1986d). *Development of Advisory Levels for Polychlorinated (PCBs) Cleanup.* Office of Health and Environmental Assessment, EPA, Washington, DC.

Environmental Protection Agency (EPA) (1986e). *Superfund Health Assessment Manual.* Office of Emergency and Remedial Response, USEPA, Washington, DC (produced by ICF. Clement Incorporated, under EPA Contract 68–01–6872).

Environmental Protection Agency (EPA) (1986f). Guidelines for the health risk assessment of chemical mixtures. *Fed. Regis.* **51** CFR 2984, 34014–34027.

Environmental Protection Agency (EPA) (1987). Risk assessment, management, communication: A guide to selected sources, update, U.S. EPA PB87–203402, Washington, DC.

Environmental Protection Agency (EPA) (1974). Proceedings of the solvent reactivity conference, (Nov.) EPA 650/3-74-010. Research Triangle Park, N.C.

Environmental Protection Agency (EPA) (1979). Toxic substances control act premanufacture testing of new chemical substances. *Fed. Regist.* **44**, 16,240–16,292.

Eschenroeder, A., Jaeger, R. J., Ospital, J. J., and Doyle, C. (1986). Health risk assessment of human exposures to soil amended with sewage sludge contaminated with polychlorinated dibenzodioxins and dibenzofurans. *Vet. Hum. Toxicol.* **28**, 356–442.

Evelyn, J. (1661). *Fumifugium or the Inconvenience of the Aer and Smoake of London Dissipated* (reprinted in *The Smoke of London*, Maxwell Reprint Co., Fairview Park, Elmsford, NY, 1969).

Fiserova–Bergerova, V. (1975). Mathematical modelling of inhalation exposure. *J. Combust. Toxicol.* **3**, 201–210.

Fischoff, B., Lichtenstein, S., Slovic, P., Derby, S., and Keeney, R. L. (1982). *Acceptable Risk.* Cambridge Univ. Press, London and New York.

Flamm, W. G., and Winbush, J. S. (1984). Role of mathematical models in assessment of risk and in attempts to define management strategy. *Fundam. Appl. Toxicol.* **4**, S395–S401.

Food Safety Council (1980). Quantitative risk assessment. In *Food Safety Assessment.* Food Safety Council, Washington, DC, chap. 11.

Fouts, J. R. (1976). Overview of the field: Environmental factors affecting chemical or drug effects in animals. *Fed. Proc., Fed. Am. Soc. Exp. Biol.* **35**, 1162.

Freed, V. H., Chiou, C. T., Schmeddling, D., and Kohnert, R. (1979). Some physical factors in toxicological assessment tests. *Environ. Health Perspect.* **30**, 75–80.

Fries, G. F. (1982). Potential polychlorinated biphenyl residues in animal products from application of contaminated sewage sludge to land. *J. Environ. Qual.* **11**, 14–20.

Fries, G. F. (1985). Bioavailability of soil-brone polybrominated biphenyls ingested by farm animals. *J. Toxicol. Environ. Health* **16**, 565–579.

Fries, G. F., and Jacobs, L. W. (1986). Evaluation of residual polybrominated biphenyl contamination present on Michigan farms in 1978. *Mich., Agric. Exp. Stn., Res. Rep.* **477**.

Fries, G. F., and Paustenbach, D. J. (1987). A critical evaluation of the factors used in assessing incinerator emissions as a potential source of TCDD in foods of animal origin. *7th Int. Dioxin Symp.*, Abstr. RC-05.

Friess, S. (1987). History of risk assessment. In *Pharmacokinetics in Risk Assessment: Drinking Water and Health*, Vol. 8. National Academy of Science, Washington, DC.

Frobisher, M., Hinsdill, R. D., Crabtree, K. T., and Goodheart, C. R. (1974). *Fundamentals of Microbiology*, 9th ed., Saunders, Philadelphia, PA, pp. 674–676.

Gargas, M. L., and Andersen, M. E. (1987). Partition co-efficients for common organic solvents. *Toxicol. Appl. Pharmacol.* **86**.

Gaylor, D. W., and Kodell, R. L. (1980). Linear interpolation algorithm for low dose risk assessment of toxic substances. *J. Environ. Pathol. Toxicol.* **4**, 305–311.

Gehring, P. J. (1984). Background exposure to 2,3,7,8-tetrachlorodibenzo-p-dioxin. In W. W. Lowrance, Ed., *Public Health Risks of the Dioxins*. Kaufmann, Inc., Los Altos, CA, pp. 151–154.

Glasson, W. A., and Tuesday, C. S. (1970). Hydrocarbon reactivities in the atmospheric photooxidation of nitric acid. *Environ. Sci. Technol.* **4**, 916–924.

Grisham, J. W. (Ed.) (1986). *Health Aspects of the Disposal of Waste Chemicals*. Pergamon, Press, Oxford.

Guthrie, F. E., and Perry, J. J. (1980). *Introduction to Environmental Toxicology*. Am. Elsevier, New York.

Guyton, A. C. (1947). Respiratory volumes of laboratory animals. *Am. J. Physiol.* **150**, 70–77.

Haggard, H. W. (1924). The absorption, distribution, and elimination of ethyl ether. II. Analysis of the mechanism of the absorption and elimination of such a gas or vapor as ethyl ether: *J. Biol. Chem.* **59**, 753–770.

Halter, M. T., and Johnson, H. E. (1977). In *Aquatic Toxicology and Hazard Evaluation*. American Society for Testing and Material, Philadelphia, PA, pp. 178–196.

Hamaker, J. W. (1975). The interpretation of soil leaching experiments. In R. Haque and V. H. Freed, Eds., *Environmental Dynamics of Pesticides*. Plenum, New York, pp. 115–133.

Hamaker, J. W., and Kerlinger, W. O. (1969). Vapor pressure of pesticides. *Adv. Chem. Ser.* **86**, 39–54.

Hamaker, J. W., and Thompson, J. H. (1972). Adsorption. In C. A. I., Goring and J. M. Haymaker, Eds. *Organic Chemicals in the Soil Environment*, Vol. 1. Dekker, New York, pp. 51–122.

Hansch, C., Quinlan, J.E., and Lawrence, G. L. (1986). The linear free energy relationship between partition coefficients and aqueous solubility of organic liquids. *J. Org. Chem.* **33**, 347–355.

Haque, R. (Ed.) (1980). *Dynamics, Exposure and Hazard Assessment of Toxic Chemicals*. Ann Arbor Science, Ann Arbor, MT.

Haque, R., and Schmedding, D. (1975). A method of measuring the water solubility of hydrophobic chemicals: Solubility of five polychlorinated biphenyls. *Bull. Environ. Contam. Toxicol.* **14**, 13–18.

Hart, W. L., Reynolds, R. C., Krasavage, W. J., Ely, T. S., Bell, R. H., and Raleigh, R. L. (1988). Evaluation of developmental toxicity data: A discussion of some pertinent factors and a proposal. *Risk Anal.* **8**, 59–70.

Hartley, H. O., and Sielken, R. L., Jr. (1977). Estimation of 'safe doses' in carcinogenic experiments. *Biometrics* **33**, 1–12.

Hartwell, J. K., Handy, R., Harris, B., and Williams, S. (1985). Heavy metal esposure in populations living around zinc and copper smelters. *Arch. Environ. Health* **38**, 284–295.

Haseman, J. K., Hoel, D. G., and Jennrich, R. I. (1981). Some practical problems arising from use of the gamma multihit model for risk estimation. *J. Toxicol. Envir. Hlth.*

Hattemer–Frey, H. A., and Travis, C. C. (1987). Human exposure to 2,3,7,8-TCDD. *Annu. Meet. Soc. Risk Anal.*, Abstr. WAM-G5.

Havender, W. (1984a). Peanut butter sandwich deadlier than muffins containing EDB. *Wall St. J.* April 4, p. 1311.

Havender, W. R. (1984b). EDB and the marigold option. *Regulation* (Jan/Feb), 13–17.

Hawley, J. (1985). Assessment of health risk from exposure to contaminated soil. *Risk Anal.* **5**, 289–302.

Hayes, A. W. (1982). *Principles and Methods of Toxicology*. Raven Press, New York.

Hayes, W. J. (1975). *Toxicology of Pesticides.* Williams & Wilkins, Baltimore, MD, pp. 130–131.

Helleiner, O. (1967). The population of Europe from the Black Death of the eve of the vital revolution. In E. E. Rich and C. H. Wilson, Eds., *The Cambridge Economic History of Europe,* Vol. 4. Cambridge Univ. Press. London and New York.

Hill, J. (1781). *Cautions Against the Immoderate Use of Snuff.* Baldwin & Jackson, London.

Himmelstein, K. J., and Lutz, R. J. (1979). A review of the applications of physiologically based pharmacokinetic modeling. *J. Pharmacokin. Biopharm.* **7,** 127–145.

Hoerger, F. (1985). Some current views on risk assessment. Presented at a seminar entitled, *Understanding Environmental Risk* sponsored by the Public Service Research and Dissemination Program, University of California at Davis, Sacramento, CA.

Hughes, J. (1975). *Ecology in Ancient Civilizations.* Univ. of New Mexico Press, Albuquerque.

Hutchinson, J. (1887). Arsenic cancer. *Br. Med. J.* **2,** 1280.

Hutt, P. (1984). Legal considerations in risk assessment under federal regulatory statutes. In J. Rodricks and R. Tardiff, Eds., *Assessment and Management of Chemical Risks.* American Chemical Society, Washington, DC, pp. 84–95.

Ikeda, M., Kozumi, A., Kasahara, N., Watanabe, T., Nakatsuka, H., and Sekita, Y. (1987). The statistical approach to the prediction of the possible presence of pollutant chemicals in the environment. *Regul. Toxicol. Pharmacol.* **7,** 321–336.

Jensen, D. J., and Hummel, R. A. (1982). Secretion of TCDD in milk and cream following the feeding of TCDD to lactating cows. *Bull. Environ. Contam. Toxicol.* **29,** 440–446.

Jensen, D. J., Getzendaner, M. E., Hummel R. A., and Turley, J. (1983). *J. Agric. Food Chem.* **31,** 118–122.

Johnson, B., and Covello, V. T. (Eds.) (1987). *Social and Cultural Construction of Risk: Essays on Risk Selection and Perception.* Reidel Pub., Hingham, MA.

Jones, D., Safe, S., Morcom, E., Coppock, C., and Ivie, W. (1986). Bioavailability of 2, 3, 7, 7-TCDD administered to Holstein dairy cows. *6th Int. Symp. Dioxins Relat. Comp.,* Abstr. BP-20.

Jury, W. A., Farmer, W. J., and Spencer, W. F. (1984). Behavior assessment model for trace organics in soil. II. Chemical classification and parameter sensitivity. *J. Environ. Qual.* **13,** 567–572.

Karickhoff, S. W., Brown, D. S., and Scott, T. A. (1979). Sorption of hydropobic pollutants on natural sediments. *Water Res.* **13,** 241–248.

Kates, R., Honenemser, C., and Kasperson, J. X. (Eds.) (1985). *Perilous Progress: Managing the Hazards of Technology.* Westview Press, Boulder, CO.

Kenaga, E. E. (1972). Guidelines for environmental study of pesticides: Determination of bioconcentration potential. *Residue Rev.* **44,** 73.

Kenaga, E. E. (1975). In R. Haque and V. H. Freed, Eds., *Environmental Dynamics of Pesticides.* Plenum Press, New York, p. 217.

Kenaga, E. E. (1979). Aquatic test organisms and methods useful for assessment of chronic toxicity of chemicals. In K. L. Dickson, A. W. Maki, and J. Cairns, Jr., Eds., *Analyzing the Hazard Evaluation Process.* American Fisheries Society, Washington, DC, pp. 101–111.

Kenaga, E. E. (1980). Correlation of bioconcentration factors of chemicals in aquatic and terrestrial organisms with their physical and chemical properties. *Ecotoxicol. Environ. Saf.* **4,** 26–38.

Kenaga, E. E. (1982a). The use of environmental toxicology and chemistry data in hazard assessment: Progress, needs, challenges. *Environ. Toxicol. Chem.* **1**(1), 69–81.

Kenaga, E. E. (1982b). Predictability of chronic toxicity from acute toxicity of chemicals in fish and aquatic invertebrates. *Environ. Toxicol. Chem.* **1**(4), 347–358.

Kenaga, E. E., and Goring, C. A. I. (1980). Relationship between water solubility, soil sorption, octanol water partitioning and concentration of chemicals in biota. *ASTM Spec. Tech. Publ.* **STP 707,** 78–115.

Kety, S. S. (1951). The theory and applications of the exchange of inert gas at the lungs and tissues. *Pharmacol. Rev.* **3**, 1–41.

Kimbrough, R., Falk, H., Stehr, P., and Fries, G. (1984). Health implications of 2, 3, 7, 8-tetrachlorodibenzo-p-dioxin (TCDD) contamination of residential soil. *J. Toxicol. Environ. Health* **14**, 47–93.

Kocher, C. W., Mahle, N. H., Hummel, R. A., Shadoff, L. A., and Getzendaner, M. E. (1978). A search for the presence of 2, 3, 7, 8-tetrachlorodibenzo-p-dioxin in beef fat. *Bull. Environ. Contam. Toxicol.* **19**, 229–236.

Kormondy, E. J. (1969). *Concepts of Ecology.* Prentice–Hall, Englewood Cliffs, NJ.

Kostecki, P. T., and Calabrese, E. J. (1987). *Petroleum Contaminated Soils: Public and Environment Health Effects.* Wiley, New York.

Krewski, D., and Van Ryzin, J. (1981). Dose response models for quantal response toxicity data. In M. Csorgo, D. Dawson, J. N. K. Rao, and E. Saleh, Eds., *Statistics and Related Topics.* North-Holland, New York, pp. 201–231.

Krewski, D., Brown, C., and Murdoch, D. (1984). Determining "safe" levels of exposure: Safety factors or mathematical models. *Fundam. Appl. Toxicol.* **4**, S383–S394.

LaGoy, P. (1987). Estimated soil ingestion rates for use in risk assessment. *Risk Anal.* **7**, 355–359.

Land, C. E. (1980). In *Perceptions of Risk.* National Council on Radiation Protection and Measurements, Washington, DC, pp. 169–185.

Lanier, M. (1985). *The History of the TLV's.* American Conference of Governmental Industrial Hygienists, Cincinnati, OH.

Lave, L., and Upton, A. C. (Eds.) (1987). *Toxic Chemicals, Health, and the Environment.* Johns Hopkins Univ. Press, Baltimore, MD.

Lee, D. R. (1980). Reference toxicants in quality control of aquatic bioassays. In A. L. Buikema, Jr. and J. Cairns, Jr., Eds., *Aquatic Invertebrate Bioassays.* American Society for Testing and Materials, Philadelphia, PA, pp. 188–199.

Lehmann, A. J., and Fitzhugh, O. G. (1954). 100-fold margin of safety. *Q. Bull.— Assoc. Food Drug Off. U.S.* **18**, 33–35.

Lehmann, A. J., Vorhes, F. A. et al. (1959). *Appraisal of the Safety of Chemicals in Foods, Drugs and Cosmetics.* Published by the Association of Food and Drug Officials of the United States, Washington, DC.

Leidel, N., and Busch, K. A. (1985). Statistical design and data analysis requirements. In *Patty's Industrial Hygiene and Toxicology*, Vol. IIIa, (2nd Ed.) E. Cralley and L. Cralley, Eds. Wiley, New York.

Leo, H., Hansch, C., and Elkins, D. (1971). Partition coefficients and their uses. *Chem. Rev.* **71**, 525–616.

Lepow, M. L., Bruckman, L., Robino, R. A., Markowitz, S., Gillette, M., and Kapish, J. (1974). Role of airborne lead in increased body burden of lead in Hartford children. *Environ. Health Perspect.* **6**, 99–101.

Lepow, M. L., Bruckman, L., Gillette, M., Markowitz, S., Robino, R., and Kapish, J. (1975). Investigations into sources of lead in the environment of urban children. *Environ. Res.* **10**, 415–426.

Leung, H. W., Murray, F. J., and Paustenbach, D. J. (1988). A proposed occupational exposure limit for 2, 3, 7, 8-TCDD. *Am. Ind. Hyg. Assoc. J* (in press).

Lippmann, M., and Schlesinger, R. B. (1979). *Chemical Contamination in the Human Environment.* Oxford Univ. Press, London and New York.

Lipsky, D. (1984). *Assessment of Potential Public Health Impacts of Predicted Emissions of PCDD and PCDF from Brooklyn Naval Yard Resource Recovery Facility.* Fred C. Hart Assoc., New York.

Lowe, L. M., and Chambers, D. B. (1983). TLV's for non-standard work schedules. *Pollut. Eng.*, November, pp. 36–37.

Lowrance, W. (1976). *Of Acceptable Risk.* Wm. Kaufman, Inc., Los Altos, CA.

Lowrance, W. (1981). *Assessment of Health Effects at Chemical Disposal Sites.* Wm. Kaufmann, Inc., Los Altos, CA.

Lowrance, W. (1985). *Modern Science and Human Values.* Oxford Univ. Press, London and New York.

Mabey, W., and Mill, T. (1978). Critical review of hydrolysis of organic compounds in water under environmental conditions. *J. Phys. Chem. Ref. Data* **7**, 383–415.

Macek, K. J., and Sleight, B. H., III (1977). Utility of toxicity tests with embryos and fry of fish in evaluating hazards associated with the chronic toxicity of chemicals to fishes. In F. L. Mayer and J. L. Hamelink, Eds., *Aquatic Toxicology and Hazard Evaluation.* American Society for Testing and Materials, Philadelphia, PA, pp. 137–146.

Macmahon, B., and Cole, P. (1969). Endocrinology and epidemiology of breast cancer. *Cancer* **24**, 1146–1151.

Macek, K. J., Buxton, K. S., Sauter, S., Gnilka, S., and Dean, J. W. (1976). *Chronic Toxicity of Atrazine to Selected Aquatic Invertebrates and Fishes,* Ecol. Res. Ser., EPA-600/3-76-047:50 p. U.S. Environmental Protection Agency, Washington, DC.

Macek, K. J., Petrocelli, S. R., and Sleight, B. H., III (1979). Consideration in assessing the potential for, and significance of, biomagnification of chemical residues in aquatic food chains. *ASTM Spec. Tech. Publ.* **STP 667**, 251–268.

Mackay, D., and Paterson, S. (1982). Calculating fugacity. *Environ. Sci. Technol.* **15**(9), 1006–1014.

Mackay, D., Paterson, S., Cheung, B., and Neely, W. B. (1985a). Evaluating the environmental behavior of chemicals with a fugacity level III model. *Chemosphere* **14**(3/4), 335–374.

Mackay, D., Paterson, S., and Cheung, B. (1985b). Evaluating the environmental fate of chemicals: The fugacity-level III approach as applied to 2, 3, 7, 8-TCDD. *Chemosphere* **14**(6/7), 859–863.

Maibach, H. I., and Gellin, G. A. (1982). *Occupational and Industrial Dermatology.* Yearbook medical publishers, Chicago.

Maki, A. (1979). An analysis of decision criteria in environmental hazard evaluation programs. In K. L. Dickson, A. W. Maki, and J. Cairns, Jr., Eds., *Analyzing the Hazard Evaluation Process.* American Fisheries Society, Washington, DC, pp. 83–100.

Maki, A. W., Dickson, K. L., and Cairns, J., Jr. (Eds.) (1980). *Biotransformation and Fate of Chemicals in the Aquatic Environment.* American Society for Microbiology, Washington, DC.

Mantel, N., and Bryan, W. R. (1961). "Safety" testing of carcinogenic agents. *J. Natl. Cancer Inst. (U.S.)* **27**, 455–460.

Mantel, N., and Schneiderman, M. A. (1975). Estimating "safe" levels, a hazardous undertaking. *Cancer Res.* **35**, 1379–1386.

Mapleson, W. W. (1963). An electric analog for uptake and exchange of inert gases and other agents. *J. Appl. Physiol.* **18**, 197–204.

Martin, W. E. (1964). Loss of Sr-90, Sr-89 and I-131 from fallout of contaminated plants. *Radiat. Bot.* **4**, 275–281.

Mayer, F. L., and Hamelink, J. L. (1977). *Aquatic Toxicology and Hazard Evaluation.* American Society of Testing and Materials, Philadelphia, PA.

McColl, R. (Ed.) (1987). *Environmental Health Risks: Assessment and Management.* Institute for Risk Research, Waterloo, Ontario.

McCord, C. P. (1937). *A Blind Hog's Acorns.* Bell Publ., Chicago, IL.

Menzel, D. (1987). Physiological pharmacokinetic modeling. *Environ. Sci. Technol.* **21**, 944–950.

Merkhofer, M. W. (1986). *Decision Science and Social Risk Management: A Comparative Evaluation of Cost-benefit Analysis, Decision Analysis, and Other Formal Decision-aiding Approaches.* Reidel Publ., Hingham, MA.

Metcalf, R. L. et al. (1975). *Arch. Environ. Contam. Toxicol.* **3**, 151–159.

Milham, S., Jr., and Strong, T. (1974). Human arsenic exposure in relation to a copper smelter. *Environ. Res.* **7**, 176–182.

Miller, G. C., and Zepp, R. G. (1979). Photoreactivity of aquatic pollutants sorbed on suspended sediments. *Environ. Sci. Technol.* **13**, 860–863.

Millican, F. K., Layman, E. M., Lourie, R. S., Takahashi, L. Y., and Dublin, C. C. (1962). The prevalance of ingestion and mouthing of nonedible substances by children. *Clin. Proc. Child. Hosp.* **28**, 207–214.

Moghissi, A. A., Marland, R. E., Congel, F. J., and Eckerman, K. F. (1980). Methodology for environmental human exposure and health risk management. In R. Haque, Ed., *Dynamics, Exposure, and Hazard Assessment of Toxic Chemicals.* Ann Arbor Sci. Press, Ann Arbor, MI, chap. 31.

Motto, H. L., Daines, R. H., Chilko, D. M., and Motto, C. K. (1970). Lead in soils and plants: Its relationship to traffic volumes and proximity to highways. *Environ. Sci. Technol.* **4**, 231–237.

Moolgavkar, S. H. (1986). Carcinogenesis modeling: From molecular biology to epidemiology. *Ann. Rev. Public. Hth.* **7**, 151–169.

Moolgavkar, S. H. (1978). The multistage theory of carcinogenesis and the age distribution of cancer in man. *J. Natl. Cancer. Inst.* **61**, 49–52.

Moolgavkar, S. H., and Knudson, A. G. (1981). Mutation and cancer: A model for human carcinogenesis. *J. Natl. Cancer. Inst.* **66**, 1037–1052.

Moolgavkar, S. H., Dewanji, A., and Venzon, D. J. (1988). A stochastic two-stage model for cancer risk assessment I: The hazard function and probability of tumor. *Risk Anal.* (in press).

Munro, I. C., and Krewski, D. R. (1981). Risk assessment and regulatory decision-making. *Food Cosmet. Toxicol.* **19**, 549–560.

National Academy of Engineering (1986). *Hazards: Technology and Fairness.* National Academy Press, Washington, DC.

National Academy of Sciences (NAS) (1983). *Risk Assessment in the Federal Government: Managing the Process.* National Academy Press, Washington, DC.

National Academy of Sciences (1987). Pharmacokinetics and risk assessment. In *Drinking Water and Health.* Vol. 8. National Academy of Science, Washington, DC.

National Research Council (NRC) (1980) *Lead in the Human Environment.* National Academy Press, Washington, DC.

Neely, W. B. (1982). Organizing data for environmental studies. *Environ Toxicol. Chem.* **1**(3), 259–266.

Neely, W. B. (1977). Material balance analysis of trichlorofluoromethane and carbon tetrachloride in the atmosphere. *Sci. Total Environ.* **8**, 267–274.

Neely, W. B., Branson, D. R., and Blau, G. E. (1974). Partition coefficients to measure bioconcentration potential of organic chemicals in fish. *Environ. Sci. Technol.* **8**, 1113–1115.

Nisbet, I. C. T., and Karch, N. (1983). *Chemical Hazards to Human Reproduction.* Noyes Data Corp., Park Ridge, NJ.

Nohl, J. (1960). *The Black Death.* Ballantine Books, Cambridge, MA.

Norberg, T. J., and Mount, D. I. (1985). A new fathead minnow (*Pimephales promelas*) subchronic toxicity test method. *Environ. Toxicol. Chem.* **4**(5), 711–718.

Office of Science and Technology Policy (OSTP) (1985). Chemical carcinogens, a review of the science and its associated principles. *Fed. Regist.* **50**(50), 10372–10442.

Oliver, B. G. (1984). Uptake of chlorinated organics from anthropogenically contaminated sediments by obigochaete worms, *Can. J. Fish Aquat. Sci.* **41**, 878–883.

Oppenheim, L. (1977). *Ancient Mesopotamia.* Univ. of Chicago Press, Chicago.

Organization for Economic Cooperation and Development (OECD) (1981). *OECD Guidelines for Testing of Chemicals,* Sect. 1: Physical Chemical Properties. 101. UV-VIS Absorption Spectra.

OECD, Paris, France (available from Publications and Information Center, 1750 Pennsylvania Ave., NW, Washington, DC 20006).

Park, C. N., and Snee, R. D. (1983). Quantitative risk assessment: State of the art for carcinogenesis. *Am. Stat.* **37**(4), 427–441.

Paustenbach, D. J. (1984). The engineer's responsibility in occupational disease prevention. In *Industrial Hygiene Aspects of Plant Operations.* Vol. II, Chap. 2, pp. 5–24.

Paustenbach, D. J. (1988). Health risk assessments in toxic tort litigation: Opportunities for improvement. *Record of the New York Bar Assn.* (in press).

Paustenbach, D. J. (1987). Assessing the potential environmental and human health risks of contaminated soil. *Comments Toxicol.* **1**, 185–220.

Paustenbach, D. J., and Langner, R. (1986). Corporate occupational exposure limits: The state of the art. *Amer. Ind. Hyg. Assn. J.* **47**, 809–818.

Paustenbach, D. J., Shu, H. P., and Murray, F. J. (1986). A critical analysis of risk assessment of TCDD contaminated soil. *Regul. Toxicol. Pharmacol.* **6**, 284–307.

Paynter, O. E., Burin, G. J., Jaeger, R. B., and Gregorio, C. A. (1988). Goitrogens and thyroid follicular cell neoplasia: Evidence for a threshold process. *Regul. Toxicol. Pharm.* **8**, 102–119.

Pearson, J. G., Foster, R. B., and Bishop, W. E. (1982). *Aquatic Toxicology and Hazard Assessment,* STP 766. American Society Testing and Materials, Philadelphia, PA.

Pennington, J. A. T. (1983). Revision of the total diet study: Food list and diets. *J. Am. Diet. Assoc.* **82**, 166–173.

Peto, R. (1978). Carcinogenic effects of chronic exposure to very low levels of toxic substances. *Environ. Health Perspect.* **22**, 155–160.

Pfeifer, K. (1984). Bioaccumulation. In *Biomonitoring Applications/Water Quality Management Seminar.* Chemical Manufacturers Association.

Piotrowski, J. (1972). Exposure tests for organic compounds in industry. National Institute of Occupational Safety and Health, Cincinnati, OH.

Poiger, H., and Schlatter, C. (1980). Influence of solvents and absorbents on dermal and intestinal absorption of TCDD. *Food Cosmet. Toxicol.* **18**, 477–481.

Pott, P. (1975). *Cancer Scroti: The Chirurgical Work of Percival Pott.* Clark & Collins, London (originally published in 1775).

Preuss, P. W., and Ehrlich, A. M. (1987). The environmental protection agency's risk assessment guidelines. *J. Am. Pol. Control Assn.* **37**, 784–791.

Rai, K. and van Ryzin, J. (1979). Risk assessment of toxic environmental substances using a generalized multi-hit dose response model. In N. Breslow and A. Whittemore, Eds., *Energy and Health.* SIAM Press, Philadelphia, PA. pp. 99–117.

Ramazzini, B. (1700). *De Morbia artificium.* Capponi, Italy, Chap XX. Ueber biasentumoren bei Fuschsinarbeitern. *Arch. Klin. Chir.* **50**, 588. Ramazzini, B. (1713). *Diseases of Workers* (Wilner Wright, transl. Classics of Medicine Library, Birmingham, AL, 1940).

Ramsey, J. C., and Andersen, M. E. (1984). A physiologically-based description of the inhaled pharmacokinetics of styrene in rats and humans. *Toxical Appl. Pharm.* **73**, 159–175.

Rand, G. M., and Petrocelli, S. R. (1985). *Fundamentals of Aquatic Toxicology.* Hemisphere Publ. Co., Washington, DC.

Rao, K. S., and Schwetz, B. A. (1981). Protecting the unborn. *Occup. Health Safety* (March) 53–61.

Rappaport, S. M., and Selvin, J. (1987). A method for evaluating the mean exposure from a log-normal distribution. *Am. Ind. Hyg. Assoc. J.* **48**, 374–379.

Rehn, L. (1895). Blasengeschwulste bei Fuchsin-Arbeitern. *Arch. Klin. Chir.* **50**, 588–800.

Reinecke, A. J., and Nash, R. G. (1984). Toxicology of TCDD and bioavailability by earthworms. *Soil Biol. Biochem.* **16**, 45–49.

Riggs, D. S. (1963). *The Mathematical Approach to Physiological Problems.* MIT Press, Cambridge, MA.

Roberts, T., Gizyn, W., and Hutchinson, T. (1974). Lead contamination of air, soil, vegetation and people in the vicinity of secondary lead smelters. *Trace Substances Environ. Health* **8**, 155–166.

Rodricks, J. V. (1988). Origins of risk assessment in food-safety decision-maxing. *J. Amer. Coll. Toxicol* (in press).

Rodricks, J. V., and Turnbull, D. (1985). Risk assessment: Biological considerations. In H. Milman and E. Weisburger, Eds., *Handbook of Carcinogen Testing.* Noyes Data Corp., Park Ridge, NJ.

Rodricks, J. V., Brett, S. N., and Wrenn, G. C. (1987). Risk decisions in federal regulatory agencies. *Regul. Toxicol. Pharmacol.* **7**, 307–320.

Roels, H., Buchet, J. P., and Lauwerys, R. R. (1980). Exposure to lead by the oral and pulmonary routes of children living in the vicinity of a primary lead smelter. *Environment* **22**, 81–94.

Romney, E. M., Lindberg, N. G., Hawthorne, H. A., Bystrom, B. B., and Larson, K. H. (1963). Contamination of plant foliage with radioactive nuclides. *Annu. Rev. Plant Physiol.* **14**, 271–279.

Ruckelshaus. W. D. (1984a). Science, risk and public policy. *Science* **221**, 1026–1028.

Ruckelshaus, W. D. (1984b). *Vital Speeches of the Day,* April 1. City News Publ. Co., Southold, NY.

Rupp, E. M., Parzyck, D. C., Walsh, P. J., Booth, R. S., Raridon, R. J., and Whitfield, B. L. (1978). Composite hazard index for assessing limiting exposures to environmental pollutants: Application through a case study. *Environ. Sci. Technol.* **12**, 802–807.

Russell, R. S. (1966). Entry of radioactive materials into plants. In R. S. Russell, Ed., *Radioactivity and Human Diet* Pergamon, New York, Chap. 5.

Sato, A., and Nakajima, T. (1979). Partition coefficients of some aromatic hydrocarbons and ketones in water, blood, and oil. *Brit. J. Ind. Med.* **36**, 231–234.

Sayre, J. W., Charney, E., Vostal, J., and Pless, B. (1974). House and hand dust as a potential source of childhood lead exposure. *Am. J. Dis. Child.* **127**, 167–170.

Schaum, J. (1984). *Risk Analysis of TCDD Contaminated Soil.* Office of Health and Environmental Assessment, U.S. Environmental Protection Agency, Washington, DC.

Scheuplein, R. J. (1987). Risk assessment and food safety: A scientist's and regulators view. *Food Drug Cosmet. Law J.* **42**, 237–250.

Schwing, R. C., and Albers, W. A., Jr. (Eds.) (1980). *Societal Risk Assessment: How Safe is Safe Enough.* Plenum Press, New York.

Schaeffer, R. (1977). A theoretical model for identifying a threshold for carcinogens. *Ill. Water Poll.* **13**, 131–139.

Sherman, B. M., and Korenman, S. G. (1974). Inadequate corpus luteum function: A pathopysiological interpretation of human breast cancer epidemiology. *Cancer (Philadelphia)* **33**, 1306–1312.

Shigan, S. S. (1976). Methods for predicting chronic toxicity parameters of substances in the area of water hygiene. *Environ. Health Perspect.* **13**, 83–89.

Shu, H. P., Paustenbach, D. J., and Murray, F. J. (1987). A critical evaluation of the use of mutagenesis, carcinogenesis, and tumor promotion data in a cancer risk assessment of 2, 3, 7, 8-tetrachlorodibenzo-p-dioxin. *Regul. Toxicol. Pharm.* **7**, 57–88.

Shu, H., Paustenbach, D., Murray, J., Marple, L., Brunck, B., Dei Rossi, D., Webb, A. S., and Tietelbaum, T. (1988a). Bioavailability of soil-bound TCDD: Oral bioavailability in the rat. *Fundam. Appl. Toxicol,* **10**, 648–654.

Shu, H., Tietelbaum, P., Webb, A. S., Marple, L., Brunck, B., Dei Rossi, D., Murray, J., and Paustenbach, D. (1988b). Bioavailability of soil-bound TCDD: Dermal bioavailability in the rat. *Fundam. Appl. Toxicol.* **10**, 335–343.

Sicherman, B. (1984). *Alice Hamilton: A Life in Letters*. Harvard Univ. Press, Cambridge, MA, pp. 158–160.

Sielken, R. L. (1985). Some issues in the quantitative modelling portion of cancer risk assessment. *Regul. Toxicol. Pharmacol.* **5**, 175–181.

Sielken, R. L. (1987a). Quantitative cancer risk assessments for 2, 3, 7, 8-TCDD. *Food Chem. Toxicol.* **25**, 257–267.

Sielken, R. L. (1987b). Statistical evaluations reflecting the skewness in the distribution of TCDD levels in human adipose tissue. *Chemosphere* **16**(8–9), 2135–2140.

Sielken, R. L. (1987c). The capabilities, sensitivity, pitfalls, and future of quantitative risk assessment. In Stephen Nicoll, Ed., *Environmental Health Risks*. Waterloo Press, Waterloo, Ontario, pp. 95–131.

Sielken, R. L. (1988). A response to Crump's evaluation of Sielken's dose-response assessment for TCDD. *Food Chem. Toxicol.* **26**, 79–83.

Silkworth, J., McMartin, D., DeCaprio, A., Rej, R., O'Keefe, P., and Kaminsky, L. (1982). Acute toxicity in guinea pigs and rabbits of soot from a polychlorinated biphenyl-containing transformer fire. *Toxicol. Appl. Pharmacol.* **65**, 425–429.

Sjöberg, L. (1986). *Risk & Society*. Allen & Unwin, Winchester, MA.

Smith, A. H. (1987). Infant exposure assessment for breast milk dioxins and furans derived from waste incineration emissions. *Risk Anal.* **7**, 347–353.

Snow, J. (1855). *On the Mode of Communication of Cholera*. Churchill, London.

Snyder, W. S. (1975). *Report of the Task Group on Reference Man*, ICRP No. 23. Pergamon, New York.

Spacie, A., and Hamelink, J. L. (1985). Bioaccumulation. In G. Rand and S. Petrocelli, Eds., *Fundamentals of Aquatic Toxicology*. Hemisphere, New York, Chap. 17, pp. 495–525.

Spencer, W. F., and Farmer, W. J. (1980). Assessment of the vapor behavior of toxic organic chemicals. In R. Hague, Ed., *Dynamics, Exposure and Hazard Assessment of Toxic Chemicals*. Ann Arbor Science, Ann Arbor, MI, pp. 143–161.

Starr, C. (1969). Social benefits versus technological risk. *Science* **165**, 1232–1238.

Starr, C. (1985). Risk management, assessment, and acceptability. *Risk Anal.* **5**, 97–102.

Stern, A. M., and Walker, C. R. (1978). Hazard assessment of toxic substances: Environmental fate testing of organic chemicals and ecological effects testing. *ASTM Spec. Tech. Publ.* **STP 657**, 81–131.

Stevens, K. R., and Gallo, M. A. (1982). Practical considerations in the conduct of chronic toxicity studies. In A. W. Hayes, Ed., *Principals and Methods in Toxicology*. Raven Press, New York.

Stokinger, H. E. (1964). Modus operandi of threshold limits committee of ACGIH *Am. Ind. Hyg. Assoc. J.* **25**, 589–594.

Stokinger, H. E. (1970). Criteria and procedures for assessing the toxic responses to industrial chemicals. In *Permissible Levels of Toxic Substances in the Working Environment*. International Labor Office, World Health Organization, Geneva.

Stokinger, H. E. (1981). Threshold limit values. Part I. In *Dangerous Properties of Industrial Materials Report*. Van Nostrand-Relmhold, New York, pp. 8–13.

Squire, R. (1981). Ranking animal carcinogens. *Science* **214**, 887–880.

Te Brake, W. (1975). Air pollution and fuel crisis in pre-industrial London, 1250–1650. *Technol. Cult.* **16**, 337–359.

Teich, A. H., and Thornton, R. (1982). *Science, Technology, and the Issues of the Eighties: Policy Outlook*. Westview Press, Boulder, CO.

Thibodeaux, L. J. (1979). *Chemodynamics, Environmental Movement of Chemicals in Air, Water and Soil*. Wiley, New York.

Thibodeaux, L. J., and Lipsky, D. (1985). *Hazard. Waste Mater.* **2**, 225–235.

Thornton, I., and Abrahams, P. (1981). Soil ingestion as a pathway of metal intake into grazing livestock. In *Proceeding of the International Conference on Heavy Metals in the Environment*, CEP Consultants, Edinburgh, pp. 167–172.

Thorslund, T. W., Brown, C. C., and Charnley, G. (1987). Biologically motivated cancer risk models. *Risk Anal.* **7**, 109–119.

Thurston, R. V., Gilfoil, T. A., Meyn, E. L., Zajdel, R. K., Aoki, T. I., and Veith, G. D. (1985). Comparative toxicity of ten organic chemicals to ten common aquatic species. *Water Res.* **19**, 1145–1155.

Tinsley, I. J. (1979). *Chemical Concepts in Pollutant Behavior.* Wiley, New York.

Travis, C. C., Richter, S. A., Crouch, C. E., Wilson, R., and Klema, E. D. (1987). Cancer risk management. *Environ. Sci. Technol.* **21**, 415–420.

Trijonis, J., Eldon, J., Gins, J., and Berglund, G. (1980). *Analysis of the St. Louis RAMS Ambient Particulate Data*, EPA Rep. 450/4-80-006a. Produced by Technology Service Corporation under EPA contract 68-02-2931 for the Office of Air, Noise, and Radiation of the U.S. Environmental Protection Agency.

Truhaut, R. (1979). An overview of the problem of thresholds for chemical carcinogens. *IARC Sci. Publ.* **25**, 191.

Tulp, M. T. M., and Hutzinger, O. (1978). Some thoughts on aqueous solubilities and partition coefficients of PCB, and the mathematical correlation between bioaccumulation and physico-chemical properties. *Chemosphere* **10**, 849–860.

U. S. Department of Health and Human Services (1986). *Determining Risks to Health: Federal Policy and Practice.* Auburn House Publ., Dover, MA.

U. S. Food and Drug Administration (USFDA) (1984). *Environmental Assessment Technical Handbook.* Center for Food Safety and Applied Nutrition and the Center for Veterinary Medicine, USFDA, Washington, DC.

Unna, P. G. (1894). *Die Histopathologie der Hautkrankheiten.* Hirschwald, Berlin.

Van den Berg, M., De Vroom, E., Van Greevenbroek, M., Olie, K., and Hutzinger, O. (1985). Bioavailability of PCDDs and PCDFs adsorbed on fly ash in rat, guinea pig and Syrian golden hamster. *Chemosphere* **14**, 865–869.

Van Ryzin, J. (1980). Quantitative risk assessment. *J. Occup. Medicine.* **22**, 321–326.

Van Ryzin, J. and Rai, K. (1979). The use of quantal response data to make prediction. In H. P. Witschi, Ed., *The Scientific Basis of Toxicity Assessment.* Elsevier/North Holland Biomedical. New York, pp. 273–290.

Veith, G. D., De Foe, D. L., and Bergstedt, B. V. (1979). Measuring and estimating the bioconcentration factor of chemicals in Fish. *J. Fish Res. Board Can.* **36**, 1040–1048.

Veith, G. C., Macek, K. J., Petrocelli, S. R., and Carroll, J. (1980). An evaluation of using water partition coefficients and water solubility to estimate bioconcentration factors for organic chemicals in fish. In J. G. Eaton, P. R. Parrish, and A. C. Hendricks, Eds., *Aquatic Toxicology.* American Society for Testing and Materials, Philadelphia, PA, pp. 116–129.

Wall Street Journal (1987). *Scaring the Public*, July 7.

Weber, J. B. (1972a). Interaction of organic pesticides with particulate matter in aquatic and soil systems. *Adv. Chem. Ser.* **111**, 55–120.

Weber, W. J. (1972b). *Physicochemical Processes for Water Quality Control.* Wiley (Interscience), New York.

Weed, S. B., and Weber, J. B. (1974). Pesticide-organic matter interactions. In W. D. Guenzi, Ed., *Pesticides in Soil and Water.* Soil Science Society of America, Madison, WI, pp. 39–66.

Weil, C. S. (1972). Statistics versus safety factors and scientific judgement in the evaluation of safety for man. *Toxicol. Appl. Pharmacol.* **21**, 454–463.

Weisburger, J. H., and Williams, G. W. (1981). The decision point approach for systematic carcinogen testing. *Food Cosmet. Toxicol.* **19**, 561–566.

Weisburger, J. H., and Williams, G. W. (1986). Chemical carcinogens. In C. D. Klaassen, J. Doull, and M. Amdur, Eds., *Casarett and Doull's Toxicology: The Basic Science of Poisons,* Macmillan, New York.

Weiss, B. (1988). Neurobehavioral toxicity as a basis for risk assessment. *Trends Pharmacolog. Sci.* **(9)**2, 59–62.

Wester, R. C., and Noonan, P. K. (1980). Relevance of animal models for percutaneous absorption. *Int. J. Pharm.* **7**, 99–110.

Whipple, C. G. (1986). Dealing with uncertainty about risk in risk management. In *Hazards: Technology and Fairness.* National Academy Press, Washington, DC.

White, L. (1967). The historical roots of our ecological crisis. *Science* **155**, 1203–1207.

Whitehead, R. G., and Paul, A. A. (1981). Infant growth and human milk requirement. *Lancet* **2**, 161–163.

Williams, D. T., LeBel, G. L., and Jenkins, E. (1984). A comparison of organochlorine residues in human adipose tissue autopsy samples from two Ontario municipalities. *J. Toxicol. Environ. Health* **13**, 19–29.

Wilson, J. (1973). Present status of drugs as teratogens in man. *Teratology* **7**, 3–16.

Wilson, R., and Crouch, E. A. C. (1987). Risk assessment and comparisons: An introduction. *Science* **236**, 267–270.

Winslow, Q. (1923). *The Evolution and Significance of the Modern Public Health Campaign.* Yale Univ. Press, New Haven, CT.

World Health Organization (1977). *Methods Used in Establishing Permissible Levels in Occupational Exposure to Harmful Agents,* Tech. Rep. 601. International Labor Office, WHO, Geneva.

Yaffee, Y., Jenkins, D., Mahon-Haft, H., et al. (1983). Epidemiological monitoring of the environmental lead exposures in California state hospitals. *Sci. Total Environ. Health* **38**, 237–245.

Yankel, A., von Lindern, I., and Walter, S. (1977). The Silver Valley lead study: The relationship between childhood blood lead levels and environmental exposure. *J. Air Pollut. Control Assoc.* **27**, 763–767.

Young, A. L. (1983). Long term studies on the persistence and movement of TCDD in a national ecosystem. In R. E. Tucker, A. L. Young, and A. P. Gray, Eds., *Human and Environmental Risks of Chlorinated Dioxins and Related Compounds.* Plenum Press, New York, pp. 173–190.

Young, A. L., and Cockerham, L. G. (1985). Fate of TCDD in field ecosystem-assessment and significance for Luran exposures. In M. A. Kamrin, and P. W. Rodgers, Eds., *Dioxins in the Environment* Hemisphere, New York, Chap. 11, pp. 153–171.

Young, A. L., Thalken, C. E., and Ward, W. E. (1975). Air Force Tech. Rep. AFATL-TR-75-142. Air Force Assessment Laboratory, Eglin AFB, FL (available from National Technical Information Services, Springfield, VA).

Young, F. A. (1987) Risk assessment: The convergence of science and the law. *Regul. Toxicol. Pharmacol.* **7**, 179–184.

Ziegler, P. (1969). *The Black Death.* Penguin Books, Middlesex, England.

Zielhuis, R. L. (1975). Permissible limits for chemical exposures. In C. Zenz, Ed., *Occupational Medicine.* Year Book Medical Publishers, Chicago, IL, pp. 579—588.

Zielhuis, R. L., and van der Kreek, F. (1979a). Calculations of a safety factor in setting health based permissible levels for occupational exposure. A proposal I. *Int. Arch. Occup. Environ. Health* **42**, 191–201.

Zielhuis, R. L., and van der Kreek, F. W. (1979b). Calculations of safety factor in setting health based permissible levels for occupational exposure. A proposal II. Comparison of extra-polated and published permissible levels. *Int. Arch. Occup. Environ. Health* **42**, 203–215.

Zinssler, H. (1935). *Rats, Lice, and History.* Atlantic Monthly Press, New York.

SUPPLEMENTAL READINGS

American Petroleum Institute (1985). *Biomonitoring: Techniques for Measuring the Biological Effects of Liquid Effluents.* Prepared by EA Engineering Science, and Technology, Inc. and Biological Monitoring, Inc. API, 1220 L Street NW, Washington, DC.

Bartman, T. R. (1982). Regulating benzene. In L. B. Lave, Ed., *Quantitative Risk Assessment in Regulation.* Brookings Institution Press, Washington, DC.

Biesinger, K. E., and Christense, G. M. (1972). Effects of various metals on survival, growth, reproduction, and metabolism of *Daphnia magna. J. Fish. Res. Board Can.* **29**, 1691–1700.

Bishop, W. E., and Maki, A. W. (1980). A critical comparison of two bioconcentration test methods. In J. G. Eaton, P. R. Parrish, and A. C. Hendricks, Eds., *Aquatic Toxicology.* American Society for Testing and Materials, Philadelphia, PA, pp. 61–77.

Blumberg, P. M., Delclos, K. B., Dunn, J. A., Jaken, S., Leach, K. L., and Yeh, E. (1983). Phorbol ester receptors and the in vivo effects of tumor promoters. *Ann. N.Y. Acad. Sci.* **407**, 303–315.

Bonaccorsi, A., di Domencio, A., Fanelli, R., Merli, F., Motta, R., Vanzati, R., and Zapponi, G. A. (1984). *Arch Toxicol., Suppl.* **7**, 431–434.

Branson, D. R., Blau, G. E., Alexander, H. C., and Neely, W. B. (1975). Bioconcentration of 2, 2′, 4, 4′-tetrachlorobiphenyl in rainbow trout as measured by an accelerated test. *Trans. Am. Fish. Soc.* **4**, 785–792.

Brungs, W. A., and Mount, D. I. (1978). Introduction to a discussion of the use of aquatic toxicity tests for evaluation of the effects of toxic substances. In J. Cairns, Jr., K. S. Dickson, and A. W. Maki, Eds., *Estimating the Hazard of Chemical Substances to Aquatic Life.* American Society for Testing and Materials, Philadelphia, PA, pp. 15–32.

Buikema, A. L., Neiderlehner, B. R., and Cairns, J., Jr. (1982). Biological monitoring. Part IV. Toxicity testing. *Water Res.* **16**, 239–262.

Clement Associates, Inc. (1986). *Endangerment Assessment for the Smuggler Mountain Site, Pitkin County, Colorado.* Prepared for the U.S. EPA (Region VIII), under Contract No. 68-01-6939.

Collins, M., and Rozengurt, E. (1982). Stimulation of DNA synthesis in murine fibroblasts by the tumor promoter teleocidin: Relationship to phorbol esters and vasopressin. *Biochem. Biophys. Res. Commun.* **104**, 1159–1166.

Cooper, M. (1957). *Pica.* Thomas, Springfield, IL, pp. 60–74.

Corn, M., and Breysse, P. N. (1985). Human exposure estimates for hazardous waste site risk assessment. In D. G. Hoel, R. A. Merrill, and F. D. Perera, Eds., *Risk Quantitation and Regulatory Policy.* Banbury Rep. No. 19. Cold Spring Harbor Laboratory, Cold Spring Harbor, New York, pp. 283–292.

Crosby, D. G., and Wong, A. S. (1977). *Science* **195**, 1337–1338.

Davidson, I. W. F., Parker, J. C., and Beliles, R. P. (1986). Biological basis for extrapolation across mammalian species. *Regul. Toxicol. Pharm.* **6**, 211–237.

Davis, J. C. (1977). Standardization and protocols of bioassays-their role and significance for monitoring research and regulatory usage. In W. R. Parker, P. E. Wells, and G. F. Westlake, Eds., *Proceedings of the Third Aquatic Toxicity Workshop,* Environ. Prot. Serv. Rep. (EPS-5-AR-771-1). Halifax, Nova Scotia, Canada, pp. 1–14.

Devine, J. M., Konishita, G. B. Peterson, R. P., and Picard, G. L. (1986). *Arch. Environ. Contam. Toxicol.* **15**, 113–119.

di Domencio, A., Silano, V., Viviano, G., and Zapponi, G. (1980). Accidental release of 2, 3, 7, 8-TCDD at Seveso, Italy. Part V. Environmental persistence of TCDD in soil. *Ecotoxicol. Environ. Saf.* **4**, 339–345.

El Sayed, E. I., Graves, J. B., and Bonner, F. L. (1967). Chlorinated hydrocarbon insecticide residues in selected insects and birds found in association with cotton fields. *J. Agric. Food Chem.* **15**(6), 1014–1017.

Environmental Protection Agency (1979). Toxic substances control act premanufacture testing of new chemical substances. *Fed. Regist.* **44**, 16240–16292.

Environmental Protection Agency (1984). *Air Quality Criteria for Lead*, Vol. 2, EPA-600/8-83-028A. USEPA, Washington, DC.

Environmental Protection Agency (1984). *National Emission Standards for Hazardous Air Pollutants; Benzene Emissions from Maleic Anhydride Plants, Ethylbenzene/Styrene Plants, and Benzene Storage Vessels; Proposed Withdrawal of Proposed Standards, Fed. Regist.* **49**, 8386, 8388. USEPA, Washington, DC ["Benzene NESHAPS Withdrawal Notice"].

Environmental Protection Agency (1984). *National Emission Standards for Hazardous Air Pollutants; Regulation of Radionuclides; Withdrawal of Proposed Standards, Fed. Regist.* **49**, 43906, 43910. USEPA, Washington, DC ["Radionuclides NESHAPS Withdrawal Notice"].

Environmental Protection Agency (1985). *Health Assessment Document for Polychlorinated Dibenzo-p-dioxins*, Final Report, EPA-600/8-84-014F. Office of Environmental Assessment, USEPA, Cincinnati, OH.

Ernst, W. (1977). Determination of the bioconcentration potential of marine organisms—A steady-state approach. *Chemosphere* **11**, 731–740.

Geckler, J. R., Horning, W. R., Neiheisel, T. M., Pickering, Q. H., and Robinson, E. L. (1976). *Validity of Laboratory Tests for Predicting Copper Toxicity in Streams*, EPA-600/3-76/1816. Office of Research and Development, Environmental Protection Agency, National Technical Information Service, Springfield, VA.

Gillette, J. W. (1983). A comprehensive prebiological screen for exotoxicologic effects. *Environ. Toxicol. Chem.* **2**(4), 463–476.

Gold, R. E., and Holcslaw, T. (1985). In *Dermal Exposure Related to Pesticide Use.* American Chemical Society, Washington, DC, pp. 253–264.

Gordus, A. A., and Bernstein, R. B. (1954). Isotope effect in continuous ultraviolet spectra: Methyl bromide-d_3 and chloroform-d. *J. Chem. Phys.* **22**, 790–795.

Henderson, C. (1957). Application factors to be applied to bioassays for the safe disposal of toxic wastes. In *Biological Problems in Water Pollution.* U.S. Department of Health, Education and Welfare, Public Health Service, Washington, DC, pp. 31–37.

Hendrix, P. F. (1982). Ecological toxicology: Experimental analysis of toxic substances in ecosystems. *Environ. Toxicol. Chem.* **1**(2), 193–199.

Hoerger, F. D., and Kenaga, E. E. (1972). Pesticide residues on plants. Correlation of representative data as a basis for estimation of their magnitude in the environment. *Environ. Qual.* **1**, 9–28.

Horning, W. B., and Weber, C. I. (1985). *Methods for Estimating the Chronic Toxicity of Effluents and Receiving Water to Freshwater Organisms.* Office of Research and Development, Cincinnati, OH.

Isensee, A. R., and Jones, G. E. (1971). Absorption and translocation of root and foliage applied 2, 4-dichlorophenol, 2, 7-dichlorodibenzo-p-diolon, and 2, 3, 7, 8-TCDD. *J. Agr. Food. Chem.* **19**, 1210–1214.

Jarvinen, A. W., and Tyo, R. M. (1979). Toxicity to minnows of endrin in food and water. *Arch. Environ. Contam. Toxicol.*

Kenaga, E. E., Whitney, W. K., Hardy, J. L., and Doty, A. E. (1965). Laboratory tests with Dursban® insecticide. *J. Econ. Entomol.* **58**(6), 1043–1050.

Kimmel, C. A., and Gaylor, D. W. (1988). Issues in qualitative and quantitative risk analysis for developmental toxicology. *Risk Anal.* **8**, 15–20.

Krishna, J. G., and Casida, J. E. (1966). Fate in rats of the radiocarbon from ten variously labelled methyl and dimethylcarbamate C^{14} insecticide chemicals and their hydrolysis products. *J. Agric. Food Chem.* **14**(2), 98–105.

Krzeminski, S. F., Gilbert, J. T., and Ritts, J. A. 1977. A pharmacokinetic model for predicting pesticide residues in fish. *Arch. Environ. Contam. Toxicol.* **5**, 157–165.

Lacher, J. R., Hummel, L. E., Bohmafalk, E. F., and Park, J. D. (1950). The near ultraviolet absorption spectra of some fluorinated derivatives of methane and ethylene. *J. Am. Chem. Soc.* **72**, 5486–5489.

Lu, P., and Metcalf, R. L. (1975). Environmental fate and biodegradability of benzene derivatives as studied in a model aquatic ecosystem. *Environ. Health Perspect.* **10**, 269–284.

Macek, K. J., Lindberg, M. A., Sauter, S., Buxton, K. S., and Costa, P. A. (1976). *Toxicity of Four Pesticides to Water Fleas and Fathead Minnows*, Ecol. Res. Ser. EPA-600/3-76-099. U.S. Environmental Protection Agency, Washington, DC.

Macek, K. J., Birge, W., Mayer, F. L., Buikema, A. L., Jr., and Maki, A. W. (1978). Discussion session synopsis of the use of aquatic toxicity tests for evaluation of the effects of toxic substances. In J. Cairns, Jr., K. L. Dickson, and A. W. Maki, Eds., *Estimating the Hazard of Chemical Substances to Aquatic Life.* American Society for Testing and Materials. Philadelphia, PA, pp. 27–32.

Maddy, K. T., Wang, R. G., Knaak, J. B., Liao, C. L., Edmission, S. C., and Winter, C. K. (1985). In *Dermal Exposure Related to Pesticide Use.* American Chemical Society, Washington, DC, pp. 445–465.

Maki, A. W. (1979). Correlations between *Daphnia magna* and fathead minnow (*Pimephales promeals*) chronic toxicity values for several classes of test substances. *J. Fish. Res. Board Can.* **36**, 411–421.

Morishima, H., Koga, T., Kawai, H., Honda, Y., and Katsurayama, K. (1977). *J. Radiat Res.* **18**, 139–150.

Mount, D. I. (1977). An assessment of application factors in aquatic toxicology. In R. A. Tubb, Ed., *Recent Advances in Fish Toxicology*, EPA-600/3-770-085. Office of Research and Development, Environmental Protection Agency, National Technical Information Service, Springfield, VA, pp. 183–190.

Mount, D. I. (1979). Adequacy of laboratory data for protecting aquatic communities. In K. L. Dickson, A. W. Maki, and J. Cairns, Jr., Eds., *Analyzing the Hazard Evaluation Process.* American Fisheries Society, Washington, DC, pp. 112–118.

Nebeker, A. V., Puglisi, F. A., and Defoe, D. L. (1974). Effect of polychlorinated biphenyl compounds on survival and reproduction of the fathead minnow and flagfish. *Trans. Am. Fish. Soc.* **103**, 562–568.

Neely, W. G., Branson, D. R., and Blau, G. E. (1974). The use of the partition coefficient to measure the bioconcentration potential of organic chemicals in fish. *Environ. Sci. Technol.* **8**, 1113–1115.

Nice, M. M. (1938). The biological significance of bird weights. *Bird-Banding* **9**(1), 1–11.

Oliver, B. G. (1984). Uptake of chlorinated organics from anthropogenically contaminated sediments by oligochaete worms. *Can. J. Fish. Aquat. Sci.* **41**, 878–883.

Oonnithan, E. S., and Casida, J. E. (1968). Oxidation of methyl and dimethylcarbamate insecticide chemicals by microsomal enzymes and anticholinesterase activity of the metabolites. *J. Agric. Food Chem.* **16**(1), 28–44.

Peltier, W., and Weber, C. I. (1985). *Methods for Measuring the Acute Toxicity of Effluents to Aquatic Organisms.* Office of Research and Development, Cincinnati, OH.

Spittler, T. M., and Feder, W. A. (1979). *Commun. Soil Sci. Plant Anal.* **9**, 1195–1210.

Sprague, J. B. (1969). Measurement of pollutant toxicity to fish. I. Bioassay methods for acute toxicity. *Water Res.* **3**, 793–821.

Sprague, J. B. (1970). Measurement of pollutant toxicity to fish. II. Utilizing and applying bioassay results. *Water Res.* **4**, 3–32.

Sprague, J. B. (1971). Measurement of pollutant toxicity to fish. III. Sublethal effects and "safe" concentrations. *Water Res.* **5**, 245–266.

Sprague, J. B. (1973). The ABCs of pollutant bioassay using fish. In J. Cairns, Jr. and K. L. Dickson, Eds., *Biological Methods for the Assessment of Water Quality.* American Society for Testing and Materials, Philadelphia, PA, pp. 6–30.

Stephan, C. E. (1977). Methods for calculating an LC50. In F. L. Mayer and J. L. Hamelink, Eds., *Aquatic Toxicology and Hazard Evaluation* American Society for Testing and Materials, Philadelphia, PA, pp. 65–85.

Stickel, W. H., Hayne, D. W., and Stickel, L. F. (1965). Effects of Heptachlor-contaminated earthworms on woodcocks. *J. Wildl. Manage.* **29**(1), 132–146.

Thalken, C. E., and Young, A. L. (1983). In R. E. Tucker, A. L. Young, and A. P. Gray, Eds., *Human and Environmental Risks of Chlorinated Dioxins and Related Compounds.* Plenum Press, New York.

Tucker, R. K., and Crabtree, D. G. (1970). *Handbook of Toxicity of Pesticides to Wildlife,* Fish Wildl. Serv., Resour. Publ. No. 84. Denver Wildlife Research Center, Denver, CO.

Travis, C. T., and White, R. K. (1988). Interspecies scaling of toxicity data. *Risk Anal.* **8**, 119–126.

U.S. Department of the Interior (1964). *Pesticide-Wildlife Studies. A review of Fish and Wildlife Service Investigations During the Calendar Year,* Circ. No. 199. Fish and Wildlife Service, U.S. Department of the Interior, Washington, DC, pp. 98–106.

U.S. Environmental Protection Agency (1984). *Air Quality Criteria for Particulate Matter and Sulfur Oxides,* Vol. 2, EPA-600-8-82-029bF. Office of Environmental Criteria and Assessment, USEPA, Research Triangle Park, NC, pp. 5–106 to 5–112.

U.S. Environmental Protection Agency (1985). *Technical Support Document for Water Quality-Based Toxics Control.* Office of Water, USEPA, Washington, DC.

Verloop, A. (1972). The use of linear free energy parameters and other experimental constants in structure activity studies. In E. J. Ariens, Ed., *Drug Design.* Vol. 3. Academic Press, New York, p. 133.

Vermeer, D. L., and Frate, D. A. (1979). *Am. J. Clin. Nutr.* **32**, 2129–2135.

Welty, J. C. (1963). *The Life of Birds.* Knopf, New York.

Williams, E., Meikle, R. W., and Redemann, C. T. (1964). Identification of metabolites of zectran insecticide in dog urine. *J. Agric. Food Chem.* **12**(5), 457–461.

Wipf, H. K., Homberger, E., Neimer, N., Ranalder, U. B., Vetter, W., and Vuilleumeir, J. P. (1982). In O. Hutzinger et al., Eds., *Chlorinated Dioxins and Related Compounds: Impact on the Environment.* Pergamon, New York, pp. 115–126.

Zepp, R. G. (1978). Quantum yields for reaction of pollutants in dilute aqueous solution. *Environ. Sci. Technol.* **12**, 327–329.

2

Risk, Uncertainty, and Causation: Quantifying Human Health Risks

Louis Anthony Cox, Jr.
US West Advanced Technologies, Englewood, Colorado

Paolo F. Ricci
Lawrence Berkeley Laboratory and University of California, Berkeley, California

1 INTRODUCTION

From their beginnings in the health, safety, and environmental impact statements and regulations of the early 1970s, health risk analyses have been concerned largely with the problem of defining *acceptable risk*. In brief, the nation has had to evaluate *what combinations of net economic benefits versus greater health and safety risks should society accept* (1, 2). Rational public management of important economic activities—activities such as the generation of electricity, transportation of hazardous chemicals, or the release, sale, and consumption of new pharmaceutical products, as well as the sale and consumption of cigarettes—requires both a set of analytic methods for quantitatively assessing the risks attributable to these activities and a set of normative decision principles for comparing the risks to the benefits. With these comparisons, acceptability can be evaluated and risk management decisions can be made.

This chapter and Chapter 3 examine a subset of the theory and practice of risk management: the portion that deals with judging the "acceptability" of economic activities that may produce chronic health risks. Unlike systems safety analysis, the art (not science) of assessing chronic health effects is still immature and lacking precision. Specialists disagree over how to define even fundamental concepts, such as *synergistic interaction* between factors, or the proportion of the health risk that should be considered "attributable" to a specific factor when many factors may interact to produce a disease such as cancer.

The development of risk assessments of chronic health effects often poses fewer technical hurdles than does assessment of *catastrophic risks* such as those from petroleum refinery fires, nuclear power plant accidents, pipeline ruptures, or industrial explosions. Statistical and epidemiological methods developed by public health scientists supplement the usual causal and mathematical engineering models typically used by risk assessors, for example, environmental fate and transport models for the dispersion and transformation of pollutants from an industrial facility, demographic and activity models for the exposure of surrounding populations to the pollutants, and pharmacokinetic and compartmental biological models for patterns of pollutant intake and uptake in the population and for effects of the doses received by individuals. The combination of empirical insights from epidemiological investigations coupled with theoretical insights from causal models sometimes allows risk assessments for chronic health effects to lead to testable estimates of risk. The uncertainties associated with such risk estimates can often be fairly well described and can be presented to risk managers, along with the other results of the risk assessment, to assist them in their decisionmaking.

Once a risk has been described as precisely as possible and the remaining uncertainties about it have been stated, a risk manager (who will often be a public decisionmaker) must decide whether to accept it or to exert further control over it. Whether a risk is acceptable generally depends not only on its objective quantitative magnitude and uncertainty but also on social and political value factors. For example, a fully informed cancer patient, cognizant of the risks and uncertainties associated with a new, unproven drug, might consider it personally acceptable. But if he works for the Food and Drug Administration (FDA), he might not find it acceptable for release to the public. Acceptability depends on the responsibilities that acceptance entails. Similarly, the extent to which society should constrain a manufacturer from offering risky products (e.g., cigarettes, laetrile) to willing, informed consumers depends on value judgments about how responsibility for deciding risk acceptability should be divided between manufacturers and consumers. What constitutes an acceptable risk for one person to offer to another depends at least in part on rights (e.g., the right to assume a risk through voluntary and informed consent) and duties (e.g., the duty not to offer an unacceptable risk to someone who might be desperate enough to accept it). At the level of specific transactions—for example, sales of products or employment transactions—the rights and duties regarding creation of known or suspected risks are governed by law—especially the law of torts (3–6).

Many potential risks, such as those from nuclear power or genetically engineered microorganisms, do not arise from private transactions. Instead, they become accepted, implicitly or explicitly, through public policy and collective decisionmaking. When the people making a risk acceptability decision are not those who primarily bear its consequences, then a political or social choice theory relating the judgment of acceptability to the preferences and judgments of those governed by it must be articulated (2, 7). Similarly, if the benefits and potential adverse consequences flowing from a risky activity fall on different subpopulations, or, more generally, if its risks and benefits are unequally distributed, then the way in which conflicts among individual interests are resolved in reaching a judgment of acceptability must be examined carefully. A claim of acceptability in this context, whatever its factual basis in objective estimates of risks and benefits, also involves an element of judgment that needs to be justified.

The purposes of this chapter are (i) to introduce the technical concepts and terminology used to describe risks quantitatively with scientific precision, (ii) to show how to calculate quantitative risk measures in simple situations, and (iii) to sensitize the reader to some important issues that arise in stating and comparing uncertain risks. Bearing these issues in mind during the conduct and presentation of a risk analysis can help the practitioner avoid misleading statements that may invite the final decisionmaker, and perhaps the analyst, to draw unsound inferences about the meaning and significance of a study. At the conclusion of this chapter, the reader should be able to convert risk-related information (e.g., survival time information about AIDS victims) into unambiguous quantitative expressions of risk and should understand the meaning and limitations of such expressions and how they allow chronic health risks to be estimated, quantified, and compared over time. Chapter 3 then discusses the legal and philosophical factors that must mediate between the factual quantitative results of risk assessments and the final policy decisions and acceptability judgments of risk managers.

2 DEFINITIONS OF RISK

To understand the results and limitations of a risk assessment, and to be able to think clearly about trade-offs among risks, costs of controlling risks, and the economic benefits of an activity, it is useful to have a clear definition of risk. As interpreted by biostatisticians and engineers, *risk* usually refers to an underlying *probability law* that generates adverse consequences (8). The actual observable consequences of a risk are only a sample realization of this probability law.

Suppose that a coin is tossed three times and that the observed sequence of outcomes is heads, heads, heads, abbreviated HHH. From this observed sequence, what can be inferred about the probability that the coin will land tails on the next toss? This is roughly analogous to a risk analysis study in which the disease state (present or absent) for an individual is monitored over time, with heads corresponding to no disease, and tails corresponding to disease. Given a history of N years without disease, what can be inferred about the probability that the disease will occur in the next year? In both the coin-tossing and the risk analysis cases, the set of empirical observations is insufficient to reveal unambiguously the underlying probability. At best, guesses or estimates can be made based on the observed sequence. Moreover, in the case of disease, unlike the coin example, it is very likely that the true underlying probability is itself changing over time. Statistical risk assessment deals with the problem of estimating probabilities from observable data.

3 INDIVIDUAL RISK: A FLOW OF PROBABILITY

Two related concepts are useful in describing risk to an individual. First is the idea of the *total risk* of a particular adverse consequence, such as death, cancer, or death from cancer. Second, a concept of *attributable risk* is needed to describe the incremental contribution to the total risk made by a particular source or cause (e.g., cigarette smoking or radiation from a nuclear power plant).

3.1 Measurement of Total Risk to an Individual

The total risk to an individual of developing some undesirable response, such as death or cancer, in a given year t may be defined as the *probability* that the individual will develop the response in that year, assuming survival until then. In other words, if he is alive and healthy at the start of year t, then the probability that he will have developed the response by the end of year t may be defined as his risk of that response in year t. (This definition is for dichotomous responses; we do not consider here the more difficult problems of defining risk for a health response that may have varying degrees of severity or that is spread out over time.) This probability is also called the individual's (discrete-time) *hazard rate* for the response in year t. Hazard rates are used by actuaries, reliability engineers, biostatisticians, and epidemiologists to describe risks (9–11). In health risk assessment, hazard rates are used to calculate probabilities of cause-specific deaths or illnesses, to derive survival time distributions, and to quantify total risks over time.

Example 1. Calculation of Hazard Rates and Probabilities of Causation

Setting. An individual is judged to be equally likely to die of cancer in any of the next 3 years and to have zero probability of surviving for more than 3 years.

(i) What is his discrete-time hazard rate for death due to cancer in each of the next 3 years if cancer is the only possible cause of death?

(ii) Suppose that the same individual is also at risk from other causes (e.g., heart disease, car accidents, suicide) and that the total mortality hazard rate from all sources *other* than his cancer is 0.1 per year. Given that he dies in year 2, what would be the probability that the cause of his death is his cancer? [This type of retrospective assessment of *probable causes* can be important in court cases when the actual cause of an event (e.g., the occurrence of a certain kind of cancer in someone exposed both to medical radiation and to radiation from nuclear weapons testing fallout) cannot be determined, but the approximate time of the occurrence can be.]

(iii) Under the same assumption of a 0.1 annual mortality rate from competing (noncancer) causes, what is the probability that the individual will *not* die of cancer? (This type of question is important to actuaries in forecasting likely claims experience for a population of policy holders known to be at risk.)

Solution

Part (i): Suppose his hazard rate is a in year 1, b in year 2, and c in year 3. By definition, the probability that he will survive year 1 is $(1 - a)$, and his probability of surviving years 1 and 2 is $(1 - a)(1 - b)$. The probability of surviving years 1, 2, and 3 is zero, by hypothesis, so $c = 1$ (i.e., there is 100% probability of death in year 3, given that he survives to the beginning of year 3). The probability that he will die in year 1 is a, by definition. The probability that he will die in year 2 is the probability that he will survive year 1 and then die in year 2; that is, it is $(1 - a)b$. The probability that he will die in year 3 is the probability that he will survive years 1 and 2; that is, it is $(1 - a)(1 - b)$. Hence, we have the system of equations $a = (1 - a)b = (1 - a)(1 - b) = 1/3$. Solving, we obtain $a = 1/3$, $b = 1/2$, and $c = 1$.

Part (ii): Given that the individual dies in year 2, the probability that the cause of his death is cancer is the ratio of the cancer hazard rate in year 2 to the total hazard rate in year 2; thus, it is $0.5/(0.5 + 0.10) = 83.33\%$. (See Section 3.2 for a general discussion of probability of causation calculations.)

Part (iii): The probability that the individual dies of a competing cause before he dies of cancer can be found by calculating the probability that he dies in each year, weighting it by the conditional probability that he dies of a noncancer cause if he does die in that year (thus obtaining the total probability that he dies of a noncancer cause in that year), and then summing over all 3 years. The probability of death in year t is given by the product $[1 - h(1)][1 - h(2)]\ldots[1 - h(t - 1)]h(t)$, where $h(i)$ denotes the total hazard rate in year i. (This is the probability of surviving all the years up through $t - 1$ and then dying in year t.)

The probability of noncancer death, given death in year t, is $0.1/h(t)$; that is, it is the ratio of the hazard rate for noncancer death in year t to the total hazard rate in year t. The prospective probability of death due to a cause other than cancer is therefore

$$(0.43)\left(\frac{0.1}{0.43}\right) + (0.57)(0.6)\left(\frac{0.1}{0.6}\right) + (0.57)(0.4)\left(\frac{0.1}{1.1}\right) = 17.8\%.$$

(It is assumed that, in year 3, cancer and noncancer causes of death compete in such a way that there is a chance of $0.1/1.1$ for the individual to die of noncancer causes before he dies of cancer.)

In summary, discrete-time hazard rates allow survival time probabilities, prospective (actuarial) probabilities of deaths or diseases due to specific causes, and retrospective (evidential) probabilities that a health effect was due to a specific cause to be calculated. Similar definitions and calculations can be made for continuous-time risks.

Example 2. Continuous-Time Hazard Functions. Suppose that a cancer patient is equally likely to die at any time between 0 and 3 years from now, and that she is certain to die within 3 years. Find her *continuous-time hazard function*, expressing instantaneous risk as a function of time.

Solution. The individual's time of death is uniformly distributed on the interval $[0, 3]$. The probability that she will survive the first t years (where t is between 0 and 3) is initially given by the *survivor function* $S(t) = 1 - t/3$. For $t > 3$, $S(t) = 0$. The initial probability that her death will arrive between t and $t + dt$ is given by $f(t)dt = dt/3$, for sufficiently small dt. [Here, $f(t) = \frac{1}{3}$ is the probability density function for her time of death. See ref. (12) for a readable introduction to elementary probability theory and statistics.] Through the use of conditional probability, the probability that her death will arrive in the next time increment dt, given that she has survived until time t, is $f(t)dt/S(t) = dt/(3 - t)$. The ratio $h(t) = f(t)/S(t)$ is defined as the individual's *continuous-time hazard function*. In the present example, $h(t) = 1/(3 - t)$.

The $h(t) = f(t)/S(t)$ definition holds in general for continuous survivor functions. Intuitively, $h(t)dt$ for small dt is the probability that the individual will die between t and $t + dt$, given that she survives until t. We shall show later that $h(t)$ is a useful and intuitive quantitative measure of instantaneous risk. For computational purposes, it is helpful to note the calculus identities $f(t) = -S'(t)$ and $h(t) = -d[\log S(t)]/dt$ (9, 10). Continuous-time hazard functions can be used just like discrete-time hazard functions to calculate survival probabilities and prospective and retrospective probabilities of causation. (See Example 7.) (Notation: In this chapter, $\log x$ denotes the natural logarithm of x.)

Defining total risk in a given year as *response probability* makes comparisons of individual risks difficult. For example, we might want to say that one individual is exposed to twice as much individual risk as another (perhaps in support of an argument about how compensation payments ought to be distributed). But probabilities do not support such comparisons. It is not true that a probability of 1 is only twice as great as a probability of 0.5; moreover, it is not clear what would be meant by a probability that is twice as great as a probability of 0.9. The probability scale is not "cardinal" is this way (13). Hazard rates provide a way of redefining risk to make such ratio comparisons meaningful.

If the probability of response in year t is p, then we may define the transformed value

$$r(p) = -\log(1-p),$$

rather than p itself, as the risk in year t. For small values of p, p and $r(p)$ are numerically very close, with $r(p)$ being only very slightly larger. For example, when $p = 0.01$, $r(p) = 0.01005$. At $p = 0$, $r(p)$ is also zero. For large probabilities, however, $r(p)$ diverges from p more and more, approaching infinity as p approaches 1. For example, $r(0.5) = 0.69$, $r(0.635) = 1$, $r(0.8) = 1.6$, $r(0.9) = 2.3$, $r(0.99) = 4.6$, and $r(0.999) = 6.91$. Interpretively, $r(p)$ is the value of the continuous-time hazard rate, which, if maintained over an interval of unit length, will produce a probability of response equal to p. This hazard rate, rather than the probability that it generates, provides the most natural quantitative measure of risk.

On the $-\log(1-p)$ hazard rate scale, unlike the probability scale, risk ratios (as well as sums and differences) can meaningfully be compared. In other words, *the continuous-time hazard rate scale is fully cardinal.*

Example 3. Comparison of Risk Ratios.
Factory A has a 90% probability of having an accident (a chemical spill) within a year. Factory B has twice as great an accident risk as factory A (so that on average, over the long run, twice as many accidents happen at factory B as at factory A per unit time.) Assume that both factories are in steady state, so that the average number of accidents per unit time remains constant at each factory. What is the probability that factory B will have an accident within a year?

Solution. An accident probability of 0.9 corresponds to a constant annual hazard rate (risk) of $-\log(1-0.9) = 2.3$. Twice this is 4.6, corresponding to an annual accident probability of $1 - \exp(-4.6) = 0.99$. Thus, factory B has a 99% probability of an accident within the next year.

Hazard rates are the appropriate measures of risk for use in risk–benefit ratios and other ratios used in risk management decisionmaking. When probabilities are very small, however, so that a probability and its corresponding hazard rate are numerically almost identical, either can be used for decisionmaking purposes.

Processes with constant hazard functions, such as those in Example 3, play a special role in risk analysis. They are called *Poisson processes* (9–11). Poisson processes provide a yardstick for measuring the instantaneous hazard rates of more general processes. The $-\log(1-p)$ measure of risk is dictated by the mathematical properties of Poisson processes. The probability of surviving for T periods with no arrivals in a Poisson process with hazard rate h can be shown to be $\exp(-hT)$. Hence, the probability of at least one response within T periods is $p = 1 - \exp(-hT)$. Setting $T = 1$ and solving for h in terms of p in this formula gives the $r(p)$ formula, $h = -\log(1-p)$.

The general importance of Poisson processes for interpreting quantitative expressions of health risks arises from the fact that any health effect occurring in an individual can be thought of as the first arrival in a random response-generating process. The risk to an individual at any moment refers to the probability of an arrival of a response (i.e., an adverse health effect) in the immediate future. In this "waiting-time" interpretation of individual risk, $h(t)$ *is the average arrival rate at time t of responses in a Poisson process with constant hazard rate equal to h(t)*. Thus, Poisson processes provide the key for interpreting hazard rates in terms of arrival rates. Specifically, $h(t)$ is measured in units of average (i.e., expected) number of responses (or arrivals) per unit time at time t. Since *expected number of arrivals per unit time* defines an absolute scale, sums, differences, and ratios of hazard rates can meaningfully be computed, solving the problems that occurred in trying to compare probabilities.

Although it is convenient to interpret risk numbers in terms of expected annual frequencies, or average times until occurrence, intuitions about these quantities can be misleading. For example, if the expected frequency of accidents in a certain type of power plant is 1 in 1000 plant-years of operation, this does *not* imply that there is a 50% chance of an accident within 500 years, nor that the probability of going for 1000 years without accident is 50%. (As the next example shows, it is only 37%.) Similarly, statements about the expected number of diseases per person-year or per lifetime of exposure can have counterintuitive implications for the lifetime probability of disease. If the leukemia hazard rate for exposure to benzene in the workplace were 1 expected case per million person-years of exposure, for example, then the probability that a randomly selected person will develop cancer from a year of exposure is not 1×10^{-6}, as might be expected, but 6.3×10^{-5}.

Example 4. Expected versus Actual Waiting Times in a Poisson Process

Setting. The continuous-time hazard rate for arrival of a catastrophic accident at an industrial plant is $0.01 = 1 \times 10E - 2$ expected accidents per year. What is the probability that the plant will survive for 50 years without an accident?

Solution. Since the hazard rate is constant over time, this is an example of a Poisson process. The probability of no arrivals in an interval of length $L = 50$ in a Poisson process with average arrival rate $h = 0.01$ is given by $\exp(-hL) = \exp[-(0.01)(50)] = \exp(-0.5) = 0.61$. [The function $\exp(-hL)$ is the survivor function for the Poisson process.] Thus, although the *expected* amount of time until an accident arrives is $1/h = 100$ plant-years, there is a 39% chance that the plant will survive less than half that long without an accident. The probability that no accident will arrive before the *expected* arrival time is only about 37% in any Poisson process. It is thus considerably more likely than not that the actual waiting time to the first arrival will be less than the average (or expected) waiting time.

In summary, Poisson processes (i.e., processes with constant hazard rates) provide a useful language for describing and comparing the magnitudes of health and safety risks. Three concepts are critical to the use of Poisson processes in risk assessment. First, the unit of risk is (expected) number of arrivals per unit time. Only for Poisson processes is the expected number of arrivals proportional to elapsed time, making the expected number of arrivals per unit time a well-defined unit. Second, for risk processes with time-varying hazard rates, the amount of risk generated between t and $t + dt$, for sufficiently small dt, namely $h(t)dt$, can be thought of as the amount of risk that would be generated by a Poisson process with average arrival rate $h = h(t)$ operating from t to $t + dt$. Thus, Poisson processes can be used to interpret general (nonconstant) hazard functions. Finally, sums, differences, and ratios of risks can meaningfully be interpreted and compared when the Poisson risk scale, that is, expected number of arrivals per unit time, is used as the measure of risk.

Example 5. Risk Sums

Setting. An 89-year old male is exposed to two sources of risk: heart attacks, which arrive according to a Poisson process with rate $h_1 = 0.1$ arrival per year, and strokes, which arrive according to an independent Poisson process with rate $h_2 = 0.15$ arrival per year.

What is the probability that he will survive for a year without experiencing either a heart attack or a stroke?

Solution. The superposition of the two risks is a Poisson process with hazard rate $h_1 + h_2 = 0.25$. The probability of surviving a year with neither sort of arrival is therefore $\exp(-0.25) = 0.78$.

Any sum of two hazard rates corresponds to a superposition of two Poisson processes. The hazard rate consisting of the sum $h_1 + h_2$ may be thought of as the risk of a health effect generated by the first arrival from either of two competing (or superimposed) Poisson processes, one with average arrival rate h_1 and the other with average arrival rate h_2.

3.2   Individual Risk Attributable to a Cause

The concept of total individual risk for a dichotomous health response at a single moment in time, say t, has now been reasonably well specified: it is the expected number of arrivals per unit time evaluated at moment t, where the first "arrival" corresponds to occurrence of the health effect. In many applications, however—for example, in the court room or in assessing the additional risk posed by a new technology or hazard—the problem is not to estimate the total risk to which an individual is exposed for some health response but to estimate the *incremental contribution to his risk* made by some particular cause or source. This is the risk that is said to be *attributable* to the source (9.14). For example, in assessing the individual risk of lung cancer attributable to cigarette smoking, we must subtract out, or otherwise adjust for, lung cancers that would have occurred even without cigarette smoking: only the incremental risk above this base line is to be attributed to cigarettes.

Example 6. *Epidemiological Calculation of Attributable Risk*

Setting. Suppose that the hazard rate for leukemia among the children in town A is 0.001 case/child-year, while in town B it is 0.002 case/child-year. If the children are thought to be identical, except that those in town B have been exposed to drinking water from a contaminated well, then what would be the quantitative risk of child leukemia attributed to drinking of the contaminated water?

Solution. The attributable risk would be $0.002 - 0.001 = 0.001$ case/child-year of exposure. Out of every thousand cases of child leukemia in town B, it is expected that 500 would have occurred even if the drinking water had not been contaminated. Thus, $500/1000 = 0.5$ is the *attributable proportion of risk* due to the contaminated well water.

Few concepts in risk analysis have occasioned as much perplexity and debate as that of the attributable risk due to a source (15, 16). By using the random arrival model of risks, we can understand the key elements of this debate. Suppose that N *sources* or *causal factors* contribute to the risk of a health response in an individual (e.g., cigarette smoking, radiation, or saccharin consumption in the causation of cancer). Each source can be thought of as firing a random stream of tiny invisible bullets, or "hits," at the exposed individual. (Hit and arrival are synonyms). The average arrival rate or *intensity* of hits from source i at time t is source i's hazard rate at time t, denoted by $h_i(t)$. As usual, the *first* hit or arrival from any source is assumed to correspond to occurrence of the health response. The source of the first hit may be identified as the *cause* of the response.

Suppose that a health response does occur at time t. Without knowing which source generated the hit that caused the response, one can still calculate *probabilities of causation* for each of the N potential causes (17).

Example 7. Probability of Causation. Suppose that a worker in a uranium mine has a hazard rate for lung cancer of 0.002 expected case/year from all nonoccupational sources, and a statistically independent hazard rate of 0.001 case/year from occupational exposure to radiation. If he does get lung cancer, then what is the probability that it was caused by occupational exposure?

Solution. Under the stated assumptions of additive hazard rates from statistically independent occupational and nonoccupational sources, the probability of causation for occupational exposure is just $0.001/(0.001 + 0.002) = 33.33\%$; that is, it is the ratio of the cause-specific hazard rate to the total hazard rate. Note that this formula, which has been proposed for use by the federal government in compensating possible victims of nuclear weapons testing fallout (18, 19), depends critically on the assumption of statistically independent, noninteracting, hazard rates. The biological realism of this assumption is open to question (15–17).

If N potential sources of a health effect are statistically independent, so that the arrival rate from one source is unaffected by the presence of other sources, then the total risk to the individual at time t from all sources is given by the sum $h(t) = h_1(t) + \cdots + h_N(t)$. The contribution to this total made by source i is $h_i(t)$, and this is the amount of risk, measured in expected arrivals per unit time, attributable to source i. Since source i contributes the fraction $h_i(t)/h(t)$ of all expected hits per unit time at time t, this is the probability that source i contributed the hit that caused the observed health response. If the time of the first hit is unknown (e.g., because the expression of its effects as an observable health response is delayed by a latency period of uncertain length), then more complicated formulas for probability of causation can be worked out (20). The basic ideas of risk attribution and probability of causation are important in tort law and legislative contexts [e.g. (18)] in which attempts are made to apply the results of quantitative risk assessments to apportion liability and/or compensation payments for injuries that may or may not have resulted from the risks created by a defendant's actions.

Example 8. Relative Risk and Probability of Causation

Setting. Let an individual's age-specific background risk of leukemia be given by a hazard function $h(t)$. According to the *relative risk hypothesis*, occupational exposure to a dose D of a leukemogen (e.g., benzene) or of radiation has the effect of multiplying the hazard function by a constant, $(1 + bD)$, where b is the potency parameter. [Dose D must be measured in biologically relevant terms; for example, see (21) for a case study involving benzene.]

(i) If the relative risk model is correct for benzene, and if a 60-year old worker develops leukemia after being exposed to 1 ppm of benzene 8 hours a day for 40 years, then what would be the probability that it was the benzene exposure that caused his leukemia?

(ii) How might a court use such information in making compensation decisions in cases where the plaintiff has suffered a probabilistic harm but is unable to offer definite "proof" of the cause of his injury (e.g., leukemia)? (For this problem, assume that tort litigation rather than Worker's Compensation is being sought as a remedy.)

Solution. (i) Under the relative risk model, the worker's background age-specific hazard rate and the age at which he develops a response (here, leukemia) are irrelevant: all that matters is the product bD at the time of response. Since leukemia has a relatively short latency period, its time of occurrence can often be estimated accurately. If the time of onset is t and the dose received as of time t is $D(t)$, then the probability that the worker's leukemia was caused by exposure to benzene (assuming competing risks) will be

$$p = \frac{bD(t)}{1 + bD(t)}.$$

If $D(t)$ and b are known, then probability of causation can be determined. In practice, application of this formula requires a biologically meaningful measure of the dose [e.g., based on a weighted cumulative dose over the 15 years prior to onset; see (21)], estimation of the potency coefficient b, and acceptance of the relative risk model for leukemogenesis. This model and an additive *absolute risk* model have been used to estimate probabilities of causation for radiogenic cancers (18).

(ii) Suppose that the court uses probabilistic evidence to try to minimize the expected error in its compensation decisions. Specifically, suppose that if the cause of the plaintiff's leukemia (benzene exposure or background) were *known*, then the defendant would be required to pay him a compensation award of C or 0, respectively. When the cause of the plaintiff's injury is uncertain, the court tries to assign a compensation amount that minimizes the expected cost of error. If the probability that benzene exposure caused the leukemia is p, and if the court awards an amount X between 0 and C, then the expected error in compensation is

$$J(X, p) = p(C - X) + (1 - p)X;$$

that is, it is the underpayment if the defendant is guilty, $C - X$, times the probability that he is guilty, p, plus the amount of overcompensation if the defendant is innocent, X, times the probability that he is innocent, $1 - p$. To minimize this expected error, the court should adopt the following rule: *if $p > 0.5$, then award full compensation, $X = C$. If $p < 0.5$, then award zero compensation.* Interestingly, this is precisely the form of compensation rule that has been traditionally used in American law under *preponderance of evidence* and related standards.

If the two types of errors (overpayment by an innocent defendant and underpayment by a guilty one) are weighted differently in the judicial process, then the above rule must be generalized. If every dollar of compensation mistakenly withheld is considered k times as bad as a dollar mistakenly awarded, then the rule becomes: award full compensation if $p > 1/(1 + k)$; otherwise, award nothing.

The above definitions of attributable risk and probability of causation are very satisfactory when the random arrival model correctly represents the nature of causation. In the epidemiological and biostatistics literature, this model is called the *competing risk model*: each source is regarded as competing with the rest to be the first to cause a health response (9, 14). If the competing risk model is assumed to hold, then the risk increments contributed by different sources can be distinguished and displayed, at least in principle, in the format shown in Table 1.

However, the competing risk model is not applicable if either (i) causes are not mutually exclusive—for example, because a response is triggered by the arrival and successful action of different kinds of hits, from different sources, within a certain time of each other;

TABLE 1. Risks that Increase Probability of Death by One Chance in a Million

Activity	Cause of Death
Smoking 1.4 cigarettes	Cancer, heart disease
Drinking $\frac{1}{2}$ liter of wine	Cirrhosis of the liver
Traveling 10 miles by bicycle	Accident
Traveling 300 miles by car	Accident
Flying 1000 miles by jet	Accident
Flying 6000 miles by jet	Cancer caused by cosmic radiation
Living 2 months in average brick building	Cancer caused by natural stone or radioactivity
One chest x-ray taken in a good hospital	Cancer caused by radiation
Living 2 months with a cigarette smoker	Cancer, heart disease
Eating 40 tablespoons of peanut butter	Liver cancer caused by aflatoxin B
Eating 100 charcoal-broiled steaks	Cancer from benzopyrene
Drinking thirty 12-oz cans of diet soda	Cancer caused by saccharin
Living 5 years at site boundary of a typical nuclear power plant in the open	
Living 20 years near PVC plant	Cancer caused by vinyl chloride (1976 standard)
Living 150 years within 20 miles of a nuclear power plant	Cancer caused by radiation
Risk of accident by living within 5 miles of a nuclear reactor for 50 years	Cancer caused by radiation

Source: Adapted from R. Wilson, Analyzing the risks of daily life, *Technology Review*, **81**, (1979). See also R. Wilson and E. A. C. Crouch, Risk assessment and comparison: an introduction, *Science*, **236**, 267–270 (1987).

or (ii) causes are not statistically independent: the average arrival rate of hits, or their success rate in doing biological damage (i.e., the *effective* hit rate), from one source depends on what other sources are present. If either exclusivity or independence of causes fails to hold, the entire notion of causation becomes problematic (17, 22). Whether these conditions are realistic for a given health effect depends on the biological damage mechanisms involved. The validity of the competing risk model, and of probability of causation calculations, cannot be decided on the basis of observed dose–response models or hazard functions but requires understanding of underlying biological processes.

Example 9. Interacting Causes. Suppose that the background hazard rate for lung cancer for a particular individual, in the absence of cigarette smoking or occupational exposure to radiation, is 0.001 expected case per year. If he smokes, this rate increases to 0.003. If he works in a uranium mine, it is 0.002. If he smokes *and* works in a uranium mine, it is 0.006: thus, smoking and exposure to radiation are assumed to interact multiplicatively in increasing his risk of lung cancer. Assuming that he does both, so that his total risk is 0.006, what is the lung cancer risk due to (i.e., attributable to) smoking?

Solution. Proceeding as in Example 6, we could say that since the risk would be only 0.002 without smoking and since it is 0.006 with smoking, the attributable risk due to smoking is $0.006 - 0.002 = 0.004$, and the attributable proportion of risk for smoking is $0.004/0.006 = 67\%$. This approach has been proposed by some risk analysts (19). One difficulty with it is that applying the same formula to the radiation exposure would give $(0.006 - 0.003)/0.006 = 50\%$ as its share in causation; the two assigned shares, of 67% and 50%, however, sum to more than 100%. Thus, this approach tends to inflate systematically the proportion of risk attributed to each factor if the factors interact synergistically (15).

An alternative approach that avoids such difficulties is to note that smoking increases risk by $0.003 - 0.001 = 0.002$ in the absence of radiation exposure, and increases it by $0.006 - 0.002 = 0.004$ in the presence of radiation exposure; its average effect, therefore, averaged over the presence and absence of the radiation factor, is to increase risk by $(0.002 + 0.004)/2 = 0.003$, and this can be defined as the risk attributable to smoking in this example (22). A similar calculation for radiation again gives 0.003 as its attributable risk; thus, each factor is assigned a 50% share in causation. More generally, if there are N factors, then averaging the incremental contribution to total hazard rate made by the ith factor over all the $N!$ possible orderings of the N factors gives a relatively satisfactory measure or definition of the risk attributable to factor i (22, 23). Reference 17 shows that in the special case of competing risks, averaging risk increments over orderings gives the same result as the probability of causation formula for the proportion of risk attributed to any specific factor.

Example 9 demonstrates that the portion of a risk that is attributed to a given cause depends on the risk-accounting convention used. In the competing risk model, there is no need for such conventions. Otherwise, for example, in the case of a cancer caused by the interaction of many chemicals and aspects of diet and lifestyle, the attribution of risk to single causes requires some (usually implicit) arbitrary risk-accounting decisions. Displaying data as in Table 1 obscures this important fact. An unknown portion of the cancer risk attributed to a "cause" such as saccharin in a table like this could equally well have been attributed to another cause, such as alcohol consumption, that interacts with it.

To illustrate this point further, suppose that occurrence of a health effect depends on whether the total number of hits received from all sources within a certain amount of time exceeds a certain threshold. Then, if a response occurs, it cannot even in principle be ascribed to any single source. Similarly, if the presence of factor A doubles the hazard from factor B, then a hit from B may partly be blamed on the presence of A. In such cases of *joint and multiple causation*, assignment of shares in causation to the different sources is as much a matter of policy as one of science. Presenting comparative risk data as in Table 1 may suggest that risk attribution is an objective scientific process. It is important for the practitioner to bear in mind that such tables require assumptions for allocating effects that are due to the interaction of multiple factors among the individual factors listed in the table. These assumptions, or conventions, should be made explicit when results are presented.

Averaging incremental effects over factor orderings, as in Example 9, provides partial guidance on the allocation of joint effects to individual causes. But it does not determine which factors (e.g., smoking, exposure to radiation) are to be considered as variables, to which risk can be attributed, and which (e.g., sex, age) are to be considered only descriptors of the population groups for which risk attributions are to be made (17). This kind of decision is a matter for policy. Policy, as well as science, determines attribution of risk in the presence of joint causes.

In summary, the total risk (defined as the expected arrival rate) of a health effect in an individual over time can be described by a hazard function. The part of this risk attributable to a specific source at any time can be expressed quantitatively as the ratio of the cause-specific hazard rate from that source to the total hazard rate, *if* the assumptions of the competing risk model (statistically independent, mutually exclusive causes) hold. Otherwise, for cases of joint causation or multiple causation, the risk analyst practitioner must work with the users of the analysis to determine what definition of attributable risk should be used.

TABLE 2. Information Used in Health Risk Assessment

I. Hazard identification
  A. Human data
    • Monitoring and surveillance (including vital statistics)
    • Epidemiologic studies
    • Clinical studies
  B. Animal data
  C. In vitro tests
  D. Molecular structure–activity relation
II. Hazard characterization
  A. Human studies
    • Epidemiologic studies
    • Clinical studies
  B. Animal studies
    • Minimal effects determination
    • Dose–response modeling
    • Special issues, including interspecies conversion and high- to low-dose extrapolation
  C. Pharmacokinetic studies (including physiologic rationale)
III. Exposure characterization
  A. Demographic information
  B. Ecologic analyses
  C. Monitoring and surveillance systems
    • Animal
    • Human
  D. Biologic monitoring of high-risk individuals
  E. Transport modeling (mathematical)
  F. Integrated exposure assessments
    • Over time
    • Over hazard (synergy)
IV. Risk determination
  A. Mathematical
    • Unit and population risk estimates
    • Threshold determination (e.g., safety factor approach, NOEL[a])
    • Statistical characterization of uncertainty
  B. Formal decision analysis
  C. Inter-risk comparisons
  D. Qualitative—panel reviews
  E. Qualitative—informal scientific advice
  F. Risk–benefit analysis

[a]NOEL = no-observed-effect level.
Source: U.S. Department of Health and Human Services (24).

4   POPULATION RISK

Hazard functions provide a way of expressing *individual* risks over time. However, risk analysts in the chronic human health and safety risk analysis area are more often concerned with quantifying risks to *populations*. One reason is that hazard rates for specific individuals usually cannot be determined from available data. In practice, hazard rates are typically estimated from epidemiological or laboratory data collected from samples of cases drawn from large populations, and only population averages or other population statistics can be estimated reliably.

Table 2, taken from a recent U.S. Department of Health and Human Services publication (24), shows the types of information most often used in health risk assessments. The hazard identification, hazard characterization, and exposure characterization steps all feature epidemiological and demographic data as key contributors to statistical risk assessments of population risks. These types of data support estimates of population risk.

A second reason for emphasizing population risk estimates is that the full impact of a technological activity or of a new regulation can only be evaluated by looking at the distribution of effects in the affected population as a whole. Quantifying the risks to appropriate target subpopulations (e.g., occupational, residential, general public, hypersensitive individuals, and future generations) is therefore one of the principal goals of health, safety, and environmental risk analyses. Combining the risks estimated for these subpopulations into a useful overall quantitative expression of total population risk is a key challenge for risk analysts, addressed in Section 4.3.

4.1   Uncertain Individual Risks as Expected Hazard Rates

Individual hazard rates for chronic health effects typically depend on both the exogenous factors to which an individual is exposed, including the extent and timing of exposure, and on endogenous factors such as the efficiency of the body's repair mechanisms, genetic predisposition to the health response, and hormonal status. While external exposures can sometimes be usefully estimated, endogenous factors mediating between exposures and health responses usually vary widely across individuals and cannot be observed. [New techniques of *molecular epidemiology*, using biological markers such as DNA adducts, promise to open more of the mediating processes and factors to direct observation, however (25–27).]

This implies that there may be substantial heterogeneity in individual responses to given exposure conditions. The consequence is that even if an individual knew his own exposure history, he would in general remain uncertain about his future hazard function, and hence about his probability of eventual response.

Uncertainty about probabilities can sometimes be incorporated into the calculation of the probabilities themselves, making it unnecessary to express risk estimates and uncertainties about the risk estimates separately.

Example 10.   Uncertain Individual Probabilities

Setting. A population in a small town consists of two types of individuals: type A = sensitive, and type B = normal. It has recently been discovered that the town's water supply has been contaminated with a carcinogenic chemical, say substance X. Now individuals of type A have a 30% probability of developing a carcinogenic response to exposure to substance X, while individuals of type B have only a 3% probability of response. Furthermore, 90% of the population is of type B, and only 10% belong to the sensitive subpopulation of type A responders. What is the true probability that a randomly selected individual from this town will develop a carcinogenic response from exposure to substance X? (This is probably the risk of greatest concern to each individual.)

Solution. Given the assumed mixture of types, a randomly selected individual will have probability $0.30 \times 0.10 + 0.03 \times 0.90 = 0.057$ of a carcinogenic response to substance X. As long as an individual has no other information, beyond these statistical proportions, about her own probable type, her *individual* risk (with respect to this information) is 0.057, just as if she belonged to a homogeneous population with identical individual risks of 0.057. However, if she gains additional information about her own probable type—for example, if "type" is genetically transmitted, and if there is a history of cancer in her family—then the individual must revise her type probabilities 0.9 and 0.1 (using Bayes' rule) to condition them on this information.

Note that in this example, even if each individual has only statistical information about the proportions of the two types in the population, so that individual risk is 0.057 for each individual, the *variance* in number of carcinogenic responses in the whole population will be smaller for this mixed population than for a homogeneous population with independent identical response probabilities (28).

This example illustrates the general point that *an individual's assessed probability of response is always conditioned on information about her*. It incorporates uncertainty about her response type as well as uncertainty due to the random nature of health responses even for a known type.

It may be tempting in Example 10 to think that any individual's "true" response probability is either 0.03 or 0.30, depending on her true (but unknown) type. But these probabilities are no truer than the 0.057: they are simply calculated with respect to improved information about the individual that incorporates knowledge of type. Arguably, the only "true" probabilities in this sense (defined as probabilities calculated with respect to perfect information) are the trivial ones of 0 and 1. Thus, any individual's response probability is actually an *expected* probability, found by aggregating over all her possible types. This realization provides the key to understanding the relation between risk and uncertainty about risk.

There is a general formula relating population risk data (proportions of different response types in the population and type-specific response probabilities or individual risks) to risks of individuals in the population. If there are M distinct types of individuals in a population, if the probability (conditioned on available information) that a particular individual is of type i is $p(i)$, for $i = 1, 2, \ldots, M$, and if the response probability for an individual of type i is $r(i)$, then the response probability for the individual (with respect to the information set $[p(1), \ldots, p(M)]$ for his probable type) is

$$r = p(1)r(1) + \cdots + p(M)r(M).$$

An analogous formula holds when $r(i)$ represents a hazard rate for individuals of type i. Types then correspond to homogeneous subpopulations in which all individuals of the same type have identical hazard functions. The use of this formula for hazard functions is illustrated in the next example.

Example 11. Uncertain Individual Hazard Functions

Setting. Assume that 50% of the people in a particular population (e.g., an occupational or residential population of interest) are permanently immune to a certain disease common among the elderly. The other 50% of the people become susceptible once they reach age 50 and have a constant hazard function of $h(t) = 0.1$ for all ages $t > 50$. What is the individual risk for a 60-year-old member of the population who does not yet have the disease and who does not know his own type?

Solution. At $t = 60$, the relevant information set consists of the fact that 10 years have passed without occurrence of the disease. It is an exercise in conditional probabilities using Bayes' rule to show that the posterior probability that an individual is immune to the disease, given that X years have passed without occurrence since he turned 50, is $1/[1 + \exp(-hX)] = 1/[1 + \exp(-0.1X)] = 0.73$ when $X = 10$. Hence, for a 60-year-old individual, the age-specific hazard rate with respect to this information set is $0.73 \times 0 + 0.27 \times 0.1 = 0.027$. The assessed hazard function continues to decrease as X increases, asymptotically approaching 0, until the disease arrives or the individual dies of other causes.

   In practice, age thresholds for onset and proportions of immune and susceptible people in the population at risk are not known with the precision used in this hypothetical example. But the qualitative point—that assessed individual risk varies predictably with passing time as beliefs about an individual's probable type are updated to reflect his survival record to date—is still valid.

   In summary, an individual's risk cannot, in general, be thought of as an objective number attached to him, like his height or age or weight. Instead, it depends on the information set on which it is based, which evolves over time. Any individual risk estimate must be seen as provisional, pending the passage of time and the acquisition of additional relevant information. The implication is that the acceptability of the information set with respect to which a risk is calculated, as well as the magnitude of the resulting number, must be considered in deciding whether the risk is "acceptable." In addition, as shown in Example 10, knowing each individual's risk (e.g., 0.057) with respect to a given set of information is insufficient to determine population risk. Two populations with identical mean individual risks may have different variances in the numbers of cases per year.

   Not only are (expected) individual risks insufficient to determine population risks, but the converse is also true: aggregate population risks, as they are sometimes measured, do not necessarily reveal anything useful about individual risks. In practice, risk statistics are usually collected and presented at very highly aggregated levels, as in Table 1. They are averaged over so many distinct individual types that they may have little relevance for any specific individual.

Example 12. An Aggregation Artifact in Population Risk

Setting. Each individual in a population belongs to exactly one of the two following exposure groups for exposure to chemical X:

   Group A (Occupational)—50% of those exposed in any year show a response, while 91% of those not exposed develop the response.

Group B (General Public)—5% of those exposed respond, while 10% of those not exposed respond.

In a sample of 2111 individuals, suppose that 1000 group A people but only 100 group B people are exposed, while 1000 group B people but only 11 group A people are unexposed. What is the aggregate population attributable risk due to exposure?

Solution. For the whole population, the observed average response probabilities will be $[(0.5)(1000) + (0.05)(100)]/1100 = 46\%$ in the exposed group and $[(0.10)(1000) + (0.91)(11)]/1011 = 11\%$ in the unexposed group. In other words, if it is determined that a randomly selected individual has not been exposed to the chemical, then the probability that she will develop a response is 11%. If it is discovered that she has been exposed, however, then the probability of response increases to 46%. Thus, the attributable risk due to exposure might conventionally be calculated as $46\% - 11\% = 35\%$. Note, however, that this obscures the fact that exposure is associated with a *decrease* in response probability for each individual. The reason that it is associated with an increase in risk at the group level is that likelihood of exposure is positively associated with membership in the high-risk (occupational) group, even though exposure itself does not cause, and in fact tends to prevent, the health effect.

The phenomenon in which exposure is associated with increased risk at the group level even though it reduces risk at the individual level is called *Simpson's paradox* (29, 30). It demonstrates that what is true for a group may not be true for any of its members. Thus, aggregate risk statistics such as those in Table 1 must be interpreted very cautiously: the causal inferences that they invite (e.g., that certain activities cause increases in risk for individuals that participate in them) may not be valid. In Section 4.3, we describe a decision-analytic approach to measuring population risk that differs substantially from the conventional approach in Example 12 and that gives potentially more useful answers that avoid Simpson's paradox.

Even when aggregation does not reverse the direction of association between exposure and health effect, it can substantially bias the numerical relation between exposure and aggregate population response. The implication is that the practitioner should always check for hidden heterogeneity before presenting aggregate population risk statistics. If heterogeneity is discovered [e.g., based on the variance in population responses over time, or based on statistical tests for *mixture distributions* (31)], then aggregate population risk statistics may be misleading. They should either be disaggregated further if possible, ideally to the level of homogeneous subpopulations, or be presented with appropriate cautions about interpreting them causally. The problem of combining risk statistics for several internally homogeneous subpopulations into a useful aggregate risk statistic for the whole population that they comprise is addressed in Section 4.3.

4.2 Individual versus Social Assessment of Population Risk

Individual risks and population risks are closely related over time when each individual initially considers himself a randomly selected member of the population and learns more about his own probable type as time passes. The purpose of this subsection is to clarify more formally these relations between individual risks and population risks and to explain how to derive one from the other.

Let $F(x, t)$ denote the number of people in a population who, at time t, have hazard rates less than or equal to x. (These hazard rates are assumed to be calculated with respect to whatever information the assessor has at time t.) For chronic health risks, individual hazard rates are assumed to be statistically independent, meaning that occurrence of the disease in one individual does not affect the probabilities or hazard rates for its occurrence in other individuals. (This is in contrast to the population risks from something like a nuclear power plant accident, where either everyone or no one in the neighboring population is affected.) With this independence assumption, $F(x, t)$ completely characterizes the population risk at time t.

If each individual in the population knows the aggregate population statistics corresponding to $F(x, t)$, but knows nothing else about his own risk, so that he considers his own hazard rate at time t to be drawn at random from the population distribution $F(x, t)$, then his assessed individual hazard rate will coincide with the mean of $F(x, t)$. In other words, *in the absence of other information, each member of the population has an assessed individual risk equal to the mean of the population risk distribution.* If an individual considers himself to be a randomly selected member of the population, then his individual risk is the expected value of the risks for all individuals in the population. This presents a paradox: if two different population risk distributions have identical means, then every individual should be indifferent between them (based on his own expected risk.) But the two distributions may not be equally desirable from a societal perspective.

Example 13. Societal versus Individual Risk Evaluation

Setting. The following "thought experiment" illustrates many of the key issues. Consider a society with only two people, and a choice between (i) a population risk in which each individual is exposed to a constant hazard rate of h and (ii) a population risk in which one of the individuals is exposed to a constant hazard rate of $2h$ and the other to a risk of 0. In the latter case, assume that neither individual knows which of them has the nonzero rate: each has a 50% chance of being the sensitive (at-risk) individual. Which (if either) of these two population risk configurations is preferable?

Discussion. In both cases, each individual assesses his own risk as h expected arrivals per unit time, at least until an occurrence of the disease is observed. In the second case, the survivor then knows in retrospect that he is no longer at risk. (Thus, the assumption of statistical independence is violated.) Would the choice between these two options (which might represent a choice between distributing a drug that exposes every taker to a small risk and distributing one that exposes sensitive individuals only to a greater risk, where no one knows his own type ex ante) be affected if the decisionmaker knew which individual had which hazard rate in the second case, even though the individuals did not? Would it change if the decisionmaker *could* find out which individual had which hazard rate, even if he chose not to? There are no scientifically "correct" answers to these questions. However, in Section 4.3 we develop an analytic framework for answering such questions for large populations with statistically independent individual risks.

Example 13, although contrived, raises several issues about value judgments and trade-offs concerning risk equity, ex ante versus ex post risk assessments, and societal attitudes toward knowledge and responsibility in the assessment of population risk distributions. Chapter 3 examines some of these philosophical issues further. The following framework suggests an approach to choosing among alternative population risk distributions in large populations.

4.3 Evaluating Population Risks: A Decision-Analytic Approach

Chronic health effect risk assessments are usually conducted for sizeable populations, involving hundreds, thousands, or millions of individuals. In such cases, statistical laws of large numbers can be applied to simplify the evaluation of population risk distributions. For example, if the population consists of several "types" of individuals, with each type corresponding to a homogeneous subpopulation of individuals having identical hazard functions for death from chronic diseases, then in each homogeneous subpopulation the amounts of time (numbers of life-years) that the members have left until death will be statistically independent, identically distributed random variables. Then statistical theory specifies that, at any time, the *total number of remaining life-years in the population, summed over all individuals now in it, will be approximately normally distributed*, with mean and variance equal to the sum of the means and variances, respectively, of the remaining life-years in each subpopulation. From a social perspective, the problem of evaluating population risk in large populations can be reduced to the problem of evaluating normal distributions for the attribute *remaining life-years in the population*.

In stating this conclusion, we are making a simplifying ethical assumption that all individuals are treated as anonymous: each life-year is equally valued, regardless of to whom it belongs. This implies that only the *sum* of individual remaining life-years (a random quantity) matters in evaluating population risk. Crucial to this criterion is the further assumption that each individual considers himself drawn at random from the set of individuals, with his own probable type being determined by relative frequencies of different types in the population. This assumed information pattern means that there are no ex ante inequities to be concerned with in the distribution of individual risks: only the sum is important.

The problem of comparing or choosing among normal distributions over a desirable attribute—in this case, remaining life-years in the population—can be solved by the methods of decision analysis. Without attempting to review the enormous decision-analytic literature that bears on risk quantification and acceptable risk decisions (7, 32–36), we can convey the flavor of the approach by the following examples.

Example 14. Decision-Analytic Comparison of Population Life Distributions. This is a simplified theoretical example that demonstrates some of the philosophy and methods of modern decision-analytic approaches to social risk management. Suppose that at time zero (the *decision date*) a decisionmaker must choose one of two risk control options: for example, building a tall stack on a new plant or building a shorter stack that will expose fewer people to greater pollutant levels. These options have different implications for the future hazard functions for deaths due to respiratory or cardiovascular illnesses of individuals in the population. Let m and v denote the mean and variance of total remaining life-years in the population under the first choice, and m' and v' denote the corresponding mean and variance under the second choice. Both life distributions will be approximately normal. Then the difference in population risk between these two distributions may, under certain decision-analytic assumptions (37), be defined as

$$k[(m - m') + (k/2)(v' - v)],$$

where the unit of measurement is *equivalent (i.e., equally desirable) deterministic number of life-years* gained or lost, depending on the sign of the expression. Here, k is a subjective parameter of *relative risk aversion* (36). A value of $k = 0$ implies that the decisionmaker considers a fifty–fifty lottery giving equal chances of an incremental gain in population life-years of 0 or 100 life-years equivalent or indifferent to a sure incremental gain of 50 years. If k is less than zero, the decisionmaker would prefer a sure gain of 50 additional life-years among the members of the population to a 50–50 chance at 0 or 100 additional life-years: she would rather not gamble. The lower is k, the lower is the number of additional life-years with certainty that the decisionmaker would accept in exchange for a probabilistic life-saving opportunity. [If k is positive, the above formula must be modified; see ref. (36, 37).]

Real decisions often involve random changes in the numbers of life-years that will be saved (or lost). For example, if the probability distribution for total remaining life-years is normal for each alternative, then the change in total remaining life-years between alternatives will also be normally distributed. Whether it is preferable to try for a larger life-year savings at the risk of falling further short is ultimately a matter of subjective judgment, as reflected in the risk attitude parameter k. This risk attitude profoundly colors the evaluation of a population risk, making the normally distributed number of remaining life-years with mean m and variance v "equivalent" to a deterministic number of only $k(m - kv/2)$ remaining life-years (or m life-years, if $k = 0$), for a decisionmaker with relative risk aversion coefficient k.

One of the principal contributions of the decision-analytic approach is that it clearly delineates the role of subjective attitudes in evaluating risks. Decisionmakers who agree on all objective statistical aspects of a risk assessment may still reach different policy conclusions if they have different risk attitudes.

Decision analysis can also be useful in evaluating uncertain risks and in clarifying fundamental trade-offs. For example, consider choosing among the following situations:

Case A (Uniform Population Risk). Each of 100 people independently is exposed to a 0.01 chance of disease.

Case B (Anonymous Sensitive Subpopulation). 10 of the 100 people are exposed to a 0.10 chance of disease. The rest have a zero chance of disease. No one knows which "type" he is unless and until he gets the disease.

Case C (Known High-Risk Population). 50 of the 100 people (e.g., those living within a certain distance of an industrial facility) are at high risk and know it. Each of these individuals independently has a 0.02 probability of disease; the remaining 50 people have zero risk.

Case D (Uncertain Individual Risks). Each individual has a random probability, independently drawn from a uniform distribution between 0 and 0.02, of getting the disease.

Case E (Uncertain Population Risk). Each individual independently has the same probability of getting the disease. The magnitude of this probability is uncertain, however; it is judged equally likely to be anywhere between 0 and 0.02.

Case F (Catastrophic Risk). There is a 0.02 chance of a catastrophic accident that will kill the 50 people nearest the facility, and a 0.98 chance of no accident and hence no deaths. Compare this to a situation where there is a 0.01 chance that all 100 people will be killed and a 0.99 probability that no one will be killed.

Imagine trying to rank these situations in terms of relative social desirability. Each of these types of trade-offs, for example, between number of people exposed and magnitude of exposure per person, between certain and uncertain risks, and between equitably distributed versus inequitably distributed risks, arises in practice, for example, in siting facilities or in regulating vaccines with uncertain or widely varying risks of undesirable side effects. Many of them can be clarified through decision-analytic methods (38–40), although decision theorists are only starting to understand how to structure and reason about decisionmaking when risks are learned or revealed increasingly accurately as time passes (41–45).

For the practitioner, perhaps the most important thing to learn from the decision-analytic perspective is that the results of a risk assessment should be presented in such a way that decision-relevant differences between certain and uncertain risks, equitably and inequitably distributed risks, or statistically independent and statistically correlated risks are not lost. The decisionmaker(s) should realize clearly when their choices of policy depend on subjective attitudes of aversion toward risk, uncertainty, inequity (both ex post and ex ante), anxiety, disappointment, or regret. Some common measures of risk, for example, *frequency–severity diagrams* and *limit lines* for catastrophic risks (8, 46–48) or average individual risks instead of frequency distributions of individual risks in the population, hide these distinctions, obscuring the need for and role of various types of subjective judgments in risk management decisionmaking. At one extreme, using expected number of illnesses or fatalities as a summary of population risk would result in the same assessment of risk (1 expected disease case or fatality) for all of the example cases A–F shown above, thus depriving the user of the risk analysis of the information needed to distinguish or choose among them. The professional risk analyst should take care not to aggregate risk information at such a high level that decision-relevant uncertainties, heterogeneities, inequities, or correlations are hidden.

Example 15. Risk Profiles

Setting. Two thousand people live near an old petroleum refinery. A risk analysis of the refinery reports that the chance (expressed as an expected annual frequency, i.e., as a hazard rate) of an accident with off-site consequences killing one or more people is 1×10^{-5} per year, the chance of an accident killing five or more people per year is 5×10^{-6} per year, the chance of an accident killing ten or more people is 1×10^{-6} per year, and soon. The report gives the entire frequency–severity curve or *risk profile* $F(N)$, showing the expected annual frequency (i.e., the hazard rate) of an accident killing N or more people, for $N = 1$–2000. Has the analyst done a good job of reporting the results of this study? What other information, if any, should she present to give decisionmakers a useful picture of the risks to the population from the refinery?.

Discussion. Presenting the $F(N)$ curve is a good beginning, but it leaves out essential information about the *distribution* of individual risks in the population. Such curves are typically built up by identifying (ideally all) accident scenarios, counting the *number* of people killed in each scenario, assessing the expected annual frequency of each scenario, and then reporting for each integer N the total probability (or hazard rate) of all scenarios in which N or more people are killed (8, 48). What this leaves out is *which* people are killed in which scenarios. For example, if the nearest neighbor to the plant is killed in every scenario where fatalities occur, then his individual risk will be much higher than if he is killed only in scenarios where the wind is blowing in his direction (and therefore away from some other people.) The $F(N)$ curve is insensitive to such differences and cross-correlations among individual risks. To correct this deficiency, the risk analyst should at a minimum supplement the $F(N)$ curve with a second curve showing the frequency distribution of individual risks in the population. This curve, say $N(x)$, would assess for each individual the total probability (annual hazard rate) of all scenarios in which that individual is killed and would then plot the number of people, $N(x)$, with fatality risk rates of x or greater for each $x > 0$. The risk to the most-threatened individual, for example, could be read directly off this curve. Thus, $N(x)$ is derived from the same information and assumptions about scenarios, scenario probabilities, and consequences as $F(N)$ but provides an additional perspective on population risk. *Risk contours* showing the risk of accident fatality at different distances around the refinery, superimposed on a map of population density, can also provide a convenient visual display of this type of information.

As a further example of the application of decision-analytic reasoning to fundamental risk management trade-offs, we show how it can clarify the choice between situations analogous to cases A and D in the list of trade-offs given above.

Example 16. Certain versus Uncertain Risks in Large Populations. Which is preferable: a population of 100 people, each with a discrete-time fatality hazard rate (= probability of death each year) of h; or a population of 100 people, each of whom is equally likely to have a hazard rate of $h/2$ or $3h/2$ each year? Assume that, in the second alternative, no individual knows his own hazard rate.

Solution. Applying the $k[(m - m') - (k/2)(v' - v)]$ formula to this problem, along with some probability calculations for the relevant means and variances, shows that for k close to zero, the second (*random risk*) option is preferable, while for extremely risk-averse decisionmakers, the first (*known risk*) option is preferable. There is no absolute basis for choosing between the known-risk and random-risk alternatives: attitude toward risk is an essential determinant of preference in this case.

There are some other worthwhile points in this example. Note that *even though the expected individual hazard rate (computed with respect to ex ante information) is identical in both cases, each individual expects to live longer in the second case*, that is, under random as opposed to known risk. The reason is that even though $0.5(h/2) + 0.5(3h/2) = h$ when only the initial information is available, as time passes, survivors will have assessed hazard rates that become closer and closer to $h/2$, and expected remaining lifetimes that become closer and closer to $2/h$ rather than $2/3h$. Survival is itself informative, providing evidence that the survivor is more likely than not of the lower-risk type: therefore, the assessed individual hazard rates will be steadily declining from their initial level of h for as long as individuals survive. Expected survival times must be calculated with respect to the information that is likely to be revealed, rather than only with respect to the initial information.

Suppose that the second case in Example 15 were modified so that *all* individuals had the same hazard rate, either $h/2$ or $3h/2$, each with 50% probability. (This would be analogous to case E.) For example, this pattern might be characteristic of a product that exposes every taker to the same risk (either $h/2$ or $3h/2$), but where the magnitude of this risk is uncertain. Then the total remaining life-years in the population would no longer be normally distributed. Instead, it would have a bimodal (two-peaked) distribution. Individual risks are no longer statistically independent from the decisionmaker's point of view, since one person's survival time is informative about the probable survival times of the others. Thus, *statistical independence is in part a property of the risk assessor's information set*, rather than an objective property of biological disease mechanism.

As a final example of the application of the decision-analytic viewpoint in risk analysis, consider the following illustration of its use in risk–benefit analysis.

Example 17. Societal versus Individual Risk–Benefit Analysis. Imagine that 600 people work in an underground coal mine. Each does roughly the same job and expects to work in the same mine for 40 years. Each initially has an occupational accident fatality hazard rate of 0.001 per year and a nonoccupational (background) hazard rate from all other sources of 0.02 per year. A proposed change in mining practices would increase the occupational fatality hazard rate to 0.002 per year, but would raise average productivity and salaries by $2000 per work-year. Each miner feels that he would be willing to accept a 0.001 increase in annual occupational hazard rate in return for an extra $2000 per year of compensation *if*, and only if, he survives for at least another 45 years to enjoy the increased wealth. Otherwise, in retrospect, he will feel that the increased risk and anxiety were not worth the increased salary. Under these assumptions, is the proposed change "acceptable"?

Discussion. Initially, each individual has an expected remaining lifetime of $1/0.021 = 47.65$ years. The proposed change would decrease *expected* remaining life to 45.45 years, which might make it just barely acceptable to each miner based on his ex ante expectations. However, the *median* survival time would only be $0.69/0.022 = 31.36$ years, due to the skewness of the exponential survivor function, which has a median equal to 0.69 times the mean. The majority of miners will therefore achieve increments in lifetime wealth and enjoyment that are insufficient in retrospect to make the increased risk worthwhile—and this is predictable in advance. There is thus a conflict between the ex ante risk projections of each individual and the statistically predictable pattern of population risk. Each individual expects to live longer than most of them actually will. Whether public decisions should be based on ex ante majority preferences for action (e.g., implementation of the proposed change) or on statistically predictable ex post majority preference for consequences is one of the policy questions confronted in the emerging field of cost–risk–benefit analysis for public policymaking (49, 50).

The idea, illustrated in Example 17, that the evaluation of a decision made today should depend on preferences at more than one point in time—not only at the decision date but also at future dates when consequences are known and regrets may be felt—has only recently started to be incorporated into the main stream of normative decision theory (44, 45). Its consequences for cost–risk–benefit analysis and for other approaches to social risk management decisionmaking have yet to be developed by economists and academic researchers. For the regulator, judge, manufacturer, or policy analyst who uses the results of a quantitative risk analysis to make or recommend decisions, however, it is essential to bear in mind that today's decisions will be evaluated retrospectively. At the decision date, it is not enough to choose the best action based on current information and preferences: retrospective preferences under different possible outcomes must also be considered.

5   SOURCES OF UNCERTAINTY IN STATISTICAL RISK ASSESSMENT

The ideas and examples in the preceding section explain the key concepts of individual risk and population risk for chronic health effects. The practice of risk assessment requires both estimating such risks from data and deciding what data to collect. In almost all cases, the resulting estimates of health risks will be highly uncertain, making relevant the kinds of considerations we have raised regarding the quantification and presentation of uncertain risks. The process of estimation itself, along with associated tests of hypotheses (e.g., that an effect on disease incidence rate or life span exists), constitutes statistical or quantitative risk assessment. Although statistical risk assessment methods are beyond the intended scope of this chapter, this section summarizes some of the most important aspects to illustrate the sources and types of uncertainties that can be expected to arise in practice.

Environmental health and safety risk assessments are usually organized around a causal chain leading from operation of a risk *source* (e.g., a power plant producing pollutants) through environmental fate and transport mechanisms to individual *exposures* and intake or uptake. Exposure, in turn, leads to a received dose, which produces a probabilistic response that can be conceptualized in terms of hazard functions. The relation between received dose and probability (or hazard function) of a health response is called the *dose–response function*: it is one of the most crucial links in the causal chain.

In practice, two statistical strategies—the *epidemiological* approach and the *experimental* (animal bioassay) approach—are most often used to estimate quantitatively human health risks from a source of exposure. The epidemiological (or quasiexperimental) approach (51, 52) focuses on statistical association between exposures and effects. The existence of an exposure–response relation in human populations is verified at some level of confidence using statistical hypothesis-testing checks applied to an exposed group and an unexposed control group. The strength of the relation may be estimated and expressed using measures such as relative risk (the ratio of the incidence rates in exposed and comparable unexposed populations) or attributable risk (the difference in incidence rates).

Example 12 illustrated some of the difficulties with the epidemiological approach. The presence of *population heterogeneity* can introduce major uncertainty about the existence as well as the sign and magnitude of health effects (68). Sound causal inference can also be hindered by a variety of other "threats to validity," including presence of *confounding factors* that might offer competing explanations for any observed association between exposure and effects, producing correlation or association in the absence of causation; *sample selection biases* that make the studied groups nonrepresentative of the larger populations for which inferences are to be drawn; and *sampling variability* that guarantees some degree of randomness in results, and hence some uncertainty about conclusions (51). In light of these difficulties, epidemiological studies must often rely on untested assumptions—for example, that there is no hidden heterogeneity or that the exposure–response relation has a particular parametric form—to reach sharp conclusions. As in Example 12, the consequence of a violation of these assumptions can be dramatically mistaken inferences about the risk relation between exposure and health responses.

The second major approach to statistical risk assessment involves controlled, designed laboratory experiments and statistical analysis of experimental data. Dose–response relations are usually the focus of such research. These relations are generally estimated by studying animal responses at high dose rates and extrapolating the resulting estimated probabilistic dose–response patterns to realistic dose level for human beings. This process involves enormous uncertainties—in the estimation of animal dose–response relations at high doses, in extrapolation of the estimates to low doses, and in extrapolation from laboratory animals to human populations.

5.1   Sampling Variability and Confidence Intervals in Risk Models

Table 2 summarized the kinds of data typically used in quantitative risk assessment (69). The following example illustrates some of the problems encountered in statistical risk assessment based on animal studies.

Example 18. *Statistical Risk Analysis of Experimental Data*

One hundred carefully matched laboratory mice are each fed d mg/day of a food additive X that is suspected of being carcinogenic. At the end of 90 days, the mice are sacrificed and inspected for tumors. Five mice are found to have tumors. In a matched control group of 100 mice, only one tumor is found.

(i) What conclusions can be drawn about the carcinogenic hazard posed by substance X?

(ii) How might the evidence from this experiment be used in setting exposure standards?

Solution

A. Hypothesis Testing and Estimation. (i) In this experiment, the time-to-tumor for each mouse is not directly observable: only the presence or absence of tumors at autopsy can be determined. Thus, sacrificing the mice after 90 days provides data that can be used to estimate directly only one point on the survival curve: the probability of surviving for 90 days without a tumor. In the exposed group a point estimate of this probability is $S(d, 90)$ = 0.95; while in the control group, it is $S(0, 90) = 0.99$. With 100 cases in each group, and assuming homogeneous populations in each group, a 95% confidence interval for the difference between the true probabilities corresponding to these sample proportions is found by the standard binomial test for differences of proportions (12) to be $(0.99 - 0.95)$ $\pm 1.96[(0.05)(0.95)/100 + (0.01)(0.99)/100]^{1/2} = 0.01 \pm 0.047$. Since this interval includes zero, we cannot reject (at the 5% significance level, i.e., the 95% confidence level) the *null hypothesis* that the true response probabilities after 90 days are identical in the exposed and unexposed populations. [This method of testing hypotheses can be found in most elementary statistics texts, including (53).] For example, the true probability of a tumor within 90 days might be 0.025 in both groups; this is quite consistent with the observed data. The basic problem is that random *sampling variability* could plausibly explain the observed difference between the two groups.

Suppose that it were *known* from past experience that the background risk level (or *spontaneous rate*) of tumors in these mice under laboratory conditions, but in the absence of exposure to substance X, is 0.01. Then the above evidence supports a much stronger conclusion. A 95% confidence interval for the 90-day response probability based on the observed 5/100 response rate is $0.05 \pm 1.96[(0.05)(0.95)/100]^{1/2} = 0.05 \pm 0.043$, falling just short of a significant difference from the background rate of 0.01. But the 90% confidence interval is $0.05 \pm 1.64[(0.05)(0.95)/100]^{1/2} = 0.05 \pm 0.036$, which does not include 0.01. Thus, we would be justified in concluding (at the 90%, but not at the 95%, confidence level) that the tumor rate after 90 days is significantly greater in the population of mice that has been exposed to substance X. The exact value of this rate is uncertain, due to sampling variability, but the 90% confidence interval is from 0.014 to 0.086.

B. Parametric Risk Modeling and Extrapolation. The analysis so far has been very limited. Only one point on the survival curve has been estimated, and even for that one point, survival probability has been estimated only for a daily dose of d mg/day of substance X; responses at higher or lower dose rates are not observed.

To extend the observed data to provide a useful basis for risk analysis, it is common practice to adopt a simple parametric statistical model that describes the dose–response relation over a wide range of values. [See, e.g. (54–56) for recent real examples.] The parameters of the model are then estimated from the observed data. For example, suppose that the simple survival time model

$$S(d, t) = \exp(-a - bdt)$$

is chosen, where $S(d, t)$ denotes the probability of surviving for at least t days without tumor, given an ingested dose of d mg/day of substance X. In this model, a and b are the parameters to be estimated. a is the base level of risk, and b reflects carcinogenic potency of X. The maximum-likelihood estimates of a and b are found by assuming that (i) the population of mice is homogeneous, so that a and b are the same for each mouse in the sample; and (ii) the sample values of $S(0, 90) = 0.99$ and $S(d, 90) = 0.95$ are exactly correct. Solving these two equations for a and b gives maximum-likelihood estimates for a and b of $a^* = 0.01$ and $b^* = 4.59 \times 10^{-4}$, respectively. The risk of tumor from any dose rate x is then extrapolated from this experiment via the fitted model

$$R(x, t) = 1 - \exp(-0.01 - 0.000459xt),$$

which is closely approximated by the linear function

$$R(x, t) = 0.01 + 0.000459xt$$

when the cumulative dose received, xt, is small. Here, $R(x, t)$ is defined as $1 - S(x, t)$, that is, as the probability of getting a tumor within t days, given a dose of x mg/day.

The risk model $R(x, t) = 0.01 + 0.000459xt$ is based on the maximum-likelihood estimates of $R(0, 90)$ and $R(d, 90)$. To obtain a *conservative* model, the upper 90% confidence bound on risk is sometimes used instead. For example, suppose that $R(0, 90)$ is known to be 0.01, but that $R(d, 90)$ has been estimated from this one experiment and has a 90% confidence interval (calculated above) of from 0.014 to 0.086. If $S(d, t)$ is assumed (conservatively) to be $1 - 0.086 = 0.914$, then repeating the calculations just performed would give the conservative risk model

$$R(d, t) = 0.01 + 0.000888xt$$

when xt is small (e.g., less than 0.1.).

C. Use of Risk Models in Risk Management. (ii) Suppose that it is decided that the incremental lifetime tumor risk to workers exposed to substance X should be less than 10^{-6}. To implement this standard, assuming that the above dose–response model is correct, one could reason as follows. Suppose that a dose of d mg/day to a mouse is assumed to correspond to a dose of $100d$ mg/day in a human being, based on the ratios of body weights and skin areas and on the assumed relative biological relevances of these two ratios for extrapolating the effects of substance X from mice to humans. (The factor of 100 is called the *interspecies dose conversion factor*.) An upper bound on occupational exposure time might be 60 years. An upper bound on lifetime might be 100 years. Incremental lifetime tumor risk is therefore probably less than $(0.000888)(0.01$ human/mouse interspecies dose conversion factor) $(100$ years) $(365$ days/year) $(x\,mg/day) = 0.323x$, which would be the risk to someone exposed to $x\,mg/day$ every day for 100 years under the conservative risk model developed above. For $0.323x$ to be less than the design goal of 1×10^{-6}, x must be less than $3.1 \times 10^{-6}\,mg/day$. This could therefore be set as an occupational exposure standard to implement the desired risk goal with high (90%) confidence, assuming that all the other assumptions made are correct.

Example 18 illustrates both the power and some of the pitfalls of quantitative risk assessment. On the positive side, it gives a formula grounded in data that can provide useful guidance for implementing public policy. This kind of quantitative reasoning is one of the chief attractions of quantitative risk assessment for policymakers who feel a need to inject a degree of scientific rigor and rationality into their decisionmaking. On the negative side, the analysis is critically dependent on assumptions that are apt to be very uncertain. These include (i) the hypothesized form of the survival function $S(x, t)$; (ii) the assumed interspecies dose conversion factor (and the more subtle assumption that a constant, rather than a function, is sufficient to make this conversion); and (iii) the assumption that all individuals have the same survival function, so that point estimates and confidence intervals can meaningfully be constructed. In practice, it may be that $S(d, 90)$, for example, is different for different members of the population. To assure that no worker will have an excess lifetime tumor risk of greater than 10^{-6}, it may then be necessary to set exposure levels so low (in order to protect the most sensitive members of the exposed population) that the activity that produces exposure to X is no longer economically feasible.

5.2 Sources of Uncertainty in Parametric Risk Models

The calculations in Example 18 have deliberately been kept very simple. However, refinements of this basic approach have been worked out in detail for many parametric risk models [e.g., see (56) for a thorough recent technical treatment] and for semiparametric models such as the class of *proportional hazard* models (57–59), in which it is assumed that the effect of exposure is to multiply the exposed individual's hazard function by a constant greater than 1. Extensions to missing and "censored" observations (e.g., to account for tumors that might have developed had not the study been ended when it was) have been made and continue to appear in the literature (57–60). Powerful general methods have been developed for large samples based on the asymptotic properties of the *log likelihood function* relating maximum-likelihood estimates of parameters to their true values (58).

Despite this sophistication in parameter estimation methods, statistical risk assessment using parametric models suffers in general from the kinds of severe practical limitations identified for Example 18. Perhaps the greatest is that *multiple models, having quite different implications at low doses, may all adequately "fit" the observed dose–response data.* The literature on cancer risk assessment, for example, is full of comparisons of Weibull, logistic, multi stage, and multihit models (often based on competing views of the underlying mechanisms of carcinogenesis), none of which can confidently be rejected on the basis of observed data (61). A complementary problem is that *none of the common parametric models may provide an adequate fit to the observed dose–response data.* Finally, *uncertainty about the parameters of a model,* as reflected in simultaneous confidence regions for the model parameters, *may translate into very wide confidence bands for hazard functions or response probabilities* (15).

5.3 Nonparametric Models

Combining uncertainty about which model to use (*model uncertainty*) with uncertainty about parameter values (*statistical uncertainty*, e.g., as captured in confidence intervals for parameters) can lead to uncertainties in predicted hazard rates and lifetime response probabilities that span three or more orders of magnitude. Partially in response to these difficulties, and partially in light of technical progress in the statistical theory of failure processes, modern methods of statistical risk assessment have more and more turned to *nonparametric methods* for analyzing survival time data (57, 58, 62). Here, the risk assessor attempts to estimate underlying hazard functions or survival functions directly from observed survival times, without going through any intervening parameters. Confidence bands are estimated for entire survival time distributions or hazard function simultaneously, rather than being constructed for parameters and then translated into corresponding confidence bands for model predictions.

Nonparametric methods based on direct maximum-likelihood estimation of survival probabilities (rather than on hypothesized underlying parameters) can accommodate a number of realistic constraints on observation conditions—for example, randomly missing or partially censored observations—and give useful estimates of survival probabilities over the region of observations. Moreover, a rich underlying mathematical theory that unifies many of the statistical methods developed by practitioners over the past 30 years is emerging (62, 63). However, even nonparametric methods cannot solve the problem of extrapolating from observed high-dose responses to probable low-dose responses. New laboratory methods based on biological markers (so-called molecular epidemiology methods) may offer a new potential for closing this gap (25–27). They may also help solve the equally challenging problems of extrapolating from a study population consisting of homogeneous laboratory animals to a target population consisting of highly heterogeneous humans (25–27; see also 65).

6 CONCLUSIONS: PRESENTING AND MANAGING UNCERTAIN RISKS

Given the inevitable and often very wide [e.g., three to six orders of magnitude (61, 66)] uncertainties in quantitative risk estimates, what steps should the authors of a risk analysis take in presenting their results to decisionmakers? Several approaches have been suggested in this chapter.

- Results should be presented in a sufficiently disaggregated form (showing risks for different subgroups) so that key uncertainties and heterogeneities are not lost in the aggregation. (See Example 12.)
- Confidence bands around the predictions of statistical models are useful, but uncertainties about the assumptions of the model itself should also be presented.
- Both individual risks (e.g., for the typical and the most-threatened individuals in the population) and population risks should be presented, so that the equity of the distribution of individual risks in the population can be taken into account.
- Any uncertainties, heterogeneities, or correlations across individual risks should be identified.

- Individual risks can be described through survival functions and hazard functions.
- Population risks can be described either at the "micro" level, in terms of frequency distributions of individual risks, or at the "macro" level, using decision-analytic models, in terms of attributes such as equivalent number of life-years.

Another part of the answer is that *sensitivity analyses* for key assumptions should be used extensively. For example, results calculated for alternative plausible animal dose–response models, interspecies conversion factors, and assumptions about response heterogeneity in the exposed human population should be presented as an integral part of the results of the analysis. If risk predictions vary substantially with the assumptions, then alternative sets of assumptions, their corresponding predictions, and an assessment of the evidence supporting each should be presented. The alternative to this very full display (which can be very difficult to work with) is to have the analyst assess the probabilities that each alternative model or set of assumptions is correct, weight the risk predictions of the different models according to these probabilities, and then present the weighted average of risks as the final result. While this Bayesian approach certainly reduces the cognitive burden on the consumer of a risk analysis by replacing a set of alternative numbers with a single composite number, it imposes the beliefs or guesses of the risk analyst on the user of the analysis. Moreover, it conceals from the user the plausible range of risks and the assumptions to which they are most sensitive.

A final suggestion on presentation is that uncertain risks can be presented in a *decision tree* format (67) showing key uncertainties about assumptions, their possible resolutions (with one branch for each alternative), and, at the tips of the tree, the resulting risk estimates. If scientific information is expected to become available that will resolve some current uncertainties, then the times at which these uncertainties will be resolved can also be presented. Displaying uncertain risks in terms of a tree of branching alternative possibilities is especially useful in clarifying how current risk management decisions may be viewed in retrospect (looking back from the tips of the tree after some current uncertainties have been resolved). This can be a very effective perspective to bring to bear on current risk management decision problems.

Assuming that the risk analyst does a good job in presenting risk assessments and uncertainties, the risk manager or decisionmaker to whom the results are presented can take one of three kinds of actions: (i) decide that the current risk level and uncertainties are acceptable, and hence do nothing (except perhaps continue to monitor); (ii) decide that the current risk level is unacceptably high and devise and implement control measures to reduce it; or (iii) decide to collect further information to reduce the uncertainties about a risk before taking any action. In choosing among these options, the risk manager must consider a variety of social, legal, political, and moral factors in addition to the technical information that the risk assessor provides. These factors are discussed in Chapter 3. The technical aspects of a risk, as described in this chapter, are prerequisites for understanding the other issues involved in managing it.

ACKNOWLEDGEMENT

We gratefully acknowledge the insights and advice of Professor Alvin W. Drake of the Massachusetts Institute of Technology.

REFERENCES

1. C. Starr, Societal benefit vs. technological risk. *Science* **165**, 1232–1238 (1969).

2. B. Fischhoff, S. Lichtenstein, R. Keeney, and S. Derby, *Acceptable Risk.* Cambridge Univ. Press, London and New York, 1981.

3. *Journal of Legal Studies,* **12** (special issue on Catastrophic Personal Injuries) (1983) (proceedings of a conference sponsored by the Hoover Institution).

4. *Journal of Legal Studies,* **14** (special issue on Tort Law Reform), 3 (1985) (proceedings of a conference sponsored by the Hoover Institution).

5. S. Shavell, A model of the optimal use of liability and safety regulation. *Rand J. Econ.* **15**(2), 271–280 (1984).

6. S. Shavell, an analysis of causation and the scope of liability in the law of torts. *J. Leg. Stud.* **9** (1980).

7. R. L. Keeney and H. Raiffa, *Decisions with Multiple Objectives.* Wiley, New York, 1976.

8. S. Kaplan and B. J. Garrick, On the quantitative definition of risk. *Risk Anal.* **1**(1), 11–26 (1981).

9. R. C. Elandt-Johnson and N. L. Johnson, *Survival Models and Data Analysis.* Wiley, New York, 1980.

10. R. E. Barlow and F. Proschan, *Statistical Theory of Reliability and Life Testing: Probability Models.* Holt, New York, 1975.

11. E. J. Henley and H. Kumamoto, *Reliability and Risk Assessment.* Prentice-Hall, Englewood Cliffs, NJ, 1981.

12. P. G. Hoel, *Elementary Statistics,* 4th ed. Wiley, New York, 1976.

13. D. H. Krantz, R. D. Luce, P. Suppes, and A. Tversky, *Foundations of Measurement,* Vol. 1. Academic Press, New York, 1971.

14. S. D. Walter, The estimation and interpretation of attributable risk in health research. *Biometrics* **32**, 829–849 (1976).

15. L. A. Cox, Statistical issues in the estimation of assigned shares for carcinogenesis liability. *Risk Anal.* **7**(1), 71–80 (1987).

16. F. A. Seiler and B. R. Scott, Mixtures of toxic agents and attributable risk calculations. *Risk Anal.* **7**(1), 81–90 (1987).

17. L. A. Cox, Probability of causation and the attributable proportion of risk. *Risk Anal.* **4**(3), 221–230 (1984).

18. *Radiation Cancer Liability,* Senate Hearing 98–1210, United States Senate, September 18, 1984.

19. S. Lagakos and F. Mosteller, Assigned shares in compensation for radiation-related cancers. *Risk Anal.* **6**, 345–375 (1986) (see also the comments that follow this paper).

20. R. E. Barlow and F. Proschan, "Importance of System Components and Fault Tree Events," Rep. ORC 73-34. Operations Research Center, University of California at Berkeley, 1974.

21. K. S. Crump and B. C. Allen Quantitative assessment of carcinogenic hazards using epidemiological data. In R. S. McColl (Ed.), *Environmental Health Risks: Assessment and Management.* Univ. of Waterloo Press, Waterloo, Ontario, Canada, 1987.

22. L. A. Cox, A new measure of attributable risk for public health applications. *Manag. Sci.* **31**, 7 (1985).

23. W. Kruskal, Relative importance by averaging over orderings. *Am. Stat.* **41**, 1 (1987).

24. U. S. Department of Health and Human Services, Task Force on Health Risk Assessment, *Determining Risks to Health: Federal Policy and Practice.* Auburn House, Dover, MA, 1986.

25. F. P. Perera, Molecular cancer epidemiology: A new tool in cancer prevention. *JNCI, J. Nat. Cancer Inst.* **78**(5), 887–898 (1987).

26. D. B. Hattis, The promise of molecular epidemiology for quantitative risk assessment. *Risk Anal.* **6**(2), 181–194 (1986).

27. F. P. Perera, New approaches in risk assessment for carcinogens. *Risk Anal.* **6**(2), 195–202 (1986).

28. W. Feller, *An Introduction to Probability Theory and Its Applications*, 2nd ed., Vol. 1. Wiley, New York, 1971.

29. C. R. Blyth, On Simpson's paradox and the sure thing principle. *J. Am. Stat. Assoc.* **67**, 364–366 (1972).

30. D. G. Saari, The source of some paradoxes from social choice theory and probability. *J. Econ. Theory* **41**, 1–22 (1987).

31. B. S. Everitt and D. J. Hand, *Finite Mixture Distributions*. Chapman & Hall, New York, 1984.

32. R. L. Keeney, *Siting Energy Facilities*. Academic Press, New York, 1980.

33. B. P. Stigum and F. Wenstop, *Foundations of Utility and Risk Theory with Applications*. Reidel Publ., Dordrecht, Netherlands, 1983.

34. R. A. Howard, On fates comparable to death. *Manage. Sci.* **30**(4), 407–422 (1984).

35. S. E. Bodily, Analysis of risks to life and limb. *Oper. Res.* **28**, 1 (1980).

36. J. S. Dyer and R. K. Sarin, Relative risk aversion. *Manage. Sci.* **28**, 875–886 (1982).

37. L. A. Cox, Comparative risk measures for heterogeneous populations. In A. Woodhead (Ed.), *Phenotypic Variation in Populations: Relevance to Risk Assessment*. Plenum Press, New York, 1987 (in press).

38. R. L. Keeney, Equity and public risk. *Oper. Res.* **28**, 527–534 (1980).

39. R. L. Keeney and R. L. Winkler, Evaluating decision strategies for equity of public risks. *Oper. Res.* **33**(5), 955–970 (1985).

40. P. C. Fishburn, Equity axioms for public risks. *Oper. Res.* **32**(4), 901–908 (1984).

41. E. Karni, *Decision Making Under Uncertainty: The Case of State-Dependent Preferences*. Harvard Univ. Press, Cambridge, MA, 1985.

42. M. Machina, Temporal risk and the nature of induced preferences. *J. Econ. Theory*, 199–231 (1984).

43. D. M. Kreps and E. L. Porteus, Dynamic choice theory and dynamic programming. *Econometrica* **47**, 91–100 (1979).

44. D. E. Bell, Risk premiums for decision regret. *Manage. Sci.* **29**, 10 (1983).

45. G. Loomes and R. Sugden, Some implications of a more general form of regret theory. *J. Econ. Theory* **41**, 270–287 (1987).

46. F. R. Farmer, Reactor safety and siting: A proposed risk criterion. *Nucl. Saf.* **8**, 539–548 (1967).

47. R. F. Griffiths (Ed.), *Dealing with Risk*. Manchester University Press, Great Britain, 1981, esp. Chap. 4.

48. A. R. Sampson and R. L. Smith, Assessing risks through the determination of rare event probabilities. *Oper. Res.* **30**(5), 839–866 (1982).

49. A. R. Ferguson and E. P. LeVeen (Eds.), *The Benefits of Health and Safety Regulation*. Ballinger, Cambridge, MA, 1981.

50. J. D. Bentkover, V. T. Covello, and J. Mumpower (Eds.), *Benefits Assessment: The State of the Art*. Reidel Publ., Boston, MA, 1986.

51. S. Anderson et al., *Statistical Methods for Comparative Studies*. Wiley, New York, 1980.

52. J. Schlesselman, *Case-Control Studies: Design, Conduct, Analysis*. Oxford Univ. Press, London and New York, 1982.

53. M. H. DeGroot, *Probability and Statistics*. Addison-Wesley, Reading, MA, 1975. [See Hoel (12) for a more elementary introduction to probability and statistics.]

54. K. G. Brown and D. G. Hoel, Statistical modeling of animal bioassay data with variable dosing regimes: Example—Vinyl chloride. *Risk Anal.* **6**(2), 155–166 (1986).

55. J. N. Rowe and J. A. Springer, Asbestos lung cancer risks: Comparison of animal and human extrapolations. *Risk Anal.* **6**(2), 171–180 (1986).

56. K. S. Crump and B. C. Allen, Quantitative assessment of carcinogenic hazards using epidemiological data. In R. S. McColl (Ed.), *Environmental Health Risks: Assessment and Management.* Univ. of Waterloo Press, Waterloo, Ontario, Canada, 1987.

57. J. D. Kalbfleish and R. L. Prentice, *The Statistical Analysis of Failure Time Data.* Wiley, New York, 1980.

58. J. F. Lawless, *Statistical Models and Methods for Lifetime Data.* Wiley, New York, 1982.

59. D. R. Cox and D. Oakes, *Analysis of Survival Data.* Chapman & Hall, New York, 1984.

60. A. Dewanji and J. D. Kalbfleisch, Nonparametric methods for survival/sacrifice experiments. *Biometrics* **42**, 325–341 (1986).

61. M. A. Schneiderman, The uncertain risks we run. In R. C. Schwing and W. A. Albers (Eds.), *Societal Risk Assessment: How Safe is Safe Enough?* Plenum Press, New York, 1980.

62. P. K. Andersen et al., Linear nonparametric tests for comparison of counting processes, with applications to censored survival data. *Int. Stat. Rev.* **50**, 219–258 (1982).

63. R. D. Gill, Understanding Cox's regression model: A martingale approach. *J. Am. Stat. Assoc.* **79**, 441–447 (1984).

64. M. Brown and S. M. Ross, The observed hazard and multicomponent systems. *Nav. Res. Logistics Q.* **29**(4), 679–683 (1982).

65. J. E. Harris and W. H. DuMouchel, Bayes methods for combining the results of cancer studies in humans and other species. *J. Am. Stat. Assoc.* **78**, 293–315 (1983).

66. R. L. Sielken, Jr., The capabilities, sensitivity, pitfalls, and future of quantitative risk assessment. In R. S. McColl (Ed.), *Environmental Health Risks: Assessment and Management.* Univ. of Waterloo Press, Waterloo, Ontario, Canada, 1987.

67. D. von Winterfeldt and W. Edwards, *Decision Analysis and Behavioral Research.* Cambridge Univ. Press, London and New York, 1987.

68. J. D. Brain et al. (Eds.), *Variations in Susceptibility to Inhaled Pollutants: Identification, Meachanisms, and Policy Implications.* Johns Hopkins Univ. Press, Baltimore, MD, 1987.

69. P. F. Ricci (Ed.) *Principles of Health Risk Assessment*, Prentice-Hall, Englewood Cliffs, N.J., (1985).

3

Epidemiology in Environmental Risk Assessment*

Maxwell W. Layard
Failure Analysis Associates, Palo Alto, California

Abraham Silvers
Electric Power Research Institute, Palo Alto, California

1 INTRODUCTION

Epidemiology can be defined as the science that describes the distribution of disease in populations and analyzes the factors that influence disease distribution. The spirit of the science is well exemplified by the methods used by John Snow in discovering the source of a cholera epidemic (1). In 1854, an epidemic of the debilitating disease cholera was killing hundreds of people in south London. Snow hypothesized that the disease entered through the alimentary system. By plotting residences of the cases on a map, Snow noticed that they were clustered around one particular public water supply, the Broad Street pump. He conjectured that water from that pump was the source of the disease and recommended that the pump be closed. This mitigation effort worked and the epidemic disappeared. Snow's procedure consisted of establishing a hypothesis, testing the hypothesis relating the exposure to disease, and then eliminating or reducing the risk factor.

In modern chronic disease epidemiology (e.g., heart disease, cancer), an intermediate step in an epidemiologic investigation is to introduce a statistical model to test the hypothesis of an association between a risk factor and disease. The elucidation of cholesterol as a risk factor for heart disease illustrates this process (2). The hypothesis is that high levels of serum cholesterol predispose an individual to coronary heart disease. Data are collected to test the hypothesis, and a statistical model, such as a linear logistic regression equation, is fitted to the data. Statistical estimation and hypothesis testing

*The views expressed here are those of the authors and do not necessarily reflect the opinions of their organizations.

methods are used to evaluate the magnitude and plausibility of the association between cholesterol level and heart disease; if the evidence provided by this assessment is sufficiently strong, an association is presumed to exist. In contemporary parlance, a hazard is identified, that is, cholestrol is a risk factor, and an association is established between disease and risk factor. Further considerations, such as consistency of an association in different studies and populations, are usually necessary to support the judgment that an association is causal (3). In this example mitigation proceeds by attempting to persuade high-risk individuals, through medical advice and public education activities, to reduce their cholesterol level by dietary means or drug therapy.

In environmental risk assessment, we are often interested in estimating a disease-specific *excess lifetime risk*, that is, the probability of dying of a certain disease caused by a specified level of environmental pollution by a toxic agent (4). The use of epidemiologic data in this risk assessment process has important advantages relative to the use of animal toxicologic data (5). Because epidemiology provides direct information from human experience, it avoids the manifold problems involved in extrapolating results from an animal species to humans. In some cases, epidemiologic studies have demonstrated the human carcinogenicity of an agent that has not been shown conclusively to be carcinogenic in animal studies (e.g., benzene). Also, human data are important in supplementing and modifying the results of animal data, because of the great variability in risk estimates from animal data arising from such factors as species differences and choice of dose–response model. Of course, in spite of their desirability, good epidemiologic data are not always available, in which case animal data must form the main basis for risk assessment.

Epidemiologic studies are difficult and costly to conduct, and there are many problems in their analysis and interpretation, some of which are discussed briefly in Section 2. Section 3 outlines some statistical approaches to analysis of epidemiologic cohort studies, and in Section 4 we give two examples of the application of epidemiologic studies to risk assessment.

2   ISSUES IN THE ANALYSIS OF EPIDEMIOLOGIC DATA

The epidemiologic investigation of human populations encompasses a variety of research methodologies, including community, occupational, and hospital studies. Although we focus on occupational studies in this chapter, the principles that are discussed here are equally valid for other types of investigation.

An epidemiologic study is an investigation of one or more human diseases, the object usually being to discover the factors associated with the diseases, such as exposure to industrial pollutants. Epidemiologic studies of exposure–disease relations are observational rather than experimental; that is, the investigator cannot control the conditions under which the study is conducted. In particular, the epidemiologist cannot randomly assign individuals to exposed and nonexposed groups if the agent under study is suspected of being disease-causing. Such random assignment is an essential feature of experimental study design. Nevertheless, properly designed and conducted epidemiologic studies can provide evidence of a causal relation between a toxic agent and disease.

Epidemiologic studies fall into two main categories: (i) prospective studies, also known as cohort studies, and (ii) retrospective studies, also known as case–control studies. The distinction between cohort and case–control studies is that in cohort studies observation proceeds forward in time, from exposure to a suspected toxic agent to disease occurrence, while in case–control studies observation is backward in time from disease occurrence to exposure history.

A cohort study consists of a group of exposed individuals, and possibly also of a group of unexposed persons called a control group. Both groups are followed for a period of time, in some cases many years, and instances of disease or death are noted in the two groups. If the study does not include a control group, then the disease or mortality experience of the exposed cohort must be compared with data from an appropriate comparison population, which might, for example, be the general U.S. population.

A case–control study has two groups, one consisting of people with a specific disease such as lung cancer (the cases), and the other, called the control group, consisting of individuals who do not have the disease but who are selected to be similar, with respect to characteristics other than exposure, to the diseased group. The histories of cases and controls are compared to see if the two groups differ in terms of exposure.

A sound epidemiologic study requires careful and workable definitions of exposure and disease. Another requirement is a set of procedures and criteria for choosing the exposed group (in the case of a cohort study) or diseased group (in a case–control study) and for choosing the control group in such a way as to avoid bias in the comparison of the groups with respect to disease or exposure. For example, bias would arise if the control group in a case–control study were chosen from people with diseases other than the one under study, and those people had exposure histories different from the exposure pattern among healthy individuals. The follow-up procedures, or methods of determining exposure history, must be well defined and applied carefully and equally to both comparison groups. Potential confounding factors—such as age—which might distort the assessment of association between exposure and disease must be identified so they can be allowed for in the statistical analysis of the study outcomes. The study groups must be large enough to provide adequate assurance that an observed association is not due to chance, if in fact there is a true association between exposure and disease.

In assessing the association between an agent and disease, a commonly used technique in epidemiologic studies is estimation of the relative risk of the disease for people who are exposed to the agent as compared to people who are not exposed. The relative risk is defined to be the ratio of the disease incidence rate among exposed people to the incidence rate among unexposed people. A disease incidence rate is typically expressed as the number of new cases per year per 100,000 persons. Relative risk is a measure of the strength of the association between exposure and disease. A relative risk of 1 corresponds to no association between the exposure agent and disease. A relative risk of 3, for example, means that exposed people in the study get the disease at three times the rate observed for unexposed people. If the exposed group consists of subgroups with different levels of exposure, then dose-specific relative risks can be calculated. Relative risk may vary with some characteristic of the study cohort, notably age, in which case it is useful to compute age-specific relative risks instead of a single summary relative risk.

In this chapter our discussion is limited to cohort studies. The excellent monograph by Breslow and Day (6) contains an extensive treatment of the analysis of case–control studies. A companion volume by the same authors (7) deals with cohort studies. As noted above, a cohort study follows an exposed group, and possibly also a nonexposed group, over a period of time. The objective of the study is to determine the rate of occurrence of one or more diseases in relation to level of exposure to a suspected toxic agent. A symbolic example of a cohort study is presented in Table 1. In this schema, the columns are levels of exposure and the rows are age ranges. As individuals in the study are followed over time, they contribute person-years to cells defined by level of exposure and age range. In the

TABLE 1. Grouped Data Layout for Cohort Study with J Age Levels and K Dose Levels

Age Level (j)	0	1	$\cdots$	K
		Exposure Level (k)		
1	y_{10} c_{10}	y_{11} c_{11}		y_{1K} c_{1K}
2	y_{20} c_{20}	y_{21} c_{21}		y_{2K} c_{2K}
$\vdots$			$y_{jk}{}^{a}$ $c_{jk}{}^{b}$	
J	y_{J0} c_{J0}	y_{J1} c_{J1}		y_{JK} c_{JK}

^{a}Number of disease occurrences.
^{b}Person-years at risk.

table, the designations inside the cells refer to the number (y_{jk}) of disease occurrences and the number of person-years at risk (c_{jk}). The disease rate per person-year in cell jk, r_{jk}, is obtained by dividing the number of disease cases by the number of person-years in cell jk; that is,

$$r_{jk} = \frac{y_{jk}}{c_{jk}}.$$

The matrix in Table 1 can be expanded to a multidimensional one in which other covariates, such as sex and socioeconomic status, are also considered.

Modern statistical approaches to the analysis of cohort data involve the selection of a quantitative model that relates disease incidence to explanatory variables such as age and dose, a subject that is taken up in Section 3. This model is used to test hypotheses and to make predictions. The hypothesis of primary interest is that increasing levels of exposure to an agent are associated with increasing occurrence rates of a disease such as cancer. In order to make predictions of disease incidence, the parameters of the model, that is, the coefficients of the explanatory variables, must be estimated.

There are many difficulties to be addressed in the analysis of cohort studies and in their application to risk assessment. Environmental exposure levels to a toxic agent for a human population are usually quite low in comparison to levels found in industrial settings in which epidemiologic studies are often conducted. Whittemore and McMillan (8), for example, noted that for radon, a cancer hazard, a working level month (WLM) is a unit measure of cumulative exposure to α radiation. An average individual living in the United States will have accumulated the equivalent of 14 WLM of radon exposure by age 70 due to exposure to ambient levels of radon in the air, whereas a typical U.S. uranium miner would have inhaled more than 3000 WLM before the establishment in 1970 of standards that were instrumental in lowering exposure levels for these workers. To establish risks associated with environmental exposures, by using data from an occupational study, it is usually necessary to perform an extrapolation from high exposures (high doses) to environmental levels (low doses). An accurate estimate of disease response at dose levels below the range of the observed data requires a reliable dose–response model as well as good estimates of its coefficients. Unfortunately, an adequate biological basis for model selection is often not available.

A frequent shortcoming of epidemiologic studies is that the levels of exposure are not well characterized. In many studies, surrogate measures are used, such as job titles or simply time employed in the industry as recalled by the individual. Establishing a dose–response relation is further complicated if exposure is intermittent or of varying intensity, which is typical in occupational studies. For example, a person may move from job to job within a company or industry and may have gaps in employment.

There are other difficult issues in the use of epidemiology for estimating disease incidence at environmental dose levels. Insufficient data may be available for adequate assessment of a hazard: the disease of interest may be rare and the study population small, making it difficult to discern significant effects. Humans live in an open society and are subject to factors that might mask the true association between exposure and disease and that may be only imperfectly measurable or not measurable at all. Different studies of the same agent may be inconsistent in their outcomes, and the reasons for the inconsistencies may be hard to identify.

The above-mentioned limitations of epidemiologic studies are often cited as reasons for discounting the value of human data in risk assessment, and conversely for the need to rely heavily on experimental animal data. But this view appears to ignore both the strengths of epidemiology and the limitations of toxicology in assessing human health risks. As noted in the introduction, epidemiologic data are directly relevant to human experience, while extrapolation of animal results to humans may be grossly erroneous. For many human diseases and toxic agents, adequate animal models are simply not available. Stallones (9) pointed out that the use of bioassay data in human risk assessment is limited almost entirely to carcinogenic agents, since this is the only case in which animal results are sufficiently analogous to human experience. The process of extrapolation from relatively high to very low doses, while certainly problematic, is common to risk assessments derived from epidemiologic occupational studies and from animal data and so cannot establish a preference for either source of information.

Whittemore (5) characterizes laboratory tests as "extremely limited tools for obtaining quantitative estimates of risk." She cites an example concerning the association between bladder cancer and saccharin ingestion, in which a single experiment with rats yielded estimates of lifetime human cancer risk due to ingestion of 12 g/day which varied by six orders of magnitude (from 0.001×10^{-6} to 5200×10^{-6}), depending on the dose and species extrapolation methods used. On the other hand, six epidemiologic case–control studies of saccharin and bladder cancer showed a consistent lack of association, which provides an upper bound on the level of human risk. Thus, epidemiology can play an important role in bracketing the risk estimates derived from animal experiments.

Epidemiologic data and analytical methods can form the basis for risk estimation by providing a model that predicts age- and dose-specific disease incidence rates. While animal experiments yield dose–response relations, they do not typically produce information that permits inferences about the dependence of human disease incidence on age. An epidemiologic model for age-specific rates, based on direct human experience, may thus provide a more reliable estimate of lifetime human disease risk at a given dose level than is available from animal data.

In the remainder of this chapter we explain how epidemiologic cohort data can be used to establish age-specific dose–response correlations between exposure and disease. We discuss the selection of a mathematical model for this purpose and statistical methods for fitting the model to the data. In two case studies we illustrate some of the considerations involved in arriving at an adequate description of the exposure–disease relation and the use of the model to develop an estimate of lifetime excess disease risk at a specified continuous level of exposure.

3   STATISTICAL APPROACHES TO PREDICTION

Suppose that we have available, from an epidemiologic cohort study, data on disease occurrence and person-years at risk for various levels of dose and age, as displayed symbolically in Table 1. In order to use these data to perform a risk assessment, we need to select a quantitative model relating disease rates to the explanatory variables and then to fit the model to the data. The model is expressed in the form of a mathematical equation, which states that the disease rate is equal to a function of the explanatory variables. As well as the values of the explanatory variables, this function involves unknown coefficients, or parameters, which must be estimated from the data. The parameter estimation process is what we mean by the phrase "fitting the model to the data." We use statistical methods to find the parameter estimates yielding rate predictions that are closest, according to a specified criterion, to the observed disease rates. In this section we discuss model selection and statistical analysis procedures for cohort studies.

First, we give a more precise definition of disease rates. The theoretical rate at which disease events occur per person per unit time at a particular instant of time t and exposure level d is a function of t and d known as the hazard rate or hazard function; we denote it by $\lambda(t, d)$. In an epidemiologic study, the hazard rate is commonly referred to as the disease incidence rate, or simply disease rate (death rate, in a mortality study). The disease rate will undoubtedly depend on factors other than age and exposure to the suspected toxicant, and to the extent that these factors are known and measurable they should be accounted for in the analysis of the study. However, in this discussion we shall for simplicity confine our attention to only two explanatory variables—age and dose level.

In cohort studies, the disease rate is often assumed to be constant in 5-year time (or age) periods (quinquennia) and is estimated for a particular quinquennium by dividing the number of newly diagnosed cases (or of deaths) by the total person-years at risk in that period. The resulting number is often very small, and it is customary to multiply it by 100,000 to yield a disease rate per 100,000 person-years. Since the time unit is a year, the rate so calculated is more accurately called the age-specific annual disease rate (or annual death rate). Another interpretation of the per-person annual disease rate is that, if it is small, it is nearly equal to the probability of a person contracting the disease in a 1-year period within a specified age quinquennium, conditional on surviving disease-free until the beginning of that year.

Referring again to Table 1, the number of disease cases in each cell, y_{jk}, is usually assumed to be an approximately Poisson-distributed random variable, and the true disease rate is modeled as a function of known covariate values and unknown parameters that are to be estimated. (The Poisson approximation is based on the disease rate in each cell being, by assumption, constant over the time period represented in the cell.) For the study represented symbolically in Table 1, a simple model called the hazard product, or multiplicative, model might be proposed. In this model the true disease rate λ_{jk} is considered to be the product of an age (row) effect ϕ_j and a dose (column) effect θ_k; that is,

$$\lambda_{jk} = \phi_j \theta_k. \tag{1}$$

Since on taking logarithms we have

$$\log \lambda_{jk} = \log \phi_j + \log \theta_k,$$

this model is also referred to as a log-linear model of age and dose effects. If θ_0, corresponding to zero dose, is set equal to 1, we see that $\phi_j = \lambda_{j0}$, and we can rewrite Eq. (1) as

$$\lambda_{jk} = \lambda_{j0}\theta_k. \tag{2}$$

It follows that under the product model the disease–rate ratio, or relative risk, for a particular dose level k relative to zero dose, does not depend on age:

$$RR_k = \frac{\lambda_{jk}}{\lambda_{j0}} = \theta_k.$$

Fitting the model to the data proceeds by finding estimates of the parameters λ_{j0} and θ_k which in some sense best fit the observed disease rates $r_{jk} = y_{jk}/c_{jk}$. (As noted below, values of the λ_{j0} are sometimes obtained from external sources, in which case only the θ_k need be estimated from the data.) If there are J age levels and K dose levels under consideration, this simple product model involves $J + K$ parameters, which must be estimated from the data or obtained from external sources.

Poisson regression methods are commonly used to fit models of disease or mortality rates to cohort data (10). The computer package GLIM (11) allows the necessary computations to be performed relatively easily. The goodness-of-fit of the models can be assessed by a measure called the deviance, which is a log likelihood ratio (12). The deviance is approximately distributed as a χ^2 random variable with degrees of freedom determined

TABLE 2. Data from U.S. Veterans Study of Cigarette Smoking and Lung Cancer Mortality

Age Group (years)		Non-smokers	Cigarettes/Day				
			Occasional	1–9	10–20	21–39	40+
35–44	Deaths	0	0	0	2	4	0
	Person-years	35,164	3,657	8,063	59,965	40,643	3,992
	(Rate per 10^5)	(0)	(0)	(0)	(3.34)	(9.84)	(0)
45–54	Deaths	0	0	0	2	10	2
	Person-years	15,134	1,283	3,129	16,392	12,839	1,928
	(Rate per 10^5)	(0)	(0)	(0)	(12.20)	(77.89)	(103.73)
55–64	Deaths	25	6	31	183	245	63
	Person-years	213,858	14,624	45,217	151,664	103,020	19,649
	(Rate per 10^5)	(11.69)	(41.03)	(68.56)	(120.66)	(237.82)	(320.63)
65–74	Deaths	49	10	44	239	194	50
	Person-years	171,211	10,053	37,130	101,731	50,045	8,937
	(Rate per 10^5)	(28.62)	(99.47)	(118.50)	(234.93)	(387.65)	(559.47)
75+	Deaths	4	1	5	15	7	3
	Person-years	8,489	512	1,923	3,867	1,273	232
	(Rate per 10^5)	(47.12)	(195.31)	(260.01)	(387.89)	(549.88)	(1,293.10)

Source: Frome and Checkoway (10). Reproduced by permission.

in a prescribed fashion. Estimates of the parameters and their estimated standard errors are also provided by GLIM.

Frome and Checkoway (10) use GLIM's Poisson regression facility to fit the product model of Eq. (1) to data from the Dorn study (13) of cigarette smoking and lung cancer among a cohort of U.S. veterans (see Table 2). The model fits the data well, the deviance being 12.5 on 20 degrees of freedom. The estimates of the λ_{j0} (age-specific nonsmoker lung cancer rates) and the θ_k (dose-specific relative risks) are displayed in Table 3.

When exposure level (dose) is treated as a continuous variable, a possibly more parsimonious product model, involving fewer parameters than the simple model of Eq. (1), is

$$\lambda(t, d) = \lambda_0(t)g(d), \tag{3}$$

where $\lambda_0(t)$ is the background or zero-dose incidence rate for the disease in question, d is dose, and g is a function that is equal to 1 when dose is zero. Forms of g that have been found useful in practice are a polynomial function

$$g(d) = 1 + \gamma_1 d + \gamma_2 d^2 + \cdots + \gamma_m d^m$$

and an exponential function

$$g(d) = \exp(\gamma d).$$

As in the case of the simple product model of Eq. (2), the relative risk for a given dose d does not depend on age:

$$RR(d) = \frac{\lambda(t, d)}{\lambda_0(t)} = g(d).$$

On the other hand, under the product model the risk difference (i.e., the disease-rate

TABLE 3. Parameter Estimates for Product Model Fit to U.S. Veterans Cohort Data

Age Group (years)	Estimated Nonsmoker Lung Cancer Death Rates/10^5 Person-Years
35–44	0.44
45–54	3.24
55–64	14.02
65–74	25.48
75 +	43.94

Cigarettes/Day	Estimated Relative Risk
None	1.00
Occasional	3.47
1–9	4.77
10–20	8.88
21–39	16.22
40 +	22.62

difference), or excess risk above background, will increase with age if $g(d) > 1$ for $d > 0$ and the background disease rate increases with age, as is usually the case:

$$\lambda(t, d) - \lambda_0(t) = \lambda_0(t) [g(d) - 1].$$

An important aspect of the product model, of Eq. (3), incorporating the function $g(d)$, is that unlike the simple model of Eq. (2), it provides a formal method for extrapolating the disease rate to dose levels due to environmental exposure, which may be much lower than the levels observed for an occupational cohort.

The background disease rate $\lambda_0(t)$ might be estimated in a number of ways. One method is to obtain $\lambda_0(t)$ from national (or regional) vital statistics. Another method is to treat the background rates as parameters which are estimated from the cohort data themselves without specifying a functional form for $\lambda_0(t)$; we have seen an example of this approach in the analysis of the U.S. veterans lung cancer data discussed above. This method is also employed in the widely used proportional hazards survival analysis model proposed by Cox (14). Using study cohort data is preferable to using external background rates if adequate data on unexposed persons are available, since the external reference population may have different characteristics from those of the study cohort. A review paper by Breslow et al. (15) discusses in detail these two approaches to estimating $\lambda_0(t)$.

A third way of estimating $\lambda_0(t)$, if an internal control group is available, is to assume a functional form for the background rates, the parameters of the function being estimated from the data. A product model of this kind arises, under certain assumptions about exposure, from the Armitage–Doll multistage theory of carcinogenesis (16), which has been found useful in describing the age distribution and exposure response to carcinogenic agents of a variety of human cancers. The simplest form of the multistage model postulates that there is, in the target tissue, a pool of cells each of which is capable of generating a malignant tumor after it has undergone a series of irreversible changes in a specific order. Thus, a cell must pass through $k - 1$ intermediate stages in its transformation from a normal state to a malignant (stage k) state. If the transition rate per unit time, in the absence of external carcinogenic exposure, from the $(i - 1)$th stage to the ith stage is α_i (independent of age), then the background age-specific disease incidence is predicted by the model to be proportional to the $(k - 1)$th power of age; that is,

$$\lambda_0(t) \propto \alpha_1 \alpha_2 \cdots \alpha_k t^{k-1}, \tag{4}$$

which more briefly can be expressed as

$$\lambda_0(t) = \alpha t^{k-1}.$$

(This assumes that the time required for a single malignant cell to grow to a detectable tumor is small relative to age t.) The log–linear relation implied by Eq. (5),

$$\log \lambda_0(t) = \log \alpha + (k - 1) \log t, \tag{5}$$

has been shown to approximate closely the form of the age distribution of adult human cancers at several different organ sites and in different populations (17). However, incidences of some cancers, notably childhood cancers and cancers of sexual organs, do not exhibit such a relation.

The effect of a carcinogen on the disease rates predicted by the multistage model depends on a number of factors, including which stages are affected by the agent and the way in which dose level influences the relevant transition rates. Regarding the latter consideration, it is frequently assumed that the transition rate of an affected stage is a linear function of dose; that is,

$$\alpha_i^* = \alpha_i + \beta_i d,$$

where α_i is the background transition rate. Referring to Eq. (4), we see that if just one stage is affected, and dose is continuous from birth at level d, then

$$\lambda(t, d) = \alpha t^{k-1}(1 + \gamma d)$$
$$= \lambda_0(t)(1 + \gamma d),$$

which is the product model of Eq. (3) with $g(d) = 1 + \gamma d$. If more than one, say m, stages are affected, then $g(d)$ is a polynomial of degree m in d:

$$g(d) = 1 + \gamma_1 d + \gamma_2 d^2 + \cdots + \gamma_m d^m,$$

where the γ_i satisfy certain constraints, notably that they are all positive.

The predictions of the Armitage–Doll multistage theory are more complicated when exposure to a carcinogen is not continuous from birth to age t. An occupational exposure, for example, begins at an age $t_0 > 0$ and might stop before the individual reaches age t. In this case the evolution of the disease rate with age depends not only on the number of stages affected but also on whether the affected stages are early or late in the sequence (18). A model of this kind is described in the arsenic example in Section 4.2.

Other multistage models of carcinogenesis are discussed in the review paper by Armitage (17), who lists many references on this topic.

In some cases the product model of Eq. (3) has been found to provide a good description of the association between disease incidence and exposure [e.g., lung cancer and cigarette smoking (19)], but for many diseases its predictions are not in accord with observed data, and different models, which may or may not have a biological rationale, must be considered. A simple possibility is an additive model,

$$\lambda(t, d) = \lambda_0(t) + f(d),$$

where $f(d) = 0$ when $d = 0$. For this model the excess risk is of course a constant independent of t, and the relative risk,

$$\mathrm{RR}(t, d) = 1 + \frac{f(d)}{\lambda_0(t)},$$

decreases with age if the background risk increases with age. For some diseases relative risk decreases with age while excess risk increases with age [an example is coronary heart disease and smoking (19)], which suggests that a model intermediate between an additive and a multiplicative model might provide an adequate description of the data. In Section 4.1 such a model is fit to data for occupational chromium exposure and lung cancer.

In this discussion we have not referred to the standardized mortality ratio (SMR), a popular summary measure of relative risk. The SMR is an appropriate summary measure when the relative risk is constant across age groups (as in the product model discussed above), but it may be misleading when that is not the case [see Whittemore (20)].

The focus of Section 4 is to illustrate how disease–rate models have been applied in environmental risk assessment. The choice of a model may be predicated on various considerations. A biological mechanism may be postulated which suggests the form of the model. An example is the Armitage–Doll multistage model of carcinogenesis discussed above. A model may also be chosen simply because it provides an adequate statistical fit to the data. For example, the model may be considered to be an additive or multiplicative function of the effects of age and dose, or a combination of such functions. The models in Section 4 illustrating these concepts are taken from reports of the U.S. EPA Cancer Assessment Group (CAG) on chromium and arsenic. These reports were used to help set federal standards for exposure to those substances.

4   APPLICATIONS

The examples presented in this section, concerning lung cancer and exposure to airborne chromium and arsenic, were selected partly because there are no good animal models available for inhalation exposure to these substances. This fact underscores the importance of the role of human epidemiologic data in risk assessment.

4.1   A Case Study: Chromium

Table 4 shows age-specific lung cancer deaths and person-years at risk for various levels of exposure to chromium (21), taken from the U.S. EPA Cancer Assessment Group (CAG) report (22). These data were derived from a study of an occupational cohort exposed to airborne chromium. The model proposed by CAG was

$$\lambda(t, d) = \lambda_0(t) + (q_1 d + q_2 d^2)t^{k-1},$$

where d and t represent dose level (in micrograms of chromium per cubic meter of air) and age, respectively, and $\lambda_0(t)$, the background rate, is estimated from 1964 U.S. vital statistics.

TABLE 4. Data from Mancuso Study of Exposure to Chromium and Lung Cancer Mortality[a]

Age	Concentration ($\mu g/m^3$)	Deaths	Person-Years	Background Rate[b]
50	5.66	3	1345	6.05×10^{-4}
50	25.27	6	931	6.05×10^{-4}
50	46.83	6	299	6.05×10^{-4}
60	4.68	4	1063	1.44×10^{-3}
60	20.79	5	712	1.44×10^{-3}
60	39.08	5	211	1.44×10^{-3}
70	4.41	2	401	1.57×10^{-3}
70	21.29	4	345	1.57×10^{-3}

[a]From U.S. EPA Health Assessment Document for Chromium (22).
[b]From 1964 U.S. Vital Statistics.

TABLE 5. Parameter Estimates for CAG Model Fit to Mancuso Chromium Data

	Parameter Estimate	Estimated Standard Error
q_1	1.15×10^{-7}	7.41×10^{-7}
q_2	1.21×10^{-9}	7.22×10^{-9}
$k-1$	1.94	1.55

TABLE 6. Estimated Correlation Matrix of Parameter Estimates for CAG Model Fit to Mancuso Chromium Data

	q_1	q_2	$k-1$
q_1	1		
q_2	0.935	1	
$k-1$	-0.997	-0.957	1

An analysis of the Mancuso (21) data using the CAG model and the GLIM computer package yielded the maximum likelihood estimates given in Table 5. They were similar to the EPA estimates. The model fits the data well, the deviance statistic being 2.2 on 5 degrees of freedom. However, the high standard errors relative to the parameter estimates indicate that the estimates are quite imprecise. The problem here is that the parameter estimates are highly interdependent, which is a consequence of the small range of $t = $ age represented in the data, namely 50–70 years, and of the correlation between d and d^2. The correlations of the parameter estimates are given in Table 6. An alternative model formulation might lead to more stable parameter estimates.

The CAG model is similar to a product model derived from the Armitage–Doll multistage model of carcinogenesis when two stages are assumed to be affected by the carcinogen, but it differs in that the background rate $\lambda_0(t)$ is obtained from external sources and is not necessarily proportional to the power of t that appears in the expression for excess risk,

$$(q_1 d + q_2 d^2)t^{k-1}.$$

Since the observed relative risk in the Mancuso data, using the external background rates, tends to decrease with age, and the excess risk tends to increase with age (see Table 7), we might consider a linear mixture of multiplicative and additive models such as that proposed by Thomas (23), using the external background rates for $\lambda_0(t)$. A multiplicative model is

$$\lambda(t, d) = \lambda_0(t)[1 + h(d)],$$

where $h(d) = 0$ when $d = 0$, and an additive model is

$$\lambda(t, d) = \lambda_0(t) + f(d),$$

where again $f(d) = 0$ when $d = 0$. In order to combine these models, we can equate them at $t = t_{min} = 50$, the lowest age represented in the data set, by setting $f(d) = h(d)\lambda_0(t_{min})$. Then

TABLE 7. Lung Cancer Mortality Relative Risks and Excess Risks for Mancuso Chromium Data

Age	Concentration ($\mu g/m^3$)	Relative Risk	Excess Risk
50	5.66	3.7	0.0016
60	4.68	2.6	0.0023
70	4.41	3.2	0.0034
50	25.27	10.7	0.0058
60	20.79	4.9	0.0056
70	21.29	7.4	0.0100
50	46.83	33.2	0.0195
60	39.08	16.5	0.0223

TABLE 8. Parameter Estimates for Mixture Model Fits to Mancuso Chromium Data

	Model with Quadratic Term		Model without Quadratic Term	
	Estimate	Standard Error	Estimate	Standard Error
q_1	0.386	0.224	0.489	0.133
q_2	0.004	0.007	—	—
α	0.374	0.411	0.321	0.376

the linear combination of the multiplicative and additive models is

$$\lambda(t, d) = \alpha\lambda_0(t)[1 + h(d)] + (1 - \alpha)[\lambda_0(t) + h(d)\lambda_0(t_{min})]$$
$$= \lambda_0(t) + h(d)[\lambda_0(t_{min}) + \alpha(\lambda_0(t) - \lambda_0(t_{min}))].$$

$\alpha = 0$ corresponds to an additive model, $\alpha = 1$ to a multiplicative model, and values of α between 0 and 1 represent models that are superadditive and submultiplicative.
Fitting this mixture model with

$$h(d) = q_1 d + q_2 d^2$$

yielded the parameter estimates and standard errors given in Table 8. A fit excluding the d^2 term indicated that its coefficient q_2 is not significantly different from zero ($\chi^2 = 0.33$ on 1 degree of freedom). The estimates from this reduced model are also given in Table 8. The fit of the model is good (deviance = 2.73 on 6 degrees of freedom). Note that the estimated standard error for q_1 is only 0.27 times the value of the parameter estimate, as compared to 6.44 times the estimate in the CAG model. Since the estimated value of α is 0.321, this analysis suggests that age and dose effects are more than additive but less than multiplicative, which is in accordance with the observed patterns of relative risk and excess risk (Table 7). However, the estimate of α has a large estimated standard error (0.376), so it is not possible to arrive at a very firm conclusion about the interaction of age and dose effects based on the small amount of data available.
For low doses, for which the quadratic term in the CAG model can be ignored, the two

models (CAG and mixture) give similar estimates of excess risk over background. At age $t = 50$, the excess risk is estimated at $0.000228 \times$ dose by the CAG model, and $0.000296 \times$ dose by the mixture model. At age $t = 70$, the excess risk is estimated to be $0.000427 \times$ dose by the CAG model and $0.000448 \times$ dose by the mixture model.

In spite of the similarity of these results, a procedure such as the mixture model formulation considered here seems preferable for these data, because it avoids the instability of the parameter estimates which results from using the term t^{k-1} when the data have only a short range of values of t. This point is important for low-dose extrapolation, for which a reliable estimate of the linear dose parameter q_1 is highly desirable.

The CAG report provides an estimate based on the Mancuso data of the *unit risk* of chromium as an air pollutant, defined as the incremental lifetime lung cancer risk over background due to continuous exposure to an atmospheric concentration of $1 \ \mu g/m^3$ of chromium. This can be interpreted as the probability of a person's dying of lung cancer due to that level of pollution, assuming, of course, that future risks remain the same as the past experience on which the estimate is based. The estimated unit risk, which takes into account probability of death from other causes, is 0.0116. If we make the reasonable assumption that excess lung cancer risk below age 40 is essentially zero, the mixture model would give roughly the same unit excess risk estimate as the CAG model. For lower than unit concentration, an excess risk estimate can be obtained by multiplying the unit excess risk estimate by the concentration in question. This procedure is referred to as linear nonthreshold low-dose extrapolation, because it assumes that there is no nonzero concentration at which excess risk is zero.

4.2   A Case Study: Arsenic

The discussion of the previous example emphasized the advantage of a strictly statistical fitting procedure to establish the model form. The next example illustrates the use of the Armitage–Doll multistage theory of carcinogenesis in selecting the model to be fit to the data. The study in question was conducted by Lee and Fraumeni (24) and concerns lung cancer deaths in a cohort of men occupationally exposed to inorganic arsenic at a Montana copper smelter. Part of the data from this study, reproduced in the CAG report on arsenic (25), is shown in Table 9. The data are classified by age at initial employment and by duration of employment. The latter is a surrogate measure for cumulative dose of arsenic.

Whittemore (18) and Day and Brown (26) show that if a multistage mechanism is assumed in which only the penultimate stage is affected by a nearly constant level of exposure to a carcinogen, then excess risk can be expressed as

$$\lambda(t,d) - \lambda_0(t) = c[(t_0 + d)^{k-1} - t_0^{k-1}], \tag{6}$$

where $t = $ age, $t_0 = $ age at start of exposure, $d = $ duration of exposure at some constant level, and c and k are parameters to be estimated. If f is the follow-up time after exposure ends, then $t = t_0 + d + f$, and the above equation indicates that excess risk at any age does not depend on f. However, if only the first stage is affected by exposure, then the multistage theory predicts that the excess risk is

$$\lambda(t,d) - \lambda_0(t) = c[(d + f)^{k-1} - f^{k-1}],$$

which does not depend on t_0, the age at initial exposure.

TABLE 9. Data from Lee–Fraumeni Study of Exposure to Arsenic and Lung Cancer Mortality—Low Exposure Level Group

Age at Initial Employment		Duration of Employment (years)				
		0–9	10–19	20–29	30–39	40+
<20	Obs[a]	0	0	1	1	3
	Exp[b]	0.056	0.117	0.478	1.59	1.57
	Pyr[c]	8524	5249	4038	3175	1376
20–29	Obs	0	0	2	5	6
	Exp	0.115	0.334	0.892	1.74	0.796
	Pyr	9951	4724	2965	2117	834
30–39	Obs	0	3	1	0	1
	Exp	0.390	0.802	0.937	0.662	0.062
	Pyr	5218	2218	1364	715	74.6
40–49	Obs	2	1	1	1	0
	Exp	1.29	1.18	0.344	0.035	0.001
	Pyr	3703	1319	386	52.7	2.00
50+	Obs	3	2	0	0	0
	Exp	1.62	0.385	0.041	0.0	0.0
	Pyr	1945	371	65.4	0.0	0.0

[a] Observed number of lung cancer deaths.
[b] Expected number of lung cancer deaths based on U.S. Vital Statistics for 1940–1965.
[c] Person-years at risk.
Source: U.S. EPA Health Assessment Document for Inorganic Arsenic (25).

Brown and Chu (27) found that the model of Eq. (6), which assumes that only the penultimate stage is affected by arsenic exposure, fitted the data from the smelter worker cohort reasonably well. The cohort was followed from 1938 through 1977. Brown and Chu excluded postemployment experience of men who ended their employment at the smelter before age 55, on the grounds that it was likely that many of these men had further employment at other copper smelters. Their analysis using GLIM produced an estimate of k equal to 6.8, which is close to the estimate of $k = 6.6$ obtained when the model

$$\lambda_0(t) = \alpha t^{k-1}$$

was fit to the U.S. lung cancer mortality statistics for 1940–1965. Workers were classified into three exposure intensity levels—*light, medium,* and *heavy*—and for these three categories the analysis produced estimates of $c \times 10^{13}$ equal to 0.603, 1.42, and 1.74, respectively. As Brown and Chu point out, the fact that the data are consistent with the model does not demonstrate the validity of the postulated biological mechanism underlying the model, but rather suggests tentative conclusions about the stage affected based on the presumption of a multistage mechanism.

The CAG report uses the Brown–Chu estimates for the light exposure category and an estimated time-weighted average atmospheric arsenic concentration of 0.291 mg As/m^3 for workers in that category to calculate a lifetime unit excess risk due to a continuous exposure of $1 \mu\text{g As/m}^3$. In this exercise the parameter c of the model is assumed to be proportional to the exposure intensity, an assumption that corresponds to a linear nonthreshold low-dose extrapolation procedure. The age-specific unit excess risk is calculated to be $9.45 \times 10^{-16} t^{5.8}$. The lifetime unit excess risk estimate is 0.000871, which

172 MAXWELL W. LAYARD AND ABRAHAM SILVERS

was arrived at by integrating the age-specific risk from 0 to 76.2 years, the latter figure being the median life span according to 1976 U.S. vital statistics. At lower than unit concentration an excess risk estimate is obtained simply by multiplying the unit risk estimate by the concentration. The lifetime excess risk can be interpreted as the probability of dying from lung cancer due to arsenic air pollution of the stated concentration.

5 CONCLUSIONS

As noted, there are many uncertainties in using data from epidemiologic studies to derive assessments of environmental risk. Inaccurate measurements of exposure, omission or inadequate measurement of other important determinants of disease, and statistical imprecision due to an insufficient study cohort size can all lead to poor estimates of dose–response relations.

Another critical area is the choice of an appropriate model for disease rates. To have some degree of confidence in extrapolating disease rates to dose levels outside the range of the observed data, it is desirable to use a model based on a plausible biological theory, and such a model is not always available.

Since we are interested in assessing excess risk above background due to a toxic agent, an accurate determination of background disease rates is clearly important. But we may not have an adequate study control group, and it is often difficult to find appropriate external reference rates; national statistics, for example, may not be applicable to groups of workers in a particular occupation and region.

In spite of these difficulties, epidemiologic information has a vital role to play in environmental risk assessment. Unlike animal data, it is directly relevant to human experience. In many instances, appropriate animal models are not available, so we must rely on epidemiologic data. Even when good animal models are available, human studies can help reduce the great uncertainty involved in the dose and species extrapolation procedures that must be applied to bioassay data.

Uncertainty is inherent in both epidemiologic and animal bioassay disease research. In both areas, different studies of the same agent often lead to widely divergent risk estimates. In the face of such uncertainty, a prudent approach is to attempt to integrate the information from all available epidemiologic and animal studies of the agent in question. This philosophy is apparent in the work of the EPA Cancer Assessment Group, exemplified in the above-cited reports, and also in the carcinogenicity review studies produced by the International Agency for Research on Cancer.

In general, environmental epidemiology is an evolving field. More complex information is being generated and more sophisticated models and analytical methodology are being developed (28). These research activities can be expected to improve the accuracy of environmental risk assessments based on epidemiologic data.

REFERENCES

1. B. McMahon and T. Pugh, *Epidemiology*. Little, Brown, Boston, MA, 1970.
2. W. B. Kannel, D. McGee, and T. Gordon, A general cardiovascular risk profile: The Framingham study. *Am. J. Cardiol.* **38**, 46–51 (1976).
3. D. G. Kleinbaum, L. L. Kupper, and H. Morgenstern, *Epidemiologic Research*. Van Nostrand-Reinhold, New York, 1982.

4. E. L. Anderson et al., Quantitative approaches in use to assess cancer risk. *Risk Anal.* **3**, 277–295 (1983).

5. A. S. Whittemore, Epidemiology in risk assessment for regulatory policy. *J. Chronic Dis.* **39**, 1157–1168 (1986).

6. N. E. Breslow and N. E. Day, *Statistical Methods in Cancer Research: Volume I—The Analysis of Case-control Studies.* IARC, Lyon, France, 1980.

7. N. E. Breslow and N. E. Day, *Statistical Methods in Cancer Research: Volume II—The Design and Analysis of Cohort Studies.* IARC, Lyon, France, 1987.

8. A. S. Whittemore and A. McMillan, Lung cancer mortality among U.S. uranium miners: A reappraisal. *J. Natl. Cancer Inst.* **71**, 489–499 (1983).

9. R. A. Stallones, Epidemiology and environmental hazards. In *Proceedings of a Symposium on Epidemiology and Health Risk Assessment.* Columbia, MD, 1985.

10. E. L. Frome and H. Checkoway, Use of poisson regression models in estimating incidence rates and ratios. *Am. J. Epidemiol.* **121**, 309–323 (1985).

11. R. J. Baker and J. A. Nelder, *The GLIM System: Release 3.* Numerical Algorithms Group, Oxford, 1978.

12. P. McCullagh and J. A. Nelder, *Generalized Linear Models.* Chapman & Hall, London 1983.

13. H. A. Kahn, The Dorn study of smoking and mortality among U.S. veterans. *Nat. Cancer Inst. Monogr.* **19** (1966).

14. D. R. Cox and D. Oakes, *Analysis of Survival Data.* Chapman & Hall, London, 1984.

15. N. E. Breslow et al., Multiplicative models and cohort analysis. *J. Am. Stat. Assoc.* **78**, 1–12 (1983).

16. P. Armitage and R. Doll, The age distribution of cancer and a multistage theory of carcinogenesis. *Br. J. Cancer* **8**, 1–12 (1954).

17. P. Armitage, Multistage models of carcinogenesis. *Environ. Health Perspect.* **63**, 195–201 (1985).

18. A. S. Whittemore, The age distribution of human cancer for carcinogenic exposures of varying intensity. *Am. J. Epidemiol.* **106**, 418–432 (1977).

19. R. Doll and R. Peto, Mortality in relation to smoking: 20 years observation on male British doctors. *Br. Med. J.* **2**, 1525–1536 (1976).

20. A. S. Whittemore, Methods old and new for analyzing occupational cohort data. *Am. J. Ind. Med.* **12**, 233–248 (1987).

21. T. F. Mancuso, Consideration of chromium as an industrial carcinogen. In T. C. Hutchinson, Ed., *Heavy Metals in the Environment.* Institute for Environmental Studies, Toronto, Canada, 1975.

22. U.S. Environmental Protection Agency, *Health Assessment Document for Chromium,* EPA-600/8-83-014F. USEPA, Research Triangle Park, NC 1984.

23. D. C. Thomas, General relative risk models for survival time and matched case-control analysis. *Biometrics* **37**, 673–686 (1981).

24. A. M. Lee and J. F. Fraumeni, Arsenic and respiratory cancer in man: An occupational study. *J. Natl. Cancer Inst.* **42**, 1045–1052 (1969).

25. U.S. Environmental Protection Agency, *Health Assessment Document for Inorganic Arsenic,* EPA-600/8-83-021F. USEPA, Washington, DC, (1984).

26. N. E. Day and C. C. Brown, Multistage models and primary prevention of cancer. *J. Natl. Cancer Inst.* **64**, 977–989 (1980).

27. C. C. Brown and K. C. Chu, Implications of the multistage theory of carcinogenesis applied to occupational arsenic exposure. *J. Natl. Cancer Inst.* **70**, 455–463 (1983).

28. S. H. Moolgavkar and R. L. Prentice (Eds.), *Modern Statistical Methods in Chronic Disease Epidemiology.* Wiley, New York, 1986.

4

A Time-to-Response Perspective on Ethylene Oxide's Carcinogenicity

Robert L. Sielken, Jr.

Sielken, Inc., Bryan, Texas

INTRODUCTION

Risk management and regulation are important activities and deserve the best possible input, including the most scientific quantitative risk assessments. Quantitative dose–response modeling and quantitative risk characterization can be valuable contributors to such risk assessments. However, the value of their contributions depends on the procedures actually used, how they are used, and an understanding of how the results of these procedures should be interpreted. Cancer risk assessments have often been unduly influenced by poorly understood, overly simplified quantitative models and risk characterizations.

There are several steps in developing a quantitative risk assessment, and several scientific disciplines are required to do a thorough assessment. This chapter focuses on only one step, the use of statistical methodology to infer and describe the animal dose–response relation (1). An extensive multistep hazard assessment of ethylene oxide (EO) is provided in ref. 2.

The primary function of the statistical methodology considered herein is *not* to determine whether a particular chemical is carcinogenic. Instead, its function is to quantify the relation between the occurrence of specified carcinogenic responses and the level of exposure to the particular chemical. This chapter considers both the modeling of the dose–response relation and the ways in which the "risks" corresponding to the resultant dose–response model are described (i.e., the risk characterizations). Statistical methodologies do not address the important biological issue of the relevance to humans of carcinogenic responses in experimental animals. This responsibility resides with the pathologists, epidemiologists, and toxicologists.

Different carcinogenic responses (e.g., liver foci, hyperplasia, and carcinoma) may have quite different dose–response relations. Furthermore, the health impacts of different carcinogenic responses may be very different (e.g., no detectable impact, mild discomfort, a severe disability, or a threat to life). Thus, it is important that the specific carcinogenic response being evaluated be defined clearly with respect to site, stage of development, and severity of the health impact. Because the health impact of an exposure is generally the ultimate concern, all of the events that are counted as the specified carcinogenic response should be of equal health consequence, such as all causing death as opposed to some causing death and some being small lesions with no perceptible effects on desired activities.

The early dose–response models like the probit, logit, one-hit, multihit, Weibull, and multistage models are called *quantal response models* because they only "count" the number of individuals which develop the specified carcinogenic response and ignore the time at which this event occurs. These models are not biological models. Instead, they are overly simplistic probabilistic representations of the complex biological phenomena involved in carcinogenesis. Quantal response models assume that essentially nothing is known about carcinogenesis except that the events in the carcinogenic process are irreversible (not repairable). Each of these models is founded on the basis of one of the following three ideas:

1. Cancer occurs if and only if a particular number of "hits" occur; hits can occur in any order and are as likely to occur at any one time as another; what constitutes a hit is unknown.
2. Cancer occurs whenever an individual's "tolerance" to a chemical is exceeded; what constitutes or determines the tolerance is unknown.
3. Cancer occurs whenever an unspecified sequence of unspecified events is completed.

(See, for example, refs. 3–5 for mathematical presentations of these foundations.)

Quantal response models do not directly incorporate time. Hence, they cannot incorporate research results on cell proliferation, tissue growth, and changes in biological processes that are age dependent. Furthermore, quantal response models must treat "dose" as a single number and not a time-dependent quantity.

Of course, since quantal response models do not include time, their risk characterizations cannot include time either. For example, quantal response models do not differentiate between an event that occurs at age 5 and an event that occurs at age 60. Quantal response models would imply that the risks from two exposures were the same if the two response frequencies were the same even though one exposure might produce cancer much earlier than the other exposure. Therefore, quantal response models may not reasonably differentiate between the health effects of two alternatives.

In brief, quantal response models cannot reflect the research that treats life as an ongoing, changing biological process, and they cannot reasonably characterize the risks for an individual who cares about the length and quality of his or her life.

Time-to-response models are dose–response models that include the time at which the carcinogenic response might occur as well its frequency (6–24). Time-to-response models are not exact biological models, but by treating life as a sequence of days, weeks, and months, the time-to-response models can be more biologically reflective than the quantal response models (13, 20–22, 24). Furthermore, the time-to-response models have the potential to incorporate explicitly time-varying dose levels, that is, the different dose levels and the times at which they occur when the dose is not at the same level throughout the lifetime (20, 21).

Time-to-response models can be used even when the time that the response occurs cannot be observed directly. There is sufficient information if the experimenter can determine whether or not the specified response has occurred by the time that the individual is last observed (i.e., at the time of death, sacrifice, or end of the experiment). Of course, if the carcinogenic response is detectable at the time when it occurs, then the time of the response would be observable and used in the model fitting. Furthermore, since health is the primary concern in risk assessments, it may not be reasonable to model a specified response unless that response is detectable, that is, unless the response causes some detectable change in the individual's health. Time-to-response models can also be extended to reflect the presence of competing risks, that is, events such as heart attacks or accidents, which may occur before the specified carcinogenic response occurs (19, 20, 25).

Although quite a number of researchers (4, 26–34) and government agencies (35, 36) have discussed the strengths and weaknesses of the most popular models for estimating the *frequency* of the response at low doses, few have focused on the critical feature of the *time of occurrence* of that adverse response (34, 37–39). Scientists involved in risk assessment should not lose sight of the purpose of their work—that is, to provide the best possible information to risk managers. An exposed individual cares about *when* a carcinogenic response might occur. Therefore, it is very important that the quantitative risk assessment for ethylene oxide inhalation make use of the available time-to-response data. Using only the quantal response data ignores the available time-to-response information, omits an important characteristic of the experimental data (i.e., the very long periods of time without any adverse carcinogenic impact), and forces the risk characterizations to not reflect the time at which an adverse effect occurs.

The quantitative impact of several of the choices involved in the quantitative risk assessments for ethylene oxide inhalation exposure will be addressed. The impacts of the choices available to the statisticians can vary the results by a few orders of magnitude (4, 32, 33, 40, 41). This chapter explains how choices, value judgments, and policy decisions can dominate some quantitative risk assessments and mask the experimental data.

The Bushy Run Research Center (BRRC) study (42, 43) and the NIOSH study (44, 45) of ethylene oxide inhalation have received the majority of the attention of toxicologists and statisticians. Both studies provided information on mononuclear cell leukemia (MCL), peritoneal mesothelioma, brain neoplasia, and survival in rats subjected to lifetime exposures. This chapter focuses on the BRRC data since both studies provided similar indications at the higher dose levels (50 ppm or more) but only the BRRC study included nonzero dose levels below 50 ppm (viz., 10 and 33 ppm).

The dose–response relation between EO inhalation and MCL in female Fischer 344 rats is analyzed in detail. Appendix A provides supplemental results for the other responses potentially associated with EO inhalation; namely, brain neoplasia in male and female rats, peritoneal mesothelioma in male rats, MCL in male rats, and time to death from any cause for both male and female rats. Some implications of the time-to-response information on EO inhalation have also been discussed in ref. 38.

Mononuclear cell leukemia in female rats was the single carcinogenic response in the federal regulatory agencies' analyses with the greatest apparent low-dose risk and hence a dominant factor in their quantitative risk assessments. A careful analysis of one dose–response relation allows the strengths and weaknesses of the different statistical methodologies to be brought out more readily and more concisely. Also, the in-depth treatment of MCL in female rats revealed that the simpler analyses done by the federal regulatory agencies may have greatly overstated the real risk of this response.

A straightforward scientific evaluation of the complete experimental data suggested that there was a very clear similarity between the effects observed in the BRRC study at 10 ppm and those observed in the two BRRC control groups and also between the effects observed at 10 ppm and those observed in historical controls. The similarity between the effects at 10 ppm and those in the controls was also apparent in the fitted time-to-response models of the dose–response relation. However, if only the quantal response data were considered and the time-to-response information were ignored, then the similarity between the behaviors at 10 and 0 ppm was obscured. Other limitations and pitfalls associated with quantal response data analysis procedures are discussed briefly in Appendix B.

The concept of using all available scientific information has recently been reinforced in the EPA's risk assessment guidelines (46). The goal of this chapter is to illustrate that, although there exist many possible statistical methods that can be used to evaluate bioassay data and numerous, often conflicting, risk characterizations that can be generated, only a few of them interpret the data using all available scientific information. Like any other complex scientific analysis, the process for predicting the dose–response curve and quantifying the risks cannot reasonably be reduced to little more than a single number generated by a computer program, which, by considering only the quantal data and ignoring the time-to-response information, is based on only a small part of the available scientific evidence. Using ethylene oxide as an example, this chapter demonstrates that for many chemicals a more accurate understanding of the potential public health risks posed by these chemicals can be ascertained from bioassay data interpreted by time-to-response analyses.

EXPERIMENTAL DATA IN RODENTS

In the BRRC study of ethylene oxide inhalation, the male and female Fischer 344 rats were exposed at 0, 10, 33, and 100 ppm for 6 hours/day, 5 days/week for approximately 2 years. In the NIOSH study of male Fischer 344 rats the dose levels were 0, 50, and 100 ppm for 7 hours/day, 5 days/week for 2 years. Because the observations in both studies at the higher concentrations were similar and because the BRRC study provides more direct experimental evidence on the effects at lower concentrations (10 and 33 ppm), this chapter focuses on the BRRC data.

An NTP bioassay is nearing completion which has 50 B6C3F1 mice of each sex exposed to air containing 0, 50, or 100 ppm EO. Exposures were 6 hours/day, 5 days/week for 102 weeks. Unfortunately, this study cannot provide direct experimental evidence on the shape of the dose–response relation below 50 ppm, the region of greatest interest and uncertainty.

After reviewing the toxicity data for EO, Dr. Golberg noted the following three major considerations on the use of the BRRC and NIOSH studies for risk assessment purposes (2, pp. 78 and 121).

First, the extent to which epizootic infections (SDA virus in the BRRC rats and *Mycoplasma* infections in the NIOSH study) influenced the final outcome of the study merits careful consideration. Interaction, if any, between the infectious agent and the test material would necessarily complicate interpretation of the ensuing experimental results.

Second, the relevance to humans of the tumorigenic effects observed in F344 rats is uncertain. The best-defined tumorigenic effect in both the BRRC and NIOSH Fischer 344 rat studies is enhancement of the incidence of mononuclear cell leukemia (MCL), a type of leukemia with a high spontaneous incidence in the Fischer 344 rat but not, for example, in the Sprague–Dawley rat or other mammals. The kinds of leukemias that were purported to be associated with exposure to EO in humans were quite distinct from MCL, both in the expression of the neoplasia and its course. It is wrong at present to equate MCL in rats with the overwhelming majority of human leukemias. Another carcinogenic endpoint observed in the animal studies—peritoneal mesothelioma (PM)—while clinically a form of cancer that is found in humans, has not been associated with exposure to EO in

TABLE 1. Quantal Response Data from Bushy Run Research Center Ethylene Oxide Inhalation Study in Rats

Dose* (ppm)	Proportion of Female Rats with Mononuclear Cell Leukemia	Proportion of Female Rats with Brain Neoplasia	Proportion of Male Rats with Mononuclear Cell Leukemia	Proportion of Male Rats with Peritoneal Mesothelioma	Proportion of Male Rats with Brain Neoplasia
Primary Data Sets: Animals that Died or Were Found in Moribund Condition[a]					
Control I	4/18 22.2%	0/20 0.0%	15/28 53.6%	0/26 0.0%	0/31 0.0%
Control II	7/18 38.9%	0/20 0.0%	10/28 35.7%	1/27 3.7%	0/29 0.0%
Controls I and II	11/36 30.6%	0/40 0.0%	25/56 44.6%	1/53 1.9%	0/60 0.0%
10 ppm	3/22 13.6%	1/25 4.0%	12/27 44.4%	2/28 7.1%	1/28 3.6%
33 ppm	10/31 32.3%	1/31 3.2%	13/39 33.3%	3/38 7.9%	3/40 7.5%
100 ppm	12/47 25.5%	1/53 1.9%	17/49 34.7%	18/49 36.7%**[b]	4/49 8.2%*
Secondary Data Sets: Animals that Died or Were Found in Moribund Condition or Were Sacrificed at the End of the Experiment[a]					
Control I	9/78 11.5%	1/81 1.2%	20/76 26.3%	1/74 1.4%	1/79 1.3%
Control II	13/74 17.6%	0/76 0.0%	18/77 23.4%	2/76 2.6%	0/78 0.0%
Controls I and II	22/152 14.5%	1/157 0.6%	38/153 24.8%	3/150 2.0%	1/157 0.6%
10 ppm	14/76 18.4%	1/79 1.3%	21/78 26.9%	3/79 3.8%	1/79 1.3%
33 ppm	24/79 30.4%**	3/79 3.8%	25/78 32.1%	6/77 7.8%*	4/79 5.1%*
100 ppm	27/73 37.0%**	3/79 3.8%	26/79 32.9%	21/79 26.6%**	7/79 8.9%**
EPA Data Sets (49, p. 9–150): Secondary Data Sets, Minus Rats that died or Were Sacrificed Before the First Tumor, Plus the Interim Sacrifices at 18 months in the 0- and 100-ppm Groups but not in the 10- and 33-ppm Groups					
Controls I and II	22/186[c] 11.8%	1/194[d] 0.5%		4/187[e] 2.1%	1/196[d] 0.5%
10 ppm	14/71 19.7%	1/95 1.1%		3/88 3.4%	1/99 1.0%
33 ppm	24/72 33.3%**	3/99 3.0%		7/82 8.5%*	5/98 5.1%*
100 ppm	28/73 38.3%**	4/99 4.0%*		22/96 22.9%**	7/99 7.1%**

[a]The proportion is the number of rats developing the response divided by the number of rats at risk and not lost to follow-up for this response (i.e., were histologically examined). It is assumed that all rats were available for follow-up for brain neoplasia.

[b]In the Fisher Exact Test for a statistically significant increase in the response proportion relative to that in Controls I and II, ** implies significance at the 1% level, *implies significance at the 5% level, and nothing implies no statistically significant increase.

[c]First tumor at 18 months.

[d]Total number of rats examined less 6- and 12-month sacrifices.

[e]First tumor at 15 months.

epidemiology studies. The appearance of primary brain neoplasms in both the BRRC and NIOSH investigations is of interest—at least at first glance. While the relevance of these tumors for humans may be greater than in the case of MCL or PM, the data satisfy only one (the dose–response relation) of six criteria for neurocarcinogenic action. Hence, it seems inappropriate to use these results in quantitative risk assessment.

Third, conclusions of the BRRC study, and presumably the NIOSH study as well, are complicated by the absence of a unique early-occurring tumor. Differences in the incidence of spontaneous tumors in senile rats do not carry the same weight in assessment of carcinogenicity as unique tumors occurring earlier in life. In addition, the wide variation in the background incidence of spontaneous tumors in the F344 rat, particularly MCL, makes interpretation difficult. It is interesting to note that after up to 26 months of exposure at the highest dose level (100 ppm), the leukemia incidence in male rats exposed in the BRRC study was lower than the reported spontaneous incidence in the male control rats in the NIOSH study.

The reports on the BRRC study contained considerable dose–response information. Table 1 indicates quantal response data for several carcinogenic responses. Three representations for the rats at risk are considered; namely, (i) the primary data set, corresponding to the female rats that were histologically examined and that died (i.e., died or found in moribund condition and killed), (ii) the secondary data set, equaling the primary data set plus the histologically examined female rats that were sacrificed at the end of the experiment, and (iii) the EPA data set, corresponding to the secondary data set *minus* the rats that died or were sacrificed prior to 18 months *plus* the 18-month scheduled sacrifices in the 0- and 100-ppm groups but not in the 10- and 33-ppm groups (47).

More detailed time-to-response data were also available. Time was measured in terms of months from the onset of exposure. The time of death was recorded for all rats that died. No further classification of the cause of death for these animals was reported.

The carcinogenic response analyzed in this chapter is defined as death *with* MCL in a female rat.

Any female rat that had MCL at the time it died or was sacrificed was considered to have had the carcinogenic response, death with MCL.

RISK CHARACTERIZATIONS EMPHASIZING TIME-TO-RESPONSE BUT NOT REQUIRING DOSE–RESPONSE MODELING

It is appropriate to characterize risk in terms of the time that a response occurs or the amount of time preceding a particular consequence (29, 36, 39). Some such characterizations can be made without having to do dose–response modeling. As shown below, these largely assumption-free, straightforward representations of the experimental data suggest a high degree of similarity between the real risks at 0 and 10 ppm.

Table 2 indicates the number of female rats that died with mononuclear cell leukemia (MCL) during each of the exposure months, the number that died without MCL, and the number that died but were lost to follow-up (i.e., not histologically examined for MCL). There were 120 female rats in each of the two identical control groups (denoted as Control I and Control II or CI and CII herein) and in each of the 10-, 33-, and 100-ppm exposure groups. The control level is referred to herein as the 0 dose level.

There were 1, 10, 10, and 20 rats randomly selected at 3, 6, 12, and 18 months, respectively, for interim sacrifice at each dose level (0, 10, 33, and 100 ppm). There was also a terminal sacrifice at approximately 24 months for all female rats. All rats are accounted

TABLE 2. Time to Death with Mononuclear Cell Leukemia among Female Rats Exposed to Ethylene Oxide Vapor in the Bushy Run Research Center Study (42)

Exposure (months)	Number of Deaths with Mononuclear Cell Leukemia[a] — Dose (ppm)					Number of Deaths without Mononuclear Cell Leukemia — Dose (ppm)					Number of Animals Lost to Follow-up[b] — Dose (ppm)				
	0, CI	0, CII	10	33	100	0, CI	0, CII	10	33	100	0, CI	0, CII	10	33	100
1	0	0	0	0	0	0	0	0	0	0	1	0	0	0	0
2	0	0	0	0	0	0	0	0	0	0	0	0	0	0	0
3	0	0	0	0	0	0	0	0	0	0	0	0/1	0/1	0/1	0/1
4	0	0	0	0	0	0	0	0	1	0	0	0	0	0	0
5	0	0	0	0	0	0	0	0	0	0	0	0	0	0	0
6	0	0	0	0	0	0/10	0/10	0	0	0/10	0	0	0/10	0/10	0
7	0	0	0	0	0	0	0	0	0	0	0	0	0	0	0
8	0	0	0	0	0	0	0	0	0	0	0	0	0	0	0
9	0	0	0	0	0	0	0	0	0	0	0	0	0	0	0
10	0	0	0	0	0	0	0	0	0	2	0	0	0	0	0
11	0	0	0	0	0	0	0	0	0	0	0	0	0	0	0
12	0	0	0	0	0	0/10	0/10	0/1	0	0/10	0	0	0/9	0/10	0
13	0	0	0	0	0	0	0	0	1	1	0	0	0	0	0
14	0	0	0	0	0	0	0/3	0	0	1	0	0	0	0	0
15	0	0	0	0	0	2	3	2	4	11	0	0	0	0	1
16	0	0	0	0	0	1	0	1	0	2	0	0	0	0	0
17	0	0	0	0	0	0	0	2	1	3	0	0	0	0	0
18	0	1	0	1	0/1	2/20	0/20	1	2	1/19	0	0	0/20	0/20	0
19	1	0	1	2	0	1	0	3	2	1	0	1	0	0	1
20	0	2	0	1	1	1	3	0	0	2	0	0	0	0	1
21	0	1	0	1	1	0	2	1	3	2	0	0	0	0	0
22	0	0	0	0	3	0	2	0	2	0	0	0	1	0	0
23	2	3	2	2	1	4	0	4	4	4	1	0	2	0	2
24	1/5	0/6	0/11	3/14	6/15	3/55	1/50	5/43	1/34	5/11	0	1	0	0	1
Column total	4/5	7/6	3/11	10/14	12/16	14/95	11/93	19/44	21/34	35/50	2/0	2/1	3/40	0/41	6/1

[a] A ratio like x/y implies that y animals were in the scheduled sacrifice group and x were not; a simple entry like x is like x/0 and implies that there were no such animals in the scheduled sacrifice group.

[b] These animals were not histologically examined for this response.

for in Table 2. The animals that were randomly selected for sacrifice at scheduled times can be distinguished in Table 2 from the other rats; in that, a table entry is a ratio like x/y if there were $y > 0$ rats that were scheduled sacrifices. For example, Table 2 implies the following:

1. There were no female rats that died with MCL (among those not lost to follow-up) before 18 months of exposure.
2. In Control II and at 33 and 100 ppm one rat died with MCL during the 18th exposure month.
3. The one rat that died with MCL at 100 ppm, during the 18th exposure month, was a scheduled sacrifice.
4. At 100 ppm there were a total of 16 female rats that died with MCL in scheduled sacrifices while 12 died with MCL by deaths that were not scheduled sacrifices.

The life table analysis estimates of the probabilities of a female rat dying with MCL following various numbers of exposure months are shown in Table 3. These estimates are straightforward nonparametric estimates in that they do not presume any model or mathematical form for how these probabilities change with dose or time. The estimates are

TABLE 3. Life Table Analysis Estimates of the Probability of a Female Rat Dying with Mononuclear Cell Leukemia by Specified Times

Specified Time (months)	Control I	Control II	Controls I and II	10 ppm	33 ppm	100 ppm
1	0.000	0.000	0.000	0.000	0.000	0.000
2	0.000	0.000	0.000	0.000	0.000	0.000
3	0.000	0.000	0.000	0.000	0.000	0.000
4	0.000	0.000	0.000	0.000	0.000	0.000
5	0.000	0.000	0.000	0.000	0.000	0.000
6	0.000	0.000	0.000	0.000	0.000	0.000
7	0.000	0.000	0.000	0.000	0.000	0.000
8	0.000	0.000	0.000	0.000	0.000	0.000
9	0.000	0.000	0.000	0.000	0.000	0.000
10	0.000	0.000	0.000	0.000	0.000	0.000
11	0.000	0.000	0.000	0.000	0.000	0.000
12	0.000	0.000	0.000	0.000	0.000	0.000
13	0.000	0.000	0.000	0.000	0.000	0.000
14	0.000	0.000	0.000	0.000	0.000	0.000
15	0.000	0.000	0.000	0.000	0.000	0.000
16	0.000	0.000	0.000	0.000	0.000	0.000
17	0.000	0.000	0.000	0.000	0.000	0.000
18	0.000	0.012	0.006	0.000	0.012	0.015
19	0.014	0.012	0.013	0.014	0.041	0.015
20	0.014	0.041	0.027	0.014	0.056	0.033
21	0.014	0.055	0.034	0.014	0.071	0.053
22	0.014	0.055	0.034	0.014	0.071	0.113
23	0.042	0.102	0.071	0.045	0.104	0.135
24	0.207	0.270	0.238	0.345	0.546	0.761

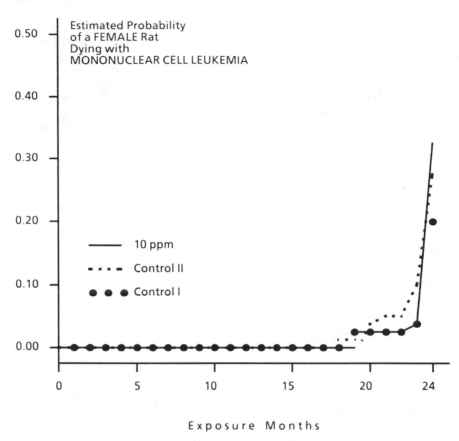

Figure 1. Life table analysis estimates of the probability of a female rat dying with mononuclear cell leukemia plotted versus the number of exposure months in the BRRC ethylene oxide inhalation study.

computed using the fairly standard technique described in ref. 48. This method incorporates all the rats and the length of time they were at risk.

There are at least two conclusions that can be drawn from Tables 2 and 3. The first is that if a response occurs at all it occurs very late relative to an average rat lifetime—mostly in the 24th month and no sooner than the 18th month in a 24-month study. The second conclusion is that the number and timing of the responses at 0 and 10 ppm are very similar. The latter conclusion is also evident in Fig. 1, which indicates the plots of the life table analysis estimates versus time for the 10-ppm exposure group and the two control groups. The plot for the 10-ppm group lies between those of the two control groups except for the very last month.

There are several other ways to characterize (i) the lateness of the MCL response in female rats, (ii) the similarity between the response times for the rats exposed to 10 ppm and the response times for the control rats, and (iii) the changes in the response times at 33 and 100 ppm relative to those at 0 and 10 ppm. For example, Table 4 indicates the number of exposure months until the proportion of animals that die with MCL reaches a prescribed percentage (1, 5, 10, or 20%). In particular, it took the same number of months

TABLE 4. Number of Months in the Bushy Run Research Center Ethylene Oxide 2-year Inhalation Study on Rats until Prescribed Percentages of Female Rats Died with Mononuclear Cell Leukemia[a]

	Prescribed Percentage of Female Rats Dying with Mononuclear Cell Leukemia			
	1%	5%	10%	20%
Control I	19	24	24	24
Control II	18	21	23	24
Controls I and II	18	23	24	24
10 ppm	19	23	24	24
33 ppm	18	20	23	24
100 ppm	18	21	22	24

[a]The table entry corresponds to the smallest number of exposure months in Table 3 such that the life table estimate of the probability of a female rat dying with MCL (expressed as a percentage and rounded to the nearest percent) is at least the prescribed percentage.

TABLE 5. Estimated Mean Number of Months without a Female Rat Dying with Mononuclear Cell Leukemia during Exposure to Ethylene Oxide in the Bushy Run Research Center Study

	Length of Experimental Period (months)	Mean Number of Months Without Dying with Mononuclear Cell Leukemia[a]	Mean Percentage of Experimental Period Without Dying with Mononuclear Cell Leukemia
Control I	24	23.70	98.7
Control II	24	23.45	97.7
Controls I and II	24	23.58	98.2
10 ppm	24	23.55	98.1
33 ppm	24	23.10	96.2
100 ppm	24	22.88	95.3

[a]Calculated using

mean number of months without dying with MCL

$$= \sum_{m=1}^{24} (m-1) \times \text{prob (dying with MCL during } m\text{th month)}$$

$$+ 24 \times \text{prob (no death with MCL during 24 months)}$$

and the life table estimates in Table 3 of the probability (prob) of a female rat dying with mononuclear cell leukemia by specified times.

(23 months) for both the 10-ppm group and the combined controls to reach a 5% incidence rate, whereas it took a noticeably shorter time at the 33 and 100 ppm levels (viz., 20 and 21 months, respectively). Throughout Table 3 the rats at 0 and 10 ppm took similar times to reach the same incidence rate (risk level); in fact, it never took less time to reach a specified incidence rate at 10 ppm than it did for the combined controls.

The average amount of time until a response occurs cannot be calculated when some individuals do not develop the response. However, the average amount of time in an experiment during which an individual has not had the response can be calculated. This latter average, called the *mean response-free period*, is not the same as the average time until the response occurs. For instance, if no rats died with MCL during a 24-month experiment, the average response-free period would be 24 months; however, the average time to death with MCL would certainly be greater than 24 months but how much greater is unknown.

Table 5 shows the average number of exposure months in the experiment that the female rats were free from the specified response, death with MCL. The maximum possible response-free period is 24 months (the length of the experiment). The female rats in the 10-ppm group averaged 23.55 months of response-free time (98.1% of the maximum response-free period). The two control groups averaged 23.45 months (97.7%) and 23.70 months (98.7%) without mortality with MCL. Hence, the average for the 10-ppm group is between the averages for the two control groups. The average for the 33 and 100 ppm groups were slightly lower [viz., 23.10 months (96.2%) and 22.88 months (95.3%), respectively] but noticeably different from that for the 10-ppm group. The similarity between the control groups and the 10-ppm group is clear. The dissimilarity between the 10-ppm group and both the 33- and 100-ppm groups is also clear.

SIMPLE STATISTICAL ANALYSIS OF TIME-TO-RESPONSE DATA

Several two-sided 95% confidence intervals on the lifetime probability of a female rat dying with MCL are shown in Table 6. Regardless of which subset of the experimental data is being considered, there is substantial overlap between the confidence intervals for the MCL response rate at 0 and at 10 ppm (see also Fig. 2). There is no statistically significant difference between the lifetime MCL response rate for the 10-ppm group and the combined controls (even at the 20% significance level). This suggests that there is no statistically detectable increase in the lifetime probability of dying with MCL from being exposed to 10-ppm EO instead of 0 ppm.

Not only is the lifetime probability of dying with MCL similar at 0 and 10 ppm, but also there is no difference between 0 and 10 ppm in *when* an individual is likely to die with MCL. In particular, being at 10 instead of 0 ppm does not appear to increase the likelihood of dying with MCL earlier. The hypothesis that there is no shifting of the likelihood of dying with MCL from one time to another (especially to an earlier time) is the hypothesis that the distribution of the time to death with MCL is the same for different dose levels. This hypothesis was tested using the available information on the length of time without a female rat dying with MCL. The statistical procedures described in ref. 49 are appropriate for this analysis and were applied to the data on the female rats that were histologically examined for MCL and that died or were sacrificed at the end of the experiment. (The procedures considered the frequency of death with MCL in three intervals: 0–18, 19–21, and 22–24 exposure months.) The hypothesis that the 0-, 10-, 33-, and 100-ppm groups had the same time-to-response distribution was rejected at the 5% significance level. The hypothesis that the 0-, 10-, and 33-ppm groups had the same time-to-response distribution was also rejected. However, the hypothesis that the controls and the 10-ppm group had the same time-to-response distribution was not rejected. These tests, which do not require any specific dose–response modeling assumptions, imply that the time-to-response distributions for the controls and the rats at 10 ppm are similar, and that the time-to-response

TABLE 6. Comparisons that Are Independent of the Dose–Response Modeling: 95% Two-Sided Confidence Intervals on the Probability of a Female Rat Dying with Mononuclear Cell Leukemia at the Control and 10-ppm Exposure Levels[a]

Experimental Group	Observed Number of Rats Dying with MCL	Number of Rats at Risk	95% Two-Sided Confidence Interval	
			Lower Bound on Probability	Upper Bound on Probability
Rats That Were Histologically Examined and Died or Were Found in Moribund Condition				
BRRC Controls I and II	11	36	0.1551	0.4560
BRRC 10 ppm	3	22	0.0000	0.2798
95% Two-sided confidence interval on the difference between the probability of death with MCL at 10 ppm and for controls			−0.3770	0.0387
Rats That Were Histologically Examined and that Died or Were Found in Moribund Condition or Were Sacrificed at the End of the Experiment				
BRRC Controls I and II	22	152	0.0888	0.2007
BRRC 10 ppm	14	76	0.0971	0.2714
95% Two-sided confidence interval on the difference between the probability of death with MCL at 10 ppm and for controls			−0.0641	0.1430
Rats That Survived the First Year of the Experiment				
BRRC Controls I and II	22	195	0.0684	0.1572
BRRC 10 ppm	14	76	0.0971	0.2714
95% Two-sided confidence interval on the difference between the probability of death with MCL at 10 ppm and for controls			−0.0572	0.1999

[a]The confidence intervals are based on the usual normal distribution approximation to the binomial distribution.

distributions at 33 and 100 ppm are different from those at 0 and 10 ppm. These results are consistent with the implications of Table 5 where the estimated mean times without a female rat dying with MCL are nearly identical at 0 and 10 ppm but smaller at 33 and 100 ppm. In short, even though the same cannot be said for the 33- and 100-ppm groups, the 10-ppm group is similar to the controls with respect to *when* and *how often* death with MCL occurs.

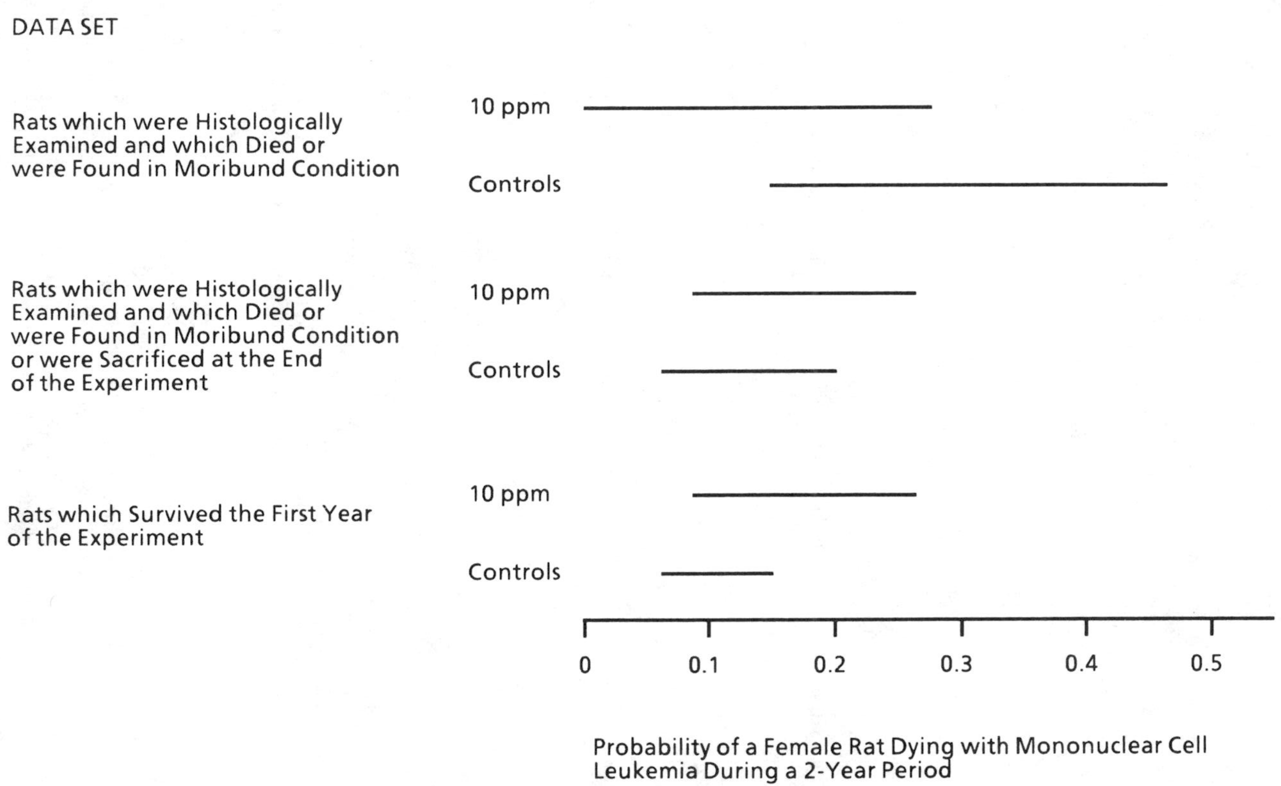

186

Figure 2. Comparisons that do not depend on dose–response modeling: the overlap between 95% two-sided confidence intervals on the probability of a female rat dying with mononuclear cell leukemia at the control and 10-ppm exposure levels.

EPA'S POSITION ON TIME-TO-RESPONSE INFORMATION

The final report (47) published by the U.S. EPA in June 1985 contains a summary of their quantitative risk assessment for EO. Their approach to estimating the risk at very low doses, like many of the past attempts by regulatory agencies, fails to reflect the available time-to-response information in either its dose–response modeling or its risk characterizations. The methodology to incorporate this additional information has been available for almost 10 years and, as discussed previously, it should be a part of most assessments if the objectives of the EPA's Cancer Risk Guidelines (46) and those of the NAS (1) are to be met.

There have frequently been several methodological shortcomings in the past quantitative risk assessments prepared by regulatory agencies for ethylene oxide, and other chemicals, in addition to the failure to reflect the available time-to-response information. Many of these shortcomings are discussed briefly in Appendix B.

EPA'S INTERPRETATION OF THE ETHYLENE OXIDE BIOASSAY DATA

The EPA's quantitative risk assessment failed to incorporate a consideration of the time-to-response information in its summary risk characterizations (47). Since 1982, the EPA has summarized the results of their risk modeling efforts in terms of what EPA calls "unit risk estimates" (although these are really *bounds* on risk and not *estimates*). These risk characterizations ignore the time-to-response information and are based solely on the proportions of animals developing the specified response at any time. Such tumor/no tumor data or response/no response data are quantal response data and do not reflect the time at which the response of concern occurs.

In EPA's description of the BRRC study, the cumulative mortality percentages versus exposure months were tabulated, and the agency noted that "at no time were significant increases in mortality observed in the 10 ppm exposure group of either sex" (47, p. 9–100). Regrettably, they did not present the corresponding tables and implications for death with MCL or other potential carcinogenic responses. Had they done so, they would have discovered that the similarity between 0 and 10 ppm observed for mortality from all causes combined extends to the specific carcinogenic responses they eventually focused on (MCL in particular). Furthermore, they would have realized that there was more to the risk characterization of EO than that suggested by the quantal response data alone.

The only time-to-response information for the carcinogenic responses which the EPA reported was a table of "Time in months to First Tumor" and "Time in months to Median Tumor." EPA summarized their interpretation of these data in the following (47, p. 9–105): "The time to first tumor for some neoplasms (but not for mononuclear cell leukemias) was decreased in the high-dose group as compared to controls, as shown in Table 9–23. Median time-to-tumor was not reduced." This information deserves more emphasis and, since they pursued no further time-to-response analyses, more discussion and follow-up. The similarity of the time-to-response behavior at 10 ppm to that at the control level was not explicitly noted by the EPA, although, as discussed previously, it would appear to be very relevant data to be considered by risk managers. Furthermore, the omission of most of the time-to-response information and implications should be included in the EPA's discussion of the uncertainties in their risk assessment.

EFFECT OF EVALUATING ONLY A PARTICULAR PORTION OF THE QUANTAL RESPONSE DATA

The inclusion or exclusion of subgroups of female rats on the basis of different factors such as sacrificed versus nonsacrificed or gross examination versus histological examination and inconsistency across the dose levels in the determination of the number of animals at risk caused the EPA risk characterization to differ markedly from the risk characterizations corresponding to alternative (and probably more reasonable) representations of the quantal response data. In most experiments there are several ways to determine which animals are included in the quantal response data and which animals are excluded (not counted). The different determinations may not be equally appropriate or equally reflective of the underlying dose–response relation. Furthermore, the same risk characteristic can differ by several orders of magnitude for different determinations of the quantal response data. The most informative determination may depend on the experimental protocol and the chemical's time-to-response behavior. The sensitivity of the risk characterization to the determination of the representation of the quantal response data should be evaluated and made clear to the risk manager.

In the primary data set the observed proportion dying with MCL did not increase as the dose increased. As indicated in Table 7, the observed percentages were 30.6, 13.6, 32.3, and 25.5% for the combined controls, 10-, 33-, and 100-ppm groups, respectively. In fact, the percentages at 10, 33, and 100 ppm are between the 22.2 and 38.9% observed in the two individual control groups. Among the female rats that died there was no increased risk of dying with mononuclear cell leukemia from a lifetime of inhalation exposure to ethylene oxide at or below 100 ppm.

In their analysis (47), the EPA evaluated a mixture of sacrificed and nonsacrificed animals. The usefulness of this analysis is questionable since there was *not* an increasing dose–response relation observed among the nonsacrificed animals, but there was one observed in the female rats sacrificed at 24 months.

The observed percentages of female rats with MCL in the 24-month sacrificed group were 9.5, 20.4, 29.2, and 57.7% in the combined controls, 10-, 33-, and 100-ppm groups, respectively. The percentage for the 24-month sacrificed group at 100 ppm is significantly greater than the percentage for the nonsacrificed group at 100 ppm (at the 1% significance level). The corresponding differences in the percentages for the 10 and 33 ppm are not significant (even at the 20% significance level). However, the percentage for the 24-month sacrificed controls is significantly decreased relative to the percentage for the nonsacrificed controls (at the 1% significance level).

The reasons for the observed differences between the nonsacrificed and 24-month sacrificed rats are not evident from the numbers themselves. However, the numbers are consistent with the hypothesis that the dose-related occurrences of MCL were "incidental" as opposed to "lethal;" that is, consistent with the dose-related occurrences not leading to an increased threat to life. The numbers are also consistent with the claim that the dose-related occurrences of MCL happen very late in the lifetime of female rats. In either case, the EPA's risk characterizations do not reflect health impact since they either are reflecting an incidental carcinogenic response and/or do not reflect the amount of a lifetime adversely affected by exposure.

The specific criteria used by EPA to select their single representation of the quantal response data did not have a consistent impact on the different dose groups. In fact, the criterion of including only histologically examined rats appears reasonable at first glance; however, it meant that the 20 female rats sacrificed at 18 months in each of the 10- and 33-

TABLE 7. Quantal Response Data from the Bushy Run Research Center Ethylene Oxide Inhalation Study on the Proportion of Female Rats with Mononuclear Cell Leukemia

Dose (ppm):	Control I	Control II	Controls I and II	10 ppm	33 ppm	100 ppm
Primary Data Set: Female Rats that Were Histologically Examined and that Died or Were Found in Moribund Condition						
Proportion	4/18	7/18	11/36	3/22	10/31	12/47
Percentage	22.2%	38.9%	30.6%	13.6%	32.3%	25.5%
Female Rats that Were Histologically Examined and Were in the 24-month Sacrifice						
Proportion	5/60	6/56	11/116	11/54	14/48	15/26
Percentage	8.3%	10.7%	9.5%	20.4%	29.2%	57.7%
Secondary Data Set: Female Rats that Were Histologically Examined and that Died or Were Found in Moribund Condition or Were in the 24-month Sacrifice						
Proportion	9/78	13/74	22/152	14/76	24/79	27/73
Percentage	11.5%	17.6%	14.5%	18.4%	30.4%	37.0%
EPA's Choice: Female Rats that Were Histologically Examined and that Survived until at Least the 18th month of the Experiment—Includes 18-Month Sacrifices at Only 0 and 100 ppm						
Proportion	9/95	13/91	22/186	14/71	24/72	28/73
Percentage	9.5%	14.3%	11.8%	19.7%	33.3%	38.4%
Female Rats that Survived until at Least the 18th month of the Experiment and Were Histologically Examined (EPA's Choice) Plus Those that Were Sacrificed at 18 months and Only Grossly Examined—Includes All 18-Month Sacrifices						
Proportion	9/95	13/91	22/186	14/91	24/92	28/73
Percentage	9.5%	14.3%	11.8%	15.4%	26.1%	38.4%
Female Rats that Were Histologically Examined and that Survived the First Year of the Experiment						
Proportion	9/98	13/97	22/195	14/76	24/78	28/91
Percentage	9.2%	13.4%	11.3%	18.4%	30.8%	30.8%
Female Rats that Were Histologically Examined and that Survived the First Year of the Experiment Plus Those that Were Sacrificed at 18 months and Only Grossly Examined						
Proportion	9/98	13/97	22/195	14/96	24/98	28/91
Percentage	9.2%	13.4%	11.3%	14.6%	24.58%	30.8%

ppm groups (i.e., about 17% of these dose groups) were excluded from the quantal response data (because they were only grossly examined) while the 40 female control rats and the 20 female rats at 100 ppm which were sacrificed at 18 months were included (because they were histologically examined). It is true that the rats in the 10- and 33-ppm groups were only grossly examined for MCL and not histologically examined; however, none of the 101 female rats that were histologically examined before 18 months had MCL, and only 1 of the 20 histologically examined female rats that were exposed to 100 ppm and sacrificed at 18 months had MCL. Thus, the female rats that were at 10 and 33 ppm and sacrificed at 18 months probably did not have MCL. Therefore, by including the 40 control rats sacrificed at 18 months and excluding the 20 rats at each of 10 and 33 ppm which were sacrificed at 18 months, EPA's choice decreased the proportion with MCL among the controls and, most likely, increased the proportion with MCL at 10 and 33 ppm. This choice exaggerates any increase in the proportion with MCL at 10 and 33 ppm relative to the controls. In short, the EPA's nonuniform treatment of the female rats sacrificed at 18 months results in biased dose–response information that inflates the risk characterization—in fact, more than doubled the implied risk.

Several alternatives to the EPA's representation of the quantal response data on female rats with MCL are indicated in Table 7. They include (i) the primary data set, (ii) the secondary data set—the primary data set plus the 24-month sacrifices, (iii) EPA's choice plus the rest of the 18-month sacrifices, (iv) all histologically examined female rats that survived the first year of the experiment, and (v) the female rats in (iv) plus the rest of the 18-month sacrifices.

In all of these alternatives, the apparent increase in the percentage of female rats with MCL between the controls and the 10-ppm group is less than the implied increase under EPA's choice. For alternative (i), the primary data set, there is no implied increase. For alternatives (ii), (iii), and (v) the implied increases are only roughly one-half of the implied increase under the EPA's choice. Alternative (iv) suffers from the same disparate treatment of the 18-month sacrifice data as EPA's choice and implies risks twice those implied by (v).

All representations of the quantal response data on MCL which combine the sacrificed and nonsacrificed female rats hide the fact that there was no observed increasing dose–response relation among the nonsacrificed rats. Of course, these representations also failed to indicate the very long period of time without evidence of a carcinogenic effect.

RISK CHARACTERIZATIONS CAN EMPHASIZE TIME TO RESPONSE

As suggested previously, a practical way to characterize the effects of a particular exposure is to describe the corresponding average amount of time in a specified observation period during which the subject is free from a specified response. This characterization has been called the *mean response-free period* or *mean free period* (36, 39). If the observation period is 24 months (as it was in the BRRC study), then the mean response-free period could be as long as 24 months. As indicated in Table 5, when the response is death with MCL, the observed mean response-free periods (observed mean numbers of months without dying with MCL) are 23.58, 23.55, 23.10, and 22.88 months for a female rat at 0, 10, 33, and 100 ppm, respectively. Thus, the risk for female rats at 10 ppm can be characterized as a decrease of 0.03 months in the mean response-free period ($0.03 = 23.58 - 23.55$).

For female rats exposed between 0 and 10 ppm, the overall observed rate of decrease in the observed mean response-free periods for dying with MCL was

$$\frac{23.58 \text{ months} - 23.55 \text{ months}}{10 \text{ ppm} - 0 \text{ ppm}} = 0.003 \text{ months/ppm}.$$

If a linear interpolation between 0 and 10 ppm is applied, this rate of decrease implies that a female rat's time span without dying with MCL during a 24-month exposure decreases approximately 0.003 months (approximately 0.09 days, 2.2 hours, or 0.0125% of a 24-month lifetime) with each 1-ppm increase in exposure from 0 to 10 ppm. The linearity assumption is almost certain to overstate the actual risks. If the mean response-free period decreased linearly with the dose level at a rate of 0.003 months/ppm, then dose levels of 2.2, 0.31, and 0.013 ppm would correspond to average reductions of approximately 0.00391, 0.00016, 0.0000027%, of a 24-month expected lifetime. These percentages correspond to approximately 1 week, 1 day, and 1 hour in a 70-year expected lifetime.

The observed mean response-free periods and estimates of dose levels corresponding to specified reductions in the mean response-free period described in the two preceding paragraphs do not take advantage of the experimental information on the shape of the dose–response relation obtained by combining the animal information from several different dose levels together. Dose–response modeling allows the information from different experimental dose levels to be combined. In addition, instead of arbitrarily assuming how risk characteristics should be interpolated between dose levels, dose–response modeling allows the experimental data themselves to imply how interpolations or extrapolations over doses and over times are to be done.

The family of multistage-Weibull time-to-response models can be used to provide reasonable models of the dose–response relations for ethylene oxide inhalation in rats. These models are generalizations of the quantal multistage model typically used by the EPA. The multistage-Weibull models can be used to extrapolate over time as well as over dose. The multistage-Weibull models fit to the available dose–response information have the probability of a specified response occurring by time t at dose d in the absence of competing risks equal to

$$P(t; d) = 1 - \exp\left[- (\alpha_0 + \alpha_1 d + \alpha_2 d^2 + \alpha_3 d^3)(t - \beta_1)^{\beta_2} \right],$$

where α_0, α_1, α_2, α_3, β_1, and β_2 are the unknown parameters whose values are to be estimated from the experimental data (12).

In such analyses, the dose scale used for modeling the dose–response relation should be the same as the dose scale that is going to be used for species extrapolation. Table 8 indicates the dose levels to which the rats in the BRRC study were exposed on the three dose scales corresponding to EO concentration in air (ppm), intake relative to body weight (mg/kg·day), and intake relative to surface area (mg/kg$^{2/3}$·day).

TABLE 8. Experimental Exposure Levels on Different Dose Scales for the BRRC Study Where Exposures Were for 6 hours/day, 5 days/week for Nearly a Lifetime and the Average Weights of Male and Female Rats Were 0.42 and 0.22 kg, respectively

Experimental Level (ppm)	Lifetime Average Concentration in Air (ppm)	Lifetime Average Intake Relative to Body Weight[a] (mg/kg·day)		Lifetime Average Intake Relative to Surface Area (mg/kg$^{2/3}$·day)	
		Male	Female	Male	Female
0	0	0	0	0	0
10	1.80	1.93	1.93	1.45	1.17
33	5.94	5.13	5.13	3.84	3.10
100	18.00	14.46	14.46	10.83	8.73

[a] Based on average intakes of 2.7 and 20.24 mg/kg·day for inhalation exposures 6 hours/day at 10 and 100 ppm, respectively (50). The average intake at 33 ppm was estimated using a linear interpolation of the average intakes at 10 and 100 ppm.

The rats in the BRRC study were exposed for 6 hours/day, 5 days/week for 2 years, which is equivalent to approximately 18% of a complete 2-year lifetime. Hence, the lifetime average exposure concentrations are 18% of the experimental concentrations (0, 10, 33, and 100 ppm). Tyler and McKelvey (50) reported that the average cumulative daily intake for male Fischer 344 rats inhaling ethylene oxide vapor for 6 hours/day was (i) 2.7 mg/kg·day when the concentration of ethylene oxide was 10 ppm and (ii) 20.24 mg/kg·day when the concentration of ethylene oxide was 100 ppm. Since the BRRC rats were exposed 5 days/week, the corresponding lifetime average exposures were 5/7 times these numbers; that is, 1.93 mg/kg·day at 10 ppm and 14.46 mg/kg·day at 100 ppm. Linear interpolation between these two numbers gives 5.13 mg/kg·day for 33 ppm. These numbers were also assumed to apply to female rats. The exposures to male and female rats can be converted from a body weight scale (mg/kg·day) to a body surface area scale (mg/kg$^{2/3}$·day) by multiplying the mg/kg·day exposures by $(0.42)^{1/3}$ and $(0.22)^{1/3}$ for males and females, respectively, where 0.42 and 0.22 kg were the average weights of male and female rats, respectively, in the BRRC study (42, 43).

The estimated dose–response relations for female rats dying with MCL were affected by the dose scale used during the model fitting. Such effects were due solely to the differences in dose scales and occur even without extrapolating across species. These effects are illustrated in Table 9 using the experimental data for the controls, the 10-ppm group, and the 33-ppm group. As shown, for a female rat inhaling EO at 1 ppm for 6 hours/day, 5 days/week for a lifetime, the fitted model values for the added probability of dying with MCL were 0.0056, 0.0028, and 0.0028 when the modeling dose scales were lifetime average concentration (ppm), intake relative to body weight (mg/kg·day), and intake relative to surface area (mg/kg$^{2/3}$·day). The corresponding decreases in the mean response-free period during the 24-month experiment were 0.0065, 0.0033, and 0.0033, respectively. Thus, for this data set the choice of the dose scale used during the model fitting made about a twofold difference in the estimated risks for female rats extrapolated from the experimental levels of 10 and 33 ppm to 1 ppm.

TABLE 9. Effects on Low-Dose Extrapolation of Modeling on Different Dose Scales[a]

Dose Scale Used in Modeling	Exposure[b] on Modeling Dose Scale	Maximum Likelihood Estimate of Risk Characteristics for Female Rats	
		Added Probability of a Response by 24 months	Mean Response-Free Period between 0 and 24 months
Lifetime average ppm	0.18	0.0056	0.0065 months
Lifetime average mg/kg·day	0.193	0.0028	0.0033 months
Lifetime average mg/kg$^{2/3}$·day	0.117	0.0028	0.0033 months

[a]Experimental data: female rats dying with mononuclear cell leukemia among histologically examined rats that were at 0, 10, or 33 ppm and died or were found in moribund condition or were sacrificed at the end of the experiment.

[b]Exposure = 1 ppm for 6 hours/day, 5 days/week for a lifetime.

The reason for these differences in estimated risk is that, when the dose scale is changed from ppm to mg/kg·day or mg/kg$^{2/3}$·day, the relative distance between the doses corresponding to 0, 10, and 33 ppm changes. On the lifetime average ppm scale, the value corresponding to 33 ppm is 3.3 times greater than that for 10 ppm, whereas on either the mg/kg·day or the mg/kg$^{2/3}$·day scale the value corresponding to 33 ppm is only about 2.7 times greater than that for 10 ppm. Thus, the increases in the proportion dying with MCL observed between 0 and 33 ppm are less nonlinear (more linear and initially more rapidly increasing) on the ppm scale than the other scales, and consequently the low-dose risks are estimated to be greater when the modeling is done on the ppm scale. There is no difference between the estimates for female rats obtained using the mg/kg·day and the mg/kg$^{2/3}$·day scales since these two scales are linearly related—here one scale is a simple constant multiple of the other.

THE BEST AVAILABLE RISK CHARACTERIZATION

The multistage-Weibull time-to-response model, when applied to the primary data on female rats dying with MCL, indicated that risks do not increase as the dose level increases. That is, based on the primary data set, the fitted time-to-response model implied that, as the dose increases between 0 and 100 ppm, the probability of a female rat dying with MCL does not increase and the mean response-free period does not decrease! These implications based on the time-to-response information are consistent with the implication of no increases in risk with increases in dose based on the quantal response data for female rats that died.

The best available risk characterization of EO based on the female rats dying with MCL is that there is no increased risk at low levels of exposure, particularly below 10 ppm. The remainder of this section considers what the risk characteristics would be if the animal data base is extended to the secondary data set, that is extended to include the *incidental* occurrence of MCL among the animals that were sacrificed at the end of the experiment. In this case the "risks" refer to an event with a more uncertain health consequence. The multistage-Weibull time-to-response models were also fit to the secondary data set. The fitted model values of several risk characteristics based on the secondary data set are shown in Table 10. These values are the maximum likelihood estimates (MLEs) based on the data in the control, 10-, and 33-ppm groups. (Maximum likelihood estimates are the model's best estimates as opposed to upper or lower bounds. The MLEs correspond to the fitted model values when the fitting is done according to the maximum likelihood criterion. This criterion is a classical fitting criterion in statistics. The corresponding fitted model maximizes the likelihood of the experiment resulting in the particular experimental data observed.) The corresponding estimates obtained by including the 100-ppm group do not differ by more than a multiple of 2 from those shown in Table 10. Including the 100-ppm group in the analysis forces the fitted model to compromise its fit in the region below 33 ppm in order to accommodate the relatively slow increases in risk observed between 33 and 100 ppm. The fitted model obtained by excluding the 100-ppm group should provide a better indication of the dose–response relation below 33 ppm.

The fitted dose–response models were obtained with the female rat's dose represented in terms of the lifetime average mg/kg·day of EO. The estimated risk characteristics in Table 10 are for female rats. Extrapolations from female Fischer 344 rats to humans are discussed in the next section. The doses in mg/kg·day in Table 10 are for female rats. For reference purposes, Table 10 also shows the ppm concentration of the ethylene oxide in air

TABLE 10. Fitted Multistage-Weibull Time-to-Response Model Values (Maximum Likelihood Estimates) of (i) Increases in the Probability of a Female Rat Dying with Mononuclear Cell Leukemia by Specified Times and (ii) the Decreases in the Mean Response-Free Period During an Expected Lifetime

Lifetime Average Dose to Female Rats (mg/kg·day)	Human Exposure (in ppm) with Same Lifetime Average Exposure (in mg/kg·day) as the Female Rats		Estimated Increases in Probability of Dying with Mononuclear Cell Leukemia by Specified Times[a]					Estimated Decreases in Mean Response-Free Period between 0 and 70 yr
	Exposure 24 h/day, 7 days/wk, 52 wk/yr for 70 yr (ppm)	Exposure 6 h/day, 5 days/wk, 51 wk/yr for 40 yr (ppm)	30 yr	40 yr	50 yr	60 yr	70 yr	
1.086	2.00	20.0	0.0[b]	0.0	0.000007	0.0008	0.02	3.6 wk
0.543	1.00	10.0	0.0	0.0	0.000003	0.0003	0.009	1.6 wk
0.2715	0.50	5.0	0.0	0.0	0.000001	0.0002	0.004	5.1 days
0.2172	0.40	4.0	0.0	0.0	0.000001	0.0001	0.003	4.0 days
0.1629	0.30	3.0	0.0	0.0	0.0000007	0.00009	0.002	2.9 days
0.1086	0.20	2.0	0.0	0.0	0.0000005	0.00006	0.002	1.9 days
0.0543	0.10	1.0	0.0	0.0	0.0000002	0.00003	0.0008	22.5 h
0.02715	0.05	0.5	0.0	0.0	0.0000001	0.00001	0.0004	11.1 h
0.00543	0.01	0.1	0.0	0.0	0.0	0.000003	0.00007	2.2 h

[a] Two years in a rat lifetime are assumed to be equivalent to 70 years in a human lifetime. All times and mean response-free periods are tabled on the 70-year lifetime scale.
[b] 0.0 means less than 0.0000001.

necessary for a 70-kg person inhaling $20\,m^3$ of air per day to receive the same dose in mg/kg·day as that indicated for the female rat. The necessary ppm concentrations are shown both for a person continuously exposed for 70 years and for a person exposed only for 6 hours/day, 5 days/week, 51 weeks/year for 40 years, which is approximately one-tenth of a 70-year lifetime.

The estimated risks in Table 10 include the increase (above the background value) in the probability of a female rat dying with MCL in each of several periods at several different exposure levels. The periods were from the beginning of the experiment (time zero) to the end of 10.2857, 13.7143, 17.1429, 20.5714, and 24 months, which for a rat with an expected 24-month lifetime are proportionally the same as from time zero to 30, 40, 50, 60, and 70 years in an expected 70-year lifetime. For example, a female rat exposed to EO and inhaling a lifetime average of 0.543 mg/kg·day has an estimated probability of dying with MCL before 20.5714 months of exposure $[20.5714 = (60/70) \times 24]$ equal to the background probability for that period plus an increase of 0.0003. The estimated increases in the female rat's probability of dying with MCL are very, very small for the periods that do not extend into the later portion of its expected lifetime and only become noticeably nonzero when the periods include a major portion of its expected lifetime. This is consistent with the other indications of the lateness of the carcinogenic effects.

The fact that the estimated increases in the probability of a female rat dying with MCL essentially only occur very late in an expected lifetime is not evident if only the increases at the end of an expected lifetime are reported. That is, the estimated increase of 0.009 for a whole expected lifetime at 0.543 mg/kg·day does not indicate that the estimated increase was only 0.0003 (30 times smaller) for 60/70 of a whole lifetime. On the other hand, *the estimated decreases in the mean response-free period do reflect the times at which the different increases in the probability occur.*

The estimated decreases in the mean response-free period from the background mean response-free period are shown in Table 10. These decreases are the decreases over an entire expected lifetime. In order to put the female rat's decreases in an expected 2-year lifetime into perspective with a 70-year expected lifetime, the table values are 35 times (35 = 70 years/2 years) the rat's actual decreases. For example, a female rat exposed to EO and inhaling a lifetime average of 0.543 mg/kg·day (e.g., exposure at approximately 2.8 ppm for 6 hours/day, 5 days/week, 51 weeks/year, for 2 years—using Table 8 and linear interpolation) has its mean number of weeks without dying with MCL decreased from its background value by 1.6 weeks/35, which is approximately 0.04% of its 2-year expected lifetime,

$$100\% \times (1.6\,\text{weeks}/35)/(2\,\text{years} \times 52\,\text{weeks/year}) = 0.044\%.$$

The lateness of ethylene oxide's carcinogenic effects is reflected in the estimated decreases in the mean response-free periods reported in Table 10. The magnitude of these decreases can be compared to what the decreases in the mean response-free period would have been if the estimated increases in probability shown in Table 10 for 70 years had been accumulated linearly over time instead of mostly in the very late portions of the 70-year period as they were in the case of EO exposure. For example, a female rat inhaling a lifetime average of 0.543 mg/kg·day of EO has a total estimated increase in probability of 0.009 over a period (24 months) proportionally equivalent to 70 years. If that probability had increased by 0.009/70 in every period proportionally equivalent to 1 year, then the decrease in the mean response-free period would have been proportional to 16.4 weeks instead of the 1.6 weeks associated with the late-occurring effects of EO. In fact, all the

TABLE 11. Rapid Disappearance of the Decreases in the Mean Response-Free Period as the Endpoint of the Period at Risk Decreases[a]

Lifetime Average Dose to Female Rats (mg/kg·day)	Human Exposure (in ppm) with Same Lifetime Exposure (in mg/kg·day)		Decreases in Mean Response-Free Period between Zero and Specified Times[b]				
	Exposure 24 h/day, 7 days/wk, 52 wk/yr for 70 yr (ppm)	Exposure 6 h/day, 5 days/wk, 51 wk/yr for 40 yr (ppm)	30 yr	40 yr	50 yr	60 yr	70 yr
1.086	2.00	20.0	0.0[c]	4.1 s	11.0 min	19.3 h	3.6 wk
0.543	1.00	10.0	0.0	1.8 s	4.7 min	8.2 h	1.6 wk
0.2715	0.50	5.0	0.0	1.0 s	2.2 min	3.8 h	5.1 days
0.2172	0.40	4.0	0.0	1.0 s	1.7 min	3.0 h	4.0 days
0.1629	0.30	3.0	0.0	0.0	1.3 min	2.2 h	2.9 days
0.1086	0.20	2.0	0.0	0.0	49.0 s	1.4 h	1.9 days
0.0543	0.10	1.0	0.0	0.0	24.1 s	41.9 min	22.5 h
0.02715	0.05	0.5	0.0	0.0	11.9 s	20.8 min	11.1 h
0.00543	0.01	0.1	0.0	0.0	2.4 s	4.1 min	2.2 h

[a] The mean response-free period is for the response defined as a female rat dying with mononuclear cell leukemia.
[b] Two years in a rat lifetime are assumed to be equivalent to 70 years in a human lifetime. All times and mean response-free periods are tabled on the 70-year lifetime scale.
[c] 0.0 means less than 1 s.

decreases in the mean response-free period shown in Table 10 would have been approximately *10 times greater* if the increases in probability shown in Table 10 had been accumulated linearly over time instead of late in the expected lifetime.

As indicated in Table 11, the decreases in the mean response-free periods diminish rapidly as the endpoint of the time frame decreases. For example, the decrease in the mean response-free period for a female rat inhaling a lifetime average of 0.543 mg/kg·day is proportional to 1.6 weeks if the interval considered ends at a time proportional to 70 years but decreases to only 8.2 hours if the interval ends at a time proportional to 60 years. The decreases in the mean response-free periods, for all the dose levels in Table 11, are over 30-fold smaller for 0–60 years than for 0–70 years. The decreases in 0–50 years are over 3000-fold smaller than those in 0–70 years.

The practical impact of the lateness of the increases in the probability of a female rat dying with MCL is that it lessens the expected proportion of a normal life span affected by EO exposure. Thus, the lateness of the increases in probability diminishes the practical consequences of any potential adverse effects associated with EO exposure.

EXTRAPOLATING FROM RATS TO HUMANS

The relevance to humans of experimental animal results depends on many factors such as the similarities in exposure patterns, pharmacokinetics, carcinogenic mechanisms,

TABLE 12. Effects on Species-to-Species Extrapolation of Assuming Dose–Response Equivalence on Different Dose Scales[a]

Dose Scale Used in Modeling and Assumed Scale for Species Equivalence	Human Exposure[b] on Dose Scale Used for Modeling and Assumed Species Extrapolation	Maximum Likelihood Estimate of Risk Characteristics		Ratio of Estimate Using Specified Dose Scale to Estimate Using mg/kg·day Scale	
		Probability of a Carcinogenic Response by the End of 70yr	Decrease in Mean Response-Free Period between 0 and 70yr	Ratio of Estimates of Probability of a Carcinogenic Response by the End of 70yr	Ratio of Estimates of Decrease in Mean Response-Free Period between 0 and 70yr
Lifetime average ppm	0.1020	0.00320	0.1310 months	4.2	4.2
Lifetime average mg/kg·day[c]	0.0554	0.00077	0.0314 months	1.0	1.0
Lifetime average mg/kg$^{2/3}$·day	0.2283	0.00586	0.2394 months	7.6	7.6

[a] Experimental data used for dose–response modeling in female rats: female rats dying with mononuclear cell leukemia among histologically examined rats that were at 0, 10, or 33 ppm and died or were found in moribund condition or were sacrificed at the end of the experiment.

[b] Human exposure = 1 ppm for 6 hours/day, 5 days/week for 40 years.

[c] A 70-kg person inhaling 20 m^3/day inhales 0.543 mg/kg·day per ppm of ethylene oxide in the air.

197

immune systems, and repair systems. The degree of relevance implied by these biological factors cannot be determined by the statistician; however, the relative quantitative behavior of different species extrapolation schemes can be determined.

The most frequently discussed candidate dose scales for the equivalence of dose–response relations across species are (i) lifetime average concentration (ppm), (ii) lifetime average milligrams per kilogram body weight per day (mg/kg·day), and (iii) lifetime average milligrams per unit body surface area per day (mg/kg$^{2/3}$·day).

Although these equivalence assumptions may appear attractive at first glance, the amount of a carcinogen that reaches its target site and its effect on the target are not necessarily simple functions of either concentration or body weight or body surface area due to the multitude and complexity of biological processes involved. It is important to remember that the equivalent human dose is intended to be *equivalent* in the sense of causing the same frequency of response in humans as observed in the animals and is not necessarily intended to be equivalent on any other physical or biological scale.

The extrapolation of low-dose risks from one species to another assumes that the dose–response relations for the two species are equal on a particular dose scale. The choice of the dose scale, which is assumed to yield equal dose–response relations, has a quantitative impact on the estimated human risks extrapolated from female rat data. That impact is illustrated in Table 12. There the estimated human risks from inhaling vapor with an EO concentration of 1 ppm for 6 hours/day, 5 days/week for 40 years have been extrapolated from the estimated dose–response relations for female rats. The three dose scales used for modeling the female rat's dose–response relation and assumed to yield an equal human dose–response relation are concentration in air (ppm), intake relative to body weight (mg/kg·day), and intake relative to surface area (mg/kg$^{2/3}$·day). Regardless of whether risk is characterized in terms of added probability or decreased mean response-free period, the estimated human risks are 4.2 and 7.6 times greater using the lifetime average ppm and mg/kg$^{2/3}$·day dose scales, respectively, than they are using the lifetime average mg/kg·day dose scale. The fitted dose–response relations are somewhat nonlinear in terms of the dose level; so that, these ratios will change slightly for different human exposure levels. If the dose–response relations would have been exactly linear in the dose level, the estimated human risks extrapolated from female rats assuming species equivalence on a surface area basis (mg/kg$^{2/3}$·day) would have been 6.8 times greater than those estimated assuming species equivalence on a body weight basis (mg/kg·day): $6.8 = (70\,\text{kg})^{1/3}/(0.22\,\text{kg})^{1/3}$.

DISCUSSION

A single number cannot realistically characterize the risks posed by exposure to a chemical. The way scientists characterize risk can markedly affect the decisions of risk managers. For example, the estimated increase in the probability of a specified response by a specified time for an increase in the dose above the background level is only one way to characterize risk. This characterization reflects only the total probability increase by a particular time and does not reflect when the increases occur. Hence, this characterization does not reflect the expected amount of time adversely impacted by an exposure. On the other hand, a mean response-free period does reflect the expected amount of time adversely impacted by an exposure. The decrease, if any, in the mean response-free period with an increase in the dose is a valuable description of the risk associated with that increased dose. Also, for some people the risk may be more easily understood if it is expressed in terms of time or lost time than in terms of a very small probability.

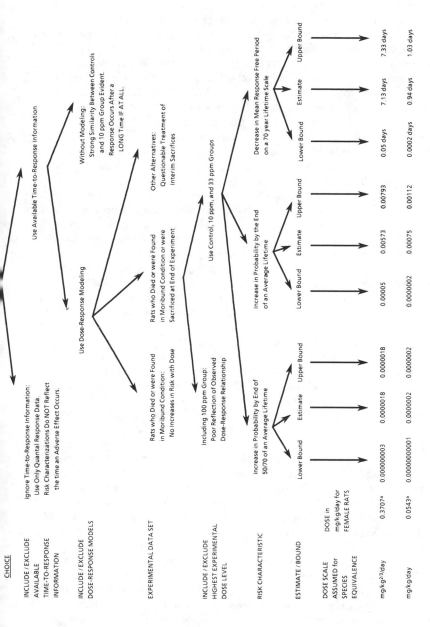

Figure 3. A choice tree for the quantitative risk assessment of ethylene oxide based on female rats dying with mononuclear cell leukemia.

[a] A 70-kg human exposed to 1 ppm EO for 6 hr/day, 5 days/week, 51 weeks/year for 40 years during a 70-year lifetime has a lifetime average exposure of 0.0543 mg/kg·day, which is equivalent to 0.3707 mg/kg·day in a female rat if species were equivalent on a surface area basis.

199

The numbers emerging from any quantitative risk assessment are not mathematical certainties. The numbers are influenced by statistical variability in the experimental outcomes and also influenced by the policy decisions, value judgments, and assumptions incorporated into the risk assessment process. The impacts of these influential factors need to be clearly displayed in order for the risk managers and regulators to put the accuracy and validity of the presented risk characterizations into their proper perspective.

The impacts of several of the choices made in the quantitative risk assessment for ethylene oxide inhalation can be represented schematically in the form of a "choice tree." Figure 3 is one such choice tree for the quantitative risk assessment of EO inhalation. A choice tree is similar to a decision tree. The risk assessment process starts at the top of the choice tree. Each level or branching point in the tree corresponds to a particular issue, which requires that one of possibly several choices must be made. The terminal risk descriptions at the end of paths and at the bottom of the tree are the result of the sequence of individual choices preceding them. The differences in a choice tree's risk descriptions indicate the impacts of the choices considered.

The choice tree in Fig. 3 reflects many of the numerous options that can be used in the EO risk assessment. The resulting risk descriptions represent a range of possible risks. Of course, the options are *not* all equally relevant and *not* all equally likely; hence, the resulting risk descriptions should *not* all be given equal weight in the decisionmaking. The validity or appropriateness of the individual choices along the path leading to a particular risk description help the risk manager determine the reasonableness, credibility, or weight to be associated with that risk description.

The next paragraph discusses the topmost branch in the tree—the choice between ignoring the available time-to-response information and using it. The next six paragraphs discuss the next six lower branches in the tree.

Since an exposed individual cares not only about whether or not he or she might develop a particular carcinogenic response, but also about when that event might occur, the initial choice in this quantitative risk assessment was whether or not to make use of the available time-to-response data. Using only the quantal response data (i) ignores the available time-to-response information, (ii) omits an important characteristic of the experimental data (i.e., the very long periods of time without any adverse carcinogenic impact), and (iii) forces the risk characterizations to *not* reflect the time at which an adverse effect occurs.

Once the decision to recognize the available time-to-response information was made, the description of the risk could have been made either with or without the use of dose–response models. Even without the use of any dose–response modeling, the similarity between the characteristics of the control groups and the 10-ppm group and the dissimilarity between these groups and the groups at 33 and 100 ppm were evident. Also, even without modeling it was clear that, if an adverse response occurred at all, it occurred very late in the time period corresponding to an average rat lifetime.

When the dose–response relations for EO were modeled, the fitted models differed substantially with the composition of the experimental data set. The differing treatment of the interim sacrificed animals at 0 and 100 ppm versus 10 and 33 ppm complicated the evaluation of all experimental animals combined. Ignoring the interim sacrificed animals at 10 and 33 ppm and including them at 0 and 100 ppm doubled the otherwise suggested risks. When only the female rats that died were considered, there was *no* increase in the risk of dying with MCL as the dose level increased.

When the dose–response models were fit to the experimental data on female rats dying with MCL among those female rats that were histologically examined and either died or were sacrificed at the end of the experiment, the fitted multistage-Weibull time-to-response model based on the control, 10-, and 33-ppm groups reflected the shape of the dose–response relation in this dose region better than the fitted model obtained by including the 100-ppm data.

The fitted time-to-response model provided estimates of several risk characteristics. Some of these risk descriptions are shown in Fig. 3 for two dose levels, 0.0543 and 0.3707 mg/kg·day. A person exposed to vapor with an EO concentration of 1.0 ppm for 6 hours/day, 5 days/week, 51 weeks/year for 40 years has a 70-year lifetime average intake of 0.0543 mg/kg·day. On a body surface area scale 0.0543 mg/kg·day for a 70-kg person is equivalent to $0.0543 \times 70^{1/3}$ mg/kg$^{2/3}$·day. For a 0.22-kg female rat $0.0543 \times 70^{1/3}$ mg/kg$^{2/3}$·day is equal to 0.3707 mg/kg·day $(0.3707 = 0.0543 \times 70^{1/3}/0.22^{1/3})$. Thus, the dose level 0.0543 mg/kg·day might be of interest to humans *if* the cancer risks for rats and humans were equivalent on a body weight basis while 0.3707 mg/kg·day might be of interest *if* species were equivalent on a surface area basis. The three risk descriptions shown in Fig. 3 are (i) the increase in the probability of a female rat dying with MCL by the end of an expected lifetime (2 years), (ii) the increase in the probability of a female rat dying with MCL by the end of 50/70 of an expected lifetime (i.e., by the end of $2 \times 50/70$ years), and (iii) the decrease in the mean response-free period—35 (i.e., 70 years/2 years) times the decrease in the length of time without the female rat dying with MCL during the 2-year experimental period.

The numerical values of the estimates of the three risk characteristics would have varied with random variations in the experimental outcomes. An indication of this variability is indicated by the lower and upper bounds that accompany each fitted model value (maximum likelihood estimate) of each risk characteristic in Fig. 3. The lower and upper values are the minimum and maximum estimated values in 10 replications of the BRRC experiment. (One replicate is the original BRRC study; the other nine replicates were simulated by sampling, with replacement, the original BRRC experimental outcomes.) When the BRRC estimates are compared to the lower and upper bounds, it is evident that the BRRC estimates would not have increased substantially with experimental variation but could have decreased to almost zero.

Figure 3 also indicates that if the risks were extrapolated from rats to humans under the assumption that the species dose–response relations are equivalent when the dose is expressed in terms of lifetime average intake relative to surface area (mg/kg$^{2/3}$·day), then the extrapolated risks would be approximately 8 times greater than they would have been if the species dose–response relations were assumed to be equivalent when the dose is expressed in terms of lifetime average intake relative to body weight (mg/kg·day). The risk characteristics in Fig. 3 do not reflect the biological uncertainty in extrapolating from rats to humans.

The carcinogenic response analyzed in this chapter has been death with mononuclear cell leukemia in a female rat. The time of the initial onset of MCL in a female rat was, like most tumors, not directly observable. In general, the appropriateness of using the time to onset as the definition of the carcinogenic response is debatable. This is particularly true when the health impact of the exposure is of primary concern. It seems much more appropriate to define the carcinogenic response as occurring only when a specified level of health consequence is reached or surpassed. This requires that the carcinogenic response refer to a detectable event—for example, discomfort, pain, disability, disfiguration, or death. Thus, the inability to analyze the onset of MCL as the specified response with the current experimental information does not appear to be a real loss as far as health-based regulatory decisionmaking is concerned.

For the rats that died with MCL it was not known whether MCL was the cause of death. If the cause of death was known, then the carcinogenic response could have been defined as death caused by MCL. However, the time to a rat's death *with* MCL is not greater than the time that MCL would have caused that rat's death. Hence, the probability of the former response (death with MCL) occurring by a specified time exceeds that for the latter response (death caused by MCL). In addition, the length of time without the former response is less than that without the latter response. Thus, when the risks are characterized in terms of either the probability of a specified response or the mean response-free period, the quantitative risks for *death with MCL* are greater than those for *death caused by MCL*. Similarly, since the sacrifice of an animal with MCL was defined herein as a death with MCL, the quantitative risk characterizations in this chapter tend to be *greater* than they would have been using a less encompassing definition of a carcinogenic response such as death caused by MCL.

When the analyses were carefully reviewed and evaluated, several conclusions became apparent. First, the available time-to-response information indicated that there was a strong similarity between the risk characteristics of the control rats and the rats at 10 ppm. Second, if an adverse carcinogenic response occurred at all, it occurred very late in the time period corresponding to an average rat lifetime.

Third, it is possible using approaches such as choice trees to make the quantitative impacts of many of the choices, options, judgments, and so on involved in a risk assessment more apparent to the risk manager and the public.

Fourth, the fitted dose–response relations were heavily influenced by the composition of the experimental data set. For the primary data set (the female rats that were histologically examined and that died), there was *no* increase in the risk of dying with mononuclear cell leukemia as the dose level increased. The interpretation of the risk descriptions for the secondary data set (the primary data set plus the animals sacrificed at the end of the experiment) is complicated by the mixing of potentially lethal occurrences of MCL with clearly nonlethal occurrences. The risk descriptions based on the data set evaluated by the EPA (the secondary data set minus the rats that died prior to the 18th month plus the 18-month interim sacrifices in the 0- and 100-ppm groups but not in the 10- and 33-ppm groups) were roughly double those for the secondary data set.

Fifth, the EPA's summaries of the risks associated with ethylene oxide inhalation ignored the available time-to-response information. If this information were utilized instead of ignored, risk descriptions could have included not only the frequency of adverse responses but also the time that they might occur. In particular, the maximum likelihood estimate of the *decrease* in the average amount of time without a carcinogenic response during an expected lifetime of 70 years was less than *1 day* for a lifetime average exposure of 0.0543 mg/kg·day of ethylene oxide. This decrease of less than 1 day in the mean response-free period reflects the very long periods of time in the BRRC study without a female rat dying with mononuclear cell leukemia. This experimental evidence was also reflected in the sharp drop in the estimated added probability of the response at 0.0543 mg/kg·day from 0.0008 for a 70-year period to 0.0000002 for a 50-year period—a 4000-fold decrease.

Sixth, risk descriptions could have been expanded to include not only very small probabilities but also characterizations in terms of response-free time that may be more readily understood by both risk managers and the public.

Finally, the usefulness of the existing and emerging time-to-response models and risk descriptions means that the time to bring a time-to-response perspective to carcinogenicity and its quantitative risk assessment is here.

APPENDIX A: ADDITIONAL TIME-TO-RESPONSE INFORMATION AND RISK CHARACTERIZATIONS FOR MONONUCLEAR CELL LEUKEMIA, PERITONEAL MESOTHELIOMA, BRAIN NEOPLASIA, AND SURVIVAL IN BOTH MALE AND FEMALE RATS

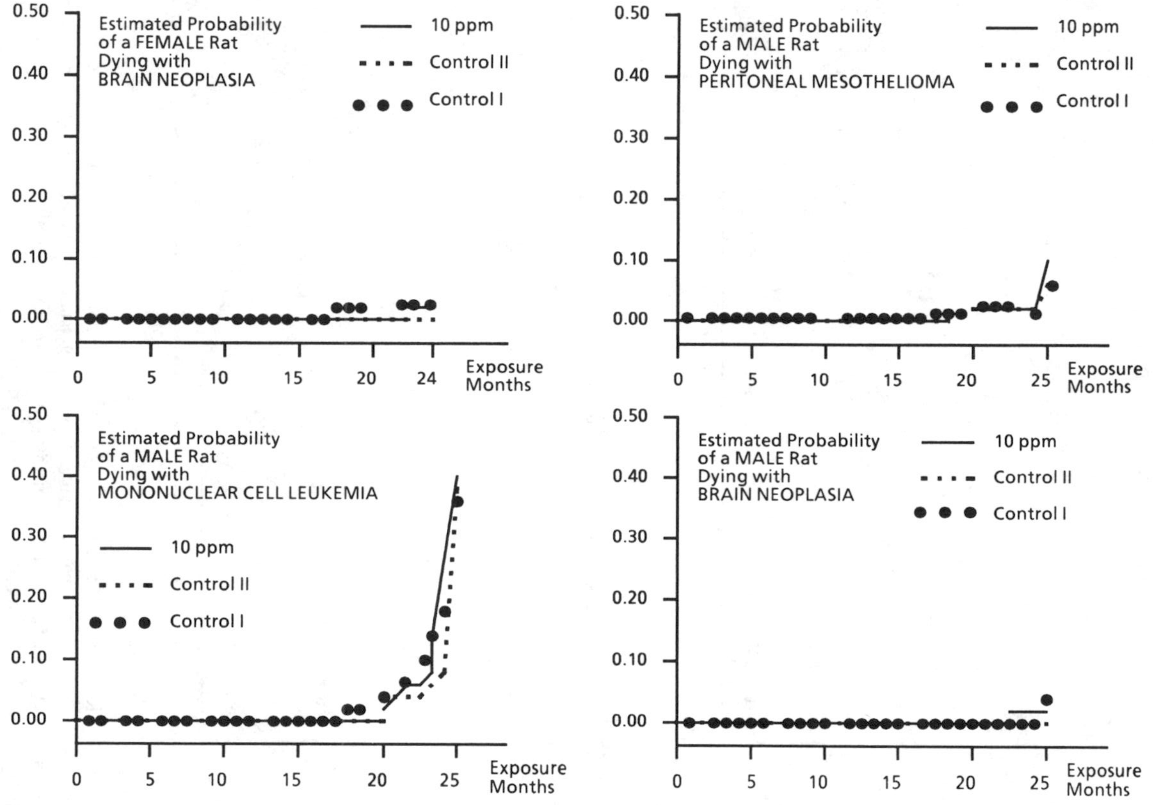

Figure A.1. Rats exposed to ethylene oxide vapor at 10 ppm in the Bushy Run Research Center study had cancer response probabilities that were virtually indistinguishable from the response probabilities for the two control groups. The life table estimates of the response probabilities for the 10-ppm group are usually in-between those for the two control groups.

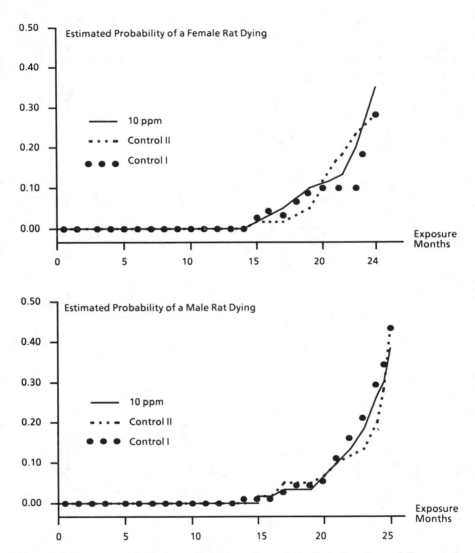

Figure A.2. Rats exposed to ethylene oxide vapor at 10 ppm in the Bushy Run Research Center study had survival probabilities that were virtually indistinguishable from the survival probabilities for the two control groups. The life table estimates of the survival probabilities for the 10-ppm group are usually in-between those for the two control groups.

TABLE A.1 Time to Death with Brain Neoplasia among Female Rats in the Bushy Run Research Center Ethylene Oxide Inhalation Study (42)

Exposure (months)	Number of Deaths with Brain Neoplasia[a] Dose (ppm)					Number of Deaths without Brain Neoplasia Dose (ppm)					Number of Animals Lost to Follow-up Dose (ppm)				
	0, CI	0, CII	10	33	100	0, CI	0, CII	10	33	100	0, CI	0, CII	10	33	100
1	0	0	0	0	0	1	0	0	0	0	0	0	0	0	0
2	0	0	0	0	0	0	0	0	0	0	0	0	0	0	0
3	0	0	0	0	0	0	0/1	0/1	0/1	0/1	0	0	0	0	0
4	0	0	0	0	0	0	0	0	1	0	0	0	0	0	0
5	0	0	0	0	0	0	0	0	0	0	0	0	0	0	0
6	0	0	0	0	0	0/10	0/10	0/10	0/10	0/10	0	0	0	0	0
7	0	0	0	0	0	0	0	0	0	0	0	0	0	0	0
8	0	0	0	0	0	0	0	0	0	0	0	0	0	0	0
9	0	0	0	0	0	0	0	0	0	0	0	0	0	0	0
10	0	0	0	0	0	0	0	0	0	2	0	0	0	0	0
11	0	0	0	0	0	0	0	0	0	0	0	0	0	0	0
12	0	0	0	0	0	0/10	0/10	0/10	0/10	0/10	0	0	0	0	0
13	0	0	0	0	0	0	0/3	0	1	1	0	0	0	0	0
14	0	0	0	0	0	0	3	0	4	1	0	0	0	0	0
15	0	0	0	0	0	2	0	2	0	12	0	0	0	0	0
16	0	0	0	0	0	1	0	1	0	2	0	0	0	0	0
17	0	0	0	0	0	0	0	2	1	2	0	0	0	0	0
18	0/1	0	0	1/2	0	2/19	1/20	1/20	2/20	1/19	0	0	0	0	0
19	0	0	0	0	0	2	1	4	4	2	0	0	0	0	0
20	0	0	0	0	0	1	5	0	1	4	0	0	0	0	0
21	0	0	0	0	0	0	3	1	4	3	0	0	0	0	0
22	0	0	0	0	0	0	2	1	2	5	0	0	0	0	0
23	0	0	1	0	0	7	3	7	6	6	0	0	0	0	0
24	0	0	0	0	0/2	4/60	2/56	5/54	4/46	11/24	0	0	0	0	0
Column totals	0/1	0/0	1/0	1/2	0/2	20/99	20/100	24/95	30/87	52/64	0	0	0	0	0

[a] A ratio like x/y implies that y animals were in the scheduled sacrifice group and x were not; a simple entry like x is like x/0 and implies that there were no such animals in the scheduled sacrifice group.

205

TABLE A.2. Time to Death with Mononuclear Cell Leukemia among Male Rats Exposed to Ethylene Oxide Vapor in the Bushy Run Research Center Study (42)

Exposure (months)	Number of Deaths with Mononuclear Cell Leukemia[a] — Dose (ppm)					Number of Deaths without Mononuclear Cell Leukemia — Dose (ppm)					Number of Animals Lost to Follow-up[b] — Dose (ppm)				
	0, CI	0, CII	10	33	100	0, CI	0, CII	10	33	100	0, CI	0, CII	10	33	100
1	0	0	0	0	0	0	0	0	0	0	0	0	0	0	0
2	0	0	0	0	0	0	0	0	0	0	0	0	0	0	0
3	0	0	0	0	0	0	0	0	0	0	0/1	0/1	0/1	0/1	0/1
4	0	0	0	0	0	0	0	0	0	0	0	0	0	0	0
5	0	0	0	0	0	1	0	0	0	0	0	0	0	0	0
6	0	0	0	0	0	0/10	0/10	0	0	0/10	0	0	0	0/10	0
7	0	0	0	0	0	0	0	0	0	0	0	0	0	0	0
8	0	0	0	0	0	0	0	0	0	0	0	0	0/10	0	0
9	0	0	0	0	0	0	0	1	1	0	0	0	0	0	0
10	0	0	0	0	0	0	0	0	0	0	0	0	0	0	0
11	0	0	0	0	0	0	0	0	1	0	0	0	0	0	0
12	0	0	0	0	0	0/10	0/10	0/1	0	1/10	0	0	0/9	0/9	0
13	0	0	0	1	0	0	0	1	1	2	0	0	0	0	0
14	0	0	0	0	0	1	0/1	0	0/1	0	0	0	0	0	0
15	0	0	0	1	0	0	2	1	1	2	0	0	0	0	0
16	0	0	0	0	0	0	0	0	2	1	0	0	0	0	0
17	2/0	0	0	0	0	1	2	1	0	2	0	0	0	0	0
18	0	0	0	0	0	0/20	1/20	0	0/2	3/20	0	0	0/20	0/18	0
19	0	0	0	0	1	0	0	0	0	1	0	0	0	0	0
20	1	0	2	1	1	2	1	2	2	0	1	0	0	0	0
21	2	2	1	2	2	0	1	1	1	4	1	0	0	0	0
22	3	0	1	2	2	1	0	2	2	3	1	1	0	0	0
23	3	0	2	2	7	0	1	1	5	6	0	0	0	0	0
24	2	3	4	2	3	3	3	1	2	2	1	0	1	1	0
25	2/5	5/8	2/9	2/12	3/9	4/43	7/41	5/42	4/27	5/21	1	0	0	1	0
Column totals	15/5	10/8	12/9	13/12	17/9	13/83	18/82	15/43	26/30	32/61	3/1	1/1	1/40	1/38	0/1

[a] A ratio like x/y implies that y animals were in the scheduled sacrifice group and x were not; a simple entry like x is like x/0 and implies that there were no such animals in the scheduled sacrifice group.

[b] These animals were not histologically examined for this response.

TABLE A.3 Time to Death with Peritoneal Mesothelioma among Male Rats Exposed to Ethylene Oxide Vapor in the Bushy Run Research Center Study (12)

Exposure (months)	Number of Deaths with Peritoneal Mesothelioma[a] Dose (ppm)					Number of Deaths without Peritoneal Mesothelioma Dose (ppm)					Number of Animals Lost to Follow-up[b] Dose (ppm)				
	0, CI	0, CII	10	33	100	0, CI	0, CII	10	33	100	0, CI	0, CII	10	33	100
1	0	0	0	0	0	0	0	0	0	0	0	0	0	0	0
2	0	0	0	0	0	0	0	0	0	0	0	0	0	0	0
3	0	0	0	0	0	0	0	0	0	0	0/1	0/1	0/1	0/1	0/1
4	0	0	0	0	0	0	0	0	0	0	0	0	0	0	0
5	0	0	0	0	0	0	0	0	0	0	1	0	0	0	0
6	0	0	0	0	0	0/10	0/10	0	0	0/10	0	0	0/10	0/10	0
7	0	0	0	0	0	0	0	0	0	0	0	0	0	0	0
8	0	0	0	0	0	0	0	1	0	0	0	0	0	0	0
9	0	0	0	0	0	0	0	0	1	0	0	0	0	0	0
10	0	0	0	0	0	0	0	0	1	0	0	0	0	0	0
11	0	0	0	0	0	0	0	0	1	0	0	0	0	0	0
12	0	0	0	0	0	0/10	0/10	0	0/1	1/10	0	0	0/10	0/9	0
13	0	0	0	0	0	0	0	0	2	0	0	0/1	0	0	0
14	0	0	0	0	0	0	0	0	0	2	1	0/1	0	0	0
15	0	0	0	0	1	0	2	0	2	3	0	0	0	0	0
16	0	0	0	0	0	0	0	1	2	0	0	0	0	0	0
17	0	0	0	0	0	1	2	1	1	0	0	0	0	0	0
18	0/1	0	0	0/1	2/1	1/19	1/20	0/10	0/12	1/19	1	0	0/10	0/7	0
19	0	1	0	0	0	0	0	0	2	1	0	0	0	0	0
20	0	1	1	0	2	3	0	3	2	3	0	0	0	0	0
21	0	0	0	1	3	2	2	2	4	2	1	1	0	1	0
22	0	0	0	0	0	4	2	3	5	2	0	0	0	0	0
23	0	0	0	0	4	3	1	3	5	9	1	0	0	0	0
24	0	0	0	0	2	5	5	6	3	3	1	1	0	1	0
25	0/1	0/1	1/1	2/3	4/3	7/47	12/48	6/50	4/36	4/27	0	0	0	0	0
Column totals	0/2	1/1	2/1	3/4	18/4	26/86	26/88	26/60	35/49	31/66	5/1	2/2	0/31	2/27	0/1

[a]A ratio like x/y implies that y animals were in the scheduled sacrifice group and x were not; a simple entry like x is like x/0 and implies that there were no such animals in the scheduled sacrifice group.

[b]These animals were not histologically examined for this response.

TABLE A.4. Time to Death with Brain Neoplasia among Male Rats in the Bushy Run Research Center Ethylene Oxide Inhalation Study (42)

Exposure (months)	Number of Deaths with Brain Neoplasia[a] — Dose (ppm)					Number of Deaths without Brain Neoplasia — Dose (ppm)					Number of Animals Lost to Follow-up — Dose (ppm)				
	0, CI	0, CII	10	33	100	0, CI	0, CII	10	33	100	0, CI	0, CII	10	33	100
1	0	0	0	0	0	0	0	0	0	0	0	0	0	0	0
2	0	0	0	0	0	0	0	0	0	0	0	0	0	0	0
3	0	0	0	0	0	0/1	0/1	0/1	0/1	0/1	0	0	0	0	0
4	0	0	0	0	0	0	0	0	0	0	0	0	0	0	0
5	0	0	0	0	0	1	0	0	0	0	0	0	0	0	0
6	0	0	0	0	0	0/10	0/10	0/10	0/10	0/10	0	0	0	0	0
7	0	0	0	0	0	0	0	0	0	0	0	0	0	0	0
8	0	0	0	0	0	0	0	0	0	0	0	0	0	0	0
9	0	0	0	0	0	0	0	1	1	0	0	0	0	0	0
10	0	0	0	0	0	0	0	0	1	0	0	0	0	0	0
11	0	0	0	0	0	0	0	0	1	0	0	0	0	0	0
12	0	0	0	0	0	0/10	0/10	0/10	0/10	1/10	0	0	0	0	0
13	0	0	0	0	0	0	0	0	2	0	0	0	0	0	0
14	0	0	0	0	0	1	0/1	0	0	2	0	0	0	0	0
15	0	0	0	0	0	0	2	0	2	4	0	0	0	0	0
16	0	0	0	0	0	0	0	1	2	0	0	0	0	0	0
17	0	0	0	0	0	1	2	1	1	0	0	0	0	0	0
18	0	0	0	0/1	3/20	2/20	1/20	0/20	0/19	3/20	0	0	0	0	0
19	0	0	0	0	1	0	0	0	2	1	0	0	0	0	0
20	0	0	0	0	4	3	1	4	2	4	0	0	0	0	0
21	0	0	0	1	5	2	3	2	4	5	0	0	0	0	0
22	0	0	1	0	0	5	1	3	6	0	0	0	0	0	0
23	0	0	0	1	12	3	1	2	4	12	0	0	0	0	0
24	0	0	0	1	5	6	6	6	2	5	0	0	0	0	0
24.5	0	0	0	0	0	4	6	4	2	4	0	0	0	0	0
25	0/1	0	0	0/1	4/27	3/47	6/49	3/51	5/38	4/27	0	0	0	0	0
Column totals	0/1	0/0	1/0	3/2	4/3	31/88	29/91	27/92	37/78	45/68	0	0	0	0	0

[a] A ratio like x/y implies that y animals were in the scheduled sacrifice group and x were not; a simple entry like x is like $x/0$ and implies that there were no such animals in the scheduled sacrifice group.

TABLE A.5. Time to Death among Female Rats Exposed to Ethylene Oxide Vapor in the Bushy Run Research Center Study (42)

Exposure (months)	Number of Deaths Dose (ppm)					Number of Rats Sacrificed at Necropsy Interval Dose (ppm)					Number of Animals Lost to Follow-up Dose (ppm)				
	0, CI	0, CII	10	33	100	0, CI	0, CII	10	33	100	0, CI	0, CII	10	33	100
1	1	0	0	0	0	0	0	0	0	0	0	0	0	0	0
2	0	0	0	0	0	0	0	0	0	0	0	0	0	0	0
3	0	0	0	0	0	0	1	1	1	1	0	0	0	0	0
4	0	0	0	1	0	0	0	0	0	0	0	0	0	0	0
5	0	0	0	0	0	0	0	0	0	0	0	0	0	0	0
6	0	0	0	0	0	10	10	10	10	10	0	0	0	0	0
7	0	0	0	0	0	0	0	0	0	0	0	0	0	0	0
8	0	0	0	0	0	0	0	0	0	0	0	0	0	0	0
9	0	0	0	0	0	0	0	0	0	0	0	0	0	0	0
10	0	0	0	0	2	0	0	0	0	0	0	0	0	0	0
11	0	0	0	0	0	0	0	0	0	0	0	0	0	0	0
12	0	0	0	0	0	10	10	10	10	10	0	0	0	0	0
13	0	0	0	1	1	0	0	0	0	0	0	0	0	0	0
14	0	0	0	0	1	0	3	0	0	0	0	0	0	0	0
15	2	3	2	4	12	0	0	0	0	0	0	0	0	0	0
16	1	0	1	0	2	0	0	0	0	0	0	0	0	0	0
17	0	0	2	1	3	0	0	0	0	0	0	0	0	0	0
18	2	1	1	3	1	20	20	20	20	20	0	0	0	0	0
19	2	1	4	4	2	0	0	0	0	0	0	0	0	0	0
20	1	5	0	1	4	0	0	0	0	0	0	0	0	0	0
21	0	3	1	4	3	0	0	0	0	0	0	0	0	0	0
22	0	2	1	2	5	0	0	0	0	0	0	0	0	0	0
23	7	3	8	6	6	0	0	0	0	0	0	0	0	0	0
24	4	2	5	4	11	60	56	54	48	26	0	0	0	0	0
Column totals	20	20	25	31	53	100	100	95	89	67	0	0	0	0	0

TABLE A.6. Time to Death among Male Rats Exposed to Ethylene Oxide Vapor in the Bushy Run Research Center Study (42)

Exposure (months)	Number of Deaths Dose (ppm)					Number of Rats Sacrificed at Necropsy Interval Dose (ppm)					Number of Animals Lost to Follow-up Dose (ppm)				
	0, CI	0, CII	10	33	100	0, CI	0, CII	10	33	100	0, CI	0, CII	10	33	100
1	0	0	0	0	0	0	0	0	0	0	0	0	0	0	0
2	0	0	0	0	0	0	0	0	0	0	0	0	0	0	0
3	0	0	0	0	0	1	1	1	1	1	0	0	0	0	0
4	0	0	0	0	0	0	0	0	0	0	0	0	0	0	0
5	1	0	0	0	0	0	0	0	0	0	0	0	0	0	0
6	0	0	0	0	0	10	10	10	10	10	0	0	0	0	0
7	0	0	0	0	0	0	0	0	0	0	0	0	0	0	0
8	0	0	0	0	0	0	0	0	0	0	0	0	0	0	0
9	0	0	1	1	0	0	0	0	0	0	0	0	0	0	0
10	0	0	0	1	0	0	0	0	0	0	0	0	0	0	0
11	0	0	0	1	0	0	0	0	0	0	0	0	0	0	0
12	0	0	0	0	1	10	10	10	10	10	0	0	0	0	0
13	0	0	0	2	0	0	0	0	0	0	0	0	0	0	0
14	1	0	0	0	2	0	1	0	0	0	0	0	0	0	0
15	0	2	0	2	4	0	0	0	0	0	0	0	0	0	0
16	0	0	1	2	0	0	0	0	0	0	0	0	0	0	0
17	1	2	1	1	0	0	0	0	0	0	0	0	0	0	0
18	2	1	0	0	3	20	20	20	20	20	0	0	0	0	0
19	0	0	0	2	1	0	0	0	0	0	0	0	0	0	0
20	3	1	4	2	5	0	0	0	0	0	0	0	0	0	0
21	2	3	2	4	5	0	0	0	0	0	0	0	0	0	0
22	5	1	3	7	2	0	0	0	0	0	0	0	0	0	0
23	3	1	3	5	13	0	0	0	0	0	0	0	0	0	0
24	6	6	6	3	5	0	0	0	0	0	0	0	0	0	0
24.5	4	6	4	2	4	0	0	0	0	0	0	0	0	0	0
25	3	6	3	5	4	48	49	51	39	30	0	0	0	0	0
Column totals	31	29	28	40	49	89	91	92	80	71	0	0	0	0	0

TABLE A.7. Life Table Analysis Estimates of Probability of a Female Rat Developing Brain Neoplasia by Specified Times

Specified Time (months)	Control I	Control II	Controls I and II	10 ppm	33 ppm	100 ppm
1	0.000	0.000	0.000	0.000	0.000	0.000
2	0.000	0.000	0.000	0.000	0.000	0.000
3	0.000	0.000	0.000	0.000	0.000	0.000
4	0.000	0.000	0.000	0.000	0.000	0.000
5	0.000	0.000	0.000	0.000	0.000	0.000
6	0.000	0.000	0.000	0.000	0.000	0.000
7	0.000	0.000	0.000	0.000	0.000	0.000
8	0.000	0.000	0.000	0.000	0.000	0.000
9	0.000	0.000	0.000	0.000	0.000	0.000
10	0.000	0.000	0.000	0.000	0.000	0.000
11	0.000	0.000	0.000	0.000	0.000	0.000
12	0.000	0.000	0.000	0.000	0.000	0.000
13	0.000	0.000	0.000	0.000	0.000	0.000
14	0.000	0.000	0.000	0.000	0.000	0.000
15	0.000	0.000	0.000	0.000	0.000	0.000
16	0.000	0.000	0.000	0.000	0.000	0.000
17	0.000	0.000	0.000	0.000	0.000	0.013
18	0.012	0.000	0.006	0.000	0.012	0.027
19	0.012	0.000	0.006	0.000	0.012	0.027
20	0.012	0.000	0.006	0.000	0.012	0.027
21	0.012	0.000	0.006	0.000	0.012	0.027
22	0.012	0.000	0.006	0.000	0.012	0.027
23	0.012	0.000	0.006	0.016	0.012	0.027
24	0.012	0.000	0.006	0.016	0.086	0.127

TABLE A.8. Life Table Analysis Estimates of Probability of a Male Rat Developing Mononuclear Cell Leukemia by Specified Times

Specified Time (months)	Control I	Control II	Controls I and II	10 ppm	33 ppm	100 ppm
1	0.000	0.000	0.000	0.000	0.000	0.000
2	0.000	0.000	0.000	0.000	0.000	0.000
3	0.000	0.000	0.000	0.000	0.000	0.000
4	0.000	0.000	0.000	0.000	0.000	0.000
5	0.000	0.000	0.000	0.000	0.000	0.000
6	0.000	0.000	0.000	0.000	0.000	0.000
7	0.000	0.000	0.000	0.000	0.000	0.000
8	0.000	0.000	0.000	0.000	0.000	0.000
9	0.000	0.000	0.000	0.000	0.000	0.000
10	0.000	0.000	0.000	0.000	0.000	0.000
11	0.000	0.000	0.000	0.000	0.000	0.000
12	0.000	0.000	0.000	0.000	0.000	0.000
13	0.000	0.000	0.000	0.000	0.011	0.000
14	0.000	0.000	0.000	0.000	0.011	0.000
15	0.000	0.000	0.000	0.000	0.021	0.000
16	0.000	0.000	0.000	0.000	0.021	0.000
17	0.000	0.000	0.000	0.000	0.032	0.000
18	0.023	0.000	0.012	0.000	0.032	0.000
19	0.023	0.000	0.012	0.000	0.032	0.015
20	0.037	0.000	0.019	0.027	0.047	0.029
21	0.064	0.028	0.046	0.040	0.076	0.061
22	0.105	0.028	0.067	0.054	0.108	0.061
23	0.147	0.028	0.088	0.083	0.142	0.185
24	0.176	0.073	0.125	0.141	0.160	0.243
25	0.362	0.398	0.382	0.415	0.552	0.607

TABLE A.9. Life Table Analysis Estimates of Probability of a Male Rat Developing Peritoneal Mesothelioma by Specified Times

Specified Time (months)	Control I	Control II	Controls I and II	10 ppm	33 ppm	100 ppm
1	0.000	0.000	0.000	0.000	0.000	0.000
2	0.000	0.000	0.000	0.000	0.000	0.000
3	0.000	0.000	0.000	0.000	0.000	0.000
4	0.000	0.000	0.000	0.000	0.000	0.000
5	0.000	0.000	0.000	0.000	0.000	0.000
6	0.000	0.000	0.000	0.000	0.000	0.000
7	0.000	0.000	0.000	0.000	0.000	0.000
8	0.000	0.000	0.000	0.000	0.000	0.000
9	0.000	0.000	0.000	0.000	0.000	0.000
10	0.000	0.000	0.000	0.000	0.000	0.000
11	0.000	0.000	0.000	0.000	0.000	0.000
12	0.000	0.000	0.000	0.000	0.000	0.000
13	0.000	0.000	0.000	0.000	0.000	0.000
14	0.000	0.000	0.000	0.000	0.000	0.000
15	0.000	0.000	0.000	0.000	0.000	0.011
16	0.000	0.000	0.000	0.000	0.000	0.011
17	0.000	0.000	0.000	0.000	0.000	0.011
18	0.012	0.000	0.006	0.000	0.013	0.047
19	0.012	0.000	0.006	0.000	0.013	0.047
20	0.012	0.014	0.013	0.013	0.013	0.075
21	0.012	0.014	0.013	0.013	0.013	0.120
22	0.012	0.014	0.013	0.013	0.030	0.120
23	0.012	0.014	0.013	0.013	0.030	0.189
24	0.012	0.014	0.013	0.013	0.030	0.228
25	0.047	0.046	0.046	0.079	0.220	0.468

TABLE A.10. Life Table Analysis Estimates of Probability of a Male Rat Developing Brain Neoplasia by Specified Times

Specified Time (months)	Control I	Control II	Controls I and II	10 ppm	33 ppm	100 ppm
1	0.000	0.000	0.000	0.000	0.000	0.000
2	0.000	0.000	0.000	0.000	0.000	0.000
3	0.000	0.000	0.000	0.000	0.000	0.000
4	0.000	0.000	0.000	0.000	0.000	0.000
5	0.000	0.000	0.000	0.000	0.000	0.000
6	0.000	0.000	0.000	0.000	0.000	0.000
7	0.000	0.000	0.000	0.000	0.000	0.000
8	0.000	0.000	0.000	0.000	0.000	0.000
9	0.000	0.000	0.000	0.000	0.000	0.000
10	0.000	0.000	0.000	0.000	0.000	0.000
11	0.000	0.000	0.000	0.000	0.000	0.000
12	0.000	0.000	0.000	0.000	0.000	0.000
13	0.000	0.000	0.000	0.000	0.000	0.000
14	0.000	0.000	0.000	0.000	0.000	0.000
15	0.000	0.000	0.000	0.000	0.000	0.000
16	0.000	0.000	0.000	0.000	0.000	0.000
17	0.000	0.000	0.000	0.000	0.000	0.000
18	0.000	0.000	0.000	0.000	0.013	0.000
19	0.000	0.000	0.000	0.000	0.013	0.000
20	0.000	0.000	0.000	0.000	0.013	0.015
21	0.000	0.000	0.000	0.000	0.013	0.015
22	0.000	0.000	0.000	0.000	0.030	0.049
23	0.000	0.000	0.000	0.015	0.048	0.068
24	0.000	0.000	0.000	0.015	0.068	0.068
24.5	0.000	0.000	0.000	0.015	0.068	0.068
25	0.039	0.000	0.019	0.015	0.110	0.219

TABLE A.11. Life Table Analysis Estimates of the Probability of a Female Rat Dying by Specified Times

Specified Time (months)	Control I	Control II	Controls I and II	10 ppm	33 ppm	100 ppm
1	0.008	0.000	0.004	0.000	0.000	0.000
2	0.008	0.000	0.004	0.000	0.000	0.000
3	0.008	0.000	0.004	0.000	0.000	0.000
4	0.008	0.000	0.004	0.000	0.008	0.000
5	0.008	0.000	0.004	0.000	0.008	0.000
6	0.008	0.000	0.004	0.000	0.008	0.000
7	0.008	0.000	0.004	0.000	0.008	0.000
8	0.008	0.000	0.004	0.000	0.008	0.000
9	0.008	0.000	0.004	0.000	0.008	0.000
10	0.008	0.000	0.004	0.000	0.008	0.018
11	0.008	0.000	0.004	0.000	0.008	0.018
12	0.008	0.000	0.004	0.000	0.008	0.018
13	0.008	0.000	0.004	0.000	0.019	0.029
14	0.008	0.000	0.004	0.000	0.019	0.039
15	0.028	0.031	0.030	0.020	0.059	0.160
16	0.038	0.031	0.035	0.030	0.059	0.180
17	0.038	0.031	0.035	0.051	0.069	0.211
18	0.061	0.043	0.052	0.062	0.103	0.222
19	0.086	0.056	0.071	0.113	0.155	0.250
20	0.099	0.123	0.110	0.113	0.168	0.304
21	0.099	0.163	0.130	0.126	0.220	0.345
22	0.099	0.189	0.143	0.139	0.246	0.413
23	0.188	0.229	0.208	0.242	0.324	0.495
24	0.283	0.280	0.282	0.360	0.421	0.727

TABLE A.12. Life Table Analysis Estimates of the Probability of a Male Rat Dying by Specified Times

Specified Time (months)	Control I	Control II	Controls I and II	10 ppm	33 ppm	100 ppm
1	0.000	0.000	0.000	0.000	0.000	0.000
2	0.000	0.000	0.000	0.000	0.000	0.000
3	0.000	0.000	0.000	0.000	0.000	0.000
4	0.000	0.000	0.000	0.000	0.000	0.000
5	0.008	0.000	0.004	0.000	0.000	0.000
6	0.008	0.000	0.004	0.000	0.000	0.000
7	0.008	0.000	0.004	0.000	0.000	0.000
8	0.008	0.000	0.004	0.000	0.000	0.000
9	0.008	0.000	0.004	0.009	0.009	0.000
10	0.008	0.000	0.004	0.009	0.018	0.000
11	0.008	0.000	0.004	0.009	0.028	0.000
12	0.008	0.000	0.004	0.009	0.028	0.010
13	0.008	0.000	0.004	0.009	0.048	0.010
14	0.019	0.000	0.009	0.009	0.048	0.030
15	0.019	0.020	0.019	0.009	0.068	0.070
16	0.019	0.020	0.019	0.019	0.088	0.070
17	0.029	0.041	0.035	0.029	0.098	0.070
18	0.051	0.052	0.052	0.029	0.098	0.104
19	0.051	0.052	0.052	0.029	0.125	0.117
20	0.090	0.065	0.078	0.081	0.151	0.182
21	0.115	0.104	0.110	0.106	0.203	0.247
22	0.179	0.117	0.149	0.144	0.294	0.273
23	0.218	0.130	0.174	0.183	0.360	0.442
24	0.295	0.208	0.252	0.259	0.399	0.507
24.5	0.346	0.286	0.316	0.310	0.425	0.559
25	0.419	0.426	0.423	0.383	0.542	0.652

TABLE A.13. Number of Months in the Bushy Run Research Center Ethylene Oxide 2-year Inhalation Study on Rats Until Prescribed Percentages of Rats Developed Particular Responses[a]

	Prescribed Precentage of Rats Developing the Particular Response							
	Female				Male			
	1%	5%	10%	20%	1%	5%	10%	20%
Response = Mononuclear Cell Leukemia								
Control I	19	24	24	24	18	21	22	25
Control II	18	21	23	24	21	24	25	25
Controls I and II	18	23	24	24	18	21	24	25
10 ppm	19	23	24	24	20	22	24	25
33 ppm	18	20	23	24	13	20	22	25
100 ppm	18	21	22	24	19	21	23	24
Response = Brain Neoplasia								
Control I	18	> 24	> 24	> 24	25	> 25	> 25	> 25
Control II	> 24[b]	> 24	> 24	> 24	> 25[b]	> 25	> 25	> 25
Controls I and II	18	> 24	> 24	> 24	25	> 25	> 25	> 25
10 ppm	23	> 24	> 24	> 24	23	> 25	> 25	> 25
33 ppm	18	24	> 24	> 24	18	23	25	> 25
100 ppm	17	24	24	> 24	20	22	25	25
Response = Peritoneal Mesothelioma								
Control I					18	25	> 25	> 25
Control II					20	25	> 25	> 25
Controls I and II					18	25	> 25	> 25
10 ppm					20	25	> 25	> 25
33 ppm					18	25	25	25
100 ppm					15	18	21	24
Response = Death								
Control I	1	18	20	24	5	18	21	23
Control II	15	19	20	23	15	18	21	24
Controls I and II	15	18	20	23	14	18	21	24
10 ppm	15	17	19	23	9	20	21	24
33 ppm	4	15	18	21	9	13	17	21
100 ppm	10	15	15	17	12	15	18	21

[a]The table entry corresponds to the smallest number of exposure months in Tables 3 and A.1–A.6 such that the life table estimate of the probability of the specified response (rounded to the nearest percent) is at least the prescribed percentage.
[b]An entry of > 24 or > 25 months implies that the percentage response was not reached by the end of the experiment.

TABLE A.14. Life Table Estimates of Mean Number of Months without a Specified Response during Exposure to Ethylene Oxide in the Bushy Run Research Center Study

	Female			Male		
	Length of Experimental Period (months)	Mean Number of Months without a Response	Mean Percentage of Experimental Period without a Response	Length of Experimental Period (months)	Mean Number of Months without a Response	Mean Percentage of Experimental Period without a Response
Response = Mononuclear Cell Leukemia						
Control I	24	23.70	98.7	25	24.06	96.3
Control II	24	23.45	97.7	25	24.45	97.8
Controls I and II	24	23.58	98.2	25	24.25	97.0
10 ppm	24	23.55	98.1	25	24.24	97.0
33 ppm	24	23.10	96.2	25	23.76	95.0
100 ppm	24	22.88	95.3	25	23.80	95.2
Response = Brain Neoplasia						
Control I	24	23.92	99.7	25	24.98	99.9
Control II	24	24.00	100.0	25	25.00	100.0
Controls I and II	24	23.96	99.8	25	24.99	100.0
10 ppm	24	23.97	99.9	25	24.95	99.8
33 ppm	24	23.84	99.3	25	24.71	98.9
100 ppm	24	23.70	98.7	25	24.64	98.6
Response = Peritoneal Mesothelioma						
Control I				25	24.87	99.5
Control II				25	24.89	99.5
Controls I and II				25	24.88	99.5
10 ppm				25	24.85	99.4
33 ppm				25	24.64	98.6
100 ppm				25	23.67	94.7
Response = Death						
Control I	24	22.86	95.3	25	23.46	93.8
Control II	24	22.82	95.1	25	23.83	95.3
Controls I and II	24	22.84	95.2	25	23.64	94.6
10 ppm	24	22.74	94.8	25	23.71	94.8
33 ppm	24	22.06	91.9	25	22.45	89.8
100 ppm	24	20.57	85.7	25	22.26	89.1

TABLE A.15. Comparisons that are Independent of Dose–Response Modeling: 95% Two-Sided Confidence Intervals on the Probability of a Rat Developing a Specified Response at the Control and 10-ppm Exposure Levels

Animal	Specified Response	Exposure Group	Observed Number of Animals with the Specified Response	Number of Animals at Risk	95% Two-Sided Confidence Interval[a] Lower Bound on Probability	Upper Bound on Probability
Female rat	Mononuclear cell leukemia	BRRC controls[b]	22	152	0.0888	0.2007
Female rat	Mononuclear cell leukemia	BRRC 10 ppm[b]	14	76	0.0971	0.2714
Female rat	Brain glioma	BRRC controls[b]	1	157	0.0000	0.0188
Female rat	Brain glioma	All BRRC controls	5	567	0.0011	0.0165
Female rat	Brain glioma	Historical controls	43	5524	0.0055	0.0101
Female rat	Brain glioma	BRRC 10 ppm[b]	1	79	0.0000	0.0373
Male rat	Mononuclear cell leukemia	BRRC controls[b]	38	153	0.1799	0.3168
Male rat	Mononuclear cell leukemia	NIOSH controls	12	39	0.1628	0.4525
Male rat	Mononuclear cell leukemia	BRRC and NIOSH controls	50	232	0.1626	0.2684
Male rat	Mononuclear cell leukemia	BRRC 10 ppm[b]	21	78	0.1708	0.3677
Male rat	Peritoneal mesothelioma	BRRC controls[b]	3	150	0.0000	0.0424
Male rat	Peritoneal mesothelioma	NIOSH controls	3	78	0.0000	0.0811
Male rat	Peritoneal mesothelioma	BRRC and NIOSH controls	7	265	0.0071	0.0457
Male rat	Peritoneal mesothelioma	BRRC 10 ppm[b]	3	79	0.0000	0.0801
Male rat	Brain glioma	BRRC controls[b]	1	157	0.0000	0.0188
Male rat	Brain glioma	All BRRC controls	7	571	0.0032	0.0213
Male rat	Brain glioma	Historical controls	57	5450	0.0078	0.0132
Male rat	Brain glioma	BRRC 10 ppm[b]	1	79	0.0000	0.0373

[a]The confidence intervals are computed using the standard normal distribution approximation to the binomial distribution.
[b]Values are based on all rats that were histologically examined for the response and that died or were found in moribund condition or were sacrificed at the end of the experiment.

219

TABLE A.16. Quantitative Impacts of Choices of Time and Response Used in Defining the Virtually Safe Dose[a]

Increase in Probability	Specified Time (months)	Estimated Virtually Safe Dose (mg/kg· day)						
		Mononuclear Cell Leukemia in Female Rats	Brain Neoplasia in Female Rats	Mononuclear Cell Leukemia in Male Rats	Peritoneal Mesothelioma in Male Rats	Brain Neoplasia in Male Rats	Death from Any Cause in Female Rats	Death from Any Cause in Male Rats
0.0001	18	2.8	0.75	1.0	>5	>5	0.014	0.44
0.0001	21	0.11	0.11	0.14	0.51	1.39	0.0068	0.28
0.0001	24	0.0073	0.021	0.24	0.029	0.083	0.0038	0.20
0.000001	18	0.056	0.0089	0.014	0.25	>5	0.0014	0.046
0.000001	21	0.0012	0.0011	0.0014	0.0055	0.019	0.000068	0.029
0.000001	24	0.000073	0.00021	0.00024	0.00029	0.00083	0.000038	0.020

[a]Estimates are based on all rats at the control, 10-, and 33-ppm dose levels which were histologically examined and which died or were found in moribund condition or were sacrificed at the end of the experiment. The modeling was done using the multistage-Weibull time-to-response model with dose expressed in mg/kg·day. The tabled estimates are the fitted model values (maximum likelihood estimates).

TABLE A.17. Maximum Likelihood Estimates of Doses Corresponding to Percentage Decreases in Mean Response-Free Periods Equivalent to 1 month, 1 week, 1 day, and 1 hour in a 70-year Lifetime[a]

Decrease in a 70-yr Lifetime	Percentage Decrease	Estimated Dose (mg/kg· day) for Each Specified Response						
		Mononuclear Cell Leukemia in Female Rats	Brain Neoplasia in Female Rats	Mononuclear Cell Leukemia in Male Rats	Peritoneal Mesothelioma in Male Rats	Brain Neoplasia in Male Rats	Death from any Cause in Female Rats	Death from any Cause in Male Rats
1.0 month	0.12	1.2	2.2	2.1	3.9	4.6	0.24	1.5
1.0 wk	0.027	0.37	0.68	0.74	1.4	2.5	0.056	0.78
1.0 day	0.0039	0.058	0.11	0.13	0.25	0.68	0.0080	0.31
1.0 h	0.00016	0.0025	0.0026	0.0055	0.011	0.031	0.00033	0.064

[a]Estimates are based on all rats at the control, 10-, and 33-ppm dose levels which were histologically examined and which died or were found in moribund condition or were sacrificed at the end of the experiment. The modeling was done using the multistage-Weibull time-to-response model with dose expressed in mg/kg·day.

TABLE A.18. Fitted Multistage-Weibull Time-to-Response Model Values (Maximum Likelihood Estimates) of (i) Increases in the Probability of a Female Rat Dying with Brain Neoplasia by Specified Times and (ii) Decreases in Mean Response-Free Period during an Expected Lifetime[a]

Lifetime Average Dose to Female Rats (mg/kg·day)	Human Exposure (in ppm) with Same Lifetime Average Exposure (in mg/kg·day) as the Female Rats		Estimated Increases in Probability of Dying with Brain Neoplasia in Female Rats by Specified Times[b]					Estimated Decreases in Mean Response-Free Period between 0 and 70 yr
	Exposure 24h/day, 7days/wk, 52 wk/yr for 70 yr (ppm)	Exposure 6h/day, 5days/wk, 51 wk/yr for 40 yr (ppm)	30 yr	40 yr	50 yr	60 yr	70 yr	
1.086	2.00	20.0	0.0[c]	0.000003	0.00008	0.0009	0.007	1.7 wk
0.543	1.00	10.0	0.0	0.000001	0.00004	0.0004	0.003	5.4 days
0.2715	0.50	5.0	0.0	0.0000006	0.00002	0.0002	0.001	2.6 days
0.2172	0.40	4.0	0.0	0.0000005	0.00001	0.0002	0.001	2.0 days
0.1629	0.30	3.0	0.0	0.0000004	0.00001	0.0001	0.0008	1.5 days
0.1086	0.20	2.0	0.0	0.0000003	0.000006	0.00007	0.0005	1.0 days
0.0543	0.10	1.0	0.0	0.0000001	0.000003	0.00004	0.0003	12.1 h
0.02715	0.05	0.5	0.0	0.0	0.000002	0.00002	0.0001	6.2 h
0.00543	0.01	0.1	0.0	0.0	0.0000003	0.000004	0.00003	1.6 h

[a] Estimates are based on all rats at the control, 10-, and 33-ppm dose levels which died or were found in moribund condition or were sacrificed at the end of the experiment. The modeling was done using the multistage-Weibull time-to-response model with dose expressed in mg/kg·day.

[b] Two years in a rat lifetime are assumed to be equivalent to 70 years in a human lifetime. All times and mean response-free periods are tabled on the 70-year lifetime scale.

[c] 0.0 means less than 0.0000001.

TABLE A.19. Fitted Multistage-Weibull Time-to-Response Model Values (Maximum Likelihood Estimates) of (i) Increases in Probability of a Male Rat Dying with Mononuclear Cell Leukemia by Specified Times and (ii) Decreases in Mean Response-Free Period during an Expected Lifetime[a]

Lifetime Average Dose to Female Rats (mg/kg·day)	Human Exposure (in ppm) with Same Lifetime Average Exposure (in mg/kg·day) as the Female Rats		Estimated Increases in Probability of Dying with Mononuclear Cell Lukemia in Male Rats by Specified Times[b]					Estimated Decreases in Mean Response-Free Period between 0 and 70 yr
	Exposure 24 h/day, 7 days/wk, 52 wk/yr for 70 yr (ppm)	Exposure 6 h/day, 5 days/wk, 51 wk/yr for 40 yr (ppm)	30 yr	40 yr	50 yr	60 yr	70 yr	
1.086	2.00	20.0	0.0[c]	0.000001	0.00005	0.0008	0.006	1.6 wk
0.543	1.00	10.0	0.0	0.0000006	0.00002	0.0003	0.003	4.9 days
0.2715	0.50	5.0	0.0	0.0000003	0.00001	0.0002	0.001	2.2 days
0.2172	0.40	4.0	0.0	0.0000002	0.000008	0.0001	0.001	1.8 days
0.1629	0.30	3.0	0.0	0.0000002	0.000006	0.00009	0.0007	1.2 days
0.1086	0.20	2.0	0.0	0.0000001	0.000004	0.00006	0.0005	20.5 h
0.0543	0.10	1.0	0.0	0.0000001	0.000002	0.00003	0.0002	10.1 h
0.02715	0.05	0.5	0.0	0.0	0.0000009	0.00001	0.0001	5.0 h
0.00543	0.01	0.1	0.0	0.0	0.0000002	0.000003	0.00002	59.6 min

[a]Estimates are based on all rats at the control, 10-, and 33-ppm dose levels which were histologically examined and which died or were found in moribund condition or were sacrificed at the end of the experiment. The modeling was done using the multistage-Weibull time-to-response model with dose expressed in mg/kg·day.
[b]Two years in a rat lifetime are assumed to be equivalent to 70 years in a human lifetime. All times and mean response-free periods are tabled on the 70-year lifetime scale.
[c]0.0 means less than 0.0000001.

TABLE A.20. Fitted Multistage-Weibull Time-to-Response Model Values (Maximum Likelihood Estimates) of (i) Increases in Probability of a Male Rat Dying with Peritoneal Mesothelioma by Specified Times and (ii) Decreases in Mean Response-Free Period during an Expected Lifetime[a]

Lifetime Average Dose to Female Rats (mg/kg·day)	Human Exposure (in ppm) with Same Lifetime Average Exposure (in mg/kg·day) as the Female Rats		Estimated Increases in Probability of Dying with Peritoneal Mesothelioma in Male Rats by Specified Times[b]					Estimated Decreases in Mean Response-Free Period between 0 and 70 yr
	Exposure 24 h/day, 7 days/wk, 52 wk/yr for 70 yr (ppm)	Exposure 6 h/day, 5 days/wk, 51 wk/yr for 40 yr (ppm)	30 yr	40 yr	50 yr	60 yr	70 yr	
1.086	2.00	20.0	0.0[c]	0.0	0.000001	0.0001	0.005	5.3 days
0.543	1.00	10.0	0.0	0.0	0.0000006	0.00007	0.002	2.3 days
0.2715	0.50	5.0	0.0	0.0	0.0000003	0.00003	0.001	1.1 days
0.2172	0.40	4.0	0.0	0.0	0.0000002	0.00002	0.0008	20.9 h
0.1629	0.30	3.0	0.0	0.0	0.0000002	0.00002	0.0006	15.5 h
0.1086	0.20	2.0	0.0	0.0	0.0000001	0.00001	0.0004	10.2 h
0.0543	0.10	1.0	0.0	0.0	0.0000001	0.000006	0.0002	5.0 h
0.02715	0.05	0.5	0.0	0.0	0.0	0.000003	0.00009	2.5 h
0.00543	0.01	0.1	0.0	0.0	0.0	0.0000006	0.00002	29.8 min

[a] Estimates are based on all rats at the control, 10-, and 33-ppm dose levels which were histologically examined and which died or were found in moribund condition or were sacrificed at the end of the experiment. The modeling was done using the multistage-Weibull time-to-response model with dose expressed in mg/kg·day.
[b] Two years in a rat lifetime are assumed to be equivalent to 70 years in a human lifetime. All times and mean response-free periods are tabled on the 70-year lifetime scale.
[c] 0.0 means less than 0.0000001.

TABLE A.21. Fitted Multistage-Weibull Time-to-Response Model Values (Maximum Likelihood Estimates) of (i) Increases in Probability of a Male Rat Dying with Brain Neoplasia by Specified Times and (ii) Decreases in Mean Response-Free Period during an Expected Lifetime[a]

Lifetime Average Dose to Female Rats (mg/kg·day)	Human Exposure (in ppm) with Same Lifetime Average Exposure (in mg/kg·day) as the Female Rats		Estimated Increases in Probability of Dying with Brain Neoplasia in Male Rats by Specified Times[b]					Estimated Decreases in Mean Response-Free Period between 0 and 70 yr
	Exposure 24 h/day, 7 days/wk, 52 wk/yr for 70 yr (ppm)	Exposure 6 h/day, 5 days/wk, 51 wk/yr for 40 yr (ppm)	30 yr	40 yr	50 yr	60 yr	70 yr	
1.086	2.00	20.0	0.0[c]	0.0	0.0	0.00004	0.002	1.8 days
0.543	1.00	10.0	0.0	0.0	0.0	0.00002	0.0007	18.6 h
0.2715	0.50	5.0	0.0	0.0	0.0	0.000008	0.0003	8.8 h
0.2172	0.40	4.0	0.0	0.0	0.0	0.000006	0.0003	7.2 h
0.1629	0.30	3.0	0.0	0.0	0.0	0.000005	0.0002	5.4 h
0.1086	0.20	2.0	0.0	0.0	0.0	0.000003	0.0001	3.6 h
0.0543	0.10	1.0	0.0	0.0	0.0	0.000002	0.00007	1.8 h
0.02715	0.05	0.5	0.0	0.0	0.0	0.0000008	0.00003	53.3 min
0.00543	0.01	0.1	0.0	0.0	0.0	0.0000002	0.000007	10.7 min

[a]Estimates are based on all rats at the control, 10-, and 33-ppm dose levels which died or were found in moribund condition or were sacrificed at the end of the experiment. The modeling was done using the multistage-Weibull time-to-response model with dose expressed in mg/kg·day.

[b]Two years in a rat lifetime are assumed to be equivalent to 70 years in a human lifetime. All times and mean response-free periods are tabled on the 70-year lifetime scale.

[c]0.0 means less than 0.0000001.

TABLE A.22. Fitted Multistage-Weibull Time-to-Response Model Values (Maximum Likelihood Estimates) of (i) Increases in Probability of a Female Rat Dying by Specified Times and (ii) Decreases in Mean Response-Free Period during an Expected Lifetime[a]

Lifetime Average Dose to Female Rats (mg/kg·day)	Human Exposure (in ppm) with Same Lifetime Average Exposure (in mg/kg·day) as the Female Rats		Estimated Increases in Probability of Female Rats Dying by Specified Times[b]					Estimated Decreases in Mean Response-Free Period between 0 and 70 yr
	Exposure 24 h/day, 7 days/wk, 52 wk/yr for 70 yr (ppm)	Exposure 6 h/day, 5 days/wk, 51 wk/yr for 40 yr (ppm)	30 yr	40 yr	50 yr	60 yr	70 yr	
1.086	2.00	20.0	0.0004	0.002	0.006	0.01	0.03	4.5 months
0.543	1.00	10.0	0.0002	0.0009	0.003	0.007	0.01	2.2 months
0.2715	0.50	5.0	0.0001	0.0005	0.001	0.004	0.007	1.1 months
0.2172	0.40	4.0	0.00008	0.0004	0.001	0.003	0.006	3.9 wk
0.1629	0.30	3.0	0.00006	0.0003	0.0009	0.002	0.004	2.9 wk
0.1086	0.20	2.0	0.00004	0.0002	0.0006	0.001	0.003	1.9 wk
0.0543	0.10	1.0	0.00002	0.00009	0.0003	0.0007	0.001	6.8 days
0.02715	0.05	0.5	0.00001	0.00005	0.0001	0.0004	0.0007	3.4 days
0.00543	0.01	0.1	0.000002	0.000009	0.00003	0.00007	0.0001	16.3 h

[a]Estimates are based on all rats at the control, 10-, and 33-ppm dose levels. The modeling was done using the multistage-Weibull time-to-response model with dose expressed in mg/kg·day.

[b]Two years in a rat lifetime are assumed to be equivalent to 70 years in a human lifetime. All times and mean response-free periods are tabled on the 70-year lifetime scale.

TABLE A.23. Fitted Multistage-Weibull Time-to-Response Model Values (Maximum Likelihood Estimates) of (i) Increases in Probability of a Male Rat Dying by Specified Times and (ii) Decreases in Mean Response-Free Period during an Expected Lifetime[a]

Lifetime Average Dose to Female Rats (mg/kg·day)	Human Exposure (in ppm) with Same Lifetime Average Exposure (in mg/kg·day) as the Female Rats		Estimated Increases in Probability of Male Rats Dying by Specified Times[b]					Estimated Decreases in Mean Response-Free Period between 0 and 70 yr
	Exposure 24 h/day, 7 days/wk, 52 wk/yr for 70 yr (ppm)	Exposure 6 h/day, 5 days/wk, 51 wk/yr for 40 yr (ppm)	30 yr	40 yr	50 yr	60 yr	70 yr	
1.086	2.00	20.0	0.00002	0.0001	0.0005	0.002	0.004	2.1 wk
0.543	1.00	10.0	0.000004	0.00003	0.0001	0.0004	0.0008	3.3 days
0.2715	0.50	5.0	0.0000009	0.000006	0.00003	0.00008	0.0002	18.6 h
0.2172	0.40	4.0	0.0000006	0.000004	0.00002	0.00005	0.0001	11.8 h
0.1629	0.30	3.0	0.0000003	0.000002	0.00001	0.00003	0.00007	6.6 h
0.1086	0.20	2.0	0.0000001	0.000001	0.000004	0.00001	0.00003	2.9 h
0.0543	0.10	1.0	0.0[c]	0.0000002	0.000001	0.000003	0.000007	42.7 min
0.02715	0.05	0.5	0.0	0.0000001	0.0000003	0.0000008	0.000002	10.6 min
0.00543	0.01	0.1	0.0	0.0	0.0	0.0	0.0000001	25.4 s

[a]Estimates are based on all rats at the control, 10-, and 33-ppm dose levels. The modeling was done using the multistage-Weibull time-to-response model with dose expressed in mg/kg·day.

[b]Two years in a rat lifetime are assumed to be equivalent to 70 years in a human lifetime. All times and mean response-free periods are tabled on the 70-year lifetime scale.

[c]0.0 means less than 0.0000001.

APPENDIX B: SOME LIMITATIONS AND PITFALLS IN MANY QUANTITATIVE RISK ASSESSMENTS THAT HAVE BEEN PREPARED BY U.S. REGULATORY AGENCIES

Quantitative risk assessments are not easy to prepare or evaluate. A checklist of 20 questions regarding the relevance of results of dose–response models has been offered in ref. 40 for risk managers and developers of quantitative risk assessments. A few additional points are listed here.

1   Quantal Response Models Are Not Detailed Biological Models for Carcinogenesis

The probit, logit, Weibull, multihit, and multistage models are the quantal response models most frequently used for high-to-low-dose extrapolations based on animal studies. These models are based on very simplified probabilistic interpretations of cancer which do not even attempt to be detailed biological models of the complex carcinogenic processes.

2   Quantal Response Models Do Not Necessarily Fit Experimental Data Well

Some quantal response models frequently do not represent a family of curves with enough flexibility (variety of shape) to reflect the observed shape in the experimental dose–response data. For example, as illustrated in Fig. B.1, the usual restrictions on the multistage model prevent it from adequately reflecting dose–response relations that are either nonincreasing or very slowly increasing at the lower experimental doses and that are very rapidly increasing at the higher experimental doses. In such situations the fitted multistage model tends to overstate greatly the risks at the lower dose levels.

3   False Impressions Can Arise from Fitting Quantal Response Models to Very High Administered Doses

The compromises inherent in curve fitting may lead to questionable fits in the dose region of primary concern. Any flattening out or leveling off of the observed dose–response relation at higher doses causes the fitted quantal response models to modify their shape in the lower-dose region in order to fit in with the relatively flat higher-dose behavior. This modification in the shape of the fitted model at the lower doses is illustrated in Fig. B.2. The use of the very-high-dose data can lead to fitted models with a false shape in the lower-dose region—frequently a false impression of linearity in the lower-dose region and an overstatement of risks or, when the true dose–response relation is linear over the lower experimental doses, an understatement of risks. These pitfalls can often be lessened by fitting the models to the observed proportions excluding the highest dose level(s).

4   Bad Fits Are Frequently Not Detected by the Chi-Square Goodness-of-fit Test

Unfortunately, proposed dose–response models are often blindly accepted whenever the chi-square goodness-of-fit test does not reject them. Although the test will not reject a true model more often than specified by the significance level, it will frequently not reject a false

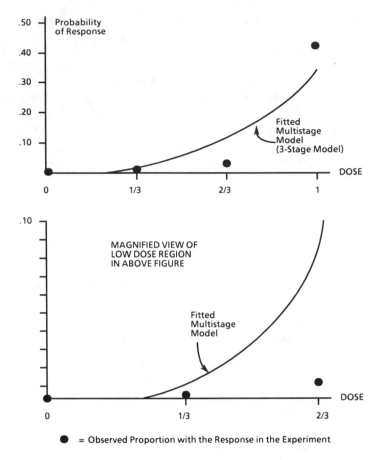

Figure B.1. Example where the usual restrictions on the multistage model prevent it from adequately reflecting the observed dose–response relation.

model either. The test's weakness stems primarily from its failure to detect patterns in the discrepancies between the fitted model's predictions and the observed experimental data. In other words, the test is weak because it does not consider the shapes of the observed and fitted dose–response relations.

5 Trend Tests Can Easily Give False Impressions about Low-Dose Behavior

In cases such as ethylene oxide inhalation where high exposures are undoubtedly carcinogenic in some animals but the region of occupational or environmental concern is the relatively low-dose levels, trend tests are not appropriate. Trend tests are primarily sensitive to changes in the response behaviors at the control level and the high-exposure levels and are quite insensitive to the relative behaviors at the control level and the low- to moderate-dose levels. To illustrate this inappropriateness of trend tests, the behavior of the Cochran–Armitage trend test (51) was simulated for an experimental design like that used in the BRRC study—namely, 240 animals at 0 ppm and 120 animals at each of 10, 33, and

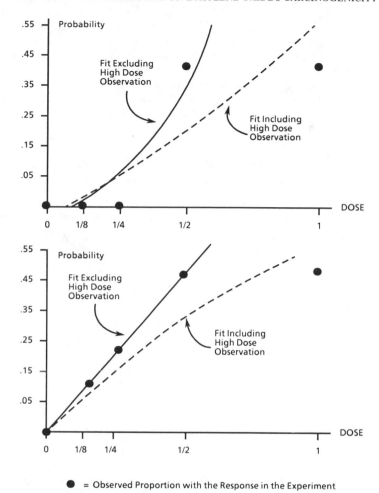

= Observed Proportion with the Response in the Experiment

Figure B.2. Examples where the fitted multistage model fails to indicate the observed dose–response relation in the lower-dose region when the model attempted also to fit a high-dose observation.

100 ppm. The true response rates in the simulation study were 0, 0, 0, and 20% at 0, 10, 33, and 100 ppm, respectively. In 100 simulations of this animal bioassay, the null hypothesis of "no trend" was rejected every time. Clearly, rejecting "no trend" does not imply that a linear trend exists or that an increasing trend over the lower doses exists.

6   The Fitted Quantal Response Models Frequently Do Not Agree on the Shape of the Dose–Response Relation

Among the quantal response models, both the probit and one-hit models have predetermined shapes for their low-dose behavior; that is, their shapes in the low-dose region are essentially unaffected by the experimental data. The probit model always approaches the background probability faster than any power of the dose, whereas the one-hit model or linear multistage model always approaches the background probability linearly and hence relatively slowly. Thus, the increased risks at very low doses are always estimated to be relatively small using probit models and relatively large using linear models like the one-hit models. Among the models without predetermined shapes like the Weibull and multistage models, there is frequent disagreement over the shape of the dose–response relation in the low-dose region. This disagreement is not just for small fractional doses but may extend over a wide range of low doses, which often includes the lower nonzero experimental dose levels.

7   The Definition of the Response May Substantially Affect the Shape of the Dose–Response Relation and the Risk Characterization

For example, for ethylene oxide inhalation the shape of the dose–response relation for mononuclear cell leukemia is different from that of peritoneal mesothelioma or brain neoplasia. The minimum required severity of the lesion (e.g., carcinoma as opposed to just hyperplasia) can also affect the shape of the dose–response relation.

8   Any Combining of Quantal Response Data for Different Responses Must Be Done Very Carefully if at All

Experimental animals should be counted only once in developing a quantal response model. Quantal response models are attempting to model the probability that an individual will develop a response during the observation period. The definition of a response may, for example, imply that an animal has responded if it has developed either leukemia or a glioma or both. However, if an animal has developed both leukemia and a glioma, then that animal represents one animal developing a response not two animals developing a response. Hence, when fitting quantal response models, it is incorrect to represent the number of animals developing a response by the total number of tumors instead of the total number of animals developing a response.

9   Defining Different Events to Be the Same Response May Result in a Misleading Quantitative Risk Assessment Unless the Events Have the Same Health Effects

If, for instance, the presence of a microscopic lesion in a sacrificed healthy animal and a death caused by a tumor are both counted as the same "response," then it is very difficult to interpret the practical consequences of the probability of a response being a particular value. Therefore, it seems reasonable only to combine events of similar practical consequences together in the definition of a response.

10   Upper Bounds on Risk Are Not Estimates of Risk

The value of the fitted model at a particular dose is an estimate of the probability of an individual developing a carcinogenic response at that dose level. That probability estimate is the estimate which is most consistent with the presumed model family. In addition to the model family's best estimate of the risk at a dose, upper and lower confidence limits on that risk can also be constructed. The purpose of these limits is to bound the true risk and not to estimate the risk. The difference between the fitted model values and the bounds on the risk may be several orders of magnitude at very small dose levels and may even be moderately large near the smaller positive experimental dose levels.

11   Upper Bounds Can be Constructed in More Than One Way and the Results Can Differ Considerably

There is more than one way to construct a bound or confidence limit, and, even for a particular model family and a given set of experimental data, the constructed bounds can differ by at least a few orders of magnitude in the low-dose region. Empirical studies of the usual confidence limit procedures for the multistage model have documented that these upper bounds frequently greatly exceed the true value when the underlying dose–response relation is sublinear.

12   Upper Bounds May Not Be Responsive to Experimental Data and Hence Fail to Differentiate Adequately between Two Different Carcinogenic Hazards

For example, empirical studies have shown that the upper bounds represented by the linearized multistage model are not very responsive to the experimental data in the sense that very different experimental outcomes still lead to very similar bounds. Fig. B.3 indicates five very different hypothetical outcomes of the BRRC study for which the linearized multistage model 95% upper confidence limits on the increased probability of a response at 1.0 ppm are all within one order of magnitude of each other (i.e., the smallest limit is no less than the largest limit divided by 10). The relatively small differences in these bounds imply that their use will portray the risks to be pretty much the same regardless of the experimental data and that dose–response relations cannot be differentiated on the basis of linearized multistage model upper confidence limits on risk.

13   Not All Values Less Than an Upper Bound Are Equally Likely to Be the True Value of the Quantity Being Bounded

If the upper bound is sufficiently small, then the risk is probably sufficiently small. However, if the upper bound is not sufficiently small, this does not mean that the risk is not sufficiently small. The true risk can be much less than its upper bound.

All values less than a 95% upper confidence limit are not equally likely to be the true value of the quantity being bounded. If the true dose–response relation is one of the curves in the model family, then the fitted model value is the most likely value of the probability of an individual developing the specified response and the values near the fitted model value are much more likely to be the true value than the values farther away.

14   The True Risk Does Not Necessarily Lie between the Smallest Upper Bound and Largest Upper Bound

The minimum of several upper bounds on the same risk is still an upper bound on that risk. Nevertheless, risk assessment documents often mistakenly refer to a range of such upper bounds as if the true value of the risk is within that range instead of below it. When different procedures are used to generate upper bounds on a specified quantity, the range from the smallest upper bound to the largest upper bound only reflects the variability in the bounding procedures; it is not a range wherein the quantity being bounded should be

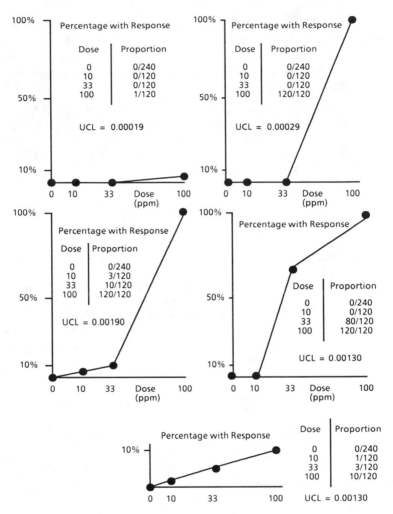

Figure B.3. Nonresponsiveness of linearized multistage model 95% upper confidence limits to experimental data: Five experimental data sets whose 95% upper confidence limits (UCL) on the increased probability of a response at 1.0 ppm differ by less than one order of magnitude.

expected to lie. The range from an upper bound to a lower bound is a range in which one would expect to find the risk being bounded.

Ranges of upper bounds are also often misinterpreted when each one of several different risks has its own individual upper bound. It is not necessarily true and may in fact be highly unlikely that the largest of the several risks exceeds the smallest of the upper bounds. For example, it is quite possible for the true risks to be 0.000001, 0.000005, and 0.00001 and the upper bounds to be 0.0002, 0.001, and 0.006, in which case the largest true risk (0.00001) is still well below the smallest upper bound (0.0002).

15   Lower Bounds on Risk Can and Should Also Be Constructed

Bounding procedures can be used to construct lower bounds as well as upper bounds. Not only do these lower bounds provide information by themselves, but the difference between the upper and lower bounds can also be informative. This difference provides an indication of how specific (tight) the bounds really are. Also, the farther apart the upper and lower bounds are using the same procedure, the less likely the true value is to being near either bound.

The relative behaviors of upper bounds, maximum likelihood estimates (fitted model values), and lower bounds are illustrated in Fig. B.4 in terms of the multistage model and the observed frequencies of peritoneal mesothelioma among the male rats in the BRRC study which were histologically examined and either died or were sacrificed at the end of the experiment. The figure only shows the lower-dose region (i.e., below 10 ppm). Two pairs of upper and lower bounds are plotted. One pair consists of the linearized multistage model values, which are upper bounds (95% upper confidence limits), and the analogous lower bounds computed using the same procedure but based on the smallest slope (instead of the largest slope), which is not statistically inconsistent with the experimental data using a likelihood ratio criterion. (The computation of these upper bounds is described in detail in ref. 52.) The second pair is determined using a bootstrap procedure; specifically, by (i) sampling (with replacement) the observed male rats to form 9 simulated replications of

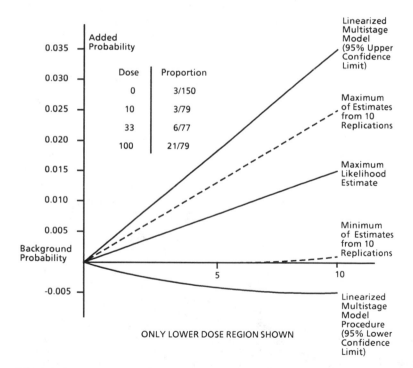

Figure B.4. Relative behaviors of upper bounds, maximum likelihood estimates (fitted model values), and lower bounds illustrated in terms of the multistage model and the observed frequencies of peritoneal mesothelioma among male rats in the BRRC study which were histologically examined and which died or were found in moribund condition or were sacrificed at the end of the experiment.

the BRRC experiment, (ii) considering the original experiment as a 10th replicate, (iii) determining the maximum likelihood estimates for each of the 10 replicates, and (iv) taking the maximum of these 10 estimates as the upper bound and the minimum as the lower bound. If each replicate had a probability of 0.5 of generating a fitted model value above the true risk and the replicates were independent, then the probability that the maximum of 5 replicates would exceed the true risk would be greater than 0.95. An analogous statement holds for the corresponding lower bounds. The replicates are not independent, so 10 replicates are used instead of five, and no specific coverage probabilities are claimed.

16   The Statistical Variability in the Quantitative Risk Assessment Caused by the Variability in the Experimental Data Should Be Distinguished, for Example, from Other Uncertainties and Policy Decisions

The bounds on risk often reflect value judgments, policy decisions, and worst case assumptions, as opposed to simply the statistical variability associated with experimental data. The amount of variability in the estimates of a particular risk that is due solely to the statistical variability (randomness) in the experimental data can be indicated in several ways. The individual simulated replications of the study and their corresponding estimates used in the bootstrap bounding procedure described in the preceding section provide one such indication. For the BRRC study, which had two control groups, the analyses can be performed using each control group alone as well as both together. For example, if the multistage model is fitted to the experimental data on female rats dying with MCL at 33 ppm, 10 ppm, and in controls, then, as shown in Table B.1, the maximum likelihood

TABLE B.1 Statistical Variation in Maximum Likelihood Estimates of the Added Probability of a Female Rat Dying with Mononuclear Cell Leukemia Due to Variation among the Controls

	Experimental Data				
Proportion with MCL[a]	Control I 9/78	Control II 13/74	Controls I and II 22/152	10 ppm 14/76	33 ppm 24/79

Fitted Multistage Model Values
Maximum Likelihood Estimates of Added Probability
Data Used in Modeling

Dose (ppm)	Control II, 10 ppm, and 33 ppm	Controls I and II, 10 ppm, and 33 ppm	Control I, 10 ppm, and 33 ppm
0.1	0.00000	0.00035	0.00064
0.25	0.00001	0.00087	0.00161
0.5	0.00003	0.00175	0.00321
0.75	0.00007	0.00263	0.00481
1.0	0.00013	0.00353	0.00641
2.0	0.00052	0.00715	0.01277
3.0	0.00117	0.01087	0.01909
4.0	0.00207	0.01469	0.02535
5.0	0.00324	0.01860	0.03159
10.0	0.01287	0.03947	0.06203

[a]Proportion with mononuclear cell leukemia among the animals that were histologically examined and that died or were found in moribund condition or were sacrificed at the end of the experiment.

estimates of the added probability for female rats at 1.0 ppm are 0.00013, 0.00353, and 0.00641 using Control II, Controls I and II combined, and Control I, respectively. In Table B.1 there seems to be considerably more variation toward smaller estimates than toward estimates that are larger than those for Controls I and II combined. For example, the maximum likelihood estimate for female rats at 1.0 ppm in Control I is less than twice that for Controls I and II combined, but the estimate for Control II is approximately 30 times smaller than that for Controls I and II combined.

REFERENCES

1. Committee on the Institutional Means for Assessment of Risks to Public Health, Commission on Life Sciences, and National Research Council, *Risk Assessment in the Federal Government: Managing the Process.* National Academy Press, Washington, DC, 1983.

2. L. Golberg, *Hazard Assessment of Ethylene Oxide.* CRC Press, Boca Raton FL, 1986.

3. Food Safety Council, Quantitative risk assessment. *Food Cosmet. Toxicol.* **18**, 711–734 (1980).

4. I. C. Munro and D. R. Krewski, Risk assessment and regulatory decision making. *Food Cosmet. Toxicol.* **19**, 549–560 (1981).

5. D. Krewski and J. Van Ryzin, Dose response models for quantal response toxicity data. In M. Csörgö, D. A. Dawson, J. N. K. Rao, and E. Saleh (Eds.), *Statistics and Related Topics.* North-Holland, Amsterdam, 1981.

6. R. E. Albert and B. Altshuler, Considerations relating to the formulation of limits for unavoidable population exposures to environmental carcinogens. In J. E. Ballou, R. H. Busch, D. D. Mahlum, and C. L. Sanders (Eds.), *Radionuclide Carcinogenesis,* AEC Symposium Series, CONF-72050, NTIS, Springfield, VA, 1973.

7. P. Armitage, The assessment of low-dose carcinogenicity. *Biometrics, Suppl.,* March, 119–129 (1982).

8. P. Armitage and R. Doll, The age distribution of cancer and a multi-stage theory of carcinogenesis. *Br. J. Cancer* **8**, 1–12 (1954).

9. P. Armitage and R. Doll, A two-stage theory of carcinogenesis in relation to the age distribution of human cancer. *Br. J. Cancer* **11**, 161–169 (1957).

10. H. O. Hartley and R. L. Sielken, Jr., Estimation of 'safe doses' in carcinogenic experiments. *Biometrics* **33**, 1–30 (1977).

11. H. O. Hartley, H. D. Tolley, and R. L. Sielken, Jr., The product form of the hazard rate model in carcinogenic testing. In M. Csorgo, D. A. Dawson, J. N. K. Rao, and E. Saleh (Eds.), *Current Topics in Probability and Statistics.* North-Holland, New York, 1981.

12. D. Krewski, K. S. Crump, J. Farmer, D. W. Gaylor, R. Howe, C. Portier, D. Salsburg, R. L. Sielken, and J. Van Ryzin, A comparison of statistical methods for low dose extrapolation utilizing time-to-tumor data. *Fundam. Appl. Toxicol.* **3**, 140–160 (1983).

13. S. H. Moolgavkar and A. G. Knudson, Jr., Mutation and cancer: A model for human carcinogenesis. *J. Nat. Cancer Inst.* **66**, 1037–1052 (1981).

14. S. H. Moolgavkar and D. J. Venzon, Two-event models for carcinogenesis: Incidence curves for childhood and adult tumors. *Math. Biosci.* **47**, 55–77 (1979).

15. R. Peto and P. N. Lee, Weibull distributions for continuous-carcinogenesis experiments. *Biometrics* **29**, 457–470 (1973).

16. R. Peto, P. N. Lee, and W. S. Paige, Statistical analysis of the bioassay of continuous carcinogens. *Br. J. Cancer* **26**, 258–261 (1972).

17. M. C. Pike, A method of analysis of a certain class of experiments in carcinogenesis. *Biometrics* **22**, 141–161 (1966).

18. R. J. Sielken, Jr., The use of the Hartley-Sielken model in low dose extrapolation. In D. Clayson, D. Krewski, and I. Munro (Eds.), *Toxicological Risk Assessment*. CRC Press, Boca Raton, FL, 1985.

19. R. J. Sielken, Jr. and L. A. Smith, Cancer dose-response models. In A. W. Hayes, R. C. Schnell, and T. S. Miya (Eds.), *Developments in the Science and Practice of Toxicology*, Elsevier Science Publishers, New York, 1983.

20. R. L. Sielken, Jr., The forthcoming merger in quantitative risk assessment. In C. W. Felix (Ed.), *Food Protection Technology*. Lewis Publishers, Chelsea, MI, 1987.

21. R. L. Sielken, Jr., Cancer dose-response extrapolations. *Environ. Sci. Technol.* **21**, 1033–1039 (1987).

22. T. W. Thorslund, C. C. Brown, and G. Charnley, Biologically motivated cancer risk models. *Risk Anal.* **7**, 109–119 (1987).

23. A. S. Whittemore, Quantitative theories of oncogenesis. *Adv. Cancer Res.* **27**, 55–88 (1978).

24. A. S. Whittemore and J. B. Keller, Quantitative theories of carcinogenesis. *SIAM Rev.* **20**, 1–30 (1978).

25. J. D. Kalbfleisch, D. R. Krewski, and J. Van Ryzin, Dose-response models for time-to-response toxicity data. *Can. J. Stat.* **11**, 25–49 (1983).

26. C. C. Brown, High-to low-dose extrapolation in animals. In J. V. Rodricks and R. G. Tardiff (Eds.), *Assessment and Management of Chemical Risks*. American Chemical Society, Washington, DC, 1984.

27. F. W. Carlborg, Multi-stage dose-response models in carcinogenesis. *Food Cosmet. Toxicol.* **19**, 361–365 (1981).

28. R. G. Cornell, R. A. Wolfe, and W. J. Butler, The analysis of animal carcinogenicity experiments. In R. G. Cornell (Ed.), *Statistical Methods for Cancer Studies*. Dekker, New York, 1984.

29. K. S. Crump, Dose response problems in carcinogenesis. *Biometrics* **35**, 157–167 (1979).

30. D. Krewski, C. Brown, and D. Murdoch, Determining 'safe' levels of exposure: Safety factors or mathematical models? *Fundam. Appl. Toxicol.* **4**, S383–S394 (1984).

31. C. N. Park and R. D. Snee, Quantitative risk assessment: State-of-the-art for carcinogenesis. In *Risk Management of Existing Chemicals*. Government Institutes, Inc., MD, 1984.

32. R. L. Sielken, Jr., Some capabilities, limitations, and pitfalls in the quantitative risk assessment of formaldehyde. In *Risk Analysis in the Chemical Industry*. Government Institutes, Inc., MD, 1985.

33. R. L. Sielken, Jr., The capabilities, sensitivity, pitfalls, and future of quantitative risk assessment. In R. S. McColl (Ed.), *Environmental Health Risks: Assessment and Management*. Univ. of Waterloo Press, Ontario, 1986.

34. R. L. Sielken, Jr., Quantitative cancer risk assessments for 2, 3, 7, 8- tetrachlorodibenzo-p-dioxin (TCDD). *Food Chem. Toxic.* **25**, 257–267 (1987).

35. E. L. Anderson and the Carcinogen Assessment Group of the U.S. Environmental Protection Agency, Quantitative approaches in use to assess cancer risk. *Risk Anal.* **3**, 277–295 (1983).

36. U.S. Interagency Staff Group on Carcinogens, Chemical carcinogens: A review of the science and its associated principles. *Environ. Health Perspect.* **67**, 201–282 (1986).

37. S. G. Austin and R. L. Sielken, Jr., Issues in assessing the carcinogenic hazards of ethylene oxide, *J. Occup. Med.* **3**, 236–245 (1988).

38. R. L. Sielken, Jr., Implications of the time-to-response information. In L. Golberg (Ed.), *Hazard Assessment of Ethylene Oxide*. CRC Press, Boca Raton, FL, 1986.

39. The SOT ED_{01} Task Force, Re-examination of the ED_{01} study: Risk assessment using time. *Fundam. Appl. Toxicol.* **1**, 88–123 (1981).

40. R. L. Sielken, Jr. Some issues in the quantitative modeling portion of cancer risk assessment. *Regul. Toxicol. Pharmacol.* **5**, 175–181 (1985).

41. T. B. Starr and R. D. Buck, The importance of delivered dose in estimating low-dose cancer risk inhalation exposure to formaldehyde. *Fundam. Appl. Toxicol.* **4**, 740–753 (1984).

42. W. M. Snellings, C. S. Weil, and R. R. Maronpot. *Final Report on Ethylene Oxide Two-Year Inhalation Study in Rats*, Proj. Rep. No. 44–20. Bushy Run Research Center, Export, PA, 1981.

43. W. M. Snellings, C. S. Weil, and R. R. Maronpot, A two-year inhalation study of the carcinogenic potential of ethylene oxide in Fischer 344 rats. *Toxicol. Appl. Pharmacol.* **75**, 105 (1984).

44. D. W. Lynch, T. R. Lewis, and W. J. Moorman, Chronic inhalation toxicity of ethylene oxide and propylene oxide in rats and monkeys—A preliminary report. *Toxicologist* **2**, 11 (1982).

45. D. W. Lynch, T. R. Lewis, W. J. Moorman, T. R. Burg, D. H. Groth, A. Kahn, L. J. Ackerman, and B. Y. Cockrell, Carcinogenic and toxicologic effects of inhaled ethylene oxide and propylene oxide in F344 rats. *Toxicol. Appl. Pharmacol.* **76**, 69 (1984).

46. Environmental Protection Agency, Guidelines for carcinogen risk assessment. *Fed. Regist.* **51**, 33993–34014 (1986).

47. U.S. Environmental Protection Agency, *Health Assessment Document for Ethylene Oxide*, Publ. No. EPA/600/8-84/009F, Final Report. USEPA, Washington, DC, 1985.

48. G. R. McKinney, J. H. Weikel, Jr., W. K. Webb, and R. G. Dick, Use of the life-table technique to estimate effects of certain steroids on probability of tumor formation in a long-term study in rats. *Toxicol. Appl. Pharmac.* **12**, 68–79 (1968).

49. R. E. Tarone, Tests for trend in life table analysis. *Biometrika* **62**, 679–682 (1975).

50. T. R. Tyler and J. A. McKelvey, *Dose-Dependent Disposition of C^{14} Labeled Ethylene Oxide in Rats*. Carnegie-Mellon Institute of Research, Pittsburgh, PA, 1980.

51. P. Armitage, Tests for linear trend in proportions and frequencies. *Biometrics* **11**, 375–386 (1955).

52. K. S. Crump, An improved procedure for low-dose carcinogenic risk assessment from animal data. *J. Environ. Path. Toxicol.* **5**, 675–684 (1982).

5

Use of Physiological Pharmacokinetics in Cancer Risk Assessments: A Study of Methylene Chloride*

Richard H. Reitz and Frederick A. Smith
Toxicology Research Laboratory, The Dow Chemical Company, Midland, Michigan

Melvin E. Andersen, Harvey J. Clewell, III, and Michael L. Gargas
Biochemical Toxicology Branch, Armstrong Aerospace Medical Research Laboratories, Wright–Patterson Air Force Base, Ohio

INTRODUCTION

Several studies of the chronic toxicity of methylene chloride (dichloromethane, DCM) have been conducted. Inhalation studies in the Syrian Golden Hamster, exposed to concentrations up to 3500 ppm for 6 h/day, did not show a tumorigenic response at any site (Burek et al., 1984). Similarly, a drinking water study sponsored by the National Coffee Association failed to reveal a dose-related statistically significant increase in tumors in the B6C3F1 hybrid mouse strain (Serota et al., 1984a) or the F344 rat (Serota et al., 1984b).

Two inhalation studies of DCM in the Sprague–Dawley rat (at doses up to 3500 and 500 ppm, respectively) revealed treatment-related effects on the levels of spontaneously occurring mammary tumors. The number of benign mammary tumors per tumor-bearing rat was increased in each of these studies (Burek et al., 1984). This observation is consistent with the observation of increased benign mammary tumors in a similar inhalation study (up to 4000 ppm) in the F344 rat [National Toxicology Program (NTP), 1985]. Low incidences of tumors in the ventral neck region in and around the salivary gland of male rats were noted in one study (Burek et al., 1984) but were not noted in the other two rat inhalation studies (Burek et al., 1984; NTP, 1985).

*Adapted from "Physiologically Based Pharmacokinetics and the Risk Assessment Process for Methylene Chloride," by M. E. Andersen, H. J. Clewell III, M. L. Gargas, F. A. Smith, and R. H. Reitz, *Toxicology and Applied Pharmacology* 87: 185–205. Copyright © 1987 by Academic Press, Inc. Reprinted by permission of the publisher.

238

Significant increases in spontaneously occurring lung and liver tumors were noted when B6C3F1 mice were exposed to 2000 or 4000 ppm of DCM. In contrast to the studies mentioned above, where DCM either failed to affect the tumor incidence or affected primarily benign tumors, the incidence of both benign and malignant tumors was elevated in this study (NTP, 1985).

The obvious question raised by these new findings is whether humans exposed to DCM are likely to develop tumors similar to those seen in mice. While there are many biological factors which must be considered in answering this question, one of the primary considerations involves differences in delivery of toxic chemicals to target tissues in the various species.

Conventional risk assessments have typically involved linear extrapolation of external dose, combined with an interspecies factor based on body surface area. By contrast, pharmacokinetic models permit the calculation of internal doses through integration of information on the administered dose, the physiological structure of the mammalian species, and the biochemical properties of the specific chemicals. Predicted internal doses can be correlated with toxicity and/or tumor incidence to yield hypotheses of the mechanisms of action of particular chemicals. Clewell and Andersen (1985) have previously discussed the reasons why the scientific basis (soundness) of the risk assessment process could be improved through the use of physiologically based pharmacokinetic (PB-PK) modeling.

To apply these principles to a DCM risk assessment, we constructed a PB-PK model of DCM disposition. This model provided quantitative descriptions of the rates of metabolism and levels of DCM in various organs of four mammalian species (rats, mice, hamsters, and humans). The PB-PK model was validated with blood concentration/time-course data from rats, mice, and humans exposed to DCM. Next, model output parameters were correlated with the tumor incidences in two chronic bioassays of DCM in the B6C3F1 mouse (NTP, 1985; Serota et al., 1984a) to formulate a hypothesis for the mechanism of tumorigenicity. Finally, relevant measures of tissue dose were calculated for use in a pharmacokinetically based risk assessment process.

METHODS

Model Structure

Ramsey and Andersen (1984) described a general PB-PK model for inhalation of volatile metabolized chemicals. This general model was modified for use with DCM (Fig. 1). Since DCM caused both liver and lung tumors, the PB-PK model developed had to include both of these tissues. Consequently, this model differed from that of Ramsey and Andersen 1984) by having a distinct, metabolically active lung compartment which was placed between the gas exchange compartment and systemic arterial blood (Fig. 1).

Transport of DCM between alveolar air and blood occurs in the gas exchange compartment in the model. Because equilibration of air with the blood in the lung occurs rapidly, it was assumed that gas/blood exchange was completed before DCM entered the lung tissue compartment. In drinking water simulations, DCM was absorbed by a zero-order process, entering the liver compartment at a constant hourly rate (mg/h) equal to $\frac{1}{24}$ the daily dose. This assumes 100% absorption of the ingested dose and is consistent with results obtained with other halogenated hydrocarbons administered in the drinking water

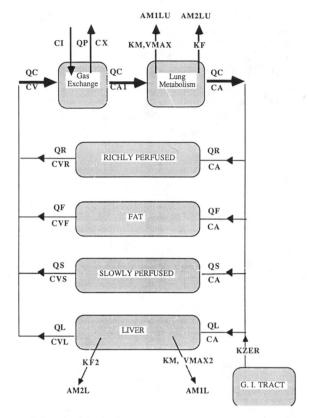

Figure 1. Diagram of the physiologically based pharmacokinetic model utilized for methylene chloride (dichloromethane, DCM). This model is an adaptation of one reported previously by Ramsey and Andersen (1984) for describing the metabolism of styrene. Tissues of the body are grouped into five compartments with similar flow and partition coefficients: Lung, fat, liver, richly perfused, and slowly perfused. Metabolism occurs in the lung and liver compartments. DCM enters the body through inhalation with absorption into pulmonary blood in the gas exchange compartment, or by ingestion with absorption directly into the liver compartment. Details of the model may be found in the appendix.

(tetrachloroethylene, Frantz and Watanabe, 1983; methylchloroform, Reitz et al., 1986, unpublished data). Intravenous administration was simulated as a very short (0.01–0.03 h) infusion of DCM directly into mixed venous blood.

Pulsatile drinking scenarios could also have been used to describe the drinking water input function. In a recent publication (National Research Council, 1986), total daily ingestion of volatile organic compounds in drinking water was described by a number of episodic inputs evenly spaced over half the day. The numbers of daily inputs examined were 72, 12, 6, and 1, the last value corresponding to bolus intubation. Only very minor differences in pharmacokinetic behavior were noted when the number of inputs was increased from 12 to 72. Zero-order input is equivalent to a very large number of pulsatile inputs and would be expected to behave very similarly to the 12- or 72-input scenario.

Mass balance differential equations for the model were similar to those of Ramsey and Andersen (1984) except for liver and lung tissue. Definitions of the algebraic constants and differential equations used for lung and liver tissue may be found in Appendix A.

Most of the simulations conducted with this model were also conducted with an alternate model in which the processes in the lung were described as occurring in a single compartment. The two formulations gave essentially equivalent results for the cases examined here. The former model was chosen for computational simplicity.

Model Parameters

To implement this physiological analysis, three major types of data are required: (i) partition coefficients (expressing the relative solubility of DCM in various tissues), (ii) physiological constants (for blood flows and tissue volumes), and (iii) biochemical constants (for important biotransformation pathways). These constants were obtained by experimentation or from the literature for each species of interest: mouse, rat, hamster, and human.

Partition Coefficients

Partition coefficients were determined with a vial equilibration technique (Sato and Nakajima, 1979) in which DCM was added to a closed vial containing test liquid. Partitioning was determined by measuring the concentration of DCM in the head space after 1 or 2 h of incubation at 37°C.

Blood/air partition coefficients were measured in samples of rat, mouse, hamster, and human blood. Tissue/air partition coefficients for liver, muscle, and fat were determined in tissues from the rat and hamster. Partition coefficients for the richly perfused nonmetabolizing tissue group and lung tissue were assumed to be equal to the measured liver/air partition coefficient. Partition coefficients for the slowly perfused tissue group were assumed to be equal to the measured muscle/air partition coefficient. Tissue/air partition coefficients for mouse and human tissue were not determined and were assumed to be equal to those measured in the rat. Tissue/blood partition coefficients were calculated by dividing the tissue/air coefficients for each tissue by the blood/air partition coefficient for that species. All partition coefficient determinations were carried out in one of our laboratories (Wright–Patterson AFB), and the values employed in the model are listed in Table 1.

Physiological Constants

Volumes of tissue and blood flows to the various tissue groups (Table 1) were taken from the literature [International Commission on Radiation Protection (ICRP), 1975; Davis and Mapleson, 1981; Caster et al., 1956] and are consistent with values used in other physiological descriptions of the pharmacokinetics of xenobiotics (Ramsey and Andersen, 1984; Gargas et al., 1986b; Fiserova-Bergerova, 1975). The lung weight is proportional to body weight (Leith, 1976) and is described by an allometric equation of the form (Adolph, 1949)

$$\text{lung weight} = 0.0115*(\text{body weight})^{0.99}.$$

Some of the ventilation rates used in this model were estimated from gas uptake studies.

TABLE 1. Kinetic Constants and Model Parameters Used in the Physiologically Based Pharmacokinetic Model for Dichloromethane

	B6C3F1[a]	F344 Rats[b]	Hamsters[b]	Human
Weights (kg)				
Body	0.0345	0.233	0.140	70.0
Lung ($\times 10^3$)	0.410	2.72	1.64	772.0
		Percentage of Body Weight		
Liver	4.0	4.0	4.0	3.14
Rapidly perfused	5.0	5.0	5.0	3.71
Slowly perfused	78.0	75.0	75.0	62.1
Fat	4.0	7.0	7.0	23.1
Flows (L/h)				
Alveolar ventilation	2.32	5.10	3.50	348.0
Cardiac output	2.32	5.10	3.35	348.0
		Percentage of Cardiac Output		
Liver	0.24	0.24	0.20	0.24
Rapidly perfused	0.52	0.52	0.56	0.52
Slowly perfused	0.19	0.19	0.19	0.19
Fat	0.05	0.05	0.05	0.05
Partition coefficients				
Blood/air	8.29	19.4	22.5	9.7
Liver/blood	1.71	0.732	0.840	1.46
Lung/blood	1.71	0.732	0.840	1.46
Rapidly perfused/blood	1.71	0.732	0.840	1.46
Slowly perfused/blood	0.960	0.408	1.196	0.82
Fat/blood	14.5	6.19	6.00	12.4
Metabolic constants				
V_{max}(mg/h)	1.054	1.50	2.047	118.9
K_m(mg/L)	0.396	0.771	0.649	0.580
KF(h^{-1})	4.017	2.21	1.513	0.53
A1	0.416	0.136	0.0638	0.00143
A2	0.137	0.0558	0.0774	0.0473

[a]Parameters correspond to the average body weight of B6C3F1 mice in the NTP bioassay (NTP, 1985).
[b]Parameters correspond to the average body weight in gas uptake studies.

In these studies, animals were placed in a small chamber with a recirculating atmosphere, chemical was injected into the chamber, and the chamber concentration decay was monitored over time. At low concentrations, with soluble well-metabolized chemicals such as DCM, the loss from the chamber appears to be dependent only on alveolar ventilation rates and chamber volume. Studies with rats and hamsters enclosed in such a chamber are consistent with a ventilation rate (QP) calculated according to the equation

$$QP = (15 \text{ L/h})(BW)^{0.74}.$$

The use of 0.74 as the exponent for body weight (BW) was proposed by Guyton (1947), based on studies with anesthetized animals. This equation predicts an alveolar ventilation of 348 L/h in a 70-kg human (total ventilation = 1.5 times alveolar ventilation or 522 L/h). This rate of ventilation is intermediate between the value reported by the ICRP (1975) for a resting human (300 L/h) and the value utilized EPA for its risk estimation (20 m^3/24 h or 833 L/h), which corresponds to humans performing mild exercise.

Cardiac output (QC) was described by a similar equation:

$$QC = (15 \text{ L/h})(BW)^{0.74}$$

and this equation gives values consistent with those reported in the medical literature (ICRP, 1975; Davis and Mapleson, 1981).

In contrast with rats and hamsters, gas uptake studies with B6C3F1 and CD1 mice indicated that QP and QC were higher than expected from the preceding equations. In the studies with DCM, as well as recent work in our laboratory with trichloroethylene, perchloroethylene, vinyl chloride, and methylcyclohexane, we have found that chamber clearance by mice is consistent with an allometric constant of approximately 28 L/h. Consequently, alveolar ventilation (QP) and cardiac output (QC) in the B63F1 mouse were calculated according to the equations

$$QP_{mouse} = (28 \text{ L/h})(BW)^{0.74}$$
$$QC_{mouse} = (28 \text{ L/h})(BW)^{0.74}.$$

Biochemical Constants (Rodents)

Dihalomethanes are metabolized via two pathways: (i) an oxidative pathway (Kubic et al., 1974) that appears to yield CO as well as considerable amounts of CO_2 (Garges et al., 1986b; Reitz et al., 1986), and (ii) a glutathione-dependent pathway (Ahmed and Anders, 1978) that produces CO_2 but no CO (Fig. 2). Both pathways release 2 mol of halide ion/mol of dihalomethane consumed. The oxidative pathway (MFO) is readily saturated at concentrations of a few hundred ppm, but the glutahione S-transferase (GST) pathway showed no indication of saturation at inhaled concentrations up to 10,000 ppm (Gargas et al., 1986b). Reactive, potentially toxic intermediates are formed in both pathways (Fig. 2).

The following procedure was employed to estimate the kinetic constants for these pathways in rodents. First, the pharmacokinetic model (Fig. 1) was adapted to describe the disposition of DCM in a closed recirculating chamber. This model included both first-order (GST) and saturable pathways (MFO), as well as all the physiological constants and partition coefficients described above. Metabolism by each pathway was apportioned between lung and liver by reference to literature data (Table 2) from Lorenz et al. (1984) who reported specific activities of MFO and GST in mouse, rat, hamster, and human tissues using model substrates for each enzyme (7-ethoxycoumarin for MFO and 2, 5-dinitrochlorobenzene for GST).

The mass balance differential equations for the liver compartment (Appendix A) contained terms for saturable oxidative metabolism (MFO) and first-order metabolism via glutathione conjugation (GST). The corresponding equations for the lung compartment contained terms A1 and A2 which represented the relative specific activities of the enzymes (Table 2) in the two tissues such that

$$A1 = MFO_{(lung)}/MFO_{(liver)}$$
$$A2 = GST_{(lung)}/GST_{(liver)}.$$

The derivation of these equations is outlined in Appendix B.

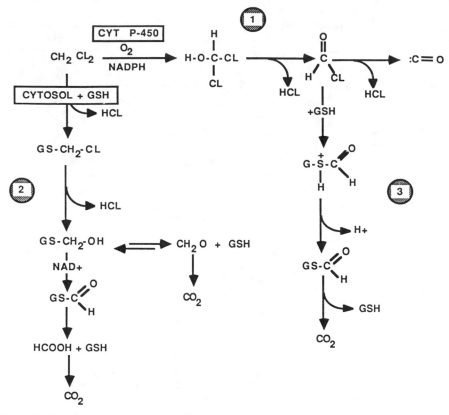

Figure 2. Proposed metabolic pathways for methylene chloride metabolism [based on Ahmed and Anders (1978) and Kubic et al. (1974)]. Potentially reactive intermediates are formed in each pathway: formyl chloride in the CYT *P*-450 (MFO) pathway, and chloromethyl glutathione in the cytosolic (GST) pathway. Either metabolic pathway can produce carbon dioxide in this scheme, but only the MFO pathway yields carbon monoxide and carboxyhemoglobin.

TABLE 2. Specific Activities of Glutathione *S*-Transferase and Mixed-Function Oxidase (Monooxygenase) in Subcellular Preparations of Rodent and Human Organs[a]

Species	Organ	Mixed-Function Oxidase	Glutathione-*S*-Transferase
Human			
	Liver	0.418 ± 0.157	1650 ± 480
	Lung	0.0006 ± 0.0003	78 ± 47
Sprague–Dawley rat			
	Liver	0.814 ± 0.118	1380 ± 110
	Lung	0.111 ± 0.035	77 ± 5
Syrian Golden hamster			
	Liver	2.570 ± 0.580	4200 ± 110
	Lung	0.164 ± 0.042	325 ± 25
NMRI mouse			
	Liver	1.760 ± 0.115	5290 ± 430
	Lung	0.732 ± 0.115	727 ± 64

[a]Specific activities are given in nmol product/min/mg protein. From Lorenz et. (1984).

Closed-chamber exposures of mice, rats, and hamsters were conducted with a variety of initial exposure concentrations. A description of this apparatus has been reported elsewhere (Gargas et al., 1986b) and a more complete description is in press (Gargas et al., 1986a). Each experiment with B6C3F1 mice employed 14 male animals, and initial concentrations were 490, 960, 2000, 3200, and 10,000 ppm DCM. Five male hamsters were employed in each experiment, with initial concentrations of 450, 1000, 1900, and 4900 ppm. Three F344 male rats were used in each exposure, with initial concentrations of 100, 500, 1000, and 3000 ppm. The concentration of DCM in the closed chamber was measured every 10 min for several hours. Optimum values of V_{max} (maximum velocity of metabolism by MFO in liver), K_m (Michaelis constant for DCM metabolism by MFO), and KF (first-order rate constant for metabolism of DCM by GST in liver) were found by minimizing the relative least squares of deviations between the actual data and the model predictions. Optimizations were performed with SIMUSOLV*, a computer program which combines numerical integration, optimization, and graphical display routines[†].

These experiments give data which are rich in information about the kinetic constants. Curves from different initial concentrations are differentially affected by the values chosen for these constants. High concentration uptake is affected predominanly by the value chosen for KF. Mid-range curves primarily reflect the influence of V_{max}, and low concentration curves are most sensitive to the value chosen for K_m.

Biochemical Constants (Humans)

Values of K_m and V_{max} needed to describe the MFO pathway in humans were estimated from studies conducted at Dow Chemical Co. in which levels of DCM and carboxyhemoglobin (HbCO) in blood and of CO and DCM in expired air were measured during and following 6-h exposures to 100 and 350 ppm DCM (R. J. Nolan and M. J. McKenna, unpublished data). These authors estimated that V_{max} in humans for the MFO pathway was 119 mg/h and K_m was 0.58 mg/L.

Gargas et al. (1986b) developed a PB-PK model for describing carboxyhemoglobin associated with metabolism of dihalomethanes to CO. This model was used in conjunction with the data of Peterson (1978) to estimate the V_{max} for the MFO pathway in humans as 137 mg/h.

These values of V_{max} agree closely with each other and with the values obtained by allometric scaling from the rat (81.4 mg/h) and hamster (158.6 mg/h). The K_m for humans is also similar to the K_m obtained in the rodent species by optimizations (Table 1).

There are no data which allow direct calculation of the kinetic constant for the nonsaturable GST pathway in humans (this would require conducting exposures of several thousand ppm in humans). However, we noted that clearance (mL/h) for the GST pathway in liver (calculated as KF * VL) appeared to possess an allometric relation in the three rodent species. This is demonstrated by the observation that the intrinsic clearance [KF * VL divided by $(BW)^{0.7}$] is quite consistent in the three species: B6C3F1 mouse, 58.5 mL/h·kg; hamster, 33.5 mL/h·kg; F344 rat, 57.1 mL/h·kg. Intrinsic clearance for humans was set equal to the highest value observed experimentally (60 mL/h·kg), and this was used to estimate the clearance in 70-kg humans as 1174 mL/h, corresponding to a KF of 0.53 h^{-1} (Table 3).

---

*SIMUSOLV is a trademark of the Dow Chemical Co.
[†]These software packages are available commercially from Mitchell and Gauthier Associates, Inc., 73 Junction Square Dr., Concord, MA 01742.

TABLE 3. Allometric Estimation of the Kinetic Constants for the GST Pathway in Humans

Species	KF^a (h^{-1})	VL^b (mL)	$KF*VL^c$ (mL/h)	BW (kg)	CLC^d (mg/h)
Mouse[e]	4.32	1.08	4.67	0.027	58.5
Hamster[e]	1.51	5.60	8.46	0.140	33.5
Rat[e]	2.21	9.32	20.6	0.233	57.1
Human	0.53[f]	2210	1174	70.0	60.0

[a]KF is the first-order rate constant obtained from the closed-chamber in vivo optimizations.
[b]VL is the estimated volume of the liver (in mL) for each of the experimental species.
[c]KF*VL is the product of columns 1 and 2.
[d]The intrinsic clearance (CLC, the clearance that would be expected in a 1-kg animal of each species if clearance were related to the 0.7 power of body weight) is calculated by dividing the clearance (KF*VL) by the body weight (BW) raised to the 0.7 power.
[e]All parameters are for the animals used in closed-chamber experiments. Mouse parameters differ from the parameters for Table 4 which were calculated for larger animals in the NTP bioassay.
[f]KF for humans was estimated by setting human CLC equal to 60.0 (approximating the highest CLC observed experimentally) and using this value to calculate KF as equal to 60 times $(70)^{0.7}$ divided by VL.

An alternate procedure for estimating the rate of metabolism of DCM by GST in humans has been described by Reitz et al. (1988). This procedure involved measuring the in vitro activity of GST in enzyme preparations from the lungs and livers of B6C3F1 mice, F344 rats, Syrian Golden hamsters, and human accident victims. Since the in vivo activity of GST in the B6C3F1 mouse was known from the gas uptake studies, it was possible to estimate the in vivo activity of GST in the other species by simple proportionality. The value of KF in humans estimated by this procedure was 0.43, which is quite close to the value of KF in humans estimated by allometric scaling.

Dose Surrogates

The PB-PK model contains a variety of information in terms of blood and tissue concentrations of DCM, exhaled DCM, and instantaneous rates of metabolism by each pathway. The parameters which were chosen as possible dose surrogates for the toxicity of DCM were (i) integrated tissue dose as area under the tissue concentration/time curve (AUCL for liver and AUCLU for lung), (ii) a virtual concentration of reactive metabolite from the MFO pathway in liver and lung tissue, and (iii) a virtual concentration of reactive metabolite from the GST pathway in liver and lung tissue. These last two measures of tissue exposure were calculated by dividing the average amount of metabolite formed per day by the volume of the organ in which it was formed. Use of this type of dose surrogate has been discussed elsewhere (NAS, 1986). The appropriate equations are

$$RISK1_{(tissue)} = AM1_{(tissue)}/V_{(tissue)}$$
$$RISK2_{(tissue)} = AM2_{(tissue)}/V_{(tissue)}.$$

The rationale for use of these particular surrogates is provided in Appendix C. These values are expected to be directly related to the area under the concentration/time curve for the reactive intermediate in the target tissues.

RESULTS

Determination of the Biochemical Constants for B6C3F1 Mice, F344 Rats, and Syrian Golden Hamsters

Closed (recirculating)-chamber exposures of rats, hamsters, and B6C3F1 mice were conducted with a variety of initial-exposure concentrations. Model predictions and experimental data are plotted for B6C3F1 mice (Fig. 3). Similar results were obtained in experiments conducted with Syrian Golden Hamsters and F344 rats (data not shown). Excellent fits were obtained for each species. The values chosen by the computer for the kinetic parameters in each species are listed in Table 1.

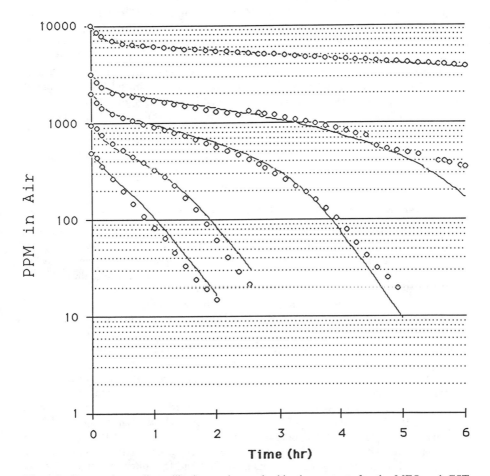

Figure 3. Gas uptake studies utilized to estimate the kinetic constants for the MFO and GST pathways in B6C3F1 mice. Data are ppm of DCM in the chamber atmosphere as a function of time. Experimental data are shown as symbols, while the computer simulation is presented as a solid line. Values of the kinetic constants obtained by computer optimization of these data are listed in Table 1.

Validation of the Model with Experimental Data

To test the reliability of the model, we have compared its predictions with several sets of blood concentration/time-course data. One of the strengths of physiological modeling is the ability to use the same model to predict the disposition of materials given by different routes of administration. Consequently, we have used data derived from intravenous studies as well as inhalation exposures.

The first data set (Fig. 4a) was from Angelo et al. (1984), who administered DCM to B6C3F1 mice intravenously at 10 and 50 mg/kg and measured the concentration in blood for periods up to 90 min postdosing. Input of DCM was simulated as a rapid infusion directly into the mixed venous blood.

In a similar fashion, the model was used to predict the blood levels of DCM in F344 rats given an intravenous dose of 10 mg/kg DCM (Fig. 4b). Blood concentrations were measured from 5 to 60 min postdosing (Andersen et al., 1984).

In addition, blood levels of DCM in F344 rats inhaling 200 or 1000 ppm DCM for 4 h were modeled (Andersen et al., 1984). Blood levels of DCM were well described by the model both during the 4-h exposure and for periods up to 120 min following cessation of exposure (Fig. 4c).

Experiments conducted with human volunteers at Dow Chemical Co. were also evaluated. In these studies, healthy volunteers were exposed to either 100 or 350 ppm of DCM for 6 h, and samples of venous blood were collected during the exposure and for periods up to 24 h after cessation of exposure. This simulation may be regarded as the ultimate test of animal extrapolation, and the predicted values for humans were in excellent agreement with the experimental data (Fig. 4d).

The model also accurately predicted the appearance and elimination of DCM metabolites (Reitz et al., 1986; Andersen et al., 1984; Gargas et al., 1986b).

Comparison of Two Studies of the Chronic Toxicity of DCM

The PB-PK model can now be used to compare the values of the relevant measures of target tissue dose during two chronic bioassays of DCM toxicity in the B6C3F1 mouse. The inhalation bioassay revealed significant increases in lung and liver tumors (NTP, 1985) while the drinking water study failed to show a dose-related increase in the incidence of either type of tumor in this same strain of mouse (Serota et al., 1984a).

Six different dose surrogates were calculated for B6C3F1 mice under the conditions of exposure in these studies: (i) area under the liver concentration/time curve (AUCL), (ii) area under the lung concentration/time curve (AUCLU), (iii) virtual concentration of metabolites derived from the MFO pathway in liver (RISK1L), (iv) virtual concentration of metabolites derived from the MFO pathway in lung (RISK1LU), (v) virtual concentration of metabolites derived from the GST pathway in liver (RISK2L), and (vi) virtual concentration of metabolites derived from the GST pathway in lung (RISK2LU).

Dose surrogates related to the MFO pathway were nearly identical in the two studies. Values of RISK1L (the liver dose surrogate) in units of mg/L per 24 h are 3575 and 3701 after exposure to 2000 and 4000 ppm, respectively, while the value of RISK1L is 5197 in mice consuming DCM in drinking water at the rate of 250 mg/kg·day. Similarly, the values of RISK1LU (the lung dose surrogate) are 1531 and 1583 after 2000 and 4000 ppm, respectively, while RISK1LU is 1227 in mice consuming DCM in drinking water at the rate of 250 mg/kg·day (Table 4).

By contrast, dose surrogates related to the activity of the GST pathway showed significant differences in the two studies. Values of RISK2L (the liver dose surrogate) are

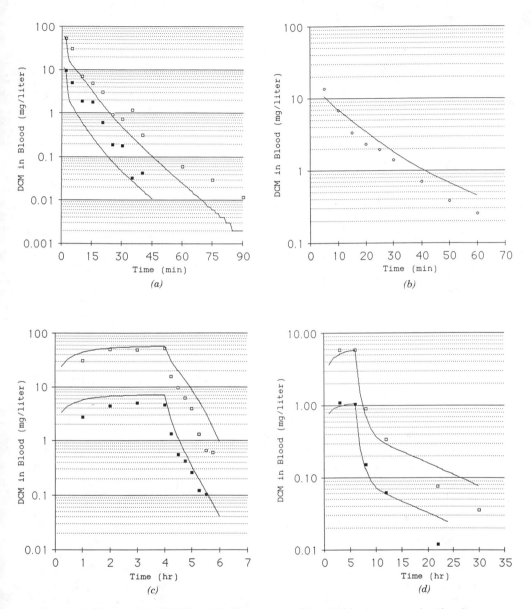

Figure 4. Validation of the PB-PK model with experimental data: (*a*) blood concentration/time data obtained in B6C3F1 mice following intravenous administration (Angelo et al., 1984); (*b*) intravenous data obtained in F344 rats; (*c*) data obtained in F344 rats during and following inhalation exposure; (*d*) data obtained in humans during and following inhalation exposure. In each case, the simulated data are presented as a solid line, while the experimental data are shown with closed or open symbols.

TABLE 4. Comparison of Average Daily Values of Dose Surrogates and Tumor Incidences in Lung and Liver Tissues of Female B6C3F1 Mice in Two Chronic Bioassays of Methylene Chloride (DCM)

	Control	Inhalation (4000 ppm)	Inhalation (2000 ppm)	Drinking Water (250 mg/kg·day)
Liver				
RISK1L[a,g]	0.0	3701.0	3575.0	5197.0
RISK2L[b,g]	0.0	1811.0	851.0	15.1
AUCL[c,h]	0.0	771.0	362.0	6.4
Tumors (%)	6.0[i]	83.0[i]	33.0[i]	6.0[i]
Lung				
RISK1LU[d,g]	0.0	1583.0	1531.0	1227.0
RISK2LU[e,g]	0.0	256.0	123.0	1.0
AUCLU[f,h]	0.0	794.0	381.0	3.1
Tumors (%)	6.0[i,j]	85.0[i,j]	63.0[i,j]	8.0[i,j]

[a]RISK1L is the dose surrogate related to MFO activity in the liver.
[b]RISK2L is the dose surrogate related to GST activity in the liver.
[c]AUCL is the dose surrogate related to concentration of DCM in the liver.
[d]RISK1LU is the dose surrogate related to MFO activity in the lung.
[e]RISK2LU is the dose surrogate related to GST activity in the lung.
[f]AUCLU is the dose surrogate related to concentration of DCM in the lung.
[g]Units are mg of DCM metabolized/liter tissue.
[h]Units are (mg/L)·h.
[i]Tumor incidence (combined benign and malignant) reported as percentage of animals examined.
[j]Combined incidence of alveolar/bronchiolar adenomas and carcinomas.

851 and 1811 after exposure to 2000 and 4000 ppm, respectively, while the value of RISK2L is only 15.1 in mice consuming DCM in drinking water at the rate of 250 mg/kg·day. Similarly, the values of RISK2LU (the lung dose surrogate) are 123 and 256 after 2000 and 4000 ppm, respectively, while RISK2LU is only 1.00 in mice consuming DCM in drinking water at the rate of 250 mg/kg·day (Table 4).

Dose surrogates related to concentrations of DCM itself in the target tissues also showed significant differences in the two studies. Values of AUCL (area under the liver concentration curve) were 362 and 771 after 2000 and 4000 ppm, respectively, and values of AUCLU (area under the lung curve) were 381 and 794, respectively, after these same exposures. By contrast, levels of these parameters were 6.4 and 3.1, respectively, in the 250 mg/kg·day drinking water study (Table 4).

The PB-PK analysis indicates that the tumor incidences observed in the two studies are inconsistent with the hypothesis that reactive intermediates from the MFO pathway are involved in the tumorigenicity of DCM, but are consistent with two other hypotheses: (i) that tumorigenicity is related to the production of reactive intermediates by the GST pathway and (ii) that tumorigenicity is related to the presence of DCM in the target organs.

Relationship of Dose Surrogate Values to Administered Dose

The PB-PK model may now be utilized to calculate the values of the toxicologically relevant chemical species in various tissues under a variety of exposure conditions. For example, the value of the liver dose surrogate related to the GST pathway (RISK2L) in

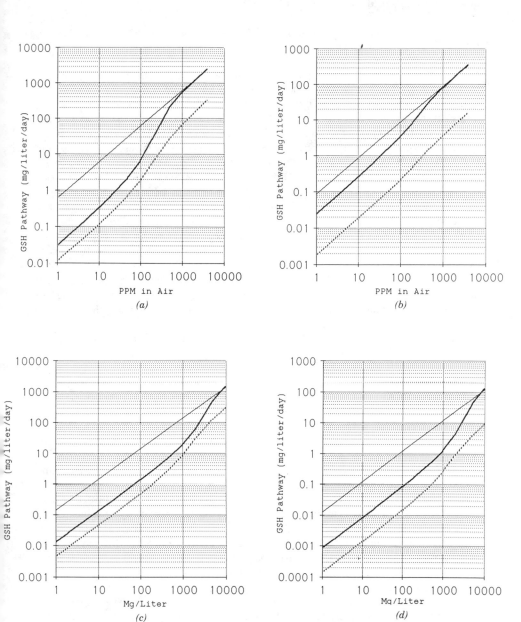

Figure 5. Predicted relationship of the dose surrogates associated with the GST pathway to external dose: (a) and (b) values of the dose surrogates in B6C3F1 mice and humans during inhalation exposure (6 h/day) in the liver and lung, respectively; (c) and (d) same dose surrogates in B6C3F1 mice and humans consuming water with DCM dissolved at various levels. Dose surrogates for mice are shown as a heavy solid line, while dose surrogates for humans are shown as a heavy dashed line. In each case, a reference line depicting a linear extrapolation from the highest administered dose of DCM is shown as a light, solid line for comparison. Units for the Y-axis are mg metabolized per liter tissue per 24 h.

B6C3F1 mice and in humans following inhalation of various concentrations of DCM for 6 h/day is plotted in Fig. 5a.

The calculated dose surrogates are displayed on a log/log plot for exposure concentrations from 1 to 4000 ppm. Dose surrogate values for B6C3F1 mice are represented by the heavy solid line, while dose surrogate values for humans are represented by the heavy dashed line. Dose surrogate values which would be obtained by linear extrapolation of data from the 4000-ppm mouse exposure are depicted as a lighter solid line in this and other figures. Dose surrogate values calculated from the PB-PK model are close to those estimated by linear extrapolation with the mouse above 1000 ppm but deviate from linearity in the region below 1000 ppm. The nonlinearity in the curve is apparent in the region where the MFO pathway saturates. Saturation of MFO makes a larger percentage of the DCM available for metabolism by the GST pathway, resulting in a disproportionate increase in RISK2L at exposure concentrations above 100 ppm. The curve for liver dose surrogate values in humans (exposed 6 h/day) also displays a nonlinearity in the region between 100 and 1000 ppm, although this is less pronounced than in mice. The values of human dose surrogates are lower than mouse dose surrogates throughout the entire exposure range.

Figure 5b presents the values of the lung dose surrogate related to GST (RISK2LU) in mice and in humans exposed to various concentrations of DCM in air. In this case, the nonlinearity in the mouse dose surrogate curve is of smaller magnitude than that in mouse liver, indicating a smaller effect of MFO on the material available for GST. As with RISK2L, the value of human RISK2LU is lower than that of mouse RISK2LU at all concentrations because of the lower activity of GST in human lung relative to that in mouse lung (Table 2).

For drinking water exposures, RISK2L and RISK2LU are plotted versus concentration of DCM present in water in milligrams/L (Fig. 5c, d). Water consumption for the two species was estimated according to the equation

$$\text{water consumption} = 0.102 * (BW)^{0.7},$$

which results in an estimated water consumption of 2.0 L/day for 70-kg humans and 9.7 mL/day for 34.5-g mice.

A nonlinearity in each of those dose surrogate curves (RISK2L and RISK2LU; mice and humans) is evident at concentrations above 1000 mg/L. Dose surrogate values for the mouse drinking water simulations with 10,000 mg/L are lower than values of the same parameter for mice inhaling 4000 ppm DCM per day (Fig. 5c, a; 5d, b). In each case, the dose surrogates for humans are lower than the dose surrogates for mice when the two species consume water with the same concentration of DCM.

Dose surrogate values for parameters related to the MFO pathway in liver (RISK1L) when DCM is present in inhaled air are displayed in Fig. 6a. Nonlinearities are apparent in the region of 100–1000 ppm. MFO products do not increase appreciably in mice above 200–400 ppm. MFO products increase, but to a less than proportionate degree, as DCM levels rise above 1000 ppm in humans due to fat storage with postexposure metabolism (Clewell and Andersen, 1985).

Dose surrogate values for parameters related to area under the liver concentration/time curve (AUCL) in animals inhaling DCM are displayed in Fig. 6b. Nonlinearities are evident in the region of 100–1000 ppm. The values of this particular dose surrogate are higher for humans than for mice, but in each case there is a marked difference between the dose surrogate values obtained by linear extrapolation from 4000 to 1 ppm and the values calculated by the PB-PK model for 1 ppm (Fig. 6b).

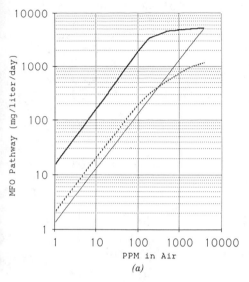
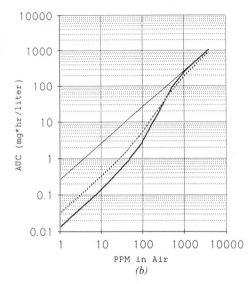

Figure 6. Predicted relationship of the dose surrogates associated with unmetabolized DCM or the MFO pathway to external dose: (*a*) dose surrogate associated with the MFO pathway in the liver (RISK1L); (*b*) dose surrogate associated with the area under the liver concentration time curve (AUCL) in mice and humans.

DISCUSSION

A great number of uncertainties are involved in the formulation of human risk estimations from the results of chronic animal studies. This chapter is not intended to be a comprehensive enumeration and discussion of all these factors. It is restricted to a discussion of the role that PB-PK models can play in relating the "external dose" of DCM to tissue doses in the target organs of various species under specific exposure scenarios.

Advantages of PB-PK

Development of a PB-PK analysis offers significant advantages over conventional pharmacokinetic analysis. In conventional pharmacokinetics, time-course curves are obtained for concentration of a parent chemical or metabolite(s) in blood or in some other body compartment. The resulting curves are then described by mathematical curve-fitting techniques, resulting in models which are more dependent on the mathematics employed than on the animal system being studied. Such descriptions are best suited to interpolation or limited extrapolation. By contrast, PB-PK models are designed to predict kinetic behavior over a broad range of doses and exposure regimens (Clewell and Andersen, 1985).

Differentiation of Metabolic Pathways

In this study gas uptake methods have been utilized to determine the kinetic constants for two pathways of dihalomethane metabolism. This approach does not unequivocally identify a particular metabolic pathway with a kinetic process. Other chemical studies are necessary to make this identification.

Such studies were reported previously by Gargas et al. (1986b), who evaluated the metabolism of five dihalomethanes. In that work, carboxyhemoglobin production (a unique product of the MFO pathway) and bromide ion liberation were correlated with the gas uptake studies. The high-affinity saturable pathway was shown to be the oxidative reaction (MFO), which produces, among other metabolites, carbon monoxide. The first-order pathway was shown to be dependent on glutathione concentration. These studies link the two uptake processes observed in vivo in the gas uptake studies with the MFO and GST pathways.

Model Validation

The goal of these experiments was to determine whether the model could successfully predict a broad range of kinetic behavior. It must be emphasized that the validation was not an exercise in curve fitting; model parameters were not "fiddled" in an attempt to hit all the data points. Nevertheless, the degree of agreement between the model predictions and the blood concentration time-course data, obtained from three laboratories and through two routes of administration, is remarkable (Fig. 4*a–d*). In particular, it is noteworthy that the disposition of DCM in humans is described accurately by the model.

Basic Assumptions

Implicit in every risk assessment procedure are some fundamental assumptions about the manner in which chemical treatments affect the carcinogenic process. In the discussion which follows it is assumed that treatments which produce equivalent average daily tissue exposures of the relevant chemical species (dose surrogates) in target organs will produce equivalent effects on the carcinogenic process in each species. Factors such as longevity of the various species and latent periods for tumor induction, which may also be biologically important, are not considered. In the PB-PK analysis, no attempt is made to incorporate a factor converting external dose to milligrams/surface area when extrapolating among species. The PB-PK model already incorporates appropriate factors for interspecies scaling. Furthermore, empirical generalizations such as converting doses to milligrams/meter^2 fail to consider the role of metabolic processes in increasing or decreasing toxicity and may lead to serious errors in interspecies extrapolation.

Hypothesis Generation

Although the PB-PK model is capable of quantitatively describing the levels of DCM and its metabolites in the body, it is not capable of determining by itself which of these parameters is likely to be related to the tumorigenicity of DCM. To make this judgment, it is necessary to incorporate pertinent biological and chemical information from other nonpharmacokinetic experiments. At the outset, we considered three possible hypotheses for the mechanism of action of DCM:

1. Tumorigenicity of DCM is related to the presence of DCM in target tissues (i.e., area under the tissue concentration/time curves).
2. Tumorigenicity of DCM is related to the production of metabolites of DCM derived from the MFO pathway in target tissues.
3. Tumorigenicity of DCM is related to the production of metabolites of DCM derived from the GST pathway in target tissues.

The first hypothesis was rejected on mechanistic considerations. The chemical reactivity of DCM is low, and there is no evidence that parent material is capable of the types of biological interactions with macromolecules which Miller and Miller (1966) have found to be prevalent in the action of chemical carcinogens. However, both metabolic pathways produce potentially reactive intermediates which might be involved in the tumorigenic process (Fig. 2).

There are several reasons for believing that metabolism by MFO is not involved in the tumorigenicity of DCM. First, it is clear that the incidence of most of the treatment-related tumors increases as the exposure concentration is raised from 2000 to 4000 ppm (Table 4). However, it has been demonstrated that HbCO, a major product of MFO activity, does not increase in rats or hamsters as exposure levels of DCM are raised above 500 ppm (McKenna et al., 1982; Burek et al., 1984).

In addition, Green (1983) has separated enzymes from the MFO and GST pathways and studied their ability to metabolically activate DCM in vitro. He found that cytosolic preparations from rat liver (containing GST) significantly increased the yield of bacterial mutations in *Salmonella typhimurium* exposed to DCM. However, rat liver microsomes rich in MFO failed to show this effect. Rannug et al. (1978) have observed that GST increases the mutagenicity of a similar compound, 1, 2-dichloroethane, in vitro studies.

Hypothesis Testing

Finally, as already discussed under Results, the PB-PK model may be utilized to compare the levels of dose surrogates from each pathway in the chronic studies of DCM administered by inhalation (NTP, 1985) or by drinking water (Serota et al., 1984a). Significant increases in the incidence of lung and liver tumors were observed in the inhalation study, but no significant increases in these tumors were seen in the drinking water study. This correlates well with the yield of the GST metabolites in the two studies (levels of GST dose surrogates were much higher in the inhalation versus the drinking water study) but is inconsistent with the activity of the MFO pathway (levels of MFO dose surrogates were equivalent in the two studies; Table 4).

These results should not be taken as indicating that the primary mechanism by which DCM increases tumorigenicity in the mouse is necessarily through direct interaction of GST metabolites with genetic material (i.e., a genotoxic effect). Genotoxicity of DCM to mammalian cells has been very low in a number of carefully conducted experiments (Schumann, 1984; Sivak, 1984). However, it does appear that the GST pathway is somehow related to the increased tumor incidences observed in B6C3F1 mice exposed to DCM.

PB-PK Risk Analysis

Quantitative risk assessments (QRA) do not provide precise estimates of human risk because of the empirical nature of the dose–response extrapolations employed. As currently practiced, QRA extrapolation procedures have been designed to protect public health through inclusion of conservative assumptions wherever uncertainty exists. Consequently, QRA has provided estimates of "plausible upper bounds" on risk. Actual risks are unknown and in many instances may be as low as zero.

Improvements will have to be made in the QRA extrapolation process before risk estimates will have value for ranking various materials for relative hazard or estimating "true" upper-bound risk in exposed populations. To do this, we need better information on chemical–tissue interaction and the mechanisms of the toxic insults. Within this framework the PB-PK model can be used to better define tissue interaction and to formulate improved human cancer risk estimations for DCM. Formulation of the risk estimation involves several steps:

1. Calculation of the *internal dose* to the target organ(s) of B6C3F1 mice under conditions which produced tumors in those animals.
2. Fitting animal tumor incidence and *internal dose* data to one or more empirical dose–response models for carcinogenesis.
3. Calculating the *internal dose* to corresponding organs of humans under defined conditions.
4. Estimating upper bounds on human risk from the dose–response model previously fitted to animal bioassay/target organ *internal dose* data.

This process differs from that used by default when pharmacokinetic data on internal dose are not available. In the absence of pharmacokinetic data, internal dose is considered to be proportional to nominal dose throughout the entire exposure range. Extrapolation from animal to man is performed by assuming that equipotent doses are expressed in milligrams of chemical per unit of surface area in the various species. It should be noted that the latter process always assumes that humans are more sensitive to a given dose of test chemical (in mg/kg·day) than rodents because of the lower surface area to volume ratio (humans are assumed to be 5–6-fold more sensitive than rats and 13-fold more sensitive than mice).

Following the default procedure for DCM (without use of PB-PK data), Singh et al. (1985) estimated that the lifetime risk for continuous exposure to a concentration of $1 \, \mu g \, DCM/m^3$ inhaled air was 4.1×10^{-6}. This estimate[1] was presented as a "plausible upper limit" on risk, along with the qualifier that "the true value is unknown and may be as low as zero.[2]" The uncertainty and upper limit aspect reflect the fact that a series of conservative assumptions were made in the face of scientific uncertainty, including uncertainty about the magnitude of the *internal dose*. Development of a unified PB-PK model for DCM permitted the reduction of uncertainty in the original risk estimation through replacement of default assumptions with results from the PB-PK model.

Internal doses for the *female* B6C3F1 mice in the drinking water and inhalation chronic bioassays were calculated with the PB-PK model and are summarized in Table 5. Tumor incidences in treated and control groups of female mice in these studies are also summarized in Table 5. (In the interest of brevity, data from male mice are not presented since these gave estimates of risk similar to those derived from female mice.)

Once internal dose had been calculated, it was necessary to choose a dose–response model to describe the animal responses. The choice of the appropriate dose–response model has been the subject of considerable discussion. Some models, including the linearized multistage (LMS) model, impose conservative assumptions on the QRA process (in this case by forcing the model to be linear at low doses). Other models such as the Probit

---

[1] 4.1×10^{-6} was the original *unit risk* estimate for DCM in the EPA document of 1985, but this estimate has subsequently been lowered by the EPA, based on use of PB-PK modeling (Balancato et al., 1987).

[2] Singh et al. estimated the risk of developing either a lung or a liver tumor, but did not estimate the risk of developing only a lung tumor or only a liver tumor.

TABLE 5. Data Used for Fitting Cancer Dose–Response Models[a]

Nominal Dose	Internal Dose Dose by PB-PK		Tumors	
	Lung	Liver	Lung	Liver
Mouse: Drinking Water				
0 mg/kg	0.0	0.0	5/100	6/100
60 mg/kg	0.395	3.00	3/100	4/99
125 mg/kg	0.902	6.77	1/50	2/50
185 mg/kg	1.46	10.8	3/50	5/50
250 mg/kg	2.19	16.0	4/50	3/50
Mouse: Inhalation				
0 ppm	0.0	0.0	3/50	3/50
2000 ppm	231.0	785.0	30/48	16/48
4000 ppm	482.0	1670.0	41/48	40/48
Human: Occupational Exposure				
1 ppm	5.36×10^{-5}	8.61×10^{-5}		
2 ppm	1.07×10^{-4}	1.73×10^{-4}		
5 ppm	2.69×10^{-4}	4.38×10^{-4}		
10 ppm	5.40×10^{-4}	8.94×10^{-4}		
20 ppm	1.09×10^{-3}	1.86×10^{-3}		
50 ppm	2.80×10^{-3}	5.34×10^{-3}		
100 ppm	5.98×10^{-3}	1.37×10^{-2}		
Human: Continuous Inhalation				
1 μg/m^3	6.16×10^{-6}	9.87×10^{-6}		
Human: Drinking Water				
1 μg/L	4.26×10^{-7}	3.66×10^{6}		

[a]The "internal dose" calculated by the PB-PK model is in average milligram equivalents of DCM metabolized by the GST pathway per day per liter volume of tissue. The values reported for mice are for exposures of 6 hr/day, 5 days/week, corrected for the fraction of a lifetime (96/102) that animals were exposed. Values reported for humans are for one year of occupational exposure, 6 hr/day, 5 days/week, corrected for the fraction of the year (48/52) that humans are in the workplace.

model make fewer assumptions about the shape of the dose–response curve. The LMS has been widely used by regulatory agencies because of the feeling that the estimates produced by this model are unlikely to underpredict the true risk. However, current regulatory practice generally includes presentation of a range of risks estimated from other models as well.

Consequently, the internal dose data were fitted to four different dose–response models currently used by the toxicological community. The models chosen were (1) the linearized multistage model (2) the Probit model, (3) the Weibull model, and (4) the Logit model. (For models (2)–(4), independence of induced tumors and background tumors was assumed.) The four models were then used to estimate risk for three specific exposure

TABLE 6. Excess Risks Calculated by Four–Response Models under Three Exposure Conditions with Nonadditive Background

	Inhal[a]	Water[b]	Occup.[c]
Risk of Lung Tumor			
LMS (w P-K)	3.0×10^{-8}	2.1×10^{-9}	1.4×10^{-5}
Logit	2.1×10^{-13}	2.3×10^{-15}	7.0×10^{-9}
Weibull	9.8×10^{-8}	8.4×10^{-9}	2.8×10^{-5}
Probit	$< 10^{-15}$	$< 10^{-15}$	$< 10^{-15}$
Geo. Mean	2.8×10^{-11}	2.5×10^{-12}	7.2×10^{-9}
Risk of Liver Tumor			
LMS (w P-K)	6.8×10^{-9}	2.5×10^{-9}	3.7×10^{-6}
Logit	2.1×10^{-26}	8.8×10^{-28}	1.2×10^{-17}
Weibull	$< 10^{-17}$	$< 10^{-17}$	$< 10^{-17}$
Probit	$< 10^{-15}$	$< 10^{-15}$	$< 10^{-15}$
Geo. Mean	3.5×10^{-17}	1.2×10^{-17}	2.6×10^{-14}
Total Risk (Lung + Liver)			
LMS (w/o P-K)[2]	4.1×10^{-6}		
LMS (w P-K)	3.7×10^{-8}	4.6×10^{-9}	1.8×10^{-5}
Logit	2.1×10^{-13}	2.3×10^{-15}	7.0×10^{-9}
Weibull	9.8×10^{-8}	8.4×10^{-9}	2.8×10^{-5}
Probit	$< 10^{-15}$	$< 10^{-15}$	$< 10^{-15}$
Geo. Mean	2.9×10^{-11}	3.1×10^{-12}	7.7×10^{-9}

[a]Continuous inhalation of 1 μg/m^3 of DCM in air for a lifetime.
[b]Consumption of 2 L water/day containing 1 μg DCM/L for a lifetime.
[c]Occupational exposure (6hr/day, 5 days/week, 48 weeks/year) to DCM at 50 ppm for one year.

scenarios: (1) lifetime exposure to 1 μg DCM/m^3 in the atmosphere (EPA's standard "Unit Risk" condition), (2) lifetime consumption of 2 L/day of water containing 1 μg DCM/L, and (3) one year's occupational exposure to DCM at the proposed Threshold Limit Value (TLV, 50 ppm).

The LMS model generally gave the highest estimates of low-dose risk for a given dose of DCM (Table 6). Low-dose risk estimates from the other three models were similar to the risk estimates from the LMS when additive backgrounds were assumed (data not shown). However, when independent backgrounds were assumed, the four models give very different predictions of low-dose risk (shown in Table 6). Although each model gave an excellent description of the observable data from the two bioassays, the models differed by 5–15 orders of magnitude in predicted risk for the exposure conditions depicted in Table 6.

The effect of incorporating pharmacokinetic principles into the risk assessment process may be visualized by comparing the total risk (lung + liver) predicted by the LMS model with and without use of the PB-PK model. Under conditions of continuous inhalation of 1 μg/m^3, the LMS predicted an upper-bound risk of 4.1×10^{-6} for lifetime exposure without PB-PK. However, use of a pharmacokinetically calculated internal dose predicted a risk more than two orders or magnitude lower: 3.7×10^{-8} (Table 6).

There are two reasons for this difference. The first is the nonlinearity in the activity of the MFO pathway. At low concentrations, most of the DCM taken up is metabolized by the MFO pathway. However, once this pathway saturates at a few hundred ppm, a disproportionate amount of DCM is metabolized by GST (which does not saturate within accessible exposure concentrations). The second reason has to do with the calculation of internal doses with the PB-PK model instead of using an empirical "surface area correction factor." Humans possess relatively lower levels of the enzyme(s) responsible for DCM toxicity, and at equivalent tissue concentrations of DCM will generate lower levels of the toxic GST metabolite than rodents.

It needs to be pointed out that use of a PB-PK model in QRA might not always result in estimation of lower risks for humans than the default procedures mentioned earlier. For instance, if a test chemical were *directly* toxic and was inactivated by metabolic enzymes, then a PB-PK model would predict risks similar to the default assumptions. Similarly, if toxicity resulted from reactive metabolite(s) produced by a saturable process, then low-dose risk extrapolated from high, saturating doses by a PB-PK model could actually be *more* than that predicted by linear extrapolations.

In summary, development of a PB-PK model for methylene chloride has provided a valuable tool for eliminating uncertainty in risk estimations for DCM. The model permitted identification of a probable mechanism of carcinogenesis for DCM and provided a quantitative basis for evaluating the effect of two competing metabolic pathways upon the production of the toxic GST metabolite in situ at various doses. We believe that risk estimations which incorporate PB-PK principles will prove significantly more reliable than risk estimations which do not consider pharmacokinetics.

APPENDIX A

Differential equations and abbreviations for the various tissue compartments utilized in the PB-PK model which are different from those reported by Ramsey and Andersen (1984) are listed below.

Gas Exchange Compartment

$$CA1 = (QC*CV + QP*CI)/(QC + QP/PB)$$

$$CX = CA1/PB$$

$$CA = CLU/PLU$$

Lung Tissue Compartment (Where Metabolism Occurs)

$$dALU \, dt = QC*(CA1 - CA) - dAM1LU - dAM2LU$$

$$dAM1LU \, dt = A1 * V_{max} * CA * (VLU/VL)/(K_m + CA)$$

$$dAM2LU \, dt = A2 * KF * CA * VLU$$

$$ALU = Integral \, (dALU \, dt)$$

$$CLU = ALU/VLU$$

$$AUCLU = Integral \, (CLU \, dt)$$

Liver Compartment

$$\mathrm{dAL}\,dt = \mathrm{QL}*(\mathrm{CA} - \mathrm{CVL}) - \mathrm{dAM1L} - \mathrm{dAM2L} + \mathrm{KZER}$$

$$\mathrm{dAM1L}\,dt = (V_{\max}*\mathrm{CVL})/(K_m + \mathrm{CVL})$$

$$\mathrm{dAM2L}\,dt = \mathrm{KF}*\mathrm{CVL}*\mathrm{VL}$$

$$\mathrm{AL} = \mathrm{Integral}\,(\mathrm{dAL}\,dt)$$

$$\mathrm{CL} = \mathrm{AL/VL}$$

$$\mathrm{CVL} = \mathrm{CL/PL}$$

$$\mathrm{AUCL} = \mathrm{Integral}\,(\mathrm{CL}\,dt)$$

Abbreviations used in the model are defined below.

Concentrations (in Milligrams/Liter)

CA1   Concentration of DCM in blood leaving gas exchange compart.
CA   Concentration of DCM in arterial blood.
CI   Concentration of DCM in inhaled air.
CL   Concentration of DCM in liver tissue.
CLU   Concentration of DCM in lung tissue.
CV   Concentration of DCM in mixed venous blood.
CVL   Concentration of DCM in venous blood leaving liver.
CX   Concentration of DCM in alveolar air.

Flows (in Liters/Hour)

QP   Alveolar ventilation rate.
QC   Cardiac output.
QL   Flow through liver compartment.

Amounts (in Milligrams of DCM)

ALU   Amount of DCM in the lung compartment.
AL   Amount of DCM in the liver compartment.
AM1L   Amount of DCM metabolized by MFO in liver.
AM2L   Amount of DCM metabolized by GST in liver.
AM1LU   Amount of DCM metabolized by GST in lung.
AM2LU   Amount of DCM metabolized by GST in lung.

Partition Coefficients

PB   Blood/air partition coefficient.
PL   Liver/blood partition coefficient.
PLU   Lung/blood partition coefficient.

Volumes (in Liters)

VL   Volume of liver.
VLU   Volume of lung.

Miscellaneous

A1   Ratio of MFO activity in lung to MFO activity in liver.
A2   Ratio of GST activity in lung to GST activity in liver.
AUCL   Area under the concentration time curve in the liver.
AUCLU   Area under the concentration time curve in the lung.
KF   First-order rate constant for GST pathway.
K_m Michaelis constant.
KZER   Zero-order rate of input of DCM to liver.
V_{max} Maximum velocity of metabolism by MFO.

APPENDIX B

Apportioning Metabolism Between Lung and Liver

Metabolism occurs by two pathways in each of two tissues: liver and lung. Total metabolism, determined by the gas uptake experiments, is apportioned between these tissues (i.e., it is assumed that metabolism in other tissues is negligibly small). In the mass balance differential equations the liver is referenced to its own metabolic constants. Lung is then referenced to the liver constants using the observed ratios of enzyme specific activities (A1 and A2) for each pathway (Lorenz et al., 1984).

Saturable (MFO) Pathway

The rate of production of metabolities in the liver is

$$dAM1L/dt = V_{max}*CVL/(K_m + CVL)$$
$$V_{max} = SA1L*VL.$$

In lung we have

$$dAM1Lu/dt = V_{max}Lu*CA/(K_m + CA)$$
$$V_{max}Lu = SA1Lu*VLu.$$

Rewriting V_{max}Lu in terms of the ratio of organ-specific activities (A1 = SA1Lu/SA1L), we obtain

$$V_{max}Lu = A1 * SA1L * VLu.$$

Substituting for SA1L in this equation, we obtain

$$V_{max}Lu = (A1 * V_{max} * VLu)/VL.$$

Assuming that K_m (the Michaelis constant) is equal in each tissue, we obtain

$$dAM1Lu/dt = A1 * (VLu/VL) * V_{max} * (CA/(K_m + CA)).$$

Glutathone-Transferase-Mediated Pathway

The rate of production of metabolites by the GST pathway in liver is

$$dAM2L/dt = V_{max}2 * CVL/(K_m2 + CVL).$$

Under first-order conditions where $K_m2 \gg CVL$, this becomes

$$dAM2L/dt = V_{max}2 * CVL/K_m2$$
$$= SA2L * VL * CVL/K_m2.$$

Defining the first-order rate constant KF as (SA2L/K_m2), we obtain

$$dAM2L/dt = KF * VL * CVL.$$

For the lung tissue compartment (again assuming equal K_m's in the two tissues), under first-order conditions where $K_m2 \gg CA$,

$$dAM2Lu/dt = V_{max}2Lu * CA/(K_m2 + CA)$$
$$= SA2Lu * VLu * CA/(K_m2 + CA)$$
$$= SA2Lu * VLu * CA/K_m2.$$

Substituting SA2Lu = (A2 * SA2L) and KF = (SA2L/K_m2), we obtain

$$dAM2Lu/dt = A2 * KF * CA * VLu.$$

APPENDIX C

Choice of Dose Surrogates

Use of the PB-PK model for risk assessment and extrapolations requires calculation of the integrated tissue dose of parent chemical and also of several reactive metabolites that are too short-lived to measure directly. These metabolites (B) can be considered as intermediates in a general metabolic scheme:

$$A \xrightarrow{\text{(1)}} B \underset{\rightarrow}{\overset{\rightarrow}{\rightleftharpoons}} \begin{matrix} C \\ D \\ E \end{matrix}$$

When all downstream reactions of B are linear with concentration, the mass balance equation for B in a tissue of volume V_t becomes

$$V_t*(dB/dt) = \text{Rate1} - (k_1*B*V_t + k_2*B*V_t + \cdots + k_i*B*V_t).$$

The concentration of a highly reactive chemical intermediate which does not accumulate will rapidly attain a steady-state condition,

$$V_t*(dB/dt) = 0,$$

allowing solution of the second equation for the steady-state concentration of B, B_{ss}.

$$B_{ss} = \text{Rate1} \bigg/ \sum_{i=1}^{n} (k_i*V_t).$$

If B is highly reactive and the $\sum k_i*V_t$ is large, this equation will be a good approximation of B_t during the entire exposure period. This equation can be integrated to give the expected integrated tissue exposure to the intermediate, B:

$$\int_0^t B_t dt = \int_0^t B_{ss} dt = \int_0^t \frac{\text{Rate 1}\ dt}{V_t}.$$

This relationship shows that integrated tissue dose of toxic metabolite is proportional to the integral of the rate of formation of B divided by tissue volume. Here, integrated rate$/V_t$ is used as a surrogate of tissue exposure to reactive intermediates. Interspecies comparisons using this dose surrogate assume that $\sum k_i*V_t$ is similar in various species.

The pathways for disappearance of B may be capacity-limited (i.e., dose dependent) at high reaction rates. Examples of this behavior occur with vinyl chloride, acetaminophen, and ethylene dichloride where reactive metabolites eventually deplete glutathione. Estimation of tissue dose with these chemicals requires that the time dependence of GSH concentrations be known or modeled. This complication is unnecessary with DCM since GSH is regenerated when DCM is metabolized by the GST pathway (Fig. 2).

REFERENCES

Adolph, E. F. (1949). Quantitative relations in the physiological constitutions of mammals. *Science* **109**, 579–585.

Ahmed, A. E., and Anders, M. W. (1978). Metabolism of dihalomethanes to formaldehyde and inorganic halide. I. *In vitro* studies. *Drug Metab. Dispos.* **4**, 357–361.

Andersen, M. E., Archer, R. L., Clewell, H. J., and MacNaughton, M. G. (1984). A physiological model of the intravenous and inhalation pharmacokinetics of three dihalomethanes. *Toxicologist* **4**, 443.

Angelo, M. J., Bischoff, K. B., Pritchard, A. B., and Presser, M. A. (1984). A physiological model for the pharmacokinetics of methylene chloride in B6C3F1 mice following i.v. administration. *J. Pharmacol. Biopharmacol.* **12**, 413–436.

Blancato, J. N., Hopkins, J., and Rhomberg, L. (1987). Update to the health assessment document and addendum for dichloromethane (methylene chloride): Pharmacokinetics, mechanism of action, and epidemiology. External Review Draft, EPA/600/8-87/030A.

Burek, J. D., Nitschke, K. D., Bell, T. J., Waskerle, D. L., Childs, R. C., Beyer, J. D., Dittenber, D. A., Rampy, L. W., and McKenna, M. J. (1984). Methylene chloride: A 2-year inhalation toxicity and oncogenicity study in rats and hamsters. *Fundam. Appl. Toxicol.* **4**, 30–47.

Caster, W. O., Poncelet, J., Simon, A. B., and Armstrong, W. D. (1956). Tissue weights of the rat. I. Normal values determined by dissection and chemical methods. *Proc. Soc. Exp. Biol. Med.* **91**, 122–126.

Clewell, H. J., and Andersen, M. E. (1985). Risk assessment extrapolations and physiological modeling. In *Advances in Health Risk Assessment for Systemic Toxicants and Chemical Mixtures.* Princeton Scientific Publishers, Princeton, NJ.

Davis, N. R., and Mapleson, W. W. (1981). Structure and quantification of a physiological model of the distribution of injected agents and inhaled anaesthetics. *Br. J. Anaesth.* **53**, 399–404.

Environmental Protection Agency (1983). *Health Assessment Document for Dichloromethane (Methylene Chloride)*, EPA-600/8-82-004B. EPA, Washington, DC.

Fiserova-Bergerova, V. (1975). Mathematical modeling of inhlation exposure. *J. Combust. Toxicol.* **3**, 201–210.

Frantz, S. W., and Watanabe, P. G., (1983). Tetrachloroethylene: Balance and tissue distribution in male Sprague-Dawley rats by drinking water administration. *Toxicol. Appl. Pharmacol.* **69**, 66–72.

Gargas, M. L., Andersen, M. E., and Clewell, H. J., III (1986a). A simulation analysis of gas uptake data. *Toxicol. Appl. Pharmacol.* **86**, 341–352.

Gargas, M. L., Clewell, H. J., and Andersen, M. E. (1986b). Metabolism of inhaled dihalomethanes *in vivo*: Differentiation of kinetic constants for two independent pathways. *Toxicol. Appl. Pharmacol.* **87**, 211–223.

Green, T. (1983). The metabolic activation of dichloromethane and chlorofluoromethane in a bacterial mutation assay using *Salmonella typhimurium. Mutat. Res.* **118**, 277–288.

Guyton, A. C. (1947). Respiratory volumes of laboratory animals. *Am. J. Physiol.* **150**, 70–77.

International Commission on Radiation Protection (ICRP) (1975). *Report of the Task Group on Reference Man*, ICRP Publ. 23. Pergamon, Elmsford, NY.

Kubic, V. L., Anders, M. W., Engel, R. R., Barlow, C. H., and Caughey, W. S. (1974). Metabolism of dihalomethanes to carbon monoxide. I. *In vivo* studies. *Drug Metab. Dispos.* **2**, 53–57.

Leith, D. E. (1976). Comparative mammalian respiratory mechanics. *Physiologist* **19**, 485–510.

Lorenz, J., Glatt, H. R., Fleischmann, R., Ferlinz, R., and Oesch, F. (1984). Drug metabolism in man and its relationship to that in three rodent species: Monooxygenase, epoxide hydroxylase, and glutathione S-transferase activities in subcellular fractions of lung and liver. *Biochem. Med.* **32**, 43–56.

McKenna, M. J., Zempel, J. A., and Braun, W. H. (1982). The pharmacokinetics of inhaled methylene chloride in rats. *Toxicol. Appl. Pharmacol.* **65**, 1–10.

Miller, E. C., and Miller, J. A. (1966). Mechanisms of chemical carcinogenesis: Nature of proximate carcinogens and interactions with macromolecules. *Pharmacol. Rev.* **18**, 805.

National Academy of Sciences (1986). "Dose Route Extrapolations: Using Inhalation Toxicity data to set Drinking Water Limits," in *Drinking Water and Health*, Vol. 6, Chapter 6, National Academy Press, Washington, DC, pp. 185–236.

National Research Council (1986). Dose route extrapolations: Using inhalation toxicity data to set drinking water limits. In R. D. Thomas (Ed.), *Drinking Water and Health*, Vol. 6. National Academy Press, Washington, DC, pp. 185–236.

National Toxicology Program (NTP) (1985). *NTP Technical Report on the Toxicology and Carcinogenesis Studies of Dichloromethane in F-344/N Rats and B6C3F1 Mice (Inhalation Studies)*, NTP-TR-306 (broard draft). NTP, Washington, DC.

Park, C. N., and Snee, R. D. (1983). Quantitative risk assessment: State of the art for carcinogenesis. *Am. Stat.* **37**, 427.

Peterson, J. E. (1978). Modeling the uptake, metabolism, and excretion of dichloromethane by man. *Am. Ind. Hyg. J.* **39**, 41–47.

Ramsey, J. R., and Andersen, M. E. (1984). A physiologically based description of the inhalation pharmacokinetics of styrene in rats and humans. *Toxicol. Appl. Pharmacol.* **73**, 159–175.

Rannug, U., Sundvall, A., and Ramel, C. (1978). The mutagenic effect of 1, 2-dichloroethane on *Salmonella typhimurium*. I. Activation through conjugation with glutathione *in vitro*. *Chem.-Biol. Interact.* **20**, 1.

Reitz, R. H., Mendrala, A. M., Park, C. N., Andersen, M. E., and Guengerich, F. P. (1988). Incorporation of in vitro enzyme data into the PB-PK model for methylene chloride (CH_2Cl_2): Implications for risk assessment. *Toxicology Letters*, (in press).

Reitz, R. H., Smith, F. A., and Andersen, M. E. (1986). *In vivo* metabolism of ^{14}C-methylene chloride (MEC). *Toxicologist* **6**, 260.

Sato, A., and Nakajima, T. (1979). Partition coefficients of some aromatic hydrocarbons and ketones in water, blood, and oil. *Br. J. Ind. Med.* **36**, 231–234.

Schumann, A. M. (1984). Inhalation Kinetics. Food Solvents Workshop I: Methylene Chloride. March 8–9, Bethesda, MD.

Serota, D., Ulland, B., and Carlborg, F. (1984a). Hazelton Chronic Oral Study in Mice. Food Solvents Workshop I: Methylene Chloride. March 8–9, Bethesda, MD.

Serota, D., Ulland, B., and Carlborg, F. (1984b). Hazleton Chronic Oral Study in Rats. Food Solvents Workshop I: Methylene Chloride. March 8–9, Bethesda, MD.

Singh, D. V., Spitzer, H. L., and White, P. D. (1985). *Addendum to the Health Assessment Document for Dichloromethane (Methylene Chloride). Updated Carcinogenicity Assessment of Dichloromethane*, EPA/600/8-82/004F. EPA, Washington, DC.

Sivak, A. (1984). Gentoxicological Assessment Food Solvents Workshop I: Methylene Chloride. March 8–9, Bethesda, MD.

6

Superfund Risk Assessments: The Process and Past Experience at Uncontrolled Hazardous Waste Sites*

Craig Zamuda

Office of Policy, Planning and Evaluation, U.S. Environmental Protection Agency, Washington, DC

INTRODUCTION

The Comprehensive Environmental Response, Compensation and Liability Act of 1980 (CERCLA) authorizes the federal government to respond directly to releases, or threatened releases, of hazardous substances that may endanger public health, welfare, or the environment (42 U.S.C. 9601 et seq.). In addition, the National Oil and Hazardous Substances Pollution Contingency Plan (NCP, 40 CFR 300 et seq.) establishes a framework for implementing CERCLA by outlining the process for developing and evaluating appropriate response actions for Superfund sites. Together, CERCLA and the NCP require that a response action be cost effective and that it be adequate to protect human health and the environment. The U.S. Environmental Protection Agency (EPA) has developed risk assessment procedures in order to address the public health concerns and to ensure that Superfund response actions limit the concentration of hazardous substances in the environment to avoid unacceptable risks to human health (USEPA, 1986a–f).

Quantitative risk assessment has received increased attention because of the recognition of both the potential threat to human health from hazardous substances and the potential for releases of hazardous substances into the environment. Hazardous waste is a problem of enormous magnitude. An estimated 247 million metric tons of hazardous waste were managed in facilities regulated by the Resource Conservation and Recovery Act (RCRA; 40 CFR 260–280) and an additional 322 million tons of waste managed in units exempt from RCRA permitted facilities in 1985 (USEPA, 1986g). RCRA regulations should prevent much of this waste from ending up in sites that will need to be addressed by CERCLA. However, waste generated before RCRA regulation may not have been

---

*The opinions and viewpoints expressed in this article are those of the author and not necessarily those of the U.S. Environmental Protection Agency.

disposed of properly and may be found at sites that could be addressed by CERCLA. Superfund may conceivably be used to clean up as many as 328,000 sites including up to 600 closed RCRA facilities, 52,000 municipal landfills, 75,000 industrial landfills, 64,000 mining waste sites, and 187,000 leaking underground storage tanks (Hayes and Mackerron, 1987). Many of these sites may be removal actions and would not require in-depth risk assessments. Nevertheless, the General Accounting Office (GAO) estimated the number of major uncontrolled hazardous waste sites at 4000 in 1985, with cleanup costs at approximately $40 billion (GAO, 1985). The Office of Technology Assessment (OTA) estimates that over 10,000 sites may be eligible for Superfund cleanup including 5000 of the 621,000 operating and closed solid waste facilities, 1000 hazardous waste facilities, 2000 sites detected because of improved site identification and selection, and the 2000 sites the EPA has projected for the NPL (OTA, 1985).

Recognizing the extent of the hazardous waste problem and the role of risk assessment, the Office of Emergency and Remedial Response of the EPA has developed risk assessment procedures that are used for a variety of purposes. Risk assessment is used for designating substances as hazardous and establishing minimum quantities for reporting releases when they would present substantial danger. In addition, risk assessment is used to evaluate the relative dangers of various sites in order to establish priorities for response actions and for developing, evaluating, and selecting appropriate response actions at Superfund sites.

This chapter describes the basic components of the Superfund risk assessment process. Although the EPA has responsibilities beyond the protection of human health, the uses of risk assessment discussed here are largely restricted to assessment of human health risk rather than the risk to the environment and/or wildlife. Specific examples of how risk assessments have been used to characterize and describe risks at several uncontrolled hazardous waste sites are presented. Much of this information comes from Public Health Evaluation documents, chapters from Remedial Investigations and Feasibility Studies, or from Endangerment Assessments of Superfund enforcement sites, all of which are generically referred to as public health evaluations or PHEs. While the focus of this chapter is on the role of risk assessment in long-term permanent remedial actions, the chapter also describes the use of risk assessment to (i) identify the nation's most hazardous waste sites, which are then designated on the National Priorities List and thereby become eligible for Superfund-financed cleanup actions and (ii) determine appropriate cleanup responses for immediate "removal" actions.

HAZARD RANKING SYSTEM AND THE NATIONAL PRIORITIES LIST

EPA uses a risk-based analysis to identify those uncontrolled or abandoned hazardous waste sites that may require long-term remedial actions under Superfund. The Hazard Ranking System (HRS) is the principal method used initially to rank the potential risks posed by the approximately 26,000 sites that have been reported to the EPA (50 Fed. Reg. 47931). These sites are located throughout the nation and vary from mine tailings to hazardous waste spills to abandoned manufacturing facilities. Sites with sufficiently high scores are considered for placement on the EPA's National Priorities List (NPL). The HRS assigns numerical scores to a variety of factors that affect the potential risk posed by a site including characteristics of waste toxicity, exposure potential, and potentially exposed populations. Scores for the groundwater pathway, surface water pathway, and air pathway are combined to get an overall score for a site. Sites on the NPL present the most serious problems among uncontrolled hazardous waste sites nationwide and are eligible for long-term remedial actions through the Superfund program.

The HRS scores a site using information collected during the preliminary assessment and site inspection. The preliminary assessment consists of a review of any available documents on the site to determine if further action is needed. If so, the site inspection is conducted and additional information about the site is obtained. This may include information on the types of soils, location and number of people in the area, location of aquifers and wells of concern, and nature and quantity of the waste (e.g., toxicity, volume, persistence) and includes limited site sampling. Based on this information three factors are used to score sites:

1. The possibility that hazardous substances will migrate offsite through groundwater, surface water, or air and reach populated areas.
2. The possibility that people will come in contact with hazardous substances.
3. The possibility of fire or explosion caused by hazardous substances.

The second and third factors are used to identify sites that require immediate removal action. Only the first factor is used to place sites on the NPL and is generally referred to as the *HRS score*.

The HRS does not determine if cleanup is technologically possible or worthwhile, or the amount of cleanup needed. These issues are addressed in the Remedial Investigation and Feasibility Study (RI/FS) process conducted at sites listed on the NPL. During the development of the RI/FS, conditions at the site are studied, problems are defined, and alternative methods to clean up the site are evaluated. The criteria for developing remedial alternatives for response action, as described in the NCP, require that at least one alternative be developed for each of the following categories, as appropriate:

- Alternative for offsite treatment or disposal.
- Alternatives that attain "applicable or relevant and appropriate" federal public health and environmental requirements.
- Alternatives that exceed "applicable or relevant and appropriate" federal public health and environmental requirements.
- Alternatives that do not attain "applicable or relevant and appropriate" public health or environmental standards, but that will "reduce the likelihood of present or future threat from the hazardous substances and that provide significant protection to public health and welfare and environment."
- A no-action alternative.

The HRS is not designed to distinguish between the risks presented by two sites whose scores are similar, but rather to provide a meaningful indicator of different levels of risks between sites with large differences. In short, it is a method for prioritizing sites so that those posing the greatest hazard receive the most timely response. The scores are weighted to increase those given to sites that threaten densely populated areas, that have greater likelihood of exposure to affected populations, or that contain large volumes of waste. Sites are placed on the NPL only if they receive a ranking score of 28.5 or more (on a scale of 0–100), except for the one state priority site that each state is allowed to designate, regardless of its ranking. Although the HRS was designed to help fulfill the CERCLA requirement that at least 400 sites warranting the highest priority for remedial action be identified, as of February 1987, the NPL contained 951 sites.

SUPERFUND REMOVAL ACTIONS

CERCLA and the NCP require that the decision for a removal action be based on an assessment that the action will prevent or mitigate risk of harm to human health or to the environment from certain specified situations. A removal action is considered a short-term action intended to stabilize or clean up an incident or site that poses a threat. Removal actions may include (i) removing and disposing of hazardous substances, (ii) controlling access to the site (e.g., constructing a fence, posting warning signs), (iii) providing a temporary alternate water supply to local residents, and (iv) temporarily relocating area residents. CERCLA [as amended by the Superfund Amendments and Reauthorization Act of 1986 (SARA)] limits removal actions to 12 months in duration and a total cost of $2 million, although exemptions may be granted.

The risk assessment process used to determine the need for action and evaluate the type and extent of response for removal action differs from that conducted for remedial actions. This difference is the result of several factors including the constraints of cost and time as established by CERCLA. Furthermore, the risk assessment for removal actions has generally focused on short-term exposure and acute/subchronic effects, rather than lifetime exposure and chronic effects considered under remedial actions. As a result, the specific health-based criteria used to determine the need for, and extent of, cleanup may also vary between removal and remedial actions.

Initially under CERCLA, a removal action could only be taken in response to an "immediate and significant threat." As a matter of policy, a removal action was triggered if contaminant levels exceeded the EPA Ten-Day Drinking Water Health Advisory.* However, as a result of revisions to the NCP, which expanded the scope of removal authority, this trigger level has been revised. The revision now allows removal actions to be taken in response to a "threat". As a result, removal actions can be taken in less urgent situations than before, and a risk assessment decision model that considers lifetime health advisory levels, in addition to short-term levels, has been established (50 FR 47912, November 20, 1985).

Even if the lifetime "action levels" are not exceeded a removal action may be taken if warranted by site-specific factors. Examples of such factors include the size of the population at risk, the duration of exposure, the presence of sensitive persons in the population, evidence that a contaminated ground water plume is moving, evidence that contaminant levels will increase (e.g., increased pumping from an aquifer anticipated during summer months), or synergistic effects resulting from multiple contaminants.

SUPERFUND REMEDIAL ACTIONS

The application of the risk assessment process to determine the eligibility of sites for potential federally-financed cleanups and for determining the appropriate extent of

---

*The Office of Drinking Water's nonregulatory health advisories are concentrations of contaminants in drinking water at which adverse effects would not be anticipated to occur. The 10-day advisory is calculated for a 10-kg child (a 1-year-old infant) assumed to drink 1 L of water per day.

remedy in emergency situations is not its central use in Agency. The primary application of quantitative risk assessment in the Superfund program is to evaluate the potential risk posed at each NPL facility so that the appropriate remedial alternative is identified. The selection of a remedy is based on a comparison of alternatives that examine not only the public health impacts, but also the environmental impacts, technological and engineering feasibility, cost and institutional factors. Although the results of a particular risk assessment are only one of several factors that are considered in making site-specific decisions, these are the most important factor in determining if a remedial action is necessary and if the proposed remedy is adequately protective of human health (Zamuda, 1986).

The NCP establishes a framework for developing and evaluating various remedial alternatives for Superfund sites. The NCP describes two major elements of the site remedial planning process: the remedial investigation (RI) and the feasibility study (FS). During the remedial investigation, field investigators obtain site characterization data necessary to determine what responses, if any, should be considered and evaluated for a site. During the feasibility study, remedial alternatives are developed to effectively address site contamination problems identified in the remedial investigation.

The Superfund Record of Decision (ROD) summarizes the information from the remedial investigation and the feasibility study. The ROD describes the remedial action chosen for a site and how it meets the requirements for consideration of public health, cost, and compliance with Federal public health and environmental standards. The RODs include specific clean-up levels for contaminated media based on health criteria and remedial alternatives for a site.

Feasibility study analyses include engineering, institutional, public health, environmental, and cost-effectiveness evaluations. Guidance for carrying out these analyses is available in the *Guidance on Remedial Investigations Under CERCLA* (U.S. EPA, 1985a) and *Guidance on Feasibility Studies Under CERCLA* (U.S. EPA, 1985b). In addition, a risk assessment process and procedures manual, the *Superfund Public Health Evaluation Manual* (U.S. EPA, 1986a) has been developed that describes how to conduct the public health evaluation. The goals of the process are to ensure that Superfund remedies adequately protect public health and that the risk assessment process is consistent among various sites. A description of the Superfund public health evaluation process, the role of public health evaluation in the Superfund remedial program, and practical application of a risk assessment follow.

THE SUPERFUND PUBLIC HEALTH EVALUATION PROCESS

The Superfund Public Health Evaluation (PHE) process is used to evaluate threats to public health posed by Superfund sites. In developing the necessary procedures, EPA recognizes that, while total consistency among users would be desirable, the evaluations cannot be reduced to simple, cookbook procedures. State-of-the-art risk assessment techniques require the use of informed scientific judgment. Each site poses its own unique set of circumstances that must be addressed on a case-by-case basis. The approach to assessment is designed to balance the need for consistency, clear guidance, and use of EPA approved methods with the need for flexibility to address potential threats from specific releases and exposure situations.

The phrase "public health evaluation" refers to that component of the risk assessment conducted at Superfund sites to generate estimates of human health risks. Although the

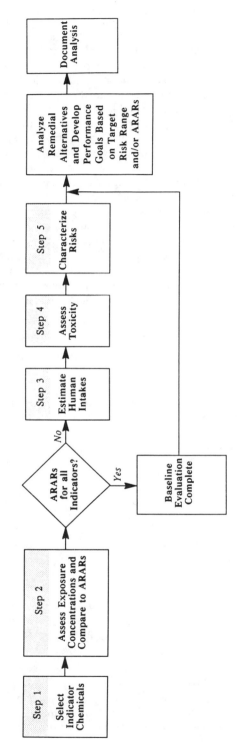

Figure 1. Flowchart of the Superfund Public Health Evaluation process.

271

actual risk assessment conducted at sites includes an environmental impact component, within the context of this chapter the phrases "risk assessment" and "public health evaluation" will be used interchangeably.

The Superfund PHE is conducted in two phases. The baseline evaluation is an assessment of risk to human health based on site conditions and projected exposure levels and examines the effects of taking no action at the Superfund sites. The assessment is initiated early in the remedial process and is complete once the assessment team has a sufficient understanding of the risks posed by the site and the chemicals and exposure pathways of most concern. At the completion of the baseline evaluation the chemicals posing a significant risk at the site will have been identified, along with the media and exposure pathways of concern. In addition, preliminary chemical-specific clean up goals, based on acceptable levels of exposure, will have been identified.

The second phase of the public health evaluation involves refining initial design ideas for remedial alternatives to address specific health concerns at the site and preliminary cleanup goals identified in the baseline evaluation, and evaluating the consequences of implementing those alternatives. Environmental concerns—especially those settings that place large numbers of fish, birds, and other wildlife or endangered species at risk—may also be important in determining the appropriate level of cleanup and may actually drive the cleanup at some sites.* Environmental considerations are made separately from the public health evaluation. A flowchart of the baseline public health evaluation process is presented in Fig. 1.

BASELINE PUBLIC HEALTH EVALUATION: ASSESSING INITIAL SITE CONDITIONS

The National Contingency Plan requires, among other things, that a public health analysis be completed for each remedial site under the assumption that no action is taken. The assessment of the initial site conditions before any remedial activity is called the *baseline public health evaluation*. The baseline evaluation may range from a relatively straightforward, uncomplicated risk assessment to a very detailed and complex one. The risk assessment process, shown in Fig. 1, consists of five steps:

1. Selection of indicator chemicals.
2. Determination of human exposures.
3. Estimation of human intakes.
4. Evaluation of toxicity.
5. Characterization of risk.

This risk assessment process is a generic one that is broadly applicable to most sites. As a consequence of attempting to cover a wide variety of sites, many of the process components, steps, and techniques do not apply at every site. Determining which elements of the process are necessary, which are desirable, and which are extraneous represents key decisions within each assessment.

*At the Burnt Fly Bog site in New Jersey (EPA/ROD/R02-83/002) (SRD, 1983d) [ROD signed November 16, 1983] (NTIS No. PB85 213676/AS], excavation of lagoons and wetland was undertaken to remove threats to public health and the environment. However, wetlands will be restored to natural contours and revegetated based on the environmental consideration of erosion control and biological restoration.

INCREASING COMPLEXITY/LEVEL OF EFFORT

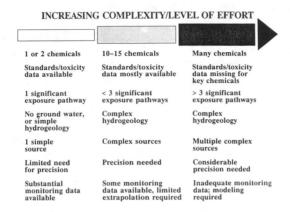

1 or 2 chemicals	10–15 chemicals	Many chemicals
Standards/toxicity data available	Standards/toxicity data mostly available	Standards/toxicity data missing for key chemicals
1 significant exposure pathway	< 3 significant exposure pathways	> 3 significant exposure pathways
No ground water, or simple hydrogeology	Complex hydrogeology	Complex hydrogeology
1 simple source	Complex sources	Multiple complex sources
Limited need for precision	Precision needed	Considerable precision needed
Substantial monitoring data available	Some monitoring data available, limited extrapolation required	Inadequate monitoring data; modeling required

Figure 2. Continuum of analytical complexity for Superfund Public Health Evaluations.

Just as variations in site conditions affect what exposure and risk calculations are relevant for a site, conditions also determine the necessary level of effort required for a site. Figure 2 illustrates the continuum of complexity and resource requirements determined by the conditions at a site. Site-specific factors affecting the level of effort include the number and identity of chemicals present; availability of appropriate requirements, standards, and/or toxicity data; number and complexity of exposure pathways; quality and quantity of available monitoring data; and the necessity for precision in the results. Sites best represented by the descriptions toward the left of the continuum in Fig. 2 correspond to a relatively low level of effort and analytical complexity, while sites consistent with the descriptions toward the right are more complex and generally require a greater level of effort. The factors that place a site somewhere in the continuum are largely independent. Thus, one factor may correspond to the need for a complex analysis while others correspond to a simple analysis (e.g., a site may have two chemicals with available standards and only one exposure pathway via groundwater but may have a complex hydrogeology that requires considerable effort to characterize).

Reviewing Existing Data

Prior to initiating a public health evaluation, available site data relevant to a detailed risk assessment are gathered, organized, and reviewed. Among the types of information collected are site background data, disposal history, types of remedial actions being considered, chemical analyses (e.g., surface water and groundwater, soil, air), site characterization data necessary for exposure assessment (e.g., topography, hydrogeology), and information on human populations. Any potential adverse effects observed in animals or humans (toxicity data) and human body burden data are also reviewed.

Limited soil and/or groundwater data for a specific site introduces varying degrees of uncertainty in characterizing the spatial and temporal extent of contamination. Adequate data should be collected not only to determine whether contaminants are present but also to identify the extent of contamination at the site. In addition, multiple sampling events may be necessary to determine whether the contamination varies on a temporal as well as a spatial basis. If the sampling history is too short it will be difficult to detect time trends, especially in groundwater, making it difficult to predict future exposure levels and health risks.

The quality of data may also be a limiting factor in conducting a quantitative risk assessment. To evaluate the quality of data, information should be obtained regarding sampling and analytical procedures. Variation in sampling procedures can result in large differences in the analytical results. For example, the results will vary significantly for heavy metal analysis depending on how a groundwater sample was filtered and preserved. If the groundwater sample is not filtered and preserved appropriately, the heavy metals may precipitate out of solution and subsequently not be detected during the analysis. The accurate sampling of contaminated soil is even more difficult since cross contamination of the sampling instruments can occur and result in false positives.

Site monitoring data should not be used in the risk assessment process without establishing proper quality assurance and quality control (QA/QC) procedures. This is particularly important if data are obtained from several different laboratories. If QA/QC cannot be verified, the data may be only appropriate for qualitative risk assessments.

Selecting Indicator Chemicals

The first step in the process is to select a subset of chemicals to be studied in depth. Since monitoring studies at hazardous waste sites often demonstrate the presence of numerous chemicals, it may be both impractical and unnecessarily time consuming to assess the risk of each one. To avoid these difficulties, the Superfund public health evaluation is based on selected chemicals, referred to as *indicator chemicals*, that pose the greatest potential health hazard at a site.

Indicator chemicals must be chosen carefully so that they represent the most toxic, mobile, and persistent chemicals, as well as those present in the largest amounts. A selection procedure based partly on numerical algorithms and partly on professional judgment is utilized by the EPA. For each chemical, toxicity is examined in light of concentrations measured in specific environmental media. In addition, various chemical and physical properties that affect the potential for a substance to migrate or persist in the environment are considered.

The following algorithm is used to score each chemical measured at the site:

$$IS_i = \sum (C_{ij} T_{ij}),$$

where IS_i = indicator score for chemical i (unitless)
$\quad\quad C_{ij}$ = concentration of chemical i in medium j at the site based on monitoring data (units in mg/L for water, mg/kg for soil, mg/m^3 in air)
$\quad\quad T_{ij}$ = a toxicity constant for chemical i in medium j (units are inverse of concentration units).

Concentration values used in this equation for a given chemical should be representative of all available site monitoring data that have been QA/QC validated. In determining the representative concentration it may be appropriate to use a geometric or arithmetic mean of some or all of the samples, or it may be more appropriate to choose a concentration that reflects a time trend occurring at the site. Consideration should also be given to detection frequency, generally giving relatively less weight to chemicals detected infrequently.

Toxicity constants (T values) are derived for each environmental medium and for carcinogenic and chronic effects (USEPA, 1985c, 1986a). Essentially, the indicator score is a ratio between measured concentration and a toxicity-based concentration benchmark that is used to rank the site chemicals. Toxicity constants for noncarcinogens are derived from the minimum effective dose for chronic effects, a severity effect factor, and standard factors for body weight and oral or inhalation intake. Toxicity constants for potential carcinogens are based on the dose at which 10% incremental carcinogenic response is obserced (ED_{10}) and the same standard intake and body weight factors. Because of the probable differences in dose–response mechanisms (nonthreshold versus threshold), potential carcinogens and noncarcinogens are scored and selected independently. It should be noted that the toxicity constants are used only for selecting indicator chemicals and are not used for characterizing the risk associated with exposure to the selected chemicals.

Although the indicator score is the initial selection factor, several additional factors are also important. These factors include five chemical properties related to exposure potential: water solubility, vapor pressure, Henry's law constant, organic carbon partition coefficient (K_{oc}), and persistence in various media. High or low values of these factors for a chemical found at a site may produce a high future exposure potential and may warrant inclusion of a particular chemical in the list of indicator chemicals despite a low indicator score.

Some additional questions that need to be answered prior to finalizing the list of indicator chemicals for a particular site include the following: (i) Have outlying data points unrealistically influenced the indicator scores? (ii) Have the temporal and spatial variabilities of the contaminants been considered? (iii) Has the presence of a contaminant in more than one medium been adequately addressed? (iv) Have "elevated" background concentrations and/or offsite sources of contamination been considered?

Although there is no strict protocol for determining the appropriate number of indicator chemicals for a site, the total number generally varies between 10 and 20. With regard to the specific hazardous substances that have been selected in the past, the analysis of PHEs from a representative sample of 32 sites indicates that 51 chemicals were chosen as indicators among these sites. Chemicals that were chosen as indicators for more than one of these are listed in Table 1. Benzene, trichloroethylene, PCBs, and tetrachloroethylene were chosen as indicator chemicals at over one-third of the sites; lead, vinyl chloride, cadmium, and chromium were chosen as indicator chemicals for one-quarter or more of the sites.

Some chemicals are chosen as indicators for only certain media but not for all media of concern at a particular site. For example, PCBs are often chosen as indicator chemicals for soil exposure pathways but not for groundwater exposure pathways because their strong hydrophobicity tends to keep them bound to soil particles preventing their leaching into groundwater. The Environmental Conservation and Chemical Company site in Zionsville, Indiana, is one site where PCBs served as an indicator chemical in the soil medium but not for other exposure media. At Laskin/Poplar Oil site in Jefferson, Ohio, PCBs, dioxins, and polynuclear aromatic hydrocarbons were chosen as indicator chemicals for soil, and benzene and chlorinated solvents were chosen as indicators for the groundwater medium. Consideration of chemical concentrations and mobility potential in various media has led to the selection of different indicator chemicals for different exposure routes.

Illustrative Example: Selecting Indicator Chemicals. This example illustrates the use of the indicator chemical scoring system used for selecting indicator chemicals. Only a limited

TABLE 1. Frequency of Hazardous Substances Selected as Indicator Chemicals at Superfund Sites

Chemical Name	Frequency[a] (site percent)
Benzene	41
Trichloroethylene	41
Polychlorinated biphenyls	38
Tetrachloroethylene	34
Lead	31
Vinyl chloride	28
Arsenic	28
Cadmium	25
Chromium	25
1,1-Dichloroethylene	16
1,1,2-Trichloroethane	13
1,2-Dichloroethane	13
Xylene	13
Polynuclear aromatic hydrocarbons	13
1,1,2,2-Tetrachloroethane	9
Chloroform	9
Ethylbenzene	9
Toluene	9
Zinc	9
Methylene chloride	6
Benzo[a]pyrene	6
2,3,7,8-TCDD (dioxin)	6
N-Nitrosodiphenylamine	6
Mercury	6
Phenol	6
Pentachlorophenol	6
Copper	6
Nickel	6

[a]Frequency based on the number of times the hazardous substance was selected as an indicator chemical for the quantitative risk assessment conducted at 34 Superfund sites. Sites surveyed included the following: Clear Creek, CO; Smuggler, CO; Coleman-Evans, FL; Hipps Road, FL; Pepper Steel, FL; Wauconda Sand and Gravel, IL; Environmental Conservation and Chemical, IN; Main Street Well Field, IN; Seymour Recycling Corp., IN; Re-Solve, MA; Croveland Wells, MA; Southern Maryland, MD; Burrows, MI; Charlevoix, MI; LeHiller/Mankato, MN; Thompson Chemical, MO; Anaconda, MT; Helen Kramer Landfill, NH; D' Imperio Property, NJ; Lang, NJ; Metaltec, NJ; Lipari Landfill, NJ; Arcanum Iron and Metal, OH; Beacon Heights Landfill, OH; Fields Brook, OH; Laskin, OH; Pristine, OH; Bruin Lagoon, PA; Mill Creek, PA; Davis Liquids, RI; Geiger, SC; Mowbray, SC; Morgantown Ordnance, WV; and Schmaltz, WI.

TABLE 2. Chemical Concentrations in Various Environmental Media

Chemical	Groundwater (µg/L)		Surface Water (µg/L)		Soil (mg/kg)	
	Range	Representative	Range	Representative	Range	Representative
Arsenic	0.01–0.46	0.075	<0.01	—	1.7–36	7
Tetachloro-ethylene	BDL[a]–67.0	3.2	BDL–0.012	0.003	BDL–13,000	2
1,2,4-Trichloro-benzene	BDL–1.2	0.11	BDL–0.026	0.002	BDL–210	15.8
Chlorobenzene	25–40	31	10–30	19	—	—

[a]BDL = below detection limit.

277

number of chemicals are presented in this hypothetical example, and in a normal Superfund situation all the chemicals would be evaluated in the public health evaluation. However, this example does illustrate what factors are considered in the selection of indicator chemicals.

The following chemicals were detected in groundwater, surface water, and soil at a site during the site inspection and remedial investigation: arsenic, tetrachloroethylene, 1, 2, 4-trichlorobenzene, and chlorobenzene. The range of concentrations and a representative concentration for each chemical is presented in Table 2. The representative concentration value was based on the geometric mean of the samples with the chemical above detection limits. Toxicity constants are provided in Table 3. Toxicity constants were determined separately for noncarcinogens and carcinogenic potential. If a chemical is a potential carcinogen, such as arsenic and tetrachloroethylene, the indicator chemical scores should be calculated for both toxicological classes.

To develop an indicator score (IS) for a chemical sum the representative concentration value (C) is multiplied by the toxicity factor (T) value across the media (Table 4). For arsenic, the carcinogenic CT value for groundwater of 0.31 (Table 4) was calculated by multiplying the representative concentration of arsenic in groundwater ($0.75 \, \mu g/L$;

TABLE 3. Toxicity Information for Scoring Indicator Chemicals

Chemical	Toxicological Class	Toxicity Constant[a]	
		Water	Soil
Arsenic	Carcinogen	4.1	2.0×10^{-4}
	Noncarcinogen	18	9.0×10^{-4}
Tetrachloroethylene	Carcinogen	8.9×10^{-3}	4.4×10^{-7}
	Noncarcinogen	9.6×10^{-3}	4.8×10^{-7}
1, 2, 4-Trichlorobenzene	Noncarcinogen	0.21	1.1×10^{-5}
Chlorobenzene	Noncarcinogen	0.143	7.14×10^{-6}

[a]Values obtained from the Superfund Public Health Evaluation Manual (USEPA, 1986a).

TABLE 4. Scoring for Indicator Chemicals: Calculation of CT and IS Values

Chemical	Ground Water CT	Surface Water CT	Soil CT	IS Value
		Carcinogen		
Arsenic	0.31	—	0.0014	0.3114
Tetrachloro-ethylene	0.028	2.6×10^{-5}	8.8×10^{-7}	0.028
		Noncarcinogen		
Arsenic	0.14	—	0.0063	0.14
Tetrachloro-ethylene	0.028	2.7×10^{-5}	9.6×10^{-6}	0.028
1, 2, 4-Trichloro-benzene	0.023	4.2×10^{-4}	1.7×10^{-9}	0.023
Chlorobenzene	0.0044	0.0027	—	0.0044

TABLE 5. Scoring for Indicator Chemical Selection: Indicator Score and Exposure Factors[a]

Chemical	IS Values		Water Solubility (mg/L)	Vapor Pressure (mm Hg)	Henry's Law (atm·m³/mole)	K_{oc}	Half-Life (daus)		
	PC[b]	NC[c]					Ground Water	Surface Water	Soil
Arsenic	0.31	0.14	1.5×10^6	0	0	—	10,000	10,000	10,000
Tetrachloro-benzene	0.28	0.28	150	18	0.026	364	264	1–30	—
1,2,4-Trichloro-benzene		0.023	30	0.29	0.0023	9,200	10,000	1.2	—
Chlorobenzene		4.4×10^{-3}	466	11.7	0.00372	330	—	0.30	—

[a]Exposure factors derived from the Superfund Public Health Evaluation Manual (USEPA, 1986a).
[b]Carcinogenic effects.
[c]Noncarcinogenic effects.

279

Table 2) times the toxicity factor in water (4.1; Table 3). The carcinogenic IS score for arsenic of 0.3114 (Table 4) represents the sum of the carcinogenic CT scores for arsenic in groundwater and soil (e.g., 0.31 groundwater $CT + 0.0014$ soil $CT = 0.3114$ IS). If a compound is present in both groundwater and surface water only the higher CT value for the two media is used to calculate the IS value. This approach for water makes the conservative assumption that all drinking water is obtained from the source giving the higher CT value. For example, in the case of chlorobenzene the noncarcinogenic IS score was based on the CT for groundwater [0.0044 rather than the CT for surface water (0.0027; Table 4)].

The IS scores for the carcinogenic and noncarcinogenic properties of each chemical, as well as relevant exposure factors, are presented in Table 5. Final selection of indicator chemicals will be based on a consideration of the indicator score in conjunction with the physicochemical properties of the chemicals that influence the exposure potential.

Determining Extent and Duration of Human Exposure

Once indicator chemicals have been selected, the extent and duration of human exposure to each contaminant can be estimated. Chronic and subchronic exposures are evaluated for each human exposure pathway identified at the site. The results of this step are estimates for long-term and short-term concentrations of indicator chemicals at all exposure points. Estimating exposure point chemical concentrations at most sites requires using both monitoring data and environmental fate modeling. Valid site sampling data indicate the identities and concentrations of chemicals present in particular locations and points in time. However, in addition to this information, environmental fate modeling may be useful in estimating concentrations at different locations and points in time.

Selection of a particular environmental fate model is dependent on many factors, including (i) appropriateness to site conditions, (ii) degree of model validation, and (iii) availability of required input data (USEPA, 1988). Models that have been commonly used in Superfund actions include the Atmospheric Transport Model (ATM), a gaussian dispersion model for estimation of pollutant concentrations released from point, area, or line sources of atmospheric contamination (Patterson et al., 1982). The ATM model is part of the Graphical Exposure Modeling Systems (GEMS), a set of computer models capable of assessing contaminant fate in air, surface water, groundwater, and soil which are integrated with pertinent data files with nationwide soil, land use, and meteorological data, as well as data on major rivers, lakes, and reservoirs. (Information on the GEMS is available through the Office of Pesticides and Toxic Substances of the EPA.) A commonly used surface water model is the Exposure Analysis Modeling System (EXAMS), which simulates the ultimate distribution and concentration of organic chemicals in aquatic systems (Burns et al., 1982). The Analytical Transient One-, Two-, and Three-Dimensional Simulation Model (AT123D) is a groundwater transport model that is designed to simulate the rate of contaminant transport and transformation in the saturated zone (Yeh, 1981).

Specific site information that describes a contaminant's behavior relative to actual site conditions may be limited. In these cases, site data may be supplemented with information concerning the behavior of specific contaminants in a general context. In addition, information may be available which describes the behavior of a structurally related chemical in conditions similar to those at the site. This approach may be helpful for examining various processes such as oxidation–reduction, photolysis, volatilization, sorption, and biologically mediated activities (e.g., bioaccumulation, biotransformation, and biodegradation).

A combination of site monitoring data and environmental modeling results may be necessary to estimate chemical concentrations at exposure points. Monitoring data must be reviewed thoroughly and used to the extent possible, particularly to assist in the selection, calibration, and verification of chemical fate models and to help in the estimation of source terms (i.e., release rates) for these models.

Appropriate choice of contaminant concentrations is important in estimating exposure doses for each medium. Typically, the EPA has used both maximum and representative contaminant concentrations found at the site to establish the "worst case" and "realistic case" site conditions. In addition to the maximum and mean information, knowledge of the frequency each contaminant was detected provides a better understanding of the site data and how realistic the worst case versus the realistic case conditions may be.

Importance of Monitoring Data. At most sites having PHEs, the evaluations indicate that monitoring data were often the major source of information for determining groundwater exposure point concentrations. Often, this method of determining groundwater exposure concentrations incorporates the assumption that chemical concentrations will not change over the course of a 70-year lifetime exposure. In those situations where modeling was not attempted, the decision was generally based on uncertainty in the appropriateness of particular models and uncertainty as to whether contaminant concentrations will increase, decrease, or remain constant over the exposure period.

At many sites having multiple exposure pathways, risk assessors used monitoring data for some pathways (e.g., soil and groundwater ingestion) and exposure modeling for other exposure routes [e.g., see Cowherd et al. (1985) for wind erosion and dust inhalation]. For example, at the Morgantown site in West Virginia, a model was developed to predict concentrations of indicator chemicals in the Monongahela River due to runoff of contaminated surface water, recharge of contaminated groundwater, and erosion of contaminated soil. Runoff, recharge, and erosion rates were generated for contaminated areas of the site and combined with contaminant concentrations in the on-site surface water and soil to estimate loading rates of contaminant into the river. Equilibrium distribution coefficients were used to determine surface water concentrations from sediment and soil concentrations. A surface water dispersion equation was then used to predict the contaminant concentrations at two exposure points, including the drinking water intake of a community downstream of the site. This analysis indicated that concentrations of contaminants at the community drinking water intake did not exceed applicable federal drinking water standards under best-estimate exposure scenarios. However, using maximum plausible exposure scenarios, mercury concentrations exceeded state water quality criteria for a potable water supply. Excess lifetime cancer risks from ingestion of river water and consumption of fish under best-estimate conditions were estimated to be on the order of 10^{-5} and 10^{-7} for arsenic and chlorinated polynuclear aromatic hydrocarbons (PAHs), respectively. Estimates based on maximum plausible exposure assumptions were on the order of 10^{-4} and 10^{-5} for arsenic and PAHs, respectively.

At the Coleman-Evans site in Whitehouse, Florida, uptake of indicator chemicals from soil by plants and subsequent ingestion by humans were estimated using models developed by Briggs et al. (1982). At the Davis Liquids site in Rhode Island, a screening model was used to evaluate the significance of exposures to indicator chemicals volatilizing from surface water. The emission rates from surface water were calculated for indicator chemicals using the model in Lyman et al. (1982) that is based on molecular diffusion across an air–water interface. The emission rate was used as input to the simple box model of Hanna et al. (1982), which calculates the ambient air concentration in a volume of air determined by the mixing height of the air column and site conditions.

The Mocubray Engineering Company site in Alabama provides an example of the use of models to evaluate the volatilization of PCBs from soil using a method derived from Shen (1982). The first step was to calculate the volumetric emission rate of PCBs coming from the soil. This emission rate is then used with the Hanna box model (Hanna et al., 1982) to estimate the air concentration in a volume of air, assuming no reduction in concentration resulting from wind dispersion or topographical features (e.g., trees or hills). For this site, the mixing volume was assumed to be applicable to onsite exposure as well as exposures up to $\frac{1}{8}$ mile offsite, at which point dispersion becomes important.

At the Lang Property site in New Jersey, a screening model was used to determine how much contaminant volatilization was likely to occur from soil. The Farmer model (Farmer et al., 1980) was used to predict emission rates of volatile contaminants from soil. The Farmer model estimates volatilization as a function of the chemical and physical properties of the material and the properties of the soil (porosity, soil density, and depth). Emission rates were then input into the Turner atmospheric dispersion model (Turner, 1970), which calculates the concentration at a downwind receptor depending on wind speed and dispersion coefficients for the appropriate atmospheric stability class, to estimate exposure to a hypothetical person who would be exposed to the site every day.

Comparing Projected Concentrations to Standards. At this point in the baseline PHE process, the projected concentrations of indicator chemicals at exposure points are compared to contaminant specific "applicable or relevant and appropriate" (ARARs) federal or state environmental or public health requirements. Examples of requirements that the EPA has determined may be applicable or relevant and appropriate for the purpose of risk assessment depending on site conditions are Safe Drinking Water Act Maximum Contaminant Levels (MCLs; 40 CFR 141.11–12, 15–16) and Clean Air Act National Ambient Air Quality Standards (NAAQS; 40 CFR 50). In addition, the Superfund Amendments and Reauthorization Act of 1986 (P.L. 99–499) Section 121(d)(A) specifies that remedial action requires a level or standard of control "which at least attains Maximum Contaminant Level Goals established under the Safe Drinking Water Act (50 FR 46880, November 13, 1985) and Water Quality Criteria (EPA 1980) established under the Clean Water Act." These additions to the list of applicable or relevant and appropriate requirements are not reflected in the PHEs completed before reauthorization of Superfund. However, even before reauthorization, consideration of a wide variety of other EPA requirements for the purpose of choosing and documenting a remedial action for a site was necessary. As a result of this policy and because of the interrelation between the Resource Conservation and Recovery Act (RCRA) and CERCLA programs, RCRA remedial standards for groundwater protection are expected to constitute the majority of applicable or relevant and appropriate requirements for Superfund response actions.

In choosing the final remedial alternative in the ROD process of risk management, a variety of other requirements may be applicable or relevant and appropriate. For example, PCB waste oils at the Laskin/Poplar Oil site in Jefferson, Ohio (EPA/ROD/RO8-9-84) [Superfund Record of Decision (SRD), 1984a] were removed and incinerated in compliance with 40 CFR 761 requirements for PCBs under the Toxic Substances Control Act (TSCA). At Triangle Chemical, Texas (EPA/ROD RO6-85-007) (SRD, 1985c), RCRA guidelines for tank closure, floodplain management under Executive Order 11988, and Clean Water Act MCLs were included in the analysis of remedies.

RCRA design and operating requirements are often the basis for remedies at Superfund sites. However, these requirements generally do not deal with the level of clean up; rather, they address appropriate methods for disposal of contamination found at CERCLA sites. RCRA addresses the design of waste piles, land treatment facilities, and landfills (40 CFR¶264, Subparts L, M, and N, respectively); the operation of incinerators and groundwater monitoring programs (40 CFR ¶ 264, Subparts O and F, respectively); and requirements for closure and post closure of facilities where CERCLA waste is disposed after remedial action (40 CFR ¶ 264, Subpart G). However, the design and operating requirements generally do not address how much removal is necessary at a site or when a site is "clean enough" to protect public health and the environment.

The Hocomonco Pond site in Massachusetts (EPA/ROD/R01-85) (SRD-1985f) provides an example of the application of RCRA design and operating requirements. Excavated sediments from a nearby pond and contaminated soil will be disposed of in an onsite facility built to RCRA standards. The onsite facility and a former lagoon at the site will be covered with one continuous cap designed to RCRA specifications. RCRA does not address how much soil or sediment must be removed. Ambient standards or risk assessment may be used for that determination. RCRA caps have also been chosen as part of the remedial action at the New Lyme site in Ohio (EPA/ROD/R09-27-85) (SRD, 1984b) to prevent further spread of wastes.

If applicable or relevant and appropriate requirements exist for all indicator chemicals, then the baseline analysis is complete by determining the extent to which chemicals exceed or fall short of their ambient requirements. The NCP requires the assessment of the extent to which federal environmental and public health requirements are applicable or relevant and appropriate to a specific site and the extent to which contamination levels exceed those requirements or other federal criteria, advisories, and guidance and state standards [40 CFR 300.68(e) (2) (xii–xiii)]. The degree to which the remedial alternative that is ultimately selected attains or does not attain applicable or relevant and appropriate requirements is discussed below in the section on Evaluating Remedial Alternatives.

Even in those situations where applicable or relevant and appropriate requirements are available for all the indicator chemicals, reliance on these requirements alone may be insufficient to assess potential risks at Superfund sites for many reasons, including the following: (i) the requirements may not be health based (e.g., MCLs are required by law to assess technological and economic feasibility as well as health effects); (ii) relevant requirements may not exist (e.g., soil contamination) or may be limited in number (e.g., ambient air quality standards); (iii) the requirements may be based on dated or obsolete toxicity information; (iv) the requirements address contamination within an individual medium rather than on a multimedia approach; and (v) the requirements address exposure to single chemicals rather than chemical mixtures.

For some Superfund sites applicable or relevant and appropriate requirements may not exist for the selected indicator chemicals and exposure pathways or media of concern. In those situations a public health evaluation will consist of a comparison of the expected environmental concentrations to the applicable or relevant and appropriate requirements for those indicators that have them, and a comparison to health-based advisory levels for the entire group of selected indicator chemicals. This latter comparison generally requires estimating human intake levels and comparing those levels to "acceptable" levels of exposure.

Estimating Human Intake

After estimating exposure point concentrations of specific chemicals through the relevant pathways, it is necessary to estimate the amount (in mg/kg·day) of a substance taken in by a person (e.g., inhalation, ingestion, dermal contact). Where exposure pathways are known or can be expected, standard assumptions about consumption of air, water, and soil are combined with representative concentrations (e.g., arithmetic or geometric mean, where appropriate) in various media to generate intake values. Human activity patterns that affect intake, such as fraction of time spent at the exposure point, are also considered. Reasonable intake assumptions should be developed if other human exposure pathways appear to be significant at the site.

The EPA has adopted or developed several standard intake assumptions for general use in public health evaluations. For adults, drinking water consumption is assumed to be 2 L/day, based on a survey of water consumption literature conducted by the National Academy of Sciences (NAS) (1977). They estimated that 1.63 L of water a day were consumed, based on review of nine articles. The higher value of 2 L/day was recommended by NAS to protect heavy water consumers (NAS, 1977). For children, drinking water consumption is assumed to be 1 L/day, assuming an average child body weight of 10 kg. EPA has estimated consumption of fresh water and estuarine fish to be 6.5 g/day. This value was determined as part of the ambient water quality criteria setting exercise under the Safe Drinking Water Act (USEPA, 1980). Some other standard assumptions such as the 70-kg human and air intake of 20 m^3 per 24-h day are based on other surveys and have been adopted as standard assumptions by the EPA (USEPA, 1980). Human activity patterns, such as fraction of time spent at the exposure point, are also considered and may be used to adjust intake values for specific sites.

Other human exposure pathways may be significant at a site. For example, intake of vegetables was considered at the Coleman-Evans site where there was a potential risk from consumption of contaminated vegetables. Dermal contact and subsequent inadvertent ingestion of soil has been considered at several sites, including Davis Liquids in Rhode Island, Anaconda in Montana, and Times Beach in Missouri. This exposure results from a person's hands coming in contact with contaminated soil and carrying it into the mouth while eating or smoking cigarettes. Several researchers have investigated this exposure route and quantified soil intakes (Kimbrough et al., 1984; Hawley, 1985; Paustenbach et al., 1986; Calabrese, 1987). Their assumptions and results are quite different and the risk assessors performing the PHEs must weigh the relevance of the assumptions made by the researchers with the conditions at the particular site.

Exposure assessments must also consider the presence of population groups with high sensitivity to chemical exposure. Sensitive subpopulations that may be at higher risk include infants and children, elderly people, pregnant women, and people with chronic illnesses. Sites may be located in areas without readily identifiable sensitive subpopulations, but if such groups are present, the number of people involved and their proximity to the point of exposure should be determined.

The most common example of a sensitive subpopulation is children. This sensitivity is due both to increased sensitivity of children to chemicals, such as lead, and their tendency to ingest soil by normal mouthing of soiled objects or by pica (direct consumption of soil and dust). These exposure routes may be primary exposure routes at sites with contaminated soil material. Children as a sensitive subpopulation have been important at mine tailing sites that are contaminated with lead because children are especially susceptible to irreversible brain damage and learning disabilities resulting from exposure to lead. At both the Smuggler Mountain site in Colorado (EPA/ROD/R08-86-005) (SRD, 1986) and the Mill Creek site in Montana remedial alternatives were selected to protect children from lead exposure.

Evaluating Toxicity and Characterizing Risk

The next step in the process is to evaluate the toxicity associated with each chemical. For many chemicals found at Superfund sites, toxicological data have been evaluated by the EPA and reference doses (RfDs) for noncarcinogenic effects and cancer potency factors for potential carcinogens have been developed (USEPA, 1987). The reference doses are developed based on a survey of current toxicological literature including animal studies and human epidemiology studies. No observed adverse effect levels (NOAELs) were determined from those studies in the literature. No observed effect levels (NOELs) and lowest effect level (LEL) are also determined if data are sufficient.

Illustrative Example: Bromomethane.   An animal study conducted by Irish et al. (1940) was considered appropriate for determining a NOAEL. In this study, researchers exposed rats, rabbits, guinea pigs, and monkeys to bromomethane by inhalation for 7.5–8 h/day, 5 days/week for 6 months or until the majority of the animals had died or exhibited severe reactions. Variable numbers of animals were exposed to bromomethane concentrations of 17, 33, 66, 100, or 200 ppm. The highest NOAELs were estimated to be 17 ppm (3.8 mg/kg·day) for rabbits, 33 ppm for monkeys, 66 ppm for rats, and 100 ppm for guinea pigs. Rabbits exposed to 33 ppm (7.4 mg/kg·day) and higher concentrations developed pulmonary damage and paralysis. Monkeys also developed paralysis, and guinea pigs and rats exhibited various types of lung pathology. Rabbits were the most sensitive to bromomethane toxicity in this study; the NOAEL and LOAEL were determined to be 3.8 and 7.4 mg/kg·day, respectively. Concentrations were converted to doses for animal inhalation data using the following equation modified from USEPA (1980):

$$NOAEL = 65 \text{ mg/m}^3 \times 2.0 \text{ m}^3/\text{day} \times 7.5 \text{ h}/24 \text{ h} \times 5 \text{ days}/7 \text{ days} \times 0.5/3.8 \text{ kg}$$

$$= 3.8 \text{ mg/kg·day}.$$

To the NOAEL, uncertainty factors and modifying factors were added to determine the EPA reference dose (RfD). Three factors of 10 were used to convert the NOAEL for bromomethane to a human reference dose, which account for extrapolation from animal data, use of a subchronic assay to determine a chronic reference dose, and for protection of sensitive human subpopulations. An additional modifying factor of 10 was also used because of both the low number of test animals at the NOAEL and because of the marked severity of effect at the LEL. A determination of confidence in the RfD is also made. In this case low confidence was put in the study, the data, and the RfD because the study indicated no control animals, no statistical analysis was performed on the data, and limited human exposure data were available.

Illustrative Example: Carbaryl. The critical study for the development of the RfD for carbaryl is Carpenter et al. (1961). Carbaryl was fed to groups of 20 CF-N rats per sex at concentrations of 0, 50, 100, 200, and 400 ppm of diet for 2 years. Food consumption and body weight records were maintained. Interim sacrifices (4–8 animals) from concurrent auxiliary groups were performed at 6, 9, and 12 months for organ weight comparisons and histopathological analysis. Hematological analyses were done at irregular intervals throughout the study. Surviving animals were sacrificed at 2 years with gross and histopathological examinations performed. Slight histopathological changes in the kidneys and liver were reported at the high-dose level. Diffuse cloudy swelling of renal tubules was observed at 1 and 2 years. A statistically significant increase in cloudy swelling of the hepatic cords was also observed after 2 years. Based on body weight and food consumption data, the lowest observed adverse effect level (LOAEL) of 400 ppm was converted to an equivalent dose of 15.6 mg/kg·day. The NOAEL established was 9.6 mg/kg·day. An uncertainty factor of 100 was applied to the NOAEL to account for interspecies and intraspecies variations. No modifying factor was necessary because of the high quality of the critical study. The RfD was set at 0.1 mg/kg·day.

A process similar to the RfD development has also been used to determine the critical toxicity values for subchronic and chronic exposures for the Health Effects Assessments (HEA) documents developed by the EPA (USEPA, 1986a).

For risk characterization, these acceptable levels are compared to estimated intake levels for potentially exposed individuals. Multiple chemical exposures are assessed using an approach based on the EPA's *"Guidelines for Health Risk Assessment of Chemical Mixtures"* (USEPA, 1986d). This approach results in the calculation of a *hazard index* and assumes that multiple, subthreshold exposures may result in an adverse effect and that these effects are additive. This approach encourages consideration of the cumulative "insult" from a number of chemicals that induce the same health effect. The final risk assessment includes both an indication of potential risk from the mixture as well as a chemical-by-chemical comparison of estimated intake levels with acceptable intake levels.

Illustrative Example: Hazard Index. In this hypothetical example residents near a Superfund site are exposed to several chemicals in their drinking water supply. The chronic daily intake (CDI) and the acceptable chronic intake levels (AIC) have been determined for the indicator chemicals at this site (Table 6). The route specific CDI:AIC ratios are calculated for each chemical. To determine the overall hazard index the total (inhalation and oral) CDI:AIC ratios are summed. In this example, the hazard index equals the sum of the oral CDI:AIC (1.0) and the inhalation CDI:AIC (4.9) or 5.9. In general, if the total is less than 1, there is probably no chronic health hazard. If the sum is greater than 1, as in this example, there is the potential for a chronic health hazard.

EVALUATING CARCINOGENS

For carcinogens, upper-bound carcinogenic potency factors have been developed by the EPA's Carcinogen Assessment Group. The potency factors are expressed as the lifetime cancer risk per mg/kg body weight per day. This factor is an estimated upper 95% confidence limit on the carcinogenic potency of the chemical. Cancer potency factors, in combination with estimated intake levels, are used to calculate upper-bound confidence

TABLE 6. Calculation of Chronic Hazard Index[a]

	Inhalation			Oral		
Chemical	CDI	AIC	CDI:AIC	CDI	AIC	CDI:AIC
Cadmium	—	—	—	0.00014	0.00029	0.48
Ethylbenzene	0.35	0.1	3.5	0.005	0.1	0.058
Xylenes	0.58	0.4	1.4	0.0046	0.01	0.46

[a]Sum of inhalation CDI:AIC = 4.9; sum of oral CDI:AIC = 1.0; sum of all ratios = 5.9.

TABLE 7. Calculation of Risk from Potential Carcinogens

Chemical	Exposure Route	CDI (mg/kg·day)	Carcinogenic Potency Factor (mg/kg·day)$^{-1}$	Route-Specific Risk
Bis(2-chloro-ethyl)ether	Oral	6.4×10^{-4}	1.1	7.0×10^{-4}
Chloroform	Oral	1.1×10^{-2}	8.1×10^{-4}	8.9×10^{-4}
			Total upper-bound Risk = 1.6×10^{-3}	

limits on carcinogenic risks. The EPA's guidelines for mixtures permit "risk additivity" to be used for carcinogens. This procedure allows a total upper-bound carcinogenic risk to be estimated by summing the risks posed by individual indicator chemicals.

Illustrative Example: Calculation of Risk from Potential Carcinogens. In this hypothetical example, bis(2-chloroethyl)ether and chloroform were detected in the drinking water supply of residents near a Superfund site. Chronic daily intakes (CDIs) were estimated from sampling data, and the carcinogenic potency factors obtained from the EPA IRIS data base (USEPA, 1987; Table 7). Route-specific risk values were estimated for each chemical by multiplying the potency factor by the CDI. For example, the route-specific risk value for chloroform of 8.9×10^{-4} was determined by multiplying the potency factor $(8.1 \times 10^{-2}$ mg/kg·day) by the CDI $(1.1 \times 10^{-2}$ g/kg·day). The chemical-specific risks of bis(2-chloroethyl)ether (7.0×10^{-4}) and chloroform (8.9×10^{-4}) were summed to give an upper-bound estimate of total incremental risk of 1.6×10^{-3}.

Carcinogenic risk tends to dominate the risk at most Superfund sites. This may be due in part to the exceedingly low environmental levels of chemical carcinogens that are believed necessary to ensure protection of human health. In a survey of 34 site PHEs conducted in the development of this chapter, 12 carcinogens [primarily Class A–human carcinogens and Class B–probable carcinogens, based on the EPA classification system (USEPA, 1986b)] were found as contaminants in the groundwater at the 20 sites having contaminated groundwater. Table 8 lists these carcinogens and the concentrations and risks associated with them. Only groundwater that is or could potentially be used as a drinking water supply was considered in this table because it is the most frequently contaminated media that is associated with the overall highest individual risks. The frequency of appearance in this survey refers to the number of times that a chemical was found as a contaminant in groundwater at a site, and its presence posed a potential threat to human health. Trichloroethylene was found in groundwater at 10 sites, almost one-third of the sites examined in the survey, and one-half of those sites with polluted groundwater. Benzene and vinyl chloride were also commonly found as groundwater contaminants.

The mean concentrations and individual risks for both "worst" (based on maximum groundwater concentration values) and "realistic" (based on mean groundwater concentration values) cases are presented in Table 8. Chemical concentrations are averaged only for those sites where elevated levels of contamination were observed. For example, arsenic was reported in groundwater at four sites. Mean concentrations were determined by averaging concentration values for those sites having data only; no zeros were averaged for those sites not reported to have arsenic. The chemical-specific cancer risks from groundwater ingestion were averaged across the 34 sites at which that chemical was

TABLE 8. Environmental Concentrations and Projected Lifetime Carcinogenic Risks for Hazardous Substances Detected in Groundwater at 34 Abandoned Hazardous Waste Sites: Values Averaged for All Sites Having that Chemical

Chemical	Frequency of Appearance[a]	Maximum Concentration (μg/L)	Maximum Individual Risk	Mean Concentration (μg/L)	Mean Individual Risk
Trichloroethylene	10	40,000	2×10^{-2}	20,000	1×10^{-2}
Vinyl chloride	9	5,500	2×10^{-1}	1,400	1×10^{-1}
Benzene	9	1,622	3×10^{-3}	280	3×10^{-4}
Tetrachloroethylene	6	12,000	2×10^{-2}	1,050	1×10^{-3}
Arsenic	4	95	2×10^{-2}	9.8	4×10^{-3}
1,2-Dichloroethane	4	9,000	2×10^{-2}	81	2×10^{-3}
Chloroform	3	2,800	7×10^{-3}	98	2×10^{-4}
PCBs	3	27	3×10^{-3}	4.0	1×10^{-3}
1,1-Dichloroethene	3	72	2×10^{-4}	5.6	2×10^{-5}
Methylene chloride	2	1.2×10^{6}	4×10^{-2}	53,000	8×10^{-4}
1,1,2-Trichloroethane	2	1,500	3×10^{-3}	23	3×10^{-4}
N-Nitrosodiphenylamine	2	90	9×10^{-7}	NR[b]	8×10^{-7}

[a]Out of a total of 34 Superfund Public Health Evaluations (PHEs). Superfund sites presented in Table 1.
[b]Mean (or representative) concentrations not reported in PHEs.

reported. Individual cancer risk values for the realistic case scenario ranged from 0.1 for vinyl chloride to 8×10^{-7} for N-nitrosodiphenylamine.

Uncertainties in Quantitative Assessments

All estimates of risk are dependent on numerous assumptions and many uncertainties that are inherent in the risk assessment process. As a result, in any evaluation of the level of risk associated with a site, it is necessary to address the level of confidence, or the uncertainty associated with the estimated level of risk.

Uncertainties are associated with both the toxicity information (e.g., hazard identification and dose–response assessment) used to establish acceptable levels of exposure, as well as the exposure assessment information used to estimate the actual or projected exposure levels for populations associated with the release of hazardous substances. Most toxicity information is derived from animal studies, for example, and reputable scientists may disagree on how to interpret these data in terms of potential human health effects. A single toxicity parameter based on an animal study does not convey the route of administration of test doses of the suspect chemicals, the organ(s) in which the response occurred, or the severity of endpoints in the animal experiment used to calculate the dose–response relation. Consequently, extrapolation to humans is a source of uncertainty. Many toxicity studies are done at high doses relative to exposures associated with waste disposal sites; extrapolation from high to low doses also increases the uncertainty of risk estimates. Exposure modeling is based on many simplifying assumptions that add to the uncertainty. Often the quality or quantity of site-specific chemical monitoring data may be limited. The additivity of toxicant risks and the additivity of doses of the same toxicant from different exposure routes are additional assumptions and additional sources of uncertainty. Consequently, those factors that may significantly increase the uncertainty of the risk assessment results should be identified and addressed in a qualitative and, if possible, quantitative manner.

EVALUATING REMEDIAL ALTERNATIVES

Once the baseline evaluation is completed, information about chemical releases, routes of exposure, human exposure points, and the level and timing of risk can be used to develop and refine proposed remedial alternatives. Remedies may include containment of wastes; removal of wastes for incineration, landfill, or treatment; provision of alternate water supplies; or institutional barriers to exposure, such as deed restrictions. A combination of these or other alternatives may be chosen as the remedy at a site depending on the needs at a specific site.

Remedies must be evaluated for the extent to which they attain applicable or relevant and appropriate environmental requirements. These standards may be design and operating requirements, such as certain landfill, liner, and cover requirements under RCRA, or they may define allowable ambient concentration levels for specific chemicals. In the absence of applicable or relevant and appropriate design requirements, design standards may vary depending on the type of remedial alternative.

Ultimately, remedial alternatives under consideration are analyzed with respect to public health and environmental protection, consistency with applicable or relevant and appropriate requirements, technical feasibility, and cost; and one alternative is selected. The NCP requires that the chosen remedy mitigate and minimize threats to and provide adequate protection to public health and the environment. The remedy providing that level of protection at the least cost will most likely be the chosen remedy. Consideration of cost is one of the important inputs to the risk management decision. For example, at the Jibboom Junkyard site in California (EPA/ROD RO9-85-008 and as amended on October 4, 1985) (SRD, 1985a), excavation and offsite disposal at a RCRA approved hazardous waste disposal facility was chosen as the selected alternative because it reduced soil lead concentrations to below 500 ppm. Removal was chosen over capping, a lower-cost alternative, because of threat of possible groundwater contamination should groundwater levels in the area rise. However, providing alternate water sources to replace contaminated wells was chosen as the remedial action at the Matthews Electroplating site in Roanoke, Virginia (ROD, 6-2-83) (SRD, 1983). This option represented the cost-effective remedy that was protective of public health and the environment. Additional action at the site (i.e., capping) was determined to be unnecessary because it provided no additional public health or environmental protection for the additional expenditure. At the McKin site in Maine (EPA/ROD RO1-85-009) (SRD, 1985d) contaminated soil will be cleaned up to levels that are protective of the ground water and other potential routes of exposure. Groundwater monitoring will be conducted to ensure no migration of contaminants during the remedial activity.

Source control options control or remove the source of contamination before it has migrated much beyond the site. These options are designed based on applicable or relevant and appropriate requirements. RCRA design and operating standards will generally be relevant, especially for source control options that result in containment of wastes. Applicable or relevant and appropriate requirements from RCRA may include requirements for land treatment, landfills, or incinerators (40 CFR 264.270–264.299, 264.300–264.339, 264.340–264.999), respectively. Other RCRA guidance and technical documents listed in 50 *Fed. Reg.* 47,950 may also be pertinent and should be considered. When applicable or relevant and appropriate requirements are unavailable, design of remedial alternatives is based on best engineering judgment. However, when source control options involve partial removal of contamination, best engineering judgment cannot help define how far to excavate what levels are allowable for residual chemicals. In these situations, a risk-based approach using target risk levels and toxicity values is used to help define performance goals for source control options.

For source control options that are designed based on best engineering judgment, there is still a requirement to consider the public health consequences of selecting those alternatives. The public health evaluation process requires that the investigator review detailed technical analyses completed for source control measures so that public health consequences of technology failure may be considered.

Management of migration options address contaminants that have migrated away from the source. These options are also designed based on applicable or relevant and appropriate requirements. When requirements are unavailable for all chemicals of interest, a risk-based approach is used. Remedial alternatives should be refined as necessary to ensure that options considered by the site manager are within a carcinogenic risk range of 10^{-4}–10^{-7}. The exact carcinogenic risk level chosen for a site will depend on a variety of factors including other environmental health factors borne by the affected population (i.e., other exposures to known air, water, or other pollutants creating a high-risk load), level of uncertainty in the data and models used in risk analysis, the expected effectiveness and reliability of manufactured systems affecting exposure (e.g., slurry walls, pumping wells), current and expected future use of the affected resource, and impacts on the environment at any surface water to which the plume will discharge. It may also be useful to determine the affected population. Regardless of what risk level is chosen, experience indicates that the health risk from potential carcinogens generally drives the development of performance goals for remedial alternatives. If noncarcinogens are present, the remedy should be designed to achieve not only the acceptable carcinogenic risk level but also the chronic and subchronic acceptable intake levels for the noncarcinogens.

Within the carcinogenic risk range of 10^{-4}–10^{-7}, the 10^{-6} carcinogenic risk is often chosen as the target risk level to be achieved by the remedial action. The following examples describe sites where a 10^{-6} risk level was chosen and others where different cleanup targets were chosen. At the Reilly Tar site, St. Louis Park, Minnesota (EPA/ROD/RO6-6-84) (SRD, 1985b) the ROD specifies that the 10^{-6} cancer risk level for polyaromatic hydrocarbons, the chemicals of chief concern at the site, be chosen as the goal for cleanup of a contaminated aquifer. The most cost-effective and technically feasible alternative meeting that goal was selected. In other situations other values in the risk range may ultimately be chosen for the remedial action. For example, at the McKin site in Gray, Maine (EPA/ROD/RO1-85-009) (SRD, 1985d) a 10^{-5} lifetime statistical cancer risk level was chosen for trichloroethylene, the chemical of highest concern, because of relatively low levels of uncertainty regarding levels of contamination in the affected aquifer following 5 years of monitoring, no known regular human use of the contaminated aquifer, consideration of natural attenuation mechanisms, and consideration of the effect of remedial action at the site.

The 10^{-5} cancer risk level was also chosen for groundwater at the Old Mill, Ohio site (EPA/ROD R05-85-018) (SRD, 1985c) because that level can be reached with 30 years of treatment, whereas the 10^{-6} cancer risk level will not be reached for 100 years. Background may be chosen as the cleanup level as was the case at Triangle Chemical in Texas (EPA/ROD/R06-85-007) (SRD, 1985c).

In addition to addressing the long-term health effects at a site, short-term effects of implementation must also be considered for all remedial alternatives. For example, it may be important to consider inhalation risks to nearby residents if installation of a particular technology involves substantial excavation and dust generation. This evaluation may be qualitative or quantitative and is used to develop management practices to control releases during construction.

Overall, the public health evaluation of remedial alternatives is an iterative process that involves refining the design of specific remedies. A risk-based approach for controlling releases can usually demonstrate that one or two chemicals in the mixture are responsible for most of the risk. These chemicals actually drive the risk assessment, and therefore drive the performance goals for remedial alternatives. Once these chemicals are sufficiently controlled, the risks from other chemicals in the mixture are likely to be negligible in comparison.

SUMMARY

In a review of the site-specific risk assessments that have been conducted by the EPA Superfund program, some general conclusions can be drawn. First, out of a wide array of possible exposure pathways (e.g., inhalation of volatilized contaminants, ingestion of contaminated soil, dermal contact) ingestion of contaminated groundwater is considered to pose the greatest risk to human health. Second, despite the presence of literally hundreds of hazardous substances found at Superfund sites, experience suggests that the majority of the risk associated with these sites is due to a few hazardous substances. Third, conservative assumptions are frequently used in the exposure and toxicity assessments (e.g., lifetime exposure, upper-bound potency estimates). However, decisions based on the use of conservative assumptions do not necessarily result in overly protective remedies. The science on which risk assessments are based is typically not sufficient to allow consideration of synergistic effects among hazardous substances, or all the potential health endpoints, or more than a fraction of the universe of hazardous substances that might pose some risk. Finally, risk assessment is an essential tool used by the EPA to address the risks to human health resulting from environmental releases of hazardous substances.

These conclusions are supported by a recent study of the Executive Scientific Panel of the Universities Associated for Research and Education in Pathology (Grisham, 1986). They conclude that while demonstrable effects may not have resulted unequivocally from exposure to chemicals released at hazardous waste sites, significant uncertainties and inherent scientific difficulties complicate these analyses. Lack of causal association between health effects and chemical exposures does not mean that such effects are not present. They also agree that the potential hazard to human health presented by many sites is significant and that monitoring of emissions, investigation of potential health risks, and site remediation should continue in order to prevent potential threats from becoming human health and environmental impairments.

Although risk assessment is an important tool for agency decisionmaking, the EPA recognizes the limitations and uncertainties associated with quantitative risk assessments and has undertaken several efforts to address these. For example, the EPA has developed guidelines for the assessment of different health endpoints, including carcinogenicity (USEPA, 1986b), mutagenicity (USEPA, 1986c), and developmental toxicity (USEPA, 1986e). Guidelines have also been developed to evaluate the effects of chemical mixtures (USEPA, 1986d) and for exposure assessments (USEPA, 1986f). In addition to these guidelines, the EPA has also established procedures for conducting site-specific risk assessments. Together, these efforts will foster consistency of approach on a nationwide basis, establish a standard for quality work, and help inform the public about how scientific judgments and assumptions have been incorporated into the risk assessment process.

The guidance development efforts of EPA assist in formulating the science policy basis of risk assessment; however, additional research efforts are also needed to address the uncertainties in quantitative assessments. As a result of the Superfund Amendments and Reauthoriztion Act of 1986, Superfund resources can be used to conduct hazardous substances research. This has enhanced EPA research efforts and will broaden our understanding not only of the physicochemical properties and behavior of hazardous substances in the environment but also of how hazardous substances cause adverse health effects. In addition to EPA research efforts, other Superfund research efforts include those of the Agency for Toxic Substances and Disease Registry of the Department of Health and Human Services (e.g., epidemiological studies at Superfund sites) and the National Toxicology Program (e.g., toxicity testing of Superfund hazardous substances). These efforts are all part of a growing effort to improve the scientific basis of risk assessment.

REFERENCES

Briggs, G. G., Bromilow, R. H., and Evans, A. A. (1982). Relationship between lipophilicity and root uptake and translation of non-ionized chemicals by barley. *Pestic. Sci.* **13**, 495–504.

Burns, L. A., Cline, D. M., and Lassiter, R. R. (1982). *Exposure Analysis Modeling System*

(EXAMS) Users Manual and System Documentation, EPA-600/3-82-023. Environmental Research Laboratory, Office of Research and Development, U.S. Environmental Protection Agency, Athens, GA.

Calabrese, E. (1987). A Quantitative Evaluation of the Amount of Soil Ingested by Toddlers. A report by the School of Public Health, University of Masschusetts, Amherst.

Carpenter, C. P., Weil, C. W., and Polin, P. E. (1961). Mammalian toxicity of 1-Naphthayl-N-methylcarbamate (seven insecticide). J. Agric. Food Chem. **9**, 30–39.

Cowherd, C., Jr., Muleski, G. E., Englehart, P. J., and Gillette, P. A. (1985). Rapid Assessment of Exposure to Particulate Emissions from Surface Contamination Sites. Office of Health and Environmental Assessment, U.S. Environmental Protection Agency, Washington, DC.

Farmer, W. J., Yang, M. S., and Feffey, J. (1980). Land Disposal of Hexachlorobenzene Wastes: Controlling Vapor Movement in Soils, EPA 600/7-80-119. U.S. Environmental Protection Agency, Washington, DC.

General Accounting Office (GAO) (1985). Cleaning Up Hazardous Waste: An Overview of Superfund Reauthorization Issues, GAO/RCED-85-69. GAO, Washington DC.

Grisham, J. W. (Ed.) (1986). Health Aspects of the Disposal of Waste Chemicals. Pergamon Press, New York.

Hanna, S. R., Briggs, G. A., and Hosker, R. P., Jr. (1982). Handbook on Atmospheric Diffusion. Atmospheric Turbulence and Diffusion Laboratory, National Oceanic and Atmospheric Administration, U.S. Department of Energy, Oak Ridge, TN.

Hawley, J. K. (1985). Assessment of health risk from exposure to contaminated soil. Risk Anal. **5**, 289–302.

Hayes, D. J., and MacKerron, C. B. (1987). Superfund II. A new mandate. A bureau of national affairs special report. Environ. Rep. **17**(42), 13.

Hazardous Site Control Division (1985). Superfund Record of Decision Update. Hocomonco Pond, MA. (approved September 30, 1985). U.S. Environmental Protection Agency, Vol. 1, No. 8. Washington, DC.

Irish, D. D., Adams, E. M., Spencer, H. C., and Rowe, V. K. (1940). The response attending exposure of laboratory animals to vapors to methyl bromide. J. Ind. Hyg. Toxicol. **22**, 218–230.

Kimbrough, R. D., Falk, H., Stehr, P., and Fries, G. (1984). Health implications of 2, 3, 7, 8-tetrachlorodibenzodioxin (TCDD) contamination of residential soil. J. Toxicol Environ. Health **14**, 47–93.

Lyman, W. S., Reehl, W. F., and Rosenblatt, D. H. (1982). Handbook of Chemical Property Estimation Methods. McGraw-Hill, New York.

National Academy of Sciences (NAS) (1977). Drinking Water and Health. National Research Council, Washington, DC.

Office of Technology Assessment (OTA) (1985). Superfund Strategy, OTA-ITE-252. OTA, Washington DC.

Patterson, M. R., Sworski, T. J., and Sjoreen, A. L. (1982). User's Manual for UTM-TOX, a Unified Transport Model (draft report), ORNL-TM-8182. Oak Ridge National Laboratory, Oak Ridge, TN: (IEG-AD-89-F-1-3999-0).

Paustenbach, D. J., Shu, H. P., and Murray, F. J. (1986). A critical examination of assumptions used in risk assessments of dioxin contaminated soil. Regul. Toxicol. Pharmacol. **6**, 284–307.

Shen, T. T. (1982). Air quality assessment for land disposal of industrial waste. Environ. Manage. **6**, 297–305.

Superfund Record of Decision (SRD) (1983). Matthews Electroplating, VA. (EPA/ROD/RO3-83) U.S. Environmental Protection Agency, Washington, DC (NTIS No. PB85 213841/AS).

Superfund Record of Decision (SRD) (1983a). Burnt Fly Bog, NJ. (EPA/ROD/RO2-83/002) U.S. Environmental Protection Agency, Washington, DC (NTIS No. PB85 213676/AS).

Superfund Record of Decision (SRD) (1984a). Laskin/Poplar Oil, OH (EPA/ROD/RO8-9-84). U.S. Environmental Protection Agency, Washington, DC (NTIS No. PB85 213924/AS).

Superfund Record of Decision (SRD) (1984b). New Lyme, OH (EPA/ROD/RO9-27-85). U.S. Environmental Protection Agency, Washington, DC (NTIS No. PB85 133907/AS).

Superfund Record of Decision (SRD) (1985a). Jibboom Junkyard, CA (EPA/ROD/RO9-85-008). U.S. Environmental Protection Agency, Washington, DC (NTIS No. PB85 229094/AS).

Superfund Record of Decision (SRD) (1985b). Reilly Tar, MN (EPA/ROD/RO6-6-84). U.S. Environmental Protection Agency, Washington, DC (NTIS No. PB85 213965/AS).

Superfund Record of Decision (SRD) (1985c). Triangle Chemical, TX (EPA/ROD/RO6-85-007). U.S. Environmental Protection Agency, Washington, DC (NTIS No. PB85 249530/AS).

Superfund Record of Decision (SRD) (1985d). McKin Site, ME (EPA/ROD/RO1-85-009). U.S. Environmental Protection Agency, Washington, DC (NTIS No. PB85 249639/AS).

Superfund Record of Decision (SRD) (1985e). Old Mill, OH (EPA/ROD/RO5-85-018). U.S. Environmental Protection Agency, Washington, DC (NTIS No. PB85 249647/AS).

Superfund Record of Decision (SRD) (1985f). Hocomonco Pond, MA (EPA/ROD/R01-85) U.S. Environmental Protection Agency, Washington, DC (NTIS No. PB86 172400/AS).

Superfund Record of Decision (SRD) (1986). Smuggler Mountain, CO (EPA/ROD/RO8-86-005). U.S. Environmental Protection Agency, Washington, DC (NTIS No. PB87 189908/AS).

Turner, D. B. (1970). *Workbook of Atmospheric Dispersion Estimates*, NTIS 8B-191-482. U.S. Department of Health, Education, and Welfare, Cincinnati, OH.

U.S. Environmental Protection Agency (USEPA) (1980). Water quality criteria documents: Availability. *Fed. Regist.* **45**, 79318–79379.

U.S. Environmental Protection Agency (USEPA) (1985a). *Guidance on Remedial Investigations Under CERCLA*, EPA/540/G-85/002. Office of Emergency and Remedial Response, USEPA, Washington, DC.

U.S. Environmental Protection Agency (USEPA) (1985b). *Guidance on Feasibility Studies Under CERCLA*, EPA/540/G-85/003. Office of Emergency and Remedial Response, USEPA, Washington, DC.

U.S. Environmental Protection Agency (USEPA) (1985c). Reportable quantity adjustments. *Fed. Regist.* **50**, 13514–13522.

U.S. Environmental Protection Agency (USEPA) (1986a). *Superfund Public Health Evaluation Manual*, EPA 540/1-86/060. Office of Emergency and Remedial Response, USEPA, Washington, DC.

U.S. Environmental Protection Agency (USEPA) (1986b). Guidelines for carcinogenic risk assessment. *Fed. Regist.* **51**, 33992–34003.

U.S. Environmental Protection Agency (USEPA) (1986c). Guidelines for mutagenicity risk assessment. *Fed. Regist.* **51**, 34006–34012.

U.S. Environmental Protection Agency (USEPA) (1986d). Guidelines for the health risk assessment of chemical mixtures. *Fed. Regist.* **51**, 34014–34025.

U.S. Environmental Protection Agency (USEPA) (1886e). Guidelines for the health assessment of suspect developmental toxicants. *Fed. Regist.* **51**, 34028–34040.

U.S. Environmental Protection Agency (USEPA) (1986f). Guidelines for exposure assessment. *Fed. Regist.* **51**, 34042–34054.

U.S. Environmental Protection Agency (USEPA) (1986g). *National Screening Survey of Hazardous Waste Treatment, Storage, and Disposal and Recycling Facilities*, Summary of Results for TSDR Facilities Active in 1985. USEPA, Washington, DC.

U.S. Environmental Protection Agency (USEPA) (1987). *Integrated Risk Information System*, EPA 600/8-86/032a. USEPA, Washington, DC.

U.S. Environmental Protection Agency (USEPA) (1988). *Superfund Exposure Assessment Manual*, OSWER Directive NO: 9285.5–1. Office of Emergency and Remedial Response, USEPA, Washington, DC.

Yeh, G. T. (1981). *AT123D, Analytical Transient One-, Two-, and Three-Dimensional Simulation of Waste Transport in the Aquifer System*, Environ. Sci. Div. Publ. No. 1939 (ORNL-5601). Oak Ridge National Laboratory, Oak Ridge, TN.

Zamuda, C. D. (1986). The superfund record of decision process: Part 1. The role of risk assessment. *Chem. Waste Litigation Rep.* **11**, 847–859.

7

A Comprehensive Methodology for Assessing the Risks to Humans and Wildlife Posed by Contaminated Soils: A Case Study Involving Dioxin*

Dennis J. Paustenbach
McLaren Environmental Engineering, Chem Risk Division, Alameda, California

INTRODUCTION

Millions of yards of soil throughout the United States have been contaminated with numerous types of liquid and solid wastes containing metals, radioactive materials, gasoline, solvents, used oils, sludges and aqueous wastes. The potential environmental hazards due to contamination of runoff water, pollution of groundwater, as well as the resulting possible adverse effects on biota, fish, and wildlife have been studied for a number of years (1, 2). The potential hazards posed by contaminated soil have received less study (3–12). In light of the thousands of hazardous waste sites that have been identified in the United States alone and the presence of contaminated soil in residential areas, a scientifically valid and generalized approach to evaluating the human and environmental health risk is needed (10, 13).

Although the health hazards of living close to a hazardous waste site have been a concern during much of the past 10 years, in the main, epidemiology studies have not shown that these sites produce adverse health effects in humans who live near them (5, 12). Certainly, under some circumstances, soil contaminated with sufficiently high levels of particular toxicants could present a hazard to humans and wildlife but such situations appear to be uncommon.

Exposure to contaminated soil can occur through skin contact, inhalation, or ingestion. Although an important route of exposure, inhalation of contaminated dust, by itself, rarely represents a significant health hazard (10). Humans can be exposed as a result of their occupation, recreational activities, or through exposure in and around the home (14, 15). Occupational exposure to contaminated soil is normally limited to those who are

*This chapter is based in part on a paper that appeared in *Comments on Toxicology*, Vol. 1, pp. 185–220. Portions are reprinted with permission of Gordon & Breach Publishers, London.

involved in the remediation of hazardous waste sites (16–19). Exposure of persons within the community can occur through the inhalation of dust derived from soil at a contaminated site, through accidental uptake via the ingestion of dust from hand-to-mouth-contact due to poor hygienic practices, and through dermal absorption of contaminated soil that has fallen out of the air onto the skin, that is, through, deposition (3, 9, 10). The direct ingestion of contaminated soil by adults is generally not a concern since most adults do not intentionally eat dirt. The ingestion of soil by children, ages 2–6, who have mouthing tendencies needs to be considered in any risk assessment; but generally toddlers do not have access to hazardous waste sites. When soil within a residential area is contaminated, its ingestion by toddlers is almost certainly the primary hazard (3, 6, 7, 13, 45).

Although some have claimed that it is difficult or impossible to estimate—either prospectively or retrospectively—the dermal, inhalation, and oral uptake of chemicals to which humans have been exposed in the environment or at work, there appears to be little basis for these claims. Admittedly, it is true that there are varying degrees of uncertainty in the estimates of likely exposure; however, there is no reason why a reasonably accurate approximation cannot be made using currently available data. In an attempt to evaluate the magnitude of the health hazard, estimates of exposure and the subsequent systemic absorption have been made for (i) pesticide applicators (20–26), (ii) children exposed to lead via dust and dirt (27–54), (iii) workers exposed to vapors and dusts (55–57), (iv) vegetation, wildlife, and humans exposed to nuclear fallout (58–61), (v) persons involved in accidental chemical releases (62), and (vi) those exposed in Vietnam (63–66) have been conducted. Each of these studies contains information that is useful for developing exposure estimates for nearly any situation.

The work conducted to date should contain a sufficient amount of information to develop exposure estimates that are within a factor of 2–10-fold (too high or too low) of the actual exposure (65). These quantitative estimates should be much more valuable in understanding the potential health risks of an activity than such routinely used descriptions as small, moderate, or large! In contrast, estimates that contain approximately one order of magnitude of uncertainty should be valuable since they considerably, narrow the range of possible values for exposure, which could span as much as 14 orders of magnitude (0.0000000000001 g/kg·day to 5 g/kg·day). In light of the apparent acceptance of the uncertainties surrounding low-dose extrapolation models used to interpret cancer bioassays, which can vary by three to four orders of magnitude (depending on the model used and the bounding technique) (63, 64), the degree of uncertainty inherent in a high-quality exposure estimate should be acceptable for most situations.

Post hoc estimates of exposure can also be valuable in interpreting and conducting epidemiological studies. In this approach, observed adverse health effects in a population can be compared against the exposure levels, and a dose–response relation can be inferred. Certainly, the procedures that have been used in attempts to understand the risk to Vietnam veterans exposed to 2, 3, 7, 8-tetrachlorodibenzo-p-dioxin (TCDD) (63–66), agricultural workers exposed to pesticides (20–26), the citizens of Seveso exposed to TCDD (62), the residents of communities whose soil or buildings were contaminated by TCDD (3, 4, 6, 12), the residents of Hiroshima and Nagasaki following their exposure to radiation (69), the miners exposed to radon (140), and environmental uptake of cadmium (70) should be adequate to distinguish insignificant versus significant exposure.

Contaminated soil can pose not only a direct hazard to humans but also indirect hazards. For example, we know that some chemicals in the soil can leach into groundwater, as well as into streams via runoff (10, 15, 72–75). The contamination of

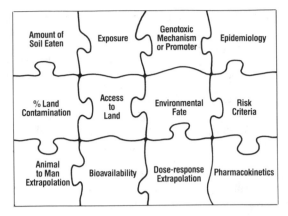

Figure 1. Environmental risk assessments of contaminated soil must consider a number of critical factors. To understand fully the risks, each of the factors, like the pieces of a puzzle, must be included. [From Paustenbach et al. (6) with modifications with permission from *Regulatory Toxicology and Pharmacology*.]

streams can pose a threat to wildlife, for example, birds, fish, deer, rabbits, and other species (73). This can be a genuine problem in areas where pesticides are incorrectly applied to farmland (74). In addition, some crops and vegetables can absorb the soil contaminant and enter the food chain.

Thus far, no U.S. federal regulatory agency has promulgated a standard for contaminated soil, but recent proposed regulations acknowledge the potential risks (76, 77). Only, five states have passed formal standards for contaminated soil while 18 others have informal clean-up levels. The Environmental Protection Agency (EPA) has suggested ways to assess the hazard posed by direct contact with contaminated soil (78, 79). The potential hazards posed by soil that has been sprayed or amended with sludges have recently received attention and approaches for evaluating it have been offered (8, 9, 80). Furthermore, contaminated soil often dictates the degree of necessary cleanup at Superfund sites. Usually, the existing land use or the use of legal restrictions to prevent certain future uses (e.g., pasture land, shopping center, industrial site, or residential area) will dictate the level of necessary cleanup.

This chapter discusses specific physical, physiological, and chemical parameters needed to estimate the uptake of a given chemical present in contaminated soil. Special emphasis is placed on the risk assessments of TCDD-contaminated soil, which were conducted by the Centers for Disease Control (CDC) (3) and, to a lesser degree, by the EPA (78), since they have become the benchmarks against which other assessments of contaminated soil are compared (4, 6, 7, 10). Alternative assumptions to those used in these assessments are discussed. Although there are many important factors to consider when evaluating the human health hazards posed by contaminated soil, this chapter addresses most of the critical ones (Fig. 1).

INGESTION OF SOIL BY CHILDREN

The exposure estimation procedure is perhaps the most important aspect of risk assessments of sites having contaminated soil. In the CDC's assessment of dioxin in soil (3),

TABLE 1. CDC Estimates of TCDD Uptake by Route of Exposure (1 ppb in Soil)

Route	Average Daily Dose (fg/kg·day)	Lifetime Uptake (%)
Ingestion of soil	606	95
Dermal uptake of soil	20	3
Uptake of soil inhaled	10	2

Source: Paustenbach et al. (6) with permission from *Regulatory Toxicology and Pharmacology.*

TABLE 2. Ingestion of Dirt^a (CDC Assumption)

Age Group	Soil Ingested (mg/day)	Lifetime Uptake (%)
0–9 months	0	0
9–18 months	1,000	2.6
1.5–3.5 years	10,000	70.0
3.5–5 years	1,000	5.2
5–70 years	100	22.6

^{a}Adjusted for seasonal variations.
Source: Paustenbach et al. (6) with permission from *Regulatory Toxicology and Pharmacology.*

their estimates indicated that the primary route of exposure for humans was soil ingestion (Table 1). The CDC predicted that, for a residential site containing soil contaminated with TCDD, about 95% of the average lifetime uptake of TCDD would occur as a result of soil ingestion; about 3% of the lifetime dose would be absorbed through the skin as a result of contact with contaminated soil (associated with gardening and poor hygiene); and no more than 2% of the total dose would be due to inhalation of TCDD-contaminated dust. Other environmental risk assessments (4, 6) have also indicated that soil ingestion by toddlers is the primary hazard in residential settings. Paustenbach (10) showed that for persons living 70 years in an area having TCDD-contaminated soil, inhalation was the predominant route of entry. For dioxin and other persistent chemicals, the primary hazard is the intake by fish of contaminated sediment from runoff and the ultimate ingestion of these fish by humans. For chemicals absorbed by plants, ingestion of vegetables would be another important exposure pathway.

In its calculations, the CDC assumed that 10,000 mg/day of soil would be ingested by children aged 1.5–3.5 years, and that during other periods ingestion would be much less, depending on age (Table 2). Persons between 5 and 10 years of age were assumed to ingest 1000 mg of soil per day, and those aged 17–70 were expected to ingest 101 mg/day through incidental exposure (3). If these assumptions are used, the resulting estimates indicate that about 80% of the entire lifetime dose of nonvolatile and non-water-soluble chemicals that are present in contaminated soil occurs during the first 5 years of life (e.g., chemicals whose environmental half-life is at least 10 years).

In light of the critical role that soil ingestion can play when estimating human exposure to contaminated soil, it is important to understand what is known about the typical amount of dust and dirt consumed by children and adults (10). The research efforts to evaluate lead uptake by children due to ingestion of contaminated soil, paint chips, dust, and plaster provides the best source of information. For example, Walter and co-workers (27) estimated that a normal child typically ingests very small quantities of dust or dirt between the ages of 0 and 2, the largest quantities between ages 2 and 7, and nearly insignificant amounts thereafter. In the classic text by Cooper (28), it was noted that the desire of children to eat dirt or place inedible objects in their mouths "becomes established in the second year of life and has disappeared more or less spontaneously by the age of four to five years." A study by Charney et al. (29) also indicated that mouthing tends to begin at about 18 months and to continue through 72 months, depending on several factors such as nutritional and economic status as well as race. Work by Sayre et al. (30) indicated that ages 2–6 years are the important years, but that "intensive mouthing diminishes after 2–3 years of age."

An important distinction that is often blurred in risk assessments involving con-taminated soil is the difference between the ingestion of small quantities of dirt due to mouthing tendencies and the disease known as pica. Children who intentionally eat large quantities of dirt, plaster, or paint chips (1–10 g/day) and, as a consequence, are at greater risk of developing health problems can be said to suffer from the disease knows as pica (28). If the craving is for dirt alone, this disease is known as geophasia. It is this disease, rather than pica, which is of primary concern in areas of contaminated soil. The incidence of pica has often been misquoted because some of the best studies were conducted in children who already suffered from lead poisioning due, in part, to pica. For example, in such populations, the incidence of pica has been reported at about 20% (28). In contrast, in the general population, actual pica occurs in about 1–10% of the population (30, 31), while geophasia is more rare. In light of the potential size of this group, for those soils where access to children is not restricted, risk estimates for those with geophasia should be identified.

In 1977, Duggan and Williams (32) summarized the literature on the amount of lead uptake due to ingestion of dust and dirt. Based on their review, they estimated that a quantity of 50 μg of lead was the best estimate for daily ingestion of dust by children. The field studies by Clausing et al. (50) and Calabrese (51) are not inconsistent with their conclusions. Assuming, on the high side, an average lead concentration of 1000 ppm, this would indicate an ingestion of 50 mg/day of soil and dust. Lepow and co-workers (33, 34) estimated a rate of ingestion equal to 100–250 mg/day (specifically, 10 mg ingested 10–25 times a day). Barltrop (35) also estimated that the potential uptake of soils and dusts by a toddler is about 100 mg/day.

One approach to estimating soil ingestion has been to wash the hands of children and then estimate the amount eventually ingested due to poor personal hygiene. In a Dutch study, the amount of lead on hands ranged from 4 to 12 ng (36). By assuming maximum lead concentrations of 500 ng/g (the levels were typically lower) and by assuming the child ingested the entire contents adsorbed to his hand on 10 separate occasions, the amount of ingested dirt would equal 240 mg. Thus, to eat 10,000 mg of soil per day, as suggested by the CDC, the child would daily have to place his hand in his mouth 410 times, a rate that seems improbable (81).

A report by the National Research Council, which addressed the hazards of lead (37), suggested a figure of 40 mg/day for daily ingestion of dust dirt and soil. Day et al. (38) suggested a figure of 100 mg/day (based on eating soiled candy), and Bryce-Smith (46) estimated 33 mg/day. In its document addressing lead in air, the EPA (47) assumed that a child ate 50 mg/day of household dust, 40 mg/day of street dust, and 10 mg/day of dust derived from their parents' clothing (i.e., a total of 100 mg/day). More recently, Hawley (4)

TABLE 3. Other Estimates for Ingestion of Soil by Humans

Age Group (years)	Lepow et al. (34)[a] (mg/day)	Duggan and Williams (32) (mg/day)	Baltrop (35) (mg/day)	Hawley (4) (mg/day)	Clausing et al. (50) (mg/day)	Calabrese et al. (51) (mg/day)
0–2	—[b]	—	—	Negligible	—	—
2–6	100	50	100	90	56	< 25
6–18	—	—	—	21	—	—
18–70	—	—	—	57	—	—

[a]Used in EPA TCDD risk assessment.
[b]Dash indicates the researchers did not discuss these age groups.
Source: Paustenbach et al. (6) with permission from *Regulatory Toxicology and Pharmacology.*

reviewed the available literature on soil ingestion and concluded that uptake by toddlers was approximately 100 mg/day, but he developed a more complex lifetime exposure schedule than had been proposed by others (Table 3). Bellinger et al. (48) suggested a figure of 20 mg/day. Based on all these data, a value of 100 mg/day was recently suggested by La Goy (52) for purposes of risk assessment.

Rather than estimate the amount of soil eaten by children through visual observations, the better approach is to measure the amount of a nonmetabolized "tracer" chemical present in the soil in the children's feces and/or urine. Binder et al. (49) conducted a preliminary or pilot study that employed a rigorous experimental approach involving the analysis of trace elements in children's stool samples. Their data indicated that children 1–3 years of age ingest about 180 mg/day of soil (geometric mean) based on the quantity of silicon, aluminum, and titanium found in the faces. The limitations of this study and the difficulties encountered in the interpretation of the titanium data have been reviewed by Clement Associates (7).

In a more recent study, Clausing et al. (50) studied the amount of soil eaten by 24 hospitalized and nursery school children. They analyzed the amount of aluminum, titanium, and acid-soluble residue in the feces of children aged 2–4. The data were normally distributed. They found an average of 105 mg/day of soil in the feces of nursery school children and 49 mg/day in those hospitalized. Even with the limited number of children in the study, the difference between the two groups was significant ($p < 0.01$). If the value for the hospitalized children is assumed to be the background due to intake of these substances from nonsoil sources (e.g., diet and toothpastes), the estimated average amount of soil ingested by this group of nursery school children would be 56 mg/day. This value is in the lower range of the estimates in the literature and supports the use of 50 to 100 mg/day as a reasonable daily average uptake of soil by toddlers (ages 2–4 or 1.5–3.5).

The most thorough and rigorous study to date recently completed by Calabrese et al. (51). They quantitatively evaluated six different tracer elements in the stools of 65 school children, ages 2–4. They attempted to evaluate children from diverse socioeconomic backgrounds. This study was more definitive than prior investigations because they analyzed the diet of the children, assayed for the presence of tracers in the diapers, assayed house dust and surrounding soil, and corrected for the pharmacokinetics of the tracer materials. The results indicate that a reasonable value for typical soil ingestion by children is about 25 mg/day. This paper presents an excellent discussion of the reasons why prior work has suggested that this figure was greater than this value.

When all this published information on soil ingestion is considered, the data indicate that a consensus estimate for soil ingestion by children (ages 1.5–3.5 or ages 2–4) is about

25–50 mg/day. The 100-mg/day figure was used by the EPA in its risk assessment (78) and in the *EPA Superfund Health Assessment Manual* (77). Depending on the situation and the chemical, as will be shown later in this chapter, the use of 50 or 100 mg/day for ages 1.5–3.5, rather than figures as high as 10,000 mg/day, can significantly change the risk estimates for contaminated areas.

SOIL INGESTION BY ADULTS

For the majority of persons beyond the age of 5–6, the daily uptake of dirt due to intentional ingestion is relatively low. With the possible exception of some lower-income persons who eat certain soils and clays, especially black women, adults do not intentionally ingest dirt or soil (53). However, adults may ingest dirt on fruits and vegetables and via poor personal hygiene. It has been shown that nearly all soil ingested from crops is due to leafy vegetables (47, 60). Interestingly, investigations at nuclear weapons trials have shown that particles which exceed 45 μm are seldom retained on leaves (58). This is consistent with the results observed with granular pesticides (59). Furthermore, the superficial contamination by the smaller particles is readily lost from leaves—usually by mechanical processes or rain, and certainly by washing (59, 60). As a result, unless the soil contaminant is absorbed into the plant, surface contamination of plants by dirt rarely presents a health hazard.

It has been estimated that the deposition rate of dust from the ambient air in rural environments is about $0.012 \, \mu g/cm^2$ day (47) based on studies of dust containing about $300 \, \mu g/g$ of lead (the substance for which these data were obtained). The EPA (47) has also estimated that even at relatively high air concentrations ($0.45 \, mg/m^3$ total dust), it is unlikely that surface deposition alone can account for more than $0.6–1.5 \, \mu g$ lead/g dust (2–$5 \, \mu g/g$ lead) on the surface of lettuce during a 21-day growing period. These data suggest that the daily ingestion of dirt and dust by adults is unlikely to exceed about 0–5 mg/day even if all the 137 g of leafy and root vegetables, sweet corn, and potatoes consumed by adult males each day were replaced by family garden products (47).

In the EPA's document on lead (47), they estimated that persons could take up $100 \, \mu g/day$ of lead from vegetables using worst-case assumptions. The actual uptake by adults from vegetables should actually be much less, and probably negligible, since this estimate assumes that all the suspended dust on vegetables is contaminated with lead, that persons do not wash the vegetables, that garden vegetables are eaten throughout the year rather than only during the growing season, and that persons actually eat only vegetables from their own gardens.

A second potential way to ingest dirt is through poor personal hygiene. It has been suggested that the primary route of uptake is through the accidental ingestion of dirt on the hands (4) and that may be of special concern to smokers who tend to have more frequent hand-to-mouth contact. It is true that before the importance of this route of entry was recognized, persons who worked in lead factories between 1890 and 1920 probably received a large portion of their body burden of this chemical due to poor hygiene; however, such conditions are now rare (83). The exposure experience of agricultural workers who apply or work with pesticide dusts should be a more useful resource for estimating the potential human exposure to soil (21–25, 55–57). Due to the frequency and degree of exposure to these chemicals during their manufacture or application, these data could be expected to overpredict the likely uptake of soil from the hands of persons who live on or near sites having contaminated soil. Most of the published studies on pesticides have involved liquids like the organophosphates rather than "soil-like" particles. However, studies of the exposure of persons who apply granular pesticides might be more useful in defining an upper bound for estimates of dermal exposure for those who are exposed to contaminated soil (20, 22) than estimates based on dusty workplaces.

In general, the available data on the incidental ingestion of contaminated soil due to poor personal hygiene indicate that this should not constitute a significant hazard. However, additional studies evaluating dust, dirt and soil uptake by adults would be useful and it is clear that poor industrial hygiene practices need to be minimized in the occupational setting. For example, Knarr and co-workers (22) showed that the maximum likely uptake of granular and liquid pesticides by applicators via all routes of exposure is in the range of 2–20 mg/day and that this was consistent with the results of the other investigators. These estimates would appear to be overestimates of actual conditions at hazardous waste sites since persons involved in remediation generally wear personal protective equipment when working with the contaminated dirt. For those persons who live offsite, the contribution of contaminated dirt from the site to the overall airborne dust level and the resulting deposition of soil or house dust onto skin should be markedly less. By analogy to the study of dusty highways, the deposition of dust decreases dramatically with distance from the road (84, 85).

In summary, even having considered the contribution of poor hygiene and soil-contaminated food, the 100-mg/day figure used by the CDC to estimate soil uptake by adolescents and adults at residential sites containing contaminated soil seems unlikely, and a figure of 2–5 mg/day seems more reasonable and justifiable based on the available, relevant data. This figure is consistent with those scientists who have inferred that adults should ingest about one-tenth the amount of soil ingested by children.

EXPOSURE FROM DERMAL CONTACT

Quantitative estimates of the dermal uptake of chemicals within dusts or soil contain more uncertainty than estimates for other routes of entry. In the CDC's assessment of TCDD-contaminated soil, they assumed that dermal exposures would follow "an age-dependent pattern of deposition similar to soil ingestion" as shown in Table 4 (3). For TCDD, the CDC assumed that dirt would remain on the hand for a period long enough to bring about 1% absorption—the percent absorption determined in rats exposed for 24 h (78, 86, 87). A 24-h duration is almost certainly longer than what is likely for humans under normal conditions; therefore, this would represent a value beyond

TABLE 4. Amount of Soil Deposited on Skin (CDC Assumption)

Age Group	Soil on Skin (day)
0–9 months	0 g
9–18 months	1 g
1.5–3.5 years	10 g
3.5–5 years	1 g
5–70 years	100 mg

Source: Paustenbach et al. (6) with permission from *Regulatory Toxicology and Pharmacology.*

"worst case." A more likely scenario is that persons would be exposed for 4–8 h/day, with some degree of washing at the end of this period. When estimating the degree of systemic absorption, it is necessary to recognize that a pure liquid chemical will be absorbed to a greater degree than when present on a carrier or medium such as soil (78, 86–94). For chemicals less strongly bound to the soil, such as those that are water soluble, the rate of release, availability, and absorption through the skin might be much greater (95, 96).

In both assessments of dioxin on soil, the CDC and EPA correctly assumed that the opportunity for dermal exposure would be affected by weather conditions, and consequently they made adjustments (3, 78). In the CDC calculations, it appears that they assumed for the Midwestern states that persons would have direct dermal contact with soil for about 180 days/year for 64 years (70–6) due to gardening and yard work. This estimate is almost certain to overestimate the actual average exposure, since (i) not everyone in the community gardens, (ii) many persons wear gloves when working intimately with dirt, (iii) gardeners work directly with the soil primarily during only planting and weeding, (iv) most people do not garden each day, and (v) the number of days of precipitation during the gardening season further diminishes the frequency of exposure.

The EPA, in its risk assessment (78), used an alternative set of assumptions for dermal exposure, which, because they were based on actual field investigations, seem more realistic than the CDC's assumptions. The EPA cited the work of Roels et al. (45), who showed that about 0.5 mg of soil per cm² of skin adheres to a child's hand after playing in and around the home. This is similar to that reported by Day et al. (38), who observed that 5–50 mg of dirt transferred from a child's hand to a sticky sweet. Sayre et al. (30) analyzed the amount of lead on children's hands due to house dust. Assuming values of 500 and 2000 μg/kg for the lead concentration in rural and urban house dust, respectively, their data indicate dust uptake due to mouthing tendencies at about 100 mg/day if all dust on both sides of the hand were ingested or absorbed through the skin. Uptake can also be estimated by multiplying the appropriate absorption rate for a given chemical and the amount of dirt on the skin using table values for skin surface area (97). This is illustrated later in the discussions of Cases I and II.

EXPOSURE FROM INHALATION

Although some persons have been concerned about inhaling dangerously high levels of chemicals from waste sites, either as a vapor or as a contaminant of ambient dust, the EPA, CDC, and numerous independent scientists have shown that inhalation usually does not constitute a route of entry that will adversely affect human health (2, 3, 6, 9, 81). It is worthwhile to note that even though a health hazard due to the inhalation of airborne chemicals may not exist at many of these sites, the presence of odorous chemicals in the soil or the water solubility of the chemical contaminants (posing a threat to groundwater) frequently dictate that some level of cleanup will be necessary. The degree of inhalation hazard is generally dictated by the volatility of the chemical, its toxicity, the proximity of the population to the waste site, and the amount of dust generated at the site (for nonvolatile contaminants). In the CDC assessment of dioxin, they assumed that the average air concentration of total suspended particulates (TSP) was 0.14 mg/m³ and that 100% of this amount (by weight) was respirable. From this, they calculated that exposure to dust containing 1 ppb of TCDD would result in an average lifetime daily uptake of 10 fg/kg·day—roughly 2% of the amount taken up by ingestion, according to the CDC calculations (Table 1).

When actual field data are considered, inhalation will usually contribute only slightly to the total absorbed dose. This is in contrast with what has often been assumed in risk assessments. For example, the EPA has collected data which indicate that the average concentration of total suspended particulates (TSP) in Missouri is about one-half the level assumed by the CDC, or about 0.070 mg/m^3 (98). For other geographical locations, concentrations of 0.15 mg/m^3 for urban environments and 0.10 mg/m^3 for rural environments are good estimates of TSP for use in risk assessment; however, site-specific information should be used whenever possible. Owing to the many surveys conducted by the EPA during the past 15 years, site-specific data are often available. In those situations where vehicular traffic on bare contaminated soil is possible, the resulting increased human exposure to higher levels of dust should be considered (85).

To assess the health hazard posed by airborne particles, three size categories should be considered: total suspended particulates (TSP) and inhalable and respirable particles. Generally, TSP are those having aerodynamic mean diameters under 30 μm. The respirable fraction are those less than 10 μm in diameter.

Only a fraction (about 30%) of the inhalable dust are respirable (aerodynamic diameter less than 10 μm) (98). Schaum (78) estimated that no more than 50% of the TSPs should be respirable and Cowherd et al. (99) confirmed that only 30% of TSPs are respirable. When conducting these estimates of dose, it is important to remember that not all airborne particles are derived from contaminated soil. In one study, about 83% of the nonrespirable particles obtained during sampling were from crustal material (e.g., soil) but only 47% of the respirable particles were from soil (98). More exhaustive studies conducted by the EPA have suggested that the portion of inhalable dust derived from soil is generally less than these figures (100). Usually, site specific data are collected during feasibility studies and these should be used in endangerment assessments.

BIOAVAILABILITY: DERMAL ABSORPTION

Bioavailability is an important parameter in any risk assessment of contaminated soil. Throughout this discussion, bioavailability is used to describe the percentage of a chemical in soil which is absorbed by humans (as suggested in animal studies) following exposure via inhalation, ingestion, or dermal contact (101). For dioxin-contaminated soil, there are a number of parameters that are likely to influence the degree of dermal and oral bioavailability including aging (time following contamination), soil type (e.g., silt, clay, and sand), co-contaminants (e.g., oil and other organics), and the concentration of contaminant on the soil (101). These factors have been shown to be relevant for most xenobiotics.

The bioavailability of a chemical on soil is very much affected by its chemical and physical properties (96). Depending on the chemical of concern and the above-mentioned variables, the dermal bioavailability of a given soil contaminant can vary between 0.05 and 50% (6, 94, 101). Large molecular weight chemicals often bind to the soil and are less water soluble, while smaller molecules are frequently water soluble, volatile, and highly bioavailable (95, 96).

Most dermal bioavailability data for contaminated soil have been obtained in animals or in vitro test systems. This introduces a significant source of uncertainty. In the interest of conservatism, safety factors have often been applied to dermal bioavailability data obtained in animals when estimating human uptake. This uncertainty factor is probably unnecessary in most cases since human skin has generally been shown for a diverse class of chemicals to be about 10-fold less permeable to xenobiotics than the skin of rabbits and rats (102, 103); the laboratory animals typically used. More recently, Shu et al. (101) have reviewed the oral bioavailability studies on TCDD and the uncertainties in the research. Few other chemicals have been studied to determine their dermal bioavailability on soil or other media.

BIOAVAILABILITY: INGESTION

The difficulties of assessing the oral bioavailability of a chemical contaminant on soil are clearly demonstrated by the research surrounding TCDD. The data of Poiger and Schlatter (86) suggested that as the time of contact between the soil and TCDD increased (known as aging) the oral bioavailability decreased. McConnell et al. (92) studied Missouri soil contaminated with TCDD, and they concluded that TCDD absorption from soil by test animals is highly efficient, but they had difficulty in arriving at an exact percentage for bioavailability. The data of Lucier et al. (93) suggested that bioavailability was dose dependent: 24% at 1 μg/kg and 50% at 5 μg/kg TCDD. In a 1985 abstract, Umbreit et al. reported the oral bioavailability of TCDD at less than 0.05% for a New Jersey manufacturing site. This work was subsequently published (94), wherein they also reported oral bioavailability of 21% for soil from a salvage yard in Newark.

More recently, Shu et al. (101) reported on a comprehensive study to evaluate oral bioavailability of TCDD on soil and showed that in the rat none of the anticipated modifying factors seemed to affect bioavailability. These authors also reviewed the oral bioavailability studies on TCDD and many of the uncertainties were discussed. The bioavailabilities of other chemicals in soil have not been studied to a great degree but inferences can be reached by evaluating soil adsorption data (74, 75, 104), volatility information (2, 72), and soil binding studies (95, 105). The oral bioavailability clearly is dependent on the media and this seems to have been illustrated in the work of Silkworth et al. (90) and Van den Berg (91) who showed that TCDD bioavailability on fly ash or soot may well be close to 1% or less.

BIOAVAILABILITY: INHALATION

The laboratory assessment of the bioavailability of inhaled particles has received very little attention since it is generally assumed that respirable particles are 100% absorbed and the contaminant systemically circulated. In the CDC analysis of TCDD (3), it was assumed that 100% of the TCDD present on all the inhaled particles would be retained and absorbed in the respiratory tract. In contrast, the EPA assessment (78) assumed that only 25% of the inhaled particles would be absorbed in the lower airways, since at least 50% of the particles would be nonrespirable (especially by weight). For most risk assessments, it is probably acceptable to assume that 100% of those particles that remain in the alveoli will be absorbed. However, it must be noted that of the total suspended particulates, usually no more than 50% are respirable (i.e., particles less than 10 μm). Of these, about 50% of the respirable particles are deposited in the upper airways and ultimately swallowed while the rest reach the alveoli or are expired.

The bioavailability of the large particles (between 10 and 50 μm) is dictated by the oral route, since they are taken up the mucociliary escalator and then swallowed (6, 78). In any assessment of soil contaminated by a chemical, the difference in bioavailability between those particles that are caught in the upper airways and swallowed versus those that reach the lower airways should be considered. For media like fly ash and soil, there will be significant effects on the predicted absorbed dose.

BIOACCUMULATION

When deciding what level of soil contamination is acceptable, it is often necessary to consider the half-life of the substance in biota and wildlife (2). For many of the persistent chemicals, the concentration present in wildlife can often exceed that detected in soil or water. For example, the presence of DDT, chlordane, and the dioxins in some fish can be sevenfold greater than the water solubility (106). Furthermore, nondetectable levels in the environment can often bioaccumulate via the food chain to detectable levels in human tissue (107). This is a particular concern for those chemicals or substances which have theoretical bioconcentration factors (BCF) in excess of 1000. Typically, the poly-halogenated cyclic substances and the metals will be of concern.

PERVASIVENESS OF CONTAMINATION

Kimbrough et al. (3) observed that of all the assumptions used in their risk analysis, the "most prominent of these is the assumption of uniform levels of contamination throughout the living space (environment)." The CDC were especially sensitive to the issue of uniformity of contamination and accessibility to the contaminated soil and generated an interesting plot that illustrates the relation between the magnitude of the risk and the percentage of the surface area of the land that has been contaminated (Fig. 2). The concept of averaging the surface soil levels when conducting the risk assessment is important in all assessments of contaminated soil, regardless of the chemical. Of course, when averaging is used, criteria should be established for defining *hot spots*. These are localized areas where the level of soil contamination is much higher than the surrounding ones. These localized areas of significantly higher-than-normal contamination should be removed before an average is calculated. The best way to describe the level of contamination at a site, for

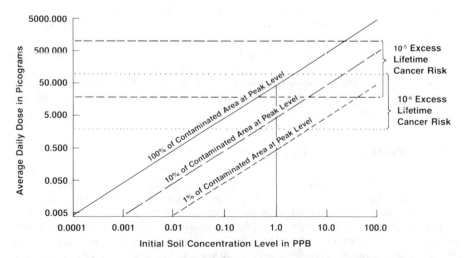

Figure 2. Effect of the degree (prevalence of dioxin soil contamination at a residential site) versus the estimated risk [from Kimbrough et al. (3).] This plot is based on an acceptable daily lifetime dose of 633 fg/kg·day (CDC's best estimate of a dose that would increase the individual cancer risk by 1 in 1,000,000).

purposes of assessing the chronic health hazard, is sample in a randomized manner and to base the exposure calculations on the geometric mean soil concentration and the geometric standard deviation (109).

SOIL SAMPLING AND DATA ANALYSIS

In most assessments of areas with potentially contaminated soil, an emphasis has been placed on locating the areas having the greatest concentration rather than obtaining a representative sampling of the site. Regrettably, the results of such subjective sampling plans are often used to develop risk assessments and remedial action plans. Since such nonrandom sampling is not representative of the average level of contamination at the site, it is virtually impossible to develop an accurate estimate of the average human exposure. The more appropriate approach to gathering data useful for conducting a health hazard assessment is to divide the contaminated site into equal quadrants (108) and to collect a statistically valid number of samples on a random basis. Samples should be collected at depths of 0–6 in., 6–18 in., and at increasing intervals until hitting bedrock unless it is shown that the chemical has not migrated below a given depth. This allows for a gross assessment of the depth and magnitude of contamination. If water-soluble chemicals are involved, 12–36-in. and 24–36″ samples are usually worth collecting during the initial survey. Once these sample have been collected and assayed, the data should be interrupted using log–normal statistics if the data are log-normally distributed (as is usually the case). This approach does not allow unusually high values to dominate the overall results and is nearly always appropriate for statistical analysis of environmental samples (109).

RESIDENTIAL VERSUS INDUSTRIAL SITES

Often, the differences in the conditions of human exposure between residential, industrial, and recreational sites are overlooked by those involved in risk assessment or those agencies responsible for setting cleanup guidelines. As noted in the CDC publication (3), "in all of these scenarios (factories, farms, residential sites), decisions must be made on a site-specific basis." The most prominent difference between a residential and an industrial setting, with respect to the hazard to human health, is the lack of access to industrial sites by the public and, in particular, by children. In the absence of such access, at least 95% of the potential exposure to relatively nonvolatile substances, such as dioxin or the heavy metals, is eliminated (Table 1). Of course, the hazard to the environment and wildlife still requires evaluation.

ENVIRONMENTAL FATE OF THE TOXICANT

It is important to recognize that the degree of human exposure (ingestion, inhalation, and dermal contact) is almost always a function of the concentration of the contaminant at the soil surface (top 0–3 cm) rather than of the concentration at lower depths. This is significant since, when exposed to sunlight, many chemicals degrade, are rapidly volatilized, or are metabolized by soil microbes. For most soil contaminants that are relatively simple organic chemicals, microbial degradation will be the critical factor at depths of 6 or more inches while depths of 0–6″ will be influenced by volatilization. The end use of the site dictates whether it is necessary to decrease the contaminant

TABLE 5. Estimated Lifetime Average Daily Dose (pg/kg·day) of TCDD as a Function of Initial Soil Concentration and Environmental Half-Life

100 ppb Soil Concentration

Exposure Period (years)	Half-life of TCDD in Soil (years)	CDC Oral Intake Schedule				Alternative Oral Intake Schedule			
		30% Oral Bioavailability		10% Oral Bioavailability		30% Oral Bioavailability		10% Oral Bioavailability	
		CDC[a]	ALT[b]	CDC	ALT	CDC	ALT	CDC	ALT
0→70	1	12	11	4.1	3.7	0.56	0.14	0.48	0.06
0→70	6	53	51	19	17	3.2	1.0	2.6	0.51
0→70	12	64	62	24	21	43	1.6	3.6	0.93
20→65	1	55×10^{-8}	55×10^{-8}	23×10^{-8}	23×10^{-8}	7.5×10^{-8}	72×10^{-8}	7.5×10^{-8}	7.2×10^{-8}
20→65	6	31×10^{-2}	0.31	0.13	0.13	0.045	0.042	0.045	0.042
20→66	12	1.8	1.8	0.79	0.77	0.27	0.25	0.27	0.25

[a]CDC (Centers for Disease Control) estimates are based on the assumptions used by Kimbrough et al. (3) for oral, dermal, and inhalation exposure and their assumptions for bioavailability. The various assumptions for the degree of oral intake and oral bioavailability used in the calculations are shown in table heading. The initial average soil concentration was 100 ppb TCDD.

[b]ALT (alternative) estimates are based on the assumptions described in this chapter for oral, dermal, and inhalation exposure and the different assumptions for bioavailability for each route of entry. The various assumptions for the degree of oral intake and oral bioavailability used in the calculations are shown in the table heading. The initial average soil concentration was 100 ppb TCDD.

concentration at depths of 3, 12, 24, or 48 in. In the case of TCDD on soil, recent research suggests that within 18 months, nearly all the TCDD in the top 1/2 cm of soil is no longer present owing to photodegradation (if in the presence of a solvent) and volatilization (110). However, dioxin that is not exposed to sunlight appears to have a half-life near to or in excess of 10–20 years (3, 13). In contrast, some volatile chemicals can persist for only hours, days or weeks at the soil surface.

A chemical's environmental half-life is important when estimating risk. The effect of environmental half-life on the anticipated lifetime exposure to TCDD on soil is illustrated in Table 5. Using the CDC's assumptions for potential oral, dermal, and inhalation exposure to soil, if the half-life at the soil surface were 1 year, the soil concentration were 100 ppb, and the bioavailability were 30%, the maximum anticipated average lifetime daily dose would be 12 pg/kg·day for 70 years of exposure. In contrast, if the half-life were 12 years, the average dose would increase to 64 pg/kg·day using the CDC's assumptions. More importantly, by using the alternative assumptions that were discussed in Case I, by using the same conditions of exposure and the average lifetime doses, and by assuming a 1- and 12-year environmental half-life for TCDD, the projected uptakes are 0.14 and 1.6 pg/kg·day, respectively. The influence of a chemical's half-life on the risk estimates is particularly important when children are not exposed to the soil (e.g., industrial site). In these settings, such as occupational exposure, the average lifetime daily uptake by adults (ages 20–65) drops dramatically with decreasing environmental half-life (Table 5). For example, using the CDC's assumptions for adult exposure (ages 20–65) to contaminated soil, the estimated uptake of TCDD is 55×10^{-8} pg/kg·day if the half-life is only 1 year, but the risk is nine orders of magnitude higher when the half-life is 12 years.

APPLYING THESE CONCEPTS

As noted in both the CDC and EPA assessments, the process of setting standards for soil cleanup should be done on a site-specific basis. This task, however, need not be a process so complex as to be impractical for regulatory agencies. Certainly, an algorithm that incorporates all the important variables could be developed, as discussed by Hawley (4), Schaum (78), and Paustenbach (10), and these calculations can easily be handled by a desktop computer.

The following case studies illustrate how the CDC methodology for evaluating contaminated soil could be applied, on a site-specific basis, incorporating data on exposure, bioavailability, percent land contamination, and environmental fate. These examples illustrate the effect of altering only a few of the critical assumptions in an environmental risk assessment and the importance of site-by-site analyses. In developing a comprehensive risk assessment, it is also important to acknowledge the uncertainties, as recommended by the National Academy of Science (111). Kimbrough et al. (3) recognized the fragility and uncertainty of many of the assumptions which they used and specifically noted that "it must be stressed that the exposure assessments used in estimating risks for carcinogenicity and reproductive health effects contain critical assumptions that are not likely to be actually encountered." Other critical issues, including the use of classic cancer risk models, as opposed to the safety factor approach to estimate carcinogenic potency in humans at low doses (depending on genotoxicity) and the incorporation of the available epidemiology data, should be examined in any comprehensive analysis of soils contaminated by suspected carcinogens (6, 11, 12).

Case I (a Residential Site)

In this example, a hypothetical residential site is evaluated. For the sake of this discussion, 10% of the soil surface in this community is assumed to be contaminated with 10 ppb TCDD. Based on the CDC analysis, 1 ppb has frequently been cited as one where remediation of a residential area should be considered (3). If only a few of the assumptions in the CDC assessment process were updated, would a thorough risk assessment suggest that cleanup is needed at this site?

Using the methods described by the CDC and the EPA, a preliminary evaluation of the need for cleanup at a given site can readily be conducted. In Case I, the CDC assessment procedure is used but a few of their values are updated. Specifically, in these calculations we used (i) a soil uptake of 100 mg/day (ages 2–6) and negligible soil ingestion for the rest of the lifetime; (ii) 10% oral and 1% dermal bioavailability; (iii) quantitative assumptions on dermal exposure; (iv) actual field data on the concentration of respirable dust in air; and (v) corrections for the differences in bioavailability between particles that are swallowed and those that are retained in the lung (Table 6).

As shown in Table 7, by using the alternate assumed values, the oral dose would not be expected to be greater than 2.8 fg/kg·day. If a 30% oral bioavailability were assumed, the average daily oral dose increases to 8.4 fg/kg·day. In contrast, the CDC's assumed values would suggest an oral uptake of about 606.5 fg/kg·day. The alternate method estimated dermal uptake of 2.7 fg/kg·day, in contrast to 20 fg/kg·day using the CDC's assumed values. Finally, the CDC assumptions would suggest that 10 fg/kg·day might be inhaled versus the 5.6 fg/kg·day value estimated using site specific data.

In summary, use of the alternative assumptions predicts that the most likely uptake of TCDD will, in this example, be 11.1 fg/kg·day. If a 30% oral bioavailability were assumed, the average daily dose increases to 16.7 fg/kg·day. In contrast, the assumptions in the CDC

TABLE 6. Exposure Assumptions Used in Case I Calculations (Lifetime Average)

Route	CDC	Alternate
Oral	0.21 g/day ingested (lifetime average)	0.0028 g/day ingested (lifetime average)
	30% absorption	10% absorption
Dermal	0.21 g/day of soil on the skin	0.5 mg soil/cm² skin
	Dose is weighted by age over lifetime	1400 cm² exposed surface
		8 h/day, 90 days/year
	1% absorption	1% absorption
Inhalation	Total suspended particulates is 0.14 mg/m³	Total suspended particulates is 0.075 mg/m³
	15 m³/day	15 m³/day
	10% in lungs	Of particles inhaled, assume 50% ingested and 50% in lungs
	100% bioavailable	Bioavailability weighted for differences in absorption for respirable and nonrespirable particles
		Only 50% of the particles are from the contaminated site

Source: Paustenbach et al. (6) with permission from *Regulatory Toxicology and Pharmacology.*

TABLE 7. Residential Site^a (Case I)

Route	TCDD Uptake (fg/kg·day)	
	CDC	Alternate
Oral	606.5	2.8
Dermal	20.0	2.7
Inhalation	10.0	5.6
Total	636.5	11.1
		$(16.7)^b$

^{a}Ten percent of land contaminated (10 ppb TCDD).
^{b}Using a 30% oral bioavailability.
Source: Paustenbach et al. (6) with permission from *Regulatory Toxicology and Pharmacology.*

assessment led to an estimate for total TCDD uptake of 636.5 fg/kg·day (which the CDC considered acceptable when recommending the 1-ppb guideline). This analysis illustrates the critical nature of certain assumptions, and it shows that remediation would not be indicated at this site; even assuming that the 636.5 fg/kg·day figure was an accurate upper limit for de minimus risk. Of course, in any isolated instances where children or adults might be exposed to TCDD soil concentrations in excess of 500–1000 ppb (e.g., hot spots), cleanup of these would need to be considered (6).

Case II (Industrial Site)

The methodology used by the CDC or by Paustenbach *et al.* (6) can also be used to assess the potential hazards at an industrial site. In this example, assume that 20% of the site has been contaminated with 100 ppb TCDD. Because it is an industrial site, children have virtually no access. Is remediation necessary? The assumptions and factors used here are shown in Table 8.

Because children are not exposed, the oral route of exposure is much less important. As shown in Table 9, calculations based on the CDC-assumed values indicate that an average dose of 590 fg/kg day TCDD could potentially be absorbed by those who work at this site (lifetime average). This value is still less than 636 fg/kg·day, the daily dose that the CDC considered acceptable (Table 1). Furthermore, use of the alternative assumptions indicates that the more likely daily uptake is 135 fg/kg·day. Since the daily intake is less than 636 fg/kg·day, these calculations suggest that 20% contamination of soil by 100 ppb TCDD is safe even using the criteria proposed by the CDC. Also, at many industrial sites, it may be acceptable to permit soils contaminated with TCDD at levels greater than 100 ppb to remain in place, especially where soil erosion is not a problem and where the contamination is at the soil surface (where it is available for photodegradation).

UPTAKE BY PLANTS

The amount of a chemical absorbed by plants grown in contaminated soil can be important in some risk assessments. The extent to which crops will take up (absorb) appreciable quantities of a xenobiotic must be evaluated on a chemical-by-chemical basis. Field studies where crops have been grown in contaminated soil have been conducted for

TABLE 8. Exposure Assumptions Used in Case II Calculations (Lifetime Average)

Route	CDC	Alternate
Oral	Not relevant	Not relevant
Dermal	Exposure is almost same as oral exposure 1% bioavailable	0.5 mg/soil 1400 cm^2 exposed skin 8 h/day, 40 years exposure 1% bioavailable
Inhalation	0.14 mg/m^3 (dust) 15 m^3/day 100% in lungs 100% bioavailable	Total suspended particulates are 0.075 mg/m^3 (Springfield, MO) 15 m^3/day Of particles inhaled, assume 50% ingested and 50% in lungs 50% of respirable particles from contaminated soil Adjust bioavailability for ingestion and inhalation

Source: Paustenbach et al. (6) with permission from *Regulatory Toxicology and Pharmacology.*

TABLE 9. Industrial Site[a] (Case II)

	TCDD Uptake (fg/kg·day)	
Route	CDC	Alternate
Oral	0	0
Dermal	390	78
Inhalation	200	57
Total	590	135

[a]Twenty percent of land contaminated (100 ppb TCDD).
Source: Paustenbach et al. (6) with permission from *Regulatory Toxicology and Pharmacology.*

numerous chemicals. Inferences for chemicals which have not been tested can be drawn based on the physical and chemical properties of the contaminant and the soil–contaminant matrix; however, actual field data are much preferred.

Interestingly, the amount of soil contaminant taken up by a plant can vary with species. For example, oats and soybean plants grown to maturity in soil contaminated with 60 ppb TCDD showed less than 1 ppb of TCDD in the seeds (112). Wipf et al. (113) failed to detect any measurable 2, 3, 7, 8-TCDD in the flesh of fruits and vegetables collected from the contaminated area in Seveso during 1977–1979, although the TCDD concentration in the soil was 10 ppb. For many chemicals, only the tubers (e.g., potatoes, carrots, onions) seem to absorb or bioconcentrate them. For other plants, the primary routes of contamination are the volatilization of the chemical from the soil with subsequent absorption by the leaves closest to the soil or, by retention of dust that has been deposited on the leaves.

If an estimate of the concentration of a chemical in a plant is known, the quantitative uptake by humans can be calculated through use of the USDA's food tables. Usually, the concentrations of xenobiotics in various plants and food for various soil levels are not available. Further, it is critical that the type of soil be understood since the relationship between absorption of a chemical by plants will be directly related to the chemicals affinity for the organic content of the soil.

Generally, common industrial solvents would not be expected to be present at significant levels in most crops due to their volatility, adsorption to soil particles, plant metabolism, or degradation in soil. Even though uptake by plants will be related to a chemicals water solubility, and this will influence the residue levels found in the animal, those chemicals that are stable or highly lipid soluble may be present and available for ingestion by those animals who eat soil while grazing. Many of the stable compounds found in soil (except perhaps the metals) which will not be present in plants, will be taken up in the fat or the liver of the animal simply due to lipid solubility or binding. Other chemicals, if present, will usually be metabolized and eliminated. Using recent estimates of the amount of fat contained in the various classes of meat in the United States and the likely uptake and retention of a substance by the animal, one can calculate the likely daily uptake by exposed persons (114, 141).

UPTAKE BY GRAZING ANIMALS

As noted by Fries (8), when the primary route of human exposure to a contaminant is through food, the persons most likely to receive the highest exposures are farmers who eat their own products, as well as their direct customers. Exposure of the general population will generally be several orders of magnitude lower because agricultural products are distributed widely, and food containing low levels of these chemicals will be diluted with uncontaminated food.

If a chemical grown in contaminated soil is absorbed by plants and not digested, it is a straightforward exercise to calculate uptake (pounds eaten per day × concentration in plant ÷ body weight). The pharmacokinetics of the chemical in the animal as well as the person consuming the meat must also be considered in the calculations since biologic half-life can markedly affect the steady-state body burdens. For dioxin and any other chemicals that are not appreciably taken up by plants, animal feed is not an important route of animal exposure. Field experience with polybrominated biphenyls (PBB) indicates that dust on the surface of plants gathered during harvest of forage crops makes an negligible contribution to residues in feed as harvested. The concentration was less than 1% of that present in soil (115).

Interestingly, the intentional ingestion of soil by grazing animals may often represent their primary route of uptake of xenobiotics introduced through environmental contamination. This phenomenon has been studied in cattle and sheep under a variety of conditions (115–127). Generally, soil ingestion is inversely related to the availability of forage. The amount is as low as 1–2% of dry matter intake during periods of lush plant growth, and it rises as high as 18% in periods when forage is sparse (8). Under New Zealand conditions, where animals can graze 365 days a year, average soil intake was about 6% of the estimated dry matter intake for cattle and 4.5% of the dry matter intake for sheep (6). In the United States, a reasonable estimate of soil uptake by grazing dairy cows is 5% of dry matter for sparse lands and less than 1% for those which are on pasture. For non lactating beef cattle, a reasonable estimate is 2% of dry matter and for a lactating cow 3% is a conservative estimate. For a non-lactating 350 kg cow, this represents soil ingestion of up to 0.6 lb/day in a diet of 20 lbs/day of feed. The amount of soil ingested is reduced more than 50% when animals are offered harvested feed as a supplement to pasture (8, 124).

Farm animals also ingest soil when they are confined to unpaved holding areas (122, 123). Under typical U.S. farm conditions, lactating cows may consume as much as 1% of their dry matter intake as soil, whereas nonlactating cattle, who have greater exposure and are less intensely fed, may consume up to 4% of their dry matter intake from this source. Pigs, due to their habit of rooting, will tend to have higher values, which can be as great as 8% of dry matter intake (123). Since pigs never subsist on pasture alone, this value may be considered an upper limit for the amount of soil ingested by pigs.

When estimating the amount of TCDD which could be present in meat or milk, several basic factors must be considered: (i) amount of soil ingested by the animal (yearly average); (ii) the fat:diet ratio is usually 5:1 for milk fat and body fat; (iii) the amount of soil ingested should be averaged over a year when animal access is less than a full year; (iv) the half-life of the chemical in growing cattle; (v) the environmental degradation of the soil contaminant in the top 2–4 cm; (vi) rate of metabolism by the animal; and (vii) soil bioavailability in the animal (122–126).

Fortunately, the practical significance of soil ingestion as a potential route of animal exposure is greatly mitigated under the U.S. agricultural conditions (8). Lactating dairy cows are rarely pastured, and some form of supplemental feeding is almost always employed. Consequently, it is unlikely that soil ingestion would ever exceed 1% of dry matter intake in actual farm situations. Fries (8) has noted that, even though cattle raised for beef might often be on pastures with little other feed, it is the general practice to fatten these animals in feedlots before slaughter. This period of time may be as long as 150 days, and animals can gain as much as 60–70% in body weight (116). During these periods, the contaminant will also be reduced by dilution in the expanding body fat pool.

Most hogs destined for slaughter are confined and would never be exposed to contaminated soil. Thus, as noted by Fries (8), only cull-breeding cattle and pigs might be expected to go directly from soil to slaughter, and these are not the animals ordinarily used for home consumption by farmers who raise them. In short, for most domestic animals in the United States, few will ever be exposed to contaminated soil without having been provided with ample feed. Because of the many factors that need to be considered, the setting of an acceptable soil level should be done on a site-specific basis (141).

RUNOFF HAZARD

For those chemicals in soil which are not rapidly degraded, the potential for accumulation in the food chain is possible (15). Specifically, soils contaminated with chemicals whose bioconcentration factors (BCF) exceed 1000 need to be assessed for the potential of the soil to enter streams or lakes via runoff. Even for those substances whose BCF is between 100 and 1000, it may be necessary to consider both the concentration, the total amount of contaminant in soil and the quantity of soil which could be eroded.

There are numerous examples of situations where even relatively small amounts of soil from sites contaminated with PCBs, dioxins, furans, DDT, kepone, and heptachlor eventually contaminated streams to a level that was easily detected in the nearby fish. Consequently, it is prudent to use existing transport models to set standards for chemical contamination of streams so as to set limits which protect aquatic life and its predators.

HUMAN BIOLOGIC HALF-LIFE

Often, chemicals that are long-lived in the environment also have long half-lives in humans. Those chemicals with biologic half-lives longer than 2–3 months may require some degree of evaluation, since it will require about 1 year for steady-state levels to be reached in living organisms. However, chemicals with half-lives of elimination in excess of 3–5 years in humans clearly require special attention since it is possible that hazardous levels could be reached following repeated exposure.

It is important to recognize that it is relatively easy to estimate the acceptable daily intake by humans of long-lived or stable chemicals using pharmacokinetic principles (19). An important consideration when assessing soil is to understand that if a contaminant has a long environmental half-life and a long biologic half-life, the chemical needs to be kept out of the food chain. For soils, this means that limited quantities of contaminated soil should be allowed to enter streams or lakes via runoff or to enter the food chain via grazing animals (8).

LEACHING INTO WATER

The possibility that water-soluble chemicals in soil can enter water via runoff or leaching has been recognized for a number of years (2, 67, 127). In general, chemicals that are water soluble are those of primary concern. Chemicals that do not bind very strongly to plants or soil represent the next most important class of chemicals. Finally, those chemicals having a long half-life in the environment are often a concern. The erosion of contaminated soil in runoff can present a special hazard for the persistent chemicals since these particles can be taken up by bottom-feeding fish and mollusks (73).

There are numerous factors to consider when water is contaminated by a liquid- or soil-bound contaminant. Some chemicals are bound to sediment and are subsequently taken up by bottom-feeding fish and mollusks. Others can pass through clay or rocklike layers of subsurface material, which often separate subsurface waters from deep aquifers (so-called drinking water aquifers). Another consideration is that fish or other aquatic organisms can take up the contaminant from the water and concentrate it in their adipose tissue or skin (2, 73). Finally, sufficiently high levels of chemicals in water can affect the chemistry and biology of lakes and streams and this can cause adverse effects on algae and other organisms.

UPTAKE BY FISH

For many of the water-soluble chemicals, the acute toxicity to fish is the major hazard (73). In contrast, for the non-water soluble chemicals, the acute and chronic toxicity to fish may be modest but their ingestion by humans can pose one of the more important routes of exposure. In recent years a number of models have been developed which allow us to predict the potential hazard to fish posed by chemicals released into the environment (2, 73), and these should be useful in assessing the potential hazard posed by contaminated soils. Fish and mollusks, because of their ability to bioconcentrate water-soluble chemicals, are usually the species most at risk if the chemical is a potent toxicant in aquatic species.

Often, the bioconcentration factor (BCF) is useful for predicting the peak steady-state level of a toxicant in fish (129, 130). Unfortunately, for those chemicals that are very poorly water soluble or very lipophilic, the simple BCF formula may break down; for example, it can dramatically underestimate or overestimate the actual bioconcentration observed in fish. Chemicals which have large BCF's need to be kept out of waterways so that fish and other aquatic species do not concentrate them in their adipose tissue and skin.

AVIAN HAZARD

Some sites, especially where contaminated soil is present over a large geographical area, may present a hazard to various bird species. When evaluating the potential avian hazard, a number of factors must be considered. Among the most important parameters is the environmental half-life of the chemical and the avian toxicity. To fully understand the hazard one must also consider the opportunity for acute and chronic exposure, the size of the contaminated area, the number of exposed species, the migratory or non-migratory nature of the birds, the biologic half-life of the substance in birds, the concentration of the contaminants within the top 2″ of soil, it's water solubility and lipid solubility, and the presence of soil dwelling insects.

Although an evaluation of the avian hazard posed by contaminated soil is a complex one, relevant information can be drawn from the avian experience with granular pesticides. Numerous poisoning incidents have been studied wherein seeds, insects, plants and other media have become contaminated with both short and long-lived pesticides. Approaches used to evaluate sites contaminated with pesticides are invaluable sources of information for developing a strategy to assess sites having contaminated soil (142–145). The historical data on chlordane, heptachlor, diazanon, and carbofuran constitute a valuable database from which one can make avian assessments.

Thorough assessments should consider birds which are both predators and seed eaters, as well as, the potential for bioconcentration by plants, insects, and other organisms in the food chain. Chemicals which have bioconcentration factors in excess of 500 are of particular concern in situations where more than a few hundred acres of land have become contaminated and run-off into waterways is possible. The rationale for conducting a screening analysis of the avian hazard in most situations involving contaminated soil is that it is possible that the site will pose no significant human or environmental hazard other than to avian species.

HAZARD TO WILDLIFE

The potential hazard of contaminated soil to deer, earthworms, birds, squirrels, and other wildlife has become a greater concern in recent years (131–133). In general, only a limited number of studies have assessed the various factors that can adversely affect the health of wildlife in the field environment, especially as a result of contaminated soil. It would appear that those chemicals that are long-lived in the environment (low water solubility, poorly metabolized, and resistant to degradation) are of primary concern. The studies of DDT and PCB in the environment probably represent the best data base for predicting the effect of rather long-lived chemicals on various wildlife.

One of the most through evaluations of the potential environmental hazards posed by contaminated soil was that conducted at Eglin Air Force Base in Florida (134, 135). In that study, over 300 biological species (plants and animals) were analyzed for TCDD. Histopathology was also conducted in the majority of the animals captured. These researchers found that the beachmouse was the best species for evaluating the maximum level of biomagnification since they lived underground, reproduced frequently, and soil ingestion (due to preening) was a major route of uptake (135). The study showed that the higher species (deer, opossum, and rabbit) usually do not eat sufficient quantities of soil to reach significant tissue levels of TCDD (soil levels less than 1 ppb). In this study, no dioxin was found in their tissues even though they spent months on soils containing about 80 ppt (geometric mean) with a range of 10–1500 ppt.

In contrast, cotton rats and beachmice water shown to have liver concentrations of 10–210 and 300–2900 ppt, respectively (30–50% of total body burden of TCDD is in liver). Numerous insects were also assayed, and these showed levels of 40–238 ppt, while birds (insect predators) had levels in the range of 50–440 ppt in the liver. Young et al. (135) concluded that for insects or animals the closeness of the relation to the soil seemed to dictate the degree of uptake. They noted that the beachmouse and cotton rat burrow in the soil, but that the deer, opossum, and rabbit do not. They were unable to identify whether the predators of insects actually received their body burdens due to ingestion of the insects or through preening of the soil with which they came into contact.

EXPOSURE/RISK CRITERIA

Although a considerable amount of effort is needed to properly identify the target species and the degree of exposure to a toxicant due to the presence of contaminated soil, the evaluation of the hazard is not complete until the absorbed dose is compared with some standard or guideline. These are usually derived from studies involving animals in experimentally exposed populations. Guidelines set for chemical carcinogens are sometimes called risk criteria.

For much of the past 50 years, the safety factor approach has been used to identify the dose at which humans would not be expected to be adversely affected (146). Until recently, the approach was also used for carcinogens, developmental toxicants and all systemic agents. Although much less complex than the mathematical models that were later developed for estimating the risk of exposure to carcinogenic agents, limits based on safety factors have generally been effective at preventing disease among exposed persons (146).

The safety or uncertainty factor approach is a simple one. Traditional toxicological procedures define a safe level of exposure for humans as some arbitrary fraction of the dose level at which no effects were observed in a group of test animals, e.g., no observed effect level (NOEL). When evaluating food additives and pesticides, where toxic effects other than cancer are a concern, an acceptable daily intake has often been established by dividing the NOEL by a safety factor of 100. The purpose of the safety factor is to account for the possibility that humans may be up to 10 times more sensitive than the animal species tested and that a 10-fold variation in sensitivity within the human population may exist (146, 147). The magnitude of this factor may be modified depending on the chemical and pharmacokinetic properties of the test compound, the severity of the adverse effect, as well as the quality of the available toxicological data.

Because genotoxic carcinogens may pose some degree of risk even at very low doses, an approach to establishing risk exposure limits or criteria other than those set through the use of safety factors was developed. These models are used to estimate the cancer risk at doses to which humans might be exposed due to water, food, air or soil contamination. The purpose of so-called cancer models is to identify a virtually safe dose (VSD) based on the extrapolation data obtained in animal tests. Because of the statistical and biological problems inherent in the identification of a true no-effect level, most mathematical models for carcinogens have eliminated the concept of a threshold e.g., a dose where no response would be expected.

The setting of standards, exposure criteria or risk criteria for contaminated soil is a difficult task since site specific factors have a significant influence on what degree of contamination would pose a hazard. For this and other reasons, only a handful of standards or regulations for contaminated soil have been established by state or federal agencies. The approximately six to ten soil standards or guidelines typically address trichloroethylene, methylene chloride, benzene, petroleum fuels, lead, PCB, and 2, 3, 7, 8-TCDD. To set such limits, the toxicological approaches discussed above should be used with consideration given to the ten or more other site-specific factors discussed throughout this paper.

DISCUSSION

Selection of the most appropriate assumptions is critical in any environmental risk assessment since often as few as one, two, or three assumptions or factors can dramatically influence the results. For example, in the health assessment of dioxin in soil, the most critical parameters are the quantity of soil ingested by children and adults, the mathematical modeling of the bioassay data, consideration of dioxin's lack of genotoxicity, and dioxin's bioavailability in a soil matrix. Other assumptions used in the assessment, while important, cannot alter the results by two to three orders of magnitude.

When evaluating the hazard posed by soil contaminated with other chemicals, numerous additional factors must be considered: Does the chemical bind tightly to soil? Does it become more difficult to desorb over time? Is the contaminant's water solubility low or high? Is it photolabile? Most importantly, is there enough contaminant present to affect the exposed animal or human population?

To date, no federal regulations governing contaminated soil have been passed. Of 22 states which claim to have set a soil clean-up level, only five consider them formal. Of the perhaps 1000 chemicals commonly used by industry, government, and homeowners which could be present in soils at excessive levels, fewer than a dozen have clean-up guidelines. Thus far, levels have been proposed for total petroleum hydrocarbons (TPH), volatile organic compounds (VOC), benzene, polynuclear aromatic hydrocarbons (PAH), trichloroethylene, polychlorinated biphenyls (PCB), ethylene dibromide (EDB), 2, 3, 7, 8-tetrachlorodibenzo-p-dioxin, toluene, and lead (11). Due to the on-going need for soil guidelines for numerous chemicals. The International Society for Regulatory Toxicology and Pharmacology established a panel of experts to begin the task of setting standards or guidelines for contaminated soil. The panel is known as the Council for the Health and Environmental Safety of Soils (CHESS).

Regulatory criteria regarding the acceptability of risk for nonubiquitous soil contaminants will probably be different from those for ubiquitous soil contaminants like lead or arsenic. For example, because fewer than 200 persons are known to live in residential areas where soil is contaminated with significant levels of dioxin, while millions live in neighborhoods having relatively high levels of lead or arsenic in the soil, higher levels of risk may be more acceptable for the former than for the latter. For example, any regulatory position regarding the risk criteria to be used for food additives (to which everyone is exposed), such as 1 in 1,000,000, would probably be inappropriate for dioxin- or PCB-contaminated soil, in light of the relatively small number of persons exposed to the latter toxins and their tendency not to migrate from the soil (assumes erosion is controlled) (136, 137).

Most environmental and occupational regulations that have been promulgated thus far accept cancer risks in the region of 1 in 1000 to 1 in 1,000,000, even where thousands of persons may be exposed (i) since it is believed that cancer risk models tend to overestimate the true risks (based on human data), (ii) because the cost–benefit criteria indicate that lower risks are impractical, or (iii) because the aggregate lifetime risk for the exposed population is close to, or less than, one additional case of cancer (136, 137). For example, the EPA has recently found the maximum individual risks and total population risks posed by a number of radionuclide and benzene sources to be too low to be considered "significant." Specifically, benzene emissions from maleic anhydride process vents created maximum individual risks of 7.6 in 100,000 and an aggregate yearly cancer incidence of 0.029 case (138). Radionuclides from facilities of the Department of Energy would expose a person who accrued lifetime exposure to a plant's most concentrated emissions to a risk of 1–8 in 10,000, such that in the aggregate, only 0.08 of an additional cancer case would be predicted to occur yearly (139). The EPA found these risks to be insignificant and eventually withdrew the proposed regulations.

The issue of the potential numbers of people affected will influence any risk management decision. Travis et al. (137) conducted a retrospective examination of the level of risk that triggered regulatory action in 132 cases. They considered three variables (i) individual risk (an upper-limit estimate of the probability that the most highly exposed individual in a population will develop cancer as a result of a lifetime exposure), (ii) population risk (an upper-limit estimate of the number of additional incidences of cancer in the exposed population), and (iii) population size. The findings of Travis et al. (137) can be summarized as follows:

1. Every situation presenting with an individual lifetime risk above 4×10^{-3} received regulatory action. Those with values below 1×10^{-6} remained unregulated.
2. For small populations, regulatory action never resulted for individual risks below 1×10^{-4}.
3. For effects resulting from exposures to the entire U.S. population, a risk level below 1×10^{-6} never triggered action; a risk level above 3×10^{-4} always did.

Consequently, regulatory agencies have taken different action, depending on the magnitude of the risk and the size of the population. Travis et al. (137) summarized their conclusion as follows:

Perhaps the most surprising aspect of our study is the consistency found among federal agencies' methods in the use of cancer risk estimates for regulatory decisions. With the possible exception of FDA decisions concerning de minimus risks, the history of federal decision making indicates that all agencies are fairly consistent in their implict definitions of de manifests and de minimum levels of risk. If the above three guidelines were adopted explicitly, consistency with past decisions would be maintained and the process of regulatory decision making would be simplified considerably.

Perhaps the most serious problem that has plagued risk assessments of the past 10 years, and one that is likely to affect assessments of contaminated soil, is the unreasonableness of some risk estimates due to the cumulative effect of conservatisms based on several worst-case assumptions for exposure. Overly zealous risk accessors have repetitively utilized parameters at the 95% level in the population. Compounding 95% confidence limits results not in a 95% confidence limit but rather in a usually much higher confidence limit. For example, if an upper bound on the intake of a chemical in drinking water were calculated assuming that the water is contaminated at the 95th percentile, and if a person drinks large quantities of water (the 95th percentile) and were physically small (the 5th percentile), then the upper bound is not a 95% upper bound but rather a much higher confidence limit. The maximum level of confidence here is 100%—specifically, $[1 - (0.05)^3] = 0.99875$.

Of course, the specific confidence level depends on the distribution of each of the various parameters. By way of illustration, if the concentration were normally distributed with means of 5.5 mg/L and variance 7.5, if drinking water consumption were normally distributed with a mean of 1 leter and variance of 0.55, if body weight were normally distributed with a mean of 78 kg and variance of 160, and if concentration, consumption, and weight were independent, then the confidence level of the corresponding upper bound would be 99.82% and not 95%. In this example, instead of 5% of the population exceeding the upper bound on intake, only 0.18% would. In other words, instead of 1 in 20 persons exceeding the upper bound on intake (the presumed goal of worst-case assumptions), only 1 person in 555 would. Applying this concept to procedures that are supposed to ensure that an individual's chance is no greater than 5% of exceeding a cancer risk of 1 in 1,000,000, the individual's actual chance is no greater than 5% of exceeding a cancer risk of 1 in 2,000,000!

In summary, soil contaminated by chemicals, including heavy metals, can pose a health hazard to exposed persons and to wildlife if the concentration and exposure are sufficiently great. However, our experience suggests that the hazard posed by direct exposure to contaminated soil, with the exception of certain well-acknowledged hazards, will frequently be quite low. When evaluating such risks, numerous factors must be considered, but special emphasis must be placed on the assumptions and factors used in estimating exposure. Because of the diversity of situations where soil is contaminated by any number of different chemicals, no generic guideline can be established for a given chemical or class of chemicals, but the procedures suggested here should be most helpful in developing a standardized process for assessing the risks to wildlife, biota, and humans.

REFERENCES

1. E. Chanlett, *Environmental Protection*. McGraw-Hill, New York, 1979, pp. 66–148.

2. H. L. Bergmann, R. A. Kimerle, and A. W. Maki, *Environmental Hazard Assessment of Effluents*. Pergamon Press, New York, 1986.

3. R. Kimbrough, H. Falk, P. Stehr, and G. Fries. Health implications of 2, 3, 7, 8-tetrachlorodibenzo-p-dioxin (TCDD) contamination of residential soil. *J. Toxicol. Environ. Health* **14**, 47–93 (1984).

4. J. Hawley. Assessment of health risk from exposure to contaminated soil. *Risk Anal.* **5**, 289–302 (1985).

5. J. W. Grisham (Ed.). *Health aspects of the Disposal of Waste Chemicals*. Pergamon Press, New York, 1986.

6. D. J. Paustenbach, H. P. Shu, and F. J. Murray. A Critical analysis of risk assessment of TCDD contaminated soil. *Regul. Toxicol. Pharmacol.* **6**, 284–307 (1986).

7. I. C. T. Nesbit, P. LaGoy, and C. Schultz, Endangerment assessment for the Smuggler Mountain Site, Pitkin County, Colorado. In D. J. Paustenbach (Ed.). *The Risk Assessment of Environmental and Human Health Hazards: A Textbook of Case Studies*. Wiley, New York, 1988.

8. G. F. Fries. Assessment of potential residues in foods derived from animals exposed to TCDD contaminated soil. *Chemosphere* **16**, 2123–2128 (1988).

9. A. Eschenroeder, R. J. Jaeger, J. J. Ospital, and C. P. Doyle, Health risk assessment of human exposures to soil amended with sewage sludge contaminated with polychlorinated dibenzodioxins and dibenzofurans. *Vet. Hum. Toxicol.* **28**, 435–442 (1986).

10. D. J. Paustenbach, Assessing the potential environmental and human health risks of contaminated soil. *Comments Toxicol.* **1**, 185–220 (1987).

11. E. J. Calabrese, and P. T. Kostecki, *Petroleum Contaminated Soils: Public and Environment Health Effects.* Wiley, New York, 1988.

12. W. Lowrance, *Assessment of Health Effects at Chemical Disposal Sites.* Wm. Kaufmann, Inc., Los Altos, CA, 1981.

13. Environmental Protection Agency, *An Approach to Estimating Exposures to 2,3,7,8-TCDD.* (draft). Office of Health and Environmental Assessment, US EPA, EPA/600/6-88-005A Washington, DC, 1988.

14. D. G. Patterson, R. E. Hoffmann, L. L. Needham, D. W. Roberts, J. L. Bagby, J. R. Pirkle, H. Falk, E. J. Sampson, and V. N. Houk, 2, 3, 7, 8-Tetrachlorodibenzo-p-dioxin levels in adipose tissue of exposed and control persons in Missouri. An interim report. *JAMA, J. Am. Med. Assoc.* **25B**, 2683–2686 (1986).

15. R. E. Menzer and J. O. Nelson, Water and soil pollutants. In *Casarett and Doull's Toxicology*, 3rd ed. C. D. Klaasan, M. O. Amdur, and J. Doull (Eds.). Macmillan, New York, 1986, pp. 825–853.

16. C. Sawyer, Contingency plans. In S. Levine (Ed.). *Protecting Personnel at Hazardous Waste Sites.* Ann Arbor Science, Ann Arbor, MI, 1985, pp. 327–349.

17. National Institute for Occupational Safety and Health, *Occupational Safety and Health Guidance Manual for Hazardous Waste Site Activities*, NIOSH Publ. 85–115. U.S. Govt. Printing Office, Washington, DC, 1985.

18. Occupational Safety and Health Administration, A proposed regulation for workers at hazardous waste sites. *Fed. Regist.* (1986).

19. H. W. Leung, F. J. Murray, and D. J. Paustenbach, A proposed occupational exposure limit for TCDD. *Am. Ind. Hyg. Assoc. J.* **49**, 466–474 (1988).

20. J. M. Devine, G. B. Konishita, R. P. Peterson, and G. L. Picard, *Arch. Environ. Contam. Toxicol.* **15**, 113–119 (1986).

21. J. Knaak, Y. Iwata, and K. T. Maddy, Evaluating the human health risks posed by exposure to pesticide treated fields. In D. J. Paustenbach (Ed.), *Risk Assessments of Environmental and Human Health Hazards: A Textbook of Case Studies.* Wiley, New York, 1988, Chap. 24.

22. R. D. Knarr, G. L. Cooper, E. A. Brian, M. G. Kleinschmidt, and D. G. Graham, Worker exposure during aerial application of a liquid and a granular formulation of ordram selective herbicide to rice. *Arch. Environ. Contam. Toxicol.* **14**, 523–527 (1985).

23. W. F. Durham, H. R. Wolfe, and J. F. Armstrong, Exposure of workers to pesticides. *Arch. Environ. Health* **14**, 622–633 (1967).

24. K. T. Maddy, R. G. Wang, J. B. Knaak, C. L. Liao, S. C. Edmiston, and C. K. Winter, Risk assessment of excess pesticide exposure to workers in California. In *Dermal Exposure Related to Pesticide Use.* American Chemical Society, Washington, DC, 1985, pp. 445–465.

25. W. J. Popendorf and R. C. Spear, Preliminary survey of factors affecting the exposure of harvesters to pesticide residues. *Am. Ind. Hyg. Assoc. J.* **35**, 374–380 (1974).

26. G. A. Wojeck, H. N. Nigg, R. S. Braman, J. H. Stamper, and R. L. Rouseff, Worker exposure to paraquat and diquat. *Arch. Environ. Contam. Toxicol.* **11**, 661–669 (1982).

27. S. D. Walter, A. J. Yankel, and I. H. von Lindern, Age specific risk factors for lead absorption in children. *Arch. Environ. Health* **35**, 53–58 (1980).

28. M. Cooper, *Pica.* Thomas, Springfield, IL, 1957, pp. 60–74.

29. E. Charney, J. Sayre, and M. Coulter, Increased lead absorption in inner city children: Where does the lead come from? *Pediatrics* **65**, 226–231 (1980).

30. J. W. Sayre, E. Charney, J. Vostal, and B. Pless, House and hand dust as a potential source of childhood lead exposure. *Am. J. Dis. Child.* **127**, 167–170 (1974).

31. F. K. Millican, E. M. Layman, R. S. Lourie, L. Y. Takahashi, and C. C. Dublin, The prevalance of ingestion and mouthing of nonedible substances by children. *Clin. Proc. Child. Hosp.* **28**, 207–214 (1962).

32. M. J. Duggan and S. Williams, Lead-in-dust in city streets. *Sci. Total Environ.* **7**, 91–97 (1977).

33. M. L. Lepow, L. Bruckman, R. A. Robino, S. Markowitz, M. Gillette, and J. Kapish, Role of airborne lead in increased body burden of lead in Hartford children. *Environ. Health Perspect.* **6**, 99–101 (1974).

34. M. L. Lepow, L. Bruckman, M. Gillette, S. Markowitz, R. Robino, and J. Kapish, Investigations into sources of lead in the environment of urban children. *Environ. Res.* **10**, 415–426 (1975).

35. D. Barltrop, Sources and significance of environmental lead for children. In *Environmental Health Aspects of Lead.* Commission of European Communities, Center for Information and Documentation, Luxembourg, 1973, pp. 675–681.

36. B. Brunekreef, D. Noy, K. Biersteker, and J. Boleij, Blood lead levels of dutch city children and their relationship to lead in the environment. *J. Air Pollut. Control Assoc.* **33**, 872–876 (1983).

37. National Research Council, *Lead in the Human Environment.* NRC, Washington, DC, 1980.

38. J. P. Day, M. Hart, and M. S. Robinson, Lead in urban street dust. *Nature (London)* **253**, 343–345 (1975).

39. A. L. Page and T. J. Ganje, (1970). Accummulation of lead in soils for regions for high and low vehicle traffic density. *Environ. Sci. Technol.* **4**, 140–142.

40. J. J. Vostal, E. J. Taves, W. Sayre, and E. Charney, Lead analysis of house dust: A method for the detection of another source of lead exposure in inner city children. *Environ. Health Perspect.* **7**, 91–97 (1974).

41. D. Barltrop, The prevalence of pica. *Am. J. Dis. Child.* **112**, 116–123 (1966).

42. S. D. Walter, A. J. Yankel, and I. H. von Lindern, Age specific risk factors for lead absorption in children. *Arch. Environ. Health* **35**, 53–58 (1980).

43. E. Calabrese, How much soil do children eat? An emerging consideration for environmental health risk assessment. *Comments Toxicol.* **1**, 229–241 (1987).

44. J. S. Lin-Fu, Vulnerability of children to lead exposure and toxicity. *N. Engl. J. Med.* **289**, 1289–1296 (1973).

45. H. Roels, J. P. Buchet, and R. R. Lauwerys, Exposure to lead by the oral and pulmonary routes of children living in the vicinity of a primary lead smelter. *Environment* **22**, 81–94 (1980).

46. D. Bryce-Smith, Lead absorption in children. *Phys. Bull.* **25**, 178–181 (1974).

47. Environmental Protection Agency, *Air Quality Criteria for Lead.* Vol. II, EPA-600/8-83/-028A. USEPA, Washington, DC, 1984.

48. D. Bellinger, A. Leviton, M. Rabinowitz, H. Needleman, and C. Waternaux, Correlates of low-level lead exposure in urban children at two years of age. *Pediatrics* (submitted for publication).

49. S. Binder, D. Sokal, and D. Maughan, Estimating soil ingestion: The use of tracer elements in estimating the amount of soil ingested by young children. *Arch. Environ. Health* **41**, 341–345 (1987).

50. O. Clausing, A. B. Brunekreef, and J. H. van Wijnen, A method for estimating soil ingestion by children. *Int. Arch. Occup. Environ. Health* **59**, 73–82 (1987).

51. E. J. Calabrese, C. E. Gilbert, P. T. Kostecki, R. Barnes, E. Stanek, P. Veneman, H. Pastides, and C. Edwards, Epidemiological Study to Estimate How Much Soil Children Eat. A report by the Division of Public Health, University of Massachusetts, Amherst, MA, 1988.

52. P. LaGoy, Estimated soil ingestion rates for use in risk assessment. *Risk Anal.* **7**, 355–359 (1987).

53. D. L. Vermeer and D. A. Frate, *Am. J. Clin. Nutr.* **32**, 2129–2135 (1979).

54. J. E. J. Gallagher, P. C. Elwood, K. M. Phillips, B. E. Davies, and D. T. Jones, Relation between pica and blood lead in areas of differing lead exposure. *Arch. Dis. Child.* **59**, 40–44 (1984).

55. H. R. Wolfe and J. F. Armstrong, Exposure of formulating plant workers to DDT. *Arch. Environ. Health* **23**, 170–176 (1971).

56. H. R. Wolfe, D. C. Armstrong, and W. F. Durham, Exposure of mosquito workers to fenthion. *Mosq. News* **34**, 263–267 (1974).

57. H. R. Wolfe, D. C. Staiff, J. F. Armstrong, and J. E. Davis, Exposure of fertilizer mixing plant workers to disulfoton. *Bull. Environ. Contam. Toxicol.* **20**, 79–86 (1978).

58. E. M. Romney, N. G. Lindberg, H. A. Hawthorne, B. B. Bystrom, and K. H. Larson, Contamination of plant foliage with radioactive nuclides. *Annu. Rev. Plant Physiol.* **14**, 271–279 (1963).

59. W. E. Martin, Loss of Sr-90, Sr-89 and I-131 from fallout of contaminated plants. *Radiat. Bot.* **4**, 275–281 (1964).

60. R. S. Russell, Entry of radioactive materials into plants. In R. S. Russell, Ed., *Radioactivity and Human Diet*, Pergamon Press, New York, 1966, Chap. 5.

61. C. F. Baes, III, R. D. Sharp, A. Sjoreen, and R. Shor, *A Review and Analysis of Parameters for Assessing Transport of Environmentally Released Radionuclides through Agriculture.* ORNL-5786. U.S. Dept. of Energy. Oak Ridge Natl. Lab. Oak Ridge, TN, 1984.

62. A. di Domencio, V. Silano, G. Viviano, and G. Zapponi, Accidental release of 2, 3, 7, 8-tetrachlorodibenzo-p-dioxin (TCDD) at Seveso, Italy. Part V. Environmental persistence of TCDD in soil. *Ecotoxicol. Environ. Saf.* **4**, 339–345 (1980).

63. K. M. Stevens, Agent Orange toxicity: A quantitative perspective. *Hum. Toxicol.* **1**, 31–39 (1981).

64. M. Gough, *Dioxin, Agent Orange: The Facts.* Plenum, New York, 1986.

65. D. J. Paustenbach, A validated approach to estimating the uptake of non-volatile chemicals by humans due to exposure to environmental contamination: Case studies involving dioxin and chloroane. *J. Toxicol. Environ. Health* (in preparation).

66. A. Young, Determination and measurement of human exposure to the dibenzo-p-dioxins. *Bull. Environ. Contam. Toxicol.* **33**, 702–709 (1984).

67. I. C. Munro and D. R. Krewski, Risk assessment and regulatory decision making. *Food Cosmet. Toxicol.* **19**, 549–560 (1981).

68. Food Safety Council, *Food Safety Assessment.* Nutrition Foundation, Washington, DC, 1980.

69. C. E. Land, in *Perceptions of Risk.* National Council on Radiation Protection and Measurements, Washington, DC, 1980, pp. 169–185.

70. E. M. Rupp, D. C. Parzyck, P. J. Walsh, R. S. Booth, R. J. Raridon, and B. L. Whitfield, Composite hazard index for assessing limiting exposures to environmental pollutants: Application through a case study. *Environ. Sci. Technol.* **12**, 802–807 (1978).

71. M. T. Halter and H. E. Johnson, in *Aquatic Toxicology and Hazard Evaluation* American Society for Testing and Material, Philadelphia, PA, 1977, pp. 178–196.

72. R. Haque (Ed.), *Dynamics, Exposure and Hazard Assessment of Toxic Chemicals.* Ann Arbor Science, Ann Arbor, MI, 1980.

73. G. M. Rand and S. R. Petrocelli, *Fundamentals of Aquatic Toxicology.* McGraw-Hill, New York, 1985.

74. G. W. Bailey and J. L. White, Factors influencing the absorption, desorption, and movement of pesticides in soil. *Residue Rev.* **32**, 29–92 (1970).

75. L. J. Thibodeaux, *Chemodynamics, Environmental Movement of Chemicals in Air, Water and Soil.* Wiley, New York, 1979.

76. U.S. Environmental Protection Agency, *Land Disposal Restrictions; Proposed Rule*, 40 CFR Part 260. Vol. 51, No. 9, January 14. USEPA, Washington, DC, 1986.

77. U.S. Environmental Protection Agency, *Superfund Health Assessment Manual*, Produced

by ICF, Clement Incorporated, under EPA Contract 68-01-6872. Office of Emergency and Remedial Response, US EPA, Washington, DC, 1986.

78. J. Schaum, *Risk Analysis of TCDD Contaminated Soil*. Office of Health and Environmental Assessment, U.S. Environmental Protection Agency, Washington, DC, 1983.

79. U.S. Environmental Protection Agency, *Endangerment Assessment Handbook*. Office of Emergency and Remedial Response, USEPA, Washington, DC, 1985.

80. R. Keenan, M. M. Sauer, F. H. Lawrence, and D. W. Crawford, Assessing the health hazard of TCDD contaminated sludge as a soil amendment. In D. J. Paustenbach (Ed.). *The Risk Assessment of Environmental and Human Health Hazards: A Textbook of Case Studies*. Wiley, New York, 1988, Chap. 28.

81. D. Lipsky, Assessment of potential health hazards associated with PCDD and PCDF emissions from a municipal waste combustor. In D. J. Paustenbach (Ed.). *The Risk Assessment of Environmental and Human Health Hazards: A Textbook of Case Studies*. Wiley, New York, 1988.

82. G. P. Markin, Translocation and fate of the insecticide Mirex within a bahia grass pasture ecosystem. *Environ. Pollut., Ser. A* **26**, 227–241 (1981).

83. B. Sicherman, *Alice Hamilton: A Life in Letters*. Harvard University Press, Cambridge, MA, 1984, pp. 158–160.

84. H. L. Cannon and J. M. Bowles, *Science* **137**, 765–766 (1962).

85. H. L. Motto, R. H. Daines, D. M. Chilko, and C. K. Motto, Lead in soils'and plants: Its relationship to traffic volumes and proximity to highways. *Environ. Sci. Technol.* **4**, 231–237 (1970).

86. H. Poiger and C. Schlatter, Influence of solvents and absorbents on dermal and intestinal absorption of TCDD. *Food Cosmet. Toxicol.* **18**, 477–481 (1980).

87. H. Shu, P. Teitelbaum, A. S. Webb, L. Marple, B. Brunck, D. Dei Rossi, J. Murray, and D. J. Paustenbach, Bioavailability of soil-bound TCDD: Dermal bioavailability in the rat. *Fundam. Appl. Toxicol.* **10**, 335–343 (1988).

88. M. Philippi, V. Krasnobagew, J. Zeyer, and R. Huetter, Microbial metabolism of TCDD under laboratory conditions. *FEMS Symp.* **12**, 2210–2233 (1981).

89. R. Huetter and M. Philippi, Studies on microbial metabolism of TCDD under laboratory conditions. In O. Hutzinger, R. W. Frei, E. Merian, and F. Pocchiari, Eds., *Chlorinated Dioxins and Related Compounds, Impact on the Environment*. Pergamon Press, New York, 1982, pp. 87–93.

90. J. Silkworth, D. McMartin, A. DeCaprio, R. Rej, P. O'Keefe, and L. Kaminsky, Acute toxicity in guinea pigs and rabbits of soot from a polychlorinated biphenyl-containing transformer fire. *Toxicol. Appl. Pharmacol.* **65**, 425–429 (1982).

91. M. Van den Berg, K. Olie, and O. Hutzinger, Uptake and selective retention in rats of orally administered chlorinated dioxins and dibenzofurans from fly-ash and fly-ash extract. *Chemosphere* **12**, 537–544 (1984).

92. E. McConnell, G. Lucier, R. Rumbaugh, P. Albro, R. D. Harvan, J. Hass, and M. Harris, Dioxin in soil: Bioavailability after ingestion by rats and guinea pigs. *Science* **223**, 1077–1079 (1984).

93. G. W. Lucier, R. C. Rumbaugh, Z. McCoy, J. Hass, R. D. Harvan, and P. Albro, Ingestion of soil contaminated with 2, 3, 7, 8 tetrachlorodibenzo-p-dioxin (TCDD) alters hepatic enzyme activities in rats. *Fundam. Appl. Toxicol.* **6**, 364–371 (1986).

94. T. H. Umbreit, E. J. Hesse, and M. A. Gallo, Acute toxicity of TCDD contaminated soil from an industrial site. *Science* **232**, 497–499 (1986).

95. E. Kenaga, Correlation of bioconcentration factors of chemicals in aquatic and terrestrial organisms with their physical and chemical properties. *Ecotoxicol. Environ. Saf.* **4**, 26–38 (1980).

96. S. M. Lambert, Functional relationship between sorption in soil and chemical structure. *J. Agric. Food Chem.* **15**, 572–576 (1967).

97. W. S. Snyder, *Report of the Task Group on Reference Man*, ICRP No. 23. Pergamon Press, New York, 1975.

98. J. Trijonis, J. Eldon, J. Gins, and G. Berglund, *Analysis of the St. Louis RAMS Ambient Particulate Data*, EPA Report 450/4-80-006a. Produced by Technology Service Corporation under EPA Contract 68-02-2931 for the Office of Air, Noise, and Radiation of the U.S. Environmental Protection Agency, Washington, DC, 1980.

99. C. Cowherd, G. Muleski, P. Englehart, and G. Gillette, *Rapid Assessment of Exposure to Particulate Emissions from Surface Contamination Sites*, EPA Control No. 68-01-6861. U.S. Environmental Protection Agency. Washington, DC, 1968.

100. U.S. Environmental Protection Agency, *Air Quality Criteria for Particulate Matter and Sulfur Oxides*, Vol. 2, EPA-600-8-82-029bF. Office of Environmental Criteria and Assessment, USEPA, Research Triangle Park, NC, 1984, pp. 5–106 to 5–112.

101. H. Shu, D. Paustenbach, J. Murray, L. Marple, B. Brunck, D. Dei Rossei, A. S. Webb, and T. Teitelbaum, Bioavailability of soil-bound TCDD: Oral bioavailability in the rat. *Fundam. Appl. Toxicol.* **10**, 648–654 (1988).

102. M. J. Bartek and J. A. LaBudde, Percutaneous absorption, in vitro. In H. Maibach, Ed., *Animal Models in Dermatology*. Churchill-Livingstone, New York, 1975, pp. 103–120.

103. R. C. Wester, and P. K. Noonan, Relevance of animal models for percutaneous absorption. *Int. J. Pharmacol.* **7**, 99–110 (1980).

104. L. S. Kaminksy, A. P. DeCaprio, J. F. Gierthy, J. B. Silkworth, and C. Tumasonis, The role of environmental matrices and experimental vehicles in chlorinated dibenzodioxin and dibenzofuran toxicity. *Chemosphere* **14**, 685–695 (1985).

105. J. W. Hamaker and J. M. Thompson, Adsorption. In C. A. I. Gorging and J. M. Haymaker, Eds., *Organic Chemicals in the Soil Environment*, Vol. 1. New York, 1972, pp. 51–122.

106. C. A. Edwards, Insecticide residues in soils. *Residue Rev.* **13**, 83–132 (1966).

107. D. T. Williams, G. L. LeBel, and E. Junkins, A comparison of organochlorine residues in human adipose tissue autopsy samples from two Ontario municipalities. *J. Toxicol. Environ. Health* **13**, 19–29 (1984).

108. M. Castanho, Methods of soil sampling. *Comments Toxicol.* **1**, 221–227 (1987).

109. S. M. Rappaport and J. Selvin, A method for evaluating the mean exposure from a log-normal distribution. *Am. Ind. Hyg. Assoc. J.* **48**, 374–379 (1987).

110. R. K. Puri, T. E. Clevenger, S. Kapila, and A. F. Yanders, Studies of the physico-chemical parameters affecting translocation of polychlorinated dibenzo-p-dioxins in soil. *7th Int. Symp. Chlorinated Dioxins Relat. Compd*, Abstract TF-09 (1987).

111. National Academy of Science, *Risk Assessment in the Federal Government: Managing the Process*. National Academy Press, Washington, DC, 1983.

112. A. R. Isensee and J. R. Jones, Absorption and translocation of root and foliage applied 2, 4-dichlorophenol, 2, 7-dichlorodibenzo-p-dioxin, and 2, 3, 7, 8-tetrachlorodibenzo-p-dioxin. *J. Agric. Food. Chem.* **19**, 1210–1214 (1971).

113. H. K. Wipf, E. Homberger, N. Neimer, U. B. Ranalder, W. Vetter, and J. P. Vuilleumeir, TCDD-levels in soil and plant samples from the Seveso area. In O. Hutzinger et al., Eds., *Chlorinated Dioxins and Related Compounds: Impact on the Environment*, Pergamon Press, New York, 1982, pp. 115–126.

114. B. C. Breidenstein, *Contribution of Red Meat to the U.S. Diet*. National Livestock and Meat Board, Chicago, IL, 1984.

115. G. F. Fries and L. W. Jacobs, Evaluation of residual polybrominated biphenyl contamination present on Michigan farms in 1978. *Mich., Agric. Exp. Stn., Res. Rep.* **477** (1986).

116. W. B. Healy, Ingestion of soil by dairy cows. *N.Z. J. Agric. Res.* **11**, 487–499 (1968).

117. W. B. Healy, T. W. Cutress, and C. Michie, Wear of sheep's teeth. IV. Reduction of soil ingestion and tooth wear by supplementing feeding. *N.Z. J. Agric. Res.* **10**, 201–209 (1967).

118. W. B. Healy and K. R. Drew, Ingestion of soil by hoggets grazing swedes. *N.Z. J. Agric. Res.* **13**, 940–944 (1970).

119. W. B. Healy and T. G. Ludwig, Wear of sheep's teeth. 1. The role of ingested soil. *N.Z. J. Agric. Res.* **8**, 737–752 (1965).

120. H. F. Mayland, A. R. Florence, R. C. Rosenau, V. A. Lazar, and H. A. Turner, Ingestion by cattle on semiarid range as reflected by titanium analysis of feces. *J. Range Manage.* **28**, 448–452 (1975).

121. I. Thornton and P. Abrahams, (1981). Soil ingestion as a pathway of metal intake into grazing livestock. In *Proceeding of the International Conference on Heavy Metals in the Environment*, CEP Consultants, Edinburgh, 1981, pp. 167–172.

122. G. F. Fries, G. S. Marrow, and P. A. Snow, Soil ingestion by dairy cattle. *J. Dairy Sci.* **65**, 611–618 (1982).

123. G. F. Fries, G. S. Marrow, and P. A. Snow, Soil ingestion by swine as a route of contaminant exposure. *Environ. Toxicol. Chem.* **1**, 201–204 (1982).

124. G. F. Fries, Potential polychlorinated biphenyl residues in animal products from application of contaminated sewage sludge to land. *J. Environ. Qual.* **11**, 14–20 (1982).

125. D. J. Jensen and R. A. Hummel, Secretion of TCDD in milk and cream following the feeding of TCDD to lactating cows. *Bull. Environ. Contam. Toxicol.* **29**, 440–446 (1982).

126. G. F. Fries, Bioavailability of soil-borne polybrominated biphenyls ingested by farm animals. *J. Toxicol. Environ. Health* **16**, 565–579 (1985).

127. D. Jones, S. Safe, E. Morcom, C. Coppock, and W. Ivie, (1986). Bioavailability of 2, 3, 7, 8 TCDD administered to Holstein dairy cows. *6th Int. Symp. Dioxins Relat. Compd* (1986), Abstr. BP-20.

128. A. L. Young, C. E. Thalken, and W. E. Ward, (1975). *Studies of the Ecological Impact of Repetitive aerial Application of Herbicides on the Ecosystem of Test Area C-52A, Eglin Air Force Base, FL*, Air Force Tech. Rep. AFATL-TR-75-142. Air Force Assessment Laboratory, Eglin AFB, FL, (1975) (available from Natl. Tech. Inf. Serv., Springfield, VA).

129. K. J. Macek, S. R. Petrocelli, and B. H. Sleight, III, Considerations in assessing the potential for, and significance of, biomagnification of chemical residues in aquatic food chains. *ASTM Spec. Tech. Publ.* **STP 667**, 251–268 (1979).

130. A. Spacie and J. Hamelink, Bioaccumulation. In G. M. Rand and S. R. Petrocelli, Eds., *Fundamentals of Aquatic Toxicology*. McGraw-Hill, New York, 1985.

131. A. J. Reinecke and R. G. Nash, Toxicology of TCDD and bioavailability by earthworms. *Soil Biol. Biochem.* **16**, 45–49 (1984).

132. A. L. Young and L. G. Cockerham, Fate of TCDD in field ecosystems: Assessment and significance for human exposures. In M. A. Kamrin and P. W. Rodges, Eds., *Dioxins in the Environment*. Hemisphere, New York, 1985, Chap. 11, pp. 153–171.

133. B. G. Oliver, Uptake of chlorinated organics from anthropogenically contaminated sediments by obigochaete worms. *Can. J. Fish Aquat. Sci.* **41**, 878–883 (1984).

134. C. E. Thalken and A. L. Young, Long-term field studies of a rodent population continuously exposed to TCDD. In R. E. Tucker, A. L. Young, and A. P. Gray, Eds., *Human and Environmental Risks of Chlorinated Dioxins and Related Compounds*. Plenum, New York, 1983.

135. A. L. Young, L. G. Cockerham, and C. E. Thalken, A long term study of ecosystem contamination with TCDD. *Chemosphere* (in press).

136. J. V. Rodricks, S. N. Brett and G. C. Wrenn, Risk decisions in federal regulatory agencies. *Regul. Toxicol. Pharmacol.* **7**, 307–320 (1987).

137. C. C. Travis, S. A. Richter, C. E. Crouch, R. Wilson, and E. D. Klema, Cancer risk management. *Environ. Sci. Technol.* **21**, 415–420 (1987).

138. Environmental Protection Agency, *National Emission Standards for Hazardous Air Pollutants; Benzene Emissions from Maleic Anhydride Plants, Ethylbenzene/Styrene Plants, and Benzene Storage Vessels; Proposed Withdrawal of Proposed Standards, Fed. Regist.*, **49**, 8386, 8388. USEPA, Washington, DC, 1984 ["Benzene NESHAPS Withdrawal Notice"].

139. Environmental Protection Agency, (1984d). *National Emission Standards for Hazardous Air Pollutants; Regulation of Radionuclides; Withdrawal of Proposed Standards, Fed. Regist.* **49**, 43906, 43910. USEPA, Washington, DC, 1984 ["Radionuclides NESHAPS Withdrawal Notice"].

140. G. Bresson, P. Pages, J. Lambard, and F. Fagnani, Occupational Radiological Risks in Uranium Mining. In International Conference on Radiation Hazards in Mining. Society of Mining Engineers, New York, 1981, pp. 111–114.

141. G. F. Fries and D. J. Paustenbach. *A Critical Evaluation of the Factors Used in Assessing Incinerator Emmissions as a Potential Source of TCDD in Food of Animal Origin.* Abstract RC-05. Seventh International Dioxin Symposium. Las Vegas, NV, 1987.

142. W. H. Stickle, D. W. Hayne, and L. F. Stickle. Effects of heptachlor-contaminated earthworms on woodcocks. *J. Wildlife Manag.* **29**, 132–146 (1965).

143. L. F. Stickle. Chemosphere pesticide residues in birds and mammals. In C. A. Edwards (Ed.). *Environmental Pollution by Pesticides.* Plenum Press, New York, 1973.

144. R. K. Tucker and D. G. Crabtree. *Handbook of Toxicity of Pesticides to Wildlife.* Fish and Wildlife Service USDI. Resource Publication #84. Denver Wildlife Research Center, Denver, CO.

145. L. R. DeWeese, L. C. McEwen, G. L. Hensler, and B. E. Petersen. Organochlorine contaminants in passeriformes and other avian prey of the peregrine falcon in the western United States. *Environ. Toxicol. Chem.* **5**, 675–693 (1985).

146. M. L. Dourson and J. F. Stara. Regulatory history and experimental support of uncertainty (safety) factors. *Regul. Toxicol. Pharmacol.* **3**, 224–238.

147. A. J. Lehman and O. G. Fitzhugh. 100-fold margin of safety. *Bull. Assoc. Food and Drug. Off.* **18**, 33–35.

148. T. M. Roberts, W. Gizyn, and T. C. Hutchinson. Lead contamination of air, soil, vegetation and people in the vicinity of secondary lead smelters. In D. D. Hemphill (Ed.), *Trace Substances in Environmental Health*, Vol. VIII. University of Missouri Press, Columbia, MO, 1974.

149. J. R. Roberts and W. K. Marshall. Retentive capacity: An index of chemical persistence expressed in terms of chemical–specific and ecosystem–specific parameters. *Ecotoxicol. Environ. Safety* **4**, 158–171 (1980).

B

ASSESSING WATER CONTAMINANTS

8

Hazard Assessment of 1, 1, 1-Trichloroethane in Groundwater

James L. Byard

James L. Byard, Toxicology Consultant, Inc., El Macero, California

INTRODUCTION

1, 1, 1-Trichloroethane (TCA) has been widely used as an industrial degreasing solvent since the mid 1950s (1, 2). Casual use practices and leaking underground tanks have resulted in contamination of soil and groundwater at a number of sites (3). One location of such sites is the Santa Clara Valley in California, also known as Silicon Valley, where the widespread use of TCA to clean microelectronic parts has led to contamination of soil and groundwater (4). The purpose of this chapter is to assess the toxicological hazards to residents of the Santa Clara Valley. They were exposed to TCA via domestic water supplies pumped from contaminated groundwater. The hazard assessment begins with a review of the physical and chemical properties of TCA.

2   PHYSICAL AND CHEMICAL PROPERTIES

TCA is a colorless liquid with a distinctive odor. Physical properties are as follows:

specific gravity $= 1.33$ (2);

boiling point $= 74°C$ (2);

vapor pressure $= 103$ mm Hg at $20°C$ (5) and 123 mm Hg at $25°C$ (6);

solubility in water $= 1300$ ppm at $25°C$ (5) and 720 ppm at $25°C$ (7);

molecular weight $= 133.4$ g (5);

1 ppm in air $= 5.4$ mg/m^3 (6);

air–water partition coefficient $= 0.68$ (6) and 1.2 (7);

$t_{1/2}$ for volatilization at room temperature ($\sim 25°C$) from water $= 20$ min (6).

TCA is stable to heat up to 260°C (8). However, TCA is unstable in the presence of aluminum and water and therefore is sold commercially with various stabilizers such as dioxane, butanol, nitromethane, and butylene oxide (5, 8). The half-life for hydrolysis in water is 7.8 months at 25°C and 36 months at 15°C (8). Sunlight does not speed the rate of breakdown. Hydrolysis products are acetic acid, hydrochloric acid, and vinylidene chloride (6, 9).

3 SITE DESCRIPTION

3.1 Surface

Land use in the Santa Clara Valley is predominantly a mixture of residential and commercial. Agriculture was once the primary land use but now occupies only a small percentage of the land surface in the valley. The Santa Clara Valley has a Mediterranean climate with warm, dry summers and cool, wet winters (10). The mean annual rainfall is 13.7 in. The average daily temperature in the valley ranges from 7 to 10°C in January to 18 to 21°C in July. The prevailing winds are from the south in the winter and are from the

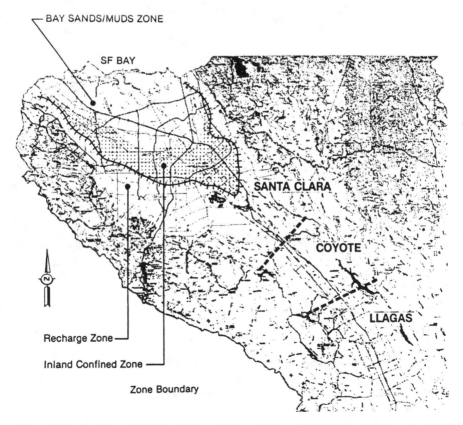

Figure 1. Surface map of the Santa Clara Valley showing the subbasins and the recharge zone. Reproduced with permission from Fig. 4–5 in ref. 4.

northwest in the summer. Average wind speeds in 1984 were 2.3 mph in January and
4.4 mph in June.

3.2   Subsurface

The Santa Clara Valley is an alluvium-filled bedrock basin draining into the southern end
of the San Francisco Bay (4). The upland areas are the recharge zone where surface water
permeates into the alluvial soils to provide the hydrostatic head for groundwater flow
toward the San Francisco Bay (Fig. 1). The aquifers in the valley are the sand and gravel
zones that provide preferred horizontal flow paths for groundwater (Fig. 2). The
intervening clay and silt zones restrict the vertical flow of groundwater.

4   CONTAMINATION AND MITIGATION

Slow releases of TCA to soil and groundwater apparently were the result, over time, of
leakage from underground piping and tanks and spills from handling TCA (4). Mitigation
has included changing work practices to prevent spills, removing buried pipes and tanks,
installing above ground tanks and pipes with secondary containment, removing contaminated soil, and pumping contaminated groundwater (10).

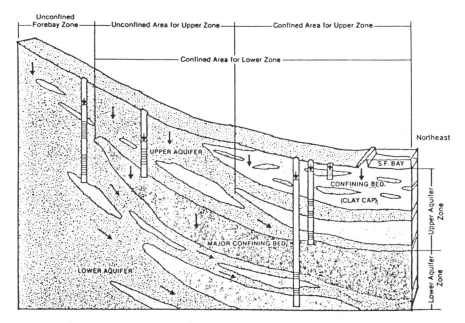

Note: Arrows indicate direction of groundwater movement without regard to quantity.

Figure 2. Hydrogeologic cross section of the Santa Clara Valley. Reproduced with permission from
Fig. 4 8 in ref. 4.

5   ENVIRONMENTAL FATE

Based on the physical and chemical properties of TCA, one would expect that solvent leaking into soil would be readily leached to groundwater where the TCA would persist with a half-life of a few years. When the groundwater is pumped to the surface, one would expect rapid volatilization into the air. Overall, the TCA in the environment would be expected to be slowly mineralized to carbon dioxide, water, and hydrochloric acid (11). Vinylidene chloride is a trace contaminant of commercial TCA (12) and is a product of the breakdown of TCA in aqueous solution (6, 9). Although the hazards of vinylidene chloride will not be dealt with in this chapter, this chemical is of concern wherever there is contamination of groundwater by TCA.

6   EXPOSURE

6.1   Domestic Wells

Approximately 20 out of 235 wells serving major water purveyors were contaminated with TCA (4). One well, located in the recharge zone, contained levels as high as 8800 ppb TCA (13). This well has been closed since late 1981 when TCA was first detected. Only a few hundred of the more than 5000 private wells and wells serving minor purveyors have been analyzed for TCA. Several of these wells are contaminated. The highest level of TCA reported was 150 ppb (4).

6.2   Routes

Based on the environmental fate of TCA, human exposure should be evaluated for each of the following routes: ingestion of contaminated water, dermal contact with contaminated water during bathing, and dermal and inhalation uptake of vapors volatilizing from the surface of contaminated water.

7   DETERMINATION OF DOSE

7.1   Ingestion

One can estimate a total human dose by making several reasonable worst case assumptions. The first assumption is that humans ingest 2 L of water per day per 70 kg body weight, and all that is ingested is absorbed from the gastrointestinal tract (3). The assumption of complete absorption is reasonable since TCA is a small molecule with both water and lipid solubility. For example, a calculated oil–water partition coefficient for TCA is 383 (14). If we assume a reference level of $1 \mu g/L$ (1 ppb) of TCA in water, the ingestion dose is

$$2 \text{ L/body weight·day} \times 1 \mu g/L \times 100\% \text{ absorption}$$
$$\times \text{ body weight}/70 \text{ kg} = 0.0286 \mu g/kg·day.$$

7.2   Toilet Bowl

Vapors of TCA can occur in the home as a result of volatilization from water surfaces. Dilling et al. (6) determined that 50% of a slowly stirred solution of 1000 ppb TCA in water volatilized in 20 min at 25°C; 90% volatilized in 69 min. Therefore, one can expect volatilization of approximately 85% TCA per hour from standing water at room temperature. For example, a toilet bowl containing 5 L of 1 ppb TCA would release 0.85/h $\times$ 1 μg/L $\times$ 5 L = 4.25 μg/h. If one assumes a bathroom that is 2 m $\times$ 3 m $\times$ 2.5 m = 15 m^3, then the airborne concentration from the toilet bowl is 4.5 μg/15 m^3 = 0.3 μg/m^3. However, the air is not static but is turning over. If we assume a turnover of 3 volumes of air per hour and a toilet that is flushed once per hour, then the maximum airborne concentration of TCA in the bathroom is 0.3 μg/m^3 $\times$ 1/3 = 0.1 μg/m^3. The actual concentration will be lower because the TCA is continuously diluted by makeup air as it volatilizes from the toilet bowl. Assuming a residence time of 1 h/day in the bathroom, a respiration rate of 18 m^3/day, a 70 kg body weight, and 30% uptake from the lungs (15), a reasonable worst case inhalation dose would be

$$0.1 \, \mu g/m^3 \times 18 \, m^3/day \times 1 \, h/24 \, h \times 1/70 \, kg \times 30\% \text{ absorption} = 0.00032 \, \mu g/kg \cdot day.$$

7.3   Shower

A similar calculation could be made for a person taking a shower or bath. The shower would probably represent the highest inhalation exposure, due to the large volume of hot water and the small air volume of a shower stall. The volatilization rate would probably be faster at shower temperatures (approximately 50°C) than at room temperature (25°C). For example, a 10-min shower with 50 L of water containing 1 ppb TCA would release approximately 25 μg TCA if the half-life for volatilization is 10 min. If the dimensions of the shower are 1 m $\times$ 1 m $\times$ 25 m = 2.5 m^3, the airborne concentration would be 25 μg/2.5 m^3 = 10 μg/m^3, assuming that the air is static. Since dermal uptake and volatilization are competing processes, and most of the water does not make direct contact with the skin, only a small fraction of the TCA in the shower water would be expected to diffuse from the water into the skin. This direct dermal absorption is estimated to be no more than 1% of the available TCA. Once TCA has volatilized, the vapor may be taken up by both the dermal and inhalation routes. A person is active when showering, so we can assume a respiration rate of 1 m^3/h or 0.167 m^3 in 10 min. If we assume that the airborne concentration of TCA is 0 μg/m^3 at the beginning of the shower and increases linearly with respect to time to 10 μg/m^3 at the end of the shower, the air does not turn over, and one shower is taken per day, then the total dose by inhalation is

$$(0 \, \mu g/m^3 + 10 \, \mu g/m^3)/2 \times 0.167 \, m^3/day \times 1/70 \, kg$$

$$\times 30\% \text{ absorption} = 0.00358 \, \mu g/kg \cdot day.$$

Dermal vapor absorption will contribute some additional TCA, estimated to be no more than 1% of the inhalation dose. The total dose of the hypothetical shower is the sum of the estimated inhalation, dermal water, and dermal vapor doses:

$$0.00358 \, \mu g/kg \cdot day + 1\% \times (50 \, \mu g - 25 \, \mu g) \times 1/70 \, kg$$

$$\times 1/day + 1\% \times 0.00358 \, \mu g/kg \cdot day = 0.0072 \, \mu g/kg \cdot day.$$

7.4   Bath

A similar calculation could be made for a bath. If we assume 100 L of water at 50°C for 20 min in a room that measures 2 m $\times$ 3 m $\times$ 2.5 m, and a half-life of volatilization of

10 min, a concentration of 1 ppb TCA will contribute a maximum of $1 \mu g/L \times 0.75 \times 100 L = 75 \mu g$ TCA to the room. Assuming three air turnovers per hour, the maximum airborne concentration of TCA will be $75 \mu g/15 m^3 \times 1/3 = 1.67 \mu g/m^3$. Assuming a respiration rate of $0.75 m^3/h$, 20 min per bath, 1 bath per day, a 70 kg body weight, and 30% uptake from the lungs, the maximum dose is

$$1.67 \mu g/m^3 \times 0.75 m^3/h \times 0.333 h$$

$$\times 1/70 \times 30\% \text{ absorption} = 0.00179 \mu g/kg \cdot day.$$

Additional amounts of TCA would come from dermal absorption of the vapor and dermal absorption from the water. Because of the greater thickness and smaller surface area of the skin relative to the lungs, dermal vapor absorption is estimated to be no more than 1% of the inhalation exposure.

Dermal absorption from the bath water is unknown, but an estimate can be made from reports of dermal uptake of toluene, xylene, ethylbenzene, and styrene from aqueous solutions (16–18). By assuming that TCA has a similar rate of dermal uptake from aqueous solutions, the dose by this route would be approximately $1 ng/cm^2 \cdot h$ by extrapolating from data by Dutkiewicz and Tyras (18) linearly to 1 ppb. Assuming a body surface area of $18,000 cm^2$, 80% immersion in the bath water, a 20 min bath once per day, and a 70 kg body weight, the dermal dose from the water would be

$$1 ng/cm^2 \cdot h \times 18,000 cm^2 \times 1/3 h \times 0.80 \times 1/day$$

$$\times 1/70 kg \times 1 \mu g/1000 ng = 0.0686 \mu g/kg \cdot day.$$

This value should be corrected for volatilization of approximately one-third of the TCA during the bath. The corrected dermal dose is therefore

$$0.0686 \mu g/kg \cdot day \times 2/3 = 0.0457 \mu g/kg \cdot day.$$

This route represents the greatest contribution to exposure, being approximately 60% higher than ingestion exposure. Since the dermal water uptake is not based on direct measurements with TCA, there may be substantial error in the estimation of this component of dose.

The total dose from the hypothetical bath described above would be the sum from inhalation, dermal vapor, and dermal water exposures:

$$0.00179 \mu g/kg \cdot day + 1\% \times 0.00179 \mu g/kg \cdot day$$

$$+ 0.0457 \mu g/kg \cdot day = 0.0475 \mu g/kg \cdot day.$$

7.5 Total Dose

A reasonable worst case bathroom exposure would be a person taking 1 bath per day and staying in the bathroom an additional 1 h each day. Under these conditions, the daily dose from the bathroom would be

$$0.0475 \mu g/kg \cdot day + 0.00032 \mu g/kg \cdot day = 0.0478 \mu g/kg \cdot day$$

for water containing 1 ppb TCA. The dose from the sum of ingestion and bathroom exposure would be

$$0.0286 \ \mu g/kg \cdot day + 0.0478 \ \mu g/kg \cdot day = 0.0764 \ \mu g/kg \cdot day$$

for water containing 1 ppb TCA. The highest inhalation exposure is for 1 h in the bathroom plus a 10-min shower and is 0.0068 $\mu g/kg \cdot day$. This value is approximately $\frac{1}{10}$th of that estimated by McKone (19) for a household inhalation dose of TCA from water. Most of this 10-fold difference can be accounted for by differences in assumptions as to uptake, volatilization rate, time of exposure, and consideration of the much lower exposure that occurs in other parts of the home.

For any level of TCA in drinking water, one can estimate the human dose by multiplying the water level in ppb times 0.0764. This dose can then be compared to doses of TCA that are known to produce toxic effects.

8 TOXICOLOGY

Several authors have summarized the toxicology of TCA (2, 3, 5, 7, 20–22). The following discussion is not a complete review of the toxicology of TCA but deals with those aspects that are important to this hazard assessment.

8.1 Fate in the Body

As previously stated, TCA is estimated to be efficiently absorbed from the gastrointestinal tract (3) and approximately 30% absorbed from the lungs (15). Once in the body, this chemical is rapidly distributed to all tissues via the bloodstream (23–27). Transient storage occurs in adipose tissue. Once exposure has ceased, residual TCA in the body is rapidly eliminated via the lungs. The potential for accumulation in the body is minimal. Only the unchlorinated carbon in TCA appears to be significantly metabolized in mammalian tissues (28, 29), ruling out a reactive metabolite. The identified metabolites are trichloroethanol, trichloroacetic acid, and their conjugates. These metabolites are excreted in the urine. Metabolism of an inhaled dose of TCA occurs to the extent of approximately 6% in rats and humans and 13% in mice (27).

8.2 Acute Toxicity

At high acute exposures, TCA acts as a narcotic on the nervous system. Stewart et al. (30) described acute symptoms in human volunteers exposed for 15 min to vapor concentrations of TCA increasing from zero to 2650 ppm. Mild eye irritation occurred at 1000–1100 ppm, throat irritation at 1900–2000 ppm, lightheadedness at 2600 ppm, and inability to stand at 2650 ppm. In animal studies, TCA was relatively nontoxic (7). LD_{50} values ranged from 6 to 12 g/kg in rabbits, mice, rats, and guinea pigs.

8.3 Subchronic Toxicity

Slight, reversible irritation at the site of application was the only observed effect in rabbits exposed dermally to 500 mg/kg·day of TCA for 90 days (7). The NOEL for subchronic inhalation exposure to rats, guinea pigs, rabbits, and monkeys was 500 ppm, 7 h/day, 5 days/week, for 26 weeks. Higher exposures produced irritation of the respiratory tract, fatty liver, and narcosis (7). McNutt et al. (31) reported that 14 weeks of continuous inhalation exposure to 250 ppm TCA produced slight lipid accumulation in the liver of mice. Prendergast et al. (32) reported that no toxicity was observed in rats, guinea pigs, rabbits, and monkeys exposed to 381 ppm TCA continuously for 90 days.

8.4   Chronic Toxicity, Including Carcinogenicity

The chronic toxicity of TCA has been evaluated by Dow Chemical (33, 34), the National Cancer Institute (35), the National Toxicology Program (36), and Maltoni et al. (37). The study by Rampy et al. (33) is a 1-year inhalation exposure in rats followed by observation to 30 months. No toxicity, including no excess cancers, were observed at the highest exposure of 1750 ppm, 6 h/day, 5 days/week. This bioassay is not fully sensitive for a chronic toxicity/carcinogenicity study, since the rats were not exposed for most of their lifetimes. The study by Quast et al. (34) is a 2-year inhalation exposure in mice. No toxicity, including no excess carcinogenicity, was observed at 1500 ppm, 6 h/day, 5 days/week. The high dose of 1500 ppm was very near a maximally tolerated dose since 2000 ppm produced toxicity in a preliminary 90-day study.

The NCI study (35) was for 90 weeks in rats. TCA exposure was for 78 weeks by oral gavage, followed by a 12-week observation period. High mortality, largely due to gavage deaths, greatly reduced the sensitivity of this study. No marked toxicity, including no marked oncogenic effect, was observed at doses up to 1500 mg/kg·day, 5 days/week. The NTP study (36) was conducted for 2 years in rats. Exposure was by oral gavage. No marked toxicity, including no marked excess cancer, was observed at 750 mg/kg·day, 5 days/week, for 2 years. Survival was poor, due in large part to gavage deaths. This study is currently being audited.

The carcinogenicity study by Maltoni et al. (37) was done in rats exposed to a single dose of 500 mg/kg·day of TCA in olive oil or olive oil alone. A single dose was given each day by oral gavage for 4–5 days/week for 104 weeks followed by an observation period of 37 weeks. Therefore, high sensitivity was attained due to the length of the observation period in this study. Forty rats of each sex were exposed to TCA and 50 rats of each sex were controls. TCA had no apparent effect on mortality or body weight. Pathology was only reported for cancers. Hence, there is no evaluation of noncancerous tissue pathology that may have been produced by TCA. Based on the NCI study (35), tissue pathology and excess cancers due to TCA would not be expected. However, Maltoni et al. (37) reported an excess of leukemias in the rats exposed to TCA (13/100 compared to 4/80). This study is contradicted by the other carcinogenicity bioassays and is far too incomplete to provide a valid indication that TCA is carcinogenic. The authors stated that further experiments are needed.

The inhalation study by Quast et al. (34) appears to be fully valid for evaluating the chronic toxicity/oncogenicity of TCA by the inhalation route. A valid chronic bioassay by the oral route has not yet been done. Little difference in toxicity between the oral and inhalation routes of exposure has been observed, probably because TCA is rapidly distributed and poorly metabolized. Therefore, toxicity by inhalation exposure should be a reasonably good estimate of toxicity by the oral route.

8.5   Genotoxicity

The mutagenicity of TCA has been evaluated in several bioassays. Most of the results have been negative. A few studies with the Ames/*Salmonella* assay have been weakly positive.

These weakly positive results can be rationalized as resulting from butylene oxide present in some commercial formulations of TCA.

In the study by Simmon et al. (38), reagents of the highest available purity were purchased from commercial suppliers. The amounts and nature of any impurities were not indicated. An approximate doubling of the background mutation rate was observed in TA100 exposed to 1 mL of TCA in a desiccator. A dose response was observed, and S-9 was not required to express the mutagenesis. In a 1980 study by Nestman et al. (39), TCA produced a dose-related increase in revertants in desiccator assays. One milliliter of TCA produced a 6-fold increase in mutagenesis in TA1535 and a 2.5-fold increase in mutagenesis in TA100. The TCA used in this study was obtained from Fisher Scientific. The Carcinogen Assessment Group of the EPA (40) later found that Fisher Scientific obtained TCA from Dow Chemical as the technical grade material containing 0.74% of butylene oxide. In a 1984 study, Nestman et al. (41) reported that TCA obtained from Fisher and from Aldrich were mutagenic. The TCA from Fisher was approximately twice as potent in TA1535 and TA100 as the TCA from Aldrich.

Domoradzki (42) compared the mutagenicity of purified and commercial TCA in the Ames/*Salmonella* assay. Both butylene oxide inhibitor and commercial TCA were mutagenic in strains TA1535 and TA100. TA1535 was more sensitive in each case. Purified TCA was negative in all strains. The potency and strain specificity of butylene oxide accounted precisely for the mutagenicity of commercial TCA. Other inhibitors of the corrosive action of TCA were found not to be mutagenic.

Shimada et al. (43) made a similar observation in the Ames/*Salmonella* assay. TCA, containing 0.45% butylene oxide, was mutagenic in strains TA100 and TA1535. Purified TCA was not mutagenic at vapor concentrations as high as 7.5%, a level that killed 96–98% of the bacteria. A vapor concentration of 10% killed 95–99% of the bacteria and produced a threefold to fourfold increase in the reversion rate. The high degree of cell killing and the lack of a dose response suggest that this apparent mutagenic effect at 10% vapor concentration is not the result of a direct genotoxic effect of TCA, but rather an indirect effect associated with cell death. In the same report, Shimada et al. (43) found that TCA does not increase the rate of DNA repair in primary cultures of rat hepatocytes.

The overall lack of genotoxicity of TCA is consistent with metabolic studies indicating that this chemical is not metabolized via a reactive metabolite (28, 29). Although this evaluation indicates that there is not a mutagenic hazard due to TCA in groundwater, the occurrence of 2, 3-butylene oxide in TCA suggests a concern that this known mutagen may also contaminate groundwater. The half-life of 1, 2-butylene oxide in water at 25°C is approximately one week (44), suggesting that the closely related structure of 2, 3-butylene oxide would degrade rapidly in groundwater.

8.6   Reproductive and Developmental Toxicity

Several investigators have found no teratogenic effects in rodents exposed to TCA (45–47). No reproductive effects were detected in these studies, except for a marginally significant decrease in fetal weight and delayed fetal development in rats exposed in utero to 2100 ppm vapors of TCA (46). Dapson et al. (48) reported an increase in cardiac abnormalities in rats exposed in utero to 10 ppm of TCA in drinking water containing 0.05% Tween 80. This finding may not be valid in light of the previous negative reports and the association of cardiac toxicity with exposure to Tween 80 (49) and the association of malformations with a related compound, Tween 20 (50). A recent NTP study (51) assessed cardiac and other visceral abnormalities in rats exposed in utero to TCA. No malformations were produced by TCA at exposures up to 30 ppm in drinking water.

The issue of cardiac abnormalities was of particular interest to residents of the Santa Clara Valley because of an apparent higher incidence in a community within the valley. Besides the negative animal studies, no association could be found between exposure to TCA and the occurrence of such abnormalities in residents of the study area (13). A retrospective epidemiological study among workers manufacturing TCA found no association between exposure and any health effect (52).

8.7   Summary of Toxicology

In summary, TCA is a relatively nontoxic chemical. Narcosis, mild organ pathology, and irritation of the respiratory tract are the major toxic effects that appear to occur only at vapor exposures of 250 ppm or greater. These effects have thresholds and are the type of effects that are reversible if the pathology is mild. At or below the threshold for toxicity, one would not expect any irreversible effects to occur. Hence, the estimation of a nontoxic dose for humans can be based on the application of appropriate safety factors to a NOEL.

9   ESTIMATION OF A NONTOXIC DOSE

9.1   No Observable Effect Level (NOEL)

The lowest NOEL for a continuous subchronic or chronic exposure to TCA can be estimated from the LOEL of 250 ppm in mice (31). A reduction of the LOEL by a factor of 5 should give a conservative estimate of the NOEL since exposure of mice to levels as high as 1500 ppm, 6 h/day, 5 days/week was without effect in a 2-year study (34). Hence, the estimated NOEL is 50 ppm. If one assumes that humans breathe $18 \, m^3/day$, humans weigh 70 kg, 30% of inhaled TCA is taken up into the body, and 1 ppm TCA is equal to $5400 \, \mu g/m^3$, then the chronic NOEL daily dose for humans is

$$50 \, ppm \times 18 \, m^3/body \cdot day \times body/70 \, kg \times 30\% \text{ absorption}$$
$$\times 5400 \, \mu g/m^3 = 21000 \, \mu g/kg \cdot day.$$

9.2   Safety Factors

A nontoxic dose can be estimated by dividing the NOEL by safety factors to account for (i) variability in species, (ii) variability in individual humans, and (iii) exposure to TCA from other sources plus exposure to other chemicals having the same mechanism(s) of action. A factor of 10 is widely used to account for each of these uncertainties. Therefore, a nontoxic dose can be calculated as

$$21000 \, \mu g/kg \cdot day \times 1/10 \times 1/10 \times 1/10 = 21 \, \mu g/kg \cdot day.$$

From our earlier estimation of a dose of $0.0764 \, \mu g/kg \cdot day$ from exposure to water containing 1 ppb TCA, one can estimate a nontoxic level in water as

$$21 \, \mu g/kg \cdot day \times 1 \, ppb/(0.0764 \, \mu g/kg \cdot day) = 270 \, ppb.$$

If one were to consider a 10-kg child ingesting 1 L of water per day, the nontoxic dose would be reduced by a factor of 3.5, to 80 ppb. The EPA (53) and the California

Department of Health Services (54) have recommended, for chronic exposure, a maximum nontoxic action level of 200 ppb TCA.

9.3   Additional Health Conservative Assumptions

The estimation of ingestion exposure ignores the volatilization of TCA from water before it is ingested. In addition to the three safety factors of 10, another health conservative assumption has been introduced into the estimate of a maximum nontoxic level in water. A LOEL from the most sensitive species has been chosen in addition to a safety factor of 10 for species variation. Workplace experience indicates that humans are not more sensitive than the mouse.

9.4   Margins of Safety

Adult residents of the Santa Clara Valley, who may have been exposed to water containing TCA measured to be as high as 8800 ppb, would not be expected to be poisoned, but the margin of safety at this level would be reduced to a factor of

$$(21000\,\mu g/kg \cdot day)/(8800\,ppb \times [0.0764\,\mu g/kg \cdot day]/ppb) = 30.$$

The next highest level measured was 150 ppb, with an estimated margin of safety of 1800.

10   CONCLUSIONS

TCA has contaminated domestic wells in the Santa Clara Valley. Detectable levels have ranged up to 8800 ppb. A review of the literature indicates that TCA is relatively nontoxic. Narcosis, mild liver injury, and irritation of the respiratory tract are the notable toxic effects that have been reported. TCA does not appear to produce irreversible injury such as mutation, terata, or cancer. Based on a lifetime continuous exposure NOEL of 21 mg/kg·day, a nontoxic level in domestic water is estimated to be 270 ppb. A maximum level of 8800 ppb found in one well is 1/30th of the estimated NOEL. Even though a level of 270 ppb is estimated to be nontoxic with a large margin of safety, when one considers the uncertainties of hazard assessment, one should strive for the lowest level that is practical.

REFERENCES

1. D. D. Irish, Methyl chloroform. In F. A. Patty, Ed., *Industrial Hygiene and Toxicology*, 2nd ed., Vol. 2. Wiley, New York, 1963.
2. T. R. Torkelson and V. K. Rowe, Halogenated aliphatic hydrocarbons containing chlorine bromine and iodine. In G. D. Clayton and F. E. Clayton, Eds., *Patty's Industrial Hygiene and Toxicology*. Wiley, New York, 1981.
3. U.S. Environmental Protection Agency, *Health Assessment Document for 1, 1, 1-Trichloroethane (Methyl Chloroform)*, Final Report. USEPA, Washington, DC, 1984.
4. U.S. Environmental Protection Agency, *Santa Clara Valley Integrated Environmental Management Project*, Revised Stage I Report. USEPA, Washington, DC, 1986.
5. International Agency for Research on Cancer, Some halogenated hydrocarbons. *IARC Monogr. Eval. Carcinog. Risk Chem. Man* **20**, 515–530 (1979).

6. W. L. Dilling, N. B. Tefertiller, and G. J. Kallos, Evaporation rates and reactivities of methylene chloride, chloroform, 1, 1, 1-trichloroethane, trichloroethylene, tetrachloroethylene, and other chlorinated compounds in dilute aqueous solutions. *Environ. Sci. Technol.* **9**, 833–838 (1975).

7. D. McKay and W. Y. Shiu, Critical review of Henry's law constants for chemicals of environmental interest. *J. Phys. Chem. Ref. Data* **10**, 1175–1199 (1981).

8. T. R. Torkelson, F. Oyen, D. D. McCollister, and V. K. Rowe, Toxicity of 1, 1, 1-trichloroethane as determined on laboratory animals and human subjects. *Am. Ind. Hyg. Assoc. J.* **19**, 353–362 (1958).

9. P. V. Cline and J. J. Delfino, Abiotic formation and degradation of 1, 1-dichloroethane (preprint extended abstract). *Am. Chem. Soc.* **27**, 577–579 (1987).

10. Harding and Lawson Associates, *Preliminary Draft of IBM Comprehensive Plan.* H & L Assoc., 1986.

11. G. McConnell, D. M. Ferguson, and C. R. Pearson, Chlorinated hydrocarbons in the environment. *Endeavour* **34**, 13–18 (1975).

12. D. Henschler, D. Reichert, and M. Metzler, Identification of potential carcinogens in technical grade 1, 1, 1-trichloroethane. *Int. Arch. Occup. Environ. Health* **47**, 263–268 (1980).

13. S. Swan, M. Deane, J. Harris, and R. Neutra, *Pregnancy Outcomes in Santa Clara County, 1980–1982.* Epidemiological Studies Section, California Department of Health Services, Sacramento, 1985.

14. A. Sato and T. Nakajima, A structure–activity relationship of some chlorinated hydrocarbons. *Arch. Environ. Health* **34**, 69–75 (1979).

15. A. C. Monster, G. Boersma, and H. Steenweg, Kinetics of 1, 1, 1-trichloroethane in volunteers; influence of exposure concentration and work load. *Int. Arch. Occup. Environ. Health* **42**, 293–301 (1979).

16. H. S. Brown, D. R. Bishop, and C. A. Rowan, The role of skin absorption as a route of exposure for volatile organic compounds (VOCs) in drinking water. *Am. J. Public Health* **74**, 479–484 (1984).

17. T. Dutkiewicz and H. Tyras, A study of the skin absorption of ethylbenzene in man. *Br. J. Ind. Med.* **24**, 330–332 (1967).

18. T. Dutkiewicz and H. Tyras, Skin absorption of toluene, styrene, and xylene by man. *Br. J. Ind. Med.* **25**, 243 (1968).

19. T. E. McKone, Human exposure to volatile organic compounds in household tap water: The indoor inhalation pathway. *Environ. Sci. Technol.* **21**, 1194–1201 (1987).

20. R. D. Stewart, The toxicology of 1, 1, 1-trichloroethane. *Ann. Occup. Hyg.* **11**, 71–79 (1968).

21. National Institute for Occupational Safety and Health, *Criteria for a Recommended Standard, Occupational Exposure to 1, 1, 1-Trichloroethane (Methyl Chloroform).* NIOSH, Cincinnati, OH, 1976.

22. National Research Council, Update. *Drinking Water Health,* pp. 74–76 (1983).

23. C. L. Hake, T. B. Waggoner, D. N. Robertson, and V. K. Rowe, The metabolism of 1, 1, 1-trichloroethane by the rat. *Arch. Environ. Health* **1**, 101–105 (1960).

24. R. D. Stewart and J. T. Andrews, Acute intoxication with methylchloroform. *JAMA, J. Am. Med. Assoc.* **195**, 904–906 (1966).

25. B. Holmberg, I. Jakobson, and K. Sigvardsson, A study on the distribution of methylchloroform and n-octane in the mouse during and after inhalation. *Scand. J. Work Environ. Health* **3**, 43–52 (1977).

26. A. C. Monster, Difference in uptake, elimination and metabolism in exposure to trichloroethylene, 1, 1, 1-trichloroethane and tetrachloroethylene. *Int. Arch. Occup. Environ. Health* **42**, 311–317 (1979).

27. A. M. Schumann, T. R. Fox, and P. G. Watanabe, [^{14}C]methyl chloroform (1, 1, 1-trichloroethane): Pharmacokinetics in rats and mice following inhalation exposure. *Toxicol. Appl. Pharmacol.* **62**, 390–401 (1982).

28. K. M. Ivanetich and L. H. Van Den Honert, "Chloroethanes: Their metabolism by hepatic cytochrome P-450 *in vitro. Carcinogenesis (London)* **2**, 697–702 (1981).

29. A. G. Salmon, R. B. Jones, and W. C. Mackrodt, Microsomal dechlorination of chlorethanes: Structure–reactivity relationships. *Xenobiotica* **11**, 723–734 (1981).

30. R. D. Stewart, H. H. Gay, D. S. Erley, C. L. Hake, and A. W. Schaffer, Human exposure to 1, 1, 1-trichloroethane vapor: Relationship of expired air and blood concentrations to exposure and toxicity. *Am. Ind. Hyg. Assoc. J.* **22**, 252–262 (1961).

31. N. S. McNutt, R. L. Amster, E. E. McConnell, and F. Morris, Hepatic lesions in mice after continuous inhalation exposure to 1, 1, 1-trichloroethane. *Lab. Invest.* **32**, 642–654 (1975).

32. J. A. Prendergast, R. A. Jones, L. J. Jenkins, and J. Siegel, Effects on experimental animals of long-term inhalation of trichloroethylene, carbon tetrachloride, 1, 1, 1-trichloroethane, dichlorodifluoromethane, and 1, 1-dichloroethylene. *Toxicol. Appl. Pharmacol.* **10**, 270–289 (1967).

33. L. W. Rampy, J. F. Quast, B. K. J. Leong, and P. J. Gehring, Results of long-term inhalation toxicity studies on rats of 1, 1, 1-trichloroethane and perchloroethylene formulations (abstract). In G. L. Plaa and W. A. M. Duncan, Eds., *Proceedings of the First International Congress on Toxicology.* Academic Press, New York, 1978, p. 562.

34. J. F. Quast, L. L. Calhoun, and M. J. McKenna, 1, 1, 1-trichloroethane formulation: A chronic inhalation toxicity and oncogenicity study in rats and mice. Part I. Results of findings in mice. *Toxicologist* **5**, Abstr. No. 55 (1985).

35. National Cancer Institute, *Bioassay of 1, 1, 1-Trichloroethane for Possible Carcinogenicity,* DHEW Publ. No. (NIH) 77–803. NCI, Washington, DC, 1977.

36. National Toxicology Program, *Draft Report on the Carcinogenesis Bioassay of 1, 1, 1-Trichloroethane in F344/N Rats and B6C3F1 Mice,* NTP Tech. Rep. No. 262. NTP, Washington, DC, 1983.

37. C. Maltoni, G. Cotti, and V. Patella, Results of long-term carcinogenicity bioassays on sprague–dawley rats of methyl chloroform, administered by ingestion. *Acta Oncol.* **7**, 101–117 (1986).

38. V. F. Simmon, K. Kauhanen, and R. G. Tardiff, Mutagenic activity of chemicals identified in drinking water. *Prog. Genet. Toxicol.* **2**, 249–258 (1977).

39. E. R. Nestman, E. G.-H. Lee et al., Mutagenicity of constituents identified in pulp and paper mill effluents using the salmonella/mammalian-microsome assay. *Mutat. Res.* **79**, 203–212 (1980).

40. U.S. Environmental Protection Agency, *The Carcinogen Assessment Group's Evaluation of the Carcinogenicity of Methyl Chloroform.* USEPA, Washington, DC, 1984.

41. E. R. Nestman, R. Otson, D. J. Kowbel, P. D. Bothwell, and T. R. Harrington, Mutagenicity in a modified *Salmonella* assay of fabric-protecting products containing 1, 1, 1-trichloroethane. *Environ. Mutagen.* **6**, 71–80 (1984).

42. J. Y. Domoradzki, *Evaluation of Chlorothene VG Solvent and its Components in the Ames' Salmonella/Mammalian Microsome Mutagenicity Assay,* Tech. Rep., Dow Chemical USA, Midland, MI, 1980.

43. T. Shimada, A. F. Swanson, P. Leber, and G. M. Williams, Activities of chlorinated ethane and ethylene compounds in the salmonella/rat microsome mutagenesis and rat hepatocyte/DNA repair assays under vapor phase exposure conditions. *Cell Biol. Toxicol.* **1** 159–179 (1985).

44. W. Mabey and T. Mill, Critical review of hydrolysis of organic compounds in water under environmental conditions. *J. Phys. Chem. Ref. Data* **7**, 383–415 (1978).

45. B. A. Schwetz, B. K. J. Leong, and P. J. Gehring, The effect of maternally inhaled trichloroethylene, perchloroethylene, methyl chloroform, and methylene chloride on embryonal and fetal development in mice and rats. *Toxicol. Appl. Pharmacol.* **32**, 84–96 (1975).

46. R. G. York, B. M. Sowry, L. Hastings, and J. M. Mason, Evaluation of teratogenicity and neurotoxicity with maternal inhalation exposure to methyl chloroform. *J. Toxicol. Environ. Health* **9**, 251–266 (1982).

47. R. W. Lane, B. L. Riddle, and J. F. Borzelleca, Effects of 1, 2-dichloroethane and 1, 1, 1-trichloroethane in drinking water on reproduction and development in mice. *Toxicol. Appl. Pharmacol.* **63**, 409–421 (1982).

48. S. C. Dapson, D. E. Hutcheon, and D. Lehr, Effect of methyl chloroform on cardiovascular development in rats. *Teratology* **29**, 25A (1984).

49. S. Nityanand and N. K. Kapoor, Effect of chronic oral administration of Tween-80 in Charles Foster rats. *Indian J. Med. Res.* **69**, 664–670 (1979).

50. U. Kocher-Becker and W. Kocher, Thalidomide-like malformations caused by a Tween surfactant in mice. *Z. Naturforsch., C. Biosci.* **36C**, 904–906 (1981).

51. R. D. George, C. J. Price, M. C. Marr, B. A. Schwetz, and R. E. Morrissey, Developmental toxicity of 1, 1, 1-trichloroethane (TCEN) in CD rats. *Toxicologist* **7**, 175 (1987).

52. C. G. Kramer, M. G. Ott, J. E. Fulkerson, and N. Hicks, Health of workers exposed to 1, 1, 1-trichloroethane: A matched-pair study. *Arch. Environ. Health* **33**, 331–342 (1978).

53. U.S. Environmental Protection Agency, *1, 1, 1-Trichloroethane*, Health Advisory, Office of Drinking Water, USEPA, Washington, DC. 1985.

54. California Department of Health Services, *Action Levels Recommended by the Department of Health Services.* CDHS, Sacramento, 1986.

9

Evaluating the Environmental Safety of Detergent Chemicals: A Case Study of Cationic Surfactants

D. M. Woltering and W. E. Bishop
The Procter & Gamble Company, Environmental Safety Department,
Ivorydale Technical Center, Cincinnati, Ohio

INTRODUCTION

In recent years much attention has been focused on assessing environmental risks resulting from the manufacture, distribution, use, and disposal of chemicals. Legislation and public concern have produced numerous regulations that continue to scrutinize the introduction of new chemicals and provide the ongoing review of existing chemicals. It has become necessary to formalize procedures for assessing hazards and for deciding whether the use of a given chemical presents an acceptable or unacceptable risk to the environment. Numerous examples of risk assessment and testing procedures (1–7) have been developed and published by regulatory agencies, by industry, and by groups or associations representing scientists from varied professional backgrounds.

Because household cleaning products are manufactured in very large quantities, used by almost all consumers, and disposed of broadly into the environment, the detergent industry has been involved in environmental risk assessment. In fact, due to a perceived need, the detergent manufacturers have taken a leadership role in the development of environmental risk assessment strategies, test methodologies, and relevant data bases. These efforts have included a number of generic approaches to safety evaluations for new and existing chemicals (5, 8–19).

Detergents are synthesized chemically from a variety of raw materials derived from petroleum, fatty acids, and other sources. They are based on surface-active agents (surfactants) that provide cleaning power and may also contain ingredients such as builders (which reduce water hardness, buffer the cleaning solution, prevent redeposition, and emulsify oils), whitening agents, suds control agents, and perfumes. A number of the major ingredients reach usage levels in the millions of pounds per year. The finished product comes in a number of forms, including granules, liquids, and crystals. These products are widely distributed and formulations vary in response to local consumer needs.

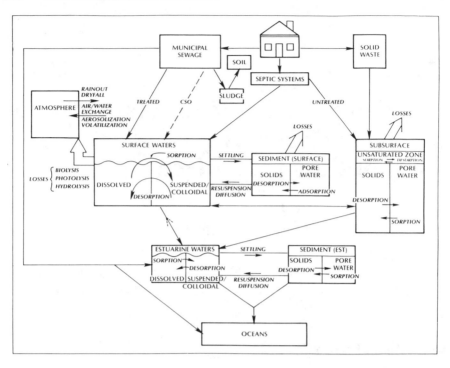

Figure 1. Predominant environmental pathways and compartments for detergent chemicals.

Detergent chemicals enter the environment primarily via the disposal of household wastewater. Typically, most of these chemicals are physically removed or degraded during sewage treatment. The remainder enter either the terrestrial environment as part of sludge disposal and home-treatment sewage effluent, or the aquatic environment as a component of municipal sewage effluent.

Figure 1 illustrates the primary routes of entry and the possible distribution of household cleaning product chemicals in the environment. The environmental loading and fate of product components will vary depending on local conditions, including such factors as the level of chemical in the product and the quantity of product marketed, household water use practices, the type of wastewater treatment and its efficiency in removing and degrading the chemical of interest, the dilution of treated effluent into a receiving water, and the posttreatment degradation and distribution of the chemical in aquatic and terrestrial compartments.

This chapter describes the environmental risk assessment approach that has evolved over many years of testing high-volume, unique-chemistry materials, which meet performance standards expected of the detergent industry. In addition, the monoalkyl quaternary surfactants (MAQs, $C_{12}-C_{18}$ alkyl chainlength), a class of specialty chemicals used in liquid and granular detergents and in fabric softener and hair conditioner products, are examined as a case study of this approach. The assessment process outlined for MAQs is applicable to most other major detergent chemicals that characteristically are produced in high volume, are well removed by conventional sewage treatment, are water soluble and biodegradable, have low potential to bioaccumulate, and are moderately toxic to sensitive species.

DETERGENT CHEMICAL RISK ASSESSMENT

Strategy and Decisionmaking

A sequential testing approach is the assessment procedure generally accepted by the scientific and regulatory communities (8, 15). The central concept is that as testing proceeds through succeeding stages, estimates of expected environmental concentrations and of the threshold concentrations producing adverse biological effects can be made with an increasing degree of accuracy and confidence. The procedure leads to the calculation of margins of safety, which can be used to decide whether additional testing is needed, and to an ultimate judgment regarding the potential environmental risk from the intended use of the chemical. The challenge is to develop the right type and amount of information to permit an informed decision to be made, while both minimizing the uncertainty in extrapolating model estimates and laboratory data to real-world situations and maximizing the use of critical time and personnel resources.

Predicted environmental concentrations of detergent chemicals are derived from a knowledge of usage level and disposal routes, and estimates of removal efficiency during wastewater treatment, effluent dilution by receiving waters, sludge application rates to soils, and subsequent degradation, partitioning, and transport of the chemical in both surface and subsurface waters and terrestrial compartments. Laboratory tests using sensitive species from relevant environmental compartments provide an estimate of inherent toxicity of the chemical as well as an indication of which species and what biological parameters are most sensitive. Potential adverse impacts of the detergent chemicals on wastewater treatment systems are also evaluated.

A comparison can then be made between the predicted environmental concentration (PEC) in relevant environmental compartments and the highest concentration at which no significant adverse biological effects were observed in the laboratory tests (i.e., NOEC or no observed effect concentration). Figure 2 represents these two concentrations by parallel lines and demonstrates that increasingly accurate estimates of these concentrations will result from a sequential series of tests. In the early phases of the risk assessment process, biological effect levels and environmental concentrations are estimated from simple exposure models, structure–activity relations, and standardized laboratory toxicity tests. Since there is a relatively high degree of uncertainty in the accuracy of these initial predictions, a wider margin between the PEC and NOEC is needed to conclude that the chemical is safe to use.

Additional data, such as *in situ* measurements of chemical concentrations and field assessments of treatment plant and ecological impact, can increase the confidence that the PEC and NOEC values are significantly different and a narrower margin of difference between the two can be tolerated. It becomes a matter of situation or chemical-specific circumstances and professional judgment to determine how much and what kind of data are needed to narrow the confidence intervals around the estimates of exposure and effect concentrations. For guidance, the USEPA has published guidelines for acceptable uncertainty factors (or assessment factors) in the aquatic environment based on the level of testing involved (1, 2, 7). The recommended "minimum margin" between the exposure and effect concentrations decreases as the data base is expanded from the results of a few, relatively simple laboratory models and screening tests to more numerous, complex, and realistic laboratory studies and exposure models. Eventually, field-scale evaluations involving measured exposures and population and/or community level responses can be performed and may be appropriate to reduce the uncertainty of extrapolation to essentially zero.

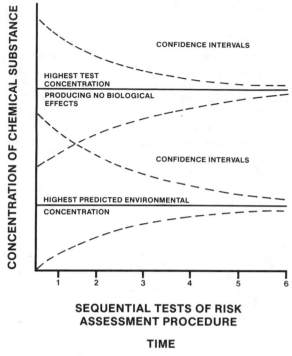

Figure 2. Diagrammatic representation of the risk assessment process, showing the increasingly narrower confidence limits for predicting environmental concentration and estimates of no adverse biological effects concentration. From Maki and Duthie (10).

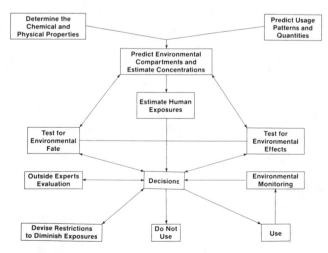

Figure 3. Flowchart for generalized environmental risk assessment. After Beck et al. (12).

A generalized environmental risk assessment program may be represented as a flowchart consisting of a number of distinct phases (12) (Fig. 3). Each phase is designed to accomplish certain scientific purposes, and all the phases are interrelated to yield an effective yet efficient assessment. In each phase, there are provisions for acquiring and organizing information and for making certain kinds of decisions. Numerous methodologies are available to estimate and/or provide measurements of the needed information. Flexibility in the choice and use of specific methods is important so that the key questions regarding a particular chemical can be addressed. For example, fate and effects tests should focus on the specific environmental compartments that will see the chemical of interest, versus conducting "all" available tests.

After initial consideration is given to the physical and chemical characteristics of the material and to the key environmental compartments where exposure is likely to occur, important fate and effects questions are identified and prioritized, and tests are selected to answer those questions. As more information is developed, a point is reached at which a decision can be made regarding the safety of a chemical given the available usage estimates. The decision may be that the material presents too high a risk, or that there is acceptable risk, or that more work needs to be carried out. Scientific judgment is used in deciding which tests to conduct and when sufficient testing has been conducted to make an overall decision on the environmental acceptability of the material. Each phase in the process of collecting sufficient data for conducting an environmental risk assessment for detergent chemicals is described briefly below. They are discussed more throughly in the case study of the monoalkyl quaternary surfactants.

Data Collection and Analysis

Physicochemical Properties. The data collection phase of the assessment begins with a consideration of the physicochemical properties of the material. They are estimated from existing information on the class of compounds or other structurally related materials, if possible, or determined in the laboratory, if necessary. The physical properties of interest usually include physical form, vapor pressure, solubility in water and in organic solvents, octanol–water partition coefficient (K_{ow}), and sorption characteristics. Chemical properties that may be relevant include ionization or dissociation properties, ion-exchange characteristics, complexation properties, and susceptibility to hydrolysis, oxidation, thermal degradation, or photolysis. This information can provide an early estimate of a chemical's exposure potential, including key environmental compartments and the form, distribution, and fate of environmentally relevant species.

These data are very useful in that they allow more complicated phenomena to be estimated. For example, octanol–water partition coefficients can be used to estimate the approximate degree to which a chemical will concentrate in aquatic organisms, relative to its ambient concentration in the surrounding water (20). A bioconcentration factor (BCF) can be predicted from the K_{ow} using an appropriate regression equation (e.g., log BCF $= 0.76 \log K_{ow} - 0.23$). The partition coefficient itself can often be calculated from molecular structure or derived from computerized data bases (21). Molecular modeling programs like the CHEMLAB-II software system (Molecular Design Ltd., 1122 B. Street, Hayward, CA 94541) allow such molecular-based calculations to be performed by computer. Use of a computer terminal with graphics capabilities allows the chemical's structure to be drawn on the terminal screen from which the K_{ow} and other molecular properties are estimated. K_{ow} can then be used to estimate BCFs, water solubility, and sorption to soils and sediments from various regression equations (20).

Predicted Use Pattern and Quantities. How the chemical will be used, and in what quantities, must be considered since usage patterns determine the routes and amounts of environmental loading and exposure. Other key considerations in this step of the assessment include the following: Will chemical usage be geographically localized or widespread? (In the detergent industry, consideration must be given to the varying use and environmental conditions between various cities, states, and countries.) Is the chemical similar enough to some other chemical already in use such that exposure and toxicity should be considered to be additive? Is the chemical replacing another material currently in use and reaching the environment? Is the chemical likely to be used by others, such that an industry-wide usage estimate and subsequent risk assessment are appropriate?

Predicting Environmental Compartments and Concentrations. Since the environmental risk assessment ultimately hinges on the comparison of exposure concentrations with those concentrations known (or at least expected) to cause a measurable and significant biological response, it is necessary that the testing program predict the concentrations in relevant environmental compartments. For these purposes, compartments are defined broadly as sewage treatment, aquatic or terrestrial, and more specifically as "sewage" influent, effluent, and digester solids, "aquatic" freshwater or marine, water or sediments, and "terrestrial" surface or subsurface, soil/groundwater, and sludge. Ultimately, these exposure estimates become part of the criteria for deciding which environmental fate and effects tests are needed to assess the potential hazard.

Focusing on the household as the primary route of disposal of detergent chemicals, and using information on anticipated use patterns, physicochemical properties, and structure–activity relations, we obtain a prediction for the environmental compartments that are most likely to contain the chemical and at what approximate levels. For example, a chemical with a high soil–sediment sorption coefficient will partition onto solids as the chemical is transported from the home through onsite or municipal wastewater treatment and into soil and sediments via sludge disposal and liquid effluent discharge.

Several equations, described below and used in the case study, are available to estimate environmental concentrations of consumer product chemicals. [Equations (1)–(6) were extracted, with permission, from STP 737, ref. 19, copyright American Society for Testing and Materials, 1916 Race Street, Philadelphia, PA 19103.] The U.S. Environmental Protection Agency (EPA) Municipal Waste Facilities Inventory (22) contains flow-rate and population-served data. This information is used to calculate *per capita wastewater flow rates* Q as

$$Q \text{ (L/capita·day)} = \frac{\text{treatment plant flow rate (L/day)}}{\text{population served}}. \tag{1}$$

The calculated median Q, based on analysis of 11,000 treatment plants and weighted by population, is 507 L/capita·day (19). The range is from 200 to 575 L and there is an indication that larger treatment plants have higher per capita wastewater flow rates.

The concentration of a detergent chemical in a *municipal wastewater influent* can be estimated by

$$C_{iw} = \frac{XP}{YQ}, \tag{2}$$

where C_{iw} = concentration of a detergent chemical in influent wastewater (mg/L)
$\quad X$ = quantity of detergent product marketed (mg/day)
$\quad P$ = detergent chemical fraction in the product (wt %/100)
$\quad Y$ = population of market area (number of people)
$\quad Q$ = per capita wastewater flow rate (L/capita·day).

[Note: Holman (19) provides additional detail on time-averaged estimates and home wastewater concentration estimates for onsite treatment.]

The concentration of a detergent chemical in a *municipal wastewater sludge* can be estimated by the generalized equation

$$C_{ds} = C_{iw} \frac{F1}{F2} (R' + R'' - D')(1 - D''), \tag{3}$$

where C_{ds} = concentration of the detergent chemical in digested sludge (mg/L)
$\quad C_{iw}$ = concentration of the detergent chemical in wastewater influent (mg/L)
$\quad F1/F2$ = ratio of municipal wastewater to digested sludge flow rates (average = 260)
$\quad R'$ = fraction of chemical removed by primary treatment (% removed/100)
$\quad R''$ = fraction of chemical removed by secondary treatment (% removed/100)
$\quad D'$ = fraction of chemical degraded in primary + secondary treatment (% degraded/100)
$\quad D''$ = fraction of chemical degraded in anaerobic digestion (%/100).

Equation (3) assumes "typical" flow rates, suspended solids levels, secondary treatment and anaerobic digestion. Again, Holman (19) provides additional details and also describes estimation procedures for atypical situations.

Sludge from wastewater treatment facilities is often used as a soil-amending agent. As a result, the chemical or its metabolites have an opportunity to enter the food chain, accumulate, or affect wildlife and/or crops. The concentration of a detergent chemical in sludge-amended soil is based on a typical application rate of 2.2 kg dry sludge solids per square meter per year (23). Assuming incorporation of the sludge to a soil depth of 15 cm and a soil bulk density of 1200 kg/m^3 yields a sludge incorporation rate of 1.22×10^{-2} kg sludge solids per kilogram soil per year. Therefore, the concentration of a detergent chemical in *sludge-amended soil* for a 1-year application can be estimated by

$$C_s = C_{ds} \times 1.22 \times 10^{-2} \frac{\text{kg sludge solids}}{\text{kg soil}} \times 1 \text{ year}, \tag{4}$$

where C_s = concentration of the chemical in sludge-amended soil (mg/kg)
$\quad C_{ds}$ = concentration of the chemical in digested sludge (mg/kg).

This estimate does not take into account possible degradation or leaching of the detergent chemical in the soil and represents only 1 year's application. Estimates of long-term steady-state soil concentrations would have to take these factors into account (19).

Municipal wastewater effluent concentrations and levels in surface waters can also be estimated using both generalized and more site-specific models. Holman (19) assumed a weighted average of primary treatment ($\sim 25\%$ of U.S. population sewered wastewater flow) and primary plus secondary treatment ($\sim 75\%$ of flow) to estimate the concentrations of detergent chemicals entering surface waters, according to

$$C_{ew} = \tfrac{1}{4}[C_{iw}(1 - R')] + \tfrac{3}{4}[C_{iw}(1 - R'')], \tag{5}$$

where C_{ew} = concentration of detergent chemical in effluent wastewater (mg/L)
$\qquad$ C_{iw} = concentration of detergent chemical in influent wastewater (mg/L)
$\qquad$ R' = fraction of chemical removed by primary treatment (% removed/100)
$\qquad$ R'' = fraction of chemical removed by secondary treatment (% removed/100).

The estimates of removal by primary and secondary treatment are developed from laboratory screening tests. The equation is based on the nationally (U.S.) weighted average of the frequency of primary and secondary treatment; other weighting factors may be used for a particular area if they differ significantly from the national values.

Approximately 84% of all municipal wastewater effluent is discharged to surface waters with the balance going to ocean outfalls, groundwater reacharge, and various types of land disposal (24). A national average approach can also be used to approximate surface water concentrations. For example, based on U.S. Geological Survey surface water records for stream flow rates (25) and on the U.S. EPA Municipal Waste Facilities Inventory for effluent discharge flow rates (22), a frequency distribution of stream dilution factors for mean flow rate conditions indicates that the national median dilution factor is approximately 100, with 90% of the dilution factors less than 1000 and 9% less than 10 (19). Obviously, dilution factors are higher during maximum stream flow conditions and lower during minimum flow conditions. An estimate of the concentration of a *chemical in a river* receiving wastewater treatment plant effluent can be obtained using

$$C_{sw} = \frac{C_{ew}}{SDF}, \tag{6}$$

where C_{sw} = concentration of the detergent chemical in surface water immediately below the outfall of a wastewater treatment plant (mg/L)
$\qquad$ C_{ew} = concentration of the chemical in wastewater effluent (mg/L)
$\qquad$ SDF = stream dilution factor, which equals the stream flow rate at the plant site divided by the effluent discharge rate.

The surface water concentration estimates based on this model use mass inputs and do not account for in-stream sorption, complexation, or degradation. Therefore, they represent an upper limit estimate for the pure chemical in the water column. For the majority of detergent chemicals these in-stream processes result in either significant changes in mass and/or in chemical form and distribution, and often in bioavailability. Water column exposure estimates should be adjusted in the risk assessment if the effect of these in-stream processes can be quantified.

Sorption of detergent chemicals, for example, on river sediments or soil, can often be adequately described by a simple linear model in which the mass or concentration of a chemical on a sorbent ($\mu g/g$) is related to its concentration in solution ($\mu g/mL$) by a sorption coefficient K_d (26).

Again, sorption can affect exposure and can indicate which environmental compartments are key to a risk assessment.

$$K_d = \frac{C_{solids}}{C_{solution}}, \tag{7}$$

where $C_{solids} = \mu g/g$ on the solids
$C_{solution} = \mu g/mL$ in solution.

Unlike sorption, which primarily results in a redistribution of material from water to soil or sediment compartments, biodegradation results in a net loss of the parent material from the environment. It is the most important fate process that results in a decrease in mass as well as exposure concentration. Several kinetic models, including modified Monod and Michaelis–Menton models, second-order, and various logistic and mixed-order models have been described in the literature to quantify biodegradation processes (27, 28). However, for a variety of different types of organic chemicals, including detergent chemicals, biodegradation rate processes can be adequately described by a simple pseudo-first-order model, in which the rate of biodegradation is directly proportional to the concentration of the chemical. Biodegradation over time can be described by the integrated form of the model:

$$\%CO_2 = A\%(1 - e^{-k_1[t-c]}), \tag{8}$$

where $A\%$ = asymptotic maximum CO_2 production
k_1 = first-order rate constant
C = lag time for biodegradation to begin.

Nonbiological degradation (e.g., hydrolysis, photolysis) should also be considered as it may be a significant transformation mechanism. In addition, partial degradation of the parent material can be an important aspect of a chemical hazard assessment, both from gradual accumulation if the chemical loading is continuous, as well as from exposure to intermediates and metabolites whose toxicity may be very different from the parent material. In practical terms, degradability and therefore persistence and accumulation of a chemical or its degradation intermediates can be viewed as the rate of degradation relative to the residence time in specific environmental compartments. Residence times vary significantly, from hours to years, depending on the compartment (e.g., surface waters, sediments, soils). The residence time concept can be used in combination with degradation rates determined at environmentally realistic concentrations and in test systems that represent the relevant environmental compartment(s). This more realistic evaluation complements, and avoids the arbitrary use of, standard CO_2 screening test results, which express the potential for biodegradability and should not be extrapolated as an absolute value to all real-world conditions. The toxicity question can be addressed by either isolating and testing persistent intermediates or by combining degradation and toxicity tests so the exposure is to all bioavailable chemical forms.

In summary, Eqs (1)–(8) provide an example of methods available for predicting environmental concentrations of consumer product chemicals that are disposed of into wastewater. Although the approach predicts only a single, average concentration on a

TABLE 1. Summary of Sewage Effluent Discharge and Dilution Factors as Function of Wastewater Treatment Type

Treatment Type	Percent of Total Number of Treatment Plants	Percent of Sewage Flow Discharge to Rivers and Streams	Dilution Factor[a]	
			50%[b]	90%[c]
Primary Clarification	6	4	1700	10
Trickling Filter	55	21	87	6
Activated Sludge	39	75	27	2
			100[d]	3[d]

[a]At mean stream flow for rivers in the United States.
[b]Greater than 50% of U.S. sewage flow will be diluted with a higher factor.
[c]Greater than 90% of U.S. sewage flow will be diluted with a higher factor.
[d]Flow weighted average for the entire United States.
Modeled from available site-specific sewage discharge and river flow data.

national basis, it has proved very useful and reliable for the detergent industry. Other chemical transport and fate assessment procedures have also been developed (29–34). Most of these procedures involve the use of physical or mathematical modeling techniques to estimate exposures.

A new environmental exposure procedure, being developed at Procter & Gamble, generates a frequency distribution prediction of U.S. stream and river concentrations for a chemical of interest (35). The analysis is based on a detailed examination of two national data bases, the 1984 U.S. EPA Needs Survey and River Reach File (36, 37). Approximately 11,500 publicly owned treatment works (POTWs) and 122,000 river miles were selected from the data bases and considered in the model. The model involves a coupling of sewage treatment type (primary clarification, trickling filters, and activated sludge) with riverine dilution under both mean and critical low (7Q10) river flow regimes. A computer program determines the frequency of concentrations in streams, just below the mixing zone after POTW discharge. With this model, it is possible to predict the fraction (%) of total POTW flow discharged to U.S. rivers and streams which will have a chemical concentration greater than any specified value, such as the threshold biological effect concentration. This predictive capability can also be applied to a more localized assessment by focusing on an identified receiving stream(s) and POTW(s) with the site-specific dilutions and treatment efficiencies.

Table 1 summarizes U.S. sewage treatment practices and dilution factors developed from the model. The analysis shows that lower dilution factors are typically associated with the more efficient types of sewage treatment. Concentrations of a chemical in the river resulting from this procedure can be displayed as a frequency distribution on the basis of treatment type, number of plants, geographical location, population served, or sewage flow. An example of how the analysis is used is included in the case study for MAQs surfactants (see Fig. 11).

Testing for Environmental Fate. A number of experimental methods are available for estimating the fate of a detergent chemical after disposal and entry into the environment.

Important questions to be addressed include removal by wastewater treatment, environmental distribution and form, and persistence. Results of environmental fate tests are used to develop refined estimates of environmental concentrations in relevant compartments. Detailed methodologies for environmental fate tests have been published (32, 38–40), and some of the most useful tests for detergent chemical assessment are briefly described below.

Persistence. The CO_2 evolution screening test (38, 41) indicates whether a chemical can be converted to carbon dioxide by microbial action and may also indicate whether it inhibits microbial activity. Radiolabeled test material or a sensitive specific analytical method can also be used to determine if partial degradation has occurred and if persistent intermediates may be present. As appropriate, more complex and realistic biodegradability tests can be conducted at realistic environmental concentrations and in appropriate (e.g., actual) environmental matrices including actual river waters (42), estuarine waters (43, 44), sediments (26), anaerobic and aerobic soils (45, 46), and groundwater (47). If there are indications that abiotic degradation mechanisms, such as hydrolysis or photolysis, are likely to be significant, rate constants can be measured and incorporated into estimates of environmental concentrations.

Degradability tests will determine the potential for the chemical to persist in the environment. Accumulation and persistence must consider the rate and extent of degradation versus the input rates and residence times in environmental compartments like water sediments, soil, and groundwater. Laboratory microcosm and *in situ* studies may also be conducted to make more refined estimates of a chemical's persistence (48). A slowly degrading or nondegradable chemical should not necessarily be judged unacceptable. Consideration should be given to usage levels and environmental sinks as well as to potential adverse effects from long-term exposure.

Treatability and Removal. Frequently used screening level methodologies include the semicontinuous activated sludge (SCAS) test (49), which measures the extent to which a chemical is removed in a simulation of the most common secondary wastewater treatment process. Removal by primary treatment can be predicted by adsorption isotherms and by settling tests (50, 51), which are appropriate for any material that will appear in influent wastewater associated with solids. The susceptibilities of the chemical to chlorination and ozonation may also be appropriate to determine.

Treatability studies with laboratory or pilot-scale models of biological treatment processes, referred to as confirmatory tests, are conducted to predict the fate and effects of the chemical in the full-scale process. Parameters measured may include primary degradation and chemical removal [continuous activated sludge (CAS) test as an example [51]), a chemical mass balance, and potential effects on both the mechanical and biological efficiency of the treatment process [anaerobic digester inhibition test as an example (52)].

Depending on the results of the laboratory tests and the need for more refined estimates of chemical fate, information on removal can also be obtained from field studies where a chemical is dosed to a treatment plant, or where the population served by the plant (e.g., a package plant for a housing development or small community) is provided with test product that contains the chemical of interest. Development of this kind of confirmatory information typically occurs at later stages in the evaluation process and requires a suitable analytical method to measure environmental concentrations. There are published reports of such detergent chemical studies for primary clarifier (51), trickling filter (51, 53), and activated sludge plants (51, 54, 55).

Distribution and Form. Treatability studies can indicate to what extent the chemical of interest will be degraded and how the remainder will be distributed in solid and liquid wastes. Tests and models to estimate the fate of the chemical in solid-phase sludge are described in previous sections. Depending on the predicted rate and extent of removal by sorption and degradation, it may also be important to estimate the distribution and form of the chemical entering the aquatic environment as part of the wastewater effluent. Relevant tests for detergent chemicals include adsorption isotherm measurements for sediments and suspended solids, measured bioconcentration factors in aquatic species if solubility and octanol–water partition coefficient data indicate the potential exists, equilibrium constants for chelation or ion exchange with trace metals if the chemical is expected to react, identification of any biologically significant metabolites or degradation products, and estimates of drinking water concentrations from surface water and groundwater sources.

Testing for Environmental Effects. An environmental assessment for most chemicals will normally require some environmental effects data. This is particularly true when the available information suggests that the chemical may be highly toxic or poorly degraded by wastewater treatment, or that it may be bioaccumulated or complex with metals or other materials. There will, however, be some chemicals for which significant additional toxicity testing may not be needed, such as those with adequate literature data or suitable structure–activity correlations, those that never reach the terrestrial or aquatic environment because of confined usage, or those that would occur only at very low levels.

Screening Level Testing. The typical effects assessment procedure for aquatic exposures involves screening level toxicity tests utilizing sensitive, or otherwise representative, species of fish, invertebrates, and algae in fresh and/or salt water. For terrestrial exposures, including sewage sludge application to agricultural land and diluted sewage effluent used for irrigation, soil invertebrates and agricultural crops are typically tested (3, 6, 56). In general, mammals and birds are unlikely to be exposed to significant concentrations of detergent chemicals, but if necessary, toxicity testing can be conducted for these species or data can be obtained from animal tests carried out to assess human safety. Microbial toxicity can also be assessed for both aquatic and terrestrial systems.

Initial Assessment and Decisions. Adverse-effect testing progresses sequentially from acute toxicity to subchronic and possibly to full life-cycle tests. The results of the toxicity tests combined with estimated environmental exposure concentrations form the basis of an initial risk assessment. If the margin of safety (i.e., the ratio of the lowest effect concentration and the estimated environmental concentration) is sufficiently large, the use of the chemical is considered safe and additional testing is typically not warranted. The decision should be made on a chemical by chemical basis taking into account all available data. The U.S. EPA has recently published guidelines for estimating concern levels for new and expanded use chemical substances in the aquatic environment (1, 2, 5). Table 2 illustrates one way to integrate exposure and effects data bases. The recommended assessment factors or minimum margins of safety decrease from 1000 to 100 to 10 as the data base is expanded from acute toxicity (e.g., an LC_{50}) for one species, to acute toxicity for several species (e.g., the lowest LC_{50}), to chronic toxicity for the most sensitive species (e.g., a chronic value from a daphnid chronic test or fish early life stage test). Well-designed field-type tests indicating the absence of population level effects significantly reduce the uncertainty inherent in the laboratory to field prediction, and therefore a direct

TABLE 2. Uncertainty Factors for Aquatic Safety Assessments Based on Integration of Exposure and Ecological Effects Data Bases[a]

		Effects Data Base				
		Single Acute	Multispecies Acute	Limited Chronic	Full Water Quality Criteria	Ecosystem
Exposure Data Base	Uncertainty Factor	1000	100	10	1	1
Model Level I	100	100,000	10,000	1,000	100	—
Model Level II	10	10,000	1,000	100	10	—
Measured	1	1,000	100	10	1	1

[a]Uncertainty is reduced as the data bases are expanded to provide a closer extrapolation to real-world conditions.
Source: Kimerle (5).

extrapolation of the results, or a safety margin of 1, is appropriate. The guidelines also recommend that further assessment is needed if a chemical's octanol–water partition coefficient predicts a bioconcentration factor of greater than 1000 (i.e., $\log K_{ow} > 4.3$).

More Realistic and Relevant Testing. Based on extensive experience with detergent chemicals, several additional considerations beyond the screening level toxicity tests may be necessary to understand fully the potential hazard posed by these chemicals. Basically, more ecologically relevant assessment techniques may be needed to reduce the extrapolation uncertainties that are inherent in using pure chemical, single-species, laboratory tests to predict significant ecological impacts in complex environmental matrices. These include studying the relevant compartment(s), chemical form and bioavailability, and target species and ecotoxicological endpoints. The rest of this section details some of these approaches.

In addition to the water and soil compartment, sediments should be considered as a potential route of exposure. If a sorptive chemical is not completely removed during wastewater treatment, it will likely partition to sediments and/or suspended solids in surface waters or will enter surface waters already sorbed to wastewater effluent solids. Methodologies for measuring the bioavailability and toxicity of sediment-sorbed chemicals have just recently become available (57–59). Exposure via both direct skin contact and ingestion should be considered. Effects can be assessed relative to measured chemical concentrations on the sediments and in interstitial and overlying water.

Attached algae, or periphyton, are the predominant group of primary producers in streams and rivers, yet this group of organisms is not typically included in most aquatic toxicity assessments. The green and to a lesser extent the blue-green phytoplanktors have been the species of choice for assessing chemical impacts on primary production. We have routinely included a diatom species in our screening tests and have conducted numerous studies in the laboratory and field to examine the effects of detergent chemicals on the growth, density, and community composition of natural river periphyton (48, 60). The results of laboratory phytoplankton assays with detergent chemicals to date have provided conservative estimates (i.e., over estimates) of the effect levels for the periphyton inhabiting streams and rivers that receive treated domestic wastewater (61, 62). We speculate that organisms in the field may be more hearty and more tolerant of some environmental stresses. Also, algal communities are typically diverse and can likely compensate for more sensitive individuals or species. This would be particularly evident when measuring functional endpoints. There is also a significant microbial community associated with the periphyton. Our studies have shown that it has a major role in the biodegradation of detergent chemicals that reach streams and rivers (48).

In addition to using the standard daphnid toxicity test to establish the relative toxicity of a chemical, we have found it useful and informative to assess toxicity to those invertebrates most likely to be exposed to detergent chemicals. Specifically, it is important to study representative invertebrates inhabiting streams and rivers below municipal sewage treatment plant discharges (63). These organisms, which include rotifers, ostracods, snails, nematodes, oligochaetes, isopods, copepods, amphipods, and insect larvae, were very often significantly (e.g., ≥ 10 times) less sensitive than the standard laboratory zooplankton test species (see Table 8). The general conclusion from these studies was that the daphnid assay overestimates the toxicity of detergent chemicals to the typical receiving water invertebrates. That is, the daphnid was consistently the most sensitive organism we have tested and therefore provides a very conservative estimate of toxicity.

Standard aquatic toxicity test endpoints including organism survival, reproduction, and growth are useful to compare effect levels and species sensitivity for different chemicals. However, unlike mammalian toxicology investigations that are focused on protecting the individual organism, environmental assessments must eventually be directed toward protecting particular populations or the structure and function of a given ecosystem. The extrapolation of a chronic no-effect level—the average response from a group of individual laboratory organisms—to predict an ecologically safe level in a receiving stream is tenuous at best. There have been relatively few studies comparing laboratory effects to field effects, and the conclusions have varied for those that have been reported. For example, in a major 5-year study, copper was added to a small stream and the effects on fish, algae, and macroinvertebrates were examined (64). It was concluded that the toxicity of copper was underestimated by the sole use of laboratory data. On the other hand, results of standard single-species laboratory tests overestimated the toxicity of the insecticide diflubenzuron, a chitin synthesis inhibitor, to complex stream communities (65).

We have attempted to address this issue of laboratory-to-field extrapolation by incorporating more relevant ecological endpoints in some of our detergent chemical risk assessments programs. Basically, this approach involved multigeneration exposures of sensitive or target populations or communities in the laboratory and/or field. Results are compared with the standard effects tests to determine the degree of similarity (predictability) in effect levels, or they are used directly as a better estimate of effects to be seen in the field. A significant finding in such studies was that the standard laboratory data typically overestimate toxicity in the field for detergent chemicals. In part, this is because the lab tests fail to account for acclimation or compensation of organisms and populations (48, 61, 62).

Finally, although most environmental risk assessments have been conducted on a single chemical or product ingredient, a detergent chemical enters the environment as part of a complex mixture of wastewater sludge or effluent. This can change the detergent's chemical form and distribution in the sediment, as well as its bioavailability and toxicity. Logical next steps to toxicity screening tests of pure compounds in high-quality laboratory water included tests in natural waters, with relevant mixtures of other chemicals, and as

TABLE 3. Acute and Chronic Toxicities of Dialkyl Cationic Surfactants in Standard Laboratory Water and River Water

Test species	Cationic surfactant	Dilution water	Effect concentration (mg/l)	95% confidence interval (mg/l)
Bluegill				
(Lepomis macrochirus)	DSDMAC	well	1.04[a]	0.74-1.45
	DTDMAC	reconstituted	0.89	0.58-1.35
	DTDMAMS	reconstituted	1.23	0.99-1.54
	DTDMAC	river	14.0	11.0-18.0
Water flea				
(Daphnia magna)	DTDMAC	well	1.06[a]	0.91-1.25
	DTDMAC	reconstituted	0.19	0.15-0.24
	DSDMAC	reconstituted	0.16	—
	DSDMAC	river	3.1	—
Fathead minnow				
(Pimephales promelas)	DTDMAC	well	0.05-0.09[b]	—
	DTDMAC	river	0.23-0.45	—

[a]The 96-h or 48-h LC_{50}.
[b]The 28-day no effect–first effect.
Source: Adapted from Lewis and Wee (14).

part of complex sewage effluents. For dialkyl cationic surfactants, as an example, toxicity studies conducted in river water showed significantly reduced acute and chronic toxicity to fish, invertebrates, and algae. The LC_{50} values and chronic no-effect levels were 4–17 times higher in standard laboratory tests, substituting river water for the typical reconstituted laboratory water medium (Table 3) (14). This observed reduction in toxicity was attributed to the insolubility of these chemicals, their strong adsorption to natural solids, and tendency to form chemical complexes with dissolved organic carbon and anionic substances (14). There is also some evidence that toxicity tests conducted in an effluent matrix are fairly predictive of *in situ* effects in receiving waters (66–68).

In summary, for the majority of commercially available detergent chemicals, the standard laboratory effects test approach has predicted a relatively large margin of safety between the estimated exposure and toxicity threshold concentrations. This gives confidence that the intended use of new chemicals will not result in adverse ecological impact. In those cases where laboratory tests indicate a low margin between exposure and chronic effects, additional testing may be warranted for further assurances of acceptable risk. Special tests beyond the normal test battery may be needed to clarify specific questions that result from a chemical's unique properties, intended use, or disposal practice. As needed, specific investigative studies should be toilored to the chemical of interest and should consider relevant environmental compartments, chemical form and bioavailability, target species, and ecologically relevant toxicological endpoints.

Environmental Monitoring. The environmental risk assessment process and the decision to use or not use a chemical are based on the integration of many estimates, predictions, and extrapolations. The uncertainties that are inherent in the estimates of toxic levels and environmental exposures are addressed through the use of *safety margins* or an acceptable level of uncertainty for predicting real-world fate and effects. When the data support the environmental safety of a chemical and the decision is made to use it in commerce, an environmental monitoring program should be considered to confirm the predicted behavior of the chemical under actual use conditions. A properly designed and conducted field study serves as a validation of the accuracy of the laboratory data and modeling process.

Chemical monitoring programs typically require a specific and sensitive analytical method to identify trace quantities of the chemical in one or more complex environmental matrices. A number of methods have been developed and utilized extensively for measuring levels of specific detergent chemicals in solid (sludge, soil, sediment) and aqueous (wastewater, river water, seawater, groundwater) compartments (69–73). Occasionally, methods must be developed for more unusual media such as fish tissues, mollusk muscle, and related substances.

Field monitoring programs for detergent chemicals have been conducted in a number of countries including the United States, Canada, Germany, France, and the United Kingdom. The programs typically involved the collection of samples of raw and treated sewage—to confirm predictions of chemical usage and loading and treatment efficiency (53–55, 70, 74–76)—and samples of surface waters receiving discharges from sewage treatment plants to confirm predictions of dilution (70, 77–79). Measured concentrations in raw sewage generally agreed within a factor of 2 with values predicted from information on usage, population, and per capita sewage flow (Table 4) (19). Removal of detergent chemicals by wastewater treatment was also reasonably predictable (Table 4). Removal

TABLE 4. Summary of Sewage Treatment Plant Monitoring for Selected Detergent Materials

Material	Concentration in Raw Sewage (a)			Ref.
	Measured mg/l	Measured to Predicted Ratio (b)	Removal (%) (a)	
NTA	0.08-3.6	0.5-1.3		[77, 78, 79]
Primary Clarification			7-34	
Trickling Filter			21-88	
Activated Sludge			81-91	
LAS	2.0-5.0	0.3-0.9		[70, 80]
Primary Clarification			29	
Trickling Filter			73-87	
Activated Sludge			96-99	
AE	0.9-4.2	0.4-0.7		[17, 80]
Primary Clarification			37	
Trickling Filter			87	
Activated Sludge			98	
C_{12-14}MAQ	0.082	1.4		[17]
Primary Clarification			29	
Trickling Filter			83	
Activated Sludge			97	
C_{16-18}MAQ	0.022-0.076	0.6		[17]
Primary Clarification			66	
Trickling Filter			48-60	
Activated Sludge			82-95	

[a]The reported ranges represent results from several locations and countries.
[b]Measured concentration divided by the predicted concentration.
Source: Woltering et al. (17).

increases as general treatment efficiency increases, and the removals were often similar to those observed for total organic matter at the same treatment plants. Results of river water monitoring below sewage outfalls can be considerably lower than the estimated exposure concentrations based only on dilution if there are substantial mass removal processes occurring in-stream. More recently, detergent monitoring programs have been expanded to include measurements in sewage sludges (70, 80, 81), sludge-amended soils (70), sediments (70), and groundwater (82).

Biological monitoring can provide an equally important confirmation of the accuracy of the risk assessment by looking at the health of the biological community that is being exposed to some finite level of chemical. Few such studies of detergent chemicals have been reported to date owing to their cost and lack of clear significance. While chemical monitoring can target individual chemicals of interest, direct biological monitoring for signs of chemical impact from treated sewage involves the evaluation of biota exposed to a complex mixture of chemicals in sludge or effluent. Cause and effect is much easier to establish when the levels of "other chemical and physical factors" are minimized versus the chemical(s) of interest. Among the biota of major interest are fish, shellfish, and other macroinvertebrates, but nearly any taxonomic group can be studied to confirm specific laboratory-based predictions.

Another useful approach involves chemical spiking into the influent of a relatively small domestic wastewater treatment plant, or spiking directly into a receiving stream, and then conducting chemical and biological monitoring downstream (48, 74). Other approaches that should provide potentially important data for confirming laboratory- and model-based fate and effects predictions include the use of realistic, large-scale experimental streams (i.e., mesocosms) that can be colonized with the appropriate biota and exposed in a dose–response design to the chemical(s) of interest in a river-water, dilute sewage-effluent matrix. Another area currently under development is the use of biological survey data for fish and invertebrates along reaches of streams and rivers that receive detergent chemical manufacturing plant effluents or predominantly domestic municipal wastewater effluents. Again, comparisons are made between specific chemical monitoring data and the condition of the biota in the receiving stream.

Biological monitoring of terrestrial systems would likely involve plant and crop assessment in areas receiving chemicals via municipal sludge amendment. We are not aware of any experimental data for detergent chemical effects on cropland; however, there is a large amount of anecdotal data on the acceptable use of municipal sewage sludge, containing detergent chemicals, for agricultural land application. Biological monitoring will continue to be important to help refine and confirm the laboratory-based predictions of effect and no-effect levels for new and expanded use chemicals in both aquatic and terrestrial compartments.

Decisionmaking Criteria. The environmental risk assessment process is intended to give the risk manager the best possible evaluation of all the scientific data so that the best decisions can be reached about the use of a chemical (83). Many decisions are made during the evaluation including the selection of tests that are appropriate given a specified use, disposal, and physicochemical properties. A good assessment will also quantitate the levels of uncertainty in the ultimate prediction of environmental fate and effects. During the data-gathering process, certain test results may have indicated that a chemical should not be used; other test data may have indicated that concern for possible effects is relieved; or the testing may indicate a need to restrict the use, either volume and/or location, in order to achieve an acceptable risk level.

Although the risk assessment approach outlined in Fig. 3 is a generic one, the scope, design of tests, and factors to be considered in developing the appropriate data base should be approached on a chemical-by-chemical basis. This flexibility will allow for efficient, yet scientifically valid, decisionmaking. Given the evolving state-of-the-art of environmental risk assessment, it is advisable to reevaluate an assessment as new, relevant information becomes available. Finally, a very effective way to be sure that the best available science is being utilized and that the assessment program has identified and adequately addressed all key issues concerning the release of a chemical into the environment is to have the risk assessment critiqued by "outside experts."

CASE STUDY: A RISK ASSESSMENT OF MAQs

A number of classes of quaternary ammonium compounds (QACs) have the potential for broadscale environmental release. For example, approximately 75 million (MM) pounds per year of dialkyldimethylammonium compounds are used in the United States as important components of fabric softeners and oil-based drilling muds. About 25 MM lb of alkyldimethylbenzelammonium compounds, another QAC, are used annually as biocides, disinfectants, and emulsifying agents. Since there are several recently published environmental risk assessments for these other QACs (14, 84, 85), this case study focuses on the C_{12}–C_{18} monoalkyl quaternary ammonium compounds (MAQs). These are considered as a class for the purpose of this assessment because of the similarities in their chemical fate and potential environmental effects.

The MAQs are cationic surfactants that work in combination with other laundry detergent ingredients to improve cleaning on grease and oil stains and to improve the dissolution of granular detergents in the wash. Small quantities are also used in fabric softener and hair conditioner products. The structure of these compounds is shown in Fig. 4.

In 1987, U.S. industry used approximately 11 MM lb of MAQs and the bulk had the potential for disposal into the environment (86). In Europe, only Germany, the United Kingdom, and France have current annual industry-wide usages of MAQs that exceed 1 MM lb; each uses ~ 1000 metric tons/yr.

Chemical and Physical Properties

Monoalkyl quaternary surfactants (MAQs) are clear, slightly viscous liquids. They are highly water soluble (>1000 mg/L) and have low octonal–water partition coefficients

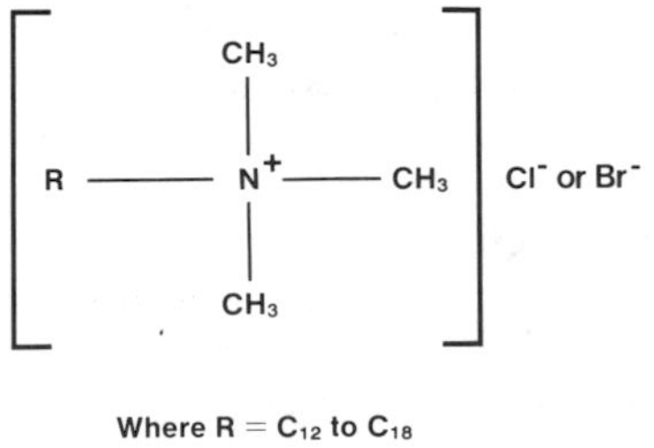

$$\left[R \text{——} N^+ \begin{matrix} CH_3 \\ | \\ \\ | \\ CH_3 \end{matrix} \text{——} CH_3 \right] Cl^- \text{ or } Br^-$$

Where R = C_{12} to C_{18}

Figure 4. Structure of monoalkyl quaternary ammonium compounds (MAQs) used in detergents.

(log K_{ow} ranges from -0.7 for C_{12} MAQ to 1.5 for C_{18} MAQ). The bioaccumulation potential of MAQs is predicted to be very low; calculated bioconcentration factors (BCFs) are less than 10.

Illustrative Example 1 (Bioconcentration Factors). A bioconcentration model (20), based on a regression equation developed for a wide variety of organic compounds, was used to calculate a bioconcentration factor (BCF) from the K_{ow} data as follows:

$$\log BCF = 0.76 \log K_{ow} - 0.23,$$

where K_{ow} ranges from -0.7 for C_{12} MAQ to 1.5 for C_{18} MAQ.

Solution

$$\log BCF = 0.76(-0.7) - 0.23 = -0.762$$
$$BCF = 0.17.$$
$$\log BCF = 0.76(1.50) - 0.23 = 1.325$$
$$BCF = 8.1.$$

MAQs ionize in aqueous solution to form organic ions with positive charge that are responsible for their surface activity. Because of their positive charge, MAQs have a strong affinity for negatively charged surfaces and for anionic compounds. Sorption to solids in the environment is predicted to be high; the measured adsorption coefficient (K_d) for MAQs and river sediment is approximately 100,000.

Illustrative Example 2 (Sorption Coefficients). Sorption of MAQs to river sediment was measured in batch test systems containing 150–900 mg dry sediment/L of water and ~ 10–1000 μg MAQ/L of water. Sorption was quantified by a sorption coefficient, K_d, where

$$K_d = \frac{[MAQ]_{solids}}{[MAQ]_{solution}} = \frac{\mu g/g}{\mu g/mL} \quad \text{(at equilibrium)}$$

Solution

$$K_d = \frac{10,500 \ \mu g/g \text{ on solids}}{0.10 \ \mu g/mL \text{ in solution}} = 105,000.$$

The average K_d for 23 combinations of varying solids and solution concentrations was $112,000 \pm 4600$. Based on this K_d, virtually all the MAQ present should be sorbed to sediments and suspended particulate matter.

Predicted Environmental Concentrations

Initial estimates of environmental concentrations of MAQs in the United States (Table 5) were made using Eq. (2)–(6) described previously. The basic assumptions for these estimates are a population of 230 MM, an average sewage flow of 507 L/capita·day, primary waste treatment for 25% of the sewage flow and secondary treatment for 75% of the sewage flow, and 132 mg of primary sludge produced/L of sewage. MAQ removal is

TABLE 5. Procedure and Estimates for Sewage Treatment Plant Loading and Subsequent Environmental Concentrations of C_{12-18} MAQs from Industry-Wide Detergent Usage

Estimated C_{12-18}MAQ Environmental Loadings and Concentrations in 1987

	France	U.K.	Germany	U.S.A.
Thousands of Metric Tons MAQ/Year	0.9	1.3	1.4	5.0
Influent Sewage (ppb)	300	423	500	110
Effluent Sewage (ppb)	117	118	150	30
Surface Water at 10:1 dilution (ppb)	12	12	15	3
Primary Sludge (ppm, dry solids)	720	950	940	220

Detailed Data Used in Making Estimates of Environmental Concentrations

	France	U.K.	Germany	U.S.A.
Population (millions)	53.5	56.0	61.4	230
Sewage Flow (L/capita/day)	150	150	150	507
Fraction 1° treatment	0.4	0.2	0.3	0.25
Fraction 1° + 2° treatment	0.6	0.8	0.7	0.75
Removal by 1° treatment[a]	0.3	0.3	0.3	0.3
Removal by 1° + 2° treatment[a]	0.9	0.9	0.9	0.9
Fraction discharged[b]	0.34	0.22	0.28	0.25
Primary sludge production (mg per liter of sewage)[c]	132	132	132	132

[a] Represent 30% removal by primary and 90% removal by primary + secondary treatment.

[b] Example calculation (Germany):

$$\text{fraction discharged} = [\text{Infl.}](1\text{-}0.3)(0.3) + [\text{Infl.}](1\text{-}0.9)(0.7)$$
$$= [\text{Infl.}](0.21) + [\text{Infl.}](0.7) = [\text{Infl.}](0.28).$$

[c] Calculated from suspended solids data from Holman (19).

estimated at 30% in primary treatment and 90% in secondary treatment. The fraction of MAQ discharged was based on these equations and equals about 25% of the total entering treatment plants.

At an annual usage of 11 MM lb (5000 metric tons), MAQ levels were estimated to be 0.110 mg/L in influent sewage, 0.028 mg/L in sewage effluent, and ~0.003 mg/L in surface waters receiving sewage effluent at a 10:1 dilution. Based on measured settling efficiencies of 30–60%, primary sludge would contain ~200 mg MAQ/kg dry solids and secondary sludge ~10 mg MAQ/kg dry solids. Assuming an application rate of 2.2 kg dry sludge solids per square meter per year, loading estimates for sludge-amended soil in 1 year would be ~2.6 mg MAQ/kg soil.

Illustrative Example 3 [Influent Sewage, Eq. (2)]. The concentration of a detergent chemical in a municipal wastewater influent can be estimated by

$$C_{iw} = \frac{\text{total daily usage of chemical}}{\text{total wastewater flow per day}}.$$

Solution. Given the information in the preceding paragraph,

$$C_{iw} = \frac{30,136 \text{ lb MAQ used per day in U.S.}}{(230 \text{ MM people})(507 \text{ L wastewater/person·day})}$$

$$= \frac{1.3669 \times 10^{10} \text{ mg/day}}{1.1661 \times 10^{11} \text{ L/day}} = 0.110 \text{ mg MAQ/L of influent.}$$

Illustrative Example 4 [Effluent Sewage, Eq. (5)]. The concentration of a detergent chemical in a municipal wastewater effluent can be estimated by

$$C_{ew} = (\% \text{ total sewage flow receiving primary treatment})$$

$$\times (\text{estimated removal efficiency})$$

$$+ [(\% \text{ sewage flow receiving secondary treatment})$$

$$\times (\text{its estimated removal efficiency})].$$

Solution. Given the information in the preceding paragraph,

$$C_{ew} = 0.25 [C_{iw}(1 - 0.30)] + 0.75 [C_{iw}(1 - 0.90)]$$

where $C_{iw} = 0.110 \text{ mg/L}$.

$$C_{ew} = 0.020 + 0.008 = 0.028 \text{ mg MAQ/L of effluent.}$$

Illustrative Example 5 [Municipal Wastewater Sludge, Eq. (3)]. The concentration of a detergent chemical in a municipal digested wastewater sludge can be estimated by

C_{ds} = (sewage influent concentration)

  × (a 260 average ratio of municipal wastewater to digested sludge flow rate)

  × (treatment removal efficiency adjusted for the fraction degraded
   —and therefore not in the sludge).

Solution. Given the information in the preceding paragraph,

C_{ds} for primary sludge = $0.110 \text{ mg/L} \times 260 \times 0.3$

$$= 8.58 \text{ mg/L, or on a dry sludge-suspended solids}$$

basis where suspended solids = 0.04 kg/L

$$= \frac{8.58 \text{ mg/L}}{0.04 \text{ kg/L}}.$$

$$C_{ds} = 214.5 \text{ mg MAQ/kg dry solids} \quad \text{(assumes no}$$

degradation in primary removal).

Illustrative Example 6 [Sludge-Amended Soil, Eq. (4)]. The concentration of a detergent chemical in sludge-amended soil for a 1-year application can be estimated by

$$C_{soil} = \text{(concentration in sludge)} \times (1.22 \times 10^{-2} \text{ kg sludge}$$

solids per kg soil per year sludge incorporation rate).

Solution. Given the information in the preceding paragraph,

$$C_s = 214.5 \text{ mg/kg} \times 1.22 \times 10^{-2}$$
$$= 2.6 \text{ mg MAQ/kg soil.}$$

(Estimates of long-term, steady-state soil concentrations would have to consider soil degradation and leaching.)

A significantly lower per capita water use in Europe resulted in predicted environmental concentrations that are approximately five times higher than those for the United States (P&G unpublished data). These estimates, shown in Table 5, included up to 0.500 mg/L MAQ in sewage influent, up to 0.150 mg/L in effluents assuming primary treatment only and a removal efficiency of 30%, and up to 0.015 mg/L in surface waters at a 10:1 effluent dilution. The highest sludge estimates were ~ 950 and ~ 35 mg MAQ/kg for primary and secondary sludges, respectively. Sludge-amended soils would contain ~ 12 mg MAQ/kg soil after a year's application.

Environmental Fate Test Results

The removal and biodegradability of monoalkyl quaternary surfactants (MAQs) were investigated using laboratory screening tests simulating wastewater treatment systems and surface waters. Essentially complete removal (99%) was observed in acclimated semicontinuous activated sludge (SCAS) units dosed at 20 mg/L MAQ over a 7-day period, based on dissolved organic carbon (DOC) analysis. Approximately 76% of theoretical CO_2 production was observed in 25-day shake flask biodegradability tests at 10–20 mg/L MAQ. Both the rate and extent of MAQ degradation were comparable to the glucose control. The conclusion was that MAQs are readily removed in wastewater treatment and have a very high potential to be rapidly and completely biodegraded.

In standard screening tests used to measure solubilization of metals by chelators, C_{12} MAQ did not solubilize metals (Cd, Cr, Cu, Fe, Mn, Ni, Pb, and Zn) from river sediment or from sewage sludge. Maximum concentrations of MAQs in these assays exceeded the maximum predicted environmental concentrations by at least 10-fold.

Environmental Effects Screening Tests

As part of an initial screen to evaluate the aquatic toxicity of MAQs, several chainlengths $(C_{12}-C_{18})$ were tested on a variety of algal species, invertebrates, and fish in a medium-hardness well water or in seawater. Test species and test methodology selection were based on the collective experience in aquatic toxicology and reflect the importance of assessing toxicity for sensitive populations and organisms of major trophic levels. The primary goal of the screening tests was to evaluate relative sensitivity of key species and the relative toxicity of the test chemical versus other well-studied materials, using standard, reproducible protocols. These studies formed the basis for decisions as to the need for more detailed follow-up studies and eventually for extrapolation to real-world conditions of chemical exposure.

Because MAQs are relatively toxic, a number of species were tested to look for significant differences in sensitivity. The 96-h EC_{50} values for green and blue-green algae and diatoms ranged from 0.12 to 0.86 mg/L MAQ. (An EC_{50} is the statistical estimate of the chemical concentration at which 50% of the test organisms would show an effect—in this case a reduction in growth.) Algistatic concentrations ranged from 0.47 to 0.97 mg/L. (The algistatic concentration is the statistical estimate of the chemical concentration that would completely inhibit growth but not cause cell death.) Daphnid 48-h EC_{50} values averaged 0.06 mg/L for five tests of various MAQs in laboratory water. The chronic no observed effect (NOEC) and first observed effect (FOEC) concentrations in 21-day laboratory tests were 0.01–0.04 mg/L MAQ. EC_{50} values for mysid and pink shrimp were 1.3 and 1.8 mg/L, respectively. The 96-h LC_{50} values for four species of freshwater fish varied with chainlength. They were 2.8–31.3 mg/L for the C_{12}–C_{14} MAQs and 0.10–0.24 mg/L for the C_{15}–C_{18} MAQs. The measured 28-day chronic NOEC/FOEC in fathead minnow egg-fry studies were 0.46–1.00 mg/L for C_{12} MAQ and 0.01–0.02 mg/L for C_{16}–C_{18} MAQs.

From the screening level aquatic toxicity tests (Table 6) it was concluded that MAQs are relatively toxic to aquatic organisms, that the invertebrates are the most sensitive

TABLE 6. Environmental Effects Data for C_{12-18} MAQs Based on Standard Aquatic and Microbial Toxicity Tests

Test	Species	Response	MAQ^a (mg/L)
Algal toxicity	green, bluegreen, diatom	96-hr EC50	0.12–0.86
	green, bluegreen, diatom	14-day algistatic	0.47–0.97
Invertebrate toxicity	Daphnia magna	48-hr EC50	0.06
	Daphnia magna	21-day NOEC-FOEC	0.01–0.04
	mysid shrimp	96-hr EC50	1.30 (C_{12})
	pink shrimp	96-hr EC50	1.80 (C_{16}-C_{18})
Fish toxicity	goldorfen, bluegill zebrafish, fathead minnow	96-hr LC50	9.50 (C_{12}-C_{14})
	goldorfen, bluegill, zebrafish, fathead minnow	96-hr LC50	0.15 C_{16}-C_{18})
	fathead minnow	early life stage NOEC-FOEC	0.46–1.00 (C_{12})
	fathead minnow	early life stage NOEC-FOEC	0.01–0.02 (C_{16}-C_{18})
Microbial toxicity	activated sludge microbes	15-min. HA_{50}	39.0
Anaerobic Digester Inhibition	digester sludge	21-day NOEC-FOEC	270–540

$^a C_{12}$–C_{18} chainlengths tested unless otherwise noted.

species to the total class of MAQs with chronic effects at ~0.025 mg/L in laboratory water, and that fish and invertebrates are equally sensitive to the lower-chainlength MAQs.

No terrestrial plant or animal toxicity studies were conducted on MAQs; however, in-house data for the related dialkyl quaternary ammonium compounds show no effects to plants at up to 1000 mg/kg in soil and 240 mg/L in solution. Soil microbial respiration studies show no inhibition at realistic levels.

Data from a standard microbial toxicity assay indicated that it takes approximately 11.3 mg MAQ/g volatile suspended solids to see a 50% reduction in the glucose uptake rate by activated sludge. These data can be used to predict whether MAQ will have an adverse affect on the activated sludge removal process. Assuming a typical activated sludge, mixed-liquor, volatile suspended solids concentration of 2500 mg/L for a municipal sewage treatment plant, the concentration predicted to cause a 50% reduction in heterotrophic activity (i.e., HA_{50}) was approximately 39 mg/L MAQ. The maximum projected environmental concentration of total MAQ in municipal wastewaters resulting from industry-wide usage was 0.5 mg/L. This concentration is well below the 39 mg/L concentration found to be inhibitory to activated sludge microorganisms, which are responsible for most of the biodegradation of organics in wastewater treatment.

Finally, a batch anaerobic digester study was conducted to determine the concentration of MAQ required to inhibit digester performance. The no observed effect concentration was 270 mg/L or 10,000 mg/kg dry sludge solids and the first observed effect concentration was 540 mg/L. Since the maximum projected total MAQ sludge concentration resulting from industry-wide usage is 950 mg/kg dry solids, no adverse effects on digester performance would be expected.

Initial Estimate of Environmental Risk

The purpose of the aforementioned testing was to obtain a general impression of the potential hazard posed by the chemical. Based on these test results and calculations, the likely environmental behavior of MAQs and the potential hazard can be summarized by the following statements (see also Table 7):

- At the maximum projected use rate, MAQs could enter municipal sewage influents at concentrations up to 0.5 mg/L. This level should not interfere with either aerobic or anaerobic treatment processes.
- At a minimum, 30–90% (primary and secondary treatment) of the MAQs should be removed during treatment and any that are not rapidly biodegraded will be sorbed to (sludge) solids.
- Sludge disposal will result in a terrestrial loading of MAQs where the compounds should undergo relatively rapid and complete biodegradation, forming no persistent or highly toxic intermediates or metabolites (assumes biodegradation kinetics are similar to those observed for aquatic systems).
- At levels anticipated in a soil–sludge matrix, MAQs should not be toxic to terrestrial species when applied to pasture or cropland.
- As much as half of the MAQ in wastewater effluent will sorb to suspended solids, sediments, or soils where they will likely continue to undergo complete biodegradation.
- There will be low ppb levels of MAQs dissolved in surface water and/or groundwater for some distance below a discharge from a municipal water treatment plant until removal or biodegradation is complete.

TABLE 7. Initial Assessment of MAQ Environmental Fate, Exposure, and Effect Levels

Fate

Bioconcentration potential	BCF estimates $\leq$ 8 (C_{12-18}MAQ)
CO_2 evolution	76% TCO_2
SCAS removal	99% efficiency based on DOC removal
Adsorption	K_d = 100,000 for sediments
Metal complexation	No mobilization of metals from sediments or sludges seen at least 10x maximum environmental levels.

Exposure (maximum)

Influent sewage (U.S./Europe)	0.110/0.500 mg/L MAQ
Effluent sewage (U.S./Europe)	0.030/0.015 mg/L MAQ assuming only primary treatment (30% removal)
Surface water (U.S./Europe)	0.003/0.015 mg/L MAQ assuming primary treatment and 10:1 river dilution and no in-stream removal
River sediments (U.S./Europe)	300/1500 mg/kg MAQ assuming K_d = 100,000 and maximum river water levels, and no degradation
Primary sludge (U.S./Europe)	~200/950 mg MAQ/kg dry solids assuming settling efficiencies of 30 to 66% and sewage influents of 0.1 to 0.5 mg/L
Secondary sludge (U.S./Europe)	~10/35 mg/kg (same assumptions as above)
Soils (U.S./Europe)	~2.5/12.0 mg/kg/yr assuming primary sludge applied at 1.22×10^{-2} kg solids per kg soil and no degradation

Effect

Microbial inhibition	HA_{50} = 39 mg/L MAQ for activated sludge microbes
Wastewater treatment inhibition	NOEC for anaerobic digester = 270 mg/L MAQ or 10,000 mg/kg dry sludge solids
Aquatic biota	Lowest chronic effect level in lab water = 0.025 mg/L MAQ (Daphnia)
Terrestrial biota	No direct measurements, but NOECs for related quats = 1000 mg/kg in soil and 240 mg/L in water

- There is a very minimal potential for bioaccumulation in fish or other aquatic species (estimated BCF < 10).
- MAQs are relatively toxic to aquatic organisms and there is a relatively small margin (~10) between the lowest chronic effect level and estimated surface water concentrations.

Based on usage information, physicochemical properties, and screening level environmental fate and effects tests, it appears that this class of chemicals has an acceptable environmental profile [i.e., not persistent, minimal potential to bioaccumulate, and very good human safety profile based on potential environmental exposure via drinking water (87)]. However, the ratio of the chronic toxicity level for the most sensitive species (*Daphnia magna*) divided by a reasonable worst case estimate for the level of MAQs in the mixing zone below a primary or secondary wastewater treatment plant could be less than

10. On this basis, the decision was made to initiate an investigative research program utilizing more realistic test systems to evaluate the fate, exposure, and effects of MAQs.

INVESTIGATIVE RESEARCH PROGRAM

A number of additional studies were conducted with the MAQs in order to reduce the uncertainty inherent in an initial assessment based on laboratory-derived screening level data and to define better the actual margin between environmental exposure levels and effect levels. The major focuses were (i) biodegradation in surface waters, sediments, soils, and groundwaters, (ii) bioavailability and toxicity in river water and sediments, (iii) fate and effects in home treatment systems, and (iv) monitoring of wastewater removals and environmental levels in key compartments. We also used this opportunity to develop and investigate novel techniques in environmental fate and effects testing and in predicting a realistic range of chemical exposures in surface waters rather than just a single average value.

Biodegradation/Toxicity Tests in River Water: Laboratory Studies

Both primary (loss of parent material) and ultimate (mineralization to CO_2) biodegradation of MAQs were rapid in river waters spiked with 0.1 and 1.0 mg/L ^{14}C-labeled MAQ. The estimated half-life for mineralization in river water was ~ 10 h at 20°C (Fig. 5). Continuously dosed river water die-away toxicity assays with *Daphnia magna* showed no evidence of the formation of intermediate products having a toxicity greater than the parent material (Fig. 6). In these 7-day tests, test material was continuously spiked into river water, and degradation and toxicity were evaluated as a function of time.

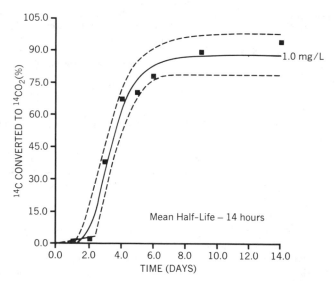

Figure 5. Biodegradation of 1 mg/L C_{12} MAQ to CO_2 in river water. Dashed contours are 95% confidence limits of the mean.

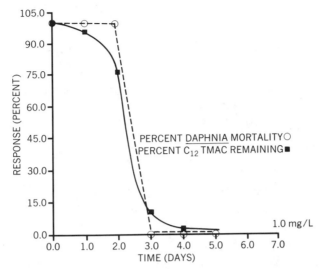

Figure 6. Continuously dosed river water die-away toxicity assay showing the biodegradation of 1 mg/L C_{12} MAQ and the corresponding toxicity profile for *Daphnia magna*.

Biodegradation in Soils and Sediments

Biodegradation in river sediments and in surface and subsurface soils followed apparent first-order kinetics at spiked concentrations approximating realistic environmental levels (i.e., < 1 up to 100 μg/g $^{14}C_{12}$ MAQ). The rate and extent of MAQ degradation was comparable to naturally occurring compounds (e.g., stearic acid control) and is sufficiently rapid to prevent accumulation of these chemicals in soil and sediment compartments. Half-lives for mineralization were approximately 1 day in sediments, 1 week in anaerobic subsurface soils, and 1 month in aerobic sludge-ammended surface soils (Fig. 7) (26). These half-lives, in relation to typical residence times in these compartments (i.e., weeks or months in sediments to years in soils), result in a prediction of extensive removal of chemical mass.

Biodegradation in Groundwater

Groundwater and subsurface soil were collected at sites in Canada and the United States using specialized procedures to avoid contamination by surface microorganisms; samples were tested for microbial activity within 24 h of collection. Biodegradation potential was assessed in aerobic slurries using 10 g soil, 10 mL groundwater, and 5 μg/L $^{14}C_{12}$ MAQ, at 20°C. MAQ was readily degraded to $^{14}CO_2$ in the test. Approximately 80% of the MAQ biodegraded in the 36-day study, with a degradation half-life estimate of 1 week [Fig. 8 and (88)].

Aquatic Species Sensitivity

Based on standard screening level toxicity tests, the lowest LC_{50} values and chronic first effect levels were for *Daphnia magna*. An acute screen of 12 typical riverine invertebrates

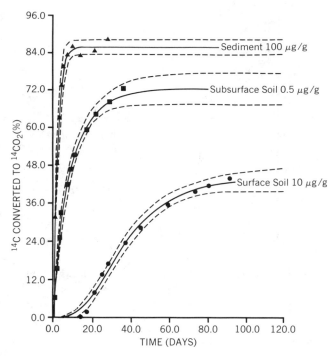

Figure 7. Biodegradation of C_{12} MAQ to CO_2 in river sediments, subsurface soils, and surface soils. Initial concentrations were 10 and $100\,\mu g/g$, 0.05 and $0.5\,\mu g/g$, and 1, 10, and $100\,\mu g/g$, respectively. Dashed contours are 95% confidence limits of the mean.

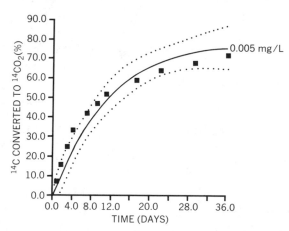

Figure 8. Biodegradation of $0.005\,mg/L$ C_{12} MAQ to CO_2 in groundwater and subsurface soil slurries. Dotted contours are 95% confidence limits of the mean.

TABLE 8. Comparative Acute Toxicity of C_{12} MAQ to Standard Invertebrate Test Species and Typical River and Stream Invertebrates

Test Species	48-h LC_{50} (mg/l C_{12}MAQ)
Standard Test Species	
Daphnia magna (Daphnid)	0.11
Typical River Species	
Cyclops sp. (Copepod)	0.75
Gammarus sp. (Amphipod)	5.10
Aeolosoma sp. (Oligochaete)	6.80
Heliosoma sp. (Snail)	9.20
Tubifex sp. (Oligochaete)	22.00
Philodina sp. (Rotifer)	28.00
Hexagenia sp. (Mayfly Larvae)	46.00
Rhabditis sp. (Nematode)	65.00
Candona sp. (Copepod)	>100.00
Paratanytarsus sp. (Midge)	160.00
Asellus sp. (Isopod)	180.00
Libellula sp. (Dragonfly Larvae)	>1000.00

(e.g., amphipod, oligochaete, snail, midge, and mayfly larvae) showed daphnids to be 7 to > 1000 times more sensitive to MAQs (Table 8). It was therefore concluded that the initial margins of safety and aquatic risk assessment for MAQs, based on daphnid toxicity results, were conservative and overestimated the threshold effect levels for typical water column organisms that inhabit rivers and streams below wastewater discharges. However, because of the economic and environmental importance of these chemicals, more information would be developed on daphnids.

Bioavailability and Toxicity in Sediments

For MAQs, sorption to suspended solids and sediment has the potential to be an important in-stream removal mechanism and is therefore a source of potentially high exposure to organisms that live in and/or ingest sediments or suspended solids. This has been shown with several xenobiotics and metals (57, 58, 89). Typical benthic organisms like oligochaetes, bivalves, amphipods, and insect larvae were at least 50 times less sensitive to MAQs than *Daphnia* based on acute LC_{50} values from water column exposures (Table 8). The chronic no-effect and first-effect levels for the midge, *Chironomus riparius*, in water only were 0.3 and 0.6 mg/L MAQ. In addition, there was no evidence of bioavailability and toxicity to aquatic midges in chronic life cycle exposures to MAQs as high as 3084 μg/kg MAQ in spiked river sediments (Table 9) (57).

Toxicity in Receiving Water Matrix: Laboratory Tests

Several acute and chronic toxicity tests with MAQs were conducted in river and lake waters to investigate whether bioavailability and toxicity are different from values in clean laboratory well water. Both acute LC_{50} values and chronic first-effect levels averaged threefold higher in surface water tests (versus laboratory water) for daphnids. The 48-h LC_{50} values were 0.1–0.5 mg/L MAQ in seven river and lake water tests. Measured

TABLE 9. Comparison of Soluble versus Sediment-Sorbed MAQ Toxicty to the Midge *Chironomus riparius* in Life Cycle Exposures

	MAQ (ppm; Mean ± S.E.)		Lifecycle Response
Sediment	Interstitial Water	Overlying Water	% Emergence
0 (Control)	0	0	98
173 ± 45	0.5 ± 0.1	0.4 ± 0.1	80
420 ± 14	1.0 ± 0.2	0.4 ± 0.1	93
427 ± 64	1.4 ± 0.1	0.5 ± 0.1	88
3084 ± 322	2.3 ± 0.1	0.5 ± 0.1	88 NOEC

Soluble MAQ

48-Hour EC50 = 6.00 mg/l
Lifecycle NOEC - FOEC = 0.32 - 0.62 mg/l

chronic NOEC and FOEC in four different surface water tests ranged from 0.05 to 0.10 mg/L MAQ. The results of two river water acute toxicity tests with bluegill and fathead minnows were comparable to the laboratory water studies—LC_{50} values of 6.0 mg/L in river water versus 2.8–31.0 for the same chainlengths in laboratory water.

Toxicity in Receiving Water Matrix: Microcosm and Field Studies

An even more realistic ecological assessment involved studies of MAQs in surface water matrices using more relevant ecological endpoints to address population and community level impacts. Basically, the approach involved both single and multigeneration exposures of sensitive or likely target populations under realistic conditions in a laboratory stream microcosm and in three *in situ* field studies. The fate, exposure, and effects of C_{12} MAQ were studied simultaneously in each system.

Microcosm Study. In the first study, the fate and effects of C_{12} MAQ were evaluated in our laboratory-stream microcosm (Fig. 9). The 20-m long artificial stream (1500 L volume) was supplied with a continuous input of river water and the bottom was covered to a depth of 1–2 cm with clean river sediment (43% clay, 29% silt, 28% sand, 1.5% total organic carbon, TOC). The first 2 m were partitioned as the "control" or upstream area, followed by a chemical dosing site and thorough mixing, and then 18 m of uninterrupted flow to an overflow drain. The rate of river water input controlled the flow rate and hydraulic retention time. An 8-h travel time was established for the MAQs study. The dosing site continuously received C_{12} MAQ at concentrations expected to be lethal to *Daphnia magna*, the most sensitive species based on the screening tests. In-stream removal processes, including biodegradation and sorption to sediments, established a concentration gradient downstream from the dosing site. Several replicate populations of *Daphnia magna*, chironomid midges, and colonized river periphyton were exposed at several distances downstream, as well as in the upstream control area, for multiple (e.g., four to six) generations of up to 4-months duration.

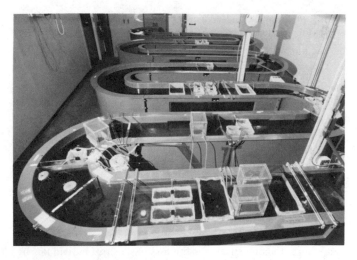

Figure 9. A 20-m long, flow-through laboratory stream microcosm used to study the aquatic fate, exposure, and population effects of MAQs.

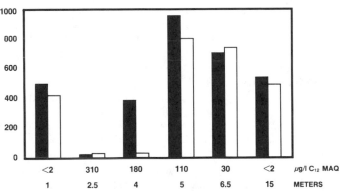

Figure 10. *Daphnia* mean population density as a function of C_{12} MAQ concentration in laboratory stream microcosm. The concentration gradient was a function of the distance downstream: 1 m is control area, 2.5 m is the first site below the point of chemical dosing, and so on. Solid bars represent the response of preexposed populations; open bars represent control-reared populations.

There were no significant differences in *Daphnia* density or biomass at up to 0.110 mg/L MAQ (Fig. 10). In fact, daphnid populations generally exceeded the control populations in size. The first effect occurred at 0.180 mg/L for populations that were exposed to MAQ for the first time. Daphnids that had been reared for several months at ~ 0.01 mg/L and then exposed to 0.180 mg/L MAQ were not affected. Significant reductions were observed for both preexposed and control-reared daphnid populations at 0.310 mg/L. There was, however, long-term survival and limited reproduction even at this highest concentration. An explanation for the observed population-level response to the chemical is the apparent

TABLE 10. Ultimate Biodegradation (Mineralization to CO_2) of MAQs in
Standard Laboratory Microcosm, and *in situ* Lake and River Test Systems

Test System	Initial MAQ Concentration (mg/l)	Approximate Half-Life (h)
Stnd. shake flask assay	0.10-1.0	10
Lab stream	0.10	2
in-situ lake plankton	0.10	20
in-situ river plankton	0.01-5.0	10
in-situ river periphyton	0.01-5.0	2
in-situ stream plankton	0.01-0.10	10
in-situ stream periphyton	0.01-0.10	30
in-situ stream sediment	0.01-0.10	115

ability of the daphnids to compensate for the loss of sensitive individuals by increases in reproduction and growth, as well as the apparent adaptation to more tolerant populations after multigeneration exposure. These results could not have been predicted from the standard *Daphnia* chronic toxicity test, which measures the average response of individual organisms using either laboratory or river water. However, acclimation, adaptation, and compensation are typical responses of many aquatic populations and are viewed as important, although underutilized, considerations when attempting to extrapolate screening level toxicity results and effect levels to surface waters (90).

Relatively high sediment concentrations of MAQ, up to 37 μg/g or about 100 times the water column concentrations, were apparently not bioavailable to midge. The midge population emergence rates and densities were comparable to the upstream controls over four generations. Finally, the periphyton communities were not adversely affected by continuous exposure to a mean of 0.513 mg/L MAQ (range 0.299–0.562 mg/L) for 5 weeks, based on measured chlorophyll, density, and species diversity.

The structure and function of microbial communities were stable for extended periods (months) and not adversely affected by chronic exposures up to ~1.0 mg/L MAQ. Rates of MAQ biodegradation were rapid in both water and periphyton fractions and were comparable to those for naturally occurring compounds like sugars and amino acids. Half-lives were less than 2 h at 0.1 mg/L MAQ (Table 10). Measurable degradation occurred in sediments, but rates were reduced owing to an apparent bioavailability factor. The development and expression of MAQ biodegradation capability showed significant dose–response relations and increased with the length of the exposure. Rapid biodegradation was observed even at trace levels of MAQ. The effect of temperature on MAQ degradation followed a typical Arrhenius relation; that is, biodegradation slowed by one-half with a 10°C drop in temperature (a $Q10$ of 2).

Field Studies. Field studies provided a real-world point of reference to evaluate the laboratory-to-field extrapolations of MAQ fate, exposure, and effects. Because of the broad-scale use of MAQs and other detergent chemicals, study sites needed to reflect the more general aspects of biological structure and function, physical habitat, and water quality in order to provide widely applicable data. We chose both river and lake ecosystems in good condition biological and receiving quantifiable amounts of treated sewage effluents. Other key considerations in site selection included accessibility, privacy

TABLE 11. MAQ Toxicity to Lake Plankton Exposed *in situ*[a]

Phytoplankton	mg/L MAQ
3-Hr. Photosynthesis (EC_{50})	2.20
21-Day Photosynthesis (First Effect)	3.87
21-Day Community Similarity (First Effect)	1.99
96-Hr. Laboratory Algal Assay (EC_{50})	0.17
Zooplankton	
21-Day Density, Number of Species and Community Similarity (First Effect)	0.40
21-Day Laboratory D. magna Assay (First Effect)	0.04

[a]Standard laboratory assay results are included for comparison.

for security of test equipment, and the ability to get permission from local authorities to intentionally add test chemicals of interest.

In the first field study with C_{12} MAQ, natural lake phytoplankton (82 species) and zooplankton (19 species including daphnids) were exposed *in situ* and effects on structural and functional parameters and biodegradation rates were measured. The experiments included 3-h light/dark bottle assays of photosynthetic activity, and 21-day exposures that were conducted in 26-L polyethylene bottles incubated in the photic zone and monitored periodically for changes in chlorophyll, community composition, and biodegradation potential.

The standard laboratory growth assays for green and blue-green algae and diatoms significantly overestimated the toxicity of MAQ (Table 11). Laboratory-derived EC_{50} values were 12–23 times less than the in situ concentration, which affected photosynthetic activity or community structure (i.e., similarity, density) (61, 62). First effects on zooplankton, including reduced numbers of species and density, occurred at 0.4 mg/L MAQ, 10 times higher than first observed effect levels in the standard 21-day *Daphnia magna* toxicity test. Biodegradation of MAQ by preexposed microbial communities was rapid and comparable to that observed for naturally occurring organic compounds (91). Turnover times (time to complete degradation) were ~ 80 h and biodegradation half-lives were ~ 20 h (Table 10). The development of MAQ degrading capability appeared to involve induction of preexisting enzymes in the general microbial population specific for MAQ degradation. This conclusion was based on the biodegradation lag time being too short to allow for gene mutation and selection.

A second field study investigated the *in situ* effects of C_{12} MAQ on river periphyton (122 species) above and below a municipal secondary treatment plant outfall. River periphyton from precolonized plexiglass slides were continuously exposed for 3 h in BOD bottles (photosynthesis assay) or for 21 days in a floating in-stream dosing apparatus. Biomass, chlorophyll, and seven community composition parameters were monitored in

TABLE 12. MAQ Toxicity to River Periphyton Exposed *in situ* above and below a Treated Sewage Effluent Outfall[a]

Most Sensitive Response	mg/L MAQ	
	River Above Sewage Outfall	River Below Sewage Outfall
3-Hr. Photosynthesis (EC_{50})	>10.0	>10.0
21-Day Photosynthesis (First Effect)	0.96	6.9
21-Day Community Similarity (First Effect)	0.96	–
21-Day Chlorophyll a (First Effect)	–	6.9

96-Hr. Laboratory Growth Assay EC_{50} = 0.17 mg/l

[a] A standard laboratory assay result is included for comparison.

the 21-day assays. The biodegradation of MAQ by periphytic bacteria was assessed by heterotrophic activity techniques.

Laboratory-derived EC_{50} values for photosynthesis and growth were an order of magnitude lower than the first-effect levels in either the 3-h or 21-day assays (Table 12). Not only was the first-effect level 10–100 times higher in the field versus the laboratory but the periphyton below the sewage outfall were less sensitive (FOEC = 6.9 mg/L) than the periphyton upstream (FOEC = 0.96 mg/L) (48). No significant adverse microbial effects were seen at up to 5 mg/L MAQ. Rates of MAQ biodegradation by periphytic and planktonic bacteria were rapid, with half-lives of ~2 h and ~10 h, respectively (Table 10). There were no significant differences in biodegradation by bacteria collected above and below the sewage outfall.

In the third field study, MAQ was dosed into a small stream in southeast Indiana that received approximately 1 million gallons per day of secondary treatment plant effluent. The dilution of effluent by the stream was only two- to three-fold during the study. The study area consisted of pools and riffles and had a sandy sediment. Stream width varied from 0.5 to 3 m with depths up to ~100 cm. Baseline biological and chemical data were collected for 1 month prior to dosing the stream. The stream was of relatively high quality based on analysis of BOD (biochemical oxygen demand, an indicator of total organic material present), dissolved oxygen, residual chlorine, and the presence of a diverse biota. For a period of 1 month, C_{12} MAQ was continuously added at a point 1.6 km below the sewage treatment plant outfall at a concentration expected to produce acute toxicity (based on *Daphnia* EC_{50}) in the mixing zone in the stream. The fate of the chemical and its effects on both indigeneous and introduced biota were monitored for 1500 m downstream, or a travel time of ~15 h in this particular stream.

Indigenous fish, macroinvertebrates, and periphyton were much less sensitive to the chemical than was the most sensitive laboratory species, *Daphnia magna*. In fact, there were no significant adverse effects noted for any of the indigenous communities, even at the dosing site, where exposure was maintained at an average of 0.27 mg/L, more than twice the acute EC_{50} for daphnids (Table 13).

TABLE 13. Response of Indigenous Organisms and Caged *Daphnia magna* in Howesville Creek, Indiana to a Continuous High Dose of C_{12} MAQ for 1 month

Creek Site (Travel Time Below Dosing Site)	C_{12}MAQ (Mean Measured Level and S.D.)	Daphnia magna Mortality (Mean and S.D.)[a]	Indigenous Organisms[b]
0 hr.	<10 μg/L	6 (7) %	Control
0.3	247 (74)	82 (4) %	No Effect
1.8	115 (33)	58 (54)	No Effect
5.1	51 (18)	6 (7)	No Effect
10.5	<10	13	No Effect
14.5	<10	4 (2)	No Effect

[a]C_{12} MAQ LC_{50} for *Daphnia magna* in laboratory test is 110 μg/L.
[b]Periphyton, macroinvertebrates, and fish.

To confirm in-stream exposures and the bioavailability of the test chemical, caged laboratory-reared daphnia, fish, and algae were exposed alongside the caged indigenous species for up to 1 week. As predicted from laboratory acute toxicity tests, 58% of the daphnids died at the site having an average exposure of 0.115 mg/L MAQ (Table 13). The in-stream MAQ was apparently in a bioavailable form, and laboratory- and field-derived acute EC_{50} values were comparable under similar exposures. [It had already been demonstrated in the laboratory stream and lake field studies that laboratory-reared daphnids did considerably better in multigeneration exposures and that naturally occurring zooplanktors (including daphnids) were much less sensitive (~ 10 times) than laboratory-reared dephanids to MAQ.] As expected, the less sensitive green and blue-green algae and fathead minnows were not affected by the MAQ even at the highest exposure site.

The stream dosing study also confirmed the rapid degradation and removal of MAQ that was predicted from the laboratory and other *in situ* studies. In-stream removal, biodegradation, and sorption to sediments resulted in a reduction of MAQ in the water column from a concentration of 0.27 mg/L in the mixing zone to less than 0.010 mg/L at a travel time of 5–10 h downstream.

C_{12} MAQ had no adverse affect on the density or activity of heterotrophic bacteria in water, sediment, or periphyton compartments of the stream. Biodegradation rates, as measured in heterotrophic activity and time course laboratory studies, were most rapid in the water column (turnover times and half-lives of ~ 40 h and ~ 10 h, respectively), followed by periphyton (turnovers of ~ 120 h and half-lives of ~ 30 h) and then sediments (turnovers of ~ 500 h and half-lives of ~ 115 h). Based on the water column measurements in the stream, the estimated half-life for MAQ was less than 2 h. This confirms the laboratory prediction of rapid biodegradation and also supports the conclusion that MAQ exposure to aquatic organisms will rapidly be reduced downstream from point sources of treated municipal wastewater.

On-Site Wastewater Treatment

A full-scale, 8-week wastewater treatment study was conducted using home aerobic and septic tank systems in households supplied with a prototype detergent product containing MAQs. Influent MAQ levels were 2–5 mg/L. Removals averaged 95% in home aerobic units and up to 50% in septic tanks. Approximately 30% of the removal can be explained by the partitioning of MAQs onto the sludge biomass. Measured adsorption coefficients for the wastewater solids averaged ~5500. There was no measurable reduction in microbial activity (MAQ and glucose uptake rates) in either system. Biodegradation of MAQ would account for the balance of the removal observed in the home aerobic units. The MAQs did not adversely affect the performance of the units based on measured operating parameters including volatile suspended solids, effluent COD (chemical oxygen demand), and MBAS (methylene blue active substances, a nonspecific measure of anionic materials).

Environmental Concentration Modeling

The probable range of "all" MAQ surface water concentrations immediately below wastewater discharges was estimated using a new Procter & Gamble developed modeling procedure (detailed in the section on Predicting Environmental Compartments and Concentrations). The model simultaneously accounts for the type of sewage treatment (i.e., the removal efficiency) and river dilution factor frequencies across the United States. Both 7Q10 (7 consecutive day, 10 year low flow) and mean river flow rates were considered. Total treatment plant discharge across the United States was evaluated considering the influent concentration of MAQs to be 0.110 mg/L (the prediction based on usage levels in *all* detergent products) and reasonable worst case removal rates of 29% by primary

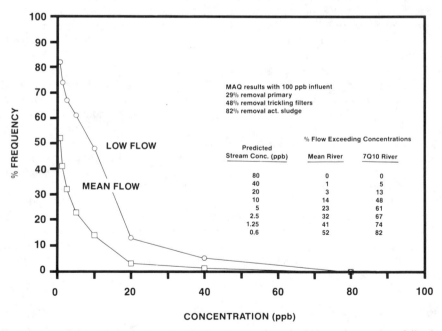

BASED ON TOTAL U.S. PLANT FLOW

MAQ results with 100 ppb influent
29% removal primary
48% removal trickling filters
82% removal act. sludge

Predicted Stream Conc. (ppb)	% Flow Exceeding Concentrations	
	Mean River	7Q10 River
80	0	0
40	1	5
20	3	13
10	14	48
5	23	61
2.5	32	67
1.25	41	74
0.6	52	82

Figure 11. Model predictions of total MAQ concentrations in U.S. surface waters following municipal wastewater treatment. The predictions are for immediately below treatment plant outfalls and consider only initial effluent dilution in reducing the downstream concentration.

clarification, 48% by trickling filter, and 82% by activated sludge plants. The model results, plotted in Fig. 11, indicated that the levels of MAQ will never be expected to exceed 0.08 mg/L under lowest flow conditions, and that for 90% of the aggregate U.S. wastewater flow, the resulting in-stream concentration would be < 0.03 mg/L at low flow and < 0.015 mg/L at mean flow for conditions of industry-wide usage. Of course, concentrations of MAQ outside the mixing zone would be expected to be much lower due to rapid biodegradation and removal via sorption to solids.

Monitoring

When possible, postmarketing chemical analysis of sampling data collected in the field is the best way to confirm the predictions of transport, fate, and exposure in the wastewater treatment process and receiving waters. Sensitive and specific analytical methods have been developed for MAQs in the relevant environmental compartments (75, 76, 92). The procedures use an HPLC (high pressure liquid chromatography) method with conductometric detection (Wescan model 212 meter and model 219–900 conductivity cell) following a concentration step involving an extraction technique. The detection limit was 2 ppb with a 100 mL environmental sample. Monitoring was done in Europe and the United States as part of premarket and test market use of new products containing MAQ.

Wastewater treatment plant and surface water monitoring programs were conducted in the United States, the United Kingdom, France, and Germany (Table 14). In the United States, the influent concentrations at three activated sludge plants sampled for 2–9 months averaged 0.069 mg/L (range 0.040–0.099). Effluents averaged 0.007 mg/L (range 0.004–0.010). Removals were therefore approximately 90%, which was the same as the average BOD removal at the plants. MAQ removal at a trickling filter plant averaged 55% (influent = 0.053 mg/L and effluent = 0.024 mg/L MAQ), somewhat less than the average BOD removal of 74%. Receiving streams immediately below these treatment plants were also monitored, and the average concentration was less than 0.002 mg/L, the detection limit of the analytical method (75).

In Europe, seven municipal treatment plants were monitored after introduction of the chemical. The wastewaters were typically sampled daily over 7 consecutive days; grab samples were used for the surface waters. In addition, grab samples of settled and digested

TABLE 14. Average Measured Concentrations and Removal Rates of C_{12-18} MAQs at Municipal Wastewater Treatment Plants in the United Kingdom, Germany, and the United States

Type of Treatment system	Wastewater Concentration (mg/L C_{12}-C_{18} MAQ)		Percent Removal
	(Influent)	(Effluent)	
U.K. (n=1)			
Trickling Filter	.082	.013	83
Activated Sludge	.082	.002	97
Germany (N=6)			
Primary	.415	.137	66
Trickling Filter	.058	.008	87
Activated Sludge	.112	.006	95
U.S.A. (N=4)			
Trickling Filter	.053	.024	55
Activated Sludge	.069	.007	90

TABLE 15. Measured River Water Concentrations of $C_{12\text{--}18}$ MAQs Immediately below Treated Sewage Outfalls in Germany, the United Kingdom, and France

Location[a]	River Stations Sampled	Average and Range of Measured MAQs (mg/L)
Germany	13 (5 Different Rivers)	0.004 (0.002 – 0.006)
U.K.	18 (11 Different Rivers)	<0.002 (<0.002 – 0.003)
France	28 (12 Different Rivers)	<0.002 (<0.002 – 0.012)

[a] Just below sewage outfalls.

sludge were taken at the plants in Germany. One German plant was used in a more extensive study to determine mass balance.

A parallel activated sludge and trickling filter system was monitored in the United Kingdom (Table 14). The influent concentration averaged 0.082 mg/L. Activated sludge and trickling filter effluents averaged 0.002 (97% removal) and 0.013 mg/L (83% removal), respectively. Removals were comparable to that for COD and total anionic surface active materials as measured by Azure-A. In six German wastewater treatment plants, average effluent concentrations were 0.137 mg/L for primary treatment ($\sim 66\%$ removal), 0.008 mg/L for trickling filters ($\sim 87\%$ removal), and 0.006 mg/L for activated sludge treatment ($\sim 95\%$ removal). Removals were slightly higher for MAQs than for BOD and COD, the typical treatment plant indicators of removal efficiency for total organic material (75).

Twenty-eight rivers were sampled in the mixing zone immediately below wastewater treatment plant outfalls in Germany, France, and the United Kingdom. The average MAQ concentrations were <0.002 mg/L in France and the United Kingdom and 0.004 mg/L in Germany (Table 15). Approximately 50% of this amount was adsorbed on the suspended solids. The highest measured concentration from the 60 samples was 0.012 mg/L in the Seine River, immediately below Paris.

In order to examine to what extent the high removal of MAQ in treatment plants was due to adsorption onto sludge and to biodegradation, a mass balance was established in one of the treatment plants in Germany. MAQ analyses were performed on samples of influent, effluent, primary, and wasted sludge, composited over a period of 1 week, a time period that has been shown to be adequate to understand a chemical's biological fate in that environment. The MAQ levels found were then combined with the average flow data. The results showed a primary removal for MAQ of 33%. Secondary removal averaged 97% and consisted of 3% adsorption onto sludge and 94% true biodegradation. This corresponded to an average biodegradation of 63% across the plant (75).

The results observed in Germany indicated that biodegradation is the major mechanism for removal of MAQ in the secondary treatment step. To determine the range of MAQ levels in sludge, grab samples were collected from all six treatment plants in Germany. The total MAQ level in aerobic sludge, taken after secondary settling, averaged $40 \pm 14 \, \mu g/g$ dry sludge and it was significantly lower than the $181 \pm 60 \, \mu g/g$ dry concentration found in digested sludge (75). All the measured values were well within the maximum estimated level of $970 \, \mu g$ MAQ/g dry solids, predicted using conservative assumptions. Overall, the monitoring data from wastewater treatment plants and rivers confirmed the predicted environmental concentrations of MAQ based on usage volumes and estimates of treatment efficiency as well as surface water dilutions.

Conclusions

The initial risk assessment for monoalkyl quaternary surfactants, based on usage information, physicochemical properties, and screening level fate and effects tests, indicated that this class of detergent chemicals had an acceptible environmental profile (i.e., not persistent, minimal potential to bioaccumulate, very good human safety profile for environmental exposure), except that the margin of safety for certain sensitive aquatic species could be less than 10. As is typical and prudent in such studies involving high-volume detergent chemicals, additional tests were initiated to reduce the level of uncertainty in extrapolating the laboratory-based assessment to the field.

The most important findings of this risk assessment, which were based on an extensive research and monitoring program of the MAQs, are summarized as follows:

1. Both laboratory microcosm and lake and river field studies confirmed the rapid and complete in-stream removal of MAQs via biodegradation and sorption. Half-lives in the water column were consistently equivalent to many naturally occurring organic compounds like sugars and amino acids. Half-lives were typically less than 10 h and often 1–2 h *in situ*.

2. There was no evidence of the formation of more toxic metabolic intermediates as a result of biodegradation.

3. The rate and extent of biodegradation in sediments, surface soils, subsurface soils, and groundwater will prevent accumulation in these compartments; half-lives of ~ 1–5 days in sediments, ~ 28 days in sludge-amended soils, ~ 7 days in anaerobic subsurface soils, and ~ 7 days in groundwater were observed.

4. MAQs were slightly less toxic (2–$3 \times$) in tests involving river water and standard test species, as compared to laboratory water toxicity tests (likely due to difference in MAQ bioavailability).

5. Laboratory and field toxicity tests demonstrated that *Daphnia magna* was significantly more sensitive to MAQs than are the typical aquatic species that live in surface waters that receive municipal wastewater effluent. Thus, a *Daphnia*-based toxicity assessment represented a very conservative model for estimating the potential impact of wastewater on rivers.

6. Laboratory microcosm and lake and river field studies demonstrated that the laboratory toxicity screening studies overestimated the effects of MAQs. Chronic-effect levels for population and community responses (including daphnids) were significantly above, that is, less hazardous, than that predicted from standard laboratory toxicity tests. First effects for invertebrates were observed at levels above 0.100 mg/L, up to 0.300–0.400 mg/L MAQ. First effects for algae were also 10 times higher than that predicted from laboratory assays.

7. Sediment-sorbed MAQs were not bioavailable or toxic to benthic organisms at levels that could realistically be expected in the environment.

8. At anticipated usage levels, MAQs will be highly removed from and have no adverse impact on home aerobic or septic tank systems.

9. Municipal wastewater treatment plant monitoring in the United States and Europe confirmed the efficient removal of MAQs ($> 90\%$ for activated sludge, $> 80\%$ for trickling

filter, and $> 60\%$ for primary treatment). Such removals were very good, comparable to that for conventional sewage parameters like BOD and COD and total surface-active anionic substances. Model predicted levels of MAQs in wastewater sludges were also consistent with the field data.

10. Surface water monitoring in the United States and Europe demonstrated that levels of MAQ are equal to, or slightly less than, those predicted using existing models. Concentrations just below wastewater treatment discharges were consistently < 0.010 mg/L. Approximately one-half of the MAQ was sorbed to suspended solids.

The information and insight gained from the more realistic and relevant follow-up program indicated that the industry-wide usage of MAQs does not pose a significant risk to the environment, and that there is a sufficient margin of safety between exposure and the threshold for adverse effects (field-derived NOEC of $\geqslant 0.100$ mg/L) to account for the remaining uncertainties even in a reasonable worst case situation. Utilizing reasonable worst case estimates of wastewater removal efficiencies for MAQs and 7Q10 low flow dilution conditions, the best available modeling techniques still show mixing zone concentrations below 0.08 mg/L MAQ for U.S. rivers. Although the data bases do not exist to do similar modeling for European conditions, even minimal dilution of the highest predicted sewage effluent concentrations (0.150 mg/L Germany versus 0.110 mg/L U.S.) results in exposures below threshold toxicity levels in the mixing zone. Again, the monitoring program confirmed that levels of MAQ are $\leqslant 0.010$ mg/L immediately below sewage discharges in the United States and Europe.

In short, MAQs that enter the environment from all current detergent sources will not adversely impact wastewater treatment systems. The relatively small fraction of MAQs that are not removed in treatment will continue to biodegrade rapidly in surface waters and groundwaters and do not pose a hazard to aquatic life or to humans. MAQs that reach the terrestrial environment as part of municipal sludge, or get to soils directly through home treatment effluent, will not accumulate, persist, or produce adverse effects.

The entire MAQ environmental assessment program, on which this case study was based, was reviewed and critiqued by a panel of four independent environmental science experts (their combined expertise covered environmental toxicology, microbiology, chemistry, engineering, and modeling). This science advisory group concluded overall: "We do not believe that MAQs constitute an environmental hazard at currently projected use rates", and that "the field data on fate and effects of MAQs provide a large measure of assurance that the laboratory data serve to overestimate probable environmental effects."

REFERENCES

1. U.S. Environmental Protection Agency, *Estimating Concern Levels for Concentrations of Chemical Substances in the Environment.* Environmental Effects Branch Position, USEPA, Washington, DC, 1984.

2. U.S. Environmental Protection Agency, *Significant New Uses of Chemical Substances: General Provisions for New Chemical Follow-up,* 40 C.F.R. Parts 721, 716 and 704 (draft). USEPA, Washington, DC, 1987.

3. Organization for Economic Cooperation and Development, *Guidelines for Testing of Chemicals: Effects on Biotic Systems.* OECD, Paris, France, 1984.

4. Organization for Economic Cooperation and Development, *Working Party on Exposure Analysis* (draft final report). Umweltbundesamt, Berlin, 1981.

5. R. A. Kimerle, Environmental risk assessment—the toxicological database and decision making. *Risk Analysis in the Chemical Industry.* Government Institutes Inc., Rockville, M. D. 1985, pp. 169–176.

6. American Society for Testing and Materials, *Working Drafts of Aquatic Toxicity Testing Practices,* Committee E47.01. ASTM, Philadelphia, PA (in preparation).

7. U.S. Environmental Protection Agency, *Technical Support Document for Water Quality-based Toxics Control.* Office of Water, USEPA, Washington, DC, 1985.

8. J. R. Duthie, The importance of sequential assessment in test programs for estimating hazard to aquatic life. *ASTM Spec. Tech. Publ.* **STP 634**, 17–35 (1977).

9. R. A. Kimerle, G. J. Levinskas, J. S. Metcalf, and L. G. Scharpf, An industrial approach to evaluating environmental safety of new products. *ASTM Spec. Tech. Publ.* **STP 634**, 36–43 (1977).

10. A. W. Maki and J. R. Duthie, Summary of proposed procedures for the evaluation of aquatic hazard. *ASTM Spec. Tech. Publ.* **STP 657**, 153–163 (1978).

11. C. M. Lee, Determination of the environmental acceptability of detergent components. In K. L. Dickson, A. W. Maki, and J. Cairns, Eds., *Analyzing the Hazard Evaluation Process.* American Fisheries Society, Washington, DC, 1979, pp. 7–22.

12. L. W. Beck, A. W. Maki, M. R. Artman, and E. R. Wilson, Outline and criteria for evaluating the safety of new chemicals. *Regul. Toxicol. Pharmacol.* **1**, 19–58 (1981).

13. N. T. deOude, Risk evaluation of new chemicals in the environment: Case studies. *Tenside Deterg.* **18**(5), 274–276 (1981).

14. M. A. Lewis and V. T. Wee, Aquatic safety assessment for cationic surfactants. *Environ. Toxicol. Chem.* **2**, 105–118 (1983).

15. A. W. Maki and W. E. Bishop, Chemical safety evaluation. In G. M. Rand and S. R. Petrocelli, Eds., *Fundamentals of Aquatic Toxicology.* Hemisphere, New York, 1985, pp. 619–649.

16. H. DeHenau, C. M. Lee, and P. A. Gilbert, The AIS approach to assessment of the environmental safety of detergents. *Tenside Deterg.* **23**(5), 267–271 (1986).

17. D. M. Woltering, R. J. Larson, W. D. Hopping, R. A. Jamieson, and N. T. deOude, Toward a more realistic assessment of the environmental fate and effects of detergent chemicals. *Tenside Deterg.* **24**(5), 286–296 (1987).

18. N. T. deOude, Environmental concentrations of detergents. *Tenside Deterg.* **20**(6), 314–316 (1983).

19. W. F. Holman, Estimating the environmental concentrations of consumer product components. *ASTM Spec. Tech. Publ.* **STP 737**, 159–182 (1981).

20. W. J. Lyman, W. F. Reehl, and D. H. Rosenblatt, *Handbook of Chemical Property Estimation Methods—Environmental Behavior of Organic Compounds.* McGraw-Hill, New York, 1982.

21. R. F. Rekker, *The Hydrophobic Fragmental Constant.* Am. Elsevier, New York, 1977.

22. U.S. Environmental Protection Agency, *Municipal Waste Facilities Inventory,* Division of Technical Support, Technical Data and Information Branch, Data and Information Service Section, USEPA, Washington, DC, 1976 (obtained on magnetic tape).

23. U.S. Environmental Protection Agency, *Sludge Treatment and Disposal,* Vol. 2, EPA625/4-78-012. USEPA, Washington, DC, 1978.

24. Metcalf and Eddy Inc., *Wastewater Engineering: Treat, Disposal, and Reuse.* McGraw-Hill, New York, 1979.

25. U.S. Department of Interior Geological Survey, *Water Resources Data, Surface Water Records.* U.S.G.S., Washington, DC, 1973, 1974.

26. R. J. Larson and R. D. Vashon, Adsorption and biodegradation of cationic surfactants in laboratory and environmental systems. *Dev. Ind. Microbiol.* **24**, 425–434 (1983).

27. R. J. Larson, Kinetic and ecological approaches for predicting biodegradation rates of zenobiotic organic chemicals in natural ecosystems. In M. J. Klug and C. A. Reddy, Eds., *Current Perspectives in Microbial Ecology.* American Society for Microbiology, Washington, DC, 1984, pp. 677–686.

28. R. M. Ventullo and R. J. Larson, Metabolic diversity and activity of heterotrophic bacteria in groundwater. *Environ. Toxicol. Chem.* **4**, 759–771 (1985).

29. G. L. Baughman and R. R. Lassiter, Prediction of environmental pollutant concentration. *ASTM Spec. Tech. Publ.* **STP 657**, 35–54 (1978).

30. D. R. Branson, Predicting the fate of chemicals in the aquatic environment from laboratory data. *ASTM Spec. Tech. Publ.* **STP 657**, 55–70 (1978).

31. A. M. Stern, A proposed approach to chemical fate assessments. *Ecotoxicol. Environ. Saf.* **4**, 404–414 (1980).

32. A. M. Stern and C. R. Walker, Hazard assessment of toxic substances: Environmental fate testing of organic chemicals and ecological effects testing. *ASTM Spec. Tech. Publ.* **STP 657**, 81–131 (1978).

33. J. L. Schoor, Modeling chemical transport in lakes, rivers and estuarine systems. *Environmental Exposure from Chemicals*, Vol. 2. CRC Press, Boca Raton, FL, 1985, pp. 55–73.

34. L. M. Games, Practical applications and comparisons of environmental exposure assessment models. *ASTM Spec. Tech. Publ.* **STP 802**, 282–299 (1983).

35. R. A. Rapaport, Prediction of consumer product chemical concentrations as a function of POTW treatment type and riverine dilution. *Environ. Toxicol. Chem.* **7**, 107–115 (1988).

36. U.S. Environmental Protection Agency, Assessment of needed publically owned wastewater treatment facilities in the United States. *1984 Needs Survey Report to Congress.* WH-546. Office of Municipal Pollution Control, USEPA, Washington, DC, 1985.

37. U.S. Environmental protection Agency, *1984 Needs Survey, U.S. EPA Office of Water Program Operations.* Priority and Needs Assessment Branch, USEPA, Washington, DC, 1983.

38. P. A. Gilbert and C. M. Lee, Biodegradation tests: Use and value. In A. W. Maki, K. L. Dickson, and J. Cairns, Eds., *Biotransformation and Fate of Chemicals in the Aquatic Environment.* American Society for Microbiology, Washington, DC, 1980, pp. 34–45.

39. Federal Register, Toxic substances control: Discussion of premanufacture testing policy and technical issues. *Fed. Regist.* **44**, No. 53, 16240–16292 (1979).

40. Organization for Economic Cooperation and Development, *Guidelines for Testing of Chemicals.* OECD, Paris, France, 1981.

41. R. J. Larson, Estimation of biodegradation potential of xenobiotic organic chemicals. *Appl. Environ. Microbiol.* **38**(6), 1153–1161 (1979).

42. R. J. Larson and L. M. Games, Biodegradation of linear alcohol ethoxylates in natural waters. *Environ. Sci. Technol.* **15**(12), 1488–1493 (1981).

43. R. J. Larson, R. D. Vashon, and L. M. Games, Biodegradation of trace concentrations of detergent chemicals in freshwater and estuarine systems. In T. A. Oxley and S. Barry, Eds., *Biodeterioration 5.* Wiley, New York, 1983, pp. 235–245.

44. F. K. Pfaender, R. J. Shimp, and R. J. Larson, Adaptation of estuarine ecosystems to the biodegradation of nitrilotriacetic acid: Effects of preexposure. *Environ. Toxicol. Chem.* **4**, 587–593 (1985).

45. T. E. Ward, Characterizing the aerobic and anaerobic microbial activities in surface and subsurface soils. *Environ. Toxicol. Chem.* **4**, 727–737 (1985).

46. T. E. Ward, Aerobic and anaerobic biodegradation of Nitrilotriacetate in subsurface soils. *Ecotoxicol. Environ. Saf.* **11**, 112–125 (1986).

47. R. M. Ventullo and R. J. Larson, Metabolic diversity and activity of heterotrophic bacteria in groundwater. *Environ. Toxicol. Chem.* **4**, 759–711 (1985).

48. M. A. Lewis, M. J. Taylor, and R. J. Larson, Structural and functional response of natural periphyton communities to a cationic surfactant with considerations on environmental fate. *ASTM Spec. Tech. Publ.* **STP 920**, 241–268 (1986).

49. C. M. Snow, A procedure and standards for the determination of the biodegradability of alkyl benzene sulfonate and linear alkylate sulfonate. *J. Am. Oil Chem. Soc.* **42**, 986 (1965).

50. W. W. Eckenfelder, *Industrial Water Pollution Control.* McGraw-Hill, New York, 1966.

51. J. E. King, W. D. Hopping, and W. F. Holman, Treatability of type A zeolite in wastewater Part I. *J. Water Pollut. Control Fed.* **52**(12), 2875–2886 (1980).

52. W. F. Holman and W. D. Hopping, Treatability of type A zeolite in wastewater Part II. *J. Water Pollut. Control Fed.* **52**(12), 2887–2905 (1980).

53. E. R. Baumann, W. D. Hopping, and F. D. Warner, Field evalution of the treatability of type A zeolite in a trickling filter plant. *J. Water Pollut. Control Fed.* **51**(9), 2301–2313 (1979).

54. R. M. Sykes, A. J. Rubin, S. A. Rath, and M. C. Chang, Treatability of a nonionic surfactant by activated sludge. *J. Water Pollut. Control Fed.* **51**(1), 71–77 (1979).

55. W. D. Hopping, Activated sludge treatability of type A zeolite. *J. Water Pollut. Control Fed.* **50**(3), 433–441 (1978).

56. U.S. Environmental Protection Agency, *Environmental Effects Test Guidelines*, EPA 560/6-32-002. USEPA, Washington, DC, 1982.

57. C. A. Pittinger, D. M. Woltering, and J. A. Masters, Bioavailability of sediment-sorbed and soluble surfactants to *Chironomus riparius* (midge). *J. Environ. Toxicol. Chem.* (in press).

58. P. S. Ziegenfuss, W. J. Renaudette, and W. J. Adams, Methodology for assessing the acute toxicity of chemicals sorbed to sediments: Testing the equilibrium partitioning theory. *ASTM Spec. Tech. Publ.* **STP 921**, 479–493 (1986).

59. W. J. Adams, P. S. Ziegenfuss, W. J. Renaudette, and R. G. Mosher, Comparison of laboratory and field methods for testing the toxicity of chemicals sorbed to sediments *ASTM Spec. Tech. Publ.* **STP 921**, 494–513 (1986).

60. M. A. Lewis, Impact of municipal wastewater effluent on water quality, periphyton and invertebrates in the Little Miami River near Xenia, Ohio. *Ohio J. Sci.* **86**(1), 2–8 (1986).

61. M. A. Lewis, Comparison of the effects of surfactants on freshwater phytoplankton communities in experimental enclosures and on algal population growth in the laboratory. *Environ. Toxicol. Chem.* **5**, 319–332 (1986).

62. M. A. Lewis, Environmental modification of the photosynthetic response of lake plankton to surfactants and significance to a laboratory-field comparison. *Water Res.* **20**(12), 1575–1582 (1986).

63. M. A. Lewis and D. Suprenant, Comparative acute toxicities of surfactants to aquatic invertebrates. *Ecotoxicol. Environ. Saf.* **7**, 313–322 (1983).

64. F. R. Geckler, W. B. Horning, T. M. Neiheisel, Q. H. Pickering, E. L. Robinson, and C. E. Stephan, *Validity of Laboratory Tests for Predicting Copper Toxicity in Streams*, EPA-600/3-76-116. USEPA, Washington, DC, 1976.

65. S. R. Hansen and R. R. Garton, Ability of standard toxicity tests to predict the effects of the insecticide diflubenzuron on laboratory stream communities. *Can. J. Fish. Aquat. Sci.* **39**, 1273–1288 (1982).

66. D. I. Mount and T. J. Norberg-King (Eds.), *Validity of Effluent and Ambient Toxicity Tests for Predicting Biological Impact, Kanawha River, Charleston, West Virginia*, EPA Res. Ser., EPA-600/3-86/006. USEPA, Washington, DC, 1986.

67. D. I. Mount, N. A. Thomas, T. J. Norberg, M. T. Barbour, T. H. Roush, and W. F. Brandes, *Effluent and Ambient Toxicity Testing and Instream Community Response on the Ottawa River, Lima, Ohio*, EPA Res. Ser., EPA-600/3-84-084. USEPA, Washington, DC, 1984.

68. D. I. Mount, and T. J. Norberg-King (Eds.), *Validity of Effluent and Ambient Toxicity Tests for*

Predicting Biological Impact, Skeleton Creek, Erid, Oklahoma, EPA Res. Ser., EPA-600/8-86/002. USEPA, Washington, DC, 1986.

69. L. M. Games, J. A. Stauback, and T. U. Kappeler, Analysis of nitrilotriacetic acid in environmental waters. *Tenside Deterg.* **18**(5), 262–265 (1981).

70. H. DeHenau, E. Matthijs, and W. D. Hopping, Linear alkylbenzene sulfonates (LAS) in sewage sludges, soils and sediments: Analytical determination and environmental safety considerations. *Int. J. Anal. Chem.* **26**, 279–293 (1986).

71. Q. W. Osburn, Analytical methodology for linear alkyl benzene sulfonate (LAS) in waters and wastes. *J. Am. Oil Chem. Soc.* **63**(2), 257–263 (1986).

72. V. T. Wee, Determination of cationic surfactants in waste- and river waters. *Water Res.* **18**(2), 223–225 (1984).

73. T. A. Neubecker, Determination of alkylethoxylated sulfates in wastewaters and surface waters. *Environ. Sci. Technol.* **19**(12), 1232–1236 (1985).

74. A. W. Maki, A. J. Rubin, R. M. Sykes, and R. L. Shank, Reduction of nonionic surfactant toxicity following secondary treatment. *J. Water Pollut. Control Fed.* **51**(9), 2301–2313 (1979).

75. E. Matthijs and H. DeHenau, Analysis of monoalkyl quaternaries and assessment of their fate in domestic wastewaters, river waters and sludges. *Vom Wasser*, **69**, 73–83 (1987).

76. V. T. Wee and J. Kennedy, Determination of trace levels of quaternary ammonium compounds in river water by liquid chromatography with conductometric detection. *Anal. Chem.* **54**, 1631–1633 (1982).

77. R. L. Anderson, W. E. Bishop, and R. L. Campbell, A review of the environmental and mammalian toxicology of nitrilotriacetic acid. *CRC Crit. Rev. Toxicol.* **15**(1), 1–102 (1985).

78. C. R. Woodiwiss, R. D. Walker, and F. A. Brownridge, Concentrations of nitrilotriacetate and certain metals in Canadian wastewater and streams: 1971–1975. *Water Res.* **13**, 599–612 (1979).

79. R. H. Wendt, A. G. Payne, and W. D. Hopping, Nitrilotriacetic acid (NTA) environmental monitoring program in Indiana; 1979–1983. *Environ. Toxicol. Chem.* **7**, 275–290 (1988).

80. R. I. Sedlak and K. A. Booman, LAS and alcohol ethoxylate: A study of their removal at a municipal wastewater treatment plant. *Soap/Cosmet., Chem. Spec.* **4**, 44–46 (1986).

81. J. McEvoy and W. Giger, Determination of linear alkylbenzene sulfonates in sewage sludge by high-resolution gas chromatography/mass spectrometry. *Environ. Sci. Technol.* **20**, 376–383 (1986).

82. E. M. Thurman, L. B. Barber, and D. LeBlanc, Movement and fate of detergents in groundwater: A field study. *J. Contam. Hydrol.* **1**, 143–161 (1986).

83. D. J. Paustenbach, Fundamentals of environmental risk assessment. *The Risk Assessment of Environmental and Human Health Hazard: A Textbook of Case Studies.* Wiley, New York, 1988.

84. R. S. Bothling, Environmental fate and toxicity in wastewater treatment of quaternary ammonium surfactants. *Water Res.* **18**(9), 1061–1076 (1984).

85. L. H. Huber, Ecological behavior of cationic surfactants from fabric softeners in the aquatic environment. *J. Am. Oil Chem. Soc.* **61**(2) 377–382 (1984).

86. SRI International, *Chemical Economics Handbook—Marketing Research Report*, SRI Int, Menlo Park, CA, 1987.

87. B. Isomaa, J. Reuter, and B. J. Djupsund. The subacute and chronic toxicity of cetyltrimethylammonium bromide (CTAB), a cationic surfactant. *Arch. Toxicol.* **35**, 91–96 (1976).

88. R. J. Larson, Biodegradation of detergent chemicals in groundwater/subsurface systems. *Household Pers. Prod. Ind.* **21**, 55–58 (1984).

89. J. P. Knezovich, F. L. Harrison, and R. G. Wilhelm, The bioavailability of sediment-sorbed organic chemicals: A review. *Water, Air, Soil Pollut.* **32**, 233–245 (1987).

90. G. A. Chapman, Do organisms in laboratory toxicity tests respond like organisms in nature? *ASTM Spec. Tech. Publ.* **STP 802**, 315–327 (1983).

91. R. M. Ventullo and R. J. Larson, Adapation of aquatic microbial communities to quaternary ammonium compounds. *Appl. Environ. Microbiol.* **51**, 356–361 (1986).

92. Q. W. Osburn, Analytical method for a cationic fabric softener in waters and wastes. *J. Am. Oil Chem. Soc.* **59**(10), 453–457 (1982).

10

Risk Assessment for Nitrilotriacetic Acid (NTA)

Robert L. Anderson and Carl L. Alden
The Procter & Gamble Company, Miami Valley Laboratories, Cincinnati, Ohio

INTRODUCTION

Nitrilotriacetic acid (NTA) is manufactured as the monohydrate of the trisodium salt ($Na_3NTA \cdot H_2O$) and it is greater than 98% pure. The impurities are mostly inorganics and probably do not contribute to the effects of NTA on mammals. NTA is a chelating agent that has many industrial uses including use in laundry detergents to complex with the calcium and magnesium in waters to aid in soil removal. NTA has been used in laundry detergents in Canada for over 15 years with continual monitoring of water levels of NTA and the potential of NTA to cause changes in sewage treatment facilities or toxicity to groundwater or surface water biota. The use of NTA in Canada is approximately 75,000,000 lb/yr and the environmental monitoring shows that the drinking water levels of NTA are in the low micrograms per liter ($\mu g/L$) range, showing that human exposure to NTA is less than 1 $\mu g/kg \cdot day$ (2.8 μg NTA/L water $\times$ 2 L H_2O/day $\div$ 70 kg body weight = 0.08 $\mu g/kg \cdot day$).

NTA is readily degraded by both anaerobic and aerobic microorganisms in sewage treatment facilities, soil, surface waters, groundwaters, and estuary waters (1). The microbial degradation of NTA is to CO_2 and NH_3, which are normal constituents in the environment (1). NTA does not affect sewage treatment facility function and it does not alter the mineral concentrations of surface waters (1). The levels of NTA in water are not toxic to any species exposed from bacteria to fish (1). In short, extensive study demonstrates that use of NTA in laundry detergents causes no environmental problems and it results in human exposure of less than 1 $\mu g/kg \cdot day$ from drinking water.

ACUTE TOXICITY OF NTA

The oral LD_{50} of $Na_3NTA \cdot H_2O$ is $\sim$ 2 g/kg for rodents and doses greater than 1 g/kg $Na_3NTA \cdot H_2O$ are emetic to the dog (2). Dermal exposure to NTA does not cause sensitization and less than 0.1% of dermal doses are absorbed (3). Subchronic inhalation of micronized NTA (6 h/day, 5 days/week for 4 weeks) at doses up to 342 $\mu g/L$ of air do not cause organ toxicity or changes in urinary mineral excretion in rats, guinea pigs, or monkeys (1).

TERATOGENICITY AND GENOTOXICITY

When tested alone or in combination with Cd or Hg NTA is not teratogenic (4–10), and reproduction studies show that NTA does not affect pup development (4). NTA has been tested in 25 separate assays for genotoxicity (1) and positive results were reported in only two assays (11, 12). Both positives occurred only at NTA concentrations greater than that of the total divalent cations in the test medium, demonstrating that the positive response was a consequence of divalent cation deprivation and not a consequence of NTA interaction with the cells (see ref. 1 for detailed discussion).

METABOLISM

When administered to a variety of animal species, including humans, NTA is not metabolized (13–15). Because of its high water solubility, it is rapidly excreted as the parent compound (unchanged) in the urine. These data, coupled with the knowledge that NTA does not contain measurable quantities of impurities, lead to the conclusion that any toxic responses must be attributed to NTA itself.

The absorption of NTA, as indicated by urinary excretion, is dependent on the medium in which it is ingested. Doses given by gavage to fasted rats are $\sim 70\%$ absorbed, NTA ingested admixed in a low-ash, semisynthetic diet is 70% absorbed, and NTA ingested admixed in high-ash, laboratory chow is 40% absorbed. There is considerable variation among species of animals in the absorption of dosed NTA (Table 1) with humans showing only 12% absorption under conditions where mice display $>90\%$ absorption. High-dose NTA absorption is decreased by dietary supplements of various divalent metals (Ni, Zn, Fe, and Mg but not Ca or Cu), probably as a consequence of NTA–metal complex formation in the gut reducing absorption. There is no difference in the systemic load of NTA when it is admixed in a chow diet as $Na_3NTA \cdot H_2O$ or H_3NTA.

At dietary doses up to $\sim 75 \,\mu$mol NTA/g diet, the absorption, tissue concentration, and urinary excretion of NTA are all zero-order processes in the rat. Rats rapidly reach a steady state (< 10 days) with any ingested dose of NTA. For example, bone NTA

TABLE 1. Species Variation in Urinary and Fecal Excretion of Orally Dosed NTA

Species	Dose (mg/kg)	% Administered Dose	
		Urine	Feces GI Wash
Mouse	180	96 ± 6	3 ± 1
Rat	10	70 ± 4	22 ± 4
Rabbit	50	23 ± 9	
Dog	20	80 ± 16	3 ± 1
Monkey	50	14	65
Human	0.15	12 ± 7	77 ± 11

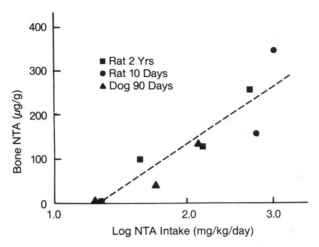

Figure 1. Concentration of NTA in the bone of rats after 10 days and 2 years and dogs after 90 days of continuous exposure to a constant dietary concentration of NTA.

concentration does not differ between day 10 and day 730 at dietary concentrations of NTA up to 20 μmol/g diet (Fig. 1). The only route of excretion of systemic NTA is via the urine as demonstrated by the fact that the stool contained no [^{14}C]NTA after 6 days of iv dosing. Renal clearance of NTA is accomplished via passive filtration; the C_{NTA}/C_{Inulin} is constant at 0.89 ± 0.01 at blood NTA concentrations up to 32 μM (1). In addition, the renal clearance of NTA is not altered by probenecid treatment or p-aminohippuric acid infusion (1).

The urine contains 200–400-fold greater concentrations of NTA than the blood, yet the bladder exposed to urine with high concentrations of NTA attained only slightly higher levels of NTA than tissues (heart and liver) exposed only to blood (Table 2). The kidney appears to contain high levels of NTA, probably due to the high NTA content of the urine in the tissue. Entrapment of only 50 μL urine/g tissue could account for all the NTA that is measured in this tissue. Furthermore, saline infusion after NTA loading shows rapid renal washout of NTA. These findings demonstrate that the measured high levels of NTA in the kidney likely represent NTA in the urine contained in the kidney for excretion and not NTA in the kidney cells.

The excretion of systemic NTA after equilibration is a relatively slow process (Fig. 2) (1). This slow excretion reflects the release of NTA bound to intracellular and plasma proteins and bone (1) (Table 2). NTA bound to plasma proteins and blood cells does not alter blood gases or plasma composition even at doses that are clearly tumorigenic. NTA bound to bone does not affect bone strength and its only effect on bone composition is to increase bone zinc in proportion to the bone NTA level (Table 3) (16). The above responses show that while NTA does enter cells and bind to protein, it has no adverse effects on their physiological function.

As would be expected for a readily absorbed, nonmetabolized chelating agent, NTA does display a dose-dependent change in the fate of ingested minerals. NTA increases urine zinc (Zn) and calcium (Ca) and it decreases the level of these minerals in the stool (17). The effect on magnesium (Mg) is the opposite; fecal levels of Mg are increased and urinary Mg excretion is decreased. Even at clearly carcinogenic doses, NTA does not reduce the net

TABLE 2. Organ/Plasma Ratio of NTA in Rats Fed Diets Containing [^{14}C]NTA to Isotope Equilibrium[a]

Organ	Fisher 344		Charles River	
	0.02%	2.0%	0.02%	2.0%
Femur	8.2	7.4	17.0	16.6
Kidney	7.3	8.3	8.0	8.1
Bladder	1.6	4.3	1.8	1.5
Liver	1.0	1.4	1.2	1.8
Lungs	0.9	1.3	1.0	1.5
Pancreas	0.5	1.0	0.6	0.9
Adrenal	1.0	1.3	2.8	1.9
Lymph node	0.6	3.3	1.3	1.3
Thymus	0.5	0.8	0.6	1.0
Spleen	0.8	1.0	0.8	1.3
Blood cells	0.2	0.1	0.4	0.3
Brain	0.1	0.1	0.1	0.2
Muscle	0.2	0.3	0.4	0.4
Testis	0.3	0.4	0.3	0.6
Heart	0.3	0.4	0.4	0.6
Carcass residue	1.0	1.3	1.9	2.1

[a]Young mature rats fed diet with indicated level of [^{14}C]NTA for 10 days. Each value is the mean of samples from three animals.

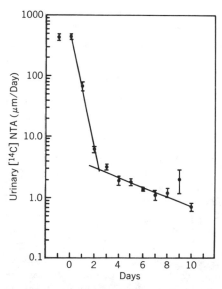

Figure 2. Urinary excretion of NTA during a 10-day period with no NTA ingestion after rats were equilibrated to [^{14}C]NTA at 75 μmol/g diet. Each value is the mean $\pm$ SEM for samples from five rats.

TABLE 3. Effect of Dietary $Na_3NTA \cdot H_2O$ Levels on Bone NTA Content and Excess Zn after 2 years of Ingestion

Dietary $Na_3NTA \cdot H_2O$ (%)	Bone NTA[a]	Zn[b]	Zn/NTA
	(nmol/g bone)		
0.03	524	627	1.20
0.15	681	841	1.23
0.50	1361	1238	0.91

[a]Determined by radioisotope dilution.
[b]Excess Zn (treatment − control).

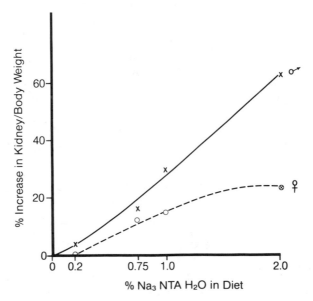

Figure 3. Effect of dietary NTA on relative kidney weight in male rats after 90 days of ingesting the indicated dietary concentrations of NTA.

retention (ingested minus excreted) of these minerals in the carcass of rapidly growing rats (17). The disposition of the trace elements, iron, manganese, and copper, are not affected by even extreme doses of NTA feeding except that urinary iron is increased in rats displaying hematuria when fed massive doses of NTA (17).

TARGET ORGAN TOXICITY

Subchronic feeding studies (3, 18) clearly demonstrate that the kidney is the primary target organ of NTA toxicity. NTA causes a dose-dependent increase in relative kidney mass (Fig. 3). Histological examination reported what was defined as hydropic degeneration (3). This lesion is characterized by foci of cytoplasmic vacuoles in the renal tubular cells of the proximal convoluted tubules. This shows that NTA at high doses is a renal tubule toxin that rapidly produces a detectable change in tissue structure.

In a 2-year feeding study (16) that included sacrifices at 6, 12, 19, and 24 months, at doses of 1.1, 5.5, and 18.2 μmol NTA/g diet, the tubular cell lesions were shown to be persistent and to lead to an NTA dose-dependent hyperplasia in the tubules containing the vacuolated cells (16). The lowest dose produced no tubular cell toxicity and the kidney was the only organ showing NTA-related toxicity.

In addition to renal toxicity, an NCI bioassay that employed doses of NTA up to 75 μmol/g diet demonstrated that NTA can cause toxicity in the transitional epithelial cells (TEC) of the renal pelvis, ureters, and bladder (19). The TEC changes have not been noted in rats fed NTA doses $\leqslant 27$ μmol NTA/g diet, and TEC toxicity does not occur in mice.

CARCINOGENICITY

NTA has been tested in six chronic exposure studies in rats and mice. The results (Fig. 4) leave little doubt that, at high doses, NTA is carcinogenic to renal tubular cells and the transitional epithelium of the renal pelvis, ureter, and bladder. A detailed discussion of each of these studies has been presented elsewhere (1) and is not repeated here. In addition, NTA has been shown to increase the tumor frequency in the kidney (20, 21) and the bladder (22) in rats dosed with an initiator for each of these sites. The results show that NTA is a promoter in the same tissues in which it is a carcinogen but only at doses that

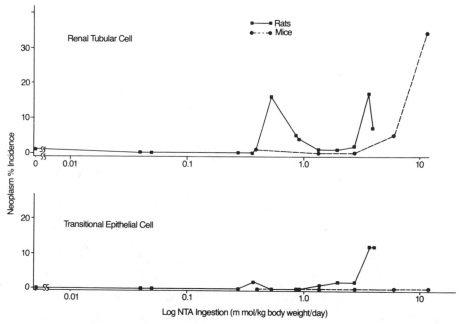

Figure 4. Incidence of neoplasms of the renal tubular cells and urothelial cells in rats and mice as a function of the log of the ingested dose of NTA. Data are the results of six chronic exposure studies. For details see ref. 1.

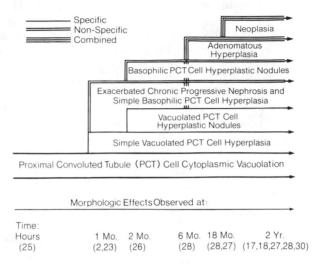

Figure 5. Sequence of events occurring in the renal cortex of the rat persistently treated with high levels of NTA in the diet. PCT = proximal tubular cell.

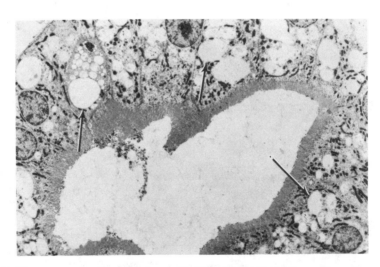

Figure 6. Ultrastructural evidence of the specific NTA toxicity-hydropic swelling of lysosomes in PCT cells (arrows).

396

induce toxicity in these tissues. The data are sufficiently convincing to define NTA as a nongenotoxic (epigenetic) carcinogen and a tumor promoter.

RENAL TUBULAR TUMOR HISTOGENESIS

Based on intensive study of urinary tract sections after acute, subchronic, and chronic exposure studies, a sequence of morphological changes that precede and accompany neoplasms of the renal tubular cells and the TEC has been described. These studies have been important in understanding the mechanism of action of NTA's carcinogenicity and thus are described in detail.

Based on time course studies, NTA at 2% in the diet (approximately 3600 μmol/kg·day) administered to Sprague–Dawley or Fischer-344 rats induces a specific sequence of morphological changes in renal cortical cells. Concomitantly, a nonspecific sequence of events occurs, as illustrated in Fig. 5. The earliest and most sensitive specific indicator of NTA toxicity is a focal swelling of the endocytic vesicles and lysosomes, a hydropic change (Fig. 6). This response develops within hours and is time- and dose-responsive in severity. Using light microscopy this lysosomal swelling is recognized as foci of clear vacuolation of proximal tubular epithelium, primarily the S2 segment (Fig. 7). These vacuoles, produced by a single dose of NTA > 73 μmol/kg, persist a maximum of 72 h (23). With continuous treatment, however, the vacuolation persists throughout the lifetime of the rat. This vacuolation response shows a distinct threshold in that only doses $\geq$ 70 μmol/kg elicit this toxic response (23, 24).

With continuation of the NTA insult over 4 weeks, the tubules with vacuolated cells become hypertrophic and then hyperplastic, while maintaining the vacuolated appearance (Figs. 8 and 9). The hyperplastic response initially appears to affect the nephron

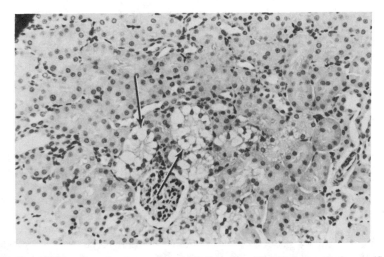

Figure 7. Vacuolation of proximal convoluted tubular cell epithelium (arrows), the specific acute manifestation of NTA injury at tumorigenic doses in rats.

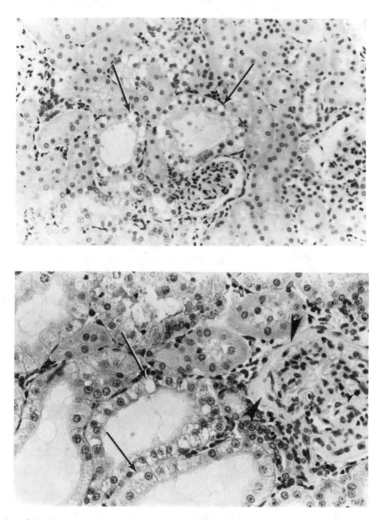

Figures 8 and 9. Simple tubular cell hyperplasia (TCH), vacuolated cell type (arrows) after 28 days of exposure and 2 years of exposure, respectively. Figure 9 also reveals glomerular sclerosis (arrow-heads), an aging change. Dosage was 2% dietary $Na_3NTA \cdot H_2O$.

uniformly, but with time the response becomes focally exaggerated, resulting in the appearance of hyperplastic tubular nodules (Fig. 10) (24, 25). After chronic exposure ($\geqslant 6$ months) affected tubules develop additional degrees of hyperplasia, designated adenomatous hyperplasia (Fig. 11). Lesions of adenomatous hyperplasia are poorly differentiable from those of early neoplasia. Finally, after 12 months or longer of exposure, incontrovertible tubular neoplasia occurs in a few rats. Kidney tumors have not been observed in moribund rats or at scheduled sacrifices prior to 12 months of continuous treatment. At the time of neoplastic transformation, the proliferative cells are no longer vacuolated and are probably no longer exposed to NTA via luminal glomerular filtrate. Only doses of NTA inducing this toxicologic vacuolar change lead to tubular tumor formation

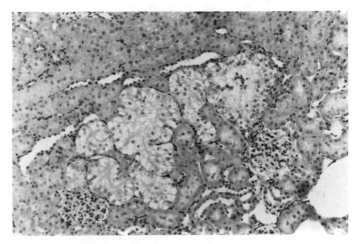

Figure 10. Tubular cell hyperplastic nodules, vacuolated cell type, occurring after 7 weeks of 2% dietary $Na_3NTA \cdot H_2O$ in rats.

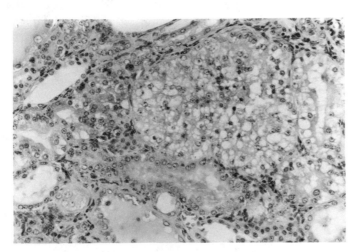

Figure 11. Adenomatous hyperplasia, vacuolated cell type occurring after 6 months of 2% dietary $Na_3NTA \cdot H_2O$.

(16, 19, 24, 26–29) but not all doses that produce tubular cell toxicity are associated with tumors even after chronic exposure.

The concomitant nonspecific sequence of events responsible for the tumors can be characterized as exacerbation of chronic progressive nephrosis (CPN) (1). CPN occurs spontaneously as an age-associated lesion in the laboratory rat kidney, probably caused by typical laboratory diet protein excess for rats at ages beyond the rapid growth phase of life. Loss of parenchyma associated with chronic progressive nephrosis is associated with tubular hyperplasia occurring as a reparative/regenerative response (Figs. 12–14). It is not

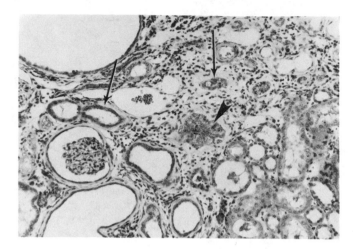

Figure 12. A rat with a moderate degree of age-related nephrosis, simple hyperplasia, basophilic cell type (arrows), and tubular hyperplastic nodules (arrowhead), basophilic cell type. All changes in this photograph are compatible with those in moderate to severe spontaneous chronic progressive nephrosis (CPN). NTA exacerbates the severity of CPN.

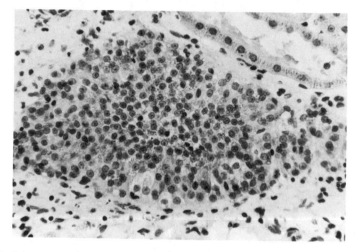

Figure 13. Adenomatous hyperplasia, basophilic cell type. In rats severely affected with age-related nephrosis, this change appears spontaneously (15). This section, however, is from a rat exposed to 2% $Na_3NTA \cdot H_2O$ for 2 years.

possible to uncouple the exacerbation of CPN from the specific toxic response since they display identical time and dose relation with respect to NTA (Fig. 15) (16, 24).

Spontaneous CPN can be associated with risk for tubular neoplasia development. Specifically, if laboratory rats are allowed to survive until the end of their natural life span, severity of CPN increases and tubular neoplasia concomitantly becomes common. Also,

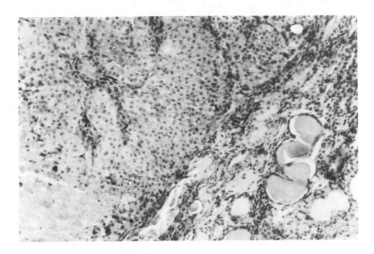

Figure 14. Solid tubular cell carcinomas, basophilic cell type. This section is from a rat treated with 2% $Na_3NTA \cdot H_2O$ for 2 years by the NCI that has severe chronic progressive nephrosis. In the NCI study controls were only mildly affected with chronic progressive nephrosis. In colonies with severe mean grades of spontaneous age-related nephrosis, tubular neoplasia also occurs (14, 15).

the spontaneous occurrence of high incidence and severe grades of CPN have been associated with increased tubular tumor incidence at 2 years in rats (27, 30).

Proliferative lesions through those designated as nodular hyperplasia are reversible if NTA exposure is stopped (Fig. 15) (24, 26). Doses of NTA that do not induce the specific toxicity do not exacerbate chronic progressive nephrosis and do not induce increases in PCT cell hyperplasia or neoplasia; thus, these represent "no effect" levels (16, 19, 24, 26, 28, 29). These findings lead to the conclusion that the toxic cell injury results in a replicative increase, or hyperplasia, which, if persistent, is causally linked with the nongenotoxic tumorigenicity. It has also been shown that NTA at toxic levels is a renal tumor promoter but not at subtoxic levels (20, 21). For NTA tubular cell vacuolation, an acute toxic response that is linked to renal tubular tumorigenesis, provides a marker for defining prerequisite biochemical events in the toxic and neoplastic event.

UROTHELIAL TUMOR HISTOGENESIS

The urothelial (transitional epithelium) changes associated with chronic NTA exposure also involve a specific sequence of events. Two percent NTA in the diet ingested by Sprague–Dawley rats rapidly results in polyuria, alkalinuria, and hematuria (17). This urine also contains massive sublight microscopic crystalluria (Fig. 16). Microscopically, the urothelium is eroded and/or ulcerated. Erosion and ulceration are evident at the light microscopic level in the pelvis and ureter after subchronic NTA exposure (Figs. 17–19). In the urinary bladder, epithelial cell injury and loss are demonstrable using scanning and transmission electron microscopy (Figs. 20–23). Erosion is associated with epithelial cell replicative increase. Replicative rate increase can be demonstrated rapidly as hyperplasia by histomorphimetry in bladders from rats in which NTA is infused directly for 72 h (Fig. 24). Infusion dosages were equivalent to those associated with NTA urinary levels in

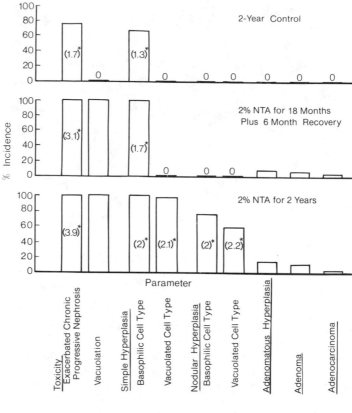

* Mean Severity 1-Minimal (<1% of parenchyma affected)
2-Mild (1-10% of parenchyma affected)
3-Moderate (11-25% of parenchyma affected)
4-Severe (>25% of parenchyma affected)

Data based on review of male rats surviving until scheduled 2-year sacrifice.

Figure 15. Renal cortical lesion index, 24-month versus 18-month NTA exposure with 6-month recovery versus untreated controls.

rats fed 2% NTA in the diet (25, 26, 31). With persistence of insult, hyperplasia of progressive severity and neoplasia occur (Figs. 25–27) (19). Thus, the tumors arise as a consequence of persistent injury and reparative hyperplasia in the target organ.

Hyperplasias of urinary bladder urothelia associated with NTA treatment are typically endophytic (growth downward into the tissue). This is in contrast to the hyperplasia associated with aniline dyes and luminal physical objects, which are exophytic in the rat (32). Consistent with the proposed mechanism of NTA injury in urothelium, growth of urinary bladder tissue sections in vitro in calcium-deficient media results in endophytic hyperplasia compared to calcium-sufficient media (33). Dosages of NTA that do not induce urothelial toxicity do not produce urothelial neoplasia (16, 19, 24, 27–29). Also consistent with the concept of urothelial toxicity being linked to replicative rate increase, endophytic hyperplasia, and tumorigenicity is the fact that NTA is positive in bladder

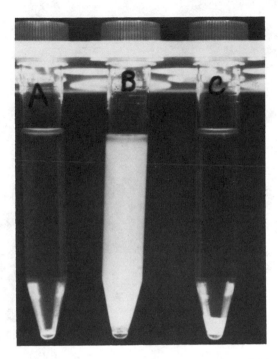

Figure 16. Urine samples from rats given 2% $Na_3NTA \cdot H_2O$ for 14 days reflecting either the turbidity of massive submicroscopic crystalluria (B) or centrifugal sediment (C) compared with a typical untreated control (A).

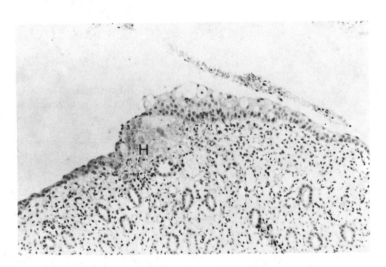

Figure 17. Ulceration and underlying hemorrhage (H) with urothelial hyperplasia peripheral to the ulcerated epithelium of the renal papilla.

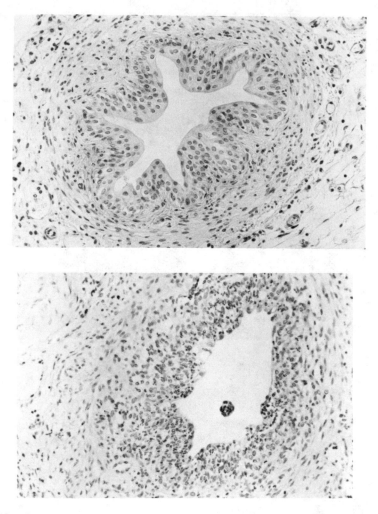

Figures 18 and 19. Ureters from a control rat (18) or rat fed a tumorigenic NTA level (2% $Na_3NTA \cdot H_2O$) for 2 weeks revealing urothelial erosion and inflammatory response.

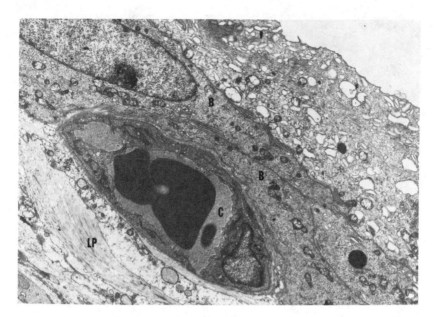

Figure 20. In this figure the transitional epithelium from a control animal bladder is approximately three cell layers thick. Portions of several basal cells (B) can be identified by their simple organization. A capillary (C) and a portion of the lamina propria (LP) are also shown. Magnification is equal to 8000 ×.

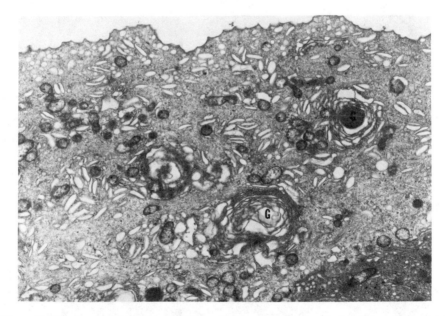

Figure 21. Subchronic (28 days) ingestion resulted in enlargement and elaboration of the Golgi apparatus (G) in superficial cells from the urinary bladder of a female rat. Magnification is equal to 12,000 ×.

405

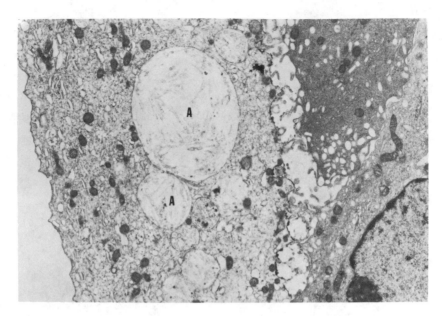

Figure 22. In more severely affected urinary bladder urothelium from rats receiving NTA for 28 days, the cytoplasm was rarified and the phagolysosomes (A) enlarged. Also notable is the widened intercellular space and the presence of electron dense deposits on the basal aspect of the superficial cell. Magnification is equal to 12,000 ×.

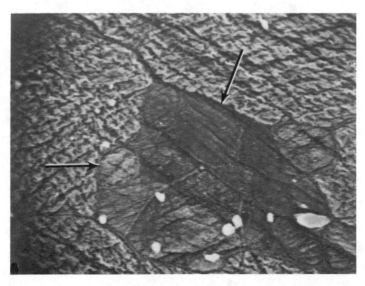

Figure 23. Bladder mucosa of a female rat subchronically treated with NTA showing a large region of superficial cell desquamation representing the area covered by 20–30 superficial cells (arrows). Magnification is equal to 8000 ×.

406

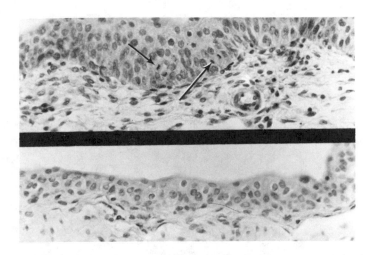

Figure 24. Urinary bladder epithelium from a rat (upper) infused for 4 days with levels of NTA comparable to urinary levels found at tumorigenic dietary dosages. Compare the treated rat with hyperplasia to the lower photograph of a control infused with saline for 4 days. Mitoses are prominent in the NTA-infused rat (arrows).

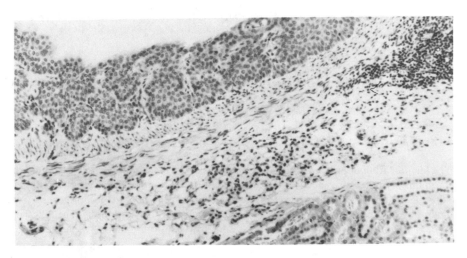

Figure 25. Renal pelvis urothelium illustrating nodular endophytic hyperplasia with dysplasia from a rat treated for 2 years with 2% dietary $Na_3NTA \cdot H_2O$.

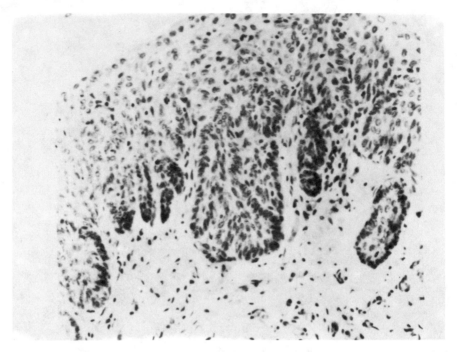

Figure 26. Urinary bladder urothelium illustrating nodular endophytic hyperplasia with dysplasia from a rat treated for 2 years with 2% $Na_3NTA \cdot H_2O$ in the diet.

promotion assays only at toxic doses (22). These toxicologic endpoints, which are linked to urinary tract tumorigenesis, provide early markers for defining the prerequisite biochemical events in the NTA-treated rat leading to tumorigenicity.

MECHANISMS OF TOXICITY

The identification of early markers of tumorigenesis provided an opportunity to study the mechanism(s) to tumorigenesis in short-term studies. The tumor incidence, as a function of NTA dose (Fig. 4), strongly suggested that the tubular cell and TEC tumorigenesis were caused by different factors. Mechanism studies confirmed this hypothesis. The following discussion considers the renal tubular cell and urothelial cell toxicities separately.

Renal Tubular Cell Toxicity

The chemical and metabolic characteristics of NTA suggest that the renal tubular cell toxicity of NTA is likely a consequence of its altering mineral disposition (17). To test this hypothesis we contrasted the effects on the kidney and urine of the forms of NTA likely to exist in the plasma of rats ingesting NTA. The various salts and metal complexes of NTA were infused iv at very high doses (6 mmol/kg·day) for up to 6 days. Infusion of the sodium or potassium salts, or the calcium or magnesium complexes, at this dose caused less renal tubular cell damage (vacuoles) than 4 days of ingesting a diet that results in a systemic dose

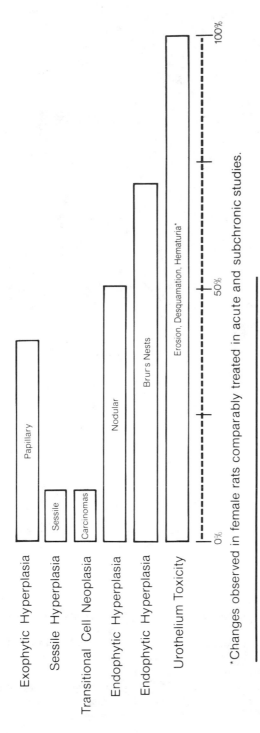

Exophytic Hyperplasia — Papillary / Sessile

Transitional Cell Neoplasia — Sessile / Carcinomas

Endophytic Hyperplasia — Nodular

Endophytic Hyperplasia — Brurs Nests

Urothelium Toxicity — Erosion, Desquamation, Hematuria*

0%   50%   100%

*Changes observed in female rats comparably treated in acute and subchronic studies.

Comparable controls included 10% of bladders with simple endophytic hyperplasia only.

All treated rat bladders affected by hyperplasia, with the exception of those with simple endophytic hyperplasia exhibited cellular atypia.

Hyperplasia and neoplasia data are derived from review of randomly selected rats from the NTP Bioassay utilizing Fischer-344 rats at the NCI.

Figure 27. Incidence of neoplastic and nonneoplastic findings in the urinary bladders of female rats fed 2% NTA in the diet for 2 years.

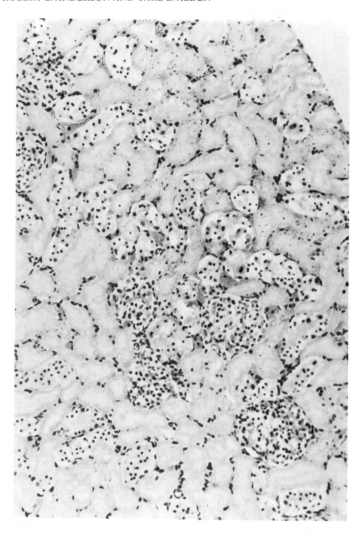

Figure 28. Photomicrograph of a kidney section of a rat infused iv with 3 mmol ZnNTA/kg for 48 h illustrating widespread tubular necrosis. Hematoxylin and eosin × 70.

of only 1.5 mmol/kg·day (75 μmol NTA/g diet). Thus, ingesting sufficient NTA to produce a total systemic NTA exposure of 6 mmol in 4 days caused more renal tubular cell toxicity than 36 mmol of the Na, K, Ca, or Mg forms dosed iv over 6 days. This finding demonstrates that none of these forms of NTA is the likely renal toxin and further that tubular cell toxicity is not solely a function of the total dose of NTA cleared by the kidney.

In contrast with the above results, when the zinc complex of NTA was infused iv at 3 mmol/kg·day, every rat died in less than 48 h (34). Thus, a total dose of < 6 mmol of ZnNTA is lethal when given iv while > 36 mmol of the other forms tested were essentially nontoxic. The rats dosed with ZnNTA showed a very consistent sequela of events in that they initially became polyuric and excreted protein, glucose, and blood in their urine in the 12–36-h period. At about 36 h the rats became anuric and were sacrificed. The kidneys from these rats displayed massive coagulative necrosis of the renal tubular cells (Fig. 28). The response to infused ZnNTA is the same as that induced by iv $HgCl_2$ and is typical of heavy metal toxicity. Figure 29 shows that when the dose of ZnNTA given iv is lowered to $\sim 2\,\mu mol/kg{\cdot}day$, the tubular cell response (vacuoles) is the same as that noted when NTA is ingested.

When the various forms were infused as $[^{14}C]NTA$, more than 90% of the infused ^{14}C dose was recovered in the urine, showing that the unique toxicity of ZnNTA is not due to a

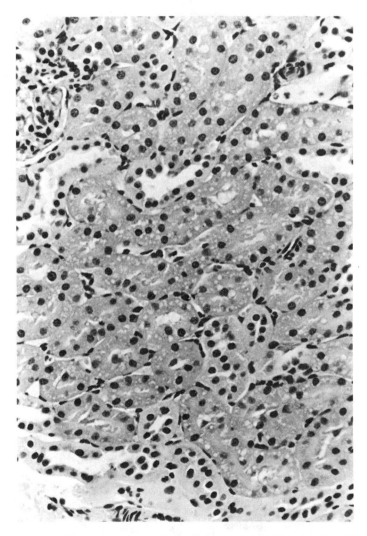

Figure 29. Photomicrograph of the kidney from a rat infused with $2.25\,\mu mol$ ZnNaNTA/day for 2 days. Note proximal convoluted tubule with vacuoles. Hematoxylin and eosin $\times 130$.

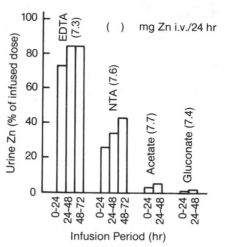

Figure 30. Urinary zinc recovery in rats infused with the same total amount of zinc as ZnEDTA, ZnNTA, and the acetate or gluconate salts of zinc.

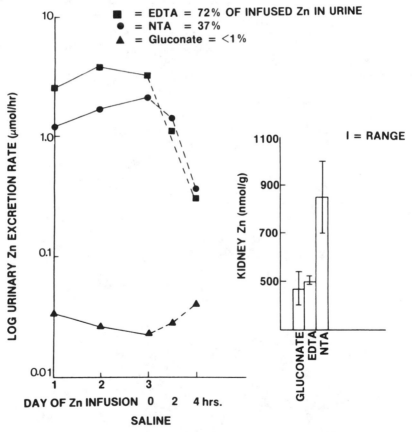

Figure 31. Urinary zinc excretion during infusion of the indicated form of zinc or saline and the concentration of zinc in kidneys after saline infusion.

TABLE 4. Concentration of NTA in the Urine of Rats Fed Various Forms of NTA

	Urinary NTA[a]		
Dietary Treatment	μmol/100 g·day	μmol/mL	% of dose
Control	0	0	—
H_3NTA	292 ± 34	42.4 ± 7.3	38 ± 5
$Na_3NTA·H_2O$	284 ± 62	26.9 ± 5.6	39 ± 8
Zn(K/Na)NTA	104 ± 27	15.3 ± 6.3	15 ± 3

[a]Mean ± SEM of five urine samples/treatment. Urine was collected during the fourth week of ingestion of diets containing various forms of NTA.

TABLE 5. Effect of Dietary Zinc Concentration on Renal Tubular Cell Damage Associated with NTA Ingestion[a]

	Incidence × Frequency		
Characteristics	8 and 14 ppm Zn	21 ppm Zn	52 ppm Zn
Kidneys examined	16	10	10
Vacuoles + simple hyperplasia	<5	15	25
Vacuoles + nodular hyperplasia	0	3	50

[a]Male rats fed semipurified diets containing the indicated levels of Zn with and without 1.2% $Na_3NTA·H_2O$ for 4 weeks. The tabular values are the product of incidence (number of kidney sections showing the particular lesion per treatment group) and frequency (mean number of tubules per kidney section showing the lesion).

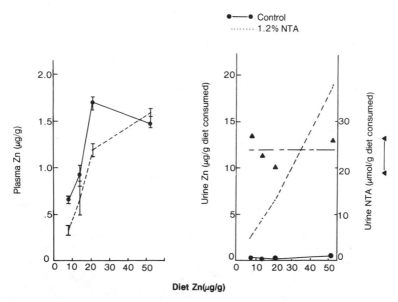

Figure 32. Plasma zinc and urine zinc and NTA in rats fed diets with the indicated zinc load with and without NTA in the diet.

cation-specific tissue uptake of the NTA. Further evidence that the toxicity is due to Zn was obtained when it was demonstrated that zinc acetate and zinc gluconate, dosed iv, produced renal tubular cell toxicity identical to that induced by ZnNTA but at lower doses of zinc. In contrast, ZnEDTA is not a very potent renal toxin. Figure 30 shows that renal toxicity is inversely proportional to the portion of the zinc dose that is recovered in the urine; that is, renal tubular toxicity is a consequence of retained zinc. These studies demonstrate that systemic ZnNTA is a potent renal toxin due to the Zn and not the NTA.

Figure 31 shows the urinary zinc output and the level of zinc in the kidneys of rats infused iv with ZnNTA, ZnEDTA, and ZnGluconate for 72 h and subsequently with saline for 4 h. This demonstrates that ZnNTA resulted in an increase in renal tissue zinc that was not mimicked by a zinc form that was mostly retained in the carcass (ZnGluconate) or by a form that was mostly excreted in the urine (ZnEDTA).

Increasing dietary zinc reduced the toxicity of a high dose of NTA because it reduces NTA absorption by $\sim 50\%$ while only slightly increasing zinc absorption (Table 4). Reducing dietary zinc at a constant high dose of dietary NTA produces renal tubular cell toxicity proportional to the reduction in the dietary level of zinc (Table 5). Analyses of plasma and urinary zinc and urinary NTA show that changing the diet zinc did not alter the systemic load of NTA, as evidenced by urinary excretion, and that the renal tubular toxicity (Table 5) was proportional to the plasma and urinary zinc (Fig. 32). These data show that dietary zinc is the limiting factor in NTA-associated renal tubular cell toxicity.

The above studies unequivocally demonstrate that renal tubular cell toxicity in animals ingesting NTA is caused by zinc and is probably a consequence of renal tissue zinc accumulation associated with increased zinc reabsorption during the renal clearance of ZnNTA present in the blood.

Since the renal clearance of NTA is via filtration, urinary NTA must arise from the low molecular weight fraction of the plasma. Therefore, we examined the effect of a clearly tumorigenic dose of NTA on the mineral composition of the total plasma and the protein-free fraction, $MW < 10,000$ (Fig. 33). The measurements were made at noon when plasma NTA is minimal and at midnight when plasma NTA is maximal, owing to the diet ingestion pattern in the rat. NTA caused no change in plasma calcium in either fraction at either time and it caused a decrease in magnesium in both fractions at both times but the effect was greater at peak blood NTA (midnight). NTA increased zinc in both fractions of the plasma at both times but the effect at midnight was statistically significant and the noon changes were not. Thus, at very high doses, NTA increases the load of zinc delivered to the renal tubular cells and the process shows a diurnal cycle that corresponds to that of the plasma NTA.

In order to determine whether the renal tubular cells reabsorbed the excess zinc in rats ingesting NTA, we compared the NTA/Zn ratio in the protein-free plasma fraction to that of the urine in rats fed three doses of NTA—0.73, 7.3, and 73 μmol/g diet (Table 6). At all three doses of NTA the ratio in the urine was approximately threefold that of the protein-free plasma fraction, showing that at all levels of ZnNTA a constant, large fraction of the filtered zinc was reabsorbed during the renal clearance of the ZnNTA. It is important to note that at the two lower doses of NTA, the plasma zinc was approximately the same and not different from that of a control plasma (data not shown), but at 73 μmol NTA/g diet the protein-free plasma zinc was increased more than fivefold. It is also important to note that when the protein-free plasma zinc was increased the urine zinc was also increased in spite of the fact that the renal tubules resorbed a large portion of the filterable zinc. Thus, it can be concluded that any dose of NTA that will increase the zinc pool in the protein-free fraction of the plasma will result in an increase in the renal tubule reabsorption of zinc and a proportional increase in urine zinc.

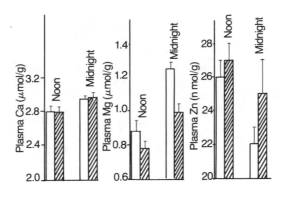

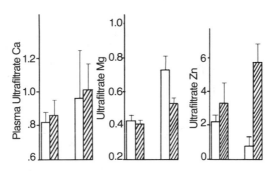

Figure 33. Plasma and protein-free fraction of plasma (ultrafiltrate = MW < 10,000) concentration of calcium, magnesium, and zinc measured at midnight and noon in control rats (open bars) and rats equilibrated to a diet containing 75 μmol NTA/g diet (shaded bars). Each value is the $\bar{x} \pm$ SEM of analyses from three rats.

TABLE 6. Effect of Dietary NTA Concentration on the Plasma Ultrafiltrate (UF) and Urinary Concentrations of NTA and Zinc[a]

Dietary NTA (μmol/g)	Plasma UF			Urine		
	Zn (neq/mL)	NTA (neq/mL)	NTA/Zn	Zn (μeq/mL)	NTA (μeq/mL)	NTA/Zn
0.73	0.79 ± 0.45	1.41 ± 0.10	2	0.06 ± 0.01	0.30 ± 0.04	5
7.3	0.77 ± 0.18	11.9 ± 0.6	15	0.07 ± 0.01	2.77 ± 0.39	40
73	3.87 ± 0.70	119 ± 11	31	0.25 ± 0.05	27.2 ± 3.8	109

[a] Each value for UF and urinary Zn and NTA is the mean $\pm$ SEM for 12 samples (6 males and 6 females at each NTA exposure rate). Three rats of each sex were fed the indicated dietary concentration of either $H_3 1\text{-}[^{14}C]NTA$ or $Na_3 1\text{-}[^{14}C]NTA\cdot H_2O$ ad libitum for 10 days. The urine values are based on a total 24-h urine collection and the UF samples were obtained between 8 and 10 a.m.

Figure 34 shows that until the protein-free plasma NTA attains a concentration of about 15 μM it has no effect on the zinc level in this fraction, but at concentrations > 15 μM there is a proportional increase in the zinc level with increasing NTA in this pool. Other studies have demonstrated that the plasma and protein-free fraction NTA concentration is a linear function of dietary NTA and it requires a NTA ingestion of ~ 100 μmol/kg each day to produce an NTA concentration of > 15 μM in the protein-free fraction of the plasma. Figure 35 shows the urinary zinc output by rats ingesting the indicated doses of NTA for 2 years. Rats fed the lowest dose (0.03% in the diet), which

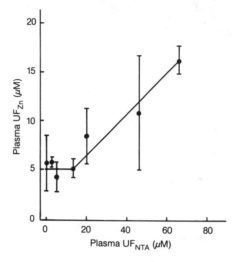

Figure 34. The concentration of zinc in the plasma ultrafiltrate (UF = MW < 10,000) as a function of the concentration of NTA in the protein-free fraction of the plasma of rats.

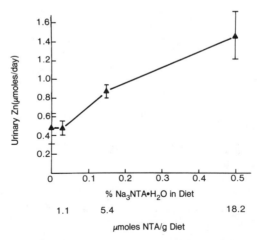

Figure 35. Urinary zinc as a function of dietary NTA concentration. Data were obtained from rats fed the indicated diet for 24 months.

caused no change in urinary zinc, produced no change in renal structure compared to the age-matched controls. The two higher doses, which increased urinary zinc in proportion to the NTA dose, induced dose-dependent changes in the tubule cells as described in the histogenesis section and there were two animals ingesting 0.5% NTA with renal tubular cell adenomas.

In summary, it has been demonstrated that renal tubular cell toxicity associated with NTA ingestion is a consequence of NTA-directed delivery of increased amounts of zinc to the renal tubules where the zinc is reabsorbed. Furthermore, until the NTA exposure exceeds a dose that will result in a protein-free plasma concentration of $\sim 15\,\mu M$ NTA, there is no change in the amount of zinc available for reabsorption and thus no change in renal tubular morphology compared to concurrent controls even after 2 years of continuous NTA ingestion. In contrast, NTA doses that do increase the pool of zinc in the protein-free fraction of the plasma do result in increased zinc resorption and tissue accumulation and these doses do cause a sequela of renal tubular cell toxicities that can result in a low incidence of tumors after chronic exposure.

TEC Toxicity

Doses of NTA that are clearly toxic to the renal tubules show no effect on the TEC even after chronic exposure as long as they are below 1 mmol/kg (Fig. 4). In spite of the fact that it requires higher doses of NTA to induce TEC tumors, the chemistry and metabolism of NTA still suggest that the response is most likely a consequence of changes in mineral disposition caused by NTA. The doses of NTA that are associated with TEC tumors are associated with increased calcium excretion in the urine (Fig. 36), while the doses that cause renal tubular cell toxicity but not TEC toxicity increase urinary zinc but not calcium (Fig. 37). The data in Fig. 33 make it certain that the increased urinary calcium cannot

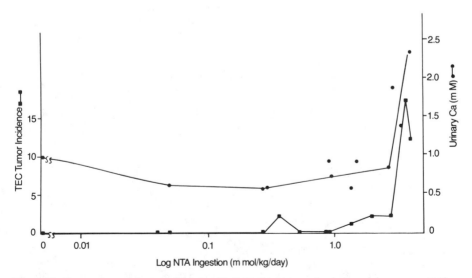

Figure 36. Comparison of the transitional epithelial cell tumors and urinary calcium concentration as a function of the ingested dose of NTA.

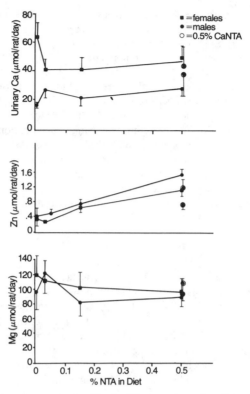

Figure 37. Urinary mineral excretion by Charles River rats ingesting diets with indicated doses of $Na_3NTA \cdot H_2O$ or CaNTA. Urine voided after 6, 12, 19, and 24 months of NTA ingestion were analyzed. Values are mean $\pm$ SEM for 16–20 analyses for each point.

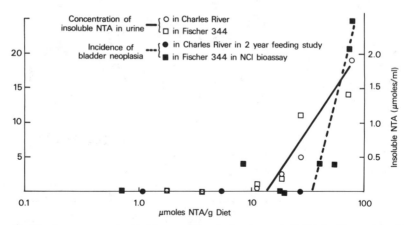

Figure 38. The dose response for bladder neoplasms in female rats fed NTA for 18 months or longer (---; Fischer 344, ■; Charles River CD, ●) compared with the dose response for the concentration of insoluble NTA in the urine in a short-term feeding study (——; Fischer-344, □; Charles River CD, ○).

418

arise from the same mechanism as the increased urinary zinc since even 73 μmol NTA/g diet does not alter the concentration of calcium in either of the plasma pools.

Urine from rats ingesting doses of NTA associated with TEC tumors contain visible quantities of insoluble material that is crystalline CaNaNTA as demonstrated by x-ray diffraction (35). A comparison of the level of crystalline CaNaNTA as a function of NTA dose to that for urothelial tumors showed great similarity (Fig. 38). It was conjectured that the urothelial tumors were a consequence of urothelial injury in response to the crystals as had been reported for several conditions associated with bladder tumors (36). Examination of the urinary tract and bladder contents has never shown the presence of CaNaNTA stones and the crystals in the urine were quite small. Thus, it seemed unlikely that the tumors resulted from the presence of crystals of CaNaNTA in the urine.

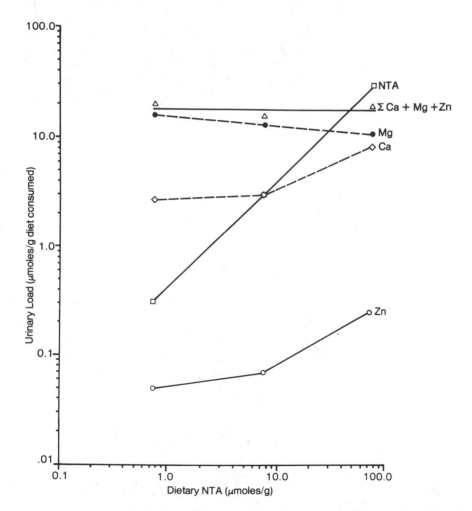

Figure 39. Urinary divalent metal and NTA excretion as a function of the dietary concentration of NTA.

Urine analyses at NTA doses that were associated with crystalline CaNaNTA and TEC tumors revealed that at these doses of NTA the urine contains more NTA than total divalent metals on a molar basis (Fig. 39). This is a unique condition to the urinary tract since at no other site, including the feces, does the concentration of NTA ever approach that of the sum of the divalent cations (Fig. 40). The fact that at doses of NTA that cause TEC tumors the urine contains uncomplexed NTA suggested that the increased calcium in the urine could arise by extraction of calcium from the urothelium by the uncomplexed NTA. Extraction of calcium from the urothelium would be expected to produce the type of response noted in the urothelial tissues, for example, loss of surface cells resulting in increased cell division leading to endophytic neoplasms.

Several tests of this hypothesis have been conducted. First, it was shown that ingestion of doses of NTA that cause TEC tumors result in a marked reduction in the concentration of calcium in the bladder while not altering the level of Na, K, Mg, or Zn (Fig. 41). This suggests that NTA can extract calcium from a readily available pool (extracellular) within the tissue while it cannot extract an intracellular cation even though NTA can form a stronger complex with that cation (Zn). The presence of an available pool of calcium was demonstrated by water washing of everted bladders. Washing bladders from controls reduced the Ca but not the Mg or Zn (Fig. 42). In contrast, washing bladders from rats fed NTA lowered Ca only slightly and to the same final concentration noted in the controls.

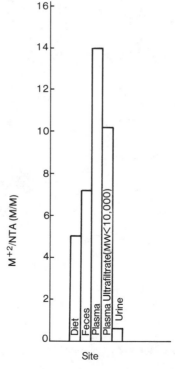

Figure 40. Ratio of divalent cation (M^{+2}) to NTA in various compartments in rats equilibrated to diets containing 75 μmol NTA/g.

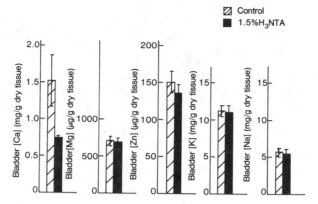

Figure 41. Effect of dietary H_3NTA (1.5%, $\sim 75\,\mu mol/g$) on the concentration of cations in the urinary bladder.

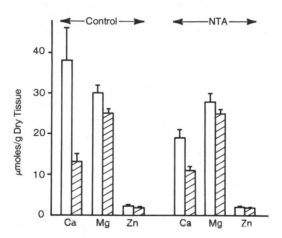

Figure 42. Effect of water washing on the concentration of divalent cations in bladder tissues from control rats and rats equilibrated with diets containing $75\,\mu mol\ NTA/g$.

Thus, the bladder does contain a pool of readily extractable calcium, which is removed in vivo in animals voiding urine with uncomplexed NTA.

NTA infused for 3 days into the bladder at a dose equivalent to the daily output of divalent cations ($200\,\mu mol/day$) did increase the urinary output of calcium and zinc but it did not significantly alter the tissue level of these metals (Fig. 43) and it did not cause bladder morphology changes different from those associated with saline infusion. However, when the dose of NTA was doubled it further increased urinary calcium but not zinc, decreased tissue calcium but not zinc (Fig. 43), and caused tissue hyperplasia and the presence of frequent mitotic figures in the bladder epithelium (Fig. 24). When the high dose was infused as the preformed $CaNH_4NTA$ complex, none of the bladder changes noted with the sodium salt occurred.

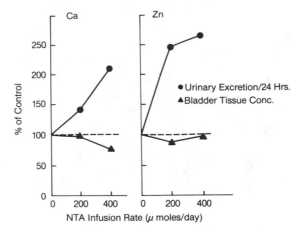

Figure 43. Effect of NTA infused directly into the bladder on urinary and bladder concentrations of calcium, magnesium, and zinc.

In summary, it has been demonstrated that at high ingestion doses of NTA the urine can attain concentrations of NTA that exceed the concentration of total divalent cations in the urine. When this state exists, the uncomplexed NTA in the urine will extract calcium from the extracellular space in the urothelium. This results in a net reduction in the tissue calcium, which allows surface cell erosion resulting in an increased mitosis that can lead to a low incidence of neoplasms after chronic exposure. The relation between NTA ingestion dose and urinary calcium excretion and bladder tumorigenicity (Fig. 36) shows that until the NTA dose exceeds ~ 2.5 mmol/kg·day neither parameter is affected; above this threshold both phenomena increase with increasing NTA dose.

RISK ASSESSMENT

The bioassay results with NTA have been used for many mathematical risk assessments. Table 7 lists some of the values obtained when different mathematical models are applied to these data (37, 38). The values are all expressed in terms of ingested NTA (μg/kg body weight per day) to allow direct comparison of the values. In all cases it was assumed that rats consume 50 g diet/kg body weight throughout their lifetimes and that water consumption is 75 g/kg body weight. The results in Table 7 show that the mathematical models of low-dose extrapolation lead to a very great difference in the virtual safe dose. Some of these values are close to the exposure that results from environmental levels of NTA (~ 3 μg/L water or 0.09 μg/kg body weight). By these criteria, NTA would pose a risk to human health.

If, however, one considers the potential risk of environmental levels of NTA based on the mechanism studies outlined in this chapter, a different conclusion will be reached. The mechanism studies clearly demonstrate that the urinary tract toxicities associated with NTA ingestion are dependent on changes in mineral distribution in the urinary tract that accompany renal clearance of systemic NTA. The conditions necessary to initiate the renal tubular cell toxicity or the urothelial toxicity are discontinuous processes that require a minimum NTA concentration in the critical compartment to initiate the toxic response.

TABLE 7. Range of Virtual Safe Dose (VSD) Calculations for NTA

VSD (μg/kg body weight·day)	Calculation Method	Reference
10^a	One-hit	40
37	Armitage–Doll	40
26×10^4	Weibull	40
40×10^4	Multihit	40
3.4^b	Linear	41
2.8	Armitage–Doll	41

[a] Virtual safe dose at risk level of 10^{-6}.
[b] The 97.5% confidence limit for 1 in 10^6 rodent tumors.

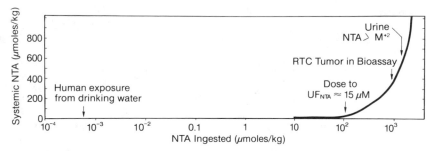

Figure 44. Systemic dose of NTA as a function of the log of ingested dose of NTA with significant points indicated.

Furthermore, the histogenesis of tumors at the two sites has been demonstrated to be the consequence of chronic toxicity, which only occur when the dose of NTA is sufficiently large to induce increased renal tubular cell zinc reabsorption of bladder epithelial calcium depletion. Doses of NTA below these critical doses (2.8×10^4 μg/kg for excess zinc delivery and 3.8×10^5 μg/kg for urine NTA/M^{2+} > 1.0) have been fed chronically to rats in four different laboratories and have shown no effects on urinary tissue morphology. For purposes of risk assessment, it can be concluded that any dose below the critical dose that results in an NTA concentration in the protein-free fraction of the plasma of < 15 μM cannot cause an increase in the amount of zinc delivered to the renal tubules (necessary condition) or increase urine NTA levels above divalent cation levels, and therefore such doses cannot induce urinary tract toxicity, which is a necessary condition to induce tissue toxicity that can result in neoplasm formation after chronic exposure.

NTA offers an unusual opportunity in the field of risk assessment in that the human exposure level can accurately be predicted because environmental levels have been monitored in Canada, where NTA-containing detergents have been sold for many years. During the entire period of NTA sales in Canada, water levels of NTA have been monitored and in 1979, following more than 10 years of use, the average drinking water NTA level was 2.82 μg/L (41). A 50-kg person who consumes 2 L of such water each day will ingest 0.1 μg NTA/kg·day. Figure 44 compares this consumption dose to that required to initiate changes in zinc disposition and bladder calcium perturbation and the lowest dose associated with urinary tract tumors. The human NTA exposure from the average drinking water in Canada is more than five orders of magnitude less than the minimal dose required to increase renal tubular zinc reabsorption. Thus, environmental concentrations of NTA pose no risk to humans because the resulting doses are at least five orders of magnitude less than the dose of NTA required to initiate the conditions necessary to induce urinary tract toxicity, which are an obligate precursor of the tumors.

The mechanism studies with NTA demonstrate the importance of determining the acute and subchronic effects of compounds in attempting to make rational judgments concerning their risk to humans. The critical examination of a mechanism is especially important when attempting to assess the significance of tumors in animals after chronic, high-dose exposure to nonmutagenic compounds.

REFERENCES

1. R. L. Anderson, W. E. Bishop, and R. L. Campbell, A review of the environmental and mammalian toxicology of nitrilotriacetic acid. *CRC Crit. Rev. Toxicol.* **15**, 1 (1985).

2. G. A. Nixon, Toxicity evaluation of trisodium nitrilotriacetate. *Toxicol. Appl. Pharmacol.* **18**, 398 (1971).

3. U.S. Environmental Protection Agency, *Potential Worker and Consumer Exposure to Nitrilotriacetic Acid in Detergents*, EPA-560/11-79-008. USEPA, Washington, DC, 1979.

4. G. A. Nolen, L. W. Klusman, D. L. Back, and E. V. Buehler, Reproduction and teratology studies of trisodium nitrilotriacetate in rats and rabbits. *Food Cosmet. Toxicol.* **9**, 509 (1971).

5. G. A. Nolen, R. L. Bohne, and E. V. Buehler, Effects of trisodium nitrilotriacetate, trisodium citrate, and a trisodium nitrilotriacetate ferric chloride mixture on cadmium and methyl mercury toxicity and teratogenesis in rats. *Toxicol. Appl. Pharmacol.* **23**, 238 (1972).

6. G. A. Nolen, E. V. Buehler, G. G. Geil, and E. I. Goldenthal, The effects of trisodium nitrilotriacetate on cadmium and methyl mercury toxicity and teratogenicity in rats. *Teratology* **5**, 264 (1972).

7. G. A. Nolen, E. V. Buehler, G. G. Geil, and E. I. Goldenthal, The effects of trisodium nitrilotriacetate on cadmium and methyl mercury toxicity and teratogenicity in rats. *Toxicol. Appl. Pharmacol.* **23**, 222 (1972).

8. H. Tjalve, A study on the distribution and teratogenicity of nitrilotriacetic acid (NTA) in mice. *Toxicol. Appl. Pharmacol.* **23**, 216 (1972).

9. L. G. Scharpf, T. D. Hill, P. L. Wright, J. B. Black, M. L. Keplinger, and J. C. Calandra, Effect of sodium nitrilotriacetate on toxicity, teratogenicity, and tissue distribution of cadmium. *Nature (London)* **239**, 231 (1972).

10. L. G. Scharpf, T. D. Hill, P. L. Wright, and M. L. Keplinger, Teratology studies on methyl mercury hydroxide and nitrilotriacetate sodium in rats. *Nature (London)* **241**, 461 (1973).

11. A. R. Malcolm, L. J. Mills, and E. J. McKenna, Inhibition of metabolic cooperation between Chinese hamster V79 cells by tumor promoters and other chemicals. In G. M. Williams, V. C. Dunkel, and V. A. Ray, Eds., *Cellular Systems for Toxicity Testing*. National Academy of Sciences, New York, 1983, p. 448.

12. K. C. Bora, Effects of nitrilotriacetic acid (NTA) on chromosome replication and structure of human cells. *Mutat. Res.* **31**, 325 (1975).

13. W. R. Michael and J. M. Wakim, Metabolism of nitrilotriacetic acid (NTA). *Toxicol. Appl. Pharmacol.* **18**, 407 (1971).

14. I. Chu, G. C. Becking. D. C. Villeneuve, and A. Viau, Metabolism of nitrilotriacetic acid (NTA) in the mouse. *Bull. Environ. Contam. Toxicol.* **78**, 417 (1978).

15. J. A. Budny and J. D. Arnold, Nitrilotriacetate (NTA): Human metabolism and its importance in the total safety evaluation program. *Toxicol. Appl. Pharmacol.* **25**, 48 (1973).

16. G. A. Nixon, E. V. Buehler, and R. J. Niewenhuis, Two-year feeding study with trisodium nitrilotriacetate and its calcium chelate. *Toxicol. Appl. Pharmacol.* **21**, 244 (1972).

17. R. L. Anderson and R. L. Kanerva, Effect of nitrilotriacetate (NTA) on cation balance in the rat. *Food Cosmet. Toxicol.* **16**, 563 (1978).

18. K. R. Mahaffey and R. A. Goyer, Trisodium nitrilotriacetate in drinking water, metabolic and renal effects in rats. *Arch. Environ. Health* **25**, 271 (1972).

19. National Cancer Institute, *Bioassays of Nitrilotriacetic Acid (NTA) and Nitrilotriacetic Acid, Trisodium Salt, Monohydrate (Na₃NTA·H₂O) for Possible Carcinogenicity (NCI-CG-TR-6)*, DHEW Publ. No. (NIH) 77–806. NCI, Bethesda, MD, 1977.

20. Y. Hiasa, Y. Kitahori, N. Konishi, N. Enoki, T. Shimoyama, and A. Miyashiro, Trisodium nitrilotriacetate monohydrate: Promoting effects on the development of renal tubular cell tumors in rats treated with N-ethyl-N-hydroxyethylnitrosamine. *JNCI, J. Natl. Cancer Inst.* **72**, 483 (1984).

21. Y. Hiasa, Y. Kitahori, N. Konishi, and T. Shimoyama, Dose-related effect of trisodium nitrilotriacetate monohydrate on renal tumorigenesis initiated with N-ethyl-N-hydroxyethylnitrosamine in rats. *Carcinogenesis (London)* **6**, 907 (1985).

22. Y. Hiasa, Y. Kitahori, N. Konishi, T. Shimoyama, and A. Miyashiro, Trisodium nitriloacetate monohydrate: Promoting effect in urinary bladder carcinogenesis in rats treated with N-butyl-N-(4-hydroxybutyl)nitrosamine. *JNCI, J. Natl. Cancer Inst.* **71**, 235 (1985).

23. J. A. Merski, Acute structural changes in renal tubular epithelium following administration of nitrilotriacetate. *Food Cosmet. Toxicol.* **19**, 463 (1981).

24. C. L. Alden and R. L. Kanerva, The pathogenesis of renal cortical tumors in rats fed 2% trisodium nitrilotriacetate monohydrate. *Food Chem. Toxicol.* **20**, 441 (1982).

25. C. L. Alden, R. L. Kanerva, R. L. Anderson, and A. G. Adkins, Short-term effects of dietary nitrilotriacetic acid in the male Charles River rat kidney. *Vet. Pathol.* **18**, 549 (1981).

26. M. C. Myers, R. L. Kanerva, C. L. Alden, and R. L. Anderson, Reversibility of nephrotoxicity induced in rats by nitrilotriacetate in subchronic feeding studies. *Food Chem. Toxicol.* **20**, 925 (1982).

27. R. A. Goyer, H. L. Falk, M. Hogan, D. D. Feldman, and W. Richter, Renal tumors in rats given trisodium nitrilotriacetic acid in drinking water for 2 years. *JNCI, J. Natl. Cancer Inst.* **66**, 869 (1981).

28. M. Greenblatt and W. Lijinsky, Carcinogenesis and chronic toxicity of nitrilotriacetic acid in Swiss mice. *J. Natl. Cancer Inst. (U.S.)* **52**, 1123 (1974).

29. W. Lijinsky, M. Greenblatt, and C. Kommineni, Brief communication: Feeding studies of nitrilotriacetic acid and derivatives in rats. *J. Natl. Cancer Inst. (U.S.)* **50**, 1061 (1973).

30. B. J. Bohen, M. R. Anver, D. H. Ringler, and R. C. Adelman, Age-associated pathological changes in male rats. *Fed. Proc., Fed. Am. Soc. Exp. Biol.* **37**, 2848 (1978).

31. R. L. Kanerva, W. R. Francis, F. R. Lefever, T. Dorr, C. L. Alden, and R. L. Anderson, Renal pelvis and ureteral dilatation in male rats ingesting trisodium nitrilotriacetate. *Food Chem. Toxicol.* **9**, 749 (1984).

32. E. Kunze, Hyperplasia, urinary bladder, rat. In T. C. Jones, U. Mohr, and R. D. Hunt, Eds., *Monographs on Pathology of Laboratory Animals: Urinary System.* Springer-Verlag, New York, 1986, p. 291.

33. D. H. Reese and R. F. Friedman, Suppression of dysplasia and hyperplasia by calcium in organ-cultured urinary bladder epithelium. *Cancer Res.* **38**, 586 (1978).

34. R. L. Anderson, The role of zinc in nitrilotriacetic (NTA)-associated renal tubular cell toxicity. *Food Cosmet. Toxicol.* **19**, 639 (1981).

35. R. L. Anderson, The relationship of insoluble nitrilotriacetate (NTA) in the urine of female rats to the dietary level of NTA. *Food Cosmet. Toxicol.* **18**, 59 (1980).

36. D. B. Clayson and E. H. Cooper, Cancer of the urinary tract. *Cancer Res.* **13**, 271 (1970).

37. Proposed System for Food Safety Assessment, Final Report of the Scientific Committee of the Food Safety Council, June, 1980.

38. D. A. Gaylor and R. L. Kodell, Linear interpolation algorithm for low dose risk assessment of toxic substances. *J. Environ. Pathol. Toxicol.* **4**, 305 (1980).

39. U. Malaiyandi, D. T. Williams, and R. O'Grady, National survey of nitrilotriacetic acid in Canadian drinking water. *Environ. Sci. Technol.* **13**, 59 (1979).

11

Assessment of the Public Health Risks Associated with the Proposed Excavation of a Hazardous Waste Site

Susan M. Brett, Joyce S. Schlesinger,
Duncan Turnbull, and Ranjit J. Machado
Environ Corporation, Washington, DC.

In recent years, excavation and removal have been the remedies frequently required by regulatory agencies for implementing source control at hazardous waste sites. A number of authors have published methodologies for determining "How clean is clean?" or for comparing the risks presented by hazardous waste sites (e.g., 1–6). Under CERCLA, the U.S. EPA directs potentially responsible parties (PRPs) to estimate and compare the public health and environmental risks associated with various proposed remedial alternatives. The available methodologies, however, do not provide sufficient guidance on how to estimate quantitatively the risks associated with the excavation of contaminated soils from hazardous waste sites.

This chapter presents a summary of the procedures used to evaluate the risks to public health associated with the proposed excavation of waste lagoons at an abandoned hazardous waste disposal facility in the northeastern United States. The major focus of this analysis is the volatilization of chemicals from the soil during the excavation process and subsequent inhalation of the vapors by residents in close proximity to the site. Guidance is provided on the selection of indicator chemicals and the derivation of an interim carcinogenic potency value for an indicator chemical found at high concentrations throughout the site. The procedures used to develop hypothetical exposure scenarios, estimate environmental concentrations, and estimate resultant human intake are described. Risk estimates are calculated for subchronic inhalation of vapor and particulates and for ingestion of particulates. Such risk estimates are based on modeling of the median concentrations of the indicator chemicals in the soil. The maximum daily doses of indicator chemicals that local residents might receive on days when the most contaminated portions of the site are excavated are also calculated and compared with derived acceptable daily intake levels for these chemicals. In addition, the risks associated with transporting the excavated material offsite are evaluated. Finally, the uncertainties and limitations in the analysis, related to the assumptions applied to assess potential toxicity and exposure, are discussed in detail.

This assessment is based on sampling data pertinent to the site, including surficial and subsurface soil investigations and the proposed excavation plan. No independent verification of provided data was conducted by the authors.

1   DESCRIPTION AND HISTORY OF THE SITE

The site is a 5-acre abandoned hazardous waste disposal facility. It is bordered to the east and west by river tributaries, to the south by a steep cliff, and to the north by a railroad switching yard. No buildings exist within the old lagoon area.

Land use in the vicinity of the abandoned disposal site includes residential, commercial, and industrial. Immediately adjacent to the site on the western border is a newly developed residential subdivision. The area south of the site is zoned residential and agricultural, while to the north, the zoning is heavy industrial. In addition, a subdivision that contains several hundred single-family dwellings is located $\frac{1}{2}$ mile southeast of the site (Fig. 1).

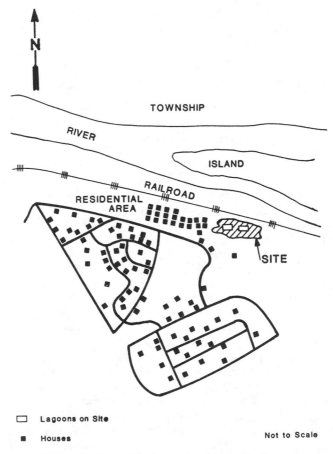

Figure 1. Elevation view of the 5-acre abandoned hazardous waste site.

The disposal site, which consisted of a series of small unlined lagoons constructed in an old sandstone quarry, was operational during the 1960s. Reportedly, liquid wastes and sludges were hauled to the site in bulk tank trucks and were disposed of in a large lagoon on the eastern portion of the site. The lagoons were filled with wastes, covered, and new lagoons were constructed. Since the lagoons were not lined, wastes were not prevented from moving down into the underlying bedrock and laterally offsite. The site was ordered closed in 1973 by the State Department of Environmental Protection and at that time the lagoons were reportedly drained, backfilled, and vegetated, and the removed liquid wastes transported offsite.

In early 1983, a citizens' complaint to regulatory agencies regarding odors emanating from the site resulted in the erection of a security fence, partial site capping, and regrading. Subsequently, a comprehensive field investigation of the site was instituted to determine the nature and extent of site contamination. Sampling conducted at the site revealed significant concentrations of various chemicals in the soil within the areas of the former lagoons and to a lesser extent outside the area of the lagoons. The onsite wastes were primarily confined to two distinct areas, which correspond to the locations of the former east and west lagoons.

The areal extent of the waste covers approximately 4000 yd^2 in the east lagoon area and 5000 yd^2 in the west lagoon area. Subsurface samples taken at various depths within the former lagoon areas showed the presence of chemical contamination within the soil column from the surface extending down to bedrock and reaching depths of over 25 ft in several areas. Sampling data indicated the presence of a variety of volatile organic chemicals (primarily xylenes, ethylbenzene, tetrachloroethylene, toluene, and 1, 2, 3-trichloropropane) in high concentrations (in excess of $10,000 \text{ mg/kg}$ in some areas) within the lagoon areas. Samples taken from a series of bedrock (deep aquifer) monitoring wells installed at the site have identified the presence of areas where nonaqueous liquid contaminants exist. This liquid, generally referred to as dense nonaqueous phase liquid (DNAPL), is located in soil beneath the former lagoons and in the bedrock between the former lagoons and the river.

Following the release of a study that evaluated the feasibility of alternative remedies, excavation of contaminated soils and wastes from the east and west lagoon areas and offsite disposal in a permitted RCRA landfill were recommended by the U.S. EPA as the onsite remedy. The decisionmakers deferred selection of remedial response measures for the underlying groundwater, the adjacent flood plain area, or the river. Consequently, this assessment addresses only the public health issues associated with onsite contamination.

2 PROPOSED EXCAVATION PLAN

The proposed remedy stipulated the excavation and offsite disposal of approximately $35,000 \text{ yd}^3$ of contaminated material. Material will be removed from the east and west lagoon areas to the extent required to reach the chemical concentrations stipulated by regulators (i.e., essentially background). An additional $20,000 \text{ yd}^3$ of uncontaminated material will be excavated and reused as fill on the site. The duration of the entire excavation operation is intended to be 5–6 months, based on a 10-h/day and 20-day/month work schedule. A preliminary excavation design was developed by a contractor, but many of the details of the excavation were left unspecified.

The excavation plan includes the design for excavating onsite contaminated soils, controlling site runoff, controlling sediment transport offsite, upgrading an existing air stripping treatment plant, and transporting contaminated materials to a secure EPA-permitted landfill. The existing site access road will be upgraded to meet the additional traffic and equipment requirements, and decontamination and transloading facilities will be constructed at the site.

Two transportation options have been considered to meet the scheduled disposal of 500 yd^3 of contaminated material per day. The road haul option specifies that material be loaded into trailers at the western edge of the active excavation pit and transported to an offsite secure landfill. The rail haul option specifies transport by rail and involves the building of a transloading facility at the disposal site since such a facility does not now exist. The excavation plan would depend on the selected transportation option. If transportation by road were selected, excavation would begin in the east pit by excavating the approximately 15,000 yd^3 of contaminated material in horizontal layers until bedrock. On completion of the east lagoon excavation and decontamination of the area, excavation operations would commence at the west lagoon. The order of excavation of the two areas would be reversed if the rail option were selected.

In the following sections, we present the methodology used to organize the above information into a framework that permits the evaluation of public health risks.

3 METHODOLOGY FOR WASTE SITE RISK ASSESSMENT

3.1 Public Health Risk Assessment Methodology

Risk assessment is the process of (i) evaluating the potential adverse health effects (toxicity) of chemicals to which people may be exposed (hazard identification); (ii) analyzing how those adverse health effects change in frequency of occurrence and in intensity with changes in the frequency, duration, and magnitude of exposure (dose–response assessment); (iii) estimating the frequency, duration, and magnitude of human exposure to the chemicals (exposure assessment); and (iv) determining the probability of health effects that may occur in individuals exposed at the levels estimated in the exposure assessment step (risk characterization). This four-step risk assessment process was developed by the National Academy of Sciences (NAS) (7) and is used by a number of groups including the U.S. Environmental Protection Agency (EPA) (8), the U.S. Food and Drug Administration (9), and other regulatory agencies.

The general approach developed to assess public health risks from excavation of the site is outlined in Table 1. This incorporates the analytical process as defined by NAS (7)

TABLE 1. Steps in Hazardous Waste Site Public Health Risk Assessment Methodology

1. Review history of site operations, available monitoring data, and proposed remedial actions.
2. Identify chemicals of concern (indicator chemicals).
3. Evaluate toxicity data on indicator chemicals.
4. Develop ADIs (acceptable daily intakes for noncarcinogens and noncarcinogenic chronic effects of carcinogens) and UCRs (unit cancer risks for carcinogens).
5. Identify populations potentially subject to exposure and develop hypothetical exposure scenarios.
6. Develop estimates of environmental concentrations and estimate resultant human intake.
7. Calculate numerical estimates of risk on the basis of estimated human intake and ADIs and UCRs.

but adds two preliminary steps that are needed in the case of assessing a hazardous waste site. The procedures used follow in general principle those outlined in the EPA's *Superfund Public Health Evaluation Manual* (10) but differ in detail. The main reason for the difference is that the Superfund manual contains no guidance for evaluating the potential risks associated with a site excavation. We have reviewed the EPA's Superfund manual and have used suggested data (e.g., toxicity factors) for risk assessment where appropriate. In a few cases, on the basis of scientific judgment, we applied values that differed from those recommended by the EPA. Such deviations from the Superfund manual are noted in the following discussion.

3.1.1 Step 1. Review of Site History, Monitoring Data, and Proposed Remedial Actions.
In the first step of the risk assessment process, the available information on the history of the hazardous waste site and its associated contamination are reviewed. Such a review is performed in order to determine the extent of contamination associated with the site (both onsite and offsite), the specific contaminants involved, and to estimate the potential for migration of these contaminants.

3.1.2 Step 2. Identification of Chemicals of Concern.
In the second step of the assessment, *indicator chemicals* may be selected from among the chemicals identified in environmental samples (10). Because of the large number of chemicals often associated with a chemical waste site, it is sometimes a practical necessity to limit the number of chemicals considered in assessing potential public health risk. The selection of such chemicals is based primarily on their measured concentration in the medium investigated (e.g., soil) and their inherent toxicities. Additional factors to be considered include physical and chemical parameters related to the chemicals, environmental mobility and persistence, which may affect the likelihood of human exposure.

In the present case, selection of indicator chemicals was based on their presence at high concentration in the soil to be excavated and their inherent toxicity. Less weight was given to chemicals whose identities were not confirmed or that were not found in more than one sample. The procedure for selection of these chemicals differed from that suggested by the EPA in its Superfund manual (10), because a major focus of this analysis was the volatilization of chemicals from the soil during the excavation process and subsequent inhalation of the vapors by individuals residing nearby. This scenario is not addressed in the EPA's procedures for selecting indicator chemicals, in which exposure to chemicals in soil is considered only in the form of ingestion. Also, the EPA's procedure emphasizes chronic exposure, while this analysis is concerned only with the subchronic exposure occurring during the several months of proposed excavation. However, the procedures used to select the indicator chemicals for this analysis do follow the general risk assessment principles endorsed by the EPA of considering both the inherent toxicity and the "representative" concentration of the contaminants in the environmental medium of concern.

3.1.3 Step 3. Evaluation of Toxicity Data on Indicator Chemicals.
In the third step of the analysis, toxicity data are identified and evaluated to determine the types of health effects or diseases that may be produced by the selected indicator chemicals. Such data are also reviewed to determine the quantitative relation between the amount of exposure to a substance and the extent of toxic injury or disease. They are generally derived from studies of humans and laboratory animals and from studies of the behavior of chemicals within the body (e.g., metabolism, pharmacokinetics).

3.1.4 Step 4. Development of Measures of Toxicity. On the basis of toxicity data, quantitative measures of potential health damage are developed in step 4 of the analysis. Different methodologies are used to develop such measures, depending on whether a chemical is a noncarcinogen or a carcinogen. In the present assessment, toxicity measures were developed to assess the health risks associated with acute (1 day) and subchronic (4 months) exposures associated with chemical releases during the period of excavation.

Since noncarcinogenic effects are thought to have a threshold dose below which the effect will not occur, one initially attempts to identify the threshold dose by determining the no-observed-effect level (NOEL) from observations of exposed people or experimental animals. In some cases, all exposures studied in the laboratory or observed in the field have produced an effect, and for these a lowest-observed-effect level (LOEL) provides the best available data for estimating the threshold. Such NOELs and LOELs are divided by safety factors (also called uncertainty factors) to obtain a chronic or subchronic acceptable daily intake (ADI) of the chemical (11). Safety factors adjust for limitations in the toxicity data and for differences between the conditions of exposure under which toxicity data were collected and the anticipated conditions of human exposure. They also adjust for variability in susceptibility in the human population and for general imprecision in extrapolating from laboratory animals to humans (12–14). This procedure for development of an ADI may also be applied to estimate chronic and subchronic noncarcinogenic risks associated with carcinogens.

For carcinogens, various threshold and no-threshold models have been assumed by different investigators in different situations. Under the no-threshold hypothesis, some decreasing level of risk is assumed to exist at all levels of exposure, declining (in proportion to the level of exposure) to zero risk at zero exposure. For this analysis we have used the no-threshold assumption in estimating risks for chemicals that have demonstrated carcinogenic effects in animals or humans.

Scientists have developed several mathematical models to estimate, by extrapolation, low-dose carcinogenic risks to humans from observed high-dose carcinogenic effects typically observed in experimental animal studies. The result of applying these models to carcinogenicity data is an estimate of the upper limit on lifetime risk per unit of dose (unit cancer risk or UCR). The mathematical model generally used by EPA and in this risk assessment to generate a UCR is the linearized multistage model. This model makes conservative assumptions about the shape of the dose–response curve and estimates the upper limit on lifetime risk per unit of dose. It consequently results in highly conservative estimates of risk; that is, the model is likely to overestimate the actual UCR for a carcinogen. In interpreting risks estimated on the basis of the application of the linearized multistage model, one must consider that the actual risk may be substantially lower than that predicted by the upper bounds of this model.

In addition, to estimate the risk of acute exposure, levels of acceptable short-term exposure may be developed. In this assessment, acute ADIs, representing the maximum 1-day exposure levels that are anticipated not to result in adverse effects in most individuals, were derived. When available, acute ADIs were based on the EPA 1-day drinking water health advisories (15) (which were converted to mg/kg·day doses). In the remaining cases, acute ADIs for the general population were derived on the basis of American Conference of Governmental Industrial Hygienists (ACGIH) Threshold Limit Values (TLVs) (16). It was assumed that the dose (in mg/kg·day) acceptable for a worker on an 8-h basis would be acceptable for an individual in the general population during occasional 1-day maximum exposure periods. The 8-h time-weighted average TLV air concentrations (in mg/m^3) were converted to acceptable maximum acute daily doses (in mg/kg·day) as follows: TLV(in mg/m^3) $\times$ (1 m^3/1000 L) $\times$ (29 L/min) $\times$ (480 min/day) $\times$ (1/70 kg) = acute ADI for general population (in mg/kg·day). Thus, the result of the fourth step of this risk assessment process is the development of acute and subchronic ADIs for noncarcinogens (and for the noncarcinogenic effects of carcinogens) and UCRs for carcinogens.

3.1.5 Step 5. Identification of Populations Potentially Subject to Exposure and Development of Hypothetical Exposure Scenarios.

In this step of the risk assessment process, populations potentially subject to exposure are identified and hypothetical exposure scenarios are developed which are specific to the site of concern. In the present assessment, scenarios were constructed to represent reasonably foreseeable acute and subchronic exposures of two subgroups (preschool children and adult females) of the local population who are anticipated to have the highest exposure to emissions generated by excavation. These scenarios account for the route of exposure, duration of exposure, and the amount of chemical absorbed into the body, as well as the characteristics of the exposed population.

3.1.6 Step 6. Development of Estimates of Environmental Concentrations and Estimation of Human Intake.

In this step of the risk assessment process estimates of environmental concentrations associated with the waste site excavation are developed and applied to estimate human exposure.

In the present assessment, the available analytical data for each indicator chemical were used to determine the median concentration in the soil to be excavated and the potential 1-day maximum soil concentration that might be encountered during the period when the most highly contaminated material is being excavated. These soil concentrations were then used in the exposure modeling. Offsite exposures were evaluated using a two-step process. First, potential chemical emission rates were estimated from the concentration of chemical in the soil matrix, physicochemical properties of both the chemicals and soil, and the nature of onsite excavation activities. Second, the calculated emission rates were used with meteorological data to predict chemical concentrations in the air at nearby residences.

The intake of volatile emissions and contaminated particulates by individuals residing at the nearby residences was then calculated based on standard body weight and respiratory parameters. In addition, dry fallout of particulate material dispersed during excavation was modeled, and incidental ingestion by children playing in and around the home was estimated. It was assumed that during site excavation the use of heavy equipment would necessitate, as a matter of safety, that security measures be taken to prevent public access. Thus, the exposure of children to onsite soils to be excavated was not modeled in this analysis.

On the basis of the exposure scenarios defined in step 5 and the estimated air concentrations, the daily intakes of each indicator chemical by each route of exposure are calculated. Where more than one route of exposure is modeled, the route-specific intakes are added to estimate the total daily intake of each indicator chemical. To assess the subchronic and chronic effects of carcinogens, the estimated average daily intake of the contaminant during the period of exposure (i.e., during the 4-month excavation period) is multiplied by the number of days of exposure and divided by the number of days in a lifetime to determine the lifetime average daily dose (LADD). For noncarcinogens, and for the noncarcinogenic effects of carcinogens, subchronic and chronic effects are assessed by applying the average daily doses (ADDs) during the exposure period directly in risk estimation.

In this assessment, for both carcinogens and noncarcinogens, average daily doses during the excavation period were determined based on the median soil concentrations of the indicator chemicals. To estimate conservatively the potential acute risks of excavation, the maximum daily dose (MDD) for each indicator chemical was calculated assuming all the soil excavated on one day contains the highest measured concentration of that chemical present in the soil onsite. The MDDs thus calculated represent upper-bound estimates since no loss or degradative processes were considered. (Further details on the methodology to estimate exposure applied in this assessment are presented in Section 4).

3.1.7 Step 7. Calculation of Estimates of Risk to Public Health. In this step of the risk assessment process, numerical estimates of risks are calculated for each indicator chemical by each potential route of exposure, on the basis of the ADIs and UCRs (step 4) and the human intakes estimated for each exposure scenario (step 6). Such estimates represent the public health risks that are postulated to result from exposure to the chemicals, at the detected concentrations, under the assumed conditions of exposure. The numerical estimate of subchronic risk for the noncarcinogens and for the noncarcinogenic effects of the carcinogens is determined by dividing the ADD (in mg/kg·day) by the acceptable daily intake (ADI, in mg/kg·day): if the ADD/ADI ratio does not exceed 1.0, then no adverse health effects would be expected to occur under the assumed conditions of exposure. Similarly, to estimate the acute risk of exposure to noncarcinogens and carcinogens, the ratio of the MDD to the acute ADI is determined and situations where this ratio exceeds 1.0 are identified. For the carcinogens the LADD (in mg/kg·day), is multiplied by the UCR (in $[\text{mg/kg·day}]^{-1}$) to calculate an upper-bound, lifetime cancer risk. For example, a lifetime increased cancer risk of 1-in-1-million (10^{-6}), calculated on the basis of the linearized multistage model, suggests that for every 1 million people exposed to that concentration of contaminant under the assumed exposure conditions, the upper bound on risk would be one new case of cancer per lifetime. Owing to the conservative nature of the model, however, the true risk may be substantially less than that predicted.

3.2 Transportation Risk Assessment Methodology

Estimates were also made of the potential number of spill incidents associated with the transportation of excavated soil from the site. Estimates were derived for the risks associated with the two options specified in the design document for the off-site disposal of contaminated material, a truck haul option and a rail haul option. The design document specified the amount of material to be hauled per day, potential landfill destinations, basic configuration of the truck and rail equipment to be used in transporting the contaminated soil, and other details concerning the truck haul and rail haul options.

Estimates of spill incidents were calculated by multiplying hazardous materials spill incident rates per vehicle mile by the total number of miles traveled over the project period (i.e., 5–6 months). Hazardous materials spill incident rates were obtained for trucks on a truck-mile and ton-mile basis, and for trains on the basis of railcar-miles and railcar-ton-miles. Release incidents for all road types (e.g., interstates, state highways) were of the order of 10^{-7} incidents per truck-mile (17). The incident rate for railcars is reported to be 2.1 $\times 10^{-6}$ incidents per railcar-mile (18). Total vehicle miles were derived by multiplying the total number of miles along the transportation route between the site and the ultimate destination, and the total number of truck or train trips needed to transport the contaminated material. Other information used in producing the estimates of transportation risks was extracted from reports published by the U.S. Department of Transportation (17), the Office of Technology Assessment (19), and an unpublished draft report of the Association of American Railroads (18).

The likelihood that human health or the environment would actually be affected by a spill incident was also examined. The risks to public health through the air pathway from a spill of contaminated material were only evaluated qualitatively. The potential risks associated with a spill of excavated material and the subsequent release of chemical contaminants into surface water were evaluated using a simple desorption model (20). In addition, for purposes of a case study, water bodies that serve as sources of municipal water supplies along one segment of a possible transportation route were identified to determine whether potable water supplies would be at risk in the event of a spill.

4   RESULTS OF APPLICATION OF RISK ASSESSMENT METHODOLOGY

4.1   Review of Monitoring Data and Selection of Indicator Chemicals (Steps 1 and 2)

A large number of chemicals have been identified in the soils of the site. Approximately 18 inorganic and 26 organic chemicals that are included on the Hazardous Substances List (HSL) under CERCLA have been detected at quantifiable levels in soils in the area of the proposed excavation. In addition, another 28 non-HSL organic chemicals were tentatively identified. The concentrations found have varied from the level of detection, generally a few parts per billion (ppb) (μg/kg soil), to several million ppb in the case of ethylbenzene, tetrachloroethylene, toluene, 1, 2, 3-trichloropropane, and 1, 2- and 1, 3-dimethylbenzenes (xylenes).

In assessing the risks associated with a hazardous waste site, it is normal practice to limit the detailed analysis to a smaller number of chemicals to prevent the analysis from becoming unwieldy, and because many of the less toxic and less prevalent chemicals would not have a substantial impact on the outcome of the analysis. Selection of indicator chemicals in the present case involved a three-stage process:

1. The onsite concentrations of the various chemicals were compared to background concentrations to determine whether the chemicals were present at elevated concentrations. This was important particularly for the inorganic chemicals, all of which were present at concentrations similar to background levels and were therefore excluded. As a check to ensure that omitting the inorganic chemicals would not significantly affect the estimate of risk, the amount of soil that would need to be in the air to exceed the American Conference of Governmental Industrial Hygienists (ACGIH) Threshold Limit Value (TLV) (16) (the maximum concentration in the air anticipated to cause no adverse effects in workers exposed 8 h/day) for each of the inorganic materials identified was calculated, assuming each chemical was present in the soil at the highest concentration at which it was found at any location onsite. These calculations showed that the contaminated dust concentrations necessary to exceed the TLV would be in excess of 100 mg/m^3 for each of the inorganic compounds. This concentration is 10 times higher than the occupational TLV for nuisance dust and is not likely to be produced at the location of the closest residence as a result of excavation. Therefore, it was concluded that these substances would not have a significant impact on the risk associated with the excavation.

TABLE 2. Selected Indicator Chemicals and Chemical Classes Represented

Chemical	Chemical Class
Chlorobenzene	Chlorobenzenes
2-Chlorophenol	Phenols
Cresol[a]	Phenols
1,2-Dichlorobenzene	Chlorobenzenes
2,4-Dimethylphenol	Phenols
Ethylbenzene	Alkylbenzenes
Nitrobenzene	Nitro/aminobenzenes
Phenol	Phenols
Tetrachloroethylene	Chloroalkenes
Toluene	Alkylbenzenes
1,2,4-Trichlorobenzene	Chlorobenzenes
1,2,3-Trichloropropane	Chloroalkanes
Xylene[b]	Alkylbenzenes

[a]Includes both o- and p-cresol (2-methylphenol and 4-methylphenol).
[b]Includes both o- and m-xylene (1,2-dimethylbenzene and 1,3-dimethylbenzene).

2. Chemicals that were present at only trace levels in the soil to be excavated and those that have not been found in more than one sample, or only tentatively identified, were likewise excluded from consideration as indicators. While their presence is undesirable, all chemicals present at low ppb levels were of relatively low inherent toxicity. They would therefore not contribute significantly to the adverse health impact of the excavation process when considered in light of the presence of several more toxic chemicals at concentrations of thousands or millions of ppb. Also, chemicals found only outside the area of the proposed excavation were likewise excluded.

3. The remaining chemicals that were clearly identified in more than one sample within the area of proposed excavation were considered in the final indicator chemical selection process.

This process yielded a final list of 13 chemicals from six chemical classes (including two pairs of isomers) that were used to estimate the risk presented by the proposed excavation (Table 2). The six classes represented are alkylbenzenes, chloroalkanes, chloroalkenes, chlorobenzenes, nitro- and aminobenzenes, and phenols. Some chemicals were excluded as indicators because more toxic members of the same chemical class were present at higher concentrations and the latter were selected as indicators for that class.

4.2 Development of Toxicity Criteria for Indicator Chemicals (Steps 3 and 4)

For each of the indicator chemicals selected we examined the available toxicity data to identify the types of acute, subchronic, and chronic health effects associated with exposure. These toxicity data were then summarized in toxicity profiles. The toxicity profiles also documented the development of acceptable acute and subchronic exposure levels (acute and subchronic ADIs) and unit cancer risks (UCRs). In this assessment, it was assumed that 4 months could be required to excavate the contaminated soil. The remainder of the period would involve the handling of noncontaminated material. Therefore, subchronic ADIs rather than chronic ADIs were applied in assessing potential risks from noncarcinogens. These subchronic ADIs were subsequently compared to the estimates of average daily dose in the exposed populations during the period of the excavation.

Acute ADIs, representing the maximum 1-day exposure levels that are anticipated not to result in adverse effects in most individuals, were derived for each indicator chemical. The EPA 1-day health advisories were available to form the basis of the acute ADIs for two indicator chemicals (ethylbenzene and xylene). The remaining acute ADIs were primarily based on American Conference of Governmental Industrial Hygienists (ACGIH) occupational threshold limit values (TLVs), which were converted to daily doses in mg/kg·day.

These acute ADIs were subsequently compared with the maximum estimated daily exposure to chemical contaminants that might occur on days when the most contaminated portions of the site would be excavated. The purpose of this comparison was to determine whether acute toxic effects would be likely to develop on those days.

For carcinogens, unit cancer risk (UCR) values were derived. Only one of the chemicals on the indicator chemical list is a known animal carcinogen, tetrachloroethylene. One other chemical, 1, 2, 3-trichloropropane, however, is suspected by the EPA of being a carcinogen and is currently under test for carcinogenicity by the National Toxicology Program (NTP). The results of this study are unavailable at this time. For purposes of this analysis, a hypothetical UCR value of $0.10 \, (\text{mg/kg·day})^{-1}$ was used for this compound for

TABLE 3. Toxicity Criteria for the Indicator Chemicals

Chemical	Acute ADI (mg/kg·day)	Subchronic ADI (mg/kg·day)	UCR (mg/kg·day)$^{-1}$	Reference
Chlorobenzene	69.6	0.04[a]		16, 21
2-Chlorophenol	3.8	0.044		16, 22
Cresols[b]	4.4	0.03		16, 23
1, 2-Dichlorobenzene	6.0	0.67		16, 24
2, 4-Dimethylphenol	3.8	0.0006		16, 25
Ethylbenzene	86.5	1.04[a]		26–28
Nitrobenzene	0.99	0.0026		16, 29
Phenol	3.8	0.02		16, 30
Tetrachloroethylene	67.6		1.7×10^{-3} (inhalation) 5.1×10^{-2} (ingestion)	16, 31
Toluene	75	1.16[a]		16, 32
1, 2, 4-Trichlorobenzene	0.8	0.02		16, 33
1, 2, 3-Trichloropropane	8.0	0.057	$(0.10)^c$	16, 34
Xylene[d]	32.3	0.0103[a]		35, 36

[a]These subchronic ADI values differ from the subchronic acceptable intake values listed in the EPA's *Superfund Public Health Evaluation Manual* (10). That for ethylbenzene is slightly higher; the others are slightly lower. The bases of the EPA's values are not described in the manual.
[b]Includes both *o*- and *p*-cresol (2-methylphenol and 4-methylphenol).
[c]Derived by analogy with other 1-to-3 carbon halogenated alkanes.
[d]Includes *o*- and *m*-xylene (1, 2-dimethylbenzene and 1, 3-dimethylbenzene).

both inhalation and ingestion. This UCR was derived by taking the geometric mean of the (oral) UCR values of five other carcinogenic halogenated alkanes (carbon tetrachloride, chloroform, 1, 2-dichloroethane, dichloromethane, and 1, 2-dibromo-3-chloropropane) that have been evaluated by the EPA's Carcinogen Assessment Group (10). The individual UCR values for those five chemicals ranged from 7.5×10^{-3} to 1.38 $(mg/kg \cdot day)^{-1}$. When the NTP bioassay is completed and the results are available, a more accurate UCR can be calculated and the conclusions of this assessment revised accordingly.

The toxicity criteria derived for the indicator chemicals are listed in Table 3 (21–36).

4.3 Identification of Populations Potentially Subject to Exposure and Development of Exposure Scenarios (Step 5)

Air emissions consisting primarily of dust and volatile organic chemicals will result from the proposed excavation activities at the site. Since excavation will necessitate removal of the surface cap and continual disturbance of the waste, the emissions of volatile organic chemicals are likely to be considerably greater than those past emissions that resulted in odor complaints from nearby residents and railroad workers during 1983.

In order to evaluate potential off site chemical exposures, eight receptor locations were selected from census blocks within $\frac{1}{2}$ mile (700 m) from the site. These include two receptor locations within a subdivision of approximately 60 single-family homes adjacent to the west side of the site, one that is the closest residence to the site (approximately 100 m) and the other that is further west, approximately halfway through the subdivision. Two additional receptor locations were selected on an island approximately 300 m north of the site. The island is presently zoned industrial and is largely deserted except for a coal-fired power plant. It was selected, however, to provide a very conservative estimate of exposures to the closest residences in a town located approximately 800 m north of the site.

To the east, the nearest residential area is located more than 1000 m from the site. Since concentrations are expected to be significantly diluted by dispersion in this 1000-m distance, no receptors were selected at the town. Finally, four receptor locations were selected to the south of the site. These were located in the nearest census blocks of an area that contained several hundred single-family homes and a recreational facility.

The overall population at risk comprises all individuals who may be exposed to vapors and dust released from the site. In estimating the public health risk that might be associated with the proposed excavation, two population groups at risk of exposure who are of particular concern were identified. These are women and young children living near the site who may spend much of their time at home. The potential exposures of these two groups were modeled in this assessment.

Other groups would also be anticipated to receive some exposure but would receive less than the two groups identified because they would likely spend less time in the neighborhood of the site. These would include residents in the area who work during the day away from their homes, railroad workers who might spend some of their time in the area of the railroad tracks adjacent to the site, hikers or hunters who might walk through the area adjacent to the site, and visitors to local residences. Workers involved in the excavation work might also be exposed, but it was assumed that they would use appropriate protective equipment (e.g., coveralls, breathing apparatus or respirators) and consequently their potential exposures and associated risks were not estimated.

In addition, for purposes of this analysis, it was assumed that individuals, particularly children, would be restricted by security measures from entering the site during

TABLE 4. Assumptions Used in Modeling Human Exposure[a]

	Adult Female	Preschool Child
Body weight (kg)	58	17
Breathing rate (m³/h)	0.875	0.333
Days per lifetime	28,105	25,550
Daily exposure (h/day)	20	20
Days of exposure during excavation of west lagoon area[a]	60	60
Days of exposure during excavation of east lagoon area[b]	60	60
Total soil ingestion (kg/day)	—	0.001
Fraction of soil contaminated[c]	—	0.1

[a]The values listed are those adopted by the Task Group on Reference Man of the International Commission on Radiological Protection (43).
[b]Although the entire excavation process is estimated to last 5–6 months, it was assumed that only 4 months will be required to excavate the contaminated soil. The remainder of the period would involve handling of noncontaminated material.
[c]Not all the soil a child might ingest would be contaminated since only some would represent dust from the excavation site. For the purpose of this assessment, it was assumed that 10% is fallout from the excavation.

excavation. Therefore, potential exposures resulting from direct contact with the contaminated soil onsite were not modeled in this assessment.

In modeling the exposure of the two groups of concern, it was assumed that both adult females and preschool children are present at their residences 20 h/day and are exposed to chemical vapors volatilized during the excavation process and to contaminated particulate material (dust) generated during excavation. In addition, children may receive additional exposure by ingestion of contaminated dust from the excavation settling in and around the home. Of the total soil ingested by a child per day, it was assumed that 10% represents fallout of contaminated dust from the site. Some exposure would also come from dermal contact with contaminated dust, but preliminary calculations indicated that exposure would be trivial by this route compared to the other routes modeled. The assumptions listed in Table 4 (43) were used in estimating the exposures of the two groups of concern.

4.4   Development of Estimates of Environmental Concentrations and Resultant Human Intake (Step 6)

The air concentrations of chemicals to which individuals residing at the eight receptor locations might be exposed during the excavation were estimated based on the concentrations of the various indicator chemicals in the soil to be excavated, knowledge of their physical and chemical properties (44) (e.g., volatility), the characteristics of the soil matrix, and weather conditions anticipated during the excavation period (i.e., wind speed, frequency, and direction, precipitation data, and temperature) (45).

Chemicals would be released in the form of vapor through two processes. First, volatilization occurs from the surface of freshly exposed excavated soil. Vapor loss by this process is enhanced by the mixing of soil as a result of onsite excavation activities. Activities such as bulldozing, front-end loading, mixing with chemical adsorbents, and transfer operations (loading and unloading) increase volatilization because of the increased air–soil contact generated by these operations. Vapor emission rates were developed for this process by using chemical-specific mass transfer coefficients (46, 47) and average areas of exposed contaminated soil based on anticipated daily soil removal rates.

The second process causing vapor loss is diffusion of chemical vapor as a result of the concentration gradient existing between the uncontaminated ambient air and the vapor in the soil pore spaces. Several authors have solved second-order differential equations to simulate the transport of vapors through soil (48, 49). The analytical solutions to these equations generally differ due to the initial and boundary conditions that are applied to the differential equations. These conditions are designated according to the specific situation being modeled (i.e., the nature and distribution of waste at the site of interest, and the variation in source concentrations with time). The following important assumptions were required for the derivation of the vapor flux due to diffusion from the contaminated soil:

1. The concentration of chemical in the air at the soil surface is negligible.
2. The chemicals are uniformly distributed through the soil column.
3. The porosity is constant in both time and space.
4. Diffusion in air is the rate-controlling step, with all other partitioning occurring instantly.
5. Adsorption is reversible.
6. No transport of chemical by water movement occurs.

Assumption 1 is generally valid, even at low wind speeds, for most chemicals except for the high molecular weight compounds (e.g., pesticides). The second assumption is a simplification since the chemical distribution at a site is rarely uniform. However, since long-term average exposures were being evaluated, assuming a uniform concentration distribution will not significantly affect overall exposure estimates. Assumption 3 is valid for the fairly homogeneous unsaturated zone above the bedrock at the site. The fourth assumption is true for most of the indicator compounds since they were generally both soluble and volatile. Adsorption (assumption 5) has been demonstrated to be a reversible process; however, recent studies have shown hysteresis to occur to some extent leaving some irreversible adsorption for certain chemicals and soil types. This was not a concern at the site since the compound contributing primarily to the risk (i.e., 1, 2, 3-trichloropropane) was present at high concentrations, and significant concentrations were expected to exist following excavation. Finally, upward transport of chemicals by water movement, often termed the *wicking effect*, is restricted to the top inch or two of soil. Chemical transport by wicking to the surface is insignificant at greater depths. Leaching of chemicals may occur to some extent; however, measures would be taken at the site to minimize infiltration (e.g., application of a tarpaulin cover at night, as well as runoff control measures).

Using these assumptions, an analytical solution for diffusional transport through soil was developed (48) and applied to estimate vapor emission rates.

Dust emissions from the site were based on the materials handling sequence as reported in the excavation plan for the site. The quantity of material to be removed daily and the nature of the equipment used for excavation were also specified in the excavation plan. For quantifying dust emissions onsite, the excavation activities were divided into eight operational categories:

TABLE 5. Important Physicochemical Properties Used in Estimating Emission Rates

Chemical	Molecular Weight (g/g mole)	Vapor Pressure (mm Hg)	Diffusion Coefficient (cm^2/s)	Henry's Law Constant (atm·m^3/mole)	Partition Coefficient (K_{oc}) (cm^3/g)
Chlorobenzene	112.56	11.8	0.0682	3.21E − 03	330
2-Chlorophenol	128.56	2.3	0.0703	8.07E − 06	73
Cresols	108.13	0.24	0.0749	6.96E − 07	21.9
1,2-Dichlorobenzene	147.01	1.5	0.0658	1.67E − 03	1,700
2,4-Dimethylphenol	122.17	0.062	0.0685	8.90E − 07	96
Ethylbenzene	106.16	7	0.0627	5.88E − 03	1,100
Nitrobenzene	123.11	0.15	0.0659	1.03E − 05	36
Phenol	94.11	0.341	0.0777	2.57E − 07	14.2
Tetrachloroethylene	165.83	14	0.0728	1.41E − 02	364
Toluene	92.15	28.6	0.0776	6.01E − 03	300
1,2,4-Trichlorobenzene	181.46	0.42	0.0621	2.02E − 03	13,000
1,2,3-Trichloropropane	147.43	1.16	0.0605	9.69E − 04	295
Xylene	106.17	3.346	0.0674	3.56E − 03	363

1. Bulldozing/front-end loading of material.
2. Wind erosion of the active excavation areas.
3. Loading into haul trucks.
4. Onsite haul by trucks.
5. Dump from haul trucks at load-out area.
6. Loading operations into haul trailers.
7. On site haul by trailers.
8. General excavation activities.

Dust emission rates corresponding to each operational category were determined from emission factors published in a U.S. EPA compilation of air pollution emission factors (50). The dust estimates were determined for short-term (10 working hours) and long-term (total duration of excavation) conditions. The short-term value applies to the anticipated daily 10 h of active operation at the site. Emissions are not expected during nonworking hours since measures to prevent dust generation (e.g., the application of a tarpaulin cover) will be instituted at the end of each working day. The long-term average emission rate was estimated from the short-term rate by factoring the nonworking hours. Since the excavation will be conducted for 10 h/day and 5 days/week (i.e., 50 working hours per week), the long-term emission rate will be lower than the short-term rate by a factor of 0.298 (i.e., 50 working hours/168 total hours per week).

The calculated long-term average emission rates, as described above, were used as inputs to the industrial source complex atmospheric dispersion model in long-term mode (ISCLT) developed by the EPA to predict vapor and particulate air concentrations at nearby residences (51). In addition, a Gaussian plume model, based on Briggs dispersion coefficients, was applied, using the short-term emission rates, in order to estimate short-term exposures that could result to downwind receptors when the excavation progressed to areas of the site containing the highest contaminant concentrations (52–54), Table 5

TABLE 6. Predicted Air Concentrations (Vapor Plus Particulates) at the Closest Residence

Chemical	Predicted Long-Term Air Concentration (mg/m^3) from Excavation		Predicted Short-Term Air Concentration (mg/m^3) from Excavation	
	West Lagoons	East Lagoons	West Lagoons	East Lagoons
Chlorobenzene	8.38E − 03	4.78E − 03	1.05E + 00	1.11E + 00
2-Chlorophenol	7.97E − 06	2.32E − 06	1.69E − 03	0.00E + 00
Cresols	3.38E − 05	7.14E − 06	1.52E − 03	1.88E − 04
1, 2-Dichlorobenzene	3.26E − 04	5.15E − 04	2.39E − 02	2.32E − 02
2, 4-Dimethylphenol	2.30E − 06	2.42E − 07	3.49E − 04	4.90E − 05
Ethylbenzene	2.50E − 01	5.77E − 02	7.23E + 00	3.31E + 00
Nitrobenzene	1.52E − 04	3.39E − 05	1.10E − 02	6.31E − 03
Phenol	4.00E − 06	4.14E − 05	8.66E − 04	3.91E − 05
Tetrachloroethylene	7.87E − 02	6.36E − 04	1.65E + 01	4.48E − 01
Toluene	7.75E − 02	1.42E − 01	1.06E + 01	8.29E + 00
1, 2, 4-Trichlorobenzene	5.30E − 05	2.39E − 04	3.38E − 03	2.70E − 02
1, 2, 3-Trichloropropane	1.84E − 01	6.26E − 02	2.61E + 00	1.18E + 00
Xylene	3.92E − 01	1.33E − 01	5.78E + 00	2.51E + 00

TABLE 7. Estimated Average and Maximum Daily Doses from Inhalation of Contaminants at the Closest Residence

Indicator Chemical	Inhalation (Vapor Plus Particulates) Average Daily Dose (ADD) (mg/kg·day, Subchronic Exposure)		Inhalation (Vapor Plus Particulates) Maximum Daily Dose (MDD) (mg/kg·day, Acute Exposure)	
	Adult Female	Preschool Child	Adult Female	Preschool Child
Chlorobenzene	2.53E − 02	3.28E − 03	1.39E − 01	1.80E − 01
2-Chlorophenol	2.40E − 06	3.12E − 06	2.12E − 04	2.76E − 04
Cresols	1.02E − 05	1.33E − 05	2.02E − 05	2.63E − 04
1, 2-Dichlorobenzene	1.55E − 04	2.02E − 04	3.00E − 03	3.89E − 03
2, 4-Dimethylphenol	6.96E − 07	9.00E − 07	3.78E − 05	4.90E − 05
Ethylbenzene	7.56E − 02	9.81E − 02	9.00E − 01	1.18E − 00
Nitrobenzene	4.58E − 05	5.95E − 05	1.39E − 03	1.80E − 03
Phenol	1.25E − 05	1.62E − 05	2.46E − 03	3.20E − 03
Tetrachloroethylene	5.25E − 05[a]	7.53E − 05[a]	2.06E − 00	2.68E − 00
Toluene	4.29E − 02	5.57E − 02	1.34E − 00	1.73E − 00
1, 2, 4-Trichlorobenzene	7.22E − 05	9.36E − 05	3.39E − 03	4.40E − 03
1, 2, 3-Trichloropropane	1.59E − 04[a]	2.27E − 04[a]	3.28E − 01	4.26E − 01
Xylene	1.18E − 01	1.53E − 01	7.33E − 01	9.53E − 01

[a]Lifetime average daily dose (for carcinogens).

presents the important physicochemical properties used in estimating emission rates and Table 6 presents the resultant long-term and short-term air concentrations of contaminants predicted at the residence in closest proximity of the site. The short-term concentrations have been averaged over a 24-h period. It was estimated that more than 90% of the tetrachloroethylene in the soil could be released into the air during excavation because of its high volatility. 1, 2, 3-Trichloropropane and xylene are less volatile, but still 20–30% and 10–15%, respectively, of the chemicals in the soil were estimated to be released into the air. If excavation and removal operations extended into warmer months, the potential for volatile emissions would be higher. Table 7 presents the average and maximum daily doses estimated by the inhalation route, for adult females and preschool children at the closest residence. Appendix A describes more fully the methodology for estimating daily doses (and risk) associated with the excavation process.

4.5   Estimation of Risks Associated with the Excavation Process (Step 7)

4.5.1   General Public Health Risk Assessment.
Potential risks to offsite populations associated with the excavation process were modeled for several routes of exposure: inhalation of vapor and contaminated particulates and ingestion of contaminated particulates. The results of these analyses are presented in the following discussion.

4.5.1.1   Subchronic Exposure

INHALATION OF VAPOR AND PARTICULATES. As described above, based on estimates of average concentrations of each indicator chemical anticipated in the vapor and particulate phases during the excavation process, human daily doses via inhalation for adult females and children were calculated (step 6). Potential cancer risks were then estimated for tetrachloroethylene and 1, 2, 3-trichloropropane. For individuals at the location of the closest residence (about 100 m west of the site), the estimated upper-bound lifetime risks from tetrachloroethylene do not exceed 10^{-6} (1 case in 1 million exposed individuals) at any of the eight locations modeled. For 1, 2, 3-trichloropropane, the upper-bound risks exceed 10^{-6} at all eight locations modeled. For both of these chemicals the vast majority (more than 99%) of the exposure, and hence the risk, comes from the vapor-phase exposure. Inhalation of chemicals attached to dust particles contributed only slightly (less than 1%) to the estimated risk.

For the noncarcinogens, xylene was the only compound for which the average daily exposure was estimated to be in excess of the subchronic ADI. Specifically, daily exposure to xylene is anticipated to be in excess of its subchronic ADI by 20-fold for inhalation by children at the closest residence and by threefold or more at the other locations modeled. In addition, if 1, 2, 3-trichloropropane is not considered to be a carcinogen, exposure to it is estimated to exceed its subchronic ADI at two of the eight locations modeled. Thus, noncarcinogenic toxic effects in local residents due to emissions resulting from the excavation process are possible. As in the case of exposure to tetrachloroethylene and 1, 2, 3-trichloropropane, exposure to the noncarcinogens was estimated to occur largely (more than 99%) as vapor.

INGESTION OF PARTICULATES. In addition to the inhalation of vapors and particulates, ingestion by children of deposited particulates has been modeled. The estimated upper-bound lifetime cancer risks for individuals at the location of the closest residence from ingestion of dust contaminated with tetrachloroethylene and 1, 2, 3-trichloropropane are 1.3×10^{-7} and 5.3×10^{-6}, respectively. In addition, the subchronic ADI for xylene is predicted to be exceeded by ninefold.

4.5.1.2   Acute Exposure. The risk estimates described above are based on the *average* concentrations of the indicator chemicals in the soil. We have also examined the maximum daily doses (MDDs) that local residents might receive on days when the most contaminated portions of the site are excavated and compared those doses to acute ADIs, as defined in Table 3. In no case did the MDD for any of the indicator chemicals exceed the corresponding acute ADI. The MDDs were less than 6% of the respective acute ADIs for all indicator chemicals, suggesting that significant acute toxic effects would not be anticipated from the excavation.

4.5.1.3   Summary of Health Risks. Table 8 lists the lifetime cancer risk estimates and average daily dose to acceptable daily intake ratios (ADD/ADI) for all the indicator chemicals for the location of the closest residence. In this table, the risks of inhalation and ingestion exposure have been combined for children. For both adults and preschool children, the estimated upper-bound total cancer risk (risks from tetrachloroethylene and 1, 2, 3-trichloropropane combined) is in excess of 10^{-6} (1 case in 1 million exposed individuals) and the predicted average daily dose for xylene exceeds its subchronic ADI. In addition, for the preschool child, the ADD/ADI ratio for 1, 2, 3-trichloropropane was exceeded by a factor of 1.5. The cancer risk estimates resulting from exposure to 1, 2, 3-trichloropropane will be revised when the results of the NTP bioassay are made available. (See Appendix A for a detailed description of methodology for estimating cancer and noncancer risks).

TABLE 8. Summary of Risk Estimates for Closest Residents[a]

	Adult Female		Preschool Child[b]	
Indicator Chemical	Cancer Risk[c]	ADD/ADI[d]	Cancer Risk[c]	ADD/ADI[d]
Chlorobenzene		6.32E − 02		8.83E − 02
2-Chlorophenol		5.46E − 05		1.32E − 04
Cresols		3.40E − 04		1.30E − 03
1, 2-Dichlorobenzene		2.32E − 04		4.60E − 04
2, 4-Dimethylphenol		1.16E − 03		7.95E − 03
Ethylbenzene		7.27E − 02		9.90E − 02
Nitrobenzene		1.76E − 02		3.29E − 02
Phenol		6.24E − 04		7.24E − 03
Tetrachloroethylene	8.93E − 08	—	2.58E − 07	—
Toluene	—	3.70E − 02	—	5.38E − 02
1, 2, 4-Trichlorobenzene	—	3.61E − 03	—	1.50E − 02
1, 2, 3-Trichloropropane	1.59E − 05	9.74E − 01	2.80E − 05	1.49E + 00
Xylene	—	1.15E + 01	—	2.03E + 01

[a]Derived using concentration estimates for coordinate, approximately 100 m west of the site.
[b]Dose estimates *combine* oral and inhalation exposures.
[c]Calculated by multiplying total lifetime average daily dose of chemical by the unit cancer risk estimate (risk = LADD × UCR).
[d]Calculated by dividing the average daily dose (ADD) received on days on which excavation occurs by the subchronic ADI. These values are based on the *higher* of the east and west lagoon air concentrations (resulting in the higher ADDs).

4.5.1.4 Odor. Although not a health concern, chemical odors that may be present during some, if not all, of the period of excavation would likely be disruptive and of concern to local residents. Besides the chemicals disposed of at the site, decomposition products such as sulfur-containing compounds are likely to be released as a result of the excavation and are a source of potential odors downwind. In order to assess the probability of chemical odors, the lowest reported odor thresholds for the indicator chemicals (55) were compared with the anticipated subchronic average concentrations and highest daily concentrations at the location of the closest residence. This comparison indicated that the lowest reported odor threshold for xylene and toluene would be exceeded by the average concentration at the closest residence throughout the excavation process. Also, 1, 2, 3-trichloropropane, which is anticipated to be present at high concentrations (up to 1.09 mg/m^3, about 0.18 ppm) in the air, is known to have a strong irritating odor at higher concentrations (50–100 ppm), though an odor threshold value was not identified.

In addition to the chemicals of greatest concern with regard to public health risks, very high proportions of several other less toxic chemicals could be released by the excavation process. On days when the most contaminated areas are excavated, the concentrations of several of the chemicals would exceed their odor thresholds; that is, unpleasant chemical odors would occur, though no acute toxic effects are predicted.

4.5.2 Assessment of Transportation Issues. In addition to assessing the risks associated with the site excavation to surrounding residents, an attempt was made to estimate the risk associated with transporting the waste offsite. It is clear that such transportation of waste will increase the number of people potentially exposed to the contaminated material. Chemical waste landfill sites in four states could potentially receive the contaminated material. An EPA-permitted landfill 600 miles from the site was modeled as the final destination of excavated material for this analysis. The contaminated waste material could be transported to the disposal site by truck or train, according to the design document.

If the truck haul option is used to transport the contaminated material, trucks would be required to drive approximately 600 miles, with each truck carrying about 14 yd^3 (20 tons) of material. About 3015 truck trips would be required to haul all the contaminated material.

If railroads were used to transport the contaminated material, trains would travel about 650 miles. Here containers of contaminated material, each containing about 20 yd^3 (28.5 tons), would be lifted by crane from railcars onto trucks. The trucks would then drive through a populated area to the landfill. According to the design document, 88 train shipments, each with 24 closed, plastic-lined "dumpster" containers on 12 open, gondola railcars would be required to transport the contaminated material.

4.5.2.1   Risks Associated with a Spill Incident. Based on rates published by the U.S. Department of Transportation, Federal Highway Administration (17), and the U.S. Congressional Office of Technology Assessment (OTA) (19), as many as eight truck spill incidents could potentially occur somewhere along the 600-mile truck haul route during the 5–6-month haul period. Applying incident rates drawn from a draft report of the Association of American Railroads (18) concerning statistical trends in rail hazardous material safety from 1978 to 1984 and data from OTA (19), it was estimated that as many as one to three train incidents involving a spill could occur during the entire series of rail shipments.

The potential human and environmental risks associated with the spill of contaminated material from the site on land are likely to be small. This is because the total amount of dust and vapors from a single spill pile that would be carried into a surrounding neighborhood would be limited and would likely be contained and cleaned up promptly. A spill on land, however, could be potentially disruptive and of concern to the residents in proximity to the site or to communities along the truck route.

A spill of excavated material (or runoff from a spill pile) into a stream or river could potentially expose fish, aquatic organisms, and humans to contaminants through dermal contact or ingestion. Specific exposures are difficult to estimate given uncertainties such as cleanup response time and the size and characteristics of the stream. To evaluate the impacts on water quality in the event of a spill in a worst-case scenario, we assumed that 14 yd^3 or 20 tons of contaminated material (a full truck trailer load) were spilled and deposited in a stream. We adopted and used as a screening tool a simple chemical desorption model (20) to estimate average concentrations of contaminants immediately downstream from a spill of contaminated material in a stream and the length of time required to deplete the contaminated material of soluble contaminants.

The model estimated that all the chemicals in the contaminated material theoretically would go into solution after being deposited in the river. Under certain circumstances, some contaminants, including xylene, 1, 2, 4-trichlorobenzene, ethylbenzene, 1, 2-dichlorobenzene, tetrachloroethylene, and 1, 2, 3-trichloropropane, could take days to desorb fully from the spill pile, if cleanup were not promptly initiated.

4.5.3   Potential for Recontamination of New Fill Soil. Following excavation of contaminated soils and waste materials, clean topsoil will be placed atop the east and west pit areas. According to the design document, two feet of clean soil will be placed over each area. Additional fill will be placed in the east pit to fill in the low areas and to provide positive drainage. The proposed excavation will not include bedrock; therefore, a large quantity of DNAPL will still exist in the bedrock above the water table beneath the former lagoons. The chemicals that comprise the DNAPL are volatile organic chemicals. Therefore, it is likely that vapors from the DNAPL in the unsaturated zone beneath the lagoon will migrate upward into the clean fill and result in contamination of the formerly clean fill material.

Vapor transport model simulations provided to the authors indicate that vapor migration and contamination of the clean fill throughout its depth will occur over a period of 0.5–25 years, depending on the thickness of the fill. Based on these simulations, the upward migration of vapors will contaminate the soil to levels greater than those specified by the original excavation plan. Hence, excavating the contaminated soil and replacing it with new soil will not result in the desired objective of eliminating contaminated soil from the site.

5 DISCUSSION

The presence of an uncontrolled hazardous waste site close to a residential area is undesirable. Although the site does not appear to present an imminent hazard to the neighboring residents, the presence of high concentrations of a variety of organic chemicals in the soil of the former lagoons provides the opportunity for future risk and some remedial action should be taken. Chemicals remaining onsite at present soil concentrations would limit future development of the site and could lead to unacceptable health risks.

Plans have been prepared for excavating the soil from the site, transporting it offsite and disposing of it in a RCRA-permitted landfill. We have attempted to assess the potential exposures and resulting public health risks associated with this proposed excavation of the contaminated soils at the site.

5.1 Summary of Findings

The following summarizes our major findings:

1. Several potential routes of exposure were identified in this risk assessment. Of the exposure routes evaluated, inhalation of vapor generated as a result of excavation activities was identified as the major contributor to public health risks.

2. Owing to the nature and toxicity of the chemicals at the site, the proposed excavation could result in carcinogenic and noncarcinogenic health risks to nearby residents. The chemicals of greatest concern at the site are tetrachloroethylene, 1, 2, 3,-trichloropropane, and xylene.

3. On the basis of estimates of releases of 1, 2, 3-trichloropropane and tetrachloro-ethylene from contaminated soil during the excavation process, the upper-bound risk of cancer to the local residents could be as high as three new cases of cancer per lifetime in 100,000 exposed individuals, or a 3×10^{-5} risk.

4. During the overall 6-month period of excavation, noncarcinogenic effects in local residents could potentially occur since average daily exposures to 1, 2, 3-trichloropropane and xylene modeled from median concentrations in soil could exceed their respective

subchronic ADIs. In the case of xylene, a 12–20-fold ADI exceedance was estimated.

5. Acute toxic effects in local residents associated with the excavation would not be expected. For all indicator chemicals, the potential maximum daily exposures that could occur on the days when the most contaminated portions of the site were excavated (modeled from maximum concentrations in soil) were less than 6% of the respective acute ADIs.

6. Based on calculations, the airborne concentrations of several of the volatile chemicals released during the excavation would exceed their odor thresholds.

7. While available transportation incident data suggest a spill incident would likely occur during the transportation of contaminated material offsite, the potential public health and environmental risks associated with such spills are estimated to be small.

8. Upward migration of vapors from the dense nonaqueous phase liquid (DNAPL) in the unsaturated bedrock beneath the former lagoons will recontaminate clean fill placed in excavated areas to levels greater than those specified in the original excavation plan. Therefore, excavating the contaminated soil and replacing it with new soil will not result in the desired objective of eliminating contaminated soil from the site.

Given these findings, we conclude that the proposed excavation at the site presents health and welfare risks to local residents which are sufficient to warrant a reevaluation of the excavation plan and consideration of alternative remedial options.

6.2 Uncertainties and Limitations in the Assessment

In attempting to assess the risks associated with the proposed excavation of a hazardous waste site, we have employed methodologies that allow for the systematic organization, analysis, and presentation of information related to the potential for releases of and human exposures to contaminants detected at the site. It should be recognized that such methodologies for risk assessment represent an inexact science, whose application is associated with limitations and uncertainties. Uncertainties arise because of the general need to make a relatively large number of assumptions and inferences to complete each of the involved steps. Some of these assumptions and inferences are needed to compensate for lack of data on the chemical of interest, or for gaps in the data available to estimate exposure. The following summarizes the major uncertainties and limitations inherent in this analysis.

5.2.1 *Limitations in Sampling Data.* In most environmental analyses, the sampling results available for estimating human exposure have limitations in quality and quantity. The shortcomings are many, including errors inherent in the sampling and analysis procedures, the failure to take an adequate number of samples to arrive at an accurate chemical distribution, and the variability of chemical concentrations in the medium under investigation. In this specific case, the sampling programs were designed to identify the overall extent of organic contamination and delineate the limits of excavation, but they were not intended to provide chemical concentration–depth profiles and distribution details desirable for conducting a risk assessment. Consequently, the results of our analysis are only as accurate as the available sampling data. In spite of the lack of ideal data, we belive the current data set is sufficient for reaching the conclusions presented.

5.2.2 *Limitations of the Excavation Plan.* In order to estimate emissions resulting from excavation we were provided details on the construction of the decontamination

area, upgrading of the existing site access road, and the quantities of contaminated material to be excavated. We were required, however, to make assumptions on some of the specifics of the excavation to estimate emissions.

In particular, in estimating vapor emissions, it was necessary to make assumptions regarding daily removal of soil in horizontal layers, the areal extent of contamination at different depths, the extent of mixing of contaminated soil and the duration of the mixing operations, the efficiency of the dust suppression practices and the control of emissions during nonworking hours, and the presence and dimensions of soil storage piles in the vicinity of the excavated area.

5.2.3   General Limitations and Uncertainties in Toxicity Data. Risk assessment involves extrapolation and inference from experimental data to predict the probability of adverse health effects under certain conditions of exposure to chemical or physical agents. Because of this need for extrapolation, there is some uncertainty in the conclusions that can be reached. This uncertainty is related primarily to limitations in the available toxicity data and in our knowledge of its applicability to the conditions of human exposure under consideration.

5.2.3.1   Limitations in the Available Toxicity Data. Limitations in toxicity data arise for several reasons. First, there are differences in our degree of knowledge of the toxic effects of different chemicals. Some chemicals have been extensively studied under a variety of conditions of exposure in several species, including humans. Others may have been little studied. This variability in the availability of toxicity data on the indicator chemicals necessitated our making a number of assumptions in the present analysis. For example, to estimate an ADI for 2, 4-dimethylphenol, it was necessary to rely on the very limited available data on a structurally related chemical, 2, 6-dimethylphenol. In the case of 1, 2, 3-trichloropropane, carcinogenicity testing is currently in progress, but the National Toxicology Program (NTP) test results are not yet available. For this assessment, a hypothetical cancer potency value was used in order to estimate the risk associated with the high concentration of this contaminant found at the site. This value will be revised after the release of the NTP results. In our judgment, such inferences were justified in order to reach initial conclusions about the risks associated with the proposed excavation.

5.2.3.2   Uncertainties in Extrapolation. Because data are unavailable that specifically identify the hazards to humans associated with the likely conditions of exposure to the various chemicals of concern, the potential hazards must be inferred by extrapolating from results obtained under other conditions of exposure, generally in experimental animals. Uncertainties are thereby introduced because the results obtained in one species must be extrapolated to another and from one set of exposure conditions to another.

5.2.4   General Limitations in Determining the Degree of Exposure

5.2.4.1   Uncertainties in Emission Estimates. The exposure concentrations were developed from a consideration of the emission sources associated with the proposed excavation. The emission data used in the present study have been derived from applicable published equations for vapor and dust emissions and the best available information on the excavation methods and characteristics of the contaminated soil. A number of assumptions about site-specific characteristics were made to carry out these calculations (e.g., soil moisture content), which necessarily introduce uncertainty into the results.

5.2.4.2 Uncertainties in the Dispersion Modeling. The long-term dispersion of particulate and vapor emissions from excavation activities was simulated in this study using the industrial source complex-long term (ISCLT) model, developed by the EPA. This model is generally recognized as being suitable for this type of application.

Although mathematical dispersion modeling is a generally accepted method of predicting exposures to airborne contaminants, the validity of the results may be affected by inaccuracies in the input data or the mathematical representation implicit in the model. Specifically in the present case, uncertainties may have been introduced due to the use of meterological data from a station 4 miles away. In order to assess the likely inaccuracies introduced by utilizing available meteorological data as representative of onsite conditions, a series of sensitivity analyses were conducted in which the effects of topographic and diurnal factors were tested. The results of the sensitivity analyses indicated relatively small variations in concentrations at the critical receptor (located approximately 100 m west of the site) as a result of possible inaccuracies in the meteorological data base. Combined with a potential model accuracy of $\pm 50\%$ (assuming representative climatology), the concentrations at the receptor could vary within a factor of approximately 2.5 of the "base case" projection. This was considered to not represent a significant change in the calculated risk of exposure to contaminants.

5.2.5 Uncertainties in Hypothetical Exposure Scenarios.

The exposure scenarios developed in this analysis were intended to model conservatively the pattern of exposure that would be associated with the proposed excavation (i.e., to result in estimates that would likely be higher than actual exposures). The scenarios depict an adult female and a preschool child who spend all but 4 h/day at home on days when excavation would occur. This scenario would clearly overestimate the exposure of individuals who work away from their home or children who attend nursery school or a day care facility distant from the site. Such individuals would be likely to spend at least 12 h/day at home, however. Thus, their exposure (at least by inhalation) would be within a factor of 2 of the scenarios modeled.

For estimating dose levels and health risks associated with inhalation, it was assumed that absorption of inhaled vapors and retention of chemicals on particulates in animal studies and in the selected human populations at risk are equivalent. Experimental and clinical data are unavailable to verify this assumption. To the extent that the volume of air breathed per minute varies according to the amount of physical work being done, and body weight varies from individual to individual, there will be some further uncertainty in the exposure estimates. These sources of uncertainty are likely smaller than many of those contributing to the overall uncertainty, however.

A greater source of uncertainty comes from the fact that the exposure model assumes that individuals will be exposed to the vapor and dust concentrations predicted by the modeling whether they are inside or outside. This may overestimate exposure for individuals spending most of their time indoors. However, since the great majority of the inhalation exposure anticipated comes from vapor, and since these vapors would be expected to infiltrate houses just as uncontaminated air does, the assumption was made that contaminant concentrations inside and outside the house would be equal.

Greater uncertainty exists in the modeling of ingestion of contaminated dust by children. The value of total soil ingestion used in this scenario, 1 g, represents a relatively low estimate of how much soil a child with pica (an abnormal desire to eat substances not normally eaten) might consume in 1 day (56). Estimates of soil consumption by children with pica have ranged up to 10 g (57). However, recent experimental data suggest that the typical ingestion of soil in preschool children is approximately 56 mg/day (56, 58). It was further assumed that 10% of total soil ingestion represents contaminated dust, on the basis that not all the soil that a child might consume would be comprised of contaminated dust. Because there is currently no firm support or guidance available in this area, this assumption was necessarily arbitrary.

The ingestion scenario also assumes that the contaminated soil that is ingested contains the average concentrations of the indicator chemicals found in the soil to be excavated. This will tend to overestimate average exposure because it does not take into consideration the loss of chemicals from the soil that will occur due to volatilization. This does not have a substantial impact on the overall risk estimate, however, because this route of exposure contributes only a small fraction of the total estimated risk.

5.2.6   Limitations in Transportation Analysis. In considering the qualitative and quantitative results of the transportation risk analysis, it should be acknowledged that uncertainties exist about the residual concentrations in the contaminated soil leaving the site. A change in the operational sequence of excavation may affect the residual concentrations in the soil and therefore affect the hazards involved in shipping the excavated soil. In addition, there is uncertainty regarding the applicability of the available transportation incident data to the case at hand. This uncertainty may have resulted in an overestimation or underestimation of the potential for a spill incident.

5.2.7   Interpretation of Results in the Context of Uncertainties. Because of the various uncertainties associated with this and most any environmental risk assessment, the results should not be considered precise predictions of risks. Rather, they represent upper-bound estimates of the potential for adverse effects in populations in the vicinity of the site under consideration. While such upper-bound risk estimates are clearly not absolute, they provide a "red flag" to regulators and decisionmakers that exposures may be unacceptable. The acceptability of risk, however, is ultimately a policy decision that in practice has tended to vary with the nature of exposure (i.e., occupational, environmental) (59, 60). In determining risk acceptability, the degree of uncertainty in the assessment should also be taken into consideration.

In the current analysis, we attempted to make explicit the assumptions applied and the reasons for their selection. While most of the techniques used for compensating for these uncertainties (e.g., the use of large safety factors and conservative extrapolation models) are designed to err on the side of safety, exceptions may exist. For example, in the case of poorly studied chemicals the possibility exists that the chemical may in fact be more toxic than anticipated. Clearly, the diversity of chemicals and potential exposure routes associated with chemical waste disposal sites make it generally necessary to apply a large number of assumptions in estimating exposure and risk. Provided that the uncertainties and limitations associated with such assumptions are carefully considered, the results of risk assessments can assist decisionmakers by providing an approximate quantification of the upper-bound of the potential risk to public health posed by anticipated releases of chemicals into the environment.

REFERENCES

1. J. V. Rodricks, Risk assessment at hazardous waste disposal sites. *Hazard. Waste* **1**(3), 333–362 (1984).

2. H. S. Brown, A critical review of current approaches to determining "How clean is clean" at hazardous waste sites. *Hazard. Waste Hazard. Mater.* **3**(3), 233–260 (1986).

3. W. W. Budd, A comparison of three risk assessment techniques for evaluating a hazardous waste landfill. *Hazard. Waste Hazard. Mater.* **3**(3), 309–320 (1986).

4. K. D. Walker and C. Hagger, Practical use of risk assessment in the selection of a remedial alternative. *Natl. Conf. Manag. Uncontrolled Hazard. Waste Sites, 5th, 1984*, pp. 321–325 (1984).

5. R. Morgan, K. Plourd, L. Smith, and T. Tyburski, Use of endangerment assessment procedures at superfund enforcement sites. *Natl. Conf. Manag. Uncontrolled Hazard. Waste Sites, 6th, 1985*, pp. 396–402 (1985).

6. C. Winklehaus, B. Turnham, and S. Golojuch, Application of U.S. EPA superfund health assessment methodology to several major superfund sites. *Natl. Conf. Uncontrolled Hazard. Waste Sites, 6th, 1985*, pp. 423–428 (1985).

7. National Research Council, *Risk Assessment in the Federal Government: Managing the Process.* National Academy Press, Washington, DC, 1983.

8. Environmental Protection Agency, Guidelines for carcinogen risk assessment. *Fed. Regist.* **51**(185), 33992–34003 (1986).

9. U.S. Food and Drug Administration, Sponsored compounds in food-producing animals: Criteria and procedures for evaluating the safety of carcinogenic residues. *Fed. Regist.* **50**, 45530–45556 (1985).

10. U.S. Environmental Protection Agency, *Superfund Public Health Evaluation Manual*, OSWER Directive 9285-4-1. Office of Emergency and Remedial Response, Office of Solid Waste and Emergency Response, USEPA, Washington, DC, 1986.

11. National Research Council, *Drinking Water and Health*, Vol. 3. National Academy Press, Washington, DC, 1980.

12. E. J. Calabrese, *Principles of Animal Extrapolation.* Wiley, New York, 1982.

13. M. L. Dourson and J. F. Starra, Regulatory history and experimental support of uncertainty (safety) factors. *Regul. Toxicol. Pharmacol.* **3**, 224–238 (1983).

14. C. S. Weil, Statistics vs. safety factors and scientific judgment in the evaluation of safety for man. *Toxicol. Appl. Pharmacol.* **21**, 454–463 (1972).

15. U.S. Environmental Protection Agency, *Health Advisories.* Office of Drinking Water, USEPA, Washington, DC, 1985.

16. American Conference of Governmental Industrial Hygienists, *Documentation of Threshold Limit Values and Biological Exposure Indices*, 5th ed. ACGIH, Cincinnati, OH, 1986.

17. U.S. Department of Transportation, Federal Highway Administration, *The Effect of Truck Size and Weight on Accident Experience*, FHWA Rep. RD-80-137. USDT, Washington, DC, 1981.

18. Association of American Railroads, *Statistical Trends in Railroad Hazardous Material Safety, 1978–1984.* AAR, Washington, DC, 1986.

19. U.S. Congress, Office of Technology Assessment, *Transportation of Hazardous Materials*, OTA-SET-304. U.S. Govt. Printing Office, Washington, DC, 1986.

20. U.S. Environmental Protection Agency, *Water Quality Assessment: A Screening Procedure for Toxic and Conventional Pollutants in Surface and Ground Water*, Part 1. EPA/600/6-85/002a, pp. 434–441. USEPA, Washington, DC, 1985.

21. J. V. Dilley, *Toxic Evaluation of Inhaled Chlorobenzene (monochlorobenzene)*, NTIS PB 276–623. NIOSH, DHEW, Cincinnati, OH, 1977 (as reported in reference 37).

22. V. D. Bubnov, F. N. Yafizov, and S. E. Ogryzkov. Toxic properties of activated o-chlorophenol for white mice and blue foxes. *Tr. VNIIVS,* **33**, 258–263 (1969) (as reported in reference 38).

23. E. R. Uzhdavini, I. K. Astafyeva, A. A. Mamayeva, and G. Z. Bakhtizina. Inhalation toxicity of

o-cresol. *Tr. Ufim Nauchno-Issled Inst. Gig. Profzabol.* **7**, 115–119 (1972) (as reported in reference 39).

24. R. L. Hollingsworth, V. K. Rowe, F. Oyen, T. R. Torkelson, and I. M. Adams, Toxicity of *o*-dichlorobenzene. Studies on animals and industrial experience. *AMA Arch. Ind. Health* **17**, 180–187 (1958) (as reported in reference 40).

25. I. K. Maazik, Dimethylphenol (xylenol) isomers and their standard content in water bodies. *Gig. Sanit.* **9**, 18 (1968) (as reported in reference 41).

26. Z. Bardodej and E. Bardodejona, Biotransformation of ethylbenzene, styrene and alpha-methylstyrene in man. *Am. Ind. Hyg. Assoc. J.* **31**, 206–209 (1970) (as reported in reference 42).

27. B. H. Chin, J. A. McKelvey, T. R. Tyler, L. J. Calisti, S. J. Kozbelt, and L. J. Sullivan, Absorption distribution and excretion of ethylbenzene, ethylcyclohexane and methyethylbenzene isomers in rats. *Bull. Environ. Contam. Toxicol.* **24**, 447–483 (1980).

28. M. A. Wolf, V. K. Rowe, D. D. McCollister, R. L. Hollingsworth, and F. Oyen, Toxicological studies of certain alkylated benzenes and benzene. *AMA Arch. Ind. Health* **14**, 387–398 (1956).

29. T. E. Hamm, Jr., M. Phelps, T. H. Raynor, and R. D. Irons, A 90-day inhalation study of nitrobenzene in F-344 rats, CD rats and B6C3F1 mice. *Toxicologist* **4**, 181 (1984).

30. C. Sandage, Tolerance criteria for continuous inhalation exposure to toxic materials. I. Effects on animals of 90-day exposure to phenol, CCl_4, and a mixture of indole, skatole, H_2S, and methyl mercaptan. *U.S. Air Force Syst. Command, Aeronaut. Syst. Div., Tech. Doc. Rep., ASD* **61–519**(1) (1961).

31. U.S. Environmental Protection Agency, *Health Assessment Document for Tetrachloroethylene (Perchloroethylene)*, EPA/600/8-82/005F, USEPA, Waxhington, DC, 1985.

32. U.S. Environmental Protection Agency, *Toluene. Health Advisory.* Office of Drinking Water, USEPA, Washington, DC, 1985.

33. P. G. Watanabe, R. J. Kociba, R. E. Hefner, Jr., A. O. Yakel, and B. K. J. Leong, Subchronic toxicity studies of 1, 2, 4-trichlorobenzene in experimental animals. *Toxicol. Appl. Pharmacol.* **45**, 322–333 (1978).

34. Hazleton Laboratories America, Inc., Final Report. 120-day toxicity gavage study of 1, 2, 3-trichloropropane in Fischer 344 rats. Submitted to *National Toxicology Program* (1983).

35. U.S. Environmental Protection Agency, *Xylenes. Health Advisory.* Office of Drinking Water, USEPA, Washington, DC, 1985.

36. E. Mirkova, C. Zaikov, G. Antov, A. Mikhailova, L. Khinkova, and I. Benchev, Prenatal toxicity of xylene. *J. Hyg., Epidemiol., Microbiol., Immunol.* **27**, 337–343 (1983).

37. U.S. Environmental Protection Agency, *Chlorobenzene—Health Advisory* (Draft). Office of Drinking Water, USEPA, Washington, DC, 1985.

38. U.S. Environmental Protection Agency, *Ambient Water Quality Criteria for 2-chlorophenol*, 440/5-80-037, PB81-117459. Office of Water Regulations and Standards, Criteria and Standards Division, USEPA, Washington, DC, 1980.

39. U.S. Environmental Protection Agency, *Research and Development. Verified Reference Doses (RFDs) of the U.S. EPA.* ADI Work Group of the Risk Assessment Forum, USEPA, Washington, DC, 1986.

40. U.S. Environmental Protection Agency, *Health Assessment Document for Chlorinated Benzenes*, EPA/600/8-84/015A. Office of Health and Environmental Assessment, USEPA, Washington, DC, 1985.

41. U.S. Environmental Protection Agency, *Ambient Water Quality Criteria for 2,4-Dimethylphenol*, 440/5-80-044, PB 81-117558. Office of Water Regulations and Standards, Criteria and Standards Division, USEPA, Washington, DC, 1980.

42. U.S. Environmental Protection Agency, Health effects and occurrence documents in support

of: National Primary Drinking Water regulations: Volatile synthetic organic chemicals. *Fed. Regist.* **50**, 46902 (1985).

43. International Commission on Radiological Protection, *Report of the Task Group on Reference Man*, ICRP Publ. No. 23. Pergamon, Oxford, 1984.

44. K. Verschueren, *Handbook of Environmental Data on Organic Chemicals*, 2nd ed. Van Nostrand-Reinhold, New York, 1983.

45. National Oceanic and Atmospheric Administration, *Comparative Climatic Data for the United States*. National Climatic Data Center, Asheville, NC, 1985.

46. S. T. Hwang, Toxic emissions from land disposal facilities. *Environ. Prog.* **1**(1), 46−552 (1982).

47. R. H. Perry and D. Green, *Perry's Chemical Engineers' Handbook*, 6th ed. McGraw-Hill, New York, 1984.

48. S. T. Hwang, J. W. Falco, and C. H. Nauman, *Development of Advisory Levels for Polychlorinated Biphenyls (PCBs) Cleanup*. Office of Health and Environmental Assessment, USEPA, Washington, DC, 1986.

49. D. C. Bomberger, J. L. Gwinn, W. R. Mabey, D. Tuse, and T. W. Chou, Environmental fate and transport at the terrestrial-atmospheric interface. Symposium on Models for Predicting Fate of Chemicals in the Environment. American Chemical Society, Division of Pesticides Chemistry, 184th National Meeting, Kansas City, MO. (1982).

50. U.S. Environmental Protection Agency, *Compilation of Air Pollution Emission Factors*, AP-42. USEPA, Research Triangle Park, NC, 1985.

51. U.S. Environmental Protection Agency, *Industrial Source Complex (ISC) Dispersion Model User's Guide*, Vols. 1 and 2. USEPA, Research Triangle Park, NC, 1979.

52. G. A. Briggs, *Diffusion Estimation for Small Emissions*, ATDL Contrib. File No. 79. Atmospheric Turbulence and Diffusion Laboratory, National Oceanic and Atmospheric Administration, Washington, DC, 1973.

53. F. Pasquill, The estimation of the dispersion of windborne materials. *Meteorol. Mag.* **90**(1063), 33−49 (1961).

54. B. D. Turner, *Workbook of Atmospheric Dispersion Estimates*. U.S. Department of Health, Education, and Welfare, Washington, DC, 1970.

55. F. A. Fazzalari (Ed.), *Compilation of Odor and Taste Threshold Values Data*. American Society for Testing and Materials, Philadelphia, PA, 1978.

56. D. J. Paustenbach, Assessing the potential environment and human health risks of contaminated soil. *Comments Toxicol.* **1**(3−4), 185−220 (1987).

57. R. D. Kimbrough, H. Falk, P. Stehr, and G. Fries, Health implications of 2,3,7,8-tetrachlorodibenzodioxin (TCDD) contamination of residential soil. *J. Toxicol. Environ. Health* **14**, 47−93 (1984).

58. P. Clausing, B. Brunekreef, and J. H. van Wijnen, A method for estimating soil ingestion by children. *Int. Arch. Occup. Environ. Health* **59**(1), 73−82 (1987).

59. J. V. Rodricks, S. M. Brett, and G. C. Wrenn, Significant risk decisions in federal regulatory agencies. *Regul. Toxicol. Pharmacol.* **7**, 307−320 (1987).

60. C. T. Travis, R. A. Richter, E. A. C. Crouch, R. Wilson, and E. D. Klema, Cancer risk management: A review of 132 federal regulatory decisions. *Environ. Sci. Technol.* **21**(5), 415−420 (1987).

APPENDIX A: METHODOLOGY FOR DOSE AND RISK ESTIMATION

A.1 Inhalation of Chemical Vapor and Particulates—Subchronic

A.1.1 Estimation of Lifetime Average Daily Dose (LADD) *and Upper-Bound Cancer Risk.* For each chemical treated as a potential carcinogen, the LADD is calculated based on the estimated air concentrations at each receptor site, together with the estimated human intake of air and duration of exposure. LADDs are calculated separately for the excavation of each former lagoon for both chemical vapor and chemicals on dust particles. These two estimates of LADD (east lagoon vapor and dust, west lagoon vapor and dust) are then added to derive the total LADD. Each individual LADD is calculated as

$$LADD = \frac{\text{(concentration)(volume inspired)(absorption)(contact/)}}{\text{(days per lifetime)(body weight)}}.$$

$$\frac{\text{(in air)}\quad\text{(per hour)}\quad\text{(from air) (lifetime)}}{}$$

For an adult female,

$$LADD = \frac{(c \text{ mg/m}^3)(0.875 \text{ m}^3/\text{h})(1)(20 \text{ h/day} \times 60 \text{ days})}{(365 \text{ days/yr} \times 77 \text{ yr/life})(58 \text{ kg})}$$

$$= (6.44 \times 10^{-4})(c)(\text{mg/kg·day})$$

for any concentration c of chemical in the air, where c is in units of mg/m^3 air. Since upper-bound risk is the product of LADD and UCR, for illustrative purposes the upper-bound lifetime risk from exposure to any concentration (c) of tetrachloroethylene is calculated as follows:

$$\text{upper-bound risk} = [(6.44 \times 10^{-4})(c) \text{ mg/kg·day}][(0.0017)(\text{mg/kg·day})^{-1}]$$

$$= (1.10 \times 10^{-6})(c)$$

for any concentration c of tetrachloroethylene.

The predicted average air concentration of tetrachloroethylene in the form of vapor and dust at the closest residence during the excavation of the east and west lagoons is $7.87 \times 10^{-2} \text{ mg/m}^3$. Therefore, the upper-bound lifetime risk from this exposure for adult women is

$$\text{upper-bound risk} = (1.10 \times 10^{-6})(7.87 \times 10^{-2})$$

$$= 8.62 \times 10^{-8}.$$

For a preschool child, the calculation would be the same, except that the child's breathing rate ($0.333 \text{ m}^3/\text{h}$) and body weight (17 kg) would be used in the equation of LADD in place of the adult female values.

A.1.2 Estimation of Average Daily Dose (ADD) *and* ADD/ADI *Ratio.* For noncarcinogens and noncarcinogenic effects of carcinogens, the ADD/ADI ratio gives an indication of whether individuals exposed to the ADD are at risk. If the ratio is greater than 1, then some risk is assumed to exist. The ADD differs from the LADD in that it is *not* averaged over a lifetime; rather, it is the average daily dose on days of exposure. The ADD is calculated as follows:

$$ADD = \frac{\overset{\text{(concentration)}}{\underset{\text{(in air)}}{}}\overset{\text{(volume inspired)}}{\underset{\text{(per hour)}}{}}\overset{\text{(absorption)}}{\underset{\text{(from air)}}{}}\overset{\text{(hours)}}{\underset{\text{(per day)}}{}}}{\text{(body weight)}}.$$

For an adult female,

$$ADD = \frac{(c\ \text{mg/m}^3)(0.875\ \text{m}^3/\text{h})(1)(20\ \text{h})}{(58\ \text{kg})}$$

$$= (3.02 \times 10^{-1})(c)\ \text{mg/kg·day}$$

for any concentration ($c\ \text{mg/m}^3$) of chemical in air.

For xylene, the average concentration at the closest residence during excavation of the west lagoon is estimated to be $3.91 \times 10^{-1}\ \text{mg/m}^3$ as vapor and 6.81×10^{-4} associated with airborne dust, for a total of $3.92 \times 10^{-1}\ \text{mg/m}^3$. The subchronic ADI of xylene is $0.0103\ \text{mg/kg·day}$. The ADD/ADI ratio for this exposure is

$$\frac{ADD}{ADI} = \frac{(3.02 \times 10^{-1})(3.92 \times 10^{-1})\ \text{mg/kg·day}}{(0.0103)\ \text{mg/kg·day}}$$

$$= 11.48.$$

A.2 Ingestion of Contaminated Dust—Subchronic (Preschool Child)

We have used the value of 1 g/day to represent the amount of dust a child with pica would ingest. Not all the soil a child living in the area of the site would ingest would consist of dust deposited from the excavation site. In the absence of knowledge of what proportion that might be, we have selected 10% as a reasonable estimate.

A.2.1 Estimation of LADD and Upper-Bound Cancer Risk.

The LADD from soil ingestion for each chemical treated as a possible carcinogen is calculated based on the concentration in the soil and the estimated human intake:

$$LADD = \frac{\overset{\text{(concentration)}}{\underset{\text{(in soil)}}{}}\overset{\text{(soil)}}{\underset{\text{(ingested/day)}}{}}\overset{\text{(fraction of)}}{\underset{\text{(soil contaminated)}}{}}\overset{\text{(gastrointestinal)}}{\underset{\text{(absorption)}}{}}\overset{\text{(contact/)}}{\underset{\text{(lifetime)}}{}}}{\text{(days/lifetime)(body weight)}}$$

$$= \frac{(c\ \text{mg/kg})(1 \times 10^{-3}\ \text{kg})(0.1)(1)(60\ \text{days/life})}{(365\ \text{days/yr} \times 70\ \text{yr/life})(17\ \text{kg})}$$

$$= (1.38 \times 10^{-8})(c)\ \text{mg/kg·day}$$

for any concentration ($c\ \text{mg/kg soil}$) of chemical in soil.

Since upper-bound risk = LADD × UCR, the upper-bound lifetime risk at any concentration of tetrachloroethylene, for example, is

$$\text{upper-bound risk} = [(1.38 \times 10^{-8})(c)\,\text{mg/kg·day}][(0.051)(\text{mg/kg·day})^{-1}]$$
$$= (7.05 \times 10^{-10})(c).$$

The average concentration of tetrachloroethylene in the west lagoon is 160 mg/kg. Therefore, the upper-bound lifetime risk to preschool children from soil ingestion during excavation of the west lagoon is

$$\text{upper-bound risk} = (7.05 \times 10^{-10})(160)$$
$$= 1.13 \times 10^{-7}.$$

A.2.2 Estimation of ADD and ADD/ADI Ratio.

A.2.2   Estimation of ADD *and* ADD/ADI *Ratio.* As noted above, the ADD is similar to the LADD except that it applies only to the period of exposure and is not averaged over a lifetime. For dust ingestion, the ADD is calculated as

$$\text{LADD} = \frac{\overset{\text{(concentration)}}{\underset{\text{(in soil)}}{}}\overset{\text{(amount of soil)}}{\underset{\text{(ingested/day)}}{}}\overset{\text{(fraction)}}{\underset{\text{(contaminated)}}{}}\overset{\text{(gastrointestinal)}}{\underset{\text{(absorption)}}{}}}{\text{(body weight)}}.$$

For the preschool child modeled,

$$\text{ADD} = \frac{(c\,\text{mg/kg})(1 \times 10^{-3}\,\text{kg/day})(0.1)(1)}{(17\,\text{kg})}$$
$$= 5.88 \times 10^{-6}(c)\,\text{mg/kg·day}$$

for any concentration (c mg/kg) of chemical in soil.

For xylene, the average soil concentration in the west lagoon is estimated as 9379 mg/kg, and the subchronic ADI is 0.0103 mg/kg·day. The ADD/ADI ratio for this exposure is

$$\frac{\text{ADD}}{\text{ADI}} = \frac{(5.88 \times 10^{-6})(9379)\,\text{mg/kg·day}}{(0.0103)\,\text{mg/kg·day}}$$
$$= 5.36.$$

A.3   Inhalation of Chemical Vapor and Particulates—Acute

The foregoing calculations considered the average exposure over the period of excavation. However, because of the nonuniform distribution of chemicals in the soil to be excavated, exposure will not be uniform from day to day during the exposure period. On days when the most contaminated portions of soil are being excavated, the exposure would be higher than the average calculated above. To determine whether those acute exposures are likely to present a risk of acute health effects, the maximum daily doses (MDDs) have been calculated and compared to acute ADIs. The MDD is calculated similarly to the ADD except that the air concentration (c) used in the equation is the concentration resulting from the highest measured soil concentration rather than the median soil concentration.

For both carcinogens and noncarcinogens the MDD/acute ADI ratio is calculated as

$$MDD = \frac{\underset{(in\ air)}{(concentration)}\ \underset{(per\ hour)}{(volume\ inspired)}\ \underset{(from\ air)}{(absorption)}\ \underset{(per\ day)}{(hours\ exposed)}}{(body\ weight)}.$$

For an adult female,

$$MDD = \frac{(c\ mg/m^3)(0.875\ m^3/h)(1)(20\ h/day)}{(58\ kg)}$$

$$= (3.02 \times 10^{-1})(c)\ mg/kg\cdot day$$

for any concentration $(c\ mg/m^3)$ of a chemical in air, where c is the highest 1-day concentration predicted on days when the most contaminated areas of soil are excavated.

For xylene, the highest 1-day concentration at the closest residence during the excavation period is predicted to be 4.91 mg/m^3 as vapor and 0.867 mg/m^3 associated with airborne dust, and the acute ADI is 32 mg/kg·day. The MDD/acute ADI ratio for this exposure is

$$\frac{MDD}{ADI} = \frac{(3.02 \times 10^{-1})(5.78)\ mg/kg\cdot day}{(32)\ mg/kg\cdot day}$$

$$= 0.05.$$

A.4   Ingestion of Contaminated Dust—Acute

Calculations similar to those for acute inhalation may be conducted for acute ingestion of dust:

$$MDD = \frac{\underset{(in\ soil)}{(concentration)}\ \underset{(ingested/day)}{(amount\ of\ soil)}\ \underset{(contaminated)}{(fraction)}\ \underset{(absorption)}{(gastrointestinal)}}{(body\ weight)}.$$

For the preschool child modeled,

$$MDD = \frac{(c\ mg/kg)(1 \times 10^{-3}\ kg/day)(0.1)(1)}{17\ kg}$$

$$= (5.88 \times 10^{-6})(c)\ mg/kg\cdot day$$

for any concentration $(c\ mg/kg$ soil) of chemical in soil.

For xylene, the highest measured soil concentration in the area to be excavated is 147,000 mg/kg, and the acute ADI is 32 mg/kg·day. The MDD/acute ADI ratio for this exposure is

$$\frac{MDD}{ADI} = \frac{(5.88 \times 10^{-6})(147,000)\ mg/kg\cdot day}{(32)\ mg/kg\cdot day}$$

$$= 0.027.$$

C

ASSESSING HAZARDOUS WASTE SITES

12

A Risk Assessment of a Former Pesticide Production Facility

Thomas C. Marshall
International Technology Corporation, Knoxville, Tennessee

Melissa Dubinsky
International Technology Corporation. Pittsburgh, Pennsylvania

Scott Boutwell
Dames and Moore, San Jose, California

1 INTRODUCTION

This risk assessment addresses the potential health and environmental risks posed by an inactive chemicals production facility that formerly manufactured dichlorodiphenyltrichloroethane (DDT), dichlorophenoxyacetic acid (2, 4-D), 2, 4, 5-trichlorophenoxyacetic acid (2, 4, 5-T), and other agricultural and industrial chemicals. The original risk assessment report was part of a remedial investigation/feasibility study (RI/FS) designed to determine what, if any, corrective action was necessary to prevent residual chemicals related to site activities from presenting a hazard to human health or the environment. A RI/FS is required by the U.S. EPA as part of meeting the regulatory goals stated in the Comprehensive Environmental Remediation and Liability Act (CERCLA, commonly referred to as the Superfund Act). The National Oil and Hazardous Substances Contingency Plan (1, 2) requires that these studies incorporate an evaluation of a number of remedial options for risk managers to consider.

The remedial investigation characterizes the environmental setting, identifies chemicals related to site activities, characterizes the extent of their presence, and collects information useful in determining the potential for offsite migration. The feasibility study is an engineering study that evaluates those alternatives that are feasible for the long-term, environmentally acceptable disposition of the site. Guidelines for conducting field studies and preparing RI/FS reports are published by the EPA (3, 4). In the RI/FS process, the risk assessment serves as a bridge that allows the process to move from the remedial investigation stage to that of a feasibility study. Guidance documents are available for risk assessment preparation in the RI/FS process (5). Although these documents were not finalized until after the present study was underway, both the guidance documents and this risk assessment were based on the EPA's risk assessment policy for environmental contamination (6). Other sources that are useful to assist in defining the scope of a health and environmental risk assessment are available (7–11).

Risk assessment involves describing both qualitatively and quantitatively the nature and magnitude of potential risks to public health and the environment. However, this is not the only purpose. A risk assessment in the RI/FS process defines site-specific remedial objectives in terms useful for evaluating reasonable alternatives. A thorough risk analysis must include a no-action alternative. The National Contingency Plan also requires that several other categories of alternatives be evaluated:

- Alternatives for offsite treatment or disposal.
- Alternatives that attain "applicable or relevant and appropriate" federal public health and environmental requirements.
- Alternatives that exceed "applicable or relevant and appropriate" federal public health and environmental requirements.
- Alternatives that do not attain "applicable or relevant and appropriate" public health or environmental standards, but that will "reduce the likelihood of present or future threat from the hazardous substances and that provide significant protection to public health and welfare and environment."

The level of detail required of a risk assessment is primarily dependent on site-specific needs to discriminate levels of performance among the various alternatives. This "practical application" approach to risk assessment may lead to certain data gaps remaining open. For example, a decision on this site to dismantle process equipment and demolish buildings precluded the need to carry out extensive monitoring to quantify their potential contribution of chemicals into the air. In other words, the no-action alternative was rejected during the risk assessment process. Therefore, the risk assessment was adequate to accomplish its intended purpose without additional data.

2   APPROACH

A baseline evaluation was conducted assuming no corrective action would be taken at the site. The overall approach to the risk assessment is similar to U.S. EPA (5) guidance and involved completion of a sequential series of tasks as follows (Fig. 1):

- Review site data.
- Select indicator chemicals.
- Estimate exposures.
- Characterize risks.
- Recommend remedial objectives and cleanup criteria.

These steps are discussed separately in the following sections. In short, the site investigation data showed that about 70 chemicals were present and the extent of their presence in the various environmental media was characterized. The indicator chemicals

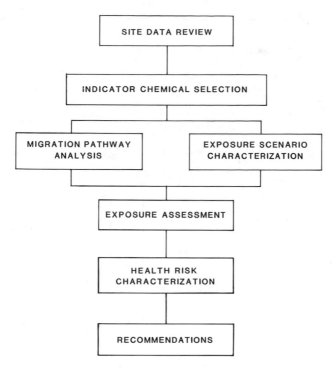

Figure 1. Flowchart of the risk assessment process.

selection process reduced the number of chemicals to be addressed to the more manageable number of 15. All pathways of migration (air, surface water, groundwater) were evaluated for the potential of these chemicals to move offsite and expose people or other receptors in the environment. These estimates of potential exposure were then compared to applicable criteria to determine if any current or future exposures might significantly exceed those associated with a very low probability to cause adverse health effects. Remedial objectives were developed to mitigate any exposure that was estimated potentially to exceed the health criteria.

3   SITE DATA REVIEW

3.1   Setting

This inactive chemical production facility formerly manufactured DDT, 2, 4-D, 2, 4, 5-T, and other agricultural and industrial chemicals. Four major and several minor structures are located on the site. In addition, several tank farms that once stored raw materials and finished products are present.

The site is nearly rectangular and occupies approximately 3.4 acres in a highly industrialized section of a major city (Fig. 2). The site was originally tidal marsh and is bounded on one side by a tidal river. The south shore of the river was filled with approximately 6–15 ft of fill to form the northernmost 30% of the property. The remainder

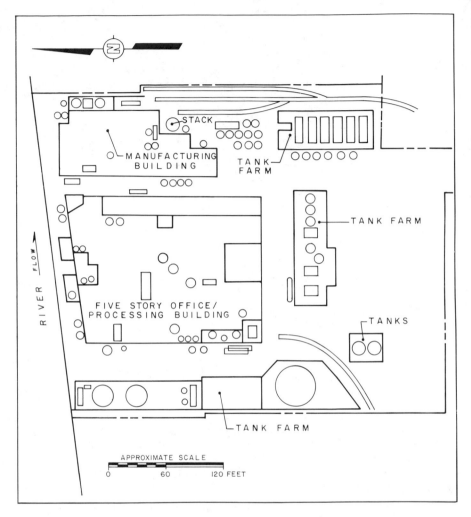

Figure 2. Facility layout prior to 1961.

of the site surface is also underlain by the granular material reportedly used to fill the previous marshland. The site lies approximately 7–10 ft above sea level. Flooding of the river at the site is controlled mainly by tidal influences. The greatest potential for inundation comes from an upstream, freshwater storm surge or tidal flooding associated with a major storm.

The bedrock underlying the site is at a depth of approximately 90 ft and consists chiefly of soft red shale and sandstone (Fig. 3). This unit is highly fractured and is the principal bedrock aquifer in the area. Above the bedrock lies approximately 80 ft of stratified sand, clay, and gravel, which forms a secondary aquifer of widely varying permeability. The fill material at the site is a limited water-bearing unit and is not a source of potable or industrial usage water. A silt layer approximately 9 ft thick separates the fill and the

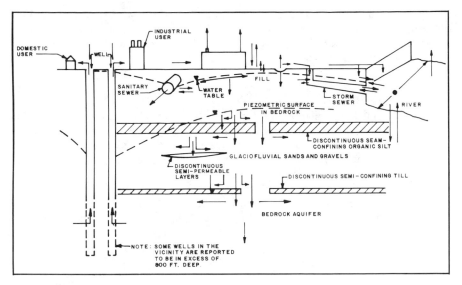

Figure 3. Schematic of surface water and groundwater migration pathways.

glaciofluvial unit and significantly retards downward flow of groundwater from the fill to the glaciofluvial sands.

About 10,000 people live within a 1-mile radius of the site based on the 1980 census data. The population potentially at risk of exposure includes employees located at adjacent businesses and people in nearby residential neighborhoods. The area has only the slightest traces of natural flora and fauna commonly found in a highly developed urban environment.

3.2   Site Activities

Modern chemical production on the site started in the mid-1940s with DDT and the phenoxy herbicides. Other products made on the site included hexachlorobenzene (HCB), Ovex (a miticide), Lindane, and β-benzene hexachloride (β-BHC).

Between 1951 and 1969 the manufacture of several products was either transferred to other locations or discontinued, leaving the phenoxy herbicides as the only products of the plant. During the late 1950s several process changes were instituted to improve the operating efficiency of the plant and an industrial sewer connecting to the city wastewater treatment line was installed in 1956.

A new process building devoted to the manufacture of sodium trichlorophenol (NaTCP), 2, 4-dichlorophenol (2, 4-DCP), monochloroacetic acid (MCA), and by-product hydrochloric acid (HCl) was erected along the river. The original chemical manufacturing building is where 2, 4-D, 2, 4, 5-T, and their esters and amines were produced. In 1967 equipment was installed to purify the NaTCP by removing 2, 3, 7, 8-tetrachlorodibenzodioxin (2, 3, 7, 8-TCDD). The facility was closed in 1969 and remained idle until it was purchased in 1971. The new owners expanded their product line by manufacturing several specialty items, but production ceased in mid-1973. Production of 2, 4-D resumed intermittently from 1974 through 1976, with a maximum monthly output of 2, 4-D of about 500,000 lb. In 1977, the plant was shut down and remained idle through 1980 when a new owner started clearing and salvaging the site. The product left in the equipment when the plant was shut down was removed and placed in 55-gal drums, of which 570 remain onsite today.

3.3 Site Investigation

Following an initial investigation that confirmed the presence of 2, 3, 7, 8-TCDD within the site boundaries, initial measures were taken to control access to the property and to restrict possible 2, 3, 7, 8-TCDD-containing material from leaving the property. The principal control measures were a fence, 24-h security guard, and coverage of the entire site, excluding areas covered by buildings and equipment, by a permeable geotextile fabric.

A detailed investigation of the site was subsequently intiated to supplement previous findings and to provide sufficient data to perform a feasibility study of remedial alternatives. This investigation was carried out in conformance with CERCLA requirements and comprised the following:

- Determination of the site's environmental setting: climate and meteorology, geology and landforms, hydrology, flora and fauna, and demography.
- Sampling: ambient air, industrial hygiene, buildings, tanks, structures and equipment, sewers and sumps, soils, groundwater, background soils, drums, river water, and river sediments.
- Laboratory analytical testing.
- Characterization of the site.

The following subsections describe the sampling and analytical testing. The term *priority pollutants* as referred to in this report is defined as the 129 compounds referred to by the U.S. EPA (12). These comprise the acid/base/neutrals (semivolatiles), volatile organic compounds (VOCs), pesticides and polychlorinated biphenyls (PCBs), herbicides, metals, total cyanide, and total phenols. Thirty-eight additional compounds on the Hazardous Substances List plus 40 additional chemicals were included (i.e., a total of 197 chemicals).

3.3.1 Ambient Air. Ambient air sampling was conducted at the site for establishing baseline conditions and for comparison of site data to data collected at other sites in the area. A single air sampling location, the roof of the office/laboratory building, was utilized for the baseline sampling. Data from this single sampling location approximately 10 m above ground level is considered representative of baseline ambient concentrations at the site because of the wind exposure at this point. The samples and monitoring data were collected over 24-h periods for 31 consecutive days in September and October so that an indication of the range of variation could be obtained.

All samples were analyzed for iron and manganese as an indicator of the proportion of the particulate air burden comprised of soil. Ten samples having the highest iron and manganese concentrations (i.e., those appearing to have the highest soil content) were subjected to the following analyses:

- Total suspended particulate (TSP) matter.
- Inhalable particulate matter (IPM).

TABLE 1. Ambient Air Results Summary for 10 Samples with Highest Iron and Manganese Concentrations

Parameters	Range of Concentration	Number of Times Detected	Median
	Metals ($\mu g/m^3$)		
Iron	0.682–1.259	10	0.926
Manganese	0.019–0.052	10	0.026
Cadmium	0.001–0.009	10	0.003
Copper	0.018–0.081	10	0.035
Nickel	0.013–0.027	10	0.022
Lead	0.364–0.399	10	0.382
Zinc	0.273–0.321	10	0.297
	Dioxins (pg/m^3)		
2, 3, 7, 8-TCDD	ND–286	2	ND
	VOC ($\mu g/m^3$)		
Methylene chloride	ND–4.27	7[a,b]	2.51
Chloroform	0.30–0.44	7[a,b]	0.37
Trichloroethene	5.60–26.67	9[b]	11.92
Benzene	1.43–7.39	9[b]	2.67
Tetrachloroethene	1.36–10.44	9[b]	3.19
Toluene	15.04–36.99	9[b]	29.33
Chlorobenzene	ND–1.58	3[b]	ND
Ethylbenzene	4.59–38.31	9[b]	7.75
m-Xylene	11.73–51.25	9[b]	21.74
o-Xylene	4.59–23.84	9[b]	9.50
p-Xylene	4.59–23.84	9[b]	9.50
1, 2-Dichlorobenzene	ND–1.85	9[b]	0.33
	Pesticides (ng/m^3)		
Hexachlorobenzene	<0.07–1.71	9	0.47
	PNA (ng/m^3)		
Benzo[a]pyrene	0.54–3.01	10	1.38
Benzo[g, h, i]perylene	0.70–2.55	10	1.63
Indeno[1, 2, 3-c, d]perylene	0.33–3.50	10	1.01
Phenanthrene	0.08–1.07	10	0.42
Benzo[b]fluoranthene	0.52–1.97	10	1.25
Anthracene	0.02–0.21	10	0.08
Fluoranthene	0.54–6.66	10	1.69
Pyrene	0.53–2.42	10	1.51
Benzo[a]anthracene	0.37–1.45	10	0.77
Chrysene	0.33–1.39	10	0.68

[a]Run partially lost.
[b]Sample broken in shipment.

TABLE 2. Summary of Detected Priority Pollutants in Near-Surface Soils

Pollutant	0–6 Inches			12–24 Inches		
	Concentration Range (μg/kg or ppb)	Number Positive Results	Number Samples Analyzed	Concentration Range (μg/kg or ppb)	Number Positive Results	Number Samples Analyzed
Base/Neutral/Acid Organics						
2,4,6-Trichlorophenol	1,500,000–1,300	5	21	1,700,000–8,700	4	21
2,4-Dichlorophenol	3,600,000–980	7	21	2,500,000–870	8	21
2,4-Dimethylphenol	—	0	21	1,700,000	1	21
Benzoic acid	1,800	1	21	—	0	21
2,4,5-Trichlorophenol	15,000,000–870	5	21	7,500,000–2,500	5	21
Acenaphthene	250	1	21	—	0	21
1,2,4-Trichlorobenzene	17,000–1,500	2	21	19,000	1	21
Hexachlorobenzene	110,000–560	13	21	720,000–3,200	9	21
1,2-Dichlorobenzene	520–230	2	21	9,000	1	21
1,3-Dichlorobenzene	—	0	21	610	1	21
1,4-Dichlorobenzene	1,400–470	3	21	1,300	1	21
Fluoranthene	6,100–330	5	21	64,000–670	6	21
Naphthalene	200	1	21	8,200	1	21
Bis(2-ethylhexyl)phthalate	1,300–310	3	21	310,000–5,100	3	21
Di-N-butylphthalate	—	0	21	370,000–2,000	2	21
Benzo[a]anthracene	4,700–910	3	21	47,000–510	5	21
Benzo[a]pyrene	4,800–1,000	3	21	44,000–560	5	21
Benzo[b]fluoranthene	7,100–2,100	3	21	71,000–940	5	21
Chrysene	12,000–2,600	2	21	120,000–1,400	6	21
Acenaphthylene	690–210	2	21	860–240	2	21
Anthracene	3,000–310	4	21	1,200–630	3	21
Benzo[g,h,i]perylene	11,000–3,300	3	21	32,000	1	21
Fluorene	320	1	21	300–250	2	21
Phenanthrene	4,100–250	5	21	61,000–440	6	21
Indeno[1,2,3,-cd]pyrene	2,500–2,200	2	21	21,000–480	2	21
Pyrene	2,200–230	6	21	78,000–280	7	21
Dibenzofuran	—	0	21	450	1	21
2-Methylnaphthalene	220	1	21	21,000	1	21

Volatile Organics

	(mg/kg or ppm)			(mg/kg or ppm)		
Benzene	21	1	21	23,000–11	3	21
Chlorobenzene	84,000–39	2	21	170,000–22	6	21
Chloroform	38	1	21	38,000–13	2	21
Ethylbenzene	—	0	21	60,000	1	21
Methylene chloride	1,500–14	21	21	130,000–21	21	21
Tetrachloroethane	860	1	21	36,000–1,300	2	21
Toluene	—	0	21	2,000,000–7	6	21
Trichloroethene	—	0	21	9	1	21
Acetone	5,000–58	13	21	2,000–68	15	21
2-Butanone	1,400–130	2	21	9,200–51	6	21
Carbon disulfide	—	0	21	7	1	21
2-Hexanone	—	0	21	36,000	1	21
Total xylenes	—	0	21	310,000	1	21

Herbicides/Pesticides/PCBs

4,4′-DDT	3,500,000–620	19	21	5,090,000–1,400	15	21
4,4′-DDE	93,000–20	14	21	37,000–1,200	8	21
4,4′-DDD	13,000–1,700	3	21	164,000–1,200	5	21
Alpha-Endosulfan	8,900	1	21	1,400	1	21
Dalapon	70,000–190	9	21	29,000–420	9	21
2,4-D	7,600–740	10	21	85,000–190	13	21
2,4,5-T	2,300–190	9	21	86,000–490	10	21

Inorganics

	(mg/kg or ppm)			(mg/kg or ppm)		
Antimony	6.6–0.09	14	21	3.0–0.10	17	21
Arsenic	23–0.13	21	21	4–0.60	21	21
Beryllium	0.85–0.22	11	21	0.84–0.25	9	21
Cadmium	3.9–0.09	12	21	26–0.08	14	21
Chromium	50–1.1	21	21	50–5.9	21	21
Copper	260–2.4	21	21	250–2.0	20	21
Lead	887–1.8	21	21	646–2.1	20	21
Mercury	39–0.1	18	21	37–0.4	16	21
Nickel	82–3.1	20	21	40–2.1	20	21
Selenium	48	1	21	2.2–0.01	3	21
Silver	1.2–0.24	7	21	11–0.25	6	21
Zinc	29,000–20	21	21	1,300–8.0	21	21
Total cyanides	1.97–0.15	19	21	2.8–0.10	19	21
Total phenols	47.8–0.28	20	21	3,378–0.10	21	21

- Metals.
- VOCs.
- Polycyclic aromatic hydrocarbons.
- Asbestos.
- 2, 3, 7, 8-TCDD.
- Pesticides and other chlorinated organics.

The analytical results for the 10 sets of samples are summarized in Table 1 and below.

The highest concentration of TSP was $254\,mg/m^3$ while the median was $134\,mg/m^3$. The highest value exceeded the secondary 24-h National Ambient Air Quality Standard (NAAQS) of $150\,mg/m^3$ for TSP but is less than the 24-h primary standard of $260\,mg/m^3$. The median IPM concentration was $77\,mg/m^3$. One IPM concentration was $196\,mg/m^3$, which is greater than the $150\,mg/m^3$ lower range for the proposed 24-h IPM NAAQS. The concentrations of all metals except iron were less than $1\,\mu g/m^3$. The iron concentration ranged from 0.682 to $1.259\,\mu g/m^3$, with the maximum occurring on the day of maximum TSP and IPM concentrations. The relative concentrations of the various metals are consistent with those measured in the city during other studies, indicating that there is no significant contribution of metals or dust to the air from the site. Measured metal concentrations in the soil are given in Table 2.

2, 3, 7, 8-TCDD was detected in 2 of the 10 samples at concentrations of 86 and $286\,pg/m^3$, respectively. No obvious relation exists between the reported 2, 3, 7, 8-TCDD levels and the meteorological conditions on the days when they occurred. It was concluded that 2, 3, 7, 8-TCDD detected may have originated from 2, 3, 7, 8-TCDD-contaminated fume hood exhaust stacks located near the rooftop sampling station.

Vinyl chloride concentrations found in five samples ranged from 0.15 to $0.33\,\mu g/m^3$, well below the occupational permissible exposure limit of $2000\,\mu g/m^3$. Vinyl chloride was never produced on site nor was it ever used as a raw material. It was not detected in any soil samples on site. These facts suggest its presence in the air originates from sources offsite. Vinyl chloride was detected in groundwater in two of eight samples at concentrations of 28 and $88\,\mu g/L$. The presence of vinyl chloride may be due to an offsite source. Alternatively, vinyl chloride may be a decomposition product of the chlorinated ethanes and ethenes that were detected onsite.

Total VOC concentrations ranged from 71 to $182\,\mu g/m^3$. Major consitutents were xylene, toluene, and ethylbenzene, which are aromatic halocarbons commonly emitted from petroleum refineries and plants manufacturing coatings and solvents. All these activities occur in the vicinity of the site. Other major constituents were trichloroethene and tetrachloroethene. The data indicate that the site probably does not contribute significantly to VOCs in air. The observed pesticide and PNA concentrations are all less than their occupational permissible exposure levels.

3.3.2 Buildings, Structures, and Equipment.

A sampling program was conducted on buildings, structures, and equipment at the site to determine the presence and levels of 2, 3, 7, 8-TCDD. These data were useful in determining the remedial alternatives to be considered and in conducting the risk–benefit analyses. A biased sampling approach was employed; that is, samples were taken at locations suspected to have high levels of 2, 3, 7, 8-TCDD. The sampling program confirmed the presence of 2, 3, 7, 8-TCDD on the interior and exterior of all the onsite structures. 2, 3, 7, 8-TCDD levels ranged as high as $41,600\,ng/m^2$ for wipe sample analysis and 1580 ppb in the structural material analyzed.

Because of the biased sampling strategy used, determination of the total amount of 2, 3, 7, 8-TCDD in the structures is not practical, and the usefulness of such data is arguable.

Another major potential source of liquid and solid waste on the site was the material stored in tanks, vessels and drums. A weighted average of all wastes determined to have positive 2, 3, 7, 8-TCDD concentrations indicated an estimated 230,000 lb of material containing 940 ppb 2, 3, 7, 8-TCDD (a total of 98 g of 2, 3, 7, 8-TCDD).

3.3.3 Soils

3.3.3.1 Near-Surface Soil Sampling. A near-surface soil sampling program was performed on the site to obtain soil samples for chemical analysis (Fig. 4). The EPA Test Methods for Evaluating Solid Waste (13) were used as guidelines for developing the sampling program. The guidelines describe how to obtain representative samples and how to estimate an appropriate number of samples to be analyzed. The objective of the sampling plan was to estimate chemical characteristics for the purpose of comparing those characteristics to applicable regulatory thresholds and to select remedial actions if required. As the guidelines state, generally, high accuracy and high precision are required if contaminants are present at a concentration close to regulatory thresholds. Alternatively, relatively low precision can be adequate if contaminants occur at levels far below or far above their applicable thresholds. A well-designed sampling program makes use of preliminary information to estimate the approximate number of samples to collect. It also analyzes such samples in a phased manner to optimize the effort. This procedure allows for analysis of the appropriate number of samples needed to evaluate remedial actions and avoids unnecessary expense. More samples can subsequently be obtained using this approach if necessary.

The near-surface soil sampling program used a systematic random sampling plan to collect data from 21 locations on the site. The approach used followed the EPA guidelines and makes use of a 50-ft by 50-ft grid. The number of locations was anticipated to provide the precision required to within the confidence interval (i.e., 80%) suggested by the guidelines.

A total of 63 samples were analyzed for 2, 3, 7, 8-TCDD from the systematic random sampling consisting of three samples for each location from 0 to 6 in., 6 to 12 in., and 12 to 24 in. (Fig. 4). A total of 42 samples were analyzed for priority pollutants consisting of two samples for each location from 0 to 6 in. and from 12 to 24 in. Each sample was a composite of the sample depth range. In addition to the systematic random sampling, other selected locations (biased samples) were taken and analyzed for 2, 3, 7, 8-TCDD only. The locations were chosen using a biased approach designed to be representative of the highest potential sources of 2, 4, 5-T and therefore were based on plant activities and functional units.

All of the 63 near-surface soil samples analyzed had identifiable 2, 3, 7, 8-TCDD concentrations. The total quantity of 2, 3, 7, 8-TCDD in the top 24 in. of soil at the 3.4-acre site was estimated to be about 96 lb.

The results of the 42 near-surface soil samples analyzed for priority pollutants are presented in Table 2. Sixty-nine semivolatile compounds were identified one or more times. Thirteen of the 38 VOCs were identified one or more times. Methylene chloride and acetone were identified most frequently. However, the concentrations are typically attributable to background levels due to handling during collection, shipping, or handling in the laboratory. Seven of the 35 herbicide, pesticide, and PCB compounds in the priority pollutant scan were detected one or more times. Of the 13 metals identified, only thallium

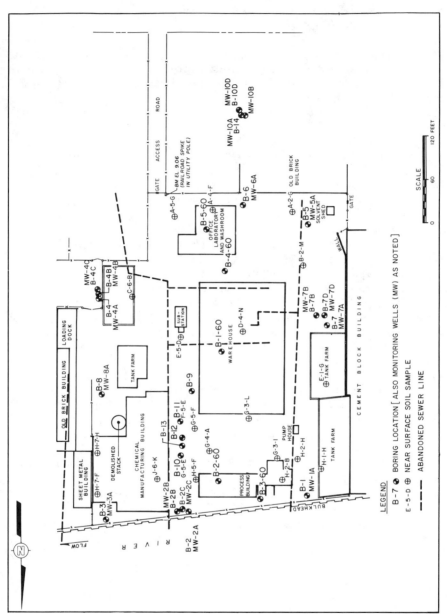

Figure 4. Locations of analytical samples and abandoned sewer lines.

472

was not detected in the near-surface samples. Cyanide and total phenols were detected in some samples.

3.3.3.2   Boring Soil Samples. Boring soil samples were collected at 13 locations onsite (Fig. 4). Of the 39 boring soil samples analyzed, 25 samples (90%) had measurable concentrations of 2, 3, 7, 8-TCDD. At depths of 0–6 in., the 2, 3, 7, 8-TCDD concentrations ranged from 19.7 to 2700 ppb. At 6–12 in., the 2, 3, 7, 8-TCDD concentrations ranged from 7.5 to 3510 ppb. At 12–24 in., the 2, 3, 7, 8-TCDD concentrations ranged from 4.7 to 830 ppb. Samples from directly above the silt had 2, 3, 7, 8-TCDD concentrations ranging from 0.36 to 71.8 ppb, with one of eight samples having no detectable 2, 3, 7, 8-TCDD. Samples from the silt zone had 2, 3, 7, 8-TCDD concentrations ranging from 0.49 to 2.8 ppb with three of seven samples having no detectable concentrations of 2, 3, 7, 8-TCDD. Knowledge of solvent use at the site, presence of solvents in the soil, and the well-documented immobility of 2, 3, 7, 8-TCDD in soil lead to the conclusion that solvents carried this material downward.

Twenty-four boring soil samples above the silt were analyzed for priority pollutants. These results are presented in Table 3. Of the 69 semivolatile compounds identified, 27 were identified one or more times. Of the 38 VOCs identified, 10 (26%) were identified one or more times. Ten (29%) of the 35 herbicides, pesticides, and PCB compounds identified were detected one or more times. Of the 13 metals identified, only selenium and thallium were not detected. All samples had positive cyanide results; phenol was positive in 7 samples.

3.3.3.3   Background Measurements in Near-Surface Soil. Samples were taken for priority pollutant and 2, 3, 7, 8-TCDD analyses at three locations offsite. There was no detectable 2, 3, 7, 8-TCDD in any of the three 0–6-in. samples. Of the 69 semivolatile compounds analyzed for, 16 were identified in the background samples one or more times. A summary of the data is provided in Table 4. Methylene chloride (concentration range 32–66 μg/kg) was the only volatile organic compound detected. DDT (200 μg/kg) and PCB-1260 (1200–1700 μg/kg) were also detected one or more times. All the inorganic parameters that were analyzed for were detected (Table 4).

3.3.4   Sewers and Sumps. Associated with the site buildings are a number of sumps and an industrial sewer system (Fig. 4). All the sumps inspected during the site investigation had previously been cleaned or emptied to some degree. Eight samples were taken from sumps and four sewer samples were collected from manholes accessible on the site. Positive 2, 3, 7, 8-TCDD results were obtained for all 12 samples, ranging from 105 to 9160 ppb in the sumps and from 19.5 to 4040 ppb in the sewers.

3.3.5   Groundwater. A series of monitoring wells were installed to evaluate the hydrogeology regime and nature of contaminants present in the groundwater. Two sets of samples were collected from each well at weekly intervals commencing 1 week after each well was installed. This protocol was intended to provide a basis of consistent data to assess the level and extent of groundwater contamination at the site.

Groundwater samples were analyzed via eight shallow monitoring wells for priority pollutants and 2, 3, 7, 8-TCDD (Fig. 4). The groundwater in the fill was found to contain a number of chemicals. 2, 3, 7, 8-TCDD ranged from 0.0059 to 10.4 ppb. A single monitoring well in the north end of the site had 2, 3, 7, 8-TCDD results significantly higher than any other groundwater sample. These very high levels of 2, 3, 7, 8-TCDD in water are probably

TABLE 3. Summary of Detected Priority Pollutants in Soil Borings

Pollutant	0–6 inches			12–24 inches			Above Silt		
	Concentration Range (μg/kg or ppb)	Number Positive Results	Number Samples Analyzed	Concentration Range (μg/kg or ppb)	Number Positive Results	Number Samples Analyzed	Concentration Range (μg/kg or ppb)	Number Positive Results	Number Samples Analyzed
				Base/Natural/Acid Organics					
2, 4, 6-Trichlorophenol	32,000–1,300	3	8	4,400–3,600	2	8	360,000–2,000	3	8
2,-Chlorophenol	2,000–230	2	8	820	1	8	6,000–1,200	2	8
2, 4-Dichlorophenol	98,000–5,900	3	8	27,000–4,700	3	8	1,400,000–1,700	5	8
Phenol	3,100	1	8	12,000–1,400	2	8	13,000–820	2	8
2, 4, 5-Trichlorophenol	20,000–1,500	4	8	16,000–1,600	3	8	270,000–12,000	4	8
Acenaphthane	2,200	1	8	4,600	1	8	0	0	8
1, 2, 4-Trichlorobenzene	1,100–430	2	8	8,500–580	2	8	14,000	1	8
Hexachlorobenzene	35,000–6,500	5	8	84,000–4,900	4	8	30,000	1	8
2-Chloronaphthalene	1,100	1	8	850	1	8	—	—	8
1, 2-Dichlorobenzene	770	1	8	8,600–570	2	8	13,000	1	8
1, 3-Dichlorobenzene	—	0	8	780	1	8	3,400	1	8
1, 4-Dichlorobenzene	2,700	1	8	49,000–960	3	8	28,000–4,600	3	8
Fluoranthene	8,700–400	5	8	20,000–3,200	4	8	1,300–560	3	8
Naphthalene	1,300	1	8	11,000	1	8	16,000–260	5	8
Bis(2-ethylhexyl)phthalate	14,000	1	8	5,100–2,600	2	8	—	0	8
Benzo[a]anthracene	—	0	8	1,900	1	8	—	0	8
Benzo[a]pyrene	—	0	8	1,600	1	8	—	0	8
Benzo[b]fluoranthene	—	0	8	7,400	1	8	1,900	1	8
Chrysene	—	0	8	4,200	1	8	—	0	8
Anthracene	950	1	8	1,200	1	8	—	0	8
Fluorene	2,100	1	8	4,200	1	8	—	0	8
Phenanthrene	3,800–230	3	8	14,000–720	5	8	2,200–350	2	8
Indeno[1, 2, 3,-cd]pyrene	—	0	8	1,400	1	8	—	0	8
Pyrene	8,100–270	5	8	18,000–1,300	5	8	460–420	2	8
Benzyl Alcohol	—	0	8	20,000	1	8	41,000	1	8
Dibenzofuran	1,300	1	8	2,100	1	8	—	0	8
2-Methylnaphthalene	2,600	1	8	8,000–850	3	8	14,000–1,600	4	8

	Range	n	N	Range	n	N	Range	n	N
Volatile Organics									
Benzene	26	1	8	1,700–680	2	8	22,000–5,600	2	8
Chlorobenzene	330	1	8	24,000–49	4	8	100,000–17	5	8
Ethylbenzene	—	0	8	100	1	8	14,000–220	2	8
Methylene chloride	410–38	8	8	1,600–6	8	8	11,000–48	8	8
Tetrachloroethane	—	0	8	15	1	8	—	0	8
Toluene	12–7	2	8	2,400–9	4	8	180,000–11	2	8
Acetone	160–57	5	8	2,300–110	7	8	4,500–85	6	8
2-Butanone	—	0	8	8,900	1	8	20,000–6,900	2	8
Carbon disulfide	—	0	8	7	1	8	13	1	8
Total xylenes	—	0	8	580	1	8	1,200	1	8
Herbicides/Pesticides/PCBs									
4,4'-DDT	830,000–17,000	5	8	3,200,000–43,000	5	8	140,000–100	4	8
4,4'-DDE	57,900–6,500	6	8	297,000–2,400	6	8	1,500–290	4	8
4,4'-DDD	78,000–2,000	5	8	182,000–3,900	5	8	370,000–42	5	8
Beta-BHC	130,000–830	2	8	120,000	1	8	100,000	1	8
Dalapon	21,000–160	6	8	94,000–300	5	8	—	0	8
Dicamba	1,700–230	3	8	1,600–100	3	8	160	1	8
2,4-D	120,000–240	8	8	16,000–110	8	8	2,800,000–140	7	8
2,4,5-T	54,000–94	8	8	14,000–95	7	8	690,000–610	5	8
2,4-DB	—	0	8	1,400	1	8	170	1	8
Dinoseb (DNBP)	590–210	2	8	—	0	8	—	0	8
Inorganics									
Antimony	11–0.2	8	8	3.5–0.1	8	8	1.1–0.1	6	8
Arsenic	20–1.0	8	8	26–2.1	8	8	120–5.7	8	8
Beryllium	—	0	8	3.7–0.2	5	8	1.4–0.1	5	8
Cadmium	3–0.5	8	8	2.5–0.3	8	8	3–0.1	6	8
Chromium	72–7.9	8	8	40–13	8	8	25–5.5	8	8
Copper	290–46	8	8	730–82	8	8	6,600–24	8	8
Lead	1,400–73	8	8	2,300–180	8	8	11,000–19	8	8
Mercury	11–0.1	8	8	7.6–0.5	8	8	95–0.2	7	8
Nickel	95–15	8	8	170–13	8	8	72–5.8	8	8
Silver	0.92–0.2	6	8	0.9–0.3	4	8	1.8–0.4	5	8
Zinc	3,900–180	8	8	1,500–190	8	8	1,300–45	8	8
Total cyanides	1.2–0.25	8	8	3.7–0.15	8	8	1.2–0.1	8	8
Total phenols	13–0.2	8	8	12–0.2	8	8	1,600–0.3	7	8

TABLE 4. Summary of Detected Compounds in Near-Surface Soils from Background Samples

| Base/Neutral/Acid Organic Compounds | Background: 0–6 inches[a] | |
	Concentration Range (μg/kg or ppb)	Number Positive Results
Di-N-butylphthalate	200	1
Benzo[a]anthracene	1,500–1,900	3
Benzo[a]pyrene	1,200–1,500	3
Benzo[a]fluoranthene	2,200–2,700	3
Chrysene	3,200–3,700	3
Acenaphthylene	250–610	3
Anthracene	580–600	3
Benzo[g, h, i]perylene	1,500–2,300	3
Fluorene	1,300–2,800	3
Phenanthrene	—	0
Indeno[1, 2, 3,-cd]pyrene	1,100–1,700	3
Pyrene	1,400–1,700	3
Dibenzofuran	—	0
2-Methylnaphthalene	—	0
2, 4, 6-Trichlorophenol	—	0
2, 4-Dichlorophenol	—	0
2, 4-Dimethylphenol	—	0
Benzoic acid	—	0
2, 4, 5-Trichlorophenol	—	0
Acenaphthene		0
1, 2, 4-Trichlorobenzene	—	0
Hexachlorobenzene	110,000–620,000	2
1, 2-Dichlorobenzene	—	0
1, 3-Dichlorobenzene	—	0
1, 4-Dichlorobenzene	—	0
Fluoranthene	2,600–3,500	3
Naphthalene	480	1
Bis(2-ethylhexyl)phthalate	670–1,700	3
Antimony	2.2–9.1	3
Arsenic	4.6–10	3
Beryllium	0.47–0.5	2
Cadmium	2.0–2.8	3
Chromium	51–98	3
Copper	127–311	3
Lead	595–1,700	3
Mercury	0.6–2.0	3
Nickel	35–74	3
Selenium	—	0
Silver	0.45–1.4	3
Zinc	428–828	3
Total cyanides	0.78–2.9	3
Total phenols	117	1

[a]Three samples analyzed for each parameter.

the result of a 2,3,7,8-TCDD-bearing solvent or other carrier in the groundwater, or 2,3,7,8-TCDD-containing colloidal soil particles suspended in the water. Groundwater samples were not filtered as per U.S. EPA protocol (14).

The priority pollutant results are summarized in Table 5. The highest concentrations of semivolatile organic and chlorinated herbicide compounds occurred in the groundwater samples from the monitoring well that had the highest 2,3,7,8-TCDD concentration results. In general, the most prevalent compounds found in the groundwater from the fill (site was originally tidal marsh as described in Section 3.1) were the chemicals associated with the manufacture that took place on the site, that is, chlorinated phenols, 4,4'-DDT, 2,4-D, and 2,4,5-T. Groundwater collected from the upper glaciofluvial sand contain fewer compounds than were found in groundwater sampled in the fill unit. The deepest well sampled contained only six organic compounds, which were present at very low concentrations. 2,3,7,8-TCDD was present in two of three water samples from the glaciofluvial sand at 0.0042 and 0.0034 ppb, respectively.

4 SELECTION OF INDICATOR CHEMICALS

The selection of indicator chemicals is an objective screening process designed to reduce the total number of chemicals found at the site to a smaller, more manageable number for exposure and risk analyses. However, it is important that the selected chemicals still represent all the chemical groups detected which could pose a significant health and environmental risk. The screening process assures that remediation objectives or cleanup criteria for indicator chemicals will meet or exceed adequate cleanup for all the chemicals detected onsite, including those that are less prevalent, toxic, and/or mobile than the indicator chemicals. The selection process is discussed in Sections 4.1 and 4.2.

4.1 Selection Methodology

The selection methodology was partially developed using draft guidance from the U.S. EPA *Superfund Public Health Evaluation Manual* (15), which was finalized recently (5). A set of selection criteria were applied to the 70 chemicals with migration potential for the purpose of obtaining a smaller group of indicator chemicals that would adequately represent the hazards posed by this site. This approach is summarized in Fig. 5 and is described below.

- The fact that some of the chemicals are isolated in a secured drum storage area prevents their environmental transport to receptors via air and water. Those chemicals that are not contained could migrate to offsite locations. Consequently, these compounds represent the "potentially mobile" chemicals.
- The 70 potentially mobile chemicals are listed with their index numbers in Table 6 and were separated into 15 different categories as listed in Fig. 5. They include 13 organic groups and two inorganic groups. Organic chemicals were grouped by toxicological characters and environmental behavior. Observed concentrations and distribution patterns were not the primary criteria in the categorization rationale.
- Where a chemical class contained only one chemical, this chemical was automatically selected as the indicator chemical.
- Those categories containing more than one chemical were evaluated for carcinogenicity. If only one chemical in a group was a known or suspected carcinogen, this

TABLE 5. Summary of Detected Priority Pollutants in Well Water Samples

Pollutant	10-09-84			10-30-84		
	Concentration Range (µg/kg or ppb)	Number Positive Results	Number Samples Analyzed	Concentration Range (µg/kg or ppb)	Number Positive Results	Number Samples Analyzed
Base/Neutral/Acid Organics						
2,4,6-Trichlorophenol	1,700–11,000	3	8	290–3,900	3	8
2-Chlorophenol	290–4,600	3	8	11–3,600	4	8
2,4-Dichlorophenol	160–48,000	5	8	370–58,000	4	8
Phenol	36–3,700	5	8	43–600	3	8
Benzoic acid	250	1	8	ND	0	8
2-Methylphenol	ND	0	8	24	1	8
4-Methylphenol	39–66	2	8	ND	0	8
2,4,5-Trichlorophenol	56–8,800	5	8	38–26,000	4	8
Acenaphthene	ND	0	8	30	1	8
1,2,4-Trichlorobenzene	200	1	8	9–890	3	8
Hexachlorobenzene	ND	0	8	770–860	2	8
2-Chloronaphthalene	ND	0	8	5	1	8
1,2-Dichlorobenzene	11–390	3	8	3–980	4	8
1,3-Dichlorobenzene	ND	0	8	13–200	2	8
1,4-Dichlorobenzene	110–590	3	8	6–1,200	4	8
Fluoranthene	15	1	8	3–120	5	8
Naphthalene	10–320	4	8	11–480	3	8
Bis(2-ethylhexyl)phthalate	55	1	8	3–75	3	8
Di-N-butylphthalate	12	1	8	8	1	8
Benzo[a]anthracene	ND	0	8	8	1	8
Anthracene	ND	0	8	4	1	8
Fluorene	10	1	8	32	1	8
Phenanthrene	2–34	2	8	3–110	5	8
Pyrene	3–19	3	8	5–46	5	8
Benzyl alcohol	8,000	1	8	4,300	1	8
2-Methylnaphthalene	7–260	4	8	3–900	6	8
Volatile Organics						
Benzene	3.0–3,900	8	8	10–7,900	7	8
Chlorobenzene	14–8,500	6	8	4–23,000	7	8
1,2-Dichloroethane	1,700	1	8	2,000	1	8
1,1,1-Trichloroethane	410	1	8	1,500	1	8

	Range (mg/kg or ppm)	n	N	Range	n	N
Chloroform	20–230	2	8	19–240	5	8
1,1-Dichloroethane	ND	0	8	53	1	8
trans-1,2-Dichloroethene	33–360	2	8	30–1,300	2	8
Ethylbenzene	44–740	3	8	43	2	8
Methylene chloride	6–12,000	8	8	3–7,400	8	8
Tetrachloroethene	2–5	2	8	2–43	3	8
Toluene	7–1,100	6	8	55–3,300	5	8
Trichloroethene	15–230	2	8	9–280	2	8
Vinyl chloride	28–88	2	8	24–220	2	8
Acetone	29–540	3	8	21–520	3	8
2-Butanone	870	1	8	180–430	2	8
Carbon disulfide	2–65	2	8	ND	0	8
4-Methyl-2-pentanone	3,300	1	8	1,800	1	8
Total xylenes	42–960	4	8	13–570	4	8
Herbicides/Pesticides/PCBs						
4,4'-DDT	17–22,000	4	8	14–2,770	4	8
4,4'-DDE	17–54	2	8	7–14	2	8
4,4'-DDD	15–13,000	5	8	7–1,390	4	8
α-Endosulfan	ND	0	8	1,240	1	8
2,4-D	6.9–27,000	6	8	74–20,000	4	8
2,4,5-T	470–5,600	4	8	68–3,500	4	8
2,4-DB	500	1	8	ND	0	8
Dinoseb (DNBP)	4.2	1	8	ND	0	8
Inorganics	(mg/kg or ppm)			(mg/kg or ppm)		
Antimony	0.003–0.151	7	8	0.001–0.024	8	8
Arsenic	0.015–0.621	8	8	0.028–0.629	8	8
Beryllium	0.003–0.008	5	8	0.002–0.010	7	8
Cadmium	0.002–0.029	8	8	0.002–0.023	8	8
Chromium	0.02–0.73	8	8	0.08–1.1	8	8
Copper	0.091–1.3	8	8	0.206–2.9	8	8
Lead	0.18–47	8	8	0.44–14	8	8
Mercury	0.001–0.16	8	8	0.002–0.066	8	8
Nickel	0.06–0.30	8	8	0.06–0.42	8	8
Selenium	ND	0	8	0.007	1	8
Silver	0.003–0.007	4	8	0.002–0.015	5	8
Zinc	0.247–17	8	8	0.864–17	8	8
Total cyanides	0.01–0.35	7	8	0.01–0.63	7	8
Total phenols	0.03–102	8	8	0.03–78	8	8

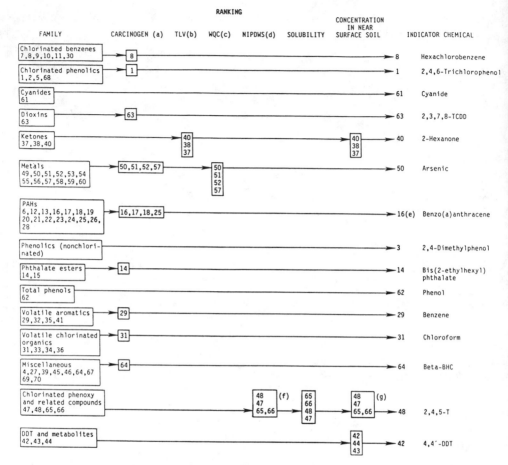

RANKING

FAMILY	CARCINOGEN (a)	TLV(b)	WQC(c)	NIPDWS(d)	SOLUBILITY	CONCENTRATION IN NEAR SURFACE SOIL	INDICATOR CHEMICAL
Chlorinated benzenes 7,8,9,10,11,30	8					8	Hexachlorobenzene
Chlorinated phenolics 1,2,5,68	1					1	2,4,6-Trichlorophenol
Cyanides 61						61	Cyanide
Dioxins 63	63					63	2,3,7,8-TCDD
Ketones 37,38,40		40 38 37				40 38 37	40	2-Hexanone
Metals 49,50,51,52,53,54 55,56,57,58,59,60	50,51,52,57		50 51 52 57				50	Arsenic
PAHs 6,12,13,16,17,18,19 20,21,22,23,24,25,26, 28	16,17,18,25						16(e)	Benzo(a)anthracene
Phenolics (nonchlori-nated)						3	2,4-Dimethylphenol
Phthalate esters 14,15	14					14	Bis(2-ethylhexyl) phthalate
Total phenols 62						62	Phenol
Volatile aromatics 29,32,35,41	29					29	Benzene
Volatile chlorinated organics 31,33,34,36	31					31	Chloroform
Miscellaneous 4,27,39,45,46,64,67 69,70	64					64	Beta-BHC
Chlorinated phenoxy and related compounds 47,48,65,66			48 47 65,66 (f)	65 66 48 47	48 47 65,66 (g)		48	2,4,5-T
DDT and metabolites 42,43,44					42 44 43		42	4,4'-DDT

(a)Carcinogenicity based on DHHS (1983) and USEPA (1984).

(b)TLVs taken from Threshold Limit Value (TLV) for Chemical Substances and Physical Agents in the Work Environment, ACGIH, 1984.

(c)USEPA Water Quality Criteria (WQC), 1980, Federal Register Vol. 45, No. 231.

(d)National Interim Primary Drinking Water Standard.

(e)Chemical No. 16 (Benzo(a)anthracene) was selected because it was the only carcinogenic PAH that was detected in the well water.

(f)Chemicals Nos. 65 and 66 do not have drinking water standards.

(g)Dicamba (No. 65) and 2,4-DB (No. 66) were not detected in the near-surface wells.

Figure 5. Indicator chemical selection.

TABLE 6. Names and Assigned Index Numbers of All Chemicals Susceptible to Offsite Transport

CAS Number[a]	Chemical Name	Risk Assessment Index Number
83-32-9	Acenaphthene	6
208-96-8	Acenaphthylene	20
67-64-1	Acetone	37
959-98-8	α-Endosulfan	45
120-12-7	Anthracene	21
	Antimony	49
	Arsenic	50
71-43-2	Benzene	29
56-55-3	Benzo[a]anthracene	16
205-99-2	Benzo[b]fluoranthene	18
191-24-2	Benzo[g, h, i]perylene	22
50-32-8	Benzo[a]pyrene	17
65-85-0	Benzoic acid	4
100-51-6	Benzyl alcohol	70
319-85-7	β-BHC (β-hexa-chlorocyclohexane)	64
	Beryllium	51
117-81-7	Bis(2-ethylhexyl)phthalate	14
78-93-3	2-Butanone	38
	Cadmium	52
75-15-0	Carbon disulfide	39
108-90-7	Chlorobenzene	30
67-66-3	Chloroform	31
91-58-7	2-Chloronaphthalene	69
95-57-8	2-Chlorophenol	68
	Chromium	53
	Copper	54
218-01-9	Chrysene	19
	Cyanide	61
94-75-7	2, 4-D (2, 4-dichlorophenoxy-acetic acid)	47
94-82-6	2, 4-DB (2, 4-dichlorophenoxy-butyric acid)	66
72-54-8	4, 4'-DDD (dichlorodiphenyl-dichloroethane)	44
72-55-9	4, 4'-DDE (1, 1-dichloro-2, 2-bis(p-chlorophenyl)-ethylene)	43
50-29-3	4, 4'-DDT (dichlorodiphenyl-trichloroethane)	42
75-99-0	Dalapon	46
132-64-9	Dibenzofuran	27
1918-00-9	Dicamba	65
95-50-1	1, 2-Dichlorobenzene	9
541-73-1	1, 3-Dichlorobenzene	10
106-46-7	1, 4-Dichlorobenzene	11
120-33-2	2, 4-Dichlorophenol	2
105-67-9	2, 4-Dimethylphenol	3
84-74-2	Di-N-butylphthalate	15

TABLE 6. (*Continued*)

CAS Number[a]	Chemical Name	Risk Assessment Index Number
88-85-7	Dinoseb (DNBP)	67
100-41-4	Ethylbenzene	32
206-44-0	Fluoranthene	12
86-73-7	Fluorene	23
118-74-1	Hexachlorobenzene	8
519-78-6	2-Hexanone	40
193-39-5	Indeno[1, 2, 3-*cd*]pyrene	25
	Lead	55
	Mercury	56
91-57-6	2-Methylnaphthalene	28
75-09-2	Methylene chloride	33
91-20-3	Naphthalene	13
	Nickel	57
85-01-8	Phenanthrene	24
108-95-2	Phenol	62
129-00-0	Pyrene	26
	Selenium	58
	Silver	59
93-76-5	2, 4, 5-T (2, 4, 5-trichloro-phenoxyacetic acid)	48
1746-01-6	2, 3, 7, 8-TCDD (2, 3, 7, 8-tetrachlorodibenzo-*p*-dioxin)	63
79-34-5	Tetrachloroethane	34
108-88-3	Toluene	36
120-82-1	1, 2, 4-Trichlorobenzene	7
79-01-6	Trichloroethene	35
95-95-4	2, 4, 5-Trichlorophenol	5
88-06-2	2, 4, 6-Trichlorophenol	1
95-47-6	Xylene	41
	Zinc	60

[a]CAS numbers are assigned by Chemical Abstracts Service (CAS) to organic compounds only.

compound was selected as the indicator. A carcinogenicity rating was based on the findings of the National Toxicology Program (NTP) as reported in the *Third Annual Report on Carcinogens* (16) and on the carcinogenic potency reported by the Carcinogen Assessment Group (17).

- Multiple chemical groups with more than one known or suspected carcinogen were then reviewed to select the compound with the highest reported carcinogenic potency.
- Multiple chemical categories with no known carcinogens were ranked according to (i) the degree of acute and chronic toxicity as indicated by the American Conference of Governmental Industrial Hygienists Threshold Limit Values (18), U.S. EPA's Ambient Water Quality Criteria or National Interim Primary Drinking Water Standards (19); (ii) water sloubility; (iii) volatility; and (iv) the reported concentration in near-surface soils.

4.2 Identification of Indicator Chemicals

As described above, a subset of potentially mobile chemicals was defined from the total analytical data base. Using the selection criteria stated above, an indicator chemical was chosen from each chemical class. The 15 representative chemicals and their index numbers (INS) are arsenic (50), benzo[a]anthracene (16), 2, 4-dimethylphenol (2, 4-DMP) (3), bis(2-ethylhexyl)phthalate (DEHP) (14), phenol (62), benzene (29), chloroform (31), 2, 4-5-T (48), 4, 4'-DDT (42), hexachlorobenzene (HCB) (8), 2, 3, 7, 8-TCDD (63), 2, 4, 6-trichlorophenol (1), 2-hexanone (40), cyanide (61), and β-BHC (64). Figure 5 illustrates the selection process and identifies these indicator chemicals.

The group of indicator chemicals was then evaluated to select subsets of chemicals for analysis in the water or air exposure pathways. The categorization of chemicals for exposure analyses via these two pathways is described below.

4.2.1 Water Exposure Pathway.
This site is located adjacent to a tidal river (i.e., this portion of the river is influenced by ocean tides). The potential transport pathways include surface water runoff into the river and leaching to groundwater systems with subsequent offsite transport. The identified significant exposure pathways are discussed in Section 5.

The proximity of the tidal river and the documented hydraulic connection between it and the groundwater systems increased the probability of offsite transport to potential receptors in the river. These receptors included finfish and benthic organisms. Both groups are susceptible to both soluble and hydrophobic or lipid-soluble contaminants.

Similarly, a number of groundwater wells were identified in proximity of the site that draw water from the glaciofluvial groundwater system. However, these wells were designated for industrial use, not for domestic use.

Exposure and risk estimations for all 15 chemicals were conducted via this pathway. The total number of indicator chemicals was chosen because of the location and sensitivity of the potential receptor groups, and the possibility of some movement with groundwater for all chemicals due to the presence of solvents.

4.2.2 Air Exposure Pathway.
Chemicals transported via the air generally exist in one of two phases, as a gas/vapor or as a particulate (sorbed to a suspended solid). The volatile indicator chemicals were ranked according to their vapor pressures and carcinogenic potencies (INs) (Table 7). The compounds 2, 4-DMP (3), DEHP (14), benzene (29), chloroform (31), and 2-hexanone (40) were ranked by decreasing vapor pressure, as a high value is indicative of greater volatility. Benzene (29) and chloroform (31) were ranked significantly higher than 2, 4-DMP (3) and DEHP (14). Benzene (29) is a human carcinogen and chloroform (31) is an animal carcinogen. Based on their relatively high vapor pressures and carcinogenicity, both benzene (29) and chloroform (31) were selected as air pathway indicator chemicals.

Chemicals that adsorb on airborne particulates under normal conditions generally have high octanol–water partition coefficients. At this site, these include 2, 4, 6-TCP (1), HCB (8), benzo[a]anthracene (16), DDT (42), 2, 4, 5-T (48), arsenic (50), cyanide (61), phenol (62), 2, 3, 7, 8-TCDD (63), and β-BHC (64). All but 2, 4, 5-T (48), cyanide (61), and phenol (62) have some reported carcinogenic potential. Because of inadequate information on the carcinogenic potency of benzo[a]anthracene, a health-protective assumption was used to rank it using the carcinogenic potency of benzo[a]pyrene, which is ranked by CAG as the most potent carcinogen of the PAHs.

Given that 2, 3, 7, 8-TCDD's carcinogenic potency index of 8, as classified by CAG, is four or more orders of magnitude higher than the other chemicals susceptible to transport

TABLE 7. Selection of Air Pathway Chemicals

Volatiles		
Ranked by Vapor Pressure[a]	Ranked by Cancer Potency[b]	Selected Chemicals
31—Chloroform (160)	31—Chloroform (8)	Chloroform
29—Benzene (76)	29—Benzene (4)	Benzene
40—2-Hexanone (2)	14—Bis(2-ethylhexyl)-	
3—2,4-Dimethylphenol (0.062)	phthalate[c]	
14—Bis(2-ethylhexyl) phthalate (2×10^{-7})		

Particulates	
Ranked by Cancer Potency[b]	Selected Chemical
63—2,3,7,8-TCDD (5×10^7)	63—2,3,7,8-TCDD
16—Benzo[a]anthracene (3×10^3)[d]	
42—4,4'-DDT (3×10^3)	
50—Arsenic (2×10^3)	
8—Hexachlorobenzene (5×10^2)	
1—2,4,6-Trichlorophenol (4)	
64—β-BHC[c]	

[a] Vapor pressure (mm Hg) in parentheses.
[b] Potency index in parentheses (17).
[c] No potency evaluation by Carcinogen Assessment Group.
[d] The carcinogenic potency of benzo[a]pyrene was used because it is higher than that of benzo[a]anthracene and thus is more health protective.

via this pathway, it was chosen as the indicator chemical to represent potential exposure to all particulate-phase chemicals.

5 EXPOSURE ASSESSMENT

The primary purpose of an exposure assessment is to determine the concentration levels over time and space in each environmental media where human and other environmental receptors may come in contact with the chemicals of concern. The four components of an exposure assessment (5, 20, 21) which are discussed in subsequent sections are (i) potential sources, (ii) significant exposure pathways, (iii) populations potentially at risk, and (iv) exposure estimates.

The approach taken in this assessment is biased toward health protective assumptions that tend to overestimate exposure. The following assumptions apply to all exposure pathways. Other pathway-specific assumptions are discussed in the respective sections on the migration pathways.

- At present the site is covered with geofabric, is fenced, and has a 24-h per day guard. This assessment assumes, for the purposes of judging exposure potential, that the present conditions will continue and there will be no further remediation of the site.

- All estimated exposure levels are based on a chemical source that is not affected by chemical adsorption to soil. However, adsorption processes are known to greatly decrease the environmental mobility of materials such as 2, 3, 7, 8-TCDD and DDT.
- The site is assumed to be the sole source of chemicals detected in environmental media during site investigation studies, even though it may not be the sole source.

5.1 Potential Sources

The potential sources of hazardous constituents were identified by a review of past operating practices at the site and by interpretation of contaminant concentration distribution in the buildings, soil, and groundwater. For the purposes of this risk assessment, the sources of contaminants were divided into the following groups for release potential: surface water, groundwater, and air.

The identification of potential sources revealed common areas of potential contaminant release or emission to an exposure pathway. This component of the exposure assessment is important because not only does it help define significant exposure pathways, but it also assists in the determination of area- or media-specific remediation objectives, should they be required.

5.1.1 *Areas Potentially Releasing Contaminants to Surface Water Runoff.* These areas include the contaminated buildings onsite because rainfall can wash contaminants off surfaces (e.g., outside walls) onto the ground (Fig. 2). These areas also include any exposed surface soil (approximately top 3 in.) where contaminants may be eroded or transported offsite in a dissolved phase. However, the exposed surface soil area onsite was extremely small due to the placement of a geofabric cover, thus negating this area as a potential source.

5.1.2 *Areas Potentially Releasing Contaminants to the Glaciofluvial Groundwater System.* As described earlier, the primary groundwater systems under the site consist of a shallow water system separated by a relatively impermeable peat-soil layer from a deeper confined glaciofluvial system. This deeper system has been identified as a source for industrial water use. The potential sources of concern were the fill above the water table, where significant contamination was detected, and the shallow groundwater system itself.

5.1.3 *Areas Potentially Releasing Contaminants into the Air.* These areas are essentially the same as those for surface runoff. Particulate emissions are most likely from buildings and any exposed surface soil, while vapor emissions are most likely to result from the soil surface. Although the site is covered with geofabric, a quantitative analysis was made for vapor emission and dispersion from the entire soil surface since the covering is not a vapor barrier.

5.2 Populations Potentially at Risk

Three primary receptor groups were identified as having the highest probability for potential exposure:

- *Workers.* The occupational population in the immediate vicinity of the site.

TABLE 8. Population Profile Information at Various Distances From the Site[a]

Distance	Number of Individuals	Cumulative Population	Number of Households
0.50	978	978	335
0.75	4,203	5,181	1,394
1.00	4,844	10,025	1,692
1.50	28,281	38,306	9,911
2.00	35,357	73,663	12,576
2.50	45,820	119,483	16,361
3.00	79,290	198,773	27,813
3.50	121,422	320,195	43,717
4.00	138,789	458,984	49,167

[a]Based on 1980 Census Tract Data.

- *Local Residents.* The closest residential population identified is approximately 200 meters offsite. The environment around the site is heavily industrialized and the population profile information provided in Table 8 reveals that about 1000 people live within a $\frac{1}{2}$-mile radius.
- *Aquatic Biota in the Tidal River.* Because of the complex nature of determining the potential magnitude of effects to aquatic biota and to humans who could eat fin fish and crustacea that have bioaccumulated chemicals, a decision was made to address the potential risks to the river in a separate project. This is presently underway. However, exposure concentrations in the river for chemicals in runoff and recharge from the site were calculated.

5.3   Significant Exposure Pathways

An exposure pathway is the potential route a hazardous substance may take to reach a susceptible human or other environmental receptor. The route of exposure and its duration will influence the impact on the receptor. Routes of exposure are usually categorized as inhalation, ingestion, and dermal exposure (direct skin contact). There may be exposure by uptake in the food chain with eventual human consumption or by dermal and inhalation exposure during recreational water use (swimming, fishing, and boating). Exposure durations are separated into two main classes: (i) acute (meaning episodic or short-time duration and frequency) and (ii) chronic [implying long-term (months and years), continuous, or frequent exposure].

A generalized exposure pathway flowchart is presented in Fig. 6. This flowchart was used to identify all potential exposure pathways. These pathways are graphically illustrated in Fig. 3. A "complete" pathway is imperative if an exposure is to occur. In other words, these factors must coincide for an exposure to occur: a source of contamination, a route of contaminant transport to a receptor, and a receptor in that path.

A thorough analysis must address all exposure pathways. To identify the potentially significant exposure pathways, the universe of possible pathways was identified and each was evaluated qualitatively for its relevance to the site. Those that were not eliminated in this manner were subjected to a quantitative analysis to provide a better characterization

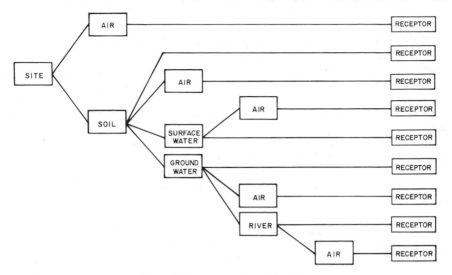

Figure 6. Exposure pathway flowchart.

of the potential for significant exposure. Based on the potential sources, potential receptor groups, and routes of potential transport at this site, three significant exposure pathways were identified:

• Transport of sorbed and dissolved chemicals via surface runoff and recharge into the adjoining tidal river, which could lead to aquatic biota exposure and human ingestion.
• Leaching of chemicals into the glaciofluvial groundwater system, with subsequent offsite transport and potential exposure via ingestion of groundwater.
• Onsite and offsite inhalation of volatile and/or particulate phase chemicals that have been released and dispersed.

Exposure estimates were conducted for these three pathways.

5.4 Exposure Estimates

The three significant exposure pathways identified above were quantitatively judged for potential exposure. Exposure estimates for each pathway are described below.

5.4.1 Surface Runoff and Recharge into the Adjoining Tidal River.   Two modes of transport of contaminants to the river were evaluated: (i) chemicals adsorbed to soil in the runoff or chemicals dissolved in the surface runoff and (ii) groundwater discharge containing chemicals from the shallow water table groundwater system. Each mode of transport is described separately.

The runoff volume from a surface during precipitation depends on the intensity and amount of rainfall, ground surface properties, and initial moisture conditions. Site-specific parameters were identified to permit calculation of the potential runoff from direct precipitation on the site.

Two scenarios were developed to set boundaries on the actual site conditions relative to these parameters. In the first case, the site was assumed to contain only pervious surfaces (soil), even though only about 50% is pervious. Direct precipitation and runoff from building gutters and surfaces will drain onto fully pervious surfaces. In other words, no runoff from the site is generated during an average storm. In this case, the precipitation rate does not exceed the infiltration capacity and all the precipitation would enter the unsaturated zone. At the opposite extreme, the second case assumes all surfaces were paved and nearly all the precipitation remains on the surface in pools and/or leaves the site as surface runoff.

Most of the runoff will enter the river directly or through storm sewers. Discharge into the river will be diluted by mixing with river water both upstream and downstream, depending on tidal conditions. A simplified dilution analysis allowed calculation of a dilution factor of approximately 10,000 for site runoff entering the river from an average storm.

Example Calculation 1 (Estimating Runoff at the Site). Discharge into the river will mix with river water both upstream and downstream depending on the tidal conditions. The mean concentration of compounds near the point of discharge in tidal rivers can be estimated using a simplified dilution analysis (22). The total flow availble for diluting the runoff (Q_d) is

$$Q_d = \frac{(Q_e + Q_f)S_o}{S_o - S},$$

where Q_e = discharge into the river [in cubic feet per second (cfs)]
$\quad\quad Q_f$ = tributary discharge from all tributaries upstream of the point of discharge into the river (cfs)
$\quad\quad S_o$ = ocean salinity
$\quad\quad S$ = salinity of the river.

The United States Geological Survey (23) has developed equations using standard regression techniques for making simplified, gross estimates of mean annual flow (Q_f). The equation for noncoastal drainages is

$$Q_f = KA^{1.0},$$

where A is the drainage area in square miles and K is a conversion factor. For this site, $K = 1.534\,\text{cfs/mi}^2$. Then

$$Q_f = (1.534\,\text{cfs/mi}^2)(920\,\text{mi})^{1.0}$$

$$= 1411\,\text{cfs}.$$

The average ocean salinity (S_o) is assumed to be 35 ppth (24). The salinity on the river about 2 miles upstream from the site from February through September 1982 ranged from 0.45 to 20 ppth. A reasonably conservative value of 10 ppth midway between the two extremes is assumed for river salinity (S). In the above equation, average runoff into the river (Q_e) is 0.19 cfs. This is insignificant when compared to the mean annual flow (Q_f) of 1411 cfs and therefore can be disregarded. The total flow available for diluting the stormwater runoff (Q_d) under average conditions can be approximated by

$$Q_d \approx \frac{(1411\,\text{cfs})(35\,\text{ppth})}{(35\,\text{ppth} - 10\,\text{ppth})} \approx 1976\,\text{cfs}.$$

The dilution factor for runoff from an average storm into the river is

$$\frac{0.19\,\text{cfs}}{10176\,\text{cfs}} = 0.0001 = 1 \times 10^{-4}.$$

Using the parameters discussed in the previous paragraphs, we find that the site's capability for adsorbing all the direct precipitation exceeds the expected precipitation from average storm events by a factor of 1.50. Therefore, in the absence of any significant hydraulic gradient, all the precipitation can move vertically through the fill. This is consistent with the assumption that the entire site area (3.4 acres) is pervious. The precipitation rate does not exceed the potential infiltration capacity of soils found at the site. Therefore, surface runoff under this scenario was not considered to be an important migration pathway for chronic, long-term exposure.

The other mode of transport of contaminants is via recharge to the river. Precipitation can move through the unsaturated zone, to the saturated groundwater system in the fill, and act as recharge to the river. Flow offsite may enter storm sewers and discharge to the river, infiltrate into sanitary sewers, travel horizontally further offsite, or move into deeper groundwater zones.

Example Calculation 2 (Estimating Water Loss to the River). A simple, steady-state water balance equation (Darcy's equation) was used to calculate discharge to the river (25):

$$Q = KiA,$$

where Q = fluid flow through a porous medium (ft^3/day)
  K = hydraulic conductivity of the porous medium (ft/day)
  i = gradient of the water table (ft/ft)
  A = cross-sectional area perpendicular to flow (ft^2).

Using site data and reasonable assumptions to derive site-specific parameter values for Darcy's equation results in a calculated discharge to the river of

$$Q = (25\,\text{ft/day})(0.02)(2100\,\text{ft}^2) = 1050\,\text{ft}^3/\text{day} = 0.012\,\text{ft}^3/\text{s}.$$

This discharge rate was then divided by the river flow Q_{7-10} (the lowest consecutive 7-day flow over a 10-year period) to obtain a health protective dilution factor:

$$(0.012\,\text{ft}^3/\text{s})/(1976\,\text{ft}^3/\text{s}) = 6.1 \times 10^{-6}.$$

Table 9 provides calculated offsite concentrations of indicator chemicals in surface water. Instream concentrations for the river were estimated by using the mean and maximum concentrations detected in the shallow wells and diluting by a factor of 6×10^6, which is the dilution factor for groundwater flow from the fill area to the river. As shown in this table, DDT concentrations are relatively high, with a mean of 1.6 ppm and a

TABLE 9. Estimated Offsite Concentrations of Indicator Chemicals in Surface Water (µg/L)

Risk Assessment Index Number	Indicator Chemical	Measured at Site		Estimated in the Adjoining River[a]	
		Mean	Maximum	Mean	Maximum
50	Arsenic	232	629	1.4×10^{-3}	3.8×10^{-3}
29	Benzene	1,063	7,900	6.4×10^{-3}	4.7×10^{-2}
16	Benzo[a]anthracene	0.5	8	3.0×10^{-6}	4.8×10^{-5}
31	Chloroform	34	240	2.0×10^{-4}	1.4×10^{-3}
42	4,4'-DDT	1,620	22,000	9.7×10^{-3}	1.3×10^{-1}
8	Hexachlorobenzene	102	860	6.1×10^{-4}	5.2×10^{-3}
63	2,3,7,8-TCDD	1.57	10.4	9.4×10^{-6}	6.2×10^{-5}
1	2,4,6-Trichlorophenol	1,481	11,000	8.9×10^{-3}	6.6×10^{-2}
40	2-Hexanone	ND[b]	ND	—	—
14	Bis(2-ethylhexyl)phthalate	10	75	6.0×10^{-5}	4.5×10^{-4}
64	β-BHC	ND	ND	—	—
48	2,4,5-T	714	5,600	4.3×10^{-3}	3.4×10^{-2}
61	Cyanide	80	630	4.8×10^{-4}	3.8×10^{-3}
62	Phenol	17,000	102,000	1.0×10^{-1}	6.1×10^{-1}
3	2,4-Dimethylphenol	ND	ND	—	—

[a]Based on dilution factor of 6.1×10^6.
[b]ND indicates not detected.

maximum of 22 ppm. This maximum concentration occurred in a monitoring well that is 3–5 ft from the bulkhead along the river. DDT is highly insoluble in water and is strongly adsorbed to soils or suspended particles containing some small carbon fraction. In the absence of cosolvents, DDT (and other hydrophobic compounds) is very immobile in soil–water systems. This was not factored into the calculations. Therefore, the estimated exposure concentrations in the river were extremely health protective and assured that the upper bound of potential risk to aquatic receptors was adequately defined.

5.4.2 Leaching of Contaminants to the Deeper Glaciofluvial Groundwater System with Subsequent Offsite Transport.
There were two primary components of groundwater transport via this pathway:

• The rate of migration of chemicals in groundwater as characterized by a plume with a moving front edge, from the fill area to the glaciofluvial sands below.
• The flux of chemicals from the glaciofluvial sand system to areas where potential exposure may take place offsite.

Each of these components is described below.

The vertical rate of migration was defined to characterize offsite migration by the groundwater pathway. The well data from the fill area and glaciofluvial sands indicated that the highest chemical concentrations were found in the fill area (Fig. 3). Relatively low concentrations were found in the sands below, indicating that the rate of migration is slow and/or that the chemicals could originate from an offsite source.

The calculated maximum vertical migration velocity of a chemical was 1 ft/yr assuming no retardation factor (i.e., the chemical moves at the same rate as the water). Using an average silt layer thickness of 9 ft, it would take a compound at least 9 years to move through the silt layer to reach the top of the sands. However, for chemicals with very low water solubility and high soil adsorption coefficients, such as DDT and 2, 3, 7, 8-TCDD and thus high retardation factors, the rate of movement will be considerably slower.

The retardation factor is an indicator of a compound's inability to move with water as the water passes through soil due to the compound's tendency to bind to soil. This is an important consideration in environmental risk assessment since it gives an indication of the rate of movement toward receptors relative to groundwater. Retardation factors based on octanol–water partitioning coefficients were estimated using site-specific organic carbon content values. The estimates were 340,000 and 38,000 for 2, 3, 7, 8-TCDD and DDT, respectively. These estimates strongly suggest that these two chemicals will move at least several thousand times slower than groundwater.

Example Calculation 3 (Estimating Retardation Factor). One equation for calculating the retardation factor (R_f) is (25)

$$R_f = 1 + \frac{\rho}{n} K_d,$$

where R_f = retardation factor
ρ = bulk density of porous media
n = porosity
K_d = distribution coefficient.

K_d can be calculated (26) as

$$K_d = K_{oc} f_{oc},$$

where K_{oc} = organic carbon partition coefficient
f_{oc} = fraction of organic carbon.

The organic carbon partition coefficient can be obtained from the relation

$$\log K_{oc} = 1.00 \log K_{ow} - 0.21,$$

where K_{ow} is the octanol–water partition coefficient.

From these equations, the retardation factor can be calculated given (26)

$$K_{ow}(DDT) = 6.19,$$

$$\rho = 1.6 \text{ g/cm}^2,$$

$$n = 0.40,$$

$$f_{oc} = 0.01.$$

(a) $\qquad \log K_{oc} = 1.00 \ (6.19) - 0.21 = 5.98;$

(b) $\qquad K_d(DDT) = (955,000)(0.01) = 9550;$

(c) $\qquad R_f(DDT) = 1 + \frac{1.6}{0.4}(9550) = 38.2.$

Although this analysis was not used to define a source or loading term for groundwater transport, it served to define the very slow potential flux of contaminants from the shallow fill to the deeper, confined glaciofluvial groundwater system. This qualitative assessment helped define the semiconfined nature of the potential source in the fill area. It also helped define the conceptual design of remedial alternatives to contain the contaminant source area.

The potential for chemicals to leach to the aquifer below the fill exists even though the vertical migration of compounds is slow. Therefore, an appraisal of chemical movement through the glaciofluvial sands and bedrock was performed to determine the potential future exposure, which may occur by ingestion of groundwater that has moved offsite.

Unlike the upper fill zone where there are few, if any, pumping wells that affect flow, the hydrology in the glaciofluvial sands and bedrock aquifers in the site vicinity may be influenced or altered by high-capacity pumping wells. To determine potential exposure from ingestion of water, a high-capacity well was identified that has a remote potential to be used as drinking water and whose cone of influence encompasses the site. Calculations for estimating potential exposure were conducted as described below.

Although groundwater below the site can potentially be drawn into the pumping wells, concentrations of compounds will be considerably attenuated. Groundwater from the site will constitute only a small portion of the total intake to the well because the total intake includes water from all radial directions. By using a simplified net flow analysis (27), an upper-bound estimate of the expected concentration of chemicals in product water was made. The supply well identified above was located approximately 600 m south of the site and was determined to be the well most likely to intercept chemical migration due primarily to its proximity to the site. A dilution factor of 1085 was estimated and was used in subsequent analyses. The mean and maximum concentrations of the indicator chemicals found in the shallow onsite well groundwater samples are shown in Table 10.

These concentrations were divided by the dilution factor to yield gross estimates of potential offsite contamination to the closest well. The maximum concentrations of compounds found in these samples represent a very conservative starting point for evaluating worst-case concentrations offsite. The mean concentrations provide a more reasonable basis for estimating offsite concentrations. Together, they provide a range of site-specific worst-case concentration estimates.

TABLE 10. Estimated Offsite Concentrations of Indicator Chemicals in Groundwater (μg/L)

Risk Assessment Index Number	Indicator Chemical	Measured at Site		Estimated in Closest Well[a]	
		Mean	Maximum	Mean	Maximum
50	Arsenic	232	629	0.21	0.58
29	Benzene	1,063	7,900	0.98	7.28
16	Benzo[a]anthracene	0.5	8	4.6×10^{-4}	7.4×10^{-3}
31	Chloroform	34	240	3.1×10^{-2}	0.22
42	4, 4'-DDT	1,620	22,000	1.49	20.3
8	Hexachlorobenzene	102	860	9.4×10^{-2}	0.79
63	2, 3, 7, 8-TCDD	1.57	10.4	1.5×10^{-3}	9.6×10^{-3}
1	2, 4, 6-Trichlorophenol	1,481	11,000	1.36	10.1
40	2-Hexanone	ND[b]	ND	NA[c]	NA
14	Bis(2-ethylhexyl)phthalate	10	75	9.2×10^{-3}	6.9×10^{-2}
64	β-BHC	ND	ND	NA	NA
48	2, 4, 5-T	714	5,600	0.66	5.2
61	Cyanide	80	630	7.4×10^{-2}	0.58
62	Phenol	17,000	102,000	15.7	94.0
3	2, 4-Dimethylphenol	ND	ND	NA	NA

[a]Based on dilution factor of 1085.
[b]ND indicates not detected.
[c]NA indicates not applicable.

Even though this well nor any well in the vicinity is permitted be to used for drinking, potential human exposure to groundwater from this well was estimated as one illustration of the potential impact on water quality.

To estimate the maximum daily exposure to chemicals from the site via groundwater, it was assumed that the ingestion rate was 1 L/day. For example, the potential daily exposure to arsenic at some time in the future could range from 0.21 to 0.58 μg/day (Table 10).

Additional exposure estimates from this illustrative approach are also listed in Table 10 as ranges, since the mean and maximum concentrations were used. These potential exposure ranges were similarly used in the selection and design of remedial alternatives. A number of health protective assumptions supplemented the quantitative analyses.

The estimates shown in Table 10 represent maximum feasible estimates of daily dose. In all likelihood, the actual daily doses will be much lower or nonexistent due to the following health protective assumptions inherent in the estimates:

- The dilution factor is underestimated since it does not consider attenuation of chemicals through biological and physiochemical reactions with the soil or attenuation due to dispersion in the groundwater. As discussed previously, these retardation and dispersion factors reduce concentrations of compounds during transport from the onsite area to the surrounding environment.

- The analysis does not consider the effects of the subsurface stratigraphy. Discontinuous layers of silt and other low-permeability layers within the glaciofluvial sands would be obstacles to the downward migration of chemicals from the near-surface soils. These would tend to slow migration to the industrial user, who is the primary groundwater user having remote opportunity for being impacted.

- The nearest well was assumed to be for drinking water even though this is an industrial well and not permitted for drinking use (nor are any wells in the vicinity permitted for drinking water).

- Estimates of exposure are based on a site that contains an ongoing source (still producing), whereas in reality the site is inactive with a finite amount of chemicals.

In short, the estimates in Table 10 are provided simply as an order-of-magnitude estimate of the degree of potential contamination rather than likely human uptake.

5.4.3 *Air Exposure Pathway.*

Two primary areas were identified as potential sources for the air exposure pathway. The covered ground surface (vapors) and the surfaces of contaminated buildings onsite (particulates). Each source/pathway is discussed separately below.

5.4.3.1 *Particulates from Buildings.*

The primary chemical of concern via particulate releases is 2, 3, 7, 8-TCDD because of its low solubility and preference for sorption onto particulates (see Section 4). These contaminated particulates may be eroded from outside building surfaces and subsequently transported by the wind to offsite receptors. The geofabric ground covering has essentially eliminated surface soil wind erosion.

Given 2, 3, 7, 8-TCDD's extremely high cancer potency index assigned by CAG, and the distribution of 2, 3, 7, 8-TCDD on most of the buildings, any required remediation objective for its cleanup would assure that cleanup objectives for less prevalent and toxic chemicals that are susceptible to particulate transport will be met as well.

Air sampling was conducted with the objective of screening for the presence or absence of 2, 3, 7, 8-TCDD. The sampling was not designed to project onsite or offsite exposures. Thirty-one 24-h air particulate samples were collected over a continuous 31-day period. Ten of the 31 air particulate samples were selected for 2, 3, 7, 8-TCDD analysis based on indications that they potentially had the highest soil content. As discussed earlier (Section 3.3.1), the results of the air sampling indicated that two samples of the 10 analyzed had detectable 2, 3, 7, 8-TCDD concentrations. No obvious relation existed between the reported the 2, 3, 7, 8-TCDD levels and the meteorological conditions on the days when they occurred. It is unlikely that the measured airborne 2, 3, 7, 8-TCDD concentrations were from fugitive emissions of 2, 3, 7, 8-TCDD-containing soil, since the site had been covered with geofabric continuously since 1983, including during the sampling. The source of the detected airborne 2, 3, 7, 8-TCDD could have been from an offsite source, from the buildings and structures on the site, or a result of some of the site investigation activities. Ample information was available to conclude that the 2, 3, 7, 8-TCDD detected originated from 2, 3, 7, 8-TCDD-contaminated fume hood exhaust stacks near the rooftop sampling station.

The sampling conducted was not designed to project onsite or offsite exposures. However, the data obtained were sufficient to conclude that the potential for occasional inhalation exposure to elevated 2, 3, 7, 8-TCDD concentration in building-related particulates might be significant. Therefore, the selected remediation should include eliminating this potential exposure, as well as potential exposure to surface soil that contained 2, 3, 7, 8-TCDD in concentrations of about 20–2000 ppb when detected.

5.4.3.2 Vapor Emissions Exposure. Although the surface soils on the site are covered with geofabric, this material is permeable to vapors, so a vapor emission and dispersion analysis was conducted. The analysis assumed that surface soil was exposed. This analysis was conducted for benzene and chloroform, which were the representative indicator chemicals for the volatilization air exposure pathway, because they were among the most volatile and most toxic.

A steady-state emission rate was calculated for each chemical (Table 11) using the equation below, which accounts for chemical diffusion from soil pores to air, relative concentration in soil, and soil cover depth, if present (28).

$$E_i = (D_i C_s A P_t)^{4/3}\left(\frac{1}{L}\right)\left(\frac{W_i}{W}\right),$$

where E_i = emission rate for the ith component (g/s)
D_i = diffusion coefficient of the ith component (cm²/s)
A = exposed area (cm²)
C_s = saturation vapor concentration of the ith component (g/cm³)
P_t = soil porosity (dimensionless)

TABLE 11. Estimated Concentrations of Indicator Chemicals for the Air Pathway (g/m³)

Risk Assessment Index Number	Indicator Chemical	Estimated Onsite		Estimated Offsite	
		Midrange	Maximum	Midrange	Maximum
29	Benzene	4.2×10^{-5}	8.3×10^{-5}	1.6×10^{-8}	3.3×10^{-8}
31	Chloroform	2.1×10^{-6}	4.2×10^{-6}	8.4×10^{-8}	1.7×10^{-7}

L = effective depth of soil cover (cm)

W_i/W = weight percent of the ith toxic component in the waste (g/g).

This type of analysis is health protective, as assumptions include (i) no sorption onto soil particles, which would retard the flux, and (ii) an infinite amount of chemical available in the soil parcel being evaluated.

The chemical source terms were then used to estimate onsite and offsite exposure concentrations. The onsite concentrations were derived by dividing the source terms by a specified volume of air over the site for a given time period. Offsite concentrations were estimated by using a steady-state gaussian dispersion equation. Assumptions used in this equation are that the wind direction is constant and always directed toward the nearest receptors and that the receptors are along the centerline of any potential plume.

The onsite concentrations were estimated to be 0.083 mg/m^3 (maximum) and 0.042 mg/m^3 (midrange) for benzene (29); and 0.0042 mg/m^3 (maximum) and 0.0021 mg/m^3 (midrange) for chloroform (31). Offsite concentrations at approximately 200 m downwind from the site were estimated to be 0.000033 mg/m^3 (maximum) and 0.000016 mg/m^3 (midrange) for benzene (29); and 0.00017 mg/m^3 (maximum) and 0.000084 mg/m^3 (midrange) for chloroform (31) (Table 11).

The air exposure pathway is considered for both onsite and offsite exposure to vapors. Onsite exposure is considered to be limited to the occupational population. Offsite exposure is developed for the closest residential population.

The following pathway-specific assumptions were used in developing the onsite occupational air exposure:

- Inhalation rate = 10 m^3/day.
- Absorption fraction = 1.0 (vapor).

The offsite air exposure estimates used the following specific assumptions for residential exposure:

- Exposure duration = 25,550 days.
- Inhalation rate = 23 m^3/day.
- Lifetime = 70 years.

A range is reported for the air pathway indicators because of the variability in chemical concentration in the soil and the range of exposure days caused by weather conditions.

Other potential emissions of volatile chemicals to secondary exposure pathways were qualitatively evaluated. They included volatilization of chemicals from groundwater and from surface water. Both of these pathways were deemed insignificant because of the estimated low concentrations of the indicator chemicals in groundwater and surface water, the limited exposure of people to groundwater from industrial wells, and the large volume of surface water in the river, allowing for rapid volatilization over a large surface area should transport to the river occur.

6   RISK CHARACTERIZATION

The objective of the risk characterization is to evaluate the significance of any potential risks posed by the site. This is accomplished by comparing the estimates of potential exposure to applicable, risk-derived criteria to determine if exposures might significantly exceed those associated with a very low probability to cause adverse health effects. The emphasis of this assessment is placed on public health risks. The populations potentially at greatest risk are the occupational population in the immediate vicinity and the closest residential population identified as being approximately 200 m offsite. The environment surrounding the site is highly industrialized, leaving the potential environmental risk relating only to the river. A separate characterization addressing potential environmental risks in the river is ongoing.

6.1   Basic Assumptions

- The U.S. EPA and Center for Disease Control (CDC) dose–response relations used to derive the carcinogenic potency index based on animal data are assumed to be valid for humans. This assumption has not been scientifically proved. Of the half-dozen equally feasible dose–response extrapolation models available, the one selected by these agencies as applied here is designed to define the highest upper-bound risk condition. The results from this model most likely overestimate the actual risk rather than underestimate it. In fact, the scientific evidence, relating to the mechanism by which 2, 3, 7, 8-TCDD induces cancer in rodents, leads to the conclusion that this chemical is a promoter and not an initiator of cancer (29–31). This renders these models invalid for application to 2, 3, 7, 8-TCDD.

- Cancer risks were estimated from projected 2, 3, 7, 8-TCDD exposures without making adjustments for bioavailability. Fries and Marrow (32) report that 50–60% of the 2, 3, 7, 8-TCDD added to feed in rat studies is absorbed by rats. However, studies by Umbreit et al. (33) suggest that as little as 0.5% of 2, 3, 7, 8-TCDD in soil may be absorbed by rats. Initially, Paustenbach et al. (34) concluded that 10% appears to be a reasonable estimate of oral bioavailability of this chemical from soil but later work by this group showed that oral bioavailability of TCDD in rodents was about 30–40% (45) and that dermal bioavailability of soil-bound TCDD was about 1% (46).

6.2   Risk Estimates

The risk estimates projected in this section are based predominantly on cancer risk. Owing to the U.S. EPA's position on the nonthreshold theory of carcinogenesis, cancer risk estimation almost always calls for the most stringent exposure criteria relative to other health effects. Therefore, by controlling human exposure to levels that protect against cancer, the hazard posed by other types of adverse health are also insignificant.

The term *cancer risk* is defined as risk in excess of existing background incidence. This "excess" is an important distinction since the estimated excess risks discussed in several of the following sections are thousands-fold lower than the U.S. human population cancer incidence of 25% or the cancer mortality of 20% (35).

The CAG (36) uses a prescribed protocol to evaluate animal data to estimate human cancer potencies. The model used is the linearized multistage extrapolation model, which provides a mathematical derivation of the dose–response slopes (37). This model is biased in that the scientific community recognizes that its use most likely overestimates the actual risk. Deliberate use of this model is a public policy decision by the EPA rather than a scientific one. No altogether conclusive evidence exists to validate selection of any of the other models that yield lower estimates of risk.

Another bias toward overestimation of the actual health risks has been adopted by the

CAG. In publishing its slope estimates, the CAG does not base the projections on the line of best fit of the data, usually referred to as the *maximum likelihood estimate*. Rather, it chooses to use the 95% confidence interval, which represents the upper bound of the risk estimate. This approach significantly exaggerates the risk related to a given dose or exposure (38, 39). Also, because the slope estimates are based on animal data, many compounds (e.g., 2, 3, 7, 8-TCDD) that have not been shown to be human carcinogens have higher potency values than those that are known human carcinogens (e.g., vinyl chloride). In short, because the models do not incorporate the role of biologic protective mechanisms or human epidemiology, they are only gross indicators that most likely overestimate potential risks. The U.S. EPA (36) and others (40) discuss these model shortcomings.

6.3   Recommended Exposure Criteria

Recommended exposure criteria for the indicator chemicals were developed separately for groundwater and air. Sample calculations for developing these criteria are discussed below. The results for all indicator chemicals are summarized in Table 12. A number of factors were considered in developing these criteria.

Example Calculation 4 (Estimating Daily Dose). The allowable daily intake was first calculated using the cancer potency slope developed by CAG (17). For the purposes of this assessment, these are assumed to be applicable for people even though this may not be the case. The cancer potency slope (q) for DDT is 8.42 $(mg/kg \cdot day)^{-1}$. The daily dose was calculated by the formula

$$D = \frac{R}{q},$$

where D is the daily dose and R is the approximate risk.
   For DDT at 10^{-5} risk,

$$D = \frac{10^{-5}}{8.42 \ (mg/kg \cdot day)^{-1}}$$

$$= 1.19 \times 10^{-6} \ mg/kg \cdot day$$

or 0.083 $\mu g/day$ for a 70-kg person. This daily dose represents the allowable dose for a residential exposure. To correct this value to an occupational exposure, the daily dose is multiplied by 2.77, which adjusts for the difference represented by a 70-year lifetime and a 38.5-year, 240-day/yr occupational lifetime.
   For DDT, the industrial exposure is $(8.3 \times 10^{-2} \ \mu g/day)(2.77) = 0.23 \ \mu g/day$. For an industrial well consumption of 1 L/day, this is equivalent to 0.23 $\mu g/L$ (Table 12).
   In this assessment, the recommended exposure criteria are based on the assumption that a lifetime incremental risk level of 1×10^{-5} (i.e., 1 in 100,000) over background is acceptable. It is important to reiterate that this represents an incremental risk, that is, an excess over the background cancer mortality frequency of one in five in the U.S. population (35). In other words, a 10^{-5} incremental risk raises the cancer mortality risk factor from 0.20000 to 0.20001. This incremental risk may be put into perspective by comparing circumstances that relate to annual mortality risks on the order of 10^{-5}.

TABLE 12. Recommended Exposure Criteria for Indicator Chemicals

			Acceptable Concentration[a] Air (mg/m³)			
			Particulates		Vapor	
Index Number	Indicator Chemical Name	Groundwater at Closest Well (μg/dL)	Onsite	Offsite	Onsite	Offsite
50	Arsenic	0.13	b	b	c	c
29	Benzene	36	b	b	30[d]	$(0.6–1.3) \times 10^{-3}$
16	Benzo[a]anthracene	0.16	b	b	c	c
31	Chloroform	28	b	b	240[d]	$(0.43–1.0) \times 10^{-3}$
42	4,4'-DDT	0.23	b	b	c	c
8	Hexachlorobenzene	1.2	b	b	c	c
63	2,3,7,8-TCDD	$(1.2–5.5) \times 10^{-5}$	$(5.3–5.4) \times 10^{-9}$	$(0.82–8.3) \times 10^{-9}$	c	c
1	2,4,6-Trichlorophenol	97	b	b	c	c
40	2-Hexanone	e	b	b	c	c
14	Bis(2-ethylhexyl)phthalate	15,000[f]	b	b	c	c
64	β-BHC	e	b	b	c	c
48	2,4,5-T	100[f]	b	b	c	c
61	Cyanide	200[f]	b	b	c	c
62	Phenol	3500[f]	b	b	c	c
3	2,4-Dimethylphenol	e	b	b	c	c

[a]Calculation based on cancer potency slopes (17) for carcinogens at the 1 in 100,000 (10^{-5}) excess risk level unless otherwise noted.

[b]Not applicable to air because it was not selected as a particulate indicator chemical.

[c]Not applicable to air because it was not selected as a vapor indicator chemical.

[d]OSHA standard for an acceptable daily exposure concentration for the occupational lifetime. Benzene ACGIH TLV = 30 mg/m³ and chloroform ACGIH TLV = 50 mg/m³.

[e]Not applicable to groundwater because none was detected in any groundwater samples.

[f]Ambient water quality criteria for noncarcinogens.

Annual risks differ from lifetime risks by a factor of 70, assuming the average life expectancy is about 70 years. For example, a 1 in 100,000 incremental cancer risk is associated with smoking 14 cigarettes (cancer, heart disease), breathing the air in New York City for 20 days, and many others that are generally regarded as acceptable (41).

This 1 in 100,000 risk level may be related directly to the site locale. The most recent census (1980) reports that within $\frac{1}{2}$ mile from the site there are less than 1000 residents (Table 8). Within a 1-mile radius there are 10,000 people. In this area, one would not be able to predict even one excess cancer incidence at these levels set for acceptable exposures. A population of 100,000 individuals spans a distance of 2.5 miles from the site. Exposure potential decreases with increasing distance from the source due to greater dilution of chemical concentrations. The potential cancer risk correspondingly decreases with increasing distance from the source. Before one would be able to project even one excess cancer, a population of about 100,000 would need to be exposed daily for a lifetime to the defined exposures on or immediately adjacent to the site.

6.4   Health Risk Estimates for Noncarcinogens

The risk associated with the noncarcinogens DEHP (14), 2, 4, 5-T (48), cyanide (61), and phenol (62) are negligible since the projected exposure concentrations (Table 10) are far lower than the recommended criteria in Table 12.

6.5   Excess Cancer Risk Estimates

6.5.1   Groundwater.   The estimated concentrations of the indicator chemicals in the closest well as shown Table 12 were taken as the potential exposure concentration for the

TABLE 13. Excess Cancer Risk Estimates

Contaminant	Airborne	Groundwater
Offsite		
2, 3, 7, 8-TCDD	a	$(9.5–800) \times 10^{-5}$
4, 4'-DDT	b	$(6.5–88) \times 10^{-5}$
Benzo[a]anthracene	b	$(2.9–46) \times 10^{-8}$
Benzene	$(1.2–5.5) \times 10^{-7}$	$(2.7–20) \times 10^{-7}$
Chloroform	$(8.4–40) \times 10^{-7}$	$(1.1–7.9) \times 10^{-8}$
2, 4, 6-Trichlorophenol	b	$(1.4–10) \times 10^{-7}$
Hexachlorobenzene	b	$(7.8–66) \times 10^{-7}$
Onsite		
2, 3, 7, 8-TCDD	a	c
4, 4'-DDT	b	c
Benzo[a]anthracene	b	c
Benzene	d	c
Chloroform	d	c

[a]Not a chemical subject to the vapor pathway.
[b]Not an indicator chemical for this pathway.
[c]No onsite receptors.
[d]Cancer risk estimation not applicable since OSHA standard applies to onsite exposure scenario. Benzene is three orders of magnitude and chloroform four orders of magnitude below their respective OSHA standards.

occupational population assuming a 1 L/day consumption rate. These data were divided by the recommended acceptable exposure criteria (Table 12) to calculate an estimated excess cancer risk above background levels that might occur without further remediation of the site (Table 13). The following assumptions were made:

- Exposure duration is 9240 days (assumed occupational lifetime of 38.5 years at 240 days/yr).
- Body weight = 70 kg.

The risk estimates are reported in ranges that reflect the ranges developed for Tables 10–12. The groundwater pathway exposure analysis projects a potential risk for 2, 3, 7, 8-TCDD (63) and DDT (42) in the offsite well. 2, 3, 7, 8-TCDD is projected to provide an excess cancer risk of 9.5×10^{-5} to 8×10^{-3} and DDT 6.5×10^{-5} to 8.8×10^{-4} (Table 13).

Since the risks for 2, 3, 7, 8-TCDD and DDT are projected to be greater than 1×10^{-5}, further evaluation of the exposure potential is in order to characterize the significance of the excess risk. As discussed in Section 5.4.2, the exposure projections, and consequently the risk estimates, are calculated without considering the reduction that adsorption has on groundwater transport of chemicals. For example, the retardation factor for 2, 3, 7, 8-TCDD was estimated to be in the range of 340,000–2,500,000. Furthermore, the calculated sorption capacity of the soil may prevent significant migration of 2, 3, 7, 8-TCDD. In other words, it is unlikely that the estimated risks could be realized even without remediation.

Cancer risks associated with arsenic (50) are considered differently from the other indicator compounds because arsenic is an element that occurs naturally in the earth's crust. Detection of arsenic onsite must be considered in relation to background levels.

Throughout the United States, arsenic levels in soils span the range from 0.1 to 40 ppm (42). The average concentration is 6 ppm. Background soil samples taken throughout the site region as part of this project show a range of 4.6–14 ppm, with a mean of 9 ppm. Forty-two surface soil samples taken onsite show a range of 0.5–23 ppm with a mean of 7 ppm. These data fall well within both the national and local background ranges.

Arsenic has been measured in a number of rivers and lakes throughout the world (43, 44). In the United States, arsenic has been found in the range of 1.6–1100 μg/L. The average is around 1.6–64 μg/L. In the groundwater on the site, arsenic was measured in the range of 15–630 μg/L, with an average of 230 μg/L. Although the groundwater concentrations onsite fall within the range for background in surface waters, the two sets of data are not strictly comparable. Arsenic is subject to changes in species, which may affect observed concentrations in groundwater. In addition, the analytical protocol specified analysis of a total sample with its associated particulate material. Therefore, the proportion of arsenic that was soluble in the groundwater samples is unknown.

Considered together, the available evidence for arsenic levels in the soils and the groundwater indicates that arsenic onsite falls within the ranges one might find elsewhere as background in the United States. Therefore, no excess risk exists due to arsenic levels recorded onsite.

6.5.2   *Air.*

Excess cancer risk estimates for the air pathway (Table 13) were determined by comparing the estimated exposure concentrations (Table 11) to the recommended acceptable exposure criteria (Table 12). The offsite acceptable exposure criteria were calculated using cancer potency slopes. The onsite exposure criteria are those set by the Occupational Safety and Health Administration (OSHA) for onsite occupational exposure. There are no excess cancer risks greater than 1×10^{-5} estimated for offsite chemical vapor exposure (Table 13). The onsite concentrations of benzene (29) and chloroform (31) are approximately three and five orders of magnitude, respectively, lower than OSHA standards for onsite occupational exposure.

6.5.3 Soil. Health risk estimates for soil were not made because the site is a secured area (fenced and provided with a 24-h/day security guard) and is covered with a geofabric. These measures have essentially eliminated direct soil contact (via dermal or inhalation routes). However, site investigation activities have confirmed the presence of elevated concentrations of 2, 3, 7, 8-TCDD in the surface soils. Since the greatest potential for human exposure associated with unremediated sites is contact with surface soils, this exposure pathway should be eliminated on a long-term basis.

6.6   Uncertainties

Health risk estimation quantitatively defines the general magnitude of human health risks posed by a defined set of circumstances. The precision of such estimates is limited by the size and quality of the data base. Often, these limitations can be overcome by defining a range of extremes. However, certain critical assumptions incorporate large uncertainties. The two critical ones are (i) the extrapolation of toxic effects observed at the high doses necessary to conduct animal studies to effects that might occur at much lower, environmentally relevant doses, and (ii) the extrapolation from animals to humans.

The approach taken in this assessment to offset uncertainties is biased toward health protective assumptions that exaggerate any risks. For example, in the estimation of potential exposures in Section 6.5, assumptions were consistently made that tend to overestimate rather than underestimate exposure whenever informational deficiencies were encountered. The health risk estimates described in this section were derived in a similar manner. This biased approach for managing uncertainties has a magnifying effect on the outcome of the risk assessment process. Since each step builds on the previous one, the overall result of biased assumptions is to overestimate risks rather than underestimate them. This approach compensates for risk assessment uncertainties and provides a margin of safety for remedial actions recommended.

This assessment provides a defensible basis for planning remediation. However, because of the inherent health protective bias, the potential risks characterized should not be perceived as representative of the actual risks posed. The actual risk is very likely much less than those projected in Table 13. In fact, the combination of all the assumptions discussed in Section 6 practically guarantee this. Furthermore, the most significant potential exposures, such as that due to 2, 3, 7, 8-TCDD in groundwater, are not projected to begin for many decades even if the health protective assumptions were realized.

7   CONCLUSIONS AND RECOMMENDATIONS

The following site-specific remedial objectives are recommended based on the findings of the risk assessment.

- The buildings and other structures onsite have the potential for particulate-associated 2, 3, 7, 8-TCDD emissions. Therefore, it is recommended that the buildings and structures be contained or demolished to prevent possible emissions of particulates.

- Since the greatest potential for human exposure to site-associated 2, 3, 7, 8-TCDD arises from contact with the surface soils, it is recommended that potential exposure to surface soils from the site be eliminated.
- The groundwater modeling coupled with the health protective assumptions project a potential for an elevated risk for 2, 3, 7, 8-TCDD (63) and DDT (42) in the closest offsite well at some time in the future. The recommendation is made that mass transport of chemicals in the groundwater be lowered to reduce the potential risk from ingestion of these compounds. The recommended conservative acceptable exposure level not to be exceeded for a 10^{-5} excess cancer risk is 5×10^{-5} μg/L for 2, 3, 7, 8-TCDD (63) and 0.23 μg/L for DDT (42).
- The worst-case modeling assumptions used in this section have resulted in a projection that estimated transport of site-associated compounds into the adjoining river (Table 9) could exceed the criteria for 2, 3, 7, 8-TCDD and DDT. It is recommended that the plans for remediation of the site include reducing mass transport of these compounds to the river.
- Remedial actions should be evaluated, selected, and implemented with appropriate consideration given to the increased potential for chemical exposure of surrounding populations that is inherent with remedial activities.

These recommendations were factored into the selection of an appropriate remedial alternative for this site. Remedial alternatives were evaluated both quantitatively and qualitatively for their risk-reduction effectiveness using the risk assessment models in this study. Other factors, such as proven technical feasibility, were also considered. The proposed remediation includes the following components to meet the objectives stated above:

- Demolish structures and facilities, spread the resulting rubble over the site, and compact. Decontaminate salvageable structural steel. Disassemble and decontaminate all salvageable tanks, vessels, and reactors.
- Construct a cap over the site that meets requirements of the Resource Conservation and Recovery Act (RCRA).
- Install, operate, and maintain a groundwater withdrawal and treatment system. Construct a slurry wall around the perimeter of the site.
- Replace the existing river bulkhead. Locate and plug inactive underground conduits (e.g. sewers) and reroute active systems.
- Implement remediation without significant risk to site workers and offsite populations.

REFERENCES

1. U.S. Environmental Protection Agency, Amendment to National Oil and Hazardous Substances Contingency Plan; the National Priorities List. *Fed. Regist.* **52**(14) 2492–2498 (1987).
2. U.S. Environmental Protection Agency, *National Oil and Hazardous Substances Pollution Contingency Plan Under the Comprehensive Environmental Response, Compensation and Liability Act of 1980.* Bureau of National Affairs, USEPA, Washington, DC, 1986.
3. U.S. Environmental Protection Agency, *Guidance on Feasibility Studies under CERCLA.* Prepared for the Office of Research and Development Cincinnati, Ohio, Office of Emergency

and Remedial Response, and Office of Waste Programs Enforcement, USEPA, Washington, DC, 1985.

4. U.S. Environmental Protection Agency, *Guidance on Remedial Investigation under CERCLA* (draft). Office of Emergency and Remedial Response, USEPA, Washington, DC, 1985.

5. U.S. Environmental Protection Agency, *Superfund Public Health Evaluation Manual*, EPA 540/1-86-060. Office of Emergency and Remedial Response, USEPA, Washington, DC, 1986.

6. R. C. Morgan, R. Clemens, B. D. Davis, T. T. Evans, J. A. Fagliano, J. A. LiBolsi, Jr., A. L. Mittelman, J. R. Murphy, J. C. Parker, and K. Partymiller, Endangerment assessments for superfund enforcement actions. *Natl. Conf. Manage. Uncontrolled Sites, 5th,* (1984).

7. F. A. Long and G. E. Schweitzer (Eds.), *Risk Assessment at Hazardous Waste Sites.* American Chemical Society, Washington, DC, 1982.

8. J. Saxena and F. Fisher (Eds.), *Hazard Assessment of Chemicals,* Vol. 1. Academic Press, New York, 1981.

9. J. Saxena (Ed.), *Hazard Assessment of Chemicals,* Vol. 3. Academic Press, Orlando, FL, 1984.

10. J. Saxena (Ed.), *Hazard Assessment of Chemicals,* Vol. 4. Academic Press, Orlando, FL, 1985.

11. R. A. Conway (Ed.), *Environmental Risk Analysis for Chemicals.* Van Nostrand, New York, 1982.

12. Guidelines for establishing test procedures for priority pollutants. *Fed. Regist.* **44**(233) (1979).

13. U.S. Environmental Protection Agency, *Test Methods for Evaluating Solid Waste,* SW-846. USEPA, Washington, DC, 1982.

14. U.S. Environmental Protection Agency, Method 613: 2, 3, 7, 8-tetrachloridibenzo-p-dioxin for dioxin in water. *Fed. Regist.* **49**(209) 43368 (1984).

15. U.S. Environmental Protection Agency, *Superfund Health Assessment Manual* (Draft), EPA Contract No. 68-01-6872. ICF Incorporated, USEPA, Washington, DC, 1985.

16. U.S. Department of Health and Human Services, *Third Annual Report on Carcinogens,* NTP 82–330. Public Health Service, USDHHS, Washington, DC, 1983.

17. U.S. Environmental Protection Agency, *Health Assessment Document for Polychlorinated Dibenzo-p-Dioxins,* EPA 600/8-84-014F. Office of Health and Environmental Assessment, USEPA, Washington, DC, 1985.

18. American Conference of Governmental Industrial Hygienists, *TLVs: Threshold Limit Values for Chemical Substances and Physical Agents in the Workroom Environment with Intended Changes for 1984-85.* ACGIH, Cincinnati, OH, 1984.

19. U.S. Environmental Protection Agency, *National Interim Primary Drinking Water Regulations.* USEPA, Washington, DC, 1982.

20. U.S. Environmental Protection Agency, *Methods for Assessing Exposure to Chemical Substances,* Vols. 1–11. Office of Toxic Substances, USEPA, Washington, DC, 1976–1987.

21. U.S. Environmental Protection Agency, *Superfund Exposure Assessment Manual* (draft), Contract No. 68-01-7090. USEPA, Washington, DC, 1986.

22. H. B. Fischer, E. J. List, R. C. Y. Koh, J. Imberger, and N. H. Brooks, *Mixing in Inland and Coastal Waters.* Academic Press, New York, 1979.

23. D. Schopp, Personal communication to IT Corporation, U.S. Geological Study, Water Resources Division, Trenton, NJ, 1987.

24. J. P. Riley and R. Chester, *Introduction to Marine Chemistry.* Academic Press, New York, 1971.

25. R. A. Freeze and J. A. Cherry, *Groundwater.* Prentice-Hall, Englewood Cliffs, NJ, 1979.

26. S. W. Karickhoff, D. S. Brown, and T. A. Scott, Sorption of hydrophobic pollutants on natural sediments. *Water Res.* **13**, 241–248 (1979).

27. V. P. Powers, *Construction Dewatering: A Guide to Theory and Practice.* Wiley, New York, 1981.

28. T. T. Shen, *Emission Estimation of Hazardous Organic Compounds from Waste Disposal Sites*, Pap. No. 80-68.8. Presented at the APCA Annual Meeting, June 1980.

29. H. P. Shu, D. J. Paustenbach, and F. J. Murray, A critical evaluation of the use of mutagenesis, carcinogenesis and tumor promotion data in a cancer risk assessment of 2, 3, 7, 8-TCDD. *Regul. Toxicol. Pharmacol.* **7**, 57–88 (1987).

30. J. D. Longstreth and J. M. Hushon, Risk assessment for 2, 3, 7, 8-TCDD. In R. E. Tucker, A. L. Young, and A. P. Gray, Eds., *Human and Environmental Risks of Chlorinated Dioxins and Related Compounds*. Plenum Press, New York, 1983, pp. 639–664.

31. J. S. Wassom, A review of the genetic toxicology of chlorinated dibenzo-p-dioxins. *Mutat. Res.* **47**, 141–160 (1977).

32. G. F. Fries and G. S. Marrow, Retention and excretion of 2, 3, 7, 8-TCDD by rats. *J. Agric. Food Chem.* **23**(2), 265–269 (1975).

33. T. H. Umbreit, E. J. Hesse and M. A. Gallo, Differential Bioavailability of dioxin from contaminated soil. In J. H. Exner, Ed., *Solving Hazardous Waste Problems Learning From Dioxins*. American Chemical Society Washington, DC. (1987), pp. 131–139.

34. D. J. Paustenbach, H. P. Shu, and F. J. Murray, A critical examination of assumptions used in risk assessments of dioxin contaminated soil. *Regul. Toxicol. Pharmacol.* **6**, 284–307 (1986).

35. S. S. Epstein, *The Politics of Cancer*. Anchor Press/Doubleday, New York, 1979.

36. U.S. Environmental Protection Agency, Guidelines for carcinogen risk assessment. *Fed. Regist.* **51**(185), 33992 (1986).

37. K. S. Crump, Methods for carcinogenic risk assessment. In P. F. Ricci, Ed., *Principles of Health Risk Assessment*. Prentice-Hall, Englewood Cliffs, NJ, 1985, pp. 279–319.

38. R. L. Sielken, F. W. Carlborg, D. J. Paustenbach, H. P. Shu, and F. J. Murray, *Alternative Approaches to Mathematically Analyzing the Bioassay Data for 2, 3, 7, 8-TCDD*. Presented at the 25th Annual Meeting of the Society of Toxicology, New Oreleans, LA, 1986, Abstr. No. 1133.

39. R. L. Sielken, Quantitative cancer risk assessment for 2, 3, 7, 8-TCDD. *Food Chem Toxicol.* **25**: 257–267. (1987).

40. D. Krewski, C. Brown, and D. Murdoch, Determining "safe" levels of exposure: Safety factors or mathematical models? *Fundam. Appl. Toxicol.* **4**, S383–S394 (1984).

41. B. Fischhoff, S. Lichtenstein, P. Slovic, S. L. Derby, and R. L. Keeney, *Acceptable Risk*. Cambridge Univ. Press, London and New York, 1981.

42. H. J. M. Bowen, *Trace Elements in Biochemistry*. Academic Press, New York, 1966.

43. J. F. Ferguson and J. Gavis, A review of the arsenic cycle in natural waters. *Water Resour.* **6**, 1259–1274 (1972).

44. R. Wagemann, Some theoretical aspects of stability and solubility of inorganic arsenic in the freshwater environment. *Water Resourc.* **12**, 139–145 (1978).

45. H. Shu, D. Paustenbach, J. Murray, L. Marple, B. Brunck, D. Dei Rossi, A. S. Webb and P. Tietelbaum. Bioavailability of soil-bound TCDD: Oral bioavailability in the rat. *Fund Appl. Toxicol.* **10**: 648–654 (1988).

46. H. Shu, P. Tietelbaum, A. S. Webb, L. Marple, B. Brunck, D. Dei Rossi, J. Murray, and D. Paustenbach. Bioavailability of soil-bound TCDD: Dermal bioavailability in the rat. *Fund. Appl. Toxicol.* **10**: 335–343 (1988).

13

The Endangerment Assessment for the Smuggler Mountain Site, Pitkin County, Colorado: A Case Study

Peter K. LaGoy* and Ian C. T. Nisbet**

ICF Clement Associates, Washington, DC

Carl O. Schulz

COSAR, Inc., Columbia, South Carolina

1 INTRODUCTION

Under the Comprehensive Environmental Response, Compensation and Liability Act of 1980, better known as the Superfund Act or CERCLA, the EPA was required by Congress to clean up (remediate) hazardous waste sites across the country. As an initial phase in this project, hazardous waste sites were ranked as to the likelihood that they could endanger public health, welfare, or the environment. The hazardous waste sites receiving the highest score were included on the National Priority List (NPL) of sites to be remediated under CERCLA.

Cleanup of a site on the NPL involves a remedial investigation (RI) to determine the extent and types of contamination present at the site and a feasibility study (FS) to determine the type of cleanup action that will be taken. Either as part of the FS or in a separate phase, the risks associated with taking no action at the site are evaluated to determine if the site presents an "imminent and substantial endangerment to public health, welfare, or the environment." This is done to determine if active remedial action is necessary and to determine the baseline risks at the site for comparison with the risk associated with the various potential remedial alternatives. It is important to note that in the context of endangerment assessment "imminent" implies an impending risk of harm. The EPA (1) states that "an imminent endangerment may exist if harm is threatened, no actual injury need have occurred or be occurring." The EPA (1) also notes that "endangerment means something less than actual harm." This chapter presents such a baseline risk assessment for a site on the EPA's NPL.

*Currently with Environmental Strategies Corporation, San Jose, California
**Currently with I. C. T. Nisbet & Company, Lincoln, Massachusetts

A site-specific risk assessment (endangerment assessment) commonly consists of the following activities:

- Detailed characterization of the site.
- Selection of the key contaminants of concern.
- Identification of potential exposure pathways.
- Review of physicochemical and toxicological properties of the chemicals of concern.
- Estimation of exposure.
- Comparison of contaminant concentrations with any applicable or relevant and appropriate standards.
- Assessment of risk.

One additional activity that should be performed in any site-specific risk assessment is an analysis of uncertainties in the assessment.

In the initial phase of the endangerment assessment, data collected during the RI are examined to determine the history, geology, hydrogeology, and climatology of the site, all of which are important in determining the potential for migration of the contaminants present at the site. Information on the level of chemicals in various environmental media are analyzed to determine representative chemical concentrations at the site. Because numerous chemicals, including naturally occurring metals, are present at any site, it is necessary to focus the assessment on key contaminants. Therefore, chemical concentrations, physiocochemical properties, toxicity, and site-specific migration potentials are evaluated to select a small group of contaminants of concern to be considered in the assessment.

Following completion of the initial data review phase of the assessment, potential exposure pathways at the site are identified and the toxicity of the chemicals of concern is examined in detail. Information on chemical concentrations in pertinent environmental media are then combined with various exposure assumptions and site-specific data to assess the likely exposure via each pathway. Finally, the exposure assessment is combined with information on the quantitative toxicity of the site contaminants to determine if the site poses a risk. As a last step, uncertainties in the assessment are outlined.

The endangerment assessment presented in this chapter is divided into four sections. In Section 2, characteristics of the site and the extent of site contamination are described and the contaminants of primary concern (the indicator chemicals) are selected. Section 3 contains a discussion of the key toxicological properties of the indicator chemicals. Section 4 includes a discussion of the potential exposure pathways and a quantitative assessment of potential exposure; then the exposure estimates are combined with the chemical-specific dose–response information from Section 3 to determine if the site contamination poses a health risk. The last section presents cleanup levels and also includes a discussion of the uncertainties in the assessment.

2   CHARACTERIZATION AND DESCRIPTION OF THE SITE

The Smuggler Mountain Site is approximately 75 acres in size and is located about 1 mile northeast of downtown Aspen, Colorado, in Pitkin County (Fig. 1). The terrain consists of a relatively steep slope forming the western side of Smuggler Mountain, which grades into gentler slopes and natural terraces between Smuggler Mountain and Roaring Fork River.

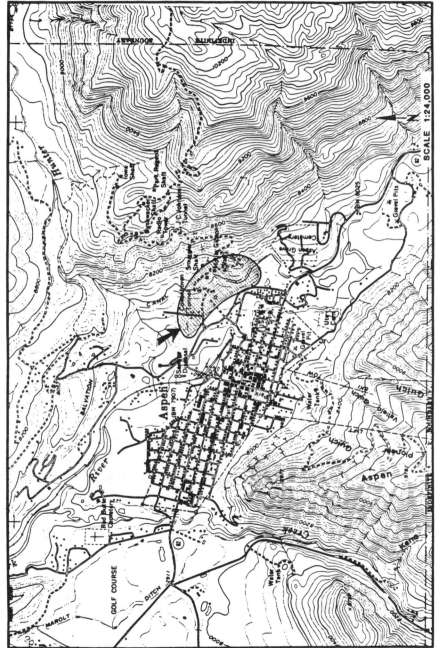

Figure 1. Approximate location of the Smuggler Mountain site.

At the base of Smuggler Mountain, tailings and other mine wastes have been placed on the gentler slopes and terraces and have subsequently been reworked by various construction projects.

The Smuggler Run Mobile Home Park is located a few hundred yards downhill from the Smuggler Mine to the southwest, and the Hunter Creek Condominiums and the Centennial Condominiums are about the same distance to the northwest. Pitkin County is also planning a recreational park on a terraced area between the trailer park and the existing mine.

Mine tailings, either covered, uncovered, or mixed with soil, comprise much of the Smuggler Mountain site (2). These mine tailings were reportedly used as fill in several local construction projects, including the mobile home park, the Hunter Creek Condominiums, and the Silver King Condominiums.

Geologically, the Smuggler site is characterized by glacial, alluvial, and colluvial sediments overlying sedimentary bedrock strata. The onsite terraces noted previously are largely glacial in origin, whereas alluvium predominates in the area adjacent to the Roaring Fork River along the southwestern site boundary. Colluvium forms an irregular thin veneer across the site and is often intermixed with tailing materials. Although bedrock is not exposed on the site itself, outcrops of limestone, dolomite, sandstone, and shale are common immediately to the east on the slopes of Smuggler Mountain. Most of the onsite native soils are derived from these strata, and the abundance of calcium carbonate allows for a natural buffering capacity.

The surface water system of the site consists primarily of the Roaring Fork River. The river flows in a northwesterly direction and serves as the ultimate receiving stream for runoff from the site. The northern portion of the site drains toward Hunter Creek, whose confluence with the Roaring Fork River is just beyond the northwestern corner of the site. Runoff from the majority of the Smuggler site occurs as overland flow.

The groundwater system of the Smuggler site is less clearly defined than the surface water regime. Based on existing data, including information from recently installed monitoring wells, groundwater is present in both the bedrock strata and the unconsolidated valley-fill sediments. Although data are lacking, the relatively low permeability of the sedimentary strata probably restricts both the occurrence and movement of groundwater. Flow is likely to be dominated by secondary permeability, that is, fracture and fault systems.

More important may be the occurrence of groundwater in the overlying unconsolidated materials. This partially saturated zone apparently receives recharge from the infiltration of precipitation and associated runoff. In the process, metal constituents within the surface and subsurface soils may be mobilized to the groundwater system. Limited data indicate that groundwater generally flows in a westerly direction, toward the center of the Roaring Fork Valley. There is no evidence that groundwater discharges to the river in the vicinity of the site; site groundwater probably merges with the alluvial system of the Roaring Fork Valley, eventually flowing in a northwesterly direction. Groundwater from this alluvial system is used for domestic purposes, including two private wells along the western edge of the site.

A total of 11 metals were initially detected in soils and mine tailings at the Smuggler Mountain site (2–4). The number of samples, average concentrations, and maximum concentrations for the detected metals are presented in Table 1.* Arsenic, cadmium,

---

*In calculating the mean concentrations found in soil, tailings, water, and air samples, a value of one-half the detection limit for a particular chemical was assigned to samples in which the chemical was not detected. This is considered unlikely to significantly over- or underestimate actual mean concentrations.

TABLE 1. Concentrations of Heavy Metals in Soil and Mine Tailings at the Smuggler Mountain Site (mg/kg)

	LD[a]	Soil			Mine Tailings			Snowmass	Background Connor and Shacklette 1975	
		No. Detected/ No. of Samples	Mean	Maximum	No. Detected/ No. of Samples	Mean	Maximum	n = 1	Mean	Range
Arsenic[b]		13/13	82[d]	303	6/6	48	80	20	5.9	2.7–15
Barium		13/13	2,240	5,620	6/6	218	425	411	630	500–1,000
Cadmium[b]		13/13	26	53	6/6	56	87	3.5	<1.0	<1–1.0
Chromium		13/13	8.3	12	6/6	7	11	4.3	40	15–100
Copper[b]		11/11	130	684	6/6	98	232	16	12	5–20
Iron		13/13	15,800	22,300	6/6	20,600	27,200	9,490	14,000	3,000–46,000
Lead[c]		13/13	4,060	8,530	6/6	8,120	13,900	191	18	15–200
Manganese		13/13	844	3,460	5/6	1,230	1,670	431	530	150–1,500
Mercury[b]	0.05	12/13	0.3	1.0	5/6	1.03	2.10	ND	0.042	0.010–0.100
Vanadium		13/13	11	17	6/6	6.7	10	8.2	42	15–70
Zinc[c]		13/13	2,330	6,990	6/6	6,810	11,100	134	42	16–74

[a]Limit of detection in mg/kg.
[b]Average soil concentrations are approximately 10 times higher than background levels.
[c]Average soil concentrations are approximately 100 times higher than background levels.
[d]The data for arsenic appeared to be geometrically distributed and the geometric mean of 50 mg/kg is probably more appropriate.
Source: Ecology and Environment Inc. (2).

TABLE 2. Airborne Concentrations of Heavy Metals and Particulates in the Vicinity of the Smuggler Mountain Site ($\mu g/m^3$)

	Concentrations Onsite			Respirable Size Particulates ($<10\,\mu$ diameter)			Background Concentrations from Snowmass			Maximum Recommended Air Concentrations
	Number Sampled	Mean	Maximum	Number Sampled	Mean	Maximum	Number Sampled	Mean	Maximum	
Total suspended particulates	66	43.5	160	18	17	44	18	36	160	260[a]
Arsenic	37	0.0003	0.0071	18	<0.0001	0.0009	18	<0.0001	0.0002	0.0001[b]
Cadmium	37	0.0012		18	0.0014	0.0043	18	0.0002	0.0018	0.0004[b]
Iron	37	1.4	7.5	18	0.58	1.8	18	0.79	3.5	30[c]
Lead	37	0.19	0.81	18	0.10	0.20	18	0.057	0.10	1.5[a]
Manganese	37	0.054	0.22	18	0.023	0.067	18	0.026	0.091	1.1[c]
Zinc	37	0.14	0.54	18	0.090	0.29	18	0.076	0.36	35[c]

[a] U.S. EPA primary air standard.
[b] Based on a 10^{-6} cancer risk, assuming a 70-kg person inhales 20 m^3 of air per day (9).
[c] Noncarcinogen: allowable chronic intake level from the HEA, assuming a 70-kg person inhales 20 m^3 of air per day (9).
Source: Ecology and Environment Inc. (5).

copper, mercury, and zinc were detected at levels that on average were about 10 times higher than the background levels of these metals in undisturbed soils in the United States, and lead was detected at a level that was about 200 times higher than U.S. background levels (4). However, later soil/tailings samples collected on or near the site during 1985 (see discussion below) suggest that the "background" levels of lead in Aspen and its vicinity may be over 200 mg/kg.

Dissolved metals were sampled in the Roaring Fork River upstream and downstream from the site. Only barium, iron, manganese, and zinc were detected in the river (2). The analytical methods used were not sensitive enough to detect levels of arsenic, cadmium, and lead that might be of concern (detection limits: arsenic, 50 μg/L; cadmium, 5 μG/L; lead, 30 μg/L). Although iron, manganese, and zinc were present at slightly higher levels downstream than upstream, the data were insufficient to make any reliable comparisons.

Groundwater samples from seven wells (three upgradient and four downgradient) in the vicinity of the Smuggler Mountain site were analyzed for metals (2). A comparison of the concentrations of metals in downgradient wells to upgradient wells was conducted to determine if the site was affecting groundwater quality. Cadmium, chromium, copper, iron, and zinc were all detected at higher concentrations in the downgradient wells than in upgradient wells, while barium was detected at higher concentrations in the upgradient wells. Cadmium and chromium were detected in the downgradient wells at levels only slightly above the detection limit. Elevated chromium and iron concentrations were found only in one downgradient well and the concentrations in the single well could be an artifact of well construction. Although the data suggest that groundwater from the site may contain elevated levels of contamination, the available data are insufficient to make any reliable comparison.

E & E took a total of 115 samples of air particulate matter from a background site and four onsite locations (5). One of the onsite locations was sampled in duplicate to determine sampler variability, and another had a second high-volume sampler designed to collect only respirable (less than 10 μm in diameter) particles. A compilation of these data is presented in Table 2. Analysis revealed that the levels of arsenic, cadmium, lead, and zinc in the air onsite were slightly elevated as compared with background concentrations near the site.

A preliminary screening for elevated levels of blood lead was conducted in Pitkin County. Of the 22 persons who volunteered for testing, 15 were children under 13 years old. In the judgment of the individuals conducting the study, only one child had an abnormally high zinc protoprophyrin level (4.2 μg/g hemoglobin; approximately equivalent to 50 μg/dL of whole blood). A sample of blood from this child was analyzed for lead and was found to have a concentration of 12 μg/dL, which is not unusual for a child of that age. The zinc protoporphyrin assay is generally considered to be indicative of blood lead levels that cause acute clinical lead intoxication (6). In addition, information on behavior was lacking. Therefore, these data are not adequate to demonstrate the presence or absence of elevated lead levels in individuals living in the vicinity of the Smuggler Mountain site.

2.1   Selection of Indicator Chemicals

Careful review of the results of the sampling and laboratory analyses indicate that the levels of lead and zinc detected in the soil and mine tailings at the site are greatly elevated compared to either a background soil sample from the same area or normal background levels. Cadmium, copper, and mercury were detected at levels approximately one order of magnitude above the expected background levels reported by Connor and Shacklette (4). Two heavy metals (barium and manganese) and a metalloid (arsenic) were somewhat elevated in conparison to the measured and expected background levels. Finally, three metals (chromium, vanadium, and iron) were only detected at the site at background levels.

Clearly, contaminants present only at background levels (chromium, vanadium, and iron) do not pose a site-specific risk and can be dropped from further consideration in the risk assessment. Several of the contaminants present at the site are toxic to humans only at fairly high levels of exposure, are not present at levels onsite that are considered likely to be of concern, and can be dropped from consideration. These include zinc, copper, barium, and manganese. One additional metal, mercury, not very toxic in inorganic form, is present at fairly low (although elevated) levels and will not be considered. Although all the metals present at elevated concentrations could be considered as indicator chemicals, experience has shown that contaminants present at these relative concentrations are unlikely to have any influence on the assessment. Therefore, in order to focus the assessment on the key contaminants, only lead, cadmium, and arsenic are considered in the risk assessment.

3   HAZARD ASSESSMENT

This section presents toxicity profiles for the indicator metals at the Smuggler Mountain site. Each profile is based on toxicological reviews published by the EPA as part of its ambient water quality criteria documents, air quality criteria documents, or health assessment documents. Each profile starts with a qualitative summary of the health effects caused by exposure to the metal, followed by a summary of the existing criteria and standards. The profiles include brief reviews of the primary studies that provide the basis for the criteria, standards, and "cancer potency factors" or "unit risks" (for the metals that have been identified as carcinogens) and of other significant studies that have been reported since preparation of the EPA's criteria documents and health assessment documents. This information is used as the basis for the risk evaluation. Because the health effects of arsenic and cadmium appear to depend on the route of exposure, the ingestion toxicity and inhalation toxicity are discussed separately for these two metals.

Many of the reported toxicological effects of the metals of concern in this report have been observed at high doses capable of causing acute responses. The potential levels of exposure at the Smuggler site are much lower and are comparable to levels that have been reported to cause chronic, long-term effects that may be difficult to detect and delayed in onset.

3.1   Arsenic

Inhalation of arsenic by humans is strongly associated with lung cancer, while ingestion of arsenic is strongly associated with a characteristic form of dermal cancer in humans and has been linked to bladder cancer, lung cancer, and hepatic angiosarcoma (7, 8). In several animal studies, arsenic has been reported to be fetotoxic, embryotoxic, and teratogenic (7). Chronic exposure to arsenic affects the nervous system and can cause dermal lesions and cardiovascular disease.

The EPA's Carcinogen Assessment Group (CAG) calculated the unit risk for lifetime exposure to arsenic in drinking water to be $4.3 \times 10^{-4} (\mu g/L)^{-1}$ and in air to be $4.3 \times 10^{-3} (\mu g/m^3)^{-1}$ based on epidemiologic studies. (7). In other words, concentrations of

1 $\mu g/L$ in drinking water or 1 $\mu g/m^3$ in air are estimated to be associated with upper-bound lifetime excess cancer risks of 4.3×10^{-4} and 4.3×10^{-3}, respectively.* The EPA has convened a Risk Assessment Forum to reevaluate the carcinogenic potency of arsenic via the oral route. Final results from this forum are not currently available. The primary drinking water standard (maximum contaminant level or MCL) for arsenic is 50 $\mu g/L$ and the Office of Drinking Water has recommended maintaining this value (9).

3.2   Cadmium

An increased incidence of lung tumors has been associated with occupational exposure to cadmium, and mice administered cadmium chloride by inhalation also developed lung tumors (10–12). Cadmium bioaccumulates in the kidneys, where it can cause renal tubular dysfunction (11, 13, 14). Chronic exposure to cadmium is also suspected of producing hypertension, anemia, sensory loss (particularly smell), endocrine alterations, and immunosuppression (11, 13).

The CAG used the epidemiological data of Thun et al. (12) to determine a best estimate of the unit cancer risk of $1.8 \times 10^{-3} (\mu g/m^3)^{-1}$ for cadmium (10). The EPA published a reference dose (RfD, formerly referred to as the allowable daily intake, or ADI) for oral exposure to cadmium of 5×10^{-4} mg/kg·day (9). The EPA established a primary drinking water standard of 10 $\mu g/L$.

3.3   Lead

The major effect of excessive exposure to lead is damage to the hematopoietic and neurological systems (15). Although an apparent threshold has been determined for the acute neurological effects seen in lead poisoning, no threshold has been determined for the effects of lead on heme synthesis or on learning ability in children (6, 15). Lead can also cause renal dysfunction, and it is known to be teratogenic to animals (15).

The EPA primary drinking water standard for lead is 50 $\mu g/L$ (9). The EPA air standard is 1.5 $\mu g/m^3$. The Centers for Disease Control (CDC) currently define *lead toxicity* in a child as a blood lead level greater than or equal to 25 $\mu g/dL$ and an erythrocyte protoporphyrin level greater than or equal to 35 $\mu g/dL$ (6). However, Bellinger et al. (16) have shown significant neurobehavioral deficits in children with blood lead levels less than 20 $\mu g/dL$ and Rabinowitz et al. (17) have shown elevated protoporphyrin levels at blood lead levels exceeding 15 $\mu g/dL$, and the EPA is considering blood lead levels below 25 $\mu g/dL$ as toxic.

4   EXPOSURE AND RISK ASSESSMENT

As discussed previously, arsenic, cadmium, and lead are present in soils in the vicinity of the Smuggler Mountain site at concentrations above background levels. In this section,

---

*The cancer risk number represents the probability of developing cancer as a direct result of exposure to the chemical agent. For example, a cancer risk of 10^{-4} means that exposure to the specified concentration of the chemical throughout a lifetime (assumed to be 70 years) may be associated with a 1 in 10,000 chance of developing cancer as a result of exposure. Generally, the unit risks are upper 95% confidence limits on the maximum likelihood estimate of the line relating exposure and dose. Because the unit risks are upper bounds, the actual risk associated with a given exposure is unlikely to be higher but may be much lower than the predicted risk.

the potential human exposure to these metals and the potential human health risks associated with that exposure are estimated.

Potential exposure pathways for humans vary at different sites and these need to be considered on a site-specific basis. The potential routes of exposure depend on the physicochemical properties of the contaminants and of the environmental media in which they are found, the characteristics of the potentially exposed population, and other factors such as climate. A discussion of the potential routes of exposure is presented below followed by the exposure and risk assessments for lead, cadmium, and arsenic. The three metals are treated somewhat differently in the assessment. For lead, toxicity is measured in terms of blood lead levels, which in turn are related not only to daily intake levels but also to concentrations of lead in various environmental media. For cadmium and arsenic, a more standard approach is used, involving comparison of an estimated daily intake or measured concentration at the site with a reference dose (RfD), available standard or criteria, or a reference concentration or unit risk.

4.1 Potential Exposure Pathways

4.1.1 Soil. The direct ingestion of contaminated soil is a potentially significant route of exposure, especially in residential areas where exposure may occur frequently and for young children who constitute the group most likely to ingest soil and dust (15). Young children may ingest contaminated dirt by normal mouthing of soiled objects and their hands or by pica, the direct consumption of dirt (18–20). Older children are less likely to eat soil or to mouth soiled objects, but they still may ingest small quantities of dirt from their hands (21, 22). Adults onsite may ingest some contaminated soil, but they are even less likely to be exposed by this route (20–22).

Dermal contact and the ingestion of locally grown vegetables are potential routes of exposure to contaminated soil, which in some areas may include mine tailings (9, 19). However, most metals are poorly absorbed through intact skin, and dermal absorption is probably an insignificant route of exposure relative to other potential routes. The consumption of vegetables grown in contaminated soils in home gardens may be a significant route of exposure but is likely to be of less importance in a mountainous region.

Airborne dispersion of contaminated soil and tailings is a potentially important route of transport and source for inhalation of suspended particulates, especially if the soils or tailings are disturbed. In general, however, the total dose due to inhalation will be small (23, 24).

4.1.2 Indoor Dust. Dust is a normal component of the indoor environment and is present both in the air and on surfaces. Exposure to indoor dust occurs via both inhalation and inadvertent ingestion. The concentrations of contaminants in indoor dust generally correlate with their concentrations in soil but other factors also influence the relation (19). Therefore, without site-specific data it is not possible to consider exposure to indoor dust as a separate exposure pathway. Assuming that indoor levels of contaminants are correlated with outdoor air and soil levels, exposure to indoor dust will be considered implicitly in the assessment, as exposure to airborne contamination is assumed to be for 24 h/day and dust ingestion most likely makes up some component of soil ingestion.

4.1.3 Surface Water. There are three potential routes of exposure to contaminants in surface water: direct ingestion, dermal contact, and consumption of aquatic organisms (fish) taken from contaminated water. The available evidence indicates that, at present, surface water is not a significant potential medium for human exposure at the Smuggler site.

4.1.4   Groundwater. The potential exists for some households downgradient of the Smuggler Mountain site to use groundwater as their sole water source but most people apparently obtain their water from a public water supply. Others may use groundwater for activities such as watering a garden. Direct ingestion of groundwater is the major route by which significant exposure to contaminated groundwater could occur.

4.1.5   Summary. The most important potential exposure pathways at the Smuggler site appear to be ingestion of contaminated soil and indoor dust, and inhalation of airborne dirt and household dust. Ingestion of vegetables grown in contaminated soil and ingestion of contaminated groundwater may also be contributing routes of exposure.

4.2   Lead

Because of the greater potential exposure of children to contaminated soil (18–20) and the evidence that young children are more sensitive to the toxic effects of lead than are adults (15), the exposure and risk assessment for lead will focus on children as the target population. Children living in the vicinity of the Smuggler Mountain site may come in direct contact with contaminated soil while playing and may be exposed to elevated levels of lead in indoor dust. Measures of lead levels in the body are believed to be more accurate correlates of the effects of lead than are daily exposure levels. Although no measured bodily levels of lead of sufficient quality for use in risk assessment were available, most health effects associated with a given exposure to lead are reported in terms of a given amount of lead in the body. Therefore, potential exposure will be presented in terms of a given bodily lead level. The most commonly used measure of bodily lead levels is the concentration of lead in the blood. As indicated earlier, levels above 25 μg/dL of lead in the blood of children are considered evidence of excessive lead absorption (6).

At present, human health criteria for lead in soil have not been established in the United States. The United Kingdom Directorate of the Environment has developed a tentative guideline of 550 mg/kg for lead in soil in residential areas (25). Vernon Houk of the Centers for Disease Control has been quoted as indicating that levels of lead in soil of 300–400 mg/kg are acceptable, based on studies of childhood lead poisoning (26). The CDC (6) stated that "in general lead in soil and dust appears to be responsible for blood lead levels in children increasing above background levels when the concentration in the soil or dust exceeds 500–1,000 ppm (mg/kg)." Yankel et al. (27) suggested that soil lead levels above 1000 mg/kg in the vicinity of a lead smelter in Idaho would pose an unacceptable health risk.

Two approaches can be used to estimate levels of lead in soil that would be safe for children at the Smuggler Mountain site. One approach makes use of the correlations between blood lead levels and lead concentrations in soil described above. The other relates the amount of lead likely to be ingested and inhaled by children exposed to contaminated soil to an acceptable daily intake for lead.

4.2.1   Blood lead–Soil Lead Correlations. The EPA has recently reviewed a number of studies that are useful in relating blood lead levels in children to levels of lead in the environment (15). Table 3 (27–30) shows the relation between blood lead levels in children

TABLE 3. Relation between Levels of Lead in Blood in Children and Airborne Lead Concentrations

Study[a]	Sample Size	Slope (μg/dL per μg/m^3)
Angle and McIntire (28): Omaha, Nebraska	1074	1.92
Roels et al. (29): Belgium	148	2.46
Yankel et al. (27) and Walter et al. (30): Idaho	879	1.52

[a]All three are population studies.
Source: Adapted from the EPA (15).

and airborne lead concentrations, as determined from three studies. These slopes range from 1.52 to 2.46 μg/dL per μg/m^3 in air. Table 4 (31–35) relates blood lead levels in children to levels of lead in soil. Here the slopes range from 0.6 to 6.8 μg/dL per 1000 mg/kg. This range of slopes is much greater than those determined for air exposure. This variability probably reflects the different characteristics of the lead in the soil, as well as other uncontrolled variables.

The studies by Angle and McIntire (28, 31), Yankel et al. (27), Walter et al. (30), and Neri et al. (35) were performed in the vicinity of lead smelters. Three other studies (32–34) were conducted in urban areas where automobile exhaust and lead paint flakes were the major contributors to lead levels in soil. Thus, none of these studies is of a population directly comparable to the population living near Smuggler Mountain.

In a recent study, Gallacher et al. (36) measured blood lead levels in 61 children between the ages of 1 and 3 living in a village in Wales where the soil was contaminated with wastes from past lead mining. These levels were compared with blood lead values for 33 similarly aged children living in a remote village in northern Wales where there was little industry or vehicular traffic. The authors measured lead concentrations in soil, indoor air, and house dust at both locations. The mean blood lead level for children in the old lead mining area was 23 μg/dL compared with 18 μg/dL for the control population. Soil lead levels had a geometric mean of 1200 mg/kg (range = 150–10,000) in the lead mining area compared to 80 mg/kg in the control area. By using only these data to calculate a slope for the relation of blood lead levels to soil lead levels, the approximate slope is 4.5 μg/dL per 1000 mg/kg lead in the soil. This value is in the middle of the range of slopes shown in Table 4. It should be noted that the average blood lead level of the control population (18 μg/dL) was considerably higher than the average blood lead level in the U.S. population [approximately 10 μg/dL (6, 37)] and was also higher than the average value (13 μg/dL) reported for children living close to the lead smelter in East Helena, Montana (38). The effect of this high background level on the relation between soil and blood lead levels is unclear, but it should be kept in mind when using these results.

By using this approach, the amount of lead in the soil that is correlated with an unacceptable blood lead level in children can be estimated using the data summarized in Tables 3 and 4 and data from the CDC studies in Montana and Idaho (38, 39). Although blood lead levels are almost certainly skewed to the right, normal statistics will be used as no information is readily available to transform the data. Use of normal rather than log–normal statistics may lead to overly conservative estimates of exposure. However, overly conservative exposure estimates will be somewhat balanced by use of a target blood lead

TABLE 4. Estimates of the Contribution of Lead in Soil to Levels of Lead in Blood

Study	Range of Lead Values in Soil ($\mu g/g$)	Depth of Sample (in.)	Estimated Slope ($\mu g/dL$ per $10^3 \mu g/g$)	Sample Size	Air Levels ($\mu g/m^3$)	Intercept ($\mu g/dL$)
Argle and McIntire (31) Study of children in Omaha, NE	16–4,792	2	6.8	1,075	NA	15.7
Stark et al. (32) Study of children in New Haven, CT	30–7,000	$\frac{1}{2}$	2.2	153	0.7–1.3	NA
	(ages 0–1) 30–7,600 (ages 2–3)		2.0	334		
Yankel et al. (27) Study of children in Kellogg, ID	50–24,600	$\frac{3}{4}$	1.1	860	1.5–30	13.2
Galke et al. (33) Study of children in Charleston, SC	9–7,890	2	1.5	194	NA	25.9
Barltrop et al. (34) Study of children in England	420–13,969	2	0.6	82	0.29–0.60	21.0
Neri et al. (35) Study of children in British Columbia	225–1,800 (group means, ages 1–3)	NA[a]	7.6	87	2.0	15.4
	225–1,800 (group means, ages 2–3)	NA	4.6	103	2.0	16.37

[a]NA: not available.
Source: Adapted from EPA (15).

517

level of 25 μg/dL, which may not be protective. The net effect is expected to be a slightly conservative (unlikely to underestimate) estimate of risk.

As indicated above, the CDC considers that blood lead levels of 25 μg/dL may be indicative of significantly elevated blood lead. Because of individual variability, in order to ensure that the majority of a given population of children (99%) has acceptable blood lead levels (below 25 μg/dL) the population mean level must be below 25 μg/dL by a factor of 2.3 standard deviations (25 μg/dL represents the 99th percentile upper confidence limit). Based on data collected by the CDC in East Helena, Montana and Kellogg, Idaho, the standard deviation of the mean for blood lead levels in areas with fairly high levels of lead in the soil is between 5 and 6, or approximately 5.5 (38, 39). Based on this standard deviation, a mean blood lead level of 12 μg/dL should ensure that at least 99% of a population of children should have blood lead levels of less than 25 μg/dL.

Based on the East Helena study (3), background exposure to lead in a rural area results in average blood lead levels of 6.6 μg/dL (38). If one assumes that the baseline blood lead level in children living in Pitkin County is also 6.6 μg/dL and that the slope of the level in blood versus the level in air is 2.0 μg/dL per μg/m³ (from Table 3), one can calculate the level of lead in soil corresponding to blood lead levels of 12 μg/dL using the equation

$$12 \ \mu g/dL = 6.6 \ \mu g/dL + 2.0 \ \mu g/dL \ \text{per} \ \mu g/m^3 \times 0.19 \ \mu g/m^3 + ky,$$

or

$$12 \ \mu g/dL - (6.6 \ \mu g/dL + 2.0 \ \mu g/dL \ \text{per} \ \mu g/m^3 \times 0.19 \ \mu g/m^3) = ky$$

or

$$5 \ \mu g/dL = ky$$

$$\frac{5 \ \mu g/dL}{k} = y,$$

where 0.19 μg/m³ is the average concentration of lead in air near the Smuggler site (Table 2), k equals the slope of the line relating blood lead levels to soil levels (Table 4), and y is the concentration of lead in soil in mg/kg. Using the slopes in Table 4 (k between 0.6 and 6.8) and solving for y, we find that the levels of lead in soil that correspond to a mean blood lead level of 12 μg/dL range from 700 to 8000 mg/kg with a mean of about 2000 mg/kg. Using the slope of 4.5 μg/dL per 1000 mg/kg in soil derived from the Gallacher et al. study (36), we find that a level of lead in soil of 1000 mg/kg would correspond to a blood lead level of 12 μg/dL. Comparison of the mean lead concentration at the Smuggler site (4000 mg/kg) to either the mean allowable level of 2000 mg/kg or the value derived from the Gallacher et al. study (36) suggests the levels of lead present at the Smuggler Mountain site may pose a health risk to children.

4.2.2   Acceptable Daily Intake. In this approach, an acceptable daily intake (ADI) for lead is used to calculate the level of lead in soil corresponding to that intake based on assumptions regarding the ingestion of soil. Mahaffey (40) indicated that a dietary level of 200–300 μg/day was probably tolerable for 2–3-year-old children but that the acceptability of this level for infants and younger children was not well established. The Food and Drug Administration is reportedly attempting to reduce daily lead intake by children younger than 5 years old to under 100 μg/day by 1988 (15). By using this number and given that the baseline exposure to lead for a young child is just slightly less than 50 μg/day (15), the daily intake of lead from other sources should be less than about 50 μg/day. The concentration of lead in soil that will result in a daily intake of 50 μg/day is 100 mg/kg if the child consumes 500 mg of soil per day yearly (reasonable maximum estimate) and 500 mg/kg if the child consumes 100 mg of soil per day for the same time period (reasonable average estimate). Comparison of the reference soil concentration derived using the ADI approach with the mean lead concentration at Smuggler (4000 mg/kg) suggests that the contamination may pose a health risk.

4.2.3 Determination of Allowable Levels of Lead in Soil at Smuggler.

The various approaches to establishing a "safe" level of lead in the soil yield widely varying results ranging from about 100 mg/kg to well over 1000 mg/kg (Table 5). The ADI approach gives relatively low safe levels in soil because safety factors are built into the ADI approach and exposure is assumed to be a daily occurrence. Use of the correlation between concentrations in soil and blood lead levels gives higher safe concentrations in soil because it is empirically based on mean values. The safe level of lead in soil is probably dependent on a number of factors, such as the source of the lead, soil particle size, and climatic conditions. The range of 500–1000 reported by the CDC appears to be reasonable, with the actual safe level dependent on site-specific conditions.

Specific considerations unique to the Smuggler Mountain site suggest that concentrations of lead close to the high end of this range may be acceptable. First, the lead at the Smuggler Mountain site is physically and chemically different from the lead present in soils in the vicinity of smelters and in urban areas where most of the studies relating concentrations in soil to body burdens have been conducted. The lead at the latter sites is generally finely divided particulate lead, lead oxides, and lead sulfate deposited from the air. The lead at the Smuggler Mountain site, in contrast, is from a natural source, appears to be present in a carbonate rock matrix, and is almost certainly less bioavailable than the lead in soil at the other sites. The EPA noted that natural lead is bound tightly within a crystalline matrix (15). Second, the Smuggler Mountain site is in an alpine environment

TABLE 5. Estimated "Safe" Levels of Lead in Soil

Source of Estimate	Level (mg/kg)	Comments
United Kingdom Directorate of the Environment (25)	500	For residential areas
Vernon Houk (26)	300–400	
CDC (6)	500–1000	Levels at which blood lead levels with increase
Yankel et al. (27)	1000	
Estimate based on correlation between soil lead and blood lead levels by EPA (15)	700–8000	Assumes slope of relation between blood lead and soil lead levels ranges from 0.6 to 6.8 μg/dL per 1000 mg/kg with a mean value of 3 μg/dL
Estimate based on Gallacher et al. (36)	1100	Slope of 4.5 μg/dL per 1000 mg/kg
Estimate based on ADI approach	100	Reasonable maximum estimate; see text
	500	Reasonable average estimate; see text

and is therefore covered by snow for as long as 6 months each year. Furthermore, when the snow is melting, the surface soil is likely to be saturated. While the snow is covering the ground or melting, the possibility of exposure to contaminated soil at the site is negligible.

For these reasons, it is concluded that concentrations of lead below 1000 mg/kg do not represent a significant human health risk at or in the vicinity of the Smuggler Mountain site. Exposure of young children to soils containing more than 1000 mg/kg lead should be prevented.

4.3   Cadmium and Arsenic

Cadmium and arsenic have been found at elevated concentrations in soil and cadmium has been found in some limited groundwater samples in the vicinity of the Smuggler Mountain site. Residents are probably exposed to cadmium and arsenic from the site through inhalation of airborne particulates and household dust, ingestion of dirt, ingestion of vegetables grown in contaminated soil, and possibly drinking of groundwater. Ingestion of vegetables and drinking of groundwater are only considered qualitatively in this assessment because information on use patterns is lacking and because they are considered unlikely to contribute substantially to exposure at the site. That is, it is recognized that these routes may contribute some small and presumably insignificant amount to exposure but the extent of their contribution is undetermined. Therefore, only exposure via ingestion of contaminated soil and inhalation of contaminated airborne particulates is considered quantitatively.

4.3.1   Ingestion Exposure.   To estimate oral uptake of a soil contaminant it is usually necessary to make certain assumptions. In these calculations, it is assumed that persons (i) weigh 70 kg (41) (ii) are exposed for half of each year for a 70-year lifetime, and (iii) ingest soil at rates presented in Table 6 (22). Using these values and the mean soil concentrations

TABLE 6.   Estimates of Soil Ingestion Rates

Age	Average Weight[a] (kg)	Maximum Case[b] (mg/day)	Average Case (mg/day)
0–1 year	10	250	50
1–6 years	15	500	100
6–11 years	30	250	50
Over 11 years	70	100	25[c]
Average[d]	70	140	30

[a]From the EPA (41).

[b]This does not include individuals who exhibit habitual pica. For them, the upper value presented in Schaum (19) of 5000 mg/day would be more appropriate.

[c]A value of 50 mg/day may be a more reasonable estimate of soil ingestion rates for adults who exhibit frequent hand-to-mouth activity (e.g., smokers) or who regularly engage in outdoor activities.

[d]The average value is a time-weighted-average intake rate assuming 5 years each at 250 and 500 mg/day (maximum) or 50 and 100 mg/day (average) and 60 years at 100 mg/day (maximum) or 25 mg/day (average). These values do not adjust for differences in body weight at different ages but are still considered to be conservative by the authors.

Source: LaGoy (22).

of arsenic and cadmium, daily uptake (chronic daily intake, CDI) can be estimated using the formula

$$CDI = \frac{C \times DI \times AR \times CF}{BW}$$

where CDI = chronic daily intake (mg/kg·day)

   C = concentration of contaminant in soil (Table 1: cadmium, 26 mg/kg; arsenic, 84 mg/kg)

   DI = daily intake from Table 6 (time-weighted-average rate of 30 or 140 mg soil/day)

   AR = annual rate of exposure (50% of each year; estimated based on site-specific considerations)

   CF = conversion factor ($1 \text{ kg}/10^6 \text{ mg}$)

   BW = average body weight (Table 6: 70 kg).

Based on these calculations, an estimate of average and reasonable maximum chronic daily intake values for cadmium are 5.6×10^{-6} and 2.6×10^{-5} mg/kg·day and for arsenic are 1.8×10^{-5} and 8.4×10^{-5} mg/kg·day, respectively.

For noncarcinogens such as cadmium, the chronic daily intake is compared to the reference dose (RfD) and if the CDI:RfD ratio is greater than 1 (i.e., if daily exposure exceeds the dose considered unlikely to be harmful), the exposure may pose a health risk. The RfD for oral exposure to cadmium is 5×10^{-4} and the CDI:RfD ratios for the reasonable average and maximum exposures are both less than 0.1. Therefore, direct ingestion of contaminated soil at the Smuggler Mountain site is considered unlikely to pose a health risk due to cadmium.

For carcinogens such as arsenic, the chronic daily intake is multiplied by the cancer potency factor to determine the upper-bound excess lifetime cancer risk. The current cancer potency factor for arsenic is 15 $(\text{mg/kg·day})^{-1}$ and multiplying this value by the CDIs indicates that upper-bound lifetime excess cancer risks of 3×10^{-4} and 1×10^{-3} are associated with exposure for a 70-year lifetime under the reasonable average and maximum scenarios, respectively.

4.3.2 Inhalation Exposure.

4.3.2 Inhalation Exposure. The assumptions used to estimate the cancer risks associated with exposure to arsenic and cadmium via inhalation are that (i) the average person breathes 20 m^3 of air per 24-h day and (ii) a person lives in the vicinity of the Smuggler Mountain site for a lifetime and is continuously exposed to contaminated airborne particulates. Only cadmium was detected in respirable airborne particulates (PM_{10} fraction) and therefore inhalation exposure to arsenic will not be considered in this assessment. The unit risk for cadmium, which is carcinogenic via inhalation, already incorporates the first assumptions. If the second assumption is correct, the cancer risk posed by the airborne particulates can be determined by multiplying the measured airborne concentration of respirable cadmium by the unit risk:

cancer risk = airborne concentration × unit risk.

The unit risk for cadmium is 1.8×10^{-3} $(\mu g/m^3)^{-1}$ and its concentration in association with respirable air particles is 0.0014 $\mu g/m^3$. Therefore, the risk associated with cadmium expsosure is

$$1.6 \times 10^{-3}\,(\mu g/m^3)^{-1} \times 0.0014\,\mu g/m^3 = 3 \times 10^{-6}.$$

The form of cadmium present in the air at the Smuggler Mountain site is probably physically and chemically different from the form of cadmium to which the workers were exposed in the studies relating cadmium inhalation to cancer. The cadmium at the latter sites is generally cadmium oxide fumes, finely divided particulate cadmium, cadmium oxides, and cadmium sulfate deposited from the air. The cadmium at the Smuggler Mountain site, in contrast, appears to be present in a carbonate rock matrix and therefore may be less bioavailable than the cadmium from industrial exposure. In addition, the Smuggler Mountain site is in an alpine environment and is therefore covered by snow for as much as 6 months each year. Furthermore, when the snow is melting, the surface soil is likely to be saturated. While the snow is covering the ground or melting, the possibility of exposure to airborne soil particulates at the site is negligible.

For these reasons, it is concluded that cadmium probably does not represent a significant human health risk at or in the vicinity of the Smuggler Mountain site. Regression analysis of the E & E data indicates that lead and cadmium levels in soil correlate quite well ($r = 0.83$; $p > 0.01$). Consequently, removing soil heavily contaminated with lead should also reduce soil cadmium concentrations.

Ingestion exposure to arsenic poses an upper-bound lifetime excess cancer risk above the commonly used EPA target risk level of 10^{-6}. Cleanup levels can be determined using an approach analogous to that used for cadmium, but the value that is derived using even the reasonable average exposure scenario (0.3 mg/kg arsenic) is well below background arsenic concentrations (approximately 20 mg/kg arsenic). Considering that concentrations of arsenic in contaminated soil are not greatly elevated above background and even though lead and arsenic concentrations in soil did not correlate particularly well, cleanup of the site for lead should decrease arsenic levels somewhat, possibly to levels equal to high background concentrations. Because cleanup to background or to EPA target risk levels is probably impractical, no specific cleanup value will be established for arsenic.

5   DISCUSSION AND CONCLUSIONS

Based on the sampling results reported in Section 2, elevated concentrations of several metals and a metalloid (arsenic) are present at the Smuggler Mountain site. The elevated concentrations of two of these elements may pose a health risk to people living in the vicinity of the site. The elevated concentrations of lead pose a risk primarily to children who may be exposed through direct or inadvertent ingestion of contaminated soil and dust. Ingestion of arsenic in soil may pose an excess cancer risk slightly above the target level (10^{-6} risk) often used by the EPA as a cleanup goal (9). There are uncertainties inherent in all the above assessments. In particular, the risk assessment for arsenic used several conservative (unlikely to underestimate exposure) assumptions. Therefore, the actual risks associated with site-specific exposure to these elements is unlikely to be higher but may be much lower than the estimated risks. However, in order to ensure that no sensitive individual is adversely affected by the contamination, it is prudent to use such conservative assumptions.

For lead, several different approaches were used to determine the likelihood of health risks. The majority of these approaches indicated that the site could pose an elevated health risk. Because of the approaches used, the uncertainties in the lead risk assessment are likely to be lower than those for cadmium and arsenic. Therefore, it is more likely that the elevated lead concentrations present at the Smuggler Mountain site pose an actual health risk to area residents. However, the fact that several factors, such as frequency of exposure (many children do not live directly adjacent to contaminated areas) and amount of direct soil contact (children may play on grassy areas rather than on areas with exposed soil), were not considered may provide some degree of conservatism to the estimates.

On the other hand, in this assessment, the effects of exposure to the toxic metals present at the Smuggler Mountain site have been considered separately and independently. However, these pollutants occur together in soil and air, and individuals will be exposed to all of them concurrently. Little specific information is available on interactions among these elements. The EPA, in their guidelines for risk assessments of chemical mixtures (42), has stated that, in the absence of such information, it is reasonable to assume that their combined effects are at least additive. This is particularly true for those compounds that affect the same targets. Thus, for example, cadmium and lead both adversely affect kidney function. Therefore, even though the estimated average daily doses of cadmium in children were below those expected to induce renal tubular disease, the added insult to the kidneys caused by higher than average lead exposures may significantly reduce the margin of safety.

Assessing the risks posed by contamination at a hazardous waste site is a complicated task. It involves the use of numerous assumptions, each of which has various degrees of inherent uncertainty. Because of the uncertainties, the estimate of risk may be quite different from the actual risk posed by the site. It is prudent, in order to protect human health, to make conservative risk estimates that are not likely to under-estimate the actual risk. However, this conservatism must be balanced in order to ensure the cleanup is not prohibitively expensive. The actual balancing of costs and benefits are a risk management concern. However, the risk assessment must present the best possible estimates of risk in order to decrease uncertainty and facilitate the risk manager's decisions.

Acknowledgements

This work was prepared in part under EPA Contract No. 68–01–6939. However, the views and opinions expressed in this chapter are solely those of the authors and do not necessarily reflect those of the Agency.

REFERENCES

1. Environmental Protection Agency, Memo from J. Winston Porter, Assistant Administrator to EPA Staff concerning Endangerment Assessment Guidance, November 22, 1985.

2. Ecology and Environment, Inc., *Interpretive Report and Health Risk Assessment of the Smuggler Mine*, TDD R8-8401-15. E&E, Aspen, CO, 1984.

3. Colorado Department of Health, *Heavy Metals in Soil—Smuggler Trailer Park, Aspen, Colorado.* Results of Analysis of Samples Collected 6/15/82 by Tom Dunlop of Pitkin County Department of Environmental Health. Division of Engineering and Sanitation, CDH, Aspen, CO, 1982.

4. J. J. Connor and H. T. Shacklette, Background geochemistry of some rocks, soils, plants, and vegetables in the conterminous United States. Statistical studies in field geochemistry. *Geol. Surv. Prof. Pap. (U.S.)* **574-F** (1975).

5. Ecology and Environment, Inc., *Report of Hi-Vol Air Sampling Activities at the Old Smuggler Mine Study Area, Aspen, Colorado.* Prepared for U.S. Environmental Protection Agency, January 24, 1985.

6. Centers for Disease Control, *Preventing Lead Poisoning in Young Children.* Public Health Services, Chronic Diseases Division, CDC, Atlanta, GA, 1985.

7. Environmental Protection Agency, *Health Assessment Document for Inorganic Arsenic,* EPA 600/8-83-021F. Office of Environmental Assessment, USEPA, Washington, DC, 1984.

8. C. Chen, Y. Chuang, S. You, T. Lin, and H. Wu, A retrospective study on malignant neoplasms of bladder, lung and liver in blackfoot disease endemic area in Taiwan. *Br. J. Cancer* **53**, 399–405 (1986).

9. Environmental Protection Agency, 1986. *Superfund Public Health Evaluation Manual,* EPA 540/1-86-060. Office of Emergency and Remedial Response, USEPA, Washington, DC, 1986.

10. Environmental Protection Agency, *Updated Mutagenicity and Carcinogenicity Assessment of Cadmium* (addendum to the Health Assessment Document for Cadmium, EPA/600/8-81/023, 1981), Final Report, EPA 600/8-83-025F. Office of Health and Environmental Assessment, USEPA, Washington, DC, 1985.

11. Environmental Protection Agency, *Drinking Water Criteria Document for Cadmium* (final draft), PB86 117934/AS. Office of Drinking Water, USEPA, Washington, DC, 1985.

12. M. J. Thun, T. M. Schnoor, A. B. Smith, W. E. Halperin, and R. A. Lemen, Mortality among a cohort of U.S. Cadmium production workers—An update. *JNCI, J. Natl. Cancer Inst.* **74**(2), 325–333 (1985).

13. Environmental Protection Agency, *Health Assessment Document for Cadmium,* EPA 600/8-81-023. Environment Criteria and Assessment Office, USEPA, Research Triangle Park, NC, 1981.

14. American Petroleum Institute, 1985. *Cadmium: Environmental and Community Health Impact,* EA Rep. API37C. API, Washington, DC, 1985.

15. Environmental Protection Agency, 1986. *Air Quality Criteria for Lead* (rev. draft), EPA 600/8-83-028F. Environmental Criteria and Assessment Office, USEPA, Research Triangle Park, NC, 1984.

16. D. Bellinger, A. Leviton, C. Waternaux, H. L. Needleman, and M. B. Rabinowitz, Longitudinal analyses of prenatal and postnatal lead exposure and early cognitive development. *N. Engl. J. Med.* **316**, 1037–1043 (1987).

17. M. B. Rabinowitz, A. Leviton, and H. L. Needleman, Occurrence of elevated protoporphyrin levels in relation to lead burden in infants. *Environ. Res.* **39**, 253–257 (1986).

18. K. R. Mahaffey, Environmental exposure to lead. In J. O. Nriagu, Ed., *The Biochemistry of Lead in the Environment,* Part B. Elsevier/North-Holland Biomedical Press, New York, 1978.

19. J. L. Schaum, *Risk Analysis of TCDD Contaminated Soil,* EPA 600/8-84-031. Office of Health and Environmental Assessment, USEPA, Washington, DC, 1984.

20. D. J. Paustenbach, Assessing the potential environmental and human health risks of contaminated soil. *Comments Toxicol.* **1**, 185–220 (1987).

21. J. K. Hawley, Assessment of health risk from exposure to contaminated soil *Risk Anal.* **5**, 289–302 (1985).

22. P. K. Lagoy, Estimated soil ingestion rates for use in risk assessment. *Risk Anal.* **7**, 355–359 (1987).

23. R. D. Kimbrough, H. Falk, D. Stehr, and G. Fries, Health implications of 2, 3, 7, 8-tetrachlorodibenzodioxin (TCDD) contamination of residential soil. *J. Toxicol. Environ. Health* **14**, 47–93 (1984).

24. D. J. Paustenbach, H. P. Shu, and F. J. Murray, A critical examination of assumptions used in risk assessments of dioxin contaminated soil. *Regul. Toxicol. Pharmacol.* **6**, 284–307 (1986).

25. M. A. Smith, *Tentative Guidelines for Acceptable Concentrations of Contaminants in Soils.* Department of the Environment, London UK, 1981.

26. H. W. Mielke, B. Blake, S. Burroughs, and N. Hassinger, Urban lead levels in Minneapolis: The case of the Hmong children. *Environ. Res.* **34**, 64–76 (1984).

27. A. J. Yankel, I. H. von Lindern, and S. D. Walter, The Silver Valley lead study: The relationship between childhood blood lead levels and environmental exposure. *J. Air Pollut. Control Assoc.* **27**, 763–767 (1977).

28. C. R. Angle and M. S. McIntire, Environmental lead and children: The Omaha study. *J. Toxicol. Environ. Health* **5**, 855–870 (1979).

29. H. A. Roels, J. P. Buchet, R. Lauwerys, P. Bruaux, F. Cleays-thoreau, A. Lafontaine, and G. Verduyn, Exposure to lead by the oral and pulmonary routes of children living in the vicinity of a primary lead smelter. *Environ. Res.* **22**, 81–94 (1980).

30. S. D. Walter, A. J. Yankel, and I. H. von Lindern, Age-specific risk factors for lead absorption in children. *Arch. Environ. Health* **35**, 53–58 (1980).

31. C. R. Angle and M. S. McIntire, Children, the barometer of environmental lead. *Adv. Pediatr.* **27**, 3–31 (1982).

32. A. D. Stark, R. F. Quah, J. W. Meigs, and E. R. DeLouise, The relationship of environmental lead to blood-lead levels in children. *Environ. Res.* **27**, 372–383 (1982).

33. W. A. Galke, D. I. Hammer, J. E. Keil, and S. W. Lawrence, Environmental determinants of lead burdens in children. *Int. Conf. Heavy Met. Environ. [Symp. Proc.], 1st, 1975,* Vol. 3, pp. 53–74 (1977) (see also EPA 600/J-78-022).

34. D. Barltrop, C. D. Strehlow, I. Thornton, and J. S. Webb, Absorption of lead from dust and soil. *Postgrad. Med. J.* **51**, 801–804 (1975).

35. L. C. Neri, H. L. Johansen, N. Schmitt, R. T. Pagan, and D. Hewitt, Blood lead levels in children in two British Columbia communities. *Trace Substances Environ. Health* **12**, 403–410 (1978).

36. J. E. J. Gallacher, P. C. Elwood, K. M. Phillips, B. E. Davies, and D. T. Jones, Relation between pica and blood lead in areas of differing lead exposure. *Arch. Dis. Child.* **59**, 40–44 (1984).

37. K. R. Mahaffey, J. L. Annest, J. Roberts, and R. S. Murphy, National estimates of blood lead levels, United States 1976–1980: Association with selected demographic and socioeconomic factors. *N. Engl. J. Med.* **307**, 573 (1982).

38. Centers for Disease Control, *East Helena, Montana, Child Lead Study, Summer 1983.* Participating Agencies include the Lewis and Clark County Health Department, Montana Department of Health and Environmental Sciences, Centers for Environmental Health— CDC, and the Environmental Protection Agency, July 1986.

39. Centers for Disease Control, *Kellogg Revisited—1983 Childhood Blood Lead and Environmental Status Report.* Participating Agencies include the Panhandle District Health Department, Idaho Department of Health and Welfare, Center for environmental Health— CDC, and the Environmental Protection Agency, July 1986.

40. K. R. Mahaffey, Quantities of lead producing health effects in humans: Sources and bioavailability. *Environ. Health Perspect.* **19**, 285–295 (1977).

41. Environmental Protection Agency, *Development of Statistical Distributions or Ranges of Standard Factors Used in Exposure Assessments,* OHEA-E-161. Office of Health and Environmental Assessment, USEPA, Washington, DC, 1985.

42. Environmental Protection Agency, Guidelines for the health risk assessment of chemical mixtures. *Fed. Regist.* **51**, 34013–34023 (1986).

14

Problems Associated with the Use of Conservative Assumptions in Exposure and Risk Analysis

L. Daniel Maxim
Everest Consulting Associates, Cranbury, N.J.

INTRODUCTION

Because many of the qualitative and quantitative factors underlying exposure and risk analyses are uncertain, it is common to choose assumptions, models, and inputs so as to minimize the likelihood that the resulting exposures or risks are understated. The maxim "better safe than sorry" succinctly summarizes the rationale for "conservative," "plausible upper-bound," or "worst-case" approaches to analysis. However, most analyses involve numerous inputs, assumptions, and/or conventions. If conservative choices are made for each, the resulting estimates may grossly exaggerate the actual risks—precluding (or at least undercutting) the development of wise public policy.

The Office of Management and Budget (OMB) in Washington, DC, recognizing that this was (in part) responsible for the less-than-optimal expenditure of some of America's resources, has expressed concern over this issue. Their concern, coupled with Executive Orders 12291 and 12498, certainly suggests that scientists involved in risk assessment make the most reasonable assumptions of exposure, rather than worst-case assumptions, in developing assessments.

This chapter is intended to provide useful guidance for the development of more realistic risk analyses. Seven specific ideas are offered which should improve the quality of risk and exposure analyses.

Most of the specific illustrations in this chapter deal with the polychlorinated biphenyls (PCBs). But our experience suggests that this class of chemicals is not atypical, so the conclusions are more broadly applicable.

The concerns regarding PCBs are due in part to their widespread use, particularly in the 1960s and 1970s, their tendency to bioaccumulate (1, 2), and studies indicating a carcinogenic potential in laboratory animals. In addition, numerous industrial and commercial sites are contaminated with these chemicals. Federal, state, and local regulatory agencies have been struggling to develop realistic policies for controlling human exposure to PCBs, so there is a large data base for examination and review. Several of these risk assessments are critically evaluated here. A critical analysis of numerous assumptions which can dramatically affect risk estimates is offered. Alternative assumptions and approaches are suggested.

THE SOURCES OF CONSERVATISM: UNCERTAINTY AND COMPLEXITY

The word *conservatism* is used here to mean the selection of assumptions, parameter estimates, models, or procedures that are designed to ensure that resulting estimates of health risks are unlikely to be understated. The wisdom of conservative choices is addressed later in this chapter, but it is first important to understand the sources of conservatism in risk and exposure analyses.

Basically, conservatism is often introduced because exposure and toxicity information are lacking and/or ambiguous. Consequently, there is often considerable uncertainty surrounding key assumptions that enter a risk analysis. For example, in the extrapolation of dose–response data from animal studies to estimate human health risks, sources of uncertainty include:

1. The selection of biological endpoint (e.g., liver tumor, lung neoplasia, total malignancies) for analysis.
2. The appropriate species-to-human dose equivalence or scaling factor (e.g., mg/kg·day, ppm in diet, surface area).
3. The relevant animal data set for analysis.
4. The statistical models and estimation procedures used for extrapolation.

Additionally, risk analysis of commercial compounds may be complicated if, as is the case with PCBs, these are mixtures of compounds rather than "pure" compounds. (Even with "pure" compounds, trace impurities may significantly affect the toxicity.)

Polychlorinated biphenyl, for example, is an operational term given to a series of chemical compounds produced industrially by chlorination of biphenyl with anhydrous chlorine and iron filings or ferric chloride as a catalyst (3). Commercially available PCB preparations contain chlorinated biphenyls with varying degrees of chlorine substitution on the biphenyl ring with the generic formula, $C_{12}H_{10-r}Cl_r$, where r is the total number of chlorine atoms per molecule. PCBs were manufactured in the United States by Monsanto under the trade name Aroclor, and by manufacturers in other countries under other trade names, including Kanechlor in Japan, and Clophen in West Germany. Table 1 shows the approximate percent composition according to degree of chlorine substitution of these commercial mixtures.

The situation is made yet more complex with PCBs than implied by Table 1, because numerous isomers of each of the chlorinated biphenyls are theoretically possible, some 209 congeners in all, and until recently congener-specific analyses were not available. The variability of composition of compounds included in the blanket term *PCB* complicates the preparation of a risk analysis because, as noted below, the various mixtures and individual congeners have different toxicities. Moreover, differing congener-specific environmental transport rates alter the composition of PCBs in environmental media.

In this chapter, the word *uncertainty* is used in a manner consistent with that employed

TABLE 1. Approximate Percentage Composition of Some Commercial PCB Products

Chlorobiphenyl	Aroclor Type or Grade							Kanechlors			Clophens	
	1016	1221	1232	1242	1248	1254	1260	KC-300	KC-400	KC-500	A 30	A 60
$C_{12}H_{10}$	<0.1	11	6	<0.1		<0.1						—
$C_{12}H_9Cl$	1	51	26	1		<0.1					1	—
$C_{12}H_8Cl_2$	20	32	29	16	2	0.5		17			21	1
$C_{12}H_7Cl_3$	57	4	24	49	18	1		60	3	5	57	2
$C_{12}H_6Cl_4$	21	2	15	25	40	21		23	33	27	17	3
$C_{12}H_5Cl_5$	1	0.5	0.5	8	36	48	12	0.6	44	55	2	20
$C_{12}H_4Cl_6$	<0.1			1	4	23	38		16	13		43
$C_{12}H_3Cl_7$				<0.1		6	41		5			25
$C_{12}H_2Cl_8$							8					5
$C_{12}H_1Cl_9$							1					
$C_{12}Cl_{10}$												
Average % chlorine	42%	21%	32%	42%	48%	54%	60%	42%	48%	54%	30%	60%

Sources: Polychlorinated Biphenyls, The National Research Council, National Academy of Sciences, Washington, DC, 1979; O. Hutzinger, S. Safe, and V. Zitko, The Chemistry of PCBs, CRC Press, Boca Raton, FL, 1980, p. 8; D. N. Paul Michael, Monsanto, personal communication; and Schaeffer et al., op cit. The figures cited for the Clophens are taken from Schaeffer.

TABLE 2. PCB Potency—Lifetime Incremental Health Effects Associated with a Lifetime Consumption of 1 gram of PCB

Risk Probability Calculation	Model	Basis for Animal to Human Conversion	Uses Upper Confidence Bound	Aroclor	Bioassay Data	Calculation
Less than 10^{-10}	Probit	ppm	No	1254	NCI liver carcinoma, adenomas, and hematopoietic system	Maxim and Harrington
3.4×10^{-8}	Logistic	$\mu g/kg$	No	1254	NCI liver carcinoma and adenomas	Maxim and Harrington
2.3×10^{-7}	Logistic	ppm	No	1254	NCI liver carcinoma and adenomas	Maxim and Harrington
3.6×10^{-7}	Extreme value	ppm	No	1254	NCI liver carcinoma and adenomas	Maxim and Harrington
3.2×10^{-6}	Logistic	ppm	No	1254	NCI hematopoietic system	Maxim and Harrington
8.7×10^{-6}	Multistage	ppm	No	1254	NCI liver carcinoma and adenomas	Maxim and Harrington
1.5×10^{-5}	One-hit	mg/kg·day	No	1260	Kimbrough hepatocellular carcinoma	OTA (Crump)
1.5×10^{-5}	One-hit	Unstated	No	1260	Kimbrough hepatocellular carcinoma	Decision Focus, Inc, based on EPA–OTS
3.2×10^{-5}	Multistage	ppm	No	1254	NCI hematopoietic system	Maxim and Harrington
3.6×10^{-5}	One-hit	ppm	No	1260	Kimbrough hepatocellular carcinoma	OTA (Crump)
4.2×10^{-5}	One-hit	ppm	99%	1254	NCI liver carcinoma and adenoma	FDA
4.2×10^{-5}	Multistage	mg/kg·day	No	1254	NCI total malignancies	EPA–OTS
6.0×10^{-5}	One-hit	ppm	99%	1260	Kimbrough liver carcinoma	FDA
6.8×10^{-5}	Multistage	mg/kg·day	95%	1254	NCI total malignancies	EPA–OTS
1.9×10^{-4}	One-hit	ppm	99%	1254	NCI total malignancies	FDA
2.5×10^{-4}	Multistage	$\mu g/(kg)^{2/3}$	No	1254	NCI total malignancies	EPA–OTS
3.2×10^{-4}	Multistage	mg/kg·day	No	1260	Kimbrough hepatocellular carcinomas and neoplastic nodules	CAL–Health, recomputed
4.1×10^{-4}	Multistage	$\mu g/(kg)^{2/3}$	95%	1254	NCI total malignancies	EPA–OTS
1.9×10^{-3}	?	Surface area	No	?	?	CAL–Health
2.2×10^{-3}	?	Surface area	?	1260	Kimbrough	EPA–OHEA
2.7×10^{-3}	?	Surface area	95%	?	?	CAL–Health
4.3×10^{-3}	Multistage	Surface area	95%	1260	Norback and Weltman	EPA cited in ATSDR

by Whipple (4): "a lack of definite knowledge, a lack of sureness; *doubt* is its closest synonym" (see also Wilson and Crouch, 5). Risk, in contrast, is used to measure the probability and severity of loss or injury. Both risk and uncertainty may be couched in probabilistic terms; the lack of predictability arises from insufficient knowledge in the case of uncertainty rather than from the probabilistic outcome of a well-understood stochastic process in the case of risk.

Real uncertainties often surround the analysis of dose–response data (points 1–4 above) in the case of most chemicals, including PCBs. The selection of the appropriate assumptions and models is often ultimately judgmental. Even the interpretation of the basic data is seldom unequivocal. Barnard (6), for example, illustrates data interpretation problems for bioassays with the case of nitrites:

> Problems of evaluation arise not only because of the mass of experimental data and questions of their validity, but also because the interpretation of the data is ultimately judgmental. A well-known example is nitrites. The original bioassay was reported to be positive; great public uproar and regulatory activity took place because nitrites are important antibacterial additives to meat. Upon full peer review of the data, the study was judged to be negative.

Dose–response model identification and estimation involve substantial uncertainty (7–11), as does the choice of scaling factors [e.g., on a weight versus a surface area basis, (12)], and the other elements above. Depending on how these uncertainties are handled, the estimates of human health risks for a chemical under investigation can differ by orders of magnitude. Table 2, for example, shows a sampling of potency values—here shown in approximate terms as the lifetime incremental health risk associated with the consumption of 1 g of PCBs—taken from the literature. For example, the 1.9×10^{-4} risk per gram estimate in Table 2 is derived as follows. Cordle, Locke, and Springer (13) estimated that 50th percentile fish eaters consumed an average of 8.46 μg PCB/day. The corresponding lifetime dose is 8.46×10^{-6} g/day times 365 days/yr times 70 yr/lifetime, or 2.16×10^{-1} g PCB/lifetime. Based on National Cancer Institute (NCI) data, Cordle et al. concluded that eaters of contaminated fish would experience an incremental lifetime health risk of 4.1 per 1000,000. Thus, the incremental lifetime risk associated with the consumption of 1 g of PCB is $4.1 \times 10^{-5}/2.16 \times 10^{-1}$ or 19×10^{-4}. This estimate used total malignancies, from the NCI study as the endpoint, a 99% statistical upper confidence estimate of the dose–response slope of a one-hit model, and based the species-to-human conversion on the assumption that equal parts per million (ppm) in the diet would produce an identical response.

The risk estimates given in Table 2 span approximately seven orders of magnitude from less than 10^{-10} to 4.3×10^{-3}. Although it may be argued that not all the estimates in Table 2 are equally likely, all have some degree of scientific credibility. Similarly broad ranges in risk have been observed for vinyl chloride, saccharin, and other compounds (14), so the estimates for PCBs should not be viewed as atypical. What then is a "reasonable" way to deal with this uncertainty? (We are mindful of Ambrose Bierce's cynical definition of reason: "to weigh probabilities in the scales of desire.")

Although numerous approaches have been proposed for quantifying and otherwise treating uncertainty, regulatory agencies have generally opted to choose the most conservative among the alternative risk estimates. For PCBs, this means (expressed in risk/gram terms) accepting a potency of the order of 10^{-3}, rather than any smaller estimate. For example, the recent Agency for Toxic Substances and Disease Registry (ATSDR) draft Toxicological Profile for PCBs (15) cites a potency (expressed in the units given in Table 2) of 4.3×10^{-3} without any mention of the fact that this estimate is the largest among many alternatives.

As noted, one of the issues that serves to complicate the selection of a potency estimate for PCBs relates to the variable composition among the commercial mixtures coupled with evidence that the toxicity varies among these mixtures. For example, an NCI study on Aroclor 1254 stated (16):

> It is concluded that under the conditons of this bioassay, Aroclor 1254 was not carcinogenic in Fischer 344 rats.

But the study generally regarded as providing the most convincing evidence of the carcinogenicity of PCBs (17) is that conducted by Kimbrough et al. (18). This Kimbrough study used Aroclor 1260, a mixture containing approximately 60% chlorine (q.v., Table 1). Moreover, the Norback and Weltman study (19) (used as the basis for EPA's recent potency estimate) also used Aroclor 1260 (of unreported purity) for its feeding studies. That these latter studies used only Aroclor 1260 is important because there is strong evidence from numerous studies that the biological activity of PCBs is a function of the degree of chlorination:

1. Feeding experiments over 224 days with Kanechlor 300, 400, and 500 in mice were conducted by Ito et al. (20). Hepatocellular carcinomas were induced only by the highest chlorinated compound, Kanechlor 500 (q.v., Table 1).

2. A study by Schaeffer et al. (21) indicated that at the end of an 800-day feeding experiment, the incidence of hepatocellular carcinoma in rats fed Clophen A 60 (similar to Aroclor 1260 q.v., Table 1) reached 48%, whereas only 3% of those fed Clophen A 30 and 0.8% of the controls were similarly affected. It is unfortunate that ATSDR remarked (p. 72) only that the Schaeffer study "demonstrates that PCB mixtures free from contamination with furans elicit a carcinogenic response." (The study reported that the Clophens were free of chlorinated dibenzofurans, but test method, level of detection, and actual results were not specified.) In fact, the Schaeffer study has much broader implications. Table 3 shows the Schaeffer data. The incidence of hepatocellular carcinoma was elevated (in a statistically significant manner) only for Clophen A 60. Thus, the results of this study not only supported other findings that PCB mixtures containing 60% chlorine by weight were associated with hepatocellular carcinoma in rats, but also indicated that PCBs containing lesser amounts of chlorine were not

TABLE 3. Frequency of Hepatocellular Alterations Induced by Chronic Feeding Studies with Clophen A 30 and Clophen A 60

	Number of Foci	Neoplastic Nodules	Hepatocellular Carcinoma
Controls	6/131	5/131	1/131
(group 1)	(4.5%)	(3.8%)	(0.8%)
Clophen A 30	63/130*	38/130*	4/130
(group 2)	(48%)	(29%)	(3%)
Clophen A 60	3/126	63/126*	61/126*
(group 3)	(2.4%)	(50%)	(48%)

Source: Schaeffer et al., as cited in Harbison et al.
*Denotes a significant difference from the control value (P = 0.05).

proven to be carcinogenic. Even if it is argued that Clophen A 30's lack of significance was solely an artifact of sample size, the raw data is consistent with the finding that the potency of A 30 is at most 1/16 that of A 60! This finding is absolutely at variance with the assumption made by EPA and ATSDR that "all PCBs have equal potency."

3. Schaeffer et al. (21) also note,

> Both the DHEW Subcommittee on Health Effects of PCBs and PBBs (1978) and Ecobichon (1975) have reported that the toxic potency of PCBs (hepatic enzyme induction, hepatocarcinogenic effect) increases with increasing chlorination and chlorine substitution in the para, ortho, meta positions, respectively.

These and other results support the notion of increasing biological hazard with increasing average degree of chlorination of PCB mixtures. Thus, Kimbrough's and Norback and Weltman's results with Aroclor 1260 have to be viewed as a "worst case," and moreover, an "unlikely worst case" as production of 1260 only accounted for a minority of total domestic PCB production (21). (According to Monsanto, production of Aroclor 1260 accounted for only 10.6% of total Aroclor production over the period 1957–1977.)

Uncertainty is not confined to potency estimates. Some of the quantities used in a risk–exposure analysis include the following:

1. Initial contaminant concentrations.
2. Physicochemical constants to describe the kinetics of contaminant transport between environmental compartments.
3. Exposure frequency of humans to contaminants in various environmental compartments.
4. Human contact (uptake) rates (e.g., soil, accretion rates, soil ingestion rates, respiration rates, consumption rates for various foodstuffs) for alternative exposure pathways.
5. Bioavailability fractions (e.g., absorption rates through skin).
6. Dose–response parameters and models.

Many of the parameters, constants, and variables in models relevant to 1–6 are not known with accuracy. As simple a quantity as soil ingestion rates—a key parameter in many PCB risk analyses—for example, admits to numerous estimates, such as are shown in Table 4. These estimates range over almost three orders of magnitude, from 25 to 10,000 mg/day.

Faced with these uncertainties and complexities, the regulatory response has generally been to avoid making choices that could potentially lead to underestimates of human health risk as illustrated above with potency estimates for PCBs. In some cases, this response has been implicit. But in others, conservative assumptions have been explicitly mandated by regulatory agency policy. For example, the carcinogen assessment guidelines employed by numerous federal and state regulatory agencies are clearly conservative, a fact acknowledged in a recent critical report by the Executive Office of the President, Office of Management and Budget (38), as shown in Table 5.

The conceptual rationale for conservatism in exposure and risk analysis is a perception among regulatory agencies that the "social cost" of "false positives" (incorrectly judging a contaminant to present a hazard) is less than that of "false negatives," a theme developed at length in a thoughtful article by Whipple (4).

TABLE 4. Estimates of Daily Soil Ingestion from Various Sources

Age	Daily Ingestion Rate (mg/day)	Source	Remarks
Toddlers	100	Barltrop (22) 1973	
?	33	Bryce-Smith 1974	Cited in Duggan and Williams (23)
4.3 years (mean)	100	Lepow et al. (24, 25) 1974, 1975	Based on observations of mouthing behavior
1–3 years	10–1,000	Day et al. (26) 1975	Based on ingestion of soil on candy
2–6 years	25	Duggan and Williams (23) 1977	Estimate of amount of street dust that urban children ingest daily
1–3 years	140–430	Mahaffey (27) 1977	Based on estimate of paint consumption by children with pica
Various	40	National Research Council (28) 1980	Recommended for the sake of exposure calculations
Various unspecified	100	EPA (29, cited in 28) 1983	Lead in air study
2–6 years	100–5,000	Schaum (30) 1984	Upper end of range represents habitual pica consumption
0–9 months	0	Kimbrough et al. (31)	Reportedly based on study of lead exposure; generally thought to be an overestimate
9–18 months	1,000		
1.5–3.5 years	10,000		
3.5–5 years	1,000		
5 years	100		
2.5 years	164	Hawley (32) 1985	Includes both soil and dust ingestion; rates calculated on 365-day/ yr basis
6 years	24		
Adults	61		
1–3 years	180	Binder et al. (33) 1985	Based on measurement of trace elements— upper 95% percentile less than 600 mg/day
0–3 years	2,500	Dime (34) 1985	Used in state of New Jersey risk analysis for PCBs
Various	100	EPA (35) 1985	Superfund health assessment manual
0–1 year	50	Clement Associates (36) 1986	Used in Smuggler Mountain endangerment assessment; meant to summarize literature estimates
1–6 years	100		
6–11 years	50		
Over 11 years	20–50		
1.5–3.5 years	100	Paustenbach et al. (37) 1986	Based on complete review of literature

TABLE 5. OMB Characterization of Cancer Assessment Models Employed by EPA and Other Federal Agencies

A few examples of these cautious or conservative assumptions are: (1) treating all benign tumors as malignant, (2) using data about only the most sensitive animal species and sex, and (3) using conservative mathematical models to extrapolate from high to low doses. Each of these three kinds of assumptions is discussed briefly below.

All benign tumors treated as malignant. In interpreting animal studies, agencies frequently interpret both benign (noncancerous) tumors and malignant (cancerous) tumors to be equally strong indications that a substance is a carcinogen. Scientists know, however, that not all benign tumors evolve into malignancies. Studies that treat benign tumors the same as malignant tumors can overstate the real risk present. Some risk assessments based on animal studies have concluded that a chemical is carcinogenic solely because of an increased number of benign tumors. Assuming that all benign tumors will become malignant will not produce a best estimate of the risk.

Use of most sensitive species and sex. Even though the results of several animal studies may be available for a particular suspected carcinogen, it is not unusual for the risk estimate to be derived only from the data for the most sensitive exposed species and sex. This conservative approach tends to overpredict the risk to humans, because it assumes that humans are as sensitive as the most sensitive animal tested even when the most sensitive animal tested is hundreds of times more sensitive than any other animal tested. Furthermore, by using the same data to derive the risk estimate and to determine the most sensitive species, the chance is increased that statistical anomalies will lead to overestimates of the risk. (If a statistical anomaly causes an upward bias in the estimated risk for a particular species, it will also increase the chance that that species will be selected as the most sensitive.) A more accurate estimate could be derived from a weighted average of all the scientifically valid, available information.

Conservative extrapolation from high doses to low doses. To determine the risks to humans from exposure to a substance, scientists must extrapolate (or estimate) from the results of high doses in animal experiments to the comparatively low doses of human exposure. This extrapolation relies upon statistical models. The risk from exposure to low doses cannot be determined with certainty. In making the extrapolation, the common practice is not to make a best estimate of the risk from human exposure to low doses, but to determine what a maximum risk would be. Often, such an extrapolation has a 95 percent chance of overstating the true risk. Usually, the explanation for using these conservative assumptions is to ensure that the actual risk is not underestimated. However, the resulting risk estimate can be over one hundred times greater than the best estimate of the risk.

Whipple suggests another factor that encourages conservatism (39):

> An additional factor encouraging conservatism is how a regulatory agency's decisions might be judged in hindsight. An overcontrolled risk will probably drop from sight once a decision is implemented and control investments made, despite continuing social costs. But an undercontrolled risk, possibly discovered through the identification of victims, is far more disturbing for a regulatory agency.

CONSERVATISM CHALLENGED: EVOLVING PERCEPTIONS AND EXECUTIVE ORDERS 12291 AND 12498

Notwithstanding the above, there appears to be a growing awareness in the regulatory community that (i) conservative assumptions can significantly overstate risks, (ii) such overstatement could actually be ultimately counterproductive, and (iii) more realistic risk estimates are appropriate.

Table 6 presents a selection of observations from regulatory personnel, environmentalists, and academics that address uncertainty, conservatism, and the consequences

TABLE 6. Uncertainty, Conservatism, and Resulting Consequences in Risk Analysis

Statement	Reference/Remarks
Historically at EPA it has been thought prudent to make what have been called conservative assumptions; that is, our values lead us, in a situation of unavoidable uncertainty, to couch our conclusions in terms of a plausible upper bound. This means that when we generate a number that expresses the potency of some substance in causing disease, we can state that *it is unlikely that the risk projected is any greater.* This is fine when the risks projected are vanishingly small; it's always nice to hear that some chemical is not a national crisis. *But when the risks estimated through such assessments are substantial, so that some action may be in the offing, the stacking of conservative assumptions one on top of another, becomes a problem for the policymaker.* If I am going to propose controls that may have serious economic and social effects, I need to have some idea how much confidence should be placed in the estimates of risk that prompted those controls. I need to know how likely real damage is to occur in the uncontrolled, partially controlled, and fully controlled cases. Only then can I apply the balancing judgments that are the essence of my job. [emphasis added]	W. D. Ruckelshaus, former EPA Administrator (40)
I'm skeptical of quantitative risk assessment, at least in the cancer field. The science is too imperfect, and the results are likely to be used literally, because all the caveats get lost.	K. Ahmed, Research Director for the Natural Resources Defense Council (41)
Milton Russell, Assistant Administrator for Policy, Planning, and Evaluation at EPA, added that "depending on which animal you use, and whether you use a model that uses surface area or weight, you can get a difference in risk of up to 39,000 times." He went on to add that uncertainties in the risk assessment process are multiplied (not added) and in the case of cancer risk this leads to extreme conservatism in the decision-making process. "If you are relatively sure of the probability of risk, like automobile accidents, the range of uncertainty is narrow, and the difference between a plausible upper bound and a maximum likelihood and a plausible lower bound is relatively small. But if you are quite uncertain (as we are in many of these health effects), the range between this upper and lower bound is very, very large. *Multiplying the large uncertainties associated with each factor in the estimate leads to cascading conservatism in decision making.*" [emphasis added]	B. Barker (41)
Often each conservative assumption is made by a different scientist or analyst responsible for a portion of the risk assessment. Each may think that erring on the side of caution or conservatism is reasonable. However, the effect of these individual conservative assumptions is compounded in the final estimate of risk presented to the decisionmaker.	OMB (42); see also Nichols and Zeckhauser (12) for a numerical example

TABLE 6. (*Continued*)

Statement	Reference/Remarks
In practice, there may be as many as 20 distinct stages in a risk assessment where conservative assumptions are made. A typical risk assessment would probably contain about 10. The final risk estimate derived from these compounded conservative assumptions may be more than a million times greater than the best estimate and may, thus, have a probability of being accurate that is virtually zero. Some combinations of these highly cautious assumptions so overstate the risk that they are unrealistic.	
More recently, EPA has adopted the multi-stage model which has a linear component at low doses (4). This model assumes that cancer is caused by a series of mutational steps, whose occurrence [sic] rest both on a dose and potency. This model also results in a conservative estimate. Most scientists accept these models as giving plausible upper limit estimates for a chemical's potency at low levels of exposure. *In other words, the potency of a substance is unlikely to be higher that* [sic] *estimated using the linear model, but could be substantially lower. Use of the linear non-threshold models reflects EPA's decision to err on the side of caution in the face of uncertainties.* The final result of the linearized extrapolation is a "unit-risk factor," which gives the estimated upper limit lifetime risk per unit of exposure. [emphasis added]	D. R. Patrick (43)
These gaps in our scientific understanding and data limitations imply that it is difficult to conduct a good risk assessment. It is no surprise that they vary in quality. The many stages where judgment must be applied make it very easy for the results to substantially overestimate or underestimate the unknown true risks. *Because a government agency's mandate typically is to protect the public, or to be safe rather than sorry, the cumulative effect of these conservative assumptions may be very large. The resulting risk estimates often are treated as plausible upper bounds.* Unless the uncertainty associated with each assumption is stated, risk managers often view these risk estimates as actual risks. [emphasis added]	A. Fisher, EPA (44)
The Agency is not alone in its concern that different assumptions and different mathematical models used can significantly alter the outcome of risk assessment. When the Occupational Safety and Health Administration (OSHA) published its cancer policy in 1980, it did detailed comparisons of how estimates of carcinogenic risk can vary with the assumptions used in developing the estimates (45 FR 5198–5200). By varying the method of low dose extrapolation used, and the toxicology or epidemiology study which formed the basis of the risk assessment commenters to the OSHA policy developed risk estimates for exposure to 1 ppm of vinyl chloride which ranged from 10^{-8} (one in one hundred million) to 10^{-1} (one in ten, or 10%). A similar exercise with saccharin by NAS, and reprinted	United States Environmental Protection Agency (45)

536

TABLE 6. (*Continued*)

Statement	Reference/Remarks
in the OSHA policy (45 FR 5200), estimated the expected number of cancer cases in the general population (exposed at 0.12 grams/day) at between 0.001 cases per million exposed, and 5200 cases per million exposed. These differing estimates were developed by using different low-dose extrapolation models and different animal-to-human extrapolation methods—all of which had some credence in the scientific community.	
Recent research has also shown a need to reevaluate the role of "conservatism" in assessing and managing risk. Making a "conservative decision" (i.e., one that is likely to be more protective of health and the environment than an alternative decision) is widely accepted as a prudent practice in risk management. *In keeping with the recommended separation of risk assessment and risk management activities, however, conservative assumptions, conservative models, conservative estimates, etc., should not be key elements in the science-based risk estimation steps. A catenation of conservative assumptions, models, and estimates throughout a risk assessment can lead to a "worst-case" (or even worst-of-the-worst-cases) prediction that may be of little value* (or possibly misleading) *to the decision maker.* Most decisions actually involve "either–or" choices between technological alternatives with different risk levels rather than a "yes–no" choice on a single risk. When dissimilar alternatives require different analysis procedures, conservatism ambiguously or inconsistently applied could lead to biased results and poor decisions—even to the choice of a technology that is less protective of human health and the environment and possibly more costly to society than an available alternative. Best estimates of the risks, costs, and benefits for the alternatives, coupled with consideration of their uncertainties (including worst-credible case considerations), should produce the optimal basis for decision making. The Council on Environmental Quality has recently noted that "rules of reason" should replace worst case analysis as the basis of regulatory decision making. [emphasis added]	Midwest Research Institute (46)

to risk and exposure assessment. It is particularly noteworthy that senior officials at EPA are beginning to understand the problems occasioned by making conservative choices at several points in the analysis and to rethink the wisdom of these procedures.

As indicated by these quotes, current thinking appears to be shifting away from the "better-safe-than-sorry" premise toward the development of models and selection of assumptions that more accurately portray the actual risks. The place for conservatism (if at all) should be in the *risk management* rather than the *risk analysis* phase of regulatory action. Raiffa (47), Chairman of the Committee on Risk and Decision Making, National Research Council, offered the following suggestion:

Probabilistic reports should not prejudice policy issues and purposely report with a prudent bias. Cascading prudent reports could result in imprudent actions, and there is a danger of double-counting competing risks. Such reporting should be honest, and not attempt to second-guess policy choices. Probabilistic reports about diverse consequences to health, for example, are very often slanted to be conservative. I believe that it is better to report honestly, and that *prudence should, more appropriately, be accounted for in the evaluation process, rather than in the assessment process.* [emphasis added]

Barnard (48) echoed these comments in an essay on the partnership between law and science in risk analysis and risk management:

It is sometimes said that the scientific evaluation of risk should be "conservative" because it deals with human health. But this puts "conservatism" in the wrong place in the regulatory structure. It is the function of the regulator to apply the social criteria of cost, safety, reasonableness, and acceptability. It is in making these decisions that "conservatism" may play a role. If a scientific evaluation is constrained in the name of "conservatism" by social values or management policy, the result will be biased in unobvious ways. Such an evaluation does not provide a sound basis for the difficult social/legal decisions a regulator must make.

Nichols and Zeckhauser (49) also address the problems resulting from blurring the distinctions between risk analysis and risk management:

In practice, the line between risk assessment and management is often blurred. Fundamental gaps in scientific knowledge and data limitations make risk assessment a highly uncertain endeavor, requiring many choices among competing models and assumptions. There is a strong temptation to have such choices reflect implicit policy judgments rather than science.

This blur is most apparent in current techniques for estimating the risks associated with carcinogens, which employ conservative assumptions that bias the estimates upward. The intent is to err on the side of safety by minimizing the chance that risks will be underestimated and thus undercontrolled. But this approach intrudes the risk assessment process into risk management. In deciding how conservative to make their estimates, risk assessors implicitly trade off risk against other factors. Unless they explicitly acknowledge these trade-offs and quantify them, their assessments will mislead others, including those charged with managing risks. For example, risk managers will be more likely to impose a costly regulation if they mistakenly believe that it can prevent ten cases of cancer than if they correctly realize that it will eliminate only one case.

Advocates of the conservative approach are likely to view this tendency toward greater control as a virtue; conservatism is intended to give extra weight to protecting public health and, under conditions of massive uncertainty, to err on the side of safety. In fact, however, conservative risk assessment is a deeply flawed approach to protecting public health. It violates the distinction between risk assessment and risk management, concealing value judgments and policy choices under a cloak of science. It creates capricious differences in the degrees of safety provided across different substances and policy areas, because degrees of conservatism vary widely. Finally, because regulators must make complex trade-offs among different risks (not only between risk and cost), conservation can lead to less rather than more safety, by misdirecting public concern and scarce agency and societal resources.

Many of the above ideas (including those given in Table 6) are addressed (explicitly or implicitly) in Presidential Executive Orders 12291 (February 17, 1981) and 12498 (January 4, 1985) directed broadly at regulatory reform. Executive Order 12291 requires benefit–cost analysis of major federal regulations. Executive Order 12498 reaffirmed these guidelines and explicitly addressed health and safety matters directly, stating (50) that "regulations that seek to reduce health or safety risks should be based upon scientific risk assessment procedures, and *should address risks that are real and significant rather than hypothetical or remote*" [emphasis added]. Such language is pointedly directed toward increasing the realism of risk analysis. Indeed, "improving coordination and consistency in risk reduction" was one of the principal themes in the recent Executive Office of the President, Office of Management and Budget (OMB) 1986–1987 Regulatory Program. In particular, this document defines the regulatory agenda for implementation of the above referenced Executive Orders. Improvements to risk assessments were a major topic of this report. OMB was strongly critical of the conservative assumptions often employed in carcinogen risk and exposure assessment (see Table 5) and highlighted the reasons why such practices were problematic (51):

> *Risk Assessments with such extreme conservative biases do not provide decisionmakers with the information they need to formulate an efficient and cost-effective regulatory strategy.* Furthermore, the inconsistency of these assumptions makes it virtually impossible to compare risks from different sources. It is particularly difficult to compare safety risk estimates, which are usually best estimates, with health risk estimates, which usually are not best estimates, because the latter embody a series of conservative assumptions. Even different estimates of health risks may not be comparable because of the different degrees of conservatism built into them. Where risk estimates for two different risks cannot be compared, it will be impossible to compare the effects of regulations controlling them.

> *A perverse and unfortunate outcome of using upper-bound estimates based on compounded conservative assumptions is that it may lead us to regulate insignificant risks and ignore more serious risks.* Furthermore, the more uncertain we are about the risk posed by a particular hazard, the higher the upper-bound risk estimate will be. Therefore, the less information we have on the risk posed by a potential hazard, the more likely we are to regulate it. Other hazards that pose certain but smaller risks are not considered as dangerous and may not be regulated. Yet, hazards with better understood risks may be more serious.

> *All the problems we have discussed resulting from compounding conservative assumptions can be addressed by developing best estimates at each stage of the risk assessment process.* Estimates of the uncertainty and the outer ranges of potential risk can be developed to supplement the best estimate. Both the best estimate and these supplementary risk indicators should be made available to decisionmakers. Then, if regulatory decisionmakers want to choose a very cautious strategy of risk control, they could do so and a margin of safety could be applied at the final decision and would be based on all the available information about its consequences and those of alternative strategies. The public and affected parties would also benefit from knowing both the expected risk and the margin of safety rather than being given only alarming and inconsistent estimates that are likely to be very different from actual risks.

> *Only when best estimates of risks and other information on the likely level of risks are presented to the decisionmaker, rather than hidden in the assumptions, can we be sure that we are issuing regulations that will make society as well off as possible.* Fortunately, more review by regulating departments and agencies and by the Executive Branch has already begun to improve consistency in risk assessment and risk management and, thereby, improve societal welfare. Executive Order No. 12291 provides a mechanism to help ensure consistency. [emphasis added]

The above quotation—and extended discussion from which it was extracted—underscores the desirability of and executive branch emphasis on the need for realism in risk analysis. It remains to identify ways to operationalize this idea. How can risk assessments be made more realistic?

SEVEN SPECIFIC SUGGESTIONS FOR IMPROVED RISK AND EXPOSURE ANALYSES

Shown below are seven suggestions to make risk and exposure assessments more useful to risk managers. The items in this list are neither exhaustive nor mutually exclusive, but experience has proven that the ideas contained are useful.

1   Emphasize Best Estimates Rather Than Extremes

As noted, many of the assumptions and numerical inputs to a risk analysis are not known with certainty. In this circumstance, it is certainly appropriate to consider "conservative" values to bound risk estimates, but it is even more important to attempt to select "best" or "most likely" sets of assumptions for risk assessment. As OMB notes (52), with respect to measures of central tendency:

> This measure is favored by statisticians, economists, and scientists because it is the most accurate measure of what, on average, is likely to happen. The use of the best estimate does not preclude the supplementary use of other measures in order to understand the variation around this average, such as the variability of the risk or its upper or lower bounds. Agencies often—and should—use these supplemental measures as well. Using the best-estimate approach along with estimates of uncertainty allows policymakers to understand the range of possible risks and to choose the margin of safety that is appropriate for specific regulations. A regulatory agency could choose to be very cautious and regulate to protect people against a risk that has a very small chance of actually occurring, i.e., a risk at the higher end of the range of uncertainty. An agency could choose to regulate so that the chances of a risk occurring are, for example, only 5 percent, 1 percent, or 0.01 percent. However, it could be very costly to regulate to this level.

> Risk assessments of health hazards—as opposed to safety hazards—particularly those based on animal tests, rarely develop a best estimate of the risk. Instead, such risk assessments of health hazards often inform the regulatory officials and the public of only the high end of the range of uncertainty of the risk, i.e., only what the most cautious estimates are. Regulations based upon these so-called upper-bound estimates may, therefore, address a risk that is almost nonexistent. When agencies focus their efforts on regulating insignificant risks, they may end up ignoring other more significant risks.

Table 2, noted earlier, shows the range of potency estimates reported for PCBs and illustrates the present emphasis on extreme rather than most likely values. The values most often employed in risk analyses of PCBs are at or near 10^{-3} in risk/gram units [equivalent to a potency of approximately 7.7 $(mg/kg \cdot day)^{-1}$]. A more reasonable estimate is likely to be nearer the neon or median of the estimates given in Table 2, say approximately 10^{-5}, yet few analyses have employed this figure.

Even when mean values are employed in an analysis, other conventions may serve to bias mean values upward, and the analyst must be careful to spot these biases. For example, a recent endangerment assessment (EA) conducted at the Northside Sanitary Landfill (NSL) based some exposure scenarios on the maximum reported contaminant concentration. Recognizing that these maximum values might overstate exposures, the analysis also estimated risks associated with mean concentrations. In calculating these mean values, the authors of the report noted (53):

> Several arbitrary conventions were used in calculating means that may bias the means. For nondetectable results, method detection limits were used for calculating the arithmetic means. Using method detection limits may bias the mean high where it is reasonable to believe contaminants were not present; however, this is consistent with current EPA policy.

Taken to its limit, such a procedure is preposterous—every site could have an arbitrarily high cancer risk by simply adding (and calculating risks for) chemicals not detected in the sampling protocol! The NSL EA did not go to this extreme, but resolved the problem by omitting calculation of means when the proportion of "nondetects" exceeded 20%—and reporting only risk estimates based on maximum values for cases where this occurred. In fact, there is a well-developed statistical theory for estimating means from truncated samples, so no such ad hoc rules are required (54). (In the future, this may be less of a problem because detection limits are generally decreasing as new analytical procedures are being developed.)

Best estimates are important in exposure calculations. OMB challenged the use of worst-case environmental conditions in exposure calculations (55):

> Use of worst-case environmental conditions. To estimate what concentrations of a contaminant reach a point at which humans might be exposed, a chemical's movement through the air, water, or soil usually must be estimated with a computer model. Movement of a chemical, for example, depends greatly on environmental conditions, such as windspeed and direction for airborne pollutants; surface water flow, acidity, and temperature for water pollutants; and groundwater velocity, flow, and soil type for chemicals that pass through the soil. Often, only one calculation is made for the entire Nation on the assumption that it is impractical to set different regulatory standards for different environmental conditions. When a single model must represent conditions for the whole Nation, agencies frequently assume the unique circumstances that together may present the greatest risk, and then assume that this circumstance exists everywhere in the Nation. For example, a gravel soil environment (rather than clay or some other soil condition) might be used in a model because chemicals in groundwater move most quickly through gravel and, thus, are likely to pose a greater risk. However, since not all soil is gravel, this assumption will overstate actual risks.

Other examples of worst-case reasoning are legion. In an occupational setting, for example, EPA, OSHA, and state agencies often assume that a worker is exposed for as much as an entire working lifetime (from age 20 to age 65) or 45 years. To illustrate, in an assessment of reentry guidelines for PCB- and TCDD-contaminated surfaces at the Binghamton (New York) State Office Building (56), it was assumed that workers would be exposed over a 30-year period. Likewise, a similar analysis by the California Department of Health Services for reentry guidelines for the One Market Plaza building (57) assumed that workers would occupy the building for 40 years. Although the possibility exists that a worker could remain at one job location for as much as a 30- or 40-year period, it cannot be termed a "most likely" value in any realistic sense. National estimates by Hall (58) suggest that only 7% of U.S. workers would hold one job—let alone to be employed at one location—for 35 years or more. The Department of Labor, Bureau of Labor Statistics (BLS), publishes data on "ongoing tenure"—and estimates of "completed tenure" have been made using these data (59). Hall (60), in particular, estimated a median completed tenure of 7.7 years for all U.S. workers in 1978, based on BLS data. Completed tenure estimates will *overstate* the expected additional years of exposure, because the completed tenure figure includes time already spent on the job (ongoing tenure) as well as the expected additional tenure. The median ongoing tenure of all workers is approximately 3.2 years (61), so to a first approximation, the likely additional tenure is 7.7−3.2 = 4.5 years, or rounded, 5 years. Five years would have been a much more realistic estimate of the likely occupational exposure for an occupant of the Binghamton or One Market Plaza office buildings. Had this and other more realistic assumptions been employed in the risk assessment at these locations, it is possible that quite different cleanup standards would have prevailed.

As a second example, a residential exposure scenario for evaluation of groundwater contamination typically posits that exposed humans ingest 2 liters of water per day—all taken from the same contaminated source—over a 70-year nominal lifetime. Yet actual studies on water consumption support figures closer to 1 liter per day (62), which includes the contained water in carbonated beverages (unlikely to contain the contaminant) and prepared hot drinks such as coffee (where heating might partially evaporate or otherwise remove or destroy contaminants). And, in any event, the assumption of 24-hour per day occupancy over a 70-year period cannot be termed plausible.

Critics might well argue with the above examples and point out that building occupants or residents who depart will be replaced by others and that, in any event, it matters little to whom the risk occurs. Even if this premise is accepted, and a person-years metric is substantial for the calculation of individual risks, the above examples cannot be dismissed lightly, particularly when considering contaminant depletion. Succeeding generations of occupants will force lower exposure levels if the contaminants decay over time as discussed below.

At least some elements within EPA are sympathetic to the need to develop more realistic exposure scenarios. For example, EPA is reportedly considering substituting a residential exposure scenario of 16 hours per day for 10 to 35 years rather than 24 hours per day for 70 years (63).

A point often overlooked in exposure analyses is pollutant depletion/removal. Over time, pollutants are depleted by a variety of mechanisms, including volatilization, erosion, dilution/dispersion, photolysis, chemical reaction, and biodegradation. These transport processes reduce the contaminant concentration and hence potential for exposure. Although some exposure and risk analyses have explicitly treated depletion (e.g., 64–66), others have omitted this phenomenon. For example, the NSL EA (67) neglected depletion entirely. Thus, contaminants present at the NSL site were assumed to remain at their initial values throughout the duration of all exposure scenarios (some lasting as long as 70 years) considered. This same analysis also posited instantaneous residential development along the periphery of the NSL site—neglecting planning, construction, and occupancy lags. No reason was given for the omission of these factors, although uncertainty about environmental half-lives may have prompted such worst-case assumptions.

Depending on the actual half-lives of the pollutants, the order of the kinetic processes involved, and the occupancy lags, the resulting overstatement in risks could be substantial. For example, assuming first-order kinetics (with decay constant k), an occupancy lag of t_1 years, and a fixed exposure endpoint at t_2 years, the average contaminant concentration C_a, as a fraction of the initial concentration C_i, can be shown by integration of the rate equation to be

$$\frac{C_a}{C_i} = \frac{\exp(-kt_1) - \exp(-kt_2)}{k(t_2 - t_1)}.$$ (1)

For first-order kinetics, the rate constant k is related to the half-life, $t_{0.5}$, by means of the well-known relation

$$k = \frac{0.6931}{t_{0.5}}.$$ (2)

Calculated exposures and risks (using customary linear models) are directly related to

TABLE 7. Average Pollutant Concentration as Fraction of Initial Value Where First-Order Removal Occurs—Including Effects of Occupancy Lag[a]

Occupancy Lag (years)	Half-Life of Pollutant (years)									
	0.5	1	1.5	2	3	5	7.5	10	15	20
	First-Order Kinetic Constant (1/years)									
	1.39E+00	6.93E−01	4.62E−01	3.47E−01	2.31E−01	1.39E−01	9.24E−02	6.93E−02	4.62E−02	3.47E−02
1	2.61E−03	1.05E−02	1.98E−02	2.96E−02	4.98E−02	9.10E−02	1.43E−01	1.93E−01	2.87E−01	3.67E−01
2	6.63E−04	5.30E−03	1.26E−02	2.12E−02	4.01E−02	8.04E−02	1.32E−01	1.83E−01	2.78E−01	3.58E−01
3	1.68E−04	2.69E−03	8.08E−03	1.52E−02	3.23E−02	7.10E−02	1.22E−01	1.73E−01	2.68E−01	3.50E−01
4	4.27E−05	1.37E−03	5.16E−03	1.09E−02	2.60E−02	6.28E−02	1.13E−01	1.64E−01	2.60E−01	3.42E−01
5	1.08E−05	6.94E−04	3.30E−03	7.85E−03	2.10E−02	5.55E−02	1.05E−01	1.55E−01	2.51E−01	3.34E−01
6	2.75E−06	3.52E−04	2.11E−03	5.64E−03	1.69E−02	4.91E−02	9.69E−02	1.47E−01	2.43E−01	3.26E−01
7	6.99E−07	1.79E−04	1.35E−03	4.05E−03	1.36E−02	4.34E−02	8.97E−02	1.39E−01	2.35E−01	3.19E−01
8	1.78E−07	9.09E−05	8.66E−04	2.91E−03	1.10E−02	3.84E−02	8.31E−02	1.32E−01	2.27E−01	3.12E−01
9	4.52E−08	4.62E−05	5.55E−04	2.09E−03	8.87E−03	3.40E−02	7.69E−02	1.25E−01	2.20E−01	3.04E−01
10	1.15E−08	2.35E−05	3.55E−04	1.50E−03	7.16E−03	3.01E−02	7.13E−02	1.18E−01	2.13E−01	2.98E−01
12	7.42E−10	6.08E−06	1.46E−04	7.78E−04	4.57E−03	2.36E−02	6.13E−02	1.06E−01	2.00E−01	2.84E−01
14	4.81E−11	1.57E−06	5.99E−05	4.03E−04	3.04E−03	1.85E−02	5.27E−02	9.56E−02	1.87E−01	2.72E−01
16	3.12E−12	4.08E−07	2.47E−05	2.09E−04	1.99E−03	1.45E−02	4.54E−02	8.61E−02	1.76E−01	2.60E−01
18	2.02E−13	1.06E−07	1.02E−05	1.08E−04	1.30E−03	1.14E−02	3.91E−02	7.75E−02	1.65E−01	2.48E−01
20	1.31E−14	2.75E−08	4.20E−06	5.64E−05	8.52E−04	9.01E−03	3.38E−02	6.99E−02	1.55E−01	2.38E−01
25	1.43E−17	9.57E−10	4.63E−07	1.11E−05	2.98E−04	5.00E−03	2.35E−02	5.42E−02	1.33E−01	2.13E−01
30	1.57E−20	3.36E−11	5.16E−08	2.20E−06	1.06E−04	2.81E−03	1.65E−02	4.23E−02	1.14E−01	1.91E−01
40	2.00E−26	4.38E−14	6.78E−10	9.18E−08	1.40E−05	9.25E−04	8.39E−03	2.63E−02	8.52E−02	1.55E−01

[a]Exposure endpoint = 70 years.

concentrations, so the ratio of the actual risk to that calculated assuming a constant pollutant concentration is equal to C_a/C_i. Table 7 shows this quantity as a function of the half-life and the occupancy lag. For example, this ratio is 2.1×10^{-2} if the exposure endpoint is 70 years, the half-life is 3 years, and the occupancy lag is 5 years, implying that the conservative model overstates risk—considering this factor alone—by a factor of approximately 48. Fortunately, these omissions are readily corrected.

2   Collect Relevant Data on Uncertain Parameters

It is sometimes taken for granted that uncertainty cannot be reduced in risk analysis because key data elements are unknown, and perhaps even unknowable—at least within the time and budget constraints generally imposed on the analyst.

Although this may be true in certain instances, it certainly does not apply across the board. Why, for example, should assumed soil ingestion rates (often a key input to risk analyses) vary as much as the estimates given in Table 4? If there is *no* basis for selection of a most likely value, additional experiments and measurements can be made—and at arguably modest cost compared to potentially inflated cleanup costs of hazardous waste sites if the current worst-case estimates continue to be used.

Other parameters of exposure or risk models that are considered to lack certainty but could easily be measured include the following:

1. Data regarding dermal contact with soils. Realistic data are lacking on human activity patterns involving soil contact. For example, who gardens? How often? What soil contact rates are appropriate? An exhibit analogous to that shown in Table 4 can be prepared for each of these important factors. Unlike some of the more esoteric aspects of potency determination, answers to these questions could be determined by relatively straightforward surveys.
2. Data regarding the absorption (bioavailability) of chemicals through ingestion, dermal contact, and respiration. Uncertainty exists for these parameters (e.g., reported dermal absorption fractions for PCBs from soils or dusts range from 7×10^{-4} to 5×10^{-1} in the literature).

A salutary development in this regard is the EPA's recent decision to sponsor additional research on soil ingestion and to suggest additional research on bioavailability (68). The value of acquiring additional information about uncertain parameters can sometimes be treated analytically using the methods of decision theory (69). These techniques can be used to identify cost–effective approaches to uncertainty reduction.

3   Risk Assessors Should Understand the Spirit of Legislative Action

A third idea is that the (interpretation of the) legislative mandates of regulatory agencies should be examined to identify potentially counterproductive aspects. With respect to PCBs, for example, the FDA established tolerance levels for PCBs in fish in the context of its statutory framework. As the FDA notes (70):

> Section 406 of the Federal Food, Drug, and Cosmetic Act ("the act"), 21 U.S.C. 346, authorizes the establishment of tolerances for poisonous or deleterious substances added to food that cannot be avoided by good manufacturing practice. PCBs are such a substance. Although *the agency's paramount concern is protection of the public health*, under section 406 *the agency must consider, in establishing a tolerance, the extent to which a contaminant is unavoidable*. In essence, the agency is

permitted to find where the proper balance lies between adequately protecting the public health and avoiding excessive losses of food to American consumers. 44 FR 38330–31. [emphasis added]

Put somewhat differently, tolerance levels are established at a level "appropriate to protect the public health" or to "provide an adequate degree of public health protection." But tolerances established by the FDA also reflect existing levels of contamination and the extent of its "avoidability" in food products to be regulated.

On first reading, the "balancing provisions" of the Food, Drug, and Cosmetic Act (Section 406 of 21 USC 346) appear quite reasonable. But on more careful examination, there are curious, and arguably perverse, consequences of the FDA's present interpretation of this legislative mandate.

Consider, for example, two hypothetical foodstuffs, A and B, each contaminated initially to an identical degree with the same hazardous substance:

1. In product A, the contamination levels are expected to remain constant over time.
2. In product B the levels of contamination are expected to decline in the future.

Assuming that products A and B are consumed in equal amounts in the human diet and are absorbed equally, the lifetime incremental health risks associated with consumption of product B are obviously smaller. Product B, by any objective standard, presents less of a health hazard than product A. Yet, there is no guarantee that FDA tolerance levels for the hazardous contaminant in product B will be larger than, or even the same as, those for product A. In fact, quite the reverse is likely to be true. This is because the risks associated with product B become progressively more "avoidable" over time—a phenomenon that allegedly justifies lower tolerance levels.

The above situation is by no means hypothetical; it has occurred with respect to PCBs in poultry and fish. In 1977, the FDA (71) proposed a reduction in the tolerance level for PCBs in poultry (later implemented) from 5 ppm (fat basis) to 3 ppm (fat basis), not because PCBs were thought to be more dangerous, but rather because elevated PCB levels were *infrequent* and *declining* in poultry:

> Because the frequency of PCB residue occurrence in feeds is low, the likelihood of residues in poultry reaching the 3 ppm (fat basis) level is very small. Moreover, data regarding PCB residues in poultry confirm this and show that PCB contamination of poultry is very sporadic and infrequent. As such, this food is not a significant source of dietary PCBs. A tolerance of 3 ppm (fat basis) will continue to provide this assurance, while also providing adequate protection for the consumer. Therefore, the Commissioner proposes to reduce the temporary tolerance for poultry from 5 ppm to 3 ppm (fat basis). As stated previously, the finished feed tolerance of 0.2 ppm cannot be reduced at this time because the analytical methodology necessary to enforce a lower tolerance is not available. The Commissioner advises that when such methodology becomes available so that the 0.2 ppm feed tolerance can be reduced, the tolerance for PCB residues in poultry will also be reevaluated.

Likewise, with respect to fish, the FDA concluded that declining PCB levels were a reason for *reducing* tolerances (72): "Based on the declining incidence of PCB contamination, which means that PCBs are now avoidable in food to a greater degree now than they were earlier... FDA decided the PCB tolerances should be reduced." Later in this same document, in response to the comment that PCB levels in fish were declining, the FDA reaffirmed its proposed standard, noting (73): "Moreover, that PCB levels are declining (i.e., that PCBs are becoming more avoidable) is a reason to consider lowering the tolerance, not a justification for leaving it unchanged." Certainly, it is time to rethink this interpretation.

4   Incorporate Consistency and Plausibility Audits into Modeling Efforts

A fourth idea is to subject candidate risk and exposure models to more searching inquiry—to conduct a consistency or plausibility audit on the model.

Although experimental measurements may be considered the ultimate validation of assumptions, these are not always possible and other approaches may be necessary. In some cases, simple material balances can furnish useful consistency and plausibility checks on the adequacy of an exposure–risk model. For example, as noted, a risk analysis was conducted to help determine appropriate reentry guidelines for PCB- and TCDD-contaminated surfaces at the Binghamton (NY) State Office Building (74). The risk analysis for contaminated surfaces assumed, among other things, that:

1. Workers (50 kg) would labor in the building for 250 days/yr over 30 years.
2. The worker's total body surface area is 1.46 m^2, with the hands accounting for 4.5% (0.066 m^2) and the arms accounting for 19% (0.28 m^2) of this total.
3. The worker is assumed to ingest the contamination from an area the size of 5% of his/her hand (0.0033 m^2) every workday.
4. The worker is assumed to make dermal (bare skin) contact with an area 25% that of his/her arms (0.0694 m^2) every workday.
5. (Unstated) All PCBs are transferred from walls upon contact with contaminated surfaces.

Given these assumptions, the daily PCB intake was calculated by Kim and Hawley (74) by the following equation (with slight differences in notation):

$$\text{intake } (\mu g/\text{day}) = C_{sr} f_{GI}(0.0033) + f_{di}(0.0694) \tag{3}$$

where C_{sr} = residual surface contamination level ($\mu g/m^2$)
   f_{GI} = gastrointestinal absorption fraction
   f_{di} = dermal absorption fraction.

The risk analysis proceeds from the exposure calculation given by equation (3).

Upon initial review, the approach appears plausible. However, a "reality check" would have revealed that it was unrealistic. A simple example illustrates the problem. Assume that the hypothetical building occupant works in a one-person office of dimensions 8 ft × 10 ft × 12 ft. The total area of the walls of this office is 352 ft^2 (327,008 cm^2). Assuming, for illustrative purposes, a 100 μg/100 cm^2 level of PCB surface contamination, the total amount of PCBs on the walls is

$$\frac{100\ \mu g}{100\ \text{cm}^2} \times 327,008\ \text{cm}^2 = 327,008\ \mu g.$$

Now according to the Kim–Hawley model, PCBs are contacted and removed by two human features, arms and hands. Using the above factors, the total amount of PCBs removed each day by incidental skin contact with the arms, denoted X, would be

$$(1.46 \, \text{m}^2 \, \text{body surface}) \times \left(\frac{0.19 \, \text{m}^2 \, \text{arm surface}}{\text{m}^2 \, \text{body surface}} \right) \times \left(\frac{0.25 \, \text{m}^2 \, \text{contacted}}{\text{m}^2 \, \text{arm}} \right)$$

$$\times (1.0 \, \text{transfer fraction}) \times (10{,}000 \, \text{cm}^2/\text{m}^2) \times \left(\frac{100 \, \mu\text{g PCB}}{100 \, \text{cm}^2} \right),$$

or

$$X = 693.5 \, \mu\text{g}.$$

Similarly, the amount of PCBs removed each day by skin contact with the hands, denoted Y, is

$$(1.46 \, \text{m}^2 \, \text{body surface}) \times \left(\frac{0.045 \, \text{m}^2 \, \text{hand}}{\text{m}^2 \, \text{body}} \right) \times (1.0 \, \text{fraction transfer})$$

$$\times \left(\frac{100 \, \mu\text{g PCB}}{100 \, \text{cm}^2} \right) = Y = 657 \, \mu\text{g}.$$

The total removed per day $= X + Y = 1350.5 \, \mu\text{g}$. It should be noted that not all of this amount of PCBs would be absorbed, but all would be removed. (The above calculation assumes that the entire surface area of the contaminated surface will be contacted. Any corrections for inaccessible areas would reduce the estimated amount of PCB uptake and removal.)

Assuming that these rates continue (as is done in the Kim–Hawley analysis), the total number of days required to exhaust the PCB contamination at the surface is $(327{,}008 \, \mu\text{g})$ $\times (1350.5 \, \mu\text{g/day}) = 242$ days. But the exposure scenario used to estimate the cancer risk assumes a 30-year period, 5 days/wk, 50 wk/yr. Clearly, the assumptions in the exposure estimate were unrealistic, and had a plausibility check been done, this could have been identified early in the analysis process.

It is interesting that the authors considered various adjustments (first-order decay) to model volatilization or other (unstated) depletion mechanisms, but no consideration was given to the process of depletion inherent in the mechanism of exposure itself. For these and other reasons, the Kim–Hawley analysis must be regarded as unrealistically conservative.

5 Use Computational Approaches That Avoid "Catch All" Assumptions

A fifth idea is to design models insofar as possible to avoid "catch all" parameters that may be ambiguous. Alternative risk and exposure models can differ in the extent to which subjective elements can enter the analysis process. Figure 1, for example, diagrams the logic of an EPA risk analysis designed to estimate appropriate cleanup levels for indoor PCB spills (75). This figure also contains the EPA's numerical estimates purporting to show that residual surface PCB contamination levels of $100 \, \mu\text{g}/100 \, \text{cm}^2$ result in lifetime incremental health risks of the order of 10^{-4}. The logic behind the model is depicted in Fig. 1.

This analysis assumed that a notional room (of area $438{,}000 \, \text{cm}^2$) has been decontaminated by replacing so-called high contact areas (area $27{,}871 \, \text{cm}^2$) and cleaning

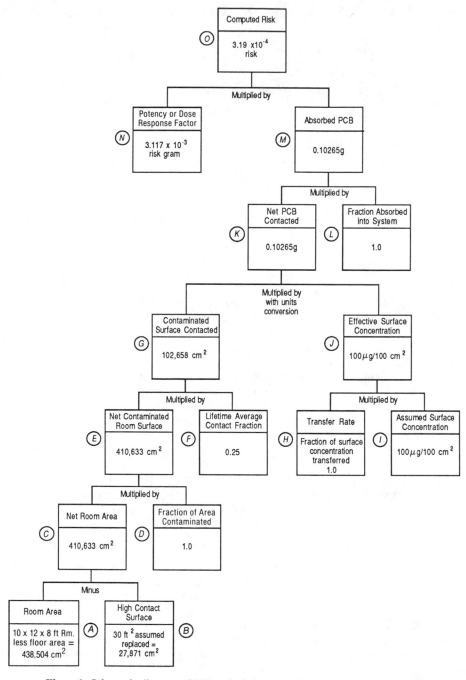

Figure 1. Schematic diagram of EPA calculation of residential exposure and risk.

the remaining surface areas to a residual PCB concentration of $100 \,\mu g/100 \,cm^2$. After cleanup, the net room area (box C in Fig. 1) is calculated as the difference between the original contaminated area (box A) and the high contact area (box B). All of this net area is assumed to be contaminated (box D), so the net contaminated room surface (box E) is the same as the original area minus the replaced high contact areas.

Human occupants are assumed to have incidental skin contact with these contaminated surfaces. Based on the assumption of an assumed residual surface PCB concentration of $100 \,\mu g/100 \,cm^2$ (box I) and the assumption that, upon contact, 100% of the surface concentration is transferred to exposed skin (box H), the potential amount of PCBs transferred (effective surface concentration, box J) per $100 \,cm^2$ contaminated surface contacted can be calculated. No surface depletion mechanisms (e.g., volatilization, penetration into wells) or effects of encapsulation (e.g., by painting) were considered in this EPA analysis.

A key computational artifice employed in the EPA model is the lifetime average contact fraction (LACF), defined as the fraction of the contaminated area that would be touched by the room's occupant in a lifetime of exposure, which was set equal to 0.25 in the analysis (box F). Multiplication of the LACF by the net contaminated room surface (box E) enables calculation of the contaminated surface contacted (box G). In turn, this quantity multiplied by the "pickup rate" or effective surface concentration (box J) estimates the net PCB contacted in a lifetime (box K), numerically equal to approximately 0.1 g. All this PCB is assumed to be absorbed (box L) even though studies (76) point to absorption fractions no more than half this amount for PCB liquids, and appreciably less for PCBs in soils or household dust (77). Finally, the potency of the PCBs is factored in (box N) using a potency value smaller than the largest given in Table 2.

The assumptions in this analysis are obviously quite conservative, but the point of introducing this example has to do with the computational construct rather than the numerical inputs. The LACF construct in the model displayed in Fig. 1 obviously simplifies the model materially. Use of this model, for example, does not require the explicit specification of human activity patterns (i.e., determination of contact frequencies) or of surface depletion mechanisms (e.g., volatilization, adsorption into interior surfaces, photolysis if exposed to sunlight). But it also leaves the analyst in a quandry when it comes to estimation of the LACF. Spend a few minutes trying to estimate your LACF for the room in which you are seated as you read this. Surely, at some time in your life, you *could* come into contact with every portion of the wall or ceiling, even those that are nominally "masked"—knocking about to retrieve your favorite pipe that fell behind the couch, replacing the ceiling light fixture, spring cleaning, mopping up a spill under the refrigerator, rehanging pictures, or painting. Nonetheless, as a practical matter, only a small portion of the room's surface area is likely to be touched with any frequency. Although the LACF concept simplifies the problem numerically, it only masks the real complexity of the physical situation being studied. The model permits the risk analyst to "doodle" and conduct a fortiori (but even if) analysis, but in the end this formulation lacks utility. Moreover, such an ambiguous construct invites a subjective rather than reasoned response. It is somewhat surprising that EPA chose a value as "low" as 0.25.

This example illustrates the linkage between the complexity of the calculated approach and that of preparing inputs. The simplistic construct depicted in Fig. 1 removes computational complexity at the expense of realism and ease of determining inputs. A balance must be struck among competing objectives, such as simplicity, realism, and availability of data, if a useful and credible risk estimate is to be produced.

6   Provide Clear Guidance to Interested Parties

If the risk anslysis community needs to emphasize realism in analysis, the users of analysis (policymakers and public) also need to understand the issue to interpret properly the results of analysis. This places a burden on the analyst to communicate clearly. As the example below shows, this is difficult.

As noted, the FDA undertook a risk analysis in support of its decision to revise the tolerance level for PCB-contaminated fish downward from 5 ppm to 2 ppm. A critique of this analysis highlighted points of conservatism and concluded that the FDA analysis was likely to have overstated risks by orders of magnitude (78). Although the FDA did not quantify the possible magnitude of overstatement of risks, it was open in acknowledging the uncertainties and the judgmentally conservative character of its resolution. For example, in the background to its 1979 ruling (79), the FDA stated the following:

> Hence, in deciding the appropriate levels for PCB tolerances under section 406, FDA *had to make some extraordinarily difficult judgments.* It has had to decide, in effect, where the proper balance lies between providing an adequate degree of public health protection and avoiding excessive losses of food to American consumers. [emphasis added]

The FDA also noted that (80) "it [FDA] also must make that judgment on the basis of *data that are incomplete, or even in dispute, and that can easily lead reasonable people to different conclusions*" [emphasis added].

The FDA acknowledged uncertainties regarding the carcinogenicity of PCBs in humans (81):

> FDA considers the question of the carcinogenicity of the PCBs unresolved. For the purposes of this risk assessment on PCBs, however, the agency treated the various PCBs as though they were carcinogenic and it considers the carcinogenicity of PCBs to be a matter worthy of further serious inquiry.

Having thus dealt with this key question by assumption, the FDA risk analysis proceeded to incorporate other conservative assumptions. These, too, were explicitly acknowledged by the FDA (82):

> The risk assessment the agency made incorporated several conservative assumptions that were designed to avoid understatement of the human risk. *Thus, it is expected that the actual risk experienced by consumers of the 12 more heavily contaminated species covered by the risk assessment is less than that estimated.* Moreover, the average consumer, who eats fish from a variety of freshwater and marine sources, will actually experience a far lower level of PCB exposure and a correspondingly lower degree of risk than those whose fish consumption is concentrated among the more heavily contaminated (predominantly freshwater) species. [emphasis added]

This statement was echoed in the 1979 *Federal Register* notice (83):

> These risk assessment methods do not purport to quantify precisely the expected human risk, but *rather attempt to estimate in quantitative terms an upper limit on the risk to humans that can be expected from a given level of exposure* to a toxic substance, assuming humans are no more susceptible to the effects of the substance than are the most susceptible members of the animal species for which toxicity data are available. These risk assessments can be useful as a means of comparing risks at various exposure levels and illustrating the toxicological judgment that a reduction in exposure will reduce risk. *Because of all the problems inherent in extrapolating from animal data to the expected human experience, however the numbers produced by a risk assessment*

must be interpreted cautiously: They are estimates of upper limits on risk and, though potentially useful for comparative purposes, *cannot be said to quantify actual human risk* precisely. These assessments attempt to avoid underestimating human risk.... [emphasis added]

and again in this same FDA document (84):

As explained in the report (Ref. 45), *the utility of this risk assessment for evaluating actual risk to humans from exposure to PCBs is extremely limited*. This is due both to difficulties inherent in making such extrapolations from animals to humans and, perhaps more importantly in this instance, to gaps and uncertainties in the data available for this particular risk assessment. For example, the toxicity studies on which the risk assessment is based used commercial preparations of PCBs, which are chemically different from the PCB residues found in fish and which contain small amounts of highly toxic impurities (e.g., dibenzofurans) not known to be present in fish residues. Also, in making the exposure estimates required for the risk assessment, it was necessary to use existing data on the numerical distribution of PCB levels in fish and rely on the assumption that the effect of a given tolerance level is to remove from commerce all fish containing PCBs exceeding the tolerances. It is possible that neither the assumption nor the data precisely reflect what actually occurs.

For these reasons and others discussed in the report (Ref. 45), the risk assessment does not provide a basis for precise quantification of the amount of risk reduction accomplished by reducing the fish tolerance. [emphasis added]

Notwithstanding such a measured appraisal of the uncertainties that clouded the standard-setting process, this standard, once established, was viewed as absolute. After a 5-ppm (now 2-ppm) standard was established, regulators, particularly in states that adopted the FDA action limit as a state standard, often acted as though consumption of fish contaminated with 4.8 ppm was "safe" but consumption of even one fish with 5.1 ppm was "unsafe." Thus, disclaimers, caveats, and qualifiers may not be sufficient to help users understand the limitations of a risk analysis. Nonetheless, it is clear that the risk analysis community needs to communicate more effectively.

Two approaches may have merit in this connection:

1. The first is what might be termed the "comparative risk" approach popularized by Crouch and Wilson (85), Ames et al. (86), and others. This approach presents estimated risks in the context of other related and everyday risks. The objective is to provide a frame of reference to help interpret the risk estimates. In my experience the comparative risk analysis is useful, but limited. The work of Slovic (87) demonstrates that public perceptions of risk are often different from that of "experts."
2. The second idea is to portray uncertainty in quantitative terms, as is illustrated below.

7 Undertake Sensitivity Analyses

It is suggested above that attention be directed toward the development of most likely or expected risks. "Conservative" estimates can be placed in perspective by making replicate computations with alternative sets of assumptions. This serves to identify the sensitivity of the calculated result to the various assumptions—and thus identify key uncertainties—as well as to bracket potential risks so that the policymaker can make a more informed choice. Other formal tools of statistics can also be applied.

Regulatory agencies appear to be increasingly receptive to sensitivity analysis or the use of multiple assumption sets. For example, in 1980, in response to comments to the Water Quality Criteria Document that other dose–response models might be considered in addition to that specified in the criteria document, EPA seemed adamantly opposed to consideration of any alternative (88):

> Comment Summary: A general discussion of alternative models is given in some of the comments. Specific models recommended include: Logistic; Probit; Multi-Hit; Mantel and Bryan; Weibull; and Pharmacokinetic.

> (EPA) Response: The inclusion of several arbitrary models in order to get a range of risk estimates would add no additional scientific information while at the same time would create confusion and thereby undermine the utility of risk estimates. The model chosen by the Agency is regarded as giving a plausible upper limit to the risk.

In the intervening years EPA has become more flexible. The guidelines for carcinogen risk assessment (89) are somewhat less rigid, permitting the use of alternative models when a biological basis exists. The guidelines for exposure assessment are yet more flexible (90) and companion EPA documents (91, 92) actively encourage sensitivity analysis and probabilistic descriptions of exposure, but to date only a few exposure analyses have been prepared that address uncertainty in an explicit fashion (93, 94).

The analyses of Paustenbach et al. (93, 94) on health risks of ingestion of TCDD-contaminated soil show the pivotal role of soil ingestion rates in developing target cleanup rates. Knowledge of which inputs are important is essential to focus analytical attention and data-gathering efforts.

Sensitivity analysis is useful in two respects: first, because key inputs can be identified, and second, because sensitivity analysis can be used to display the possible range of uncertainty of final risk or exposure estimates. To accomplish the latter, sets of assumptions are bundled into scenarios and the risk/exposure associated with these scenarios is displayed to provide estimates of uncertainty. (Where sufficient information is available, Monte Carlo or "bootstrap" methods can be used to provide a probability distribution of risk.)

Although the above may be an obvious suggestion, analyses that focus on a single (generally "plausible upper bound") estimate are sufficiently common that risk ranging was again identified as an essential practice in a recent AAAS symposium (95).

But mere use of sensitivity, or risk-ranging analysis, of course, does not guarantee that any of the exposure scenarios will be realistic. For example, the Focused Feasibility Study of a PCB-contaminated site in the state of Washington (96) purported to provide alternative estimate of risk.

The analysis provided three risk estimates, described as follows (97):

> Conservative assumptions are traditionally used in a health risk assessment to ensure maximum protection of human health. Such worst-case analyses provide valuable information because they tend to estimate an absolute upper limit of risk; however, it is highly probable that the true risk is overestimated. Therefore, each exposure pathway was analyzed separately and additional cases were structured to provide mid-range and low-range risk estimates. The data used included sample results specific to the site, toxicity data from the scientific literature, and values for model variables (e.g., ingestion rates) from a number of sources. The selection of appropriate information for model parameters is subject to a degree of uncertainty, thereby retaining conservatism even in the low-range risk estimates.

It is hard to know exactly what is being said in the above paragraph. If even the low-range risk estimate is conservative, what is the utility of the ranging? In fact, each of the exposure

TABLE 8. How Conservative is Conservative

Assumption	Tetra-Tech Worst Case	Alternative	Remarks
PCB soil concentration (ppm)	2,000	100	2000 ppm was an isolated hot spot; over 90% of area had PCB concentration of 100 ppm
Surface soil depletion	Not assumed	2-year half-life	Depletion of surface layers by photolysis and volatilization likely; overall, this assumption reduced computed risks by a factor of about 2.7 compared to the "no depletion" case
Fraction absorbed	1.0	0.2	1.0 is likely to be high, even for PCB in foods; ingestion from soils is better estimated as 0.2
Age-specific ingestion rates mg/day (yr)			Tetra-Tech's assumptions are among the largest reported in the literature; alternative assumptions are much more consistent with the estimates given in Table 2 and more recent EPA guidance expressed in recent CERCLA endangerment assessment
0–1	5,000	50	
1–2	5,000	100	
2–6	10,000	100	
6–11	1,000	50	
11–18	1,000	0	
18–70	100	0	
Body weight adjustments	Comparable	Comparable	
Potency/g for 70-kg adult	2.43×10^{-3}	1.5×10^{-5}	Figure at far left is based on potency of $4.34 (mg/kg \cdot day)^{-1}$ used by EPA in some cases; alternative is based on report prepared for OTA
Computed lifetime risk	5.4×10^{-1}	3.7×10^{-9}	

scenarios was based on highly conservative assumptions. The calculated risks from ingestion of PCB-contaminated soils at this site were 5.4×10^{-1}, 5.4×10^{-3}, and 1.8×10^{-6} for the three cases. Table 8 contrasts the worst-case calculation with what is a more likely description of actual exposure and risk. As shown, even the low-range risk estimate is likely to overstate the actual risks by three orders of magnitude.

A second example of the use of multiple exposure scenarios was prepared in connection with an Endangerment Assessment of the Picillo Site in Coventry, Rhode Island (98). A portion of this site (the "PCB pile") contained PCBs in varying concentrations from beneath detectability to 180 ppm, with an average level of 36.8 ppm. The generic exposure scenario assumed that skin contact with PCBs by teenagers and young adults was the principal route of exposure. Two specific exposure scenarios were considered a "most likely" and a "realistic worst case." The realistic worst case assumed a young male between the ages of 10 and 16 would break through the perimeter fencing and have contact with the PCB-contaminated soil 10 days/yr over a 6-year period. The amount of soil contacted per day in the realistic worst case was set at 10 g, using estimates by Kimbrough (99). It was further assumed that, in each and every contact, the portion of the pile having the greatest PCB level (180 ppm) was encountered. Bioavailability for skin contact was assumed to equal 1% for the most likely case and 5% in the realistic worst case. Other assumptions included potency and weight of humans.

Although several assumptions of this realistic worst case can be called to question, three are particularly worthy of note:

1. The assumption of 10 g/day contact attributed to Kimbrough was specified in Kimbrough's original work to apply to children in the age group from 1.5 to 3.5 years old, and not to teenagers. The contact rate applicable to children between 10 and 16 years of age would be 0.1 g/day. [Kimbrough, in another memorandum (100), considers soil contact rates as high as 10 g but concluded that each exposure to PCB-contaminated soil at concentrations of 50 ppm does not involve an unreasonable health risk.]
2. Some 92 samples were taken from the PCB pile, of which only 2 had concentrations of as much as 180 ppm. The assumption that each contact is with the most contaminated portion of the pile cannot be excluded. Nonetheless, if the youths were to contact portions of the pile at random, the probability that all 60 contacts would involve the most contaminated portion of the pile can be calculated as $(2/92)^{60}$, a number vanishingly small.
3. The bioavailability estimate for both the most likely and the realistic worst-case scenarios is too high. As noted by Paustenbach (101) in a critique of a CDC analysis of TCDD-contaminated soil (similar bioavailabilities should obtain for PCBs):

> CDC assumed that dirt would remain on the hand for a period long enough to bring about 1% absorption (Poiger and Schlatter, 1980)—the percentage absorption determined in rates exposed for 24 hours. A 24-hour duration is almost certainly longer than what is likely for humans under normal conditions. Secondly, human skin has generally been shown for a diverse class of chemicals to be less permeable to xenobiotics than the skin of rabbits and rats (Bartek and LaBudde, 1975; Wester and Noonan, 1980).

and later in this same paper (102):

> Poiger and Schlatter (1980) have conducted the only published study on dermal bioavailability. They dosed rats dermally with laboratory contaminated soil and observed that as the dose increased, the liver concentration of TCDD increased from 0.05 to 2.2%. The authors did not estimate a value for dermal bioavailability. On the basis of this study, Kimbrough and co-workers estimated a dermal bioavailability of 1% for humans (Kimbrough et al., 1980). The use of a 1% dermal bioavailability almost certainly overestimates the likely uptake by humans since rodent skin is often 3–10 times more permeable than human skin and the bioavailability of dioxin in soil appears to get smaller with decreasing concentration.

For these and other reasons it is difficult to justify the phrase "realistic worst case" to describe this exposure scenario.

So "risk ranging" provides no guarantee of realism, but it can be helpful, nonetheless. As William D. Ruckleshaus noted (103), when discussing the *first* of several principles for more reasonable discussion about risk:

> First, we must insist on risk calculations being expressed as distributions of estimates and not as magic numbers that can be manipulated without regard to what they really mean. We must try to display more realistic estimates of risk to show a range of probabilities. To help do this we need new tools for quantifying and ordering sources of uncertainty and for putting them in perspective.

CONCLUDING COMMENTS

In most lines of scientific inquiry, observation and experiment act as the ultimate "reality check." Over time, theories and predictions can be tested and, if found wanting, improved. But in the area of computation of exposure and human health risks, predictions are exceedingly difficult to verify, because the estimated probabilities are low by design. For example, the sample size for a simple comparative test of proportions to distinguish between a 20–25% chance of dying from cancer (the current U.S. average) and an alternative hypothesis that these are 10^{-6} higher would exceed the present population of the world.

For this reason, particular attention has to be paid to other, less direct means to help ensure realistic estimates. The ideas ventured here are all steps in the right direction — these are certainly not unique and may not even be the best ideas. But some steps need to be taken if more realistic models are to evolve.

Perhaps most important, it is necessary to change our *attitude* toward conservatism in risk analysis. Historically, the utility of conservative assumptions was taken to be almost self-evident: this approach demonstrated a serious concern for human health and was "above reproach." Now it is becoming clear that there is a dark side to conservatism — the potential misallocation of regulatory attention. In the end, there is little justification for pretending that things are different from the way they really are. If regulatory priorities are to be set wisely, they must be based on realistic estimates.

With respect to PCBs in particular, this chapter shows the many conservative assumptions that enter a typical risk analysis. Assumptions that all PCBs are as toxic as Aroclor 1260, conservative choices for dose-response models and species-to-human scaling factors, choice of the animal experiment that yields the highest potency, calculation of statistical upper bounds on dose-response slopes, treating all tumors as malignant, using high estimates of bioavailability, and other conservative choices for an exposure scenario (e.g., the largest soil ingestion rates, eating uncooked fish, contaminated water the sole source, neglect of environmental depletion) may be arguable individually, but collectively they are so implausible as to remove all meaning from the word *plausible* in the offen-used phrase "plausible upper-bound risk."

REFERENCES

1. *Polychlorinated Biphenyls*, NRCC No. 16077, ISNN 0316-0114. (National Research Council, Canada, 1978).

2. *Polychlorinated Biphenyls*. National Research Council, National Academy of Sciences, Washington, DC, 1979.

3. O. Hutzinger, S. Safe, and V. Zitko, *The Chemistry of PCBs*. CRC Press, Boca Raton, FL, 1980.

4. C. G. Whipple, Dealing with uncertainty about risk in risk management. 46.

5. R. Wilson and E. A. C. Crouch, Risk assessment and comparisons: An introduction. *Science* **236**, 267 (1987).

6. R. C. Barnard, Science, policy, and the law: A developing partnership in reducing the risk of cancer. *Reducing the Carcinogenic Risks in Industry.* Dekker, New York, 1986. pp. 216–242.

7. *Criteria for a Recommended Standard...Occupational Exposure to Polychlorinated Biphenyls (PCBs).* U.S. Department of Health, Education, and Welfare, NIOSH, 1977.

8. K. S. Crump and M. D. Masterman, *Assessment of Carcinogenic Risks from PCBs in Food.* Prepared for United States Congress, Office of Technology Assessment, April 1979.

9. D. W. Gaylor. The use of safety factors for controlling risk. *J. Toxicol. Environ. Health* **11**, 329–336 (1983).

10. L. D. Maxim and L. Harrington, A review of the Food and Drug Administration risk analysis for polychlorinated biphenyls in fish. *Regul. Toxicol. Pharmacol.* **4**(2), 192–219 (1984).

11. D. J. Paustenbach, H. J. Clewell, III, M. L. Gargas, and M. E. Andersen, *Development of Physiologically-Based Pharmacokinetic Model for Multiday Inhalation of Carbon Tetrachloride.* Presented at the National Academy of Sciences Workshop on Pharmacokinetics in Risk Assessment, Washington, DC, October 7–9, 1986.

12. A. L. Nichols, and R. J. Zeckhauser, The dangers of caution: Conservatism in assessment and the mismanagement of risk. In V. Kerry Smith, Ed., *Advances in Applied Micro-Economics* **4**, 55–82 (1986).

13. F. Cordle, R. Locke, and J. Springer, Risk assessment in a federal regulatory agency: An assessment of risk associated with the human consumption of some species of fish contaminated with PCB's. *Environ. Health Perspect.* **45**, 177–182 (1982).

14. U.S. Environmental Protection Agency, *Risk Assessment and Management: Framework for Decision Making*, EPA 600/9-85-002, USEPA. Washington, DC, 1984.

15. U.S. Public Health Service, ATSDR *Draft Toxicological Profile for Selected PCB (Aroclor − 1260, − 1254, − 1248, − 1242, − 1232, − 1221, and − 1016)* (1987).

16. National Cancer Institute, *Bioassay of Aroclor 1254 for Possible Carcinogenicity*, NCI Carcinogenesis Technical Report, Series No. 38, CAS No. 27323-18-8, NCl-CG-TR-38 (1978).

17. K. S. Crump, and M. D. Masterman, *Assessment of Carcinogenic Risk from PCBs in Food.* Prepared for United States Congress, Office of Technology Assessment, 1979, p. 24.

18. R. D. Kimbrough et al., 'Induction of liver tumors in Sherman strain female rats by polychlorinated biphenyls Aroclor 1260. *Journal National Cancer Institute* **55**, 1453 et seq. (1975).

19. D. H. Norback, and R. H. Weltman, Polychlorinated biphenyl induction of hepatocellular carcinoma in the Sprague-Dawley rat. *Environ. Health Perspect.* **60**, 97–105 (1985).

20. N. Ito, et al., Histopathologic studies on liver tumorigenesis induced in mice by technical polychlorinated biphenyls and its promoting effect on liver tumors induced by benzene Hexachloride. *Journal National Cancer Institute* **51**, 1637 et seq. (1973).

21. E. Schaeffer, et al., Pathology of chronic polychlorinated biphenyls (PCB) feeding in rats. *Toxicology and Applied Pharmacology* **75**, 278–288 (1984).

22. D. Barltrop, *Sources and Significance of Environmental Lead for Children*, Proc. Int. Symp. Envrion. Health Aspects of Lead. Commission of European Communities. Center for Information and Documentation, Luxembourg, 1973.

23. M. J. Duggan and S. Williams, Lead-in-dust in city streets. *Sci. Total Environ.* **7**, 91–97 (1977).

24. M. L. Lepow, L. Bruckman, R. A. Rubino, S. Markowitz, M. Gillette, and J. Kapish, Role of airborne lead in increased body burden of lead in Hartford children. *Environ. Health Perspect.* **7**, 99–102 (1974).

25. M. L. Lepow, L. Bruckman, R. A. Rubino, S. Markowitz, M. Gillette, and J. Kapish, Investigations into sources of lead in the environment of urban children. *Environ. Res.* **10**, 415–426 (1975).

26. J. P. Day, M. Hart, and M. S. Robinson, Lead in urban street dust. **Nature (London) 253**, 343–345 (1975).

27. K. R. Mahaffey, Quantities of lead producing health effects in humans: Sources and bioavailability. *Environ. Health Perspect.* **19**, 285–295 (1977).

28. Clement Associates, Inc., *Endangerment Assessment for the Smuggler Mountain Site, Pitkin Country, Colorado*, Contract 68-01-6939, Work Assignment No. 49-8L41. Prepared for

the U.S. Environmental Protection Agency, Region VIII, Montana Office, Helena Mountain, May 5, 1986.

29. U.S. Environmental Protection Agency, *Air Quality Criteria for Lead*, EPA 600/8-83-028A, II, USEPA, Washington, DC, 1983.

30. J. L. Schaum, *Risk Analysis of TCDD Contaminated Soil*, EPA 600/8-84-031, 29. Office of Health and Environmental Assessment, USEPA, Washington, DC, 1984.

31. R. D. Kimbrough, H. Falk, P. Stehr, and G. Fries, Health implications of 2,3,7,8-tetrachlorodibenzodioxin (TCDD) contamination of residential soil. *J. Toxicol. Environ. Health* **14**, 47–93 (1984).

32. J. K. Hawley, Assessment of health risk from exposure to contaminated soil. *Risk Anal.* **5**, 289–302 (1985).

33. S. Binder, D. Sokal, and D. Maughan, *Estimating the Amount of Soil Ingested by Young Children Through Tracer Elements* (draft report). Centers for Disease Control, Atlanta, GA, 1985.

34. R. A. Dime, *PCB Cleanup Levels*, memorandum to Dr. J. H. Berkowitz, Administrator. Hazardous Site Mitigation Administration, State of New Jersey, Department of Environmental Protection, March 7, 1985.

35. *Superfund Health Assessment Manual* (draft). Submitted to the Office Emergency and Remedial Response, U.S. Environmental Protection Agency, produced by ICF, Inc., under EPA Contract 68-01-6872. USEPA, Washington, DC, 1986.

36. Clement Associates, Inc., *Endangerment Assessment for the Smuggler Mountain Site, Pitkin County, Colorado*, Contract 68-01-6939, Work Assignment No. 49-8L41. Prepared for the U.S. Environmental Protection Agency, Region VIII, Montana Office, Helena Mountain, May 5, 1986.

37. D. J. Paustenbach, H P. Shu, and F. J. Murray, A critical examination of assumptions used in risk analysis of dioxin contaminated soil. *Regul. Toxicol. Pharmacol.* **6**, 284–307 (1986).

38. Executive Office of the President, *Regulatory Program of the United States Government*. Office of Management and Budget, Washington, DC, 1986–1987, p. xxiv.

39. C. G. Whipple, Dealing with uncertainty about risk in risk management. 50.

40. W. D. Ruckelshaus (former EPA Administrator), Risk in a free society. *Risk Anal.* **4**(3), 157 et seq. (1984).

41. K. Ahmed (Research Director for the Natural Resources Defense Council), as quoted by B. Barker, Cancer and the problems of risk assessment. *EPRI J.*   , 30 (1984).

42. Executive Office of the President, *Regulatory Program of the United States Government*. Office of Management and Budget, Washington, DC, 1986–1987, pp. xxv et seq.

43. D. R. Patrick (EPA), Environmental Protection Agency's risk management policy. *Environ. Progr.* **4**(1), 20–22 (1985).

44. A. Fisher (EPA), *Using Risk Assessment in Policy Decisions* (draft EPA doc.). USEPA, Washington, DC, 1986, pp. 13–14.

45. U.S. Environmental Protection Agency, *Risk Assessment: Framework for Decision Making*, EPA 600/9-85-002, 16, USEPA, Washington, DC, 1984.

46. Midwest Research Institute, *Risk Assessment Methodology for Hazardous Waste Management* (draft final report). Prepared for EPA under Contract No. EQ4C15, 1–2. MRI, 1986.

47. H. Raiffa, Science and policy: Their separation and integration in risk analysis. In H. C. Kunreuther and E. V. Ley, Eds., *The Risk Analysis Controversy: An Institutional Perspective*. Springer-Verlag, Berlin and New York, 1982. pp. 32–33.

48. R. C. Barnard, Science, policy, and the law: A developing partnership in reducing the risk of cancer. *Reducing the Carcinogenic Risks in Industry*. Dekker, New York, 1986, p. 222.

49. A. L. Nichols, and R. J. Zeckhauser, The dangers of caution: Conservatism in assessment

and the mismanagement of risk. In V. Kerry Smith, Ed., *Advances in Applied Micro-Economics* **4**, 55–82 (1986).

50. Executive Office of the President, *Regulatory Program of the United States Government*. Office of Management and Budget, Washington, DC, 1986–1987, p. xiii.

51. Executive Office of the President, *Regulatory Program of the United States Government*. Office of Management and Budget, Washington, DC, 1986–1987, pp. xxv et seq.

52. Executive Office of the President, *Regulatory Program of the United States Government*, Office of Management and Budget, Washington, DC, 1986–1987, p. xxiii.

53. CH$_2$M Hill, Ecology and Environment, *Final Remedial Investigation Report, Northside Sanitary Landfill, Indiana*, WA95.5LH2.0, Contract No. 68-01-6692, 6–29. E&E, 1986.

54. R. O. Gilbert, *Statistical Methods for Environmental Pollution Monitoring*. Von Nostrand Reinhold, New York, 1987.

55. Executive Office of the President, *Regulatory Program of the United States Government*. Office of Management and Budget, Washington, DC, 1986–1987, pp. xxiv et seq.

56. N. K. Kim and J. Hawley, *Re-entry Guidelines: Binghamton State Office Building*. Bureau of Toxic Substance Assessment, Division of Environmental Health Assessment, New York State Department of Health, Albany, NY, 1985.

57. N. Gravitz et al., *Interim Guidelines for Acceptable Exposure Levels in Office Settings Contaminated with PCB and PCB-Combustion Products*. Epidemiological Studies Section, California Department of Health Services, Berkeley, 1983.

58. R. E. Hall, The importance of lifetime jobs in the U.S. economy. *Am. Econ. Rev.* **72**(4), 720 (1982).

59. Dr. Francis Horvath, Personal communication, Bureau of Labor Statistics, Washington, DC, 1986.

60. R. E. Hall, The importance of lifetime jobs in the U.S. Economy. *Am. Econ. Rev.* **72**(4), 716 et seq. (1982).

61. F. W. Horvath, Job tenure of workers in January 1981. *Job Tenure and Occupational Change, 1981*, Bull. No. 2162. U.S. Department of Labor, Bureau of Labor Statistics, Washington, DC, 1983.

62. A. T. Pennington, Revision of the total diet study food list and diets. *Journal of the American Dietetic Association* **82**(2), (1983). See also *Health Assessment Document for Beryllium (Review draft)*. U.S. Environmental Protection Agency, Washington, DC, PB 86-183944, 1986.

63. EPA may change assumptions to reduce overestimates of risk, official tells AAAS, *Chemical Regulation Reporter*, 1806 (1988).

64. R. D. Kimbrough, H. Falk, P. Stehr, and G. Fries, Health implications of 2, 3, 7, 8-tetrachlorodibenzodioxin (TCDD) contamination of residential soil. *J. Toxicol. Environ. Health* **14**, 47–93 (1984).

65. N. K. Kim and J. Hawley, *Re-entry Guidelines: Binghamton State Office Building*. Bureau of Toxic Substance Assessment, Division of Environmental Health Assessment, New York State Department of Health, Albany, NY, 1985.

66. J. L. Schaum, *Risk Analysis of TCDD Contaminated Soil*, EPA 600/8-84-031, II et seq. Office of Health and Environmental Assessment, USEPA, Washington, DC, 1984.

67. CH$_2$M Hill, Ecology and Environment, *Final Remedial Investigation Report, Northside Sanitary Landfill, Indiana*, WA95.5LH2.0, Contract No. 68-01-6692, 6–58, E&E, 1986.

68. Exposure Assessment Group, *Estimating Exposures to 2, 3, 7, 8-TCDD*, USEPA, Washington, DC, 1987, pp. iv-29 and 1–7.

69. A. M. Finkel, and J. S. Evans, Evaluating the benefits of uncertainty reduction in environmental health risk management. *JAPCA* **37**, 1164–1171 (1987).

70. *Federal Register*, **49**, No. 100, 21514 (1984).
71. *Federal Register*, **42**, No. 63, 17491–17492 (1977).
72. *Federal Register*, **44**, No. 127, 38331 (1979).
73. *Federal Register*, **44**, No. 127, 38337 (1979).
74. N. K. Kim and J. Hawley, *Re-entry Guidelines: Binghamton State Office Building*. Bureau of Toxic Substance Assessment, Division of Environmental Health Assessment, New York State Department of Health, Albany, NY, 1985, pp. 6 et seq.
75. K. A. Hammerstrom, Memorandum, Exposure Assessment Branch, to Jane Kim, Chemical Regulation Branch, USEPA, subject: Cleanup of PCB Levels Located Indoors. USEPA, Washington, DC, 1986.
76. R. C. Webster, D. A. W. Bucks, H. I. Maibach, and J. Anderson, Polychlorinated biphenyls (PCBs): Dermal absorption, systemic elimination, and dermal wash efficiency. *J. Toxicol. Environ. Health* **12**, 511–519 (1983).
76. R. C. Webster, D. A. W. Bucks, H. I. Maibach, and J. Anderson, Polychlorinated biphenyls (PCBs): Dermal absorption, systemic elimination, and dermal wash efficiency. *J. Toxicol. Environ. Health* **12**, 511–519 (1983).
77. J. K. Hawley, Assessment of health risk from exposure to contaminated soil. *Risk Anal.* **5**, 289–302 (1985).
78. L. D. Maxim and L. Harrington, A review of the Food and Drug Administration risk analysis for polychlorinated biphenyls in fish. *Regul. Toxicol. Pharmacol.* **4**(2), 192–219 (1984).
79. *Federal Register*, **44**, No. 127, 38330 et seq. (1979).
80. *Federal Register*, **44**, No. 127, 38331 et seq. (1979).
81. *Federal Register*, **44**, No. 127, 38338 et seq. (1979).
82. *Federal Register*, **44**, No, 127, 38334 et seq. (1979).
83. *Federal Register*, **44**, No. 127, 38332 et seq. (1979).
84. *Federal Register*, **44**, No. 127, 38333 et seq. (1979).
85. E. A. C. Crouch and R. Wilson, *Risk/Benefit Analysis*, Ballinger, Cambridge, MA, 1982, pp. 165 et seq.
86. B. N. Ames, R. Magaw, and L. S. Gold, Ranking possible carcinogenic risks. *Science* **236**, 271–280 (1987).
87. P. Slovic, Perception of risk. *Science* **236**, 280–285 (1987).
88. *Federal Register*, **45**, No. 231, 79376 (1980).
89. *Federal Register*, **49**, 46294 et seq. (1984).
90. *Federal Register*, **49**, 46304 (1984).
91. A. L. Nichols et al., *The value of Acquiring Information Under Section 8(a) of TSCA: A Decision Theoretic Approach*. Harvard University, Cambridge, MA, 1983.
92. R. W. Whitmore, *Methodology for Characterizing Uncertainty in Exposure Assessments*. Research Triangle Institute, Research Triangle Park, NC, 1984.
93. D. J. Paustenbach, Assessing the potential environmental and human health risks of contaminated soil. *Comments Toxicol.* (1987).
94. D. J. Paustenbach, H. J. Clewell, III, M. L. Gargas, and M. E. Andersen, *Development of Physiologically-Based Pharmacokinetic Model for Multiday Inhalation of Carbon Tetrachloride*. Presented at the National Academy of Sciences Workshop on Pharmacokinetics in Risk Assessment, Washington, DC, October 7–9, 1986; D. J. Paustenbach, H. P. Shu, and F. J. Murray, A critical examination of assumption used in risk analysis of dioxin contaminated soil. *Regul. Toxicol. Pharmacol.* **6**, 284–307 (1986).
95. N. K. Kim and J. Hawley, *Re-entry Guidelines: Binghamton State Office Building*. Bureau of Toxic Substance Assessment, Division of Environmental Health Assessment, New York State Department of Health, Albany, NY, 1985.

96. Tetra Tech, Inc., *Strandley Scrap Metal/Manning Property Focused Feasibility Study*, TC 3075. Prepared for Seattle City Lights, Seattle, WA, July 1985.

97. Tetra Tech, Inc., *Strandley Scrap Metal/Manning Property Focused Feasibility Study*, TC 3075. Prepared for Seattle City Lights, Seattle, WA, July 1985.

98. *Endangerment Assessment and Feasibility Study, Picillo Site, Coventry, Rhode Island* (draft final report), Vol. 1. Contract No. 68-01-6769. Prepared by GCA Corporation, Bedford, MA, for U.S. Environmental Protection Agency, Office of Waste Program Enforcement, Washington, DC, April 1985.

99. R. D. Kimbrough, H. Falk, P. Stehr, and G. Fries, Health implications of 2, 3, 7, 8-tetrachlorodibenzodioxin (TCDD) contamination of residential soil, *J. Toxicol. Environ. Health* **14**, 47–93 (1984).

100. R. Kimbrough, Memorandum to Ms. Georgi Jones, Chief, Superfund Implementation Group, Subject: Request from L. Fabinski, EPA Region V, LaSalle Electrical Utilities in Illinois Residential Sample Review, March 5, 1985.

101. D. J. Paustenbach, H. P. Shu, and F. J. Murray, A criticial examination of assumptions used in risk analysis of dioxin contaminated soil. *Regul. Toxicol. Pharmacol.* **6**, 291 (1986).

102. W. D. Ruckleshaus, Risk in a free society. *Risk Anal.* **4**(3), 161 (1984).

15

Risk Analyses of Buried Wastes from Electricity Generation*

Bernard L. Cohen

Department of Physics, University of Pittsburgh, Pittsburgh, Pennsylvania

1 INTRODUCTION

The straightforward way to do a probabilistic risk analysis (PRA) is to identify all possible sequences of events that can lead to deaths among the public (or to some other targeted endpoint), estimate the probability for each event, multiply these probabilities for all events in a sequence to determine the total probability for that sequence, and finally add up the probabilities for all sequences. Interdependencies of events (common mode failures) must be taken into account, which can add greatly to the complication and uncertainty (1). Such a PRA involves development of a large program run on a digital computer.

This type of PRA has been carried out for systems like aircraft and nuclear power plants where there is complete knowledge of construction details and failure-rate experience with every component. But even in these cases, many approximations must be made, and uncertainties are quite large. If one were to apply this technique to wastes buried in the ground, the difficulties would be enormously greater because knowledge of the system is much less complete and is changing with time. Geochemistry is a much more complex subject than mechanical or electrical design of machines, and it is sensitive to a number of factors on which there is limited information.

An alternative approach is to replace the digital computer with an analog computer. Constructing such an analog computer would be a tremendous project, and it would be enormously expensive. However, that analog computer is now available, and we are all free to use it. It is our earth itself.

This chapter describes how such an approach can be used. For example, to study how waste converted into rock behaves, how ordinary rock behaves will be reviewed. Several cases of this type directed at the analysis of wastes generated by nuclear and by coal-burning power plants are presented.

*Portions of this chapter have been published previously in *American Journal of Physics*, Vol. 54, p. 38 (1986). Copyright © 1986 by the American Association of Physics Teachers.

2   NUCLEAR HIGH-LEVEL WASTE (HLW)

High-level waste (HLW) is the residue of spent nuclear fuel after it has been removed from reactors. One plan for its disposal is to convert it into a rocklike material and bury it in the natural habitat of rocks, about 600 m underground.

It is generally agreed that the principal concern is that buried HLW will be contacted by groundwater, dissolved, transported to the surface, and thereby get into our food and water supplies. We are therefore concerned with the health effects, principally the cancer risk, of this material entering human stomachs. The potential risks associated with this hazard are presented in Fig. 1; the following discussion reviews its derivation.

2.1   Risk if Material Enters Human Stomachs

Consider the risk of one particular type of cancer, liver cancer, from eating 1 millicurie (mCi)—3.7×10^7 radioactive decays per second—of one particular radioactive isotope, plutonium-239 (^{239}Pu). Ingested plutonium has a 10^{-4} probability for transmission through the walls of the gastrointestinal tract into the bloodstream; once in the blood it has a 45% chance of becoming deposited in the liver (1a). Thus, 0.45×10^{-4} or 45×10^{-6} mCi gets into the liver where it remains for an average of 40 years (1a). The number of alpha (α) particles emitted into the liver is then $(45 \times 10^{-6} \text{ mCi}) \times (3.7 \times 10^7 \text{ } \alpha/\text{s·mCi}) \times (3 \times 10^7 \text{ s/yr}) \times (40 \text{ yr}) = 2 \times 10^{12}$. Since the alpha particle energy is 4.8 MeV, the radiation energy absorbed by the liver is $(2 \times 10^{12}) \times (4.8) \times (1.6 \times 10^{-13} \text{ J/MeV}) = 1.5 \text{ J}$.

Radiation dose in rads is defined as 0.01 J of radiation energy deposited per kg of body

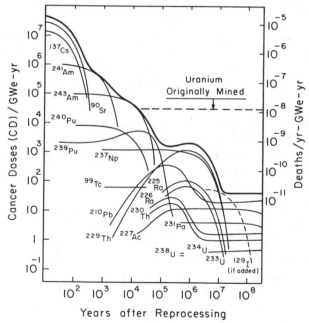

Figure 1. Cancer doses and predicted deaths per year vs. years after reprocessing of high-level radioactive waste.

organ. Since the average weight of a human liver (2) is 1.8 kg, the dose to the liver from eating 1 mCi of ^{239}Pu is $(1.5 \text{ J}/1.8 \text{ kg}) \times (1 \text{ rad}/0.01 \text{ J/kg}) = 80 \text{ rads}$.

Estimating the cancer risk from a given radiation dose is principally the realm of the National Academy of Science's Committee on Biological Effects of Ionizing Radiation (BEIR) and the United Nations Scientific Committee on Effects of Atomic Radiation (UNSCEAR).

The latest BEIR (3) and UNSCEAR (4) reports estimate the cancer risk due to alpha particle bombardment of liver principally from studies of German, Japanese, Danish, and Portugese patients injected with colloidal thorium dioxide as an x-ray contrast medium: there were 301 liver cancers versus only six normally expected among them. These studies derive a risk of 300×10^{-6} per rad. Applying this to our calculation, we find the liver cancer risk to be $(80 \times 300 \times 10^{-6}) = 0.024$ per mCi of ^{239}Pu ingested.

However, ingested plutonium may also get into the bone and cause bone cancer or into the bone marrow and cause leukemia; calculations similar to the above give these risks to be 0.011 and 0.0006/mCi, respectively (5). In addition, the 99.99% of the ^{239}Pu that does not get through the gastrointestinal tract spends about 24 h radiating its inner walls before it is excreted, thereby causing (5) an intestinal cancer risk of 0.002. Summing the results for all types of cancer gives the risk as $(0.024 + 0.011 + 0.0006 + 0.002) = 0.038/\text{mCi}$ of ^{239}Pu ingested.

If the ingestion of 1 mCi is shared among N people, each will have an average risk of $0.038/N$, making the risk of a cancer within the group $(N \times 0.038/N) = 0.038$. Thus, the number of cancers caused by ingestion of 1 mCi of ^{239}Pu is independent of N, the number of people among whom it is shared. This is a consequence of the linear, no-threshold dose–response relation used for estimating radiation risk.

The radioactive waste produced by a 1-GW ($= 1,000,000 \text{ kW}$) output electric power plant in 1 year (1 GWe-yr), after reprocessing, contains $6 \times 10^4 \text{ mCi}$ of ^{239}Pu. Thus, if all

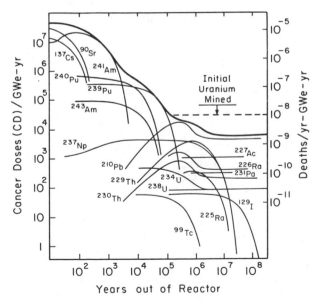

Figure 2. Cancer doses and predicted deaths per year vs. years after the high-level wastes leave the reactor.

the ^{239}Pu in 1 GWe-yr of this HLW were fed to people, we could expect $(6 \times 10^4) \times (0.038)$ = 2300 fatal cancers. We refer to this as the number of cancer doses (CD)/GWe-yr.

This result is shown on the curve labeled ^{239}Pu in Fig. 1, which is a plot of CD versus time after removal from the reactor (5). We see that it increases in the first 20,000 years as ^{243}Am decays into ^{239}Pu, but after that time it decreases due to the 24,000-year half-life of ^{239}Pu.

Of course, ^{239}Pu is not the only radioactive species in the HLW. Results of similar treatments for all other important species are also shown in Fig. 1, and they are summed to obtain the heavy curve. Its initial value of 4×10^7 means that if all the waste from 1 GWe-yr were fed to people after 10 years, we could expect 40 million cancers; on the other hand, if this feeding were delayed for 100,000 years, there would be only 1300.

If the waste is not reprocessed, but rather is buried as spent fuel, the corresponding results are shown in Fig. 2. We see that the effects in the early years are little changed, but after 100,000 years the toxicity is 30 times higher.

2.2   Probability/Year of Transfer from Rock into Groundwater

Now that we know the toxicity of the waste, the remaining problem is to estimate the probability versus time for an atom of buried waste to be dissolved in groundwater, carried with the latter back toward the surface, and eventually to reach a human stomach. Since the waste is in the form of a rock, it seems reasonable to assume that it will behave somewhat like a normal rock—we consider the validity of this assumption later. We proceed by calculating the release probability for an atom of average rock 600 m underground, which is a typical burial depth planned for the waste.

From the rate at which rivers carry dissolved and suspended material into the oceans, it is straightforward to calculate that the surface of the United States is eroding away at an average rate of 4.5×10^{-5} m/yr (6), or 1 m/22,000 yr. About 28% of this is in solution (6) (the rest is suspended particles), about 15% of the water flow in rivers is derived from groundwater (7, 8) (the rest is from surface runoff), and groundwater contains about twice the solute concentration of river water (9). Applying these corrections leads to the conclusion that groundwater dissolves and removes a total of $(4.5 \times 10^{-5}) \times (0.28) \times (0.15) \times (2) = 3.8 \times 10^{-6}$ m/yr.

We next seek the fraction of this total that is derived from 1 m of depth 600 m below ground level, that is, from between a depth of 599 and 600 m. If the groundwater flow were equal at all depths down to 600 m and zero below 600 m, this would be 1/600 of the total; but that is obviously an overestimate because there is some flow below 600 m and, more important, the flow between 599 and 600 m is much less than the average for the flow between 0 and 600 m. With an elaborate calculation (9) the flow between 599 and 600 m comes out 1/4000 of the total. Thus, $(3.6 \times 10^{-6}/4000) \approx 10^{-9}$ m/yr of depth is removed from between 599 and 600 m. This means that the average probability per year for an atom at this depth to be removed is 1.0×10^{-9}.

We now present an alternative derivation (10, 11) of this key result which is essentially completely independent of the above derivation.

A typical aquifer reaching to the waste burial depth of 600 m is about 100 km long and its flow velocity is about 100 m/yr. For a typical porosity of 10%, the water discharged from it annually per square meter of cross-sectional area is 10% of a volume 1 m² in cross section and 100 m long, or 10 m³. Chemical analyses of groundwater (6) indicate that it typically contains 30 mg/L of calcium so the 10^4 kg of water in this 10 m³ would carry 0.3 kg/m²·yr of calcium into the river it feeds. This is the first entry in column 2 of Table 1,

TABLE 1. Calculation of Fractional Removal per Year of Rock Materials by a Typical Aquifer

Element	Amount of Element $(kg/m^2 \cdot yr)$ Discharged with Water	Amount of Element (kg/m^2) in Rock ($\times 10^6$)	Fraction of Element Removed per year ($\times 10^{-8}$)
Ca	0.3	15	2
Mg	0.03	3	1
K	0.02	3	0.7
Fe	0.003	9	0.03
U	3×10^{-6}	8×10^{-4}	0.3
SiO_2	0.2	150	0.13
CO_3	1.5	18	8

and other entries in column 2 are obtained analogously. The volume of rock traversed by the aquifer is $10^5 \, m^3/m^2$, which weighs about $3 \times 10^8 \, kg/m^2$. Typical rock contains (10, 11) about 5% calcium, so the calcium content in the rock traversed by the aquifer is about (0.5) $\times (3 \times 10^8) = 15 \times 10^6 \, kg/m^2$. This is the first entry in column 3 of Table 1, and the other entries in that column are obtained analogously. If the rock contains $15 \times 10^6 \, kg/m^2$ of calcium, and $0.3 \, kg/m^2$ of calcium are removed each year, the fractional removal of calcium is $(0.3/15 \times 10^6) = 2 \times 10^{-8}$ per year. This is the first entry in column 4 of Table 1 and from this example we see that column 4 is obtained as column 2 ÷ column 3, which then allows us to determine the other entries in column 4.

From the results in column 4 it is apparent that for most elements the fractional removal per year is less than 10^{-8}. The elements most similar chemically to the important components in the waste are uranium and iron for which removal rates are much less than $10^{-8}/yr$, and the important waste components bear little chemical similarity to CO_3 ions, the only material removed at a rate appreciably higher than $10^{-8}/yr$.

We conclude that average rock, traversed by an aquifer, is removed at a rate somewhat less than $10^{-8}/yr$, perhaps something like $4 \times 10^{-9}/yr$. But only about one-fourth of all rock is traversed by an aquifer at a given time. Thus, average rock is removed at a rate of about $(\frac{1}{4}) \times (4 \times 10^{-9}) = 1 \times 10^{-9}$ per year. This is the same as the result obtained above by a very different method.

2.3   Probability for Transfer from Groundwater into Human Stomachs

To complete our exposure and risk estimates, we need the probability for an atom dissolved in groundwater, which would eventually discharge into a river, to enter a human stomach. The most important contribution to this probability is from the use of wells for potable water supplies. The total water flow in U.S. rivers (6) is $1.7 \times 10^{15} \, L/yr$ and the water flow in shallow aquifers is 16% of this (7), or $2.8 \times 10^{14} \, L/yr$. About 45% of the U.S. population (12), 1.05×10^8 people, ingest an average of 1.95 L/day (2) from these wells, a total of $(1.95) \times (365) \times (1.05 \times 10^8) = 7.4 \times 10^{10} \, L/yr$. The probability for a given atom dissolved in this water to be ingested is then $(7.5 \times 10^{10}/2.8 \times 10^{14}) = 2.6 \times 10^{-4}$. There are additional contributions from the use of rivers for potable water supplies, the eating of fish, and the use of rivers for irrigation, which bring the total probability to 4×10^{-4} (13).

2.4   Numbers of Deaths Expected

If the probability for an atom of rock to be transferred from rock at 600-m depth to a river is $1 \times 10^{-9}/yr$, and the probability that it will get into a human stomach from this process is 4×10^{-4}, the total probability per year for transfer from the rock into human stomachs is the product of these, or 4×10^{-13}/yr. An alternative independent derivation of this quantity has been developed (13), and it gives essentially the same result. We then apply this probability per year to the waste. Multiplying the ordinates in Figs. 1 and 2 by 4 $\times 10^{-13}$ only requires a shift in the ordinate scale, as shown by the scales on the right side of each of Figs. 1 and 2. This gives the deaths/yr·GWe-yr. To find the total number of eventual deaths, we must integrate these curves over time.

This raises the question of the time period over which integration is to be performed. For example, if it is the first million years, the result is 0.0026 and 0.021 deaths/GWe-yr from HLW and spent fuel, respectively. Another reasonable upper limit would be the time when the toxicity of the waste reaches that of the uranium originally mined because after that time, more lives would be saved by removal of the uranium (preventing it from entering human stomachs via groundwater release) than would be lost to the waste. That time is 14,000 years for HLW and 120,000 years for spent fuel, up to which the integrations yield 0.0018 and 0.014 deaths/GWe-yr, respectively. To carry the calculation beyond 1 million years requires a more complex treatment, taking into account the reducing depth of the waste as overlying material is eroded away, and assuming that when the material reaches the surface it becomes dissolved in rivers. The final results (9–11), are 0.006 and 0.021 deaths/GWe-yr for HLW and spent fuel, respectively, not including the effects of the uranium in the waste since that material was originally in the ground before it was mined out to produce reactor fuel.

2.5   Differences between Buried High-Level Waste and Average Rock

Before these results can be applied to HLW, however, we must take into account differences between buried waste and the average rock we have been discussing. There are basically three ways in which the waste is less secure than average rock:

1. To bury the waste, it is necessary to dig shafts down from the surface; this raises the possibility that these shafts may serve as entries for water or escape paths for the waste. The resolution of this problem depends on our ability to seal these shafts. The experts in that technology (of which I am not one) seems confident that they can seal the shafts to make them as secure as the original rock (14)—they often say more secure.

2. The radioactivity of the waste generates substantial amounts of heat, and there have been worries that this might crack the rock and thereby compromise the security of the waste. This problem has been extensively studied (15) and all indications are that rock fracture does not become a problem until temperatures reach 350°C. Since current designs for repositories limit temperatures to little more than 150°C, rock cracking seems not to be a problem. If more conservatism is desired, lower temperatures can be achieved either by spreading the waste over larger areas or by delaying burial. Heat generation declines by a factor of 10 after 100 years and by a factor of 100 after 200 years.

There are also concerns that if groundwater should contact the waste, the elevated temperature would accelerate its dissolution. However, present plans are to seal the waste in a leach-resistant casing (16) that virtually guarantees isolation from groundwater during the period of elevated temperatures.

3. Glass is thermodynamically less stable than other rocks and hence is more easily dissolved. Actually, however, the difference in dissolution rates found in tests is relatively small; the rate for waste glass is similar to that for basalt and is only about 10 times higher than that for the most durable rock materials (17). These data correlate well with thermodynamic expectations; the ratios are therefore expected to apply, at least roughly,

in a wide variety of conditions. Research on this matter is continuing, and if it is decided that glass is much less secure than average rock, other waste forms such as synroc, which chemically is effectively identical to average rock, are available.

It thus seems apparent that there are no very important ways in which buried waste is less secure than the average rock with which it is compared. On the other hand, there are several ways in which it is more secure:

1. The waste will be emplaced in a carefully selected rock formation, which is presumably more secure than the "average" location of our average rock.
2. The leach-resistant casing in which waste packages will be sealed gives a complete backup safety system that should prevent escape of the waste even if everything else goes wrong (16). This casing is obviously not available to average rock.
3. If waste should escape, the elevated radioactivity would easily be detected by routine monitoring of river and well water in plenty of time to avert health impacts.

Considering all the differences between the buried waste and the average rock with which it is compared, the former seems to be comparable in security to the latter.

2.6   Conclusions on the Burial of High-Level Wastes

Reprocessing of spent fuel involves removal of 99.5% of the uranium and plutonium for use as fuel in future reactors. It could be argued that it is unfair to consider reprocessed HLW because its burial still leaves the plutonium, which has to be disposed. Our treatment of spent fuel includes this plutonium. If nuclear power has a long-term future, it will be burned up in breeder reactors, making the spent fuel treatment an overestimàe of the danger. Nevertheless, we use the result for spent fuel, 0.02 deaths/GWe-yr, as the effects of HLW in further discussion. Note that even for the case of spent fuel burial, we must still consider the residues from uranium mining and milling and the depleted uranium left at the isotope enrichment plant; these are discussed later.

It is interesting to compare the health impact of HLW—0.02 deaths/GWe-ye—with that of the best known waste from coal-burning power plants—air pollution. Typical estimates for air pollution from coal burning are about 50 deaths/GWe-yr (18) with present practice; even giving credit for improvement due to tightening of environmental regulations would probably not reduce this below 20 deaths/GWe-yr, 1000 times the toll from nuclear HLW. Note that we are not considering the nonfatal illnesses caused by this air pollution, once estimated to be 60,000 càses/GWe-yr (18).

It should be recognized that the calculations presented here (and in the remainder of this chapter) do not address the problem of individual, peculiar, or unusual situations. They average over all possible situations, weighting each with its probability for occurrence.

3   CHEMICAL CARCINOGENS FROM COAL BURNING AND PHOTOVOLTAIC POWER (19)

3.1   Risk if Material Enters Human Stomachs

A consortium of U.S. government agencies—the Environmental Protection Agency (EPA), the Consumer Product Safety Commission, the Department of Health and

TABLE 2. Calculation of Deaths/GWe-yr Due to Carcinogenic Elements Released in Coal Burning, Integrated over 10^5 Years and over $\sim 10^7$ Years

Element	Deaths/g Ingested	Probability Ground → Stomachs	Deaths/t in Ground	Coal Deaths/GWe-yr 10^5 yr	10^7 yr
Cd	0.0013	0.013	8	20	5
Be	0.0053	0.0005	2.9	13	16
Cr	0.001	0.00002	0.19	7	39
Ni	0.00008	0.0006	0.047	1.4	8
As	0.0001	0.0024	0.24	10	1.3
			Total	50	70

Source: Reference 19.

Welfare, the Food and Drug Administration, the Department of Agriculture, and the Occupational Safety and Health Administration—have adopted the linear, no-threshold dose–response relation for chemical carcinogens (20). They have also established a Carcinogen Assessment Group within the EPA to determine the "slopes" of these linear relations, the risk/unit exposure. Unfortunately, this group only makes particular assessments when requested to do so by a government agency, so it is sometimes necessary to extend their work. For example, cadmium inhalation has been judged to cause prostate cancer with a risk of 0.0038/g inhaled (21). In order to cause prostate cancer, the cadmium must be transported from the lung to the prostate gland by the bloodstream. Since orally ingested cadmium can also get into the bloodstream, it must also present a cancer risk. Studies show that 15% of inhaled cadmium, versus 5% of orally ingested cadmium, gets into the bloodstream (1a). This implies that the cancer risk of orally ingesting cadmium is 5%/15% = 1/3 that of inhaling it, or 0.0013/g ingested. Risks from the other established everlasting chemical carcinogens—beryllium, arsenic, chromium, and nickel—are similarly available (19) and are listed in Table 2.

3.2   Probability of Transfer from the Ground into Human Stomachs

Consider the fate of a cadmium atom located randomly in the ground. The principal process for its removal is erosion followed by river transport into the oceans. Rivers carry 10^{15} g/yr of U.S. soil into the oceans (6); since cadmium is present in the ground at 0.19 ppm, about $(0.19 \times 10^{-6}) \times (10^{15}) = 1.9 \times 10^8$ g/yr of cadmium is removed from U.S. soil by this process.

From chemical analysis of food, it is estimated (22) that per capita dietary intake of cadmium is 3×10^{-5} g/day in the United States. The quantity of cadmium entering U.S. male stomachs each year—prostate cancer is a male disease—is then $(3 \times 10^{-5}$ g/day$) \times (365 \text{ days/yr}) \times (1.1 \times 10^8 \text{ men}) = 1.2 \times 10^6$ g/yr. The probability for a cadmium atom randomly located in the ground to enter a male stomach before being washed into the oceans is therefore $(1.2 \times 10^6/1.9 \times 10^8) = 0.6\%$.

3.3   Deaths Expected from Coal Burning

The number of cancers eventually expected per metric tonne (t) of cadmium in the ground can now be calculated to be $(0.0013 \text{ deaths/g}) \times (10^6 \text{ g/t}) \times (0.006) = 8$ deaths/t. A coal-burning power plant consumes 3×10^6 t/GWe-yr of coal, with an average cadmium content of 0.8 ppm. Since this cadmium eventually ends up in the ground, coal burning will cause $(3 \times 10^6) \times (0.8 \times 10^{-6}) \times (8 \text{ deaths/t}) = 20$ deaths/GWe-yr. Similar analyses for other carcinogenic elements are listed in Table 2; we see that their effects total 50 deaths/GWe-yr.

The 1×10^{15} g/yr of U.S. soil carried into the oceans corresponds to an erosion rate of 1 m of depth per 22,000 years. Assuming that the ashes from coal burning are distributed through the top 5 m of soil, the time scale for these 50 deaths/GWe-yr is about 10^5 years. If we extend our consideration to multimillion-year time periods, it could be argued that the coal will eventually reach the surface by erosion of overlying material, so the cadmium in the coal would be released even if the coal were not mined and burned. That nullifies the health effects of the cadmium in the coal but introduces another cadmium source.

Burning coal makes the carbon in it disappear permanently from the ground: the carbon dioxide product becomes distributed largely between the atmosphere and the oceans. When erosion eventually brings the coal near to the surface, the carbon in the coal will be replaced by average rock. However, this carbon contains no cadmium—the cadmium in the coal has already been taken into account—whereas its replacement does contain cadmium as a trace element impurity. This cadmium in the replacement rock represents an additional health hazard. It causes $(3 \times 10^6 \text{ t rock/GWe-yr}) \times (0.19 \times 10^{-6} \text{ t Cd/t rock}) \times (8 \text{ deaths/t Cd}) = 5$ deaths/Gwe-yr. Effects of other carcinogenic elements are similarly calculated in Table 2, from which we see that the total is 70 deaths/GWe-yr.

3.4   Deaths Expected from Photovoltaic Power

It is interesting to point out that deployment of a photovoltaic array for solar electricity requires a great deal of steel, glass, cement, and perhaps aluminum. Producing these requires about 3% as much coal burning as would be required to generate the same amount of electrical energy by direct coal burning (19). Thus, photovoltaics should be charged with 3% of the health effects of coal burning: $(3\% \times 70) = 2.1$ deaths/GWe-yr. Since coal or nuclear plants require at least an order of magnitude less materials, we ignore this problem for them.

One option for photovoltaics under serious consideration is the use of CdS photovoltaic cells. These require about 10 t/GWe-yr of cadmium; if this material ends up in the ground, it will cause $(10 \text{ t/GWe-yr}) \times (8 \text{ deaths/t}) = 80$ deaths/GWe-yr. Since most cadmium used in the United States is imported, this represents a net increase in health impacts here even in the very long term. Deep burial can postpone these health effects but cannot reduce them because, unlike radioactive waste, the cadmium does not decay away.

4   RADON PROBLEMS

The principal decay chain for uranium-238 (^{238}U) is shown in Fig. 3. When uranium decays into thorium (Th), or when thorium decays into radium (Ra), there is no movement of the material, but when radium decays into radon (Rn) the situation is very different: radon is a noble gas and thus can often diffuse away from its original location. If it is near the surface of the soil, it can percolate up into the atmosphere where it and its short half-life decay daughters can be inhaled by people. The radon itself is rapidly exhaled, but the decay

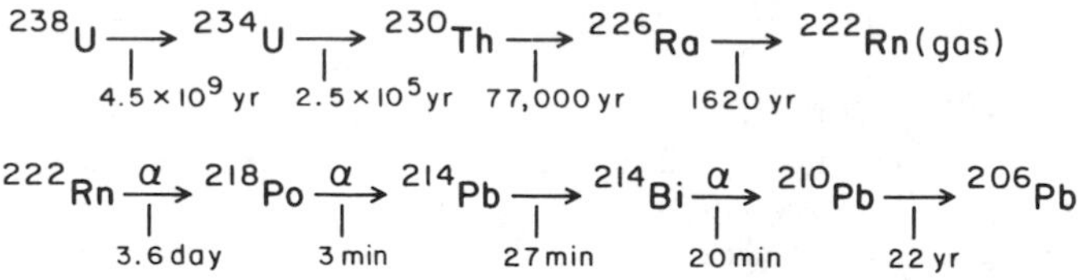

$$^{238}U \xrightarrow{} {}^{234}U \xrightarrow{} {}^{230}Th \xrightarrow{} {}^{226}Ra \xrightarrow{} {}^{222}Rn(gas)$$

4.5 × 10⁹ yr   2.5 × 10⁵ yr   77,000 yr   1620 yr

$$^{222}Rn \xrightarrow{\alpha} {}^{218}Po \xrightarrow{\alpha} {}^{214}Pb \xrightarrow{} {}^{214}Bi \xrightarrow{\alpha} {}^{210}Pb \xrightarrow{} {}^{206}Pb$$

3.6 day   3 min   27 min   20 min   22 yr

Figure 3. Decay schemes for uranium-238 and radon-222.

daughters—^{218}Po, ^{214}Pb, and ^{214}Bi—stick to the surfaces of our bronchial tubes and bombard the latter with alpha particles, which can cause lung cancer. Since uranium is present in all soil, there is radon in the air everywhere, causing a significant health hazard.

The health effects of radon have been investigated intensively among miners who worked in poorly ventilated mines and were therefore exposed to high levels of radon (3). Among one group of 4000 U.S. uranium miners so exposed, there were 159 fatal lung cancers up to 1974, versus only 25 normally expected. When this problem was first recognized in the late 1960s, ventilation was dramatically improved to the point where exposure to radon is of relatively negligible importance relative to the other hazards in mining.

It is worthwhile to point out that reducing air leakage in buildings in order to conserve fuel traps radon inside and therefore increases human exposure. Using the data from studies of miners coupled with measurements of radon levels in houses, it is straightforward to calculate that radon is now causing about 10,000 deaths/yr in the United States; the tightening of homes now recommended will cause an additional several thousand deaths per year (23). By comparison, the average number of deaths per year expected from nuclear power is generally estimated to be about 10 by government reports, or a few hundred according to the antinuclear activist organization Union of Concerned Scientists (24). Thus energy conservation is by far the most dangerous energy strategy from the standpoint of radiation hazards!

4.1   Uranium Mill Tailings

The best-known radon problem connected with the nuclear industry is the uranium-ore-processing mill tailings. After the ore is mined, it is carried to a nearby mill, where the uranium is chemically separated out and all remaining materials, known as tailings, are left at the site in a form resembling a sandy beach. We see from Fig. 3 that this includes the ^{230}Th and all of its decay products, so it continues producing radon as before, decreasing only with the 77,000-year half-life of ^{230}Th. Since without mining this radon would have been formed underground and therefore would have been much less accessible to the atmosphere, this represents a hazard created by uranium mining. Analysis (25) indicates that this will eventually cause 300 deaths/GWe-yr integrated over the 77,000-year half-life. Fortunately, however, there is an easy solution to this problem: covering the tailings with a few meters of soil reduces the emissions by a factor (26) of 20—diffusion through this layer allows time for decay of the 3.8-day half-life of radon. This is now legally required (27), and it reduces the effects to 300/20 = 15 deaths/GWe-yr. Note that this is still almost 1000 times higher than our estimated effects from HLW: if we are worried about radioactive waste from the nuclear industry we should worry about mill tailings much more than about HLW.

4.2 Uranium Mining

A more important radon consideration is the lives saved by mining uranium out of the ground to fuel nuclear power plants (28). Most of the health effects of radon are due to uranium (and its daughters) in the top 1 m of the ground. Since the area of the United States is $8 \times 10^{12} \, m^2$, and the ground has a density of $2.7 \, t/m^3$ and contains 2.7 ppm of uranium, the total quantity of uranium involved is $(1 \, m) \times (8 \times 10^{12} \, m^2) \times (2.7 \, t/m^3) \times (2.7 \times 10^{-6}) = 6 \times 10^7 \, t$. It is this uranium that is causing 10,000 deaths/yr in the United States, and it will continue to do so for 22,000 years, the average time required for 1 m of depth to erode away. Thus, this $6 \times 10^7 \, t$ of uranium will eventually cause $10,000 \times 22,000 = 22 \times 10^7$ deaths, or 3.7 deaths/t. Of course, only a tiny fraction of the uranium mined is from the top 1 m of the ground, but as erosion proceeds, essentially all uranium in the ground will eventually spend its average 22,000-years in the top 1 m, causing 3.7 deaths/t.

Fueling 1 GWe-yr of nuclear power requires mining 160 t of uranium and therefore saves $160 \times 3.7 = 590$ lives. However, this 1 m/22,000 yr erosion rate applied to mill tailings and their covers causes 29% of that number of deaths (28): about 170. Thus, the net effect of the radon from mining and milling uranium is to save $590 - 170 = 420$ lives.

Before we can count these lives as saved, we must trace what happens to the uranium that is mined. Some of it ends up with the HLW, but 80% of it is left as depleted uranium (99.8% ^{238}U, 0.2% ^{235}U) at the enrichment plant. If nuclear power has a long-range future, it will be burned up as fuel for breeder reactors. However, a viable alternative would be to dump it in oceans, where it has an average residence time of about 1 million years before becoming incorporated into the bottom sediments. Essentially all uranium in the ground is destined eventually to be eroded into the oceans and spend its million years therein, so dumping it in the oceans now has no long-term net health effects.

4.3 Radon Exposure from Coal Burning

There is still one other radon problem to be discussed; coal contains an average of 1 ppm of uranium (some coals contain as much as 40 ppm) and after the coal is burned, this uranium and its decay daughters ends up in the top few meters of the ground, serving as a source of radon (28). This causes $(3 \times 10^6 \, t \, coal/GWe\text{-}yr) \times (1 \times 10^{-6} \, t \, U/t \, coal) \times (3.7 \, deaths/t) = 11 \, deaths/Gwe\text{-}yr$. These deaths will occur over the next 10^5 years. Over a multimillion-year period, the coal with its uranium would have reached the surface by erosion of overlying materials, but as for the chemical carcinogens discussed above, the fact that the carbon in the coal will have effectively disappeared and will be replaced by average rock means that the uranium in this replacement rock is an additional source of radon. Since average rock contains 2.7 ppm of uranium, this will cause $(3 \times 10^6 \, t/GWe\text{-}yr) \times (2.7 \times 10^{-6} \, t \, U/t) \times (3.7 \, deaths/t \, U) = 30 \, deaths/GWe\text{-}yr$.

5 LOW-LEVEL WASTE (LLW)

The nuclear industry generates large amounts of low-level radioactive wastes including resins from demineralizers used to clean the reactor cooling water; filter elements from air and water cleaning; reactor components made radioactive by exposure to neutrons; and contaminated gloves, clothing, tools, instruments, and equipment. This material is appropriately packaged and buried in 6-m deep trenches at carefully selected sites governed by extensive regulations (29).

A risk analysis requires estimation of the transfer probability per year, T, from the ground into human stomachs. To do this (30), we assume that the buried waste becomes randomly distributed through the ground between the surface and depth D, and then we assume that an atom of this waste has the same transfer rate T as an atom of the same element in that soil. For example, we assume that T for ^{137}Cs is the same as T for natural Cs in the soil. The latter quantity is readily calculated as $T = q_1/q_2$, where q_1 is the quantity of Cs entering human stomachs each year, known from chemical analyses of food (2), and q_2 is the quantity of Cs in U.S. soil down to depth D, calculated from the measured abundance of Cs in soil (31).

Before proceeding, a value for D must be chosen. The new regulations (29) require that the water table be far below the trench bottoms and that there be good drainage downward from the trench to the water table, so the trenches cannot be flooded. Under these conditions, waste mobilized by water percolating through can only move downward until it reaches the top of the water table. We thus choose D to be the latter depth; a typical value is 20 m. The results are just proportional to D, so they would not be greatly changed by any other reasonable choice of its value.

Average daily dietary intake for cesium is 1×10^{-5} g/day (2); hence, $q_1 = (1 \times 10^{-5}$ g/day$) \times (365$ days/yr$) \times (2.3 \times 10^8$ population$) = 8.2 \times 10^5$ g/yr. The density of soil is 2 g/cm^3 and it contains 7 ppm of cesium; hence, q_2, the quantity of cesium in the top 20 m of U.S. soil, is $(20$ m$) \times 8 \times 10^{12}$ m^2 area$) \times (2.0 \times 10^6$ g/m$^3) \times (7 \times 10^{-6}) = 2.2 \times 10^{15}$ g. Thus, $T = (8.2 \times 10^5/2.2 \times 10^{15}) = 3.6 \times 10^{-10}$/yr. Since the half-life of ^{137}Cs is 30 years, its average lifetime is 43 years; hence, the total probability for transfer of ^{137}Cs from the soil into human stomachs is $(3.6 \times 10^{-10}) \times (43) = 1.6 \times 10^{-8}$. The LLW from 1 GWe-yr (32) contains 11 Ci of ^{137}Cs; a calculation analogous to that given for ^{239}Pu in our discussion of HLW indicates that we may expect 5.8 cancers/Ci of ^{137}Cs ingested by humans (5). The number of cancers expected from the ^{137}Cs in LLW is therefore (5.8 cancers/Ci$) \times (11$ Ci$) \times (1.6 \times 10^{-8}) = 1.0 \times 10^{-6}$. Analogous calculations are shown for other components in LLW in Table 3. For transuranics, transfer probabilities T were obtained from systematics versus position in the periodic table. All materials remaining after 10^5 years were assumed to be released into rivers by erosion, with a 10^{-4} probability for human ingestion.

TABLE 3. Calculation of Deaths/GWe-yr from Principal Components of Low-Level Waste (7.5E4 means 7.5×10^4)

Radionuclide	Half-Life (yr)	Ci/GWe-yr	T (Prob. yr)	Total Probability	Deaths/Ci Ingested	Deaths/ GWe-yr
^{59}Ni	7.5E4	1.9	1.8E − 9	2.4E − 4	0.018	6.0E − 6
^{60}Co	5.2E0	1600	7.1E − 9	5.5E − 8	0.67	5.9E − 5
^{129}I	1.7E7	0.0012	4.3E − 8	4.4E − 3	65	3.4E − 4
^{137}Cs	3.0E1	11	3.6E − 10	1.6E − 8	5.8	1.0E − 6
^{238}U	4.4E9	0.0062	2.2E − 10	1.2E − 4	8	6.0E − 6
^{239}Pu	2.4E4	0.016	7.9E − 10	3.4E − 5	38	2.1E − 5
^{240}Pu	6.6E3	0.008	7.9E − 10	7.5E − 6	38	2.2E − 6
^{241}Am	4.6E2	0.078	7.9E − 10	5.1E − 7	180	7.2E − 6
^{243}Am	7.7E3	0.0012	7.9E − 10	8.7E − 6	180	1.9E − 6
					Total	4.0E − 4

Source: Reference 30.

The deaths/GWe-yr for each radionuclide listed in Table 3 sum to a total of 4×10^{-4} deaths/GWe-yr. This is our estimate of the health consequences of LLW burial.

The principal questionable assumption in this risk analysis is that an atom of LLW is no more easily picked up by plant roots than an atom of the same element that is part of the mineral structure of soil. As a test of this assumption, we may refer to experiments in which T is determined by injecting radioactive tracers of various elements into the soil and later measuring the amount of radioactivity in the edible parts of plants grown in that soil. Numerous experiments of this type have been reported (32), and values of T obtained from them average about the same as values of T obtained from the ratio of dietary intake to concentration in soil described above (30). This confirms that atoms artificially inserted into the soil (like LLW) are no more easily taken up by plants than atoms of the same element in the mineral structure of the soil.

6 REVIEW OF THE VARIOUS RISKS ASSOCIATED WITH POWER GENERATION

The results of the risk analyses we have presented and two others are summarized in Table 4 in the column headed Eventual. The analysis for routine emissions of radioactivity from nuclear plants is by the United Nations Scientific Committee (4) and the analysis for transport of HLW is by a group from Sandia Laboratory (33).

We seen from Table 4 that there are three different types of waste from coal burning, *each* of which is at least a thousand times more harmful to human health than the wastes from nuclear power that draw so much public concern. Clearly, this public concern is very much misdirected.

While public discussion of hazards of buried waste usually centers on the very-long-term risks listed in Table 4 as "eventual," there are many good reasons to limit our consideration only to the next few hundred years (34). That is *not* because the lives of people living many thousands of years from now are less valuable than those of people living now, but because of the following considerations:

TABLE 4. Summary of Deaths/GWe-yr from Wastes Produced in Electricity Generation

Source	First 500 yr	Eventual
Nuclear		
High-level waste	0.0005	0.02
Radon problems	−0.065	−420
Routine emissions	0.05	0.3
Transport (radiation only)	0.0001	0.0001
Low-level waste	<0.0001	0.0004
Coal burning		
Air pollution	20	20
Chemical carginogens	0.5	70
Radon	0.11	30
Photovoltaics		
Coal for materials	0.6	4
Add if CdS	0.8	80

1. There is an excellent chance that a cure for cancer will be developed within the next few hundred years, in which case the projected deaths will never materialize.
2. Historically, money has drawn at least 3% real interest (after allowing for inflation) continuously for at least 5000 years. If the money spent to protect our distant progeny from our wastes were invested at even 1% interest, it would make available to them tremendous sums of money that could be spent to save enormous numbers of their lives. Simply not spending this money and thereby reducing the national debt would be essentially equivalent to this, giving our distant progeny more money to spend on themselves.
3. Spending money now on biomedical research is enormously more effective for saving future lives than spending money to protect them from our wastes.

In view of these considerations, Table 4 also contains risk estimates for the various wastes added up over only the next 500 years. In arriving at these estimates, effects of materials deposited in the top layers of soil are taken as 1% of those expected over the next 100,000 years (there is more deposit in the upper layers of soil). Lives saved by uranium mining are those due to surface mining. For high-level radioactive waste, one order of magnitude credit is given for the many important time delays associated with release scenarios.

Clearly, as shown in this 500-year perspective, the three types of waste from coal burning are *each* many times more harmful to human health than the nuclear wastes.

7   USEFULNESS OF PUBLIC EDUCATION REGARDING RELATIVE RISK

In order for the public, regulators, and other scientists to make rational decisions regarding various choices involving technological issues, it might be useful to educate them regarding risks associated with activities which they understand. One approach to the process is to compare activities by assuming that all the eventual deaths occur now, or what is equivalent, that current waste generation rates and disposal practices continue for millions of years, and consider the effects of all accumulated wastes. Certainly, it would be useful to first present the risks posed by the nuclear HLW and other energy or natural radiation related hazards.

For HLW, Table 4 lists 0.02 deaths/GWe-yr, and U.S. electricity generation (assumed to be all nuclear) is 250 GWe-yr/yr; hence, the total annual effect is $0.02 \times 250 = 5$ deaths/yr. If the U.S. population had a stable age distribution, there would be 3×10^6 deaths/yr (actually there are 2×10^6); hence, the average person's risk of dying from HLW is $\frac{5}{3} \times 10^{-6} = 1.7 \times 10^{-6}$. The average person who does die from the HLW loses about 20 years of life; hence, the average loss of life expectancy is $(1.7 \times 10^{-6}) \times (20 \,\text{yr}) \times (365 \,\text{days/yr}) = 0.012$ days, or 18 min.

The educational process could then proceed into a discussion of relative risks. It was shown during Ruckelshaus' most recent tenure as head of the EPA that by comparing some environmental risks posed by certain activities with risks deemed acceptable by the public, the EPA was able to dismiss demands to regulate trivial hazards so that they could focus on higher-priority issues. One approach that is easily understood is to discuss the risks that reduce life expectancy by about 18 min:

• A regular cigarette smoker smoking $1\frac{1}{2}$ extra cigarettes in his or her lifetime.

- An overweight person eating 120 extra calories in his or her lifetime.
- An overweight person increasing body weight by 0.006 ounces.
- Driving an extra $\frac{1}{2}$ mile every year (35).

Hopefully, such efforts will help educate the public so that they will be able to make more rational decisions as we move into a period when such decisions will be too frequent to address in only an emotional, uninformed manner.

REFERENCES

1. U.S. Nuclear Regulatory Commission, *Reactor Safety Study*, Doc. WASH-1400, or NUREG 75/014. USNRC, Washington, DC, 1975.

1a. International Commission on Radiological Protection, *Limits for Intakes of Radionuclides by Workers*, ICRP Publ. No. 30. ICRP, Pergamon, Oxford, 1979.

2. International Commission on Radiological Protection, *Report of the Task Group on Reference Man*, ICRP Publ. No. 23. Pergamon, Oxford, 1975.

3. National Academy of Sciences, Committee on Biological Effects of Ionizing Radiation (BEIR), *The Effects on Populations of Exposure to Low Levels of Ionizing Radiation.* NAS, Washington, DC, 1980.

4. United Nations Scientific Committee on Effects of Atomic Radiation, *Sources and Effects of Ionizing Radiation*, United Nations, New York, 1977.

5. B. L. Cohen, Effects of ICRP-30 and BEIR-III on hazard estimates for high level radioactive waste. *Health Phys.* **42**, 133 (1983); Effects of recent neptunium studies of high level waste hazard assessments, *ibid.* **44**, 567 (1983).

6. R. M. Garrels and F. T. MacKenzie, *Evolution of Sedimentary Rocks.* Norton, New York, 1971.

7. D. K. Todd, *Groundwater Hydrology.* Wiley, New York, 1980.

8. Ad Hoc Panel on Hydrology, Scientific Hydrology, Federal Council for Science and Technology, Washington, DC, 1962.

9. B. L. Cohen, A simple probabilistic risk analysis for high level waste repositories. *Nucl. Technol.* **69**(1), 73 (1985).

10. B. L. Cohen, Analysis, critique, and re-evaluation of high level waste repository water intrusion scenarios studies. *Nucl. Technol.* **48**, 63 (1980).

11. D. E. White, J. D. Hein, and G. A. Waring, Chemical composition of subsurface waters. In *Data of Geochemistry.* U.S. Geol. Surv., Washington, DC, 1963, Chap. F.

12. F. Byrne, *Earth and Man.* Brown, Dubuque, IA, 1974.

13. B. L. Cohen, Probability for human intake of an atom randomly released into ground, rivers, oceans, and air. *Health Phys.* **47**, 281 (1984); A generic probabilistic risk analysis of high level waste repositories. *Ibid.* **51**, 519 (1986).

14. Office of Nuclear Waste Isolation, *The Status of Borehole Plugging and Shaft Sealing for Geologic Isolation of Radioactive Waste*, ONWI-15. Battelle Mem. Inst., Columbus, OH, 1979; *Repository Sealing Field Testing Workshop*, ONWI-239. Battelle Mem. Inst., Columbus, OH, 1980; D. M. Roy, M. W. Grutzeck, and P. H. Licastro, *Evaluation of Cement Borehole Plug Longevity*, ONWI-30. Battelle Mem. Inst., Columbus, OH, 1979.

15. P. A. Witherspoon, N. G. W. Cook, and J. E. Gale, progress with field investigations at Stripa. *Lawrence Berkeley Lab.* [Rep.] **LBL-10550** (1980).

16. J. A. Ruppen, M. A. Molecke, and R. S. Glass, Titanium utilization in long term nuclear waste storage. *Sandia* [Tech. Lab. Rep.] **SAND81-2466** (1981).

17. M. J. Plodinec, G. M. Jantzen, and G. G. Wicks, *A Thermodynamic Approach to Prediction of Stability of Proposed Rad Waste Glasses.* Am. Ceram. Soc., Washington, DC, 1984.

18. U.S. Senate Committee on Public Works, *Air Quality and Stationary Source Emission Controls.* Washington, DC, 1975; R. Wilson, S. D. Colome, J. D. Spengler, and D. G. Wilson, *Health Effects of Fossil Fuel Burning.* Ballinger, Cambridge, MA, 1980; Harvard University Energy and Environmental Policy Center, *Epidemiological Assessments Relevant to Health Effect of Exposures to Airborne Particles.* Harvard University, Cambridge, MA, 1982; M. G. Morgan, S. C. Morris, A. K. Meier, and D. L. A. Schenk, A probabilistic methodology for estimating air pollution health effects from coal-fired power plants. *Energy Syst. Pol.* **2**, 287 (1978); L. D. Hamilton, Comparative risks from different energy systems. *I.A.E.A. Bull.* **22**, 35 (1980).

19. B. L. Cohen, Long term consequences of the linear no threshold dose-response relationship for chemical carcinogens. *Risk Anal.* **1**, 267 (1982).

20. U.S. Consumer Product Safety Commission, U.S. Environmental Protection Agency, U.S. Department of Health, Education, and Welfare, U.S. Food and Drug Administration, and U.S. Department of Agriculture, Scientific bases for identification of potential carcinogens and estimation of risks. *Fed. Regist.* **44**, 39858 (1979) (see p. 39873); see also *ibid.* **40**, 28242; **41**, 21402; **43**, 25658; U.S. Environmental Protection Agency, National emission standards for identifying, assessing, and regulating airborne substances posing a risk of cancer. *ibid.* **44**, 58642 (1979) (see p. 58649); U.S. Occupational Safety and Health Administration, Identification, classification, and regulation of potential occupational carcinogens. *ibid.* **45**, 5002 (1980).

21. Carcinogen Assessment Group, *Assessment of Carcinogenic Risk from Population Exposure to Cadmium in the Ambient Air.* USEPA, Washington, DC, 1978.

22. J. A. Ryan, H. R. Pahren, and J. B. Lucas, Controlling cadmium in the food chain: A review and rationale based on health effects. *Environ. Res.* **28**, 261 (1982).

23. B. L. Cohen, Health effects of radon from insulation of buildings. *Health Phys.* **39**, 937 (1980).

24. Union of Concerned Scientists, *The Risks of Nuclear Power Reactors.* Cambridge, MA, 1977).

25. C. C. Travis et al., *Radiological Assessment of Radon-222 Released from Uranium Mills and Other Natural and Technologically Enhanced Sources,* NUREG/CR-0573. U.S. Nuclear Regulatory Commission, Washington, DC, 1979; B. L. Cohen, Health effects of radon emissions from uranium mill tailings. *Health Phys.* **42**, 695 (1982).

26. U.S. Nuclear Regulatory Commission, *Final Generic Environmental Impact Statement of Uranium Milling,* NUREG-0706. USNRC, Washington, DC, 1980.

27. U.S. Code of Federal Regulations, Title 10, Part 40, Appendix A. Washington, DC. 1980.

28. B. L. Cohen, The role of radon in comparisons of effects of radioactivity releases from nuclear power, coal burning, and phosphate mining. *Health Phys.* **40**, 19 (1981).

29. U.S. Code of Federal Regulations, Title 10, Part 61. Washington, DC, 1981, Federal Register, Licensing requirements for land disposal of radioactive waste. *Fed. Regist.* **46**(142), 38096ff (1981).

30. B. L. Cohen, A generic probabilistic risk assessment for low level waste burial grounds. *Nucl. Chem. Waste Manage.* **5**, 39 (1984).

31. H. J. Rosler and H. Lange, *Geochemical Tables Am.* Elsevier, New York, 1972.

32. C. F. Baes, III, R. D. Sharp, A. Sjoreen, and R. W. Shor, A review and analysis of parameters for assessing transport of environmentally released radionuclides through agriculture. *Oak Ridge Natl. Lab.* [Rep.] **ORNL-5876** (1983).

33. U.S. Nuclear Regulatory Commission, *Final Environmental Statement on the Transportation of Radioactive material by Air and Other Modes,* Doc. NUREG-0170. USNRC, Washington, DC, 1977.

34. B. L. Cohen, Discounting in assessment of future radiation risks. *Health Phys.* **45**, 687 (1983).

35. B. L. Cohen and I. S. Lee, A catalog of risks. *Health Phys.* **36**, 707 (1979).

16

Assessment of a Waste Site Contaminated with Chromium

Robert J. Golden and Nathan J. Karch

Karch & Associates, Inc., Washington, DC

1 INTRODUCTION

Evaluation of the potential health risk associated with hazardous waste sites is currently of major societal concern. However, too often the actual threats to human health are not based on a careful analysis of the chemicals present at a site or on a realistic appraisal of the most relevant route of potential exposure. Because of the uncertainties inherent in the risk assessment process, it is necessary that each site be assessed individually in order to derive the most accurate estimates of potential risks. A variety of major legislative statutes have been enacted to respond more effectively to the need to control the disposal of hazardous wastes. In this regard, the two critical laws are the Resource Conservation and Recovery Act (RCRA) of 1976 and the Comprehensive Environmental Response, Compensation, and Liability Act (CERCLA) of 1980 (1).

Hazardous waste disposal sites can pose potential problems as a result of contamination of soil, groundwater or surface water, or air. Such multimedia contamination can then result in potential exposure to humans via ingestion, inhalation, or dermal contact. However, despite a growing concern for potential hazards associated with such sites, a recent comprehensive review by Grishan et al. (1) concluded that "there are few published scientific reports of health effects clearly attributable to chemicals from uncontrolled disposal sites."

The range of chemicals that have been detected at hazardous waste sites is impressively large and there are clearly a number of chemicals to which exposure may have adverse consequences. Risk assessment has become the primary method for estimating the potential for adverse health effects following exposure to chemicals. However, too often risk assessments make too many assumptions concerning the toxicological hazards posed by some chemicals. Specifically, these assumptions do not incorporate a thorough understanding of biological feasibility, species differences, or metabolism or account for the different effects following different routes of exposure. In addition, with respect to metals and metal-induced carcinogenesis, there is often insufficient consideration of toxicity data associated with different valence states.

In the past dozen years there has been an increased awareness that metals comprise an important class of occupational carcinogens and that environmental exposure may also pose a threat to human health. This concern about metal-induced carcinogenesis has prompted increased research activity to explain mechanistically why certain metals, but not others, are carcinogens. This effort has been of special interest to toxicologists because several carcinogenic metals are essential nutrients for rodents and humans.

Humans need some metals such as iron, potassium, and sodium in rather large quantities and there is a wide tolerance between persons. In contrast, other metals such as copper, chromium, manganese, and cobalt are required for specialized biochemical functions but can also be toxic when present at higher levels (2). While the biochemical functions of these metals is reasonably well understood, it is much less clear why small amounts are essential and larger amounts are toxic.

Those metals that are carcinogenic, yet must be present in the diet to sustain life, offer toxicologists a rare opportunity to investigate the presence of thresholds. While current regularity philosophy dictates that thresholds (either practical or otherwise) for carcinogens do not exist, this is clearly not the case for certain metals. Logically, there must be a threshold dose below which the likelihood of producing tumors is no greater than the background rate. Some have suggested that even essential levels of these metals are associated with some risk of cancer and this is somehow the price the human species must pay for the metabolic benefits derived from these elements. However, this is similar to arguing that dying is the price we must pay for living and the usefulness of such an argument is questionable.

There are several theories that attempt to explain the mechanism of metal carcinogenesis (3). The most prevalent involves the impairment by metals of the fidelity of DNA replication as mediated by DNA polymerase (3). Other theories include interactions between metals and nucleic acids, inhibitory effects of metals on nuclei acids, somatic mutations, or neoplastic transformations (3). A wide variety of in vitro test systems have been used to investigate metal carcinogenesis, but metals present special problems because of solubility and a general lack of the need for metabolic activation. It is beyond the scope of this chapter to provide an in-depth evaluation of the mechanistic evidence for metal carcinogenicity. This subject is reviewed in depth by Sunderman (3).

This chapter illustrates an approach to evaluating possible health risk which was presented by an inactive wastewater treatment residue basin that was part of an industrial plant in the Midwest. The basin was found to contain chromium, and measurements indicated that some of the groundwater under the plant site contained trace levels of chromium. This chapter reviews the toxicity, possible exposures, and potential risk to human health from the ingestion of chromium. This assessment is organized into six sections: (i) a description of the site; (ii) the basic chemistry of chromium and chromium compounds; (iii) the fate of chromium in the body; (iv) the potential toxicities of chromium; (v) the potential human exposure to chromium in groundwater from the vicinity of the basin; and (vi) the potential risks that these exposures might present.

2   BACKGROUND: WASTEWATER TREATMENT SITE

The plant associated with the wastewater treatment basin was originally constructed and operated to manufacture chrome-plated automobile bumpers. Wastewater treatment residues typical of such facilities were discharged into a large settling basin adjacent to the plant. A smaller basin, which contained comparable residues, was also present onsite.

Such overflow basins are relatively common. The wastewater containing chromium resulted from plating operations, as well as from cleaning and painting operations. The purpose of these wastewater treatment processes was to remove chromium, and other metals, from the wastewater streams and a waste slurry containing these metals was pumped to the basin for settling.

A preliminary evaluation of the site showed that chromium (but not other metals present in the basin residues) was leaching from the basin at a level that could affect groundwater. On the basis of this preliminary survey, groundwater studies were undertaken in the vicinity of the settling basins. The groundwater studies involved extensive analysis of primary and secondary drinking water pollutants, priority pollutants, and other substances. Chromium was the only substance identified at a concentration that could be considered a potential concern in groundwater.

Total chromium was detected downgradient from the large basin initially at concentrations of approximately 0.17–0.32 mg/L in shallow groundwater. These levels exceeded the EPA's primary drinking water standard of 0.05 mg/L for total chromium (since raised to 0.12 mg/L), which is applicable only to public water supplies (4). Subsequent measurements confirmed the presence of chromium in groundwater and a maximum concentration of 0.37 mg/L was identified in one of the monitoring wells that surrounded the site. The form of chromium present in groundwater was found to be predominantly chromium(VI).

The main settling basin, approximately 6 acres in size, was located on the western section of the industrial site. Groundwater rain beneath the basin from north to south. In the evaluation of such sites, it is important to determine depth, breadth, and extent of the chromium plume, the concentration gradient of the plume, and the changes in these parameters over time. This characterization of the groundwater plume helps define the exposed population and the frequency, duration, and level of exposure. The route of exposure by which residents could be exposed to chromium from drinking water was ingestion of contaminated water. Inhalation or skin contact to chromium at the site was presumed to be insignificiant.

An extensive hydrogeological survey of the site revealed that the aquifer system beneath the site was composed of sand and gravel outwash sediments interbedded with silt and clay sediments. The outwash deposits were 100–250 ft thick, overlying shale bedrock. The sand and gravel aquifer was the primary source of public and private water supply in the vicinity. Stabilized water levels indicated that the water table sloped from 24 ft beneath the ground surface at the north end of the site to 34 ft at the south end of the facility. The major direction of groundwater flow was south with some indication of lesser amounts of flow toward the southwest. The groundwater flow was essentially horizontal with little or no vertical gradient beneath the site. Analysis also revealed that groundwater flow was also being influenced by offsite sources. There was also a possibility that groundwater could have been influenced by pumping of various industrial or private wells near the site.

3   CHEMISTRY OF CHROMIUM IN ANIMALS AND HUMANS

Chromium is widely distributed throughout the natural environment, although chromium ores are relatively scarce. Chromium is a mixture of four stable isotopes with mass numbers 50, 52, 53, and 54 (4).

The inorganic chemistry of chromium has been extensively studied, but the forms in which chromium is incorporated into biological systems have not been well characterized (5). Although inorganic chromium compounds occur in valence states ranging from -2 to $+6$, chromium(III) and chromium(VI) are the most stable forms and are therefore the forms typically found in the environment.

Chromium(III) is the most stable form (5). It forms polynuclear compounds in neutral and basic solutions by linking chromium atoms through hydroxy or oxo bridges, and it forms stable complexes with amino acids and peptides. The ability of chromium(VI) to oxidize organic materials and the tendency of the resulting chromium(III) to form stable complexes with biological substances, such as proteins, provide one mechanism by which chromium interacts with mammalian macromolecules (5).

The assessment of the toxicity of chromium is complicated by the fact that it is an essential element in humans at low levels (5–8). Data on older individuals, diabetics, pregnant women, and malnourished children suggest that chromium deficiency does occur in humans (8). Offspring or siblings of diabetics and individuals with early coronary heart disease are also prone to chromium deficiency (5). Reported symptoms in humans are glucose intolerance, weight loss, and confusion (5). In one case, cited in a review by the National Academy of Sciences (8), chromium deprivation led to glucose intolerance, inability to utilize glucose for energy, neuropathy with normal insulin levels, a low respiratory quotient, and abnormal metabolism of nitrogen. In animals maintained on a low chromium diet, the reported effects of chromium deficiency have included decreased fertility, corneal opacity, and aortic plagues (5).

Chromium supplementation has been shown to improve or normalize the impaired glucose tolerance of some diabetics, elderly people, and malnourished children, but no others (6). Although these findings indicate that chromium deficiency may not be the sole cause for glucose intolerance, the results are difficult to interpret because the bioavailability of inorganic chromium in foods is low.

The most biologically active form is glucose tolerance factor (GTF). GTF is a complex and as-yet-unidentified biological material that can be isolated from yeast and pork kidney. GTF contains chromium(III), can cross biological membranes with relative ease, and is readily absorbed from the intestine (9). The inability of chromium(III) in other forms to cross biological barriers and the limited transport of chromium(VI) are discussed in the next section.

4   TOXICOLOGY AND PHARMACOKINETICS OF CHROMIUM

Because of the considerable differences between chromium(III) and chromium(VI), it is important to distinguish between inhalation and oral exposures. While there are considerable data on the absorption of chromium compounds via inhalation, it was not a route of entry in the risk evaluation of this site. The need to understand thoroughly the toxicology of a compound, whenever possible, is illustrated in this case study. For many systemic toxicants, the differences in biologic response are independent of the route of entry and this assumption is often made in the evaluation of hazardous waste sites.

4.1   Absorption of Chromium by Ingestion

The amount of chromium absorbed from the gastrointestinal (GI) tract depends on its valence state. Although there are conflicting data regarding which of the valence states

TABLE 1. Excretion in Feces and Urine of Radiolabelled Chromium Chloride [Chromium(III)] and Sodium Chromate [Chromium(VI)] by Fasted Human Volunteers and Rats

	Fasted Human Volunteers			
	Oral Administration		Duodenal Administration	
	Feces	Urine	Feces	Urine
Chromium(III)	99.6%	0.5%	93.7%	0.6%
Chromium(VI)	89.4%	2.1%	56.5%	10.6%

	Rats			
	Gastric Administration		Jejunal Administration	
	Feces	Urine	Feces	Urine
Chromium(III)	98.0%	1.4%	91.6%	4.3%
Chromium(VI)	97.7%	0.8%	76.4%	16.5%

Source: Adapted from Donaldson and Barreras (10).

is most easily absorbed when administered orally, it is clear that neither chromium(III) nor chromium(VI) is absorbed to an appreciable degree (5).

Studies by Donaldson and Barreras (10) in fasting humans indicated that the normal absorption of chromium(III) or chromium(VI) by the GI tract is low but is increased when chromium is administered directly to the intestines bypassing the gastric juices. However, the relevance of this method of dosing is questionable when drinking water is the mode of exposure. Table 1 contains data on the absorption and excretion of radiolabeled chromium chloride and sodium chromate in fasted human volunteers and rats (10).

Two routes of administration have been studied in humans and in rats. These compounds were administered orally to humans and by gastric intubation in rats (10). The oral study permitted contact with gastric juices, to the degree that they were present (the level of gastric juices are reduced by fasting). In the rodent study, radiolabeled chromium compounds were placed directly in the intestines by doudenal intubation in humans and by jejunal intubation in rats (10). This experimental procedure avoids the gastric juices altogether. The level of radioactivity was measured in feces and urine. The amount in feces was considered an indication of the amount of chromium that was extreted unchanged. The amount in urine was considered (by the authors) as a rough indication of the amount absorbed through the gastrointestinal tract.

The data in Table 1 indicate that chromium(III) is absorbed poorly (e.g., low bioavailability) in humans and rats and that gastric juices have only a small effect on such absorption. In humans, oral administration suggests that, based on data on fecal and urinary excretion, less than 10% of chromium(VI) is absorbed. Absorption in fasted humans is greater than in rats.

Donaldson and Barreras (10) confirmed the observation that gastric acidity has a dramatic effect on the absorption of chromium(VI) in patients with pernicious anemia, a disease in which one of the symptoms is a virtual absence of gastric acidity. The absorption of radioactive chromium(VI) was enhanced in these patients. Because the species of chromium(VI) is dependent on the pH, at the acidic pH levels of the gastric juices, the chromium(VI) is likely to be present primarily as dichromate and to a lesser extent as hydrochromate. At the neutral to basic pH levels of the intestine, chromium(VI) is likely to be present primarily as the chromate. These different forms of chromium(VI) are likely to differ in their binding affinities to cellular macromolecules, which would also affect absorption.

Donaldson and Barreras (10) attributed the effect of the gastric juices on absorption to the reduction of chromium(VI) to chromium(III), as well as to the effect of pH. The effect of the human gastric juices in reducing chromium(VI) to chromium(III) appears to be incomplete, but the results are difficult to interpret because Donaldson and Barreras(10) did not report the length of time that the humans had fasted. They reported that the rats had fasted overnight, and reduction of chromium(VI) to chromium(III) appears to be more complete than in the humans. However, when human gastric juices were mixed with sodium chromate before administration, absorption of chromium(VI) was reported to be completely inhibited, which suggests that the gastric juices are capable of converting virtually all the chromium(VI) to chromium(III).

MacKenzie et al. (11) administered potasium chromate [chromium(VI)] and chromic chloride [chromium(III)] to rats in their drinking water at levels between 0.45 and 25 ppm for 1 year. At concentrations up to 5 ppm chromium(VI), relatively little chromium was found in any of the body tissues examined. With the animals received 5 and 10 ppm chromate ion in the water, an appreciable increase in tissue chromium(VI) levels was observed. In the rats given water containing 25 ppm of chromium(VI), the tissue levels were up to nine times greater than the rats given 25 ppm chromium(III). This suggested that at this level (25 ppm), chromium(VI) was absorbed to a much greater extent than chromium(III). In addition, these findings indicate that conversion of chromium(VI) to chromium(III) by gastric juices is incomplete in rats because of the differences noted in absorption of chromium following administration of chromium(VI) and chromium(III).

Another study involving rats indicated that the absorption of a single oral dose (via stomach tube) of 0.1 mg/kg of either radioactive chromium chloride or sodium chromate was below 1% (12). In this study, the amount of radioactivity retained in the body after 30 days was greater for chromium(III) (0.3%) than for chromium(VI) (0.1%), which means either that more chromium(III) was absorbed or that it was less efficiently excreted.

MacKenzie et al. (13) administered radioactive sodium chromate [chromium(VI)] by stomach tube to both fasted and fed rats at a single dose of 0.19 mg/kg. The quantity of chromium administered was similar to the amount a rat would receive per day while drinking water containing 2 ppm chromium. The results indicated that absorption was greater in the fasted rats than in the nonfasted rats. Based on excretion of chromium in the urine, the authors estimated that absorption was approximately 6% in the fasted rats and approximately 3% in the nonfasted rats.

The available data indicate that chromium(III) is essentially not absorbed from the gastroinstestinal tract unless the gastric juices are absent or impaired. The proportion of chromium(VI) absorbed by the gastrointestinal tract is complicated and appears to depend on two major factors: (i) the acidity of the gastric juice and (ii) the efficiency of gastric juice in reducing chromium(VI) to chromium(III). The solubility and binding affinity of the form of chromium(VI) to substances in food or present in the stomach will depend on pH. Although the value of 5% absorption for chromium(VI) appears to represent a valid and reasonable upper bound for absorption following ingestion, the absorption of chromium(VI) may be as high as 10.6% in fasted subjects when the chromium is administered by a route in which the gastric juices are artificially avoided.

However, administration in this manner cannot be considered a reasonable route of exposure.

4.2 Dermal Absorption

The absorption of chromium through the skin (percutaneous) also may be related to the valence state of the compound, but solubility and the concentration applied appear to be more significant factors (14).

Dutkiewicz (15) investigated the absorption of 0.01, 0.1, and 0.2 M sodium chromate (Chromium(VI)] by intact human skin. The results indicated that (i) the amount of chromium(VI) absorbed was highest with the 0.01 M solution and lowest with the 0.2 M solution and (ii) the rate of absorption decreased as time of exposure increased. These results are consistent with observations made in absorption studies with rats. Studies with guinea pig skin also demonstrated no significant difference between the absorption of chromium(III) and chromium(VI) at concentrations up to 0.239 M, whereas in the concentration range 0.261–0.398 M, the amount of chromium(VI) absorbed as approximately twice that of chromium(III) (16). In vitro studies by Mali et al. (17) investigated the rates of diffusion of chromium(III) and chromium(VI) salts using skin from cadavers. Their results (using concentrations ranging up to 1%) indicated that neither compound passively diffused through intact, isolated epidermal membranes. It should be noted that the concentrations used in all these studies are unlikely to be encountered in nonoccupational settings.

While a variety of animal and human studies demonstrate that chromium (VI) may be absorbed through the skin, there is little evidence to suggest that dermal absorption contributes in any significant way to total body burden of chromium, especially as a result of environmental exposure. Furthermore, in most of the studies in which the dermal absorption of either chromium(III) or chromium(VI) was measured, the concentrations employed were often orders of magnitude larger than would ever be encountered as a result of even elevated environmental exposures.

4.3 Distribution in the Body

In addition to being poorly absorbed, chromium(III) compounds are rapidly cleared from the blood plasma although they are more slowly cleared from other tissues. Chromium(VI) is cleared less rapidly because it is bound to red blood cells. Although a number of studies describe the distribution of chromium, only those pertaining to oral exposures were considered. In most of the other studies, chromium was adminstered to the animals by intravenous injection. This route of administration, while convenient, avoids the dynamics that are involved during normal gastrointestinal absorption and therefore does not represent a useful surrogate.

MacKenzie et al. (13) administered a single oral dose (57 µg) of radioactive sodium chromate [chromium(VI)] to fasted and nonfasted rats by stomach tube. The quantity of chromium administered was similar to the amount that a rat would receive per day while drinking water containing 2 ppm chromium. The liver showed the most uptake, about 1% of the administered dose, while the kidney, blood, and spleen contained from 0.1–0.2%. In general, more chromium appeared in the tissues of the fasted animals than in the tissues of the nonfasted animals. The levels in all organs declined rapidly during 14 days, although it appeared that the chromium in the spleens of the fasted animals may have been more tightly bound than in other tissues. This may have resulted from the fact that red blood cells are normally cleared by the spleen. Considerably more chromium(VI) than chromium(III) was bound to whole blood, plasma, and red blood cells.

The distribution of chromium has also been investigated with respect to its ability to cross the placenta and affect the developing fetus. There appears to be only one relevant study in which chromium was administered orally. Mertz (6) administered radioactive chromium as chromium acetate [chromium(III)] to rats by gavage at mating. Repeated doses were given either by daily intubation during gestation or by administration in the drinking water at a concentration of 2 mg/L. No radioactivity was detected in the young at birth following a single oral (or even intravenous) dose. Repeated doses by gavage during gestation resulted in labeled chromium levels in the litters at birth of 0.5–1.5% of the mother's total body radioactivity. This may have been a function of red blood cell binding in placental blood. No transfer of maternal radioactivity was observed in the litters from dams drinking water containing chromium.

In contrast to the above observations, when radioactive chromium was administered in the form of glucose tolerance factor by stomach tube during gestation, there was a transfer of from 20 to 50% of maternal radioactivity into the fetuses. This is consistent with the role of chromium as an essential trace element. The significance of these observations is discussed in Section 5.6.

Since chromium of either valence state is so poorly absorbed from the gastrointestinal tract, Visek et al. (18) investigated the ability of intravenous injections of radioactive chromium(III) or chromium(VI) to cross the placenta. Insignificant amounts of radioactivity were found to cross the placenta of rats in the 24 h following intravenous administration of the chromium compounds, regardless of the chemical form of the isotope, its valence state, the gestational state of the animal, or the number of fetuses per litter. In no case did the recovery of radioactive chromium per total litter exceed 0.13% of the injected dose. In an abstract, Danielsson et al. (19) indicated that radioactive chromium(VI) crosses the placenta of rats in significant concentrations, whereas chromium(III) apparently does so to a far less degree.

4.4   Excretion from the Body

As with the distribution studies, only studies involving oral exposures were considered. Sayato et al. (12) administered both radioactive chromium cloride [chromium(III)] and sodium chromate [chromium(VI)] to rats by stomach tube and followed the excretion of radioactivity for 30 days. For both compounds, retention was less than 1% of the administered dose 2 days following administration and decreased with time. After 30 days the retentions of chromium(III) and chromium(VI) were about 0.3 and 0.1%, respectively. The biological half-lives were calculated to be 92 days for chromium(III) and 22 days for chromium(VI). About 99% of the oral dosage was excreted in the feces between 2 and 20 days following administration, while less than 1% of each compound was excreted in the urine.

4.5   Metabolism

Following the administration of a dose of radioactive chromium(III) or chromium(VI) to either the stomach or intestine of rats, various degrees of binding occur to red blood cells and plasma proteins (13). The degree of binding is determined by the valence state of the chromium compound. More chromium(VI) is bound to whole blood, plasma, and red blood cells than chromium(III). This was observed when absorption was from either the stomach or intestine.

Chromium(VI) readily crosses the red blood cell membrane, where it is reduced to chromium(III). It remains in this form until the red blood cell is normally destroyed. The reduction appears to be mediated by the presence of glutathione (GSH), which is present at high levels in the liver and in red blood cells as well as other cells (20). Because of the lack of equilibrium between chromium in plasma and red blood cells, blood levels of chromium will tend to be higher than tissue levels. Consequently, blood levels cannot be used as an indicator of total body burden of chromium.

Preparations of rat liver microsomes also are effective in reducing chromium(VI) to chromium(III). This has been observed in studies of the bacterial mutagenicity of various chromium compounds. Preparations of rat liver microsomes (as well as GSH, ascorbic acid, and red blood cell lysates) effectively inhibited the mutagenicity of chromium(VI) compounds by reducing chromium(VI) to chromium(III). Microsome preparations from lung or muscle tissue were not able to deactivate chromium(VI) mutagenicity (21). Similar observations have been made by other investigators (5).

Isolated rat liver mitochondria can rapidly accumulate chromium(VI). The mitochondria are apparently able to accumulate and trap chromium(VI) by first reducing chromium(VI) to chromium(III) and subsequently binding chromium(III) to proteins. Chromium(III) was taken up to a much lower degree than chromium(VI) due to its limited ability to cross cellular membranes. The presence of glutathione (GSH) in the incubation medium reduced the mitochondrial uptake of both chromium(III) and chromium(VI) (22).

4.6 Kinetics—General Impressions

Based on studies in both humans and animals, it is reasonable to assume that, at most, only 5% of an orally administered dose of chromium(VI) is absorbed, whereas chromium(III) is essentially nonabsorbable. This probably represents an overestimate of the actual absorbed amount of chromium(VI) since it may be absorbed less than this as a result of reduction of chromium(VI) to chromium(III) by acidic gastric juice. Following absorption, chromium(VI) binds to red blood cells and other plasma proteins. Chromium(VI) that actually enters the red blood cells is reduced to chromium(III), where it remains unavailable for transfer to other tissues. Most of the chromium that is not sequestered in the red blood cells is subsequently transferred to other organs, with the greatest retention by the liver, spleen, and bone marrow.

Oral exposure does not result in significant retention by the lung. Liver microsomes, but not microsomes from lung or muscle, also are capable of reducing chromium(VI) to chromium(III) although the degree of conversion is unclear. Liver mitochondria can also accumulate significant quantities of chromium(VI), which would make it unavailable to interact with other parts of the cell. Estimated half-lives for orally administered chromium(III) and chromium(VI) are 92 and 22 days, respectively, in humans. At the levels of chromium compounds to which humans may be exposed environmentally, the steady-state levels are not significant or hazardous in spite of the half-life.

5 TOXICITY OF CHROMIUM

5.1 Acute Toxicity

The acute oral toxicity of chromium(III) compounds is very low. Some oral LD_{50} values for the rat are: chromic chloride, 1.87 g/kg; chromium accetate, 11.26 g/kg; and chromium nitrate, 3.25 g/kg. The oral LD_{50} for chromium trioxide in mice and rats is 135–177 mg/kg and 80–114 mg/kg, respectively (5).

The acute oral toxicity of chromium(VI) is somewhat greater than that of chromium(III). Oral administration of high doses results in gastric corrosion due to the ability of chromium(VI) to oxidize tissue. The oral LD_{50} of sodium dichromate in humans has been reported to be 50 mg/kg (5). There do not appear to be any relevant (i.e., oral dosing) studies of acute toxicity of chromium(VI) in animals. Studies in which chromium compounds were administered by a variety of other routes indicate that the kidney is the primary target organ for toxicity, with lesser effects noted in the liver and brain (5).

5.2   Chronic Toxicity

Orally administered chromium compounds failed to demonstrate any significant toxicity in a number of chronic studies. Ivankovic and Preussmann (23) observed no toxic or carcinogenic effects after subacute and chronic oral administration to rats of high doses of chromic oxide [chromium(III)] pigment. In this study, the chromium compound was administered in the feed to both male and female rats at concentrations of 1, 2, or 5% of the diet for 2 years. There were no signs of chronic toxicity and body weights of the treated animals were not significantly different from controls. No histologic postmortem findings could be attributed to treatment with the chromium compound.

In a subacute study (90 days), the only striking observation was a dose-dependent reduction in the weights of the liver and spleen (23). These reductions in organ weights were not associated with any histological or pathological changes. Also in the 90-day study, no differences were noted between treated and control animals in red and white blood cells counts, hemoglobin levels, blood serum protein and sugar levels, or blood, sugar, protein, bilirubin, or sediment in the urine.

In another chronic study, MacKenzie et al. (11) administered potassium chromate [chromium(VI)] to rats in drinking water at concentrations of 0, 0.45, 2.2, 4.5, 7.7, 11.0, and 25 ppm for 1 year. Another group of rats also was given chromium chloride [chromium(III)] in drinking water at 25 ppm. In microscopic studies of the spleen, kidneys, liver, and bone, no significant changes were found that could be associated with exposure to any dose level of chromium. There were also no differences between these groups and controls with respect to body weight, food and water consumption, or blood analyses.

Groups of dogs were treated chronically with potassium chromate [chromium(VI)] in drinking water for 4 years at concentrations of 0.45, 2.25, 4.5, 6.75, and 11.2 ppm (24). None of the groups of dogs differed from controls with respect to weight, food consumption, growth rate, organ weights (liver, spleen, and kidney), urine analysis (albumin, acetone, bile pigments, glucose, and red blood cells), and blood analyses (hemoglobin, red blood cells, white blood cells, and differential white counts).

Schroeder and Mitchener (25) administered 5 ppm of an unspecified chromium(VI) compound in the drinking water of mice from weaning until natural death. They noted a decreased growth rate based on body weight for some time intervals measured during the course of the study, but these decreases were not consistent in all measured intervals. The female mice exhibited more of the weight decrements than the males. There were no differences from the controls in either mortality or survival. Malignant tumors were noted in the animals exposed to chromium (27.6%), however, the incidence of tumors in the controls was nearly identical (26.8%).

The statistical sensitivity is greatly reduced in studies in which the tumor incidence in controls is as high as observed by Schroeder and Mitchener (25). Even if the tumor incidence in the controls were greatly lower than the 26.8% observed, a difference in milignant tumors between treated and control animals of 0.8% only could be distinguished from chance in a study involving thousands of animals. Despite this, Hammond and Beliles (26) reported that the incidences of malignant tumors in the study by Schroeder and Mitchener (25) were slightly elevated. Given the statistical power of the study, the incidences in treated and control animals are indistinguishable.

Kanisawa and Schroeder (27) administered chromium(III) acetate to rats for their lifetimes at 5 ppm in the drinking water. Compared to controls, there were no significant differences in either spontaneous tumors or malignant tumors in any organ. Also, there were no differences in growth rates or survival between the animals exposed to chromium and the controls.

Gross and Heller (28) performed a chronic (10 months) oral toxicity study using mice, rats, and rabbits. The mice received potassium chromate [chromium(VI)] in the drinking water at levels of 100, 200, 300, 400, and 500 ppm. Another group of mice received zinc chromate [chromium(VI)] in their diet at 1%. The general health of all animals was normal and no abnormal characteristics were noted.

In young rats, no effects were noted at 300 ppm, but there was a slight roughness of the coat at 500 ppm (28). There were no adverse effects in the rats at dietary levels of 0.125%, but a general deterioration in their fur and subnormal general condition were observed at 0.25% in the diet. At higher levels in the diet (0.5 and 1%), their general condition was reported as subnormal with diarrhea, and sterility was reported.

Dietary administration of zinc chromate led to somewhat more severe toxicity at comparable levels in the diet than did potassium chromate (28). The utilization of food by rabbits at 500 ppm was unaffected. The authors concluded that for rats the maximum nontoxic level of chromium(VI) in drinking water is 500 ppm.

5.3   Toxicity—General Impressions

The acute oral toxicity of both chromium(III) and chromium(VI) is very low. Chronic oral studies have also indicated that neither valence state of chromium is associated with any appreciable toxicity. While several studies have indicated that chromium(VI) appears to be absorbed to a greater extent than chromium(III), there is no evidence that increased concentrations of chromium in the liver, kidney, spleen, or bone are associated with any adverse effects. One inadequate chronic study indicated that chromium(VI) in the diet at a concentration of 0.25% produced weight loss and a generalized subnormal condition in rats. No adverse effects were observed when chromium(VI) was present in the drinking water at a concentration of 500 ppm.

5.4   Carcinogenicity

Inhalation of chromium compounds is associated with lung cancer in humans (5, 29). The carcinogenicity of these compounds is directly related to the route of exposure and the solubility of the compound. The evidence for a carcinogenic effect is based on several epidemiological studies (29), which clearly establish a high risk of lung cancer from occupational exposure to chromium compounds in various chromate plants in the United States and Great Britain.

The identity of the specific compounds responsible for the noted effects is unknown, although it is assumed that the chromium compounds involved are predominantly insoluble chromium(VI) compounds. The conclusions of IARC (29, p. 119) are relevant:

> There is an excessive risk of lung cancer among workers in the chromate-producing industry. It is likely that exposure to one or more chromium compounds is responsible, but the identity of this or these is not known. There is no evidence that non-occupational exposure to chromium constitutes a cancer hazard.

In experimental animals, chromium(III) compounds have not produced lung tumors after inhalation, intratracheal instillation, or intrapleural implantation (5, 29). Similarly, chromium(VI) compounds administered by inhalation or intratracheal instillation were not carcinogenic in experimental animals. Some chromium(VI) compounds have produced tumors following intrabronchial or intrapleural implantation, although limitations in these studies make it difficult to draw conclusions about the carcinogenic potency of these compounds. Some chromium(VI) compounds are carcinogenic following subcutaneous injection, although implantation site tumors have only been demonstrated consistently after intramuscular implantation (5). The chromium compounds (calcium chromate, chromic chromate, zinc chromate, and strontium chromate) that have produced tumors following the above routes are either insoluble or slightly soluble in aqueous solutions.

Based on epidemiological evidence, the International Agency for Research on Cancer (IARC) has determined that there is "sufficient" evidence for the carcinogenicity of chromium in humans. The evidence for carcinogenicity in animals is also "sufficient." However, IARC accepts data from routes of exposure that are not normally encountered. Consequently, the animal data that are judged to be sufficient are based on injection or implantation studies. All such routes of administration are designed to deliver a much higher dose of a chemical to a potentially susceptible population of cells than would be delivered by more conventional routes of exposure. In short-term tests, IARC classifies the evidence as sufficient for chromium(VI) compounds, but inadequate for chromium(III) compounds (29, 30).

5.4.1 Carcinogenicity—General Impressions.
Chromium(VI) and chromium(III) are not carcinogenic following oral ingestion. IARC reviewed only two oral ingestion studies when it reached its original conclusion. Schroeder et al. (31, 32) observed no adverse effects when mice and rats received 5 ppm of a chromium(III) compound in drinking water for life. These studies were considered by IARC to be inadequate because the dose levels were low. Additional chronic ingestion studies reviewed in this analysis either were available in the literature, but not reviewed by IARC, or were published after the IARC report. In addition, very little of the extensive information on metabolism was available to IARC at the time of its review.

The results of intramuscular or intrapleural implantation studies are of questionable relevance in assessing potential human risks following oral exposures to chromium compounds. Microsomes isolated from muscle and lung are not capable of reducing chromium(VI) to chromium(III), although microsomes isolated from the liver are capable of such a reduction.

5.5 Mutagenicity

Mutagenicity tests generally are used to estimate the potential for a chemical to produce cancer through a genetic mechanism. The tests are suggestive, and not predictive, because there are instances of both false positives and false negatives. While the evidence from such tests is presumptive, there is rather good correlation between the results of a battery of such in vitro tests and the results of long-term feeding studies in animals. The following brief discussion divides the evidence for the mutagenicity of various chromium compounds into the results from tests on mammalian cells and bacterial test systems.

5.5.1   Mammalian Test Systems.

As compared to tests in bacterial test systems, the results of mutagenicity testing in mammalian in vitro test systems may approximate more closely a mammalian in vivo situation, because of the greater similarity between the cell types. Both valence states of chromium have been shown to induce various kinds of mutational events in a number of in vitro mammalian test systems.

Both 0.1 M chromium(III) and chromium(VI) can interact and bind with RNA and DNA, producing a variety of intramolecular cross-links and other effects (33). In human lymphocytes tested in vitro there was a dose-dependent increase in the frequency of sister chromatid exchanges (SCEs) induced by chromium(VI), with a 2.5-fold increase observed with 10^{-5} M potassium chromate. Chromium(III) was inactive at all concentrations tested (34). Chromium(VI), but not chromium(III), produced chromosomal aberrations and morphological transformation in hamster embryonic cells (35). The effects were reduced by the addition of a reducing agent, which presumably converted the chromium(VI) to chromium(III).

Other studies also demonstrate that chromium(VI) compounds were capable of producing cytotoxicity, chromosomal aberrations, and clastogenic effects (SCE) in cultured hamster cell lines (35). Chromium(III) compounds, while cytotoxic only at extremely high concentrations, were unable to induce SCE but did induce chromosomal aberrations (36). Additional cytogenetic effects observed in other in vitro systems as a result of treatment with chromium(VI) compounds include infidelity of DNA replication in vitro (37), stimulation of DNA repair synthesis in mammalian cell cultures (38), and in vitro cell transformation (39). It has been suggested that for many, if not all, of the observed genotoxic effects, chromium(III) actually may be the predominant intracellular chromium species as a result of the rapid reduction of absorbed chromium(VI) by intracellular components.

5.5.2   Bacterial Test Systems.

A number of bacterial in vitro mutagenicity tests have been conducted with both chromium(III) and chromium(VI) compounds. The most striking characteristic of all these tests, using a variety of bacterial test systems, is the lack of mutagenic activity in the presence of a metabolic activating system that is able to convert chromium(VI) to chromium(III).

The mutagenicity of a variety of chromium(VI) compounds has been tested in *S. typhimurium*, the *B. subtilis* rec-assay, *E. coli*, and *S. cerevisiae* and all were mutagenic in the absence of microsomes prepared from rat liver (S-9 mix) (5, 21, 40–42). However, the mutagenicity was abolished in the presence of S-9 mix prepared from rat liver or in the presence of various complexing or chelating agents. Little or no loss of mutagenicity occurred when the S-9 mix added to the plates was prepared from lung or muscle tissue. Chromium(III) compounds were nonmutagenic (5, 21, 41, 42). The activities of chromium(III) in these tests always were considerably less than chromium(VI). Thus, although some mutagenic activity is associated with both valence states of chromium, the vast majority of activity in in vitro bacterial test systems is associated with chromium(VI) (5).

5.5.3 Conclusion. In studies with mammalian cells, both chromium(VI) and chromium(III) have demonstrated mutagenic effects in addition to other indicators of DNA damage. In general, chromium(VI) is more active than chromium(III) in these in vitro test systems. While chromium(VI) has consistently demonstrated positive mutagenicity in a number of bacterial in vitro test systems, this mutagenicity always has been seen in the absence of a metabolic activation system. In the presence of a metabolic activation system (S-9 mix) prepared from mammalian liver cells, the mutagenic activity of chromium(VI) disappears. A plausible explanation for these observations is that the liver enzymes are able to reduce chromium(VI) to chromium(III), which shows little, if any, mutagenic activity in any bacterial test system. It also may be significant that metabolic activation systems prepared from either lung or muscle tissue do not cause the mutagenic activity to disappear.

5.6 Reproductive Effects

The review of reproductive effects includes teratogenicity, sterility, growth retardation, and other adverse birth outcomes as well as the ability of chromium to cross the placental barrier. However, effects observed in conjunction with maternal toxicity are discounted because the appearance of maternal toxicity tends to compromise the possible attribution of teratogenic effects to the agent, since adverse fetal effects are a well-known consequence of maternal toxicity. As previously noted, chromium does not readily cross the placenta and virtually no orally ingested chromium reaches the fetus.

Gross and Heller (28) administered potassium chromate [chromium(VI)] to both mice and rats at levels up to 500 ppm in drinking water, and both potassium chromate and zinc chromate in the diet at levels up to 1%. No adverse reproductive effects were observed in mice. Sterility was reported in rats after administration of potassium chromate at levels of 0.5 and 1% in the diet and after administration of all doses of zinc chromate (0.125, 0.25, 0.5, and 1% of the diet). These findings are difficult to interpret because of the lack of detail in the article. Neither the sex of the animals in which sterility occurred nor the incidence in the various dose groups was reported. The article contained no report of histopathological examination, and it is not possible to determine the nature of the sterility because stunted growth and other overt signs of toxicity were reported at most of the doses at which sterility occurred.

Ivankovic and Preussmann (23) administered chromic oxide, a chromium(III) pigment compound, to male and female rats in the diet at concentrations of 2 and 5% for 90 days. Mating was permitted following 60 days on these diets. All the females became pregnant, the gestation period was normal, and the young showed no malformations or adverse effects. The litter sizes also were normal. Some of the offspring were retained for lifetime observation, and after 600 days no tumors or other pathologies were observed.

A number of studies have demonstrated the capacity of chromium salts to produce a variety of fetal malformations, including cleft palate, hydrocephaly, and skeletal defects (5). In all studies in which these effects were observed, concurrent maternal toxicity was also observed. No adverse fetal effects occurred in studies in which maternal toxicity was not observed. This strongly indicates that the observed fetal malformations are indirectly induced by maternal toxicity and are not due to any direct teratogenic effects of the chromium. Furthermore, in these studies, chromic oxide (chromium(III)], was administered by routes (intravenous, intraperitoneal, and subcutaneous) that probably would lead to higher blood concentrations than could be achieved by ingestion.

5.6.1   Conclusion. Studies on placental transfer indicate that very little chromium(VI) or chromium (III), administered either intravenously or orally, crosses the placenta. The weight of the evidence demonstrates that chromium compounds are not associated with adverse reproductive effects. Only one dated and poorly documented study suggests any potential adverse reproductive effects from ingestion of chromium(VI). However, the sterility reported among rats (sex unstated) in this study is accompanied by apparent concurrent toxicity, and it is more than likely that the sterility was due to malnutrition.

5.7   Dermal Effects

Various chromium compounds have been implicated in causing allergic dermatitis associated with varying degrees of eczema (5). In almost all cases, the contact with the chromium compounds was associated with occupational exposure. Dermal sensitivity results from an initial occupational exposure that triggers an allergic reaction, and subsequent exposure in sensitive individuals produces symptoms. The confirmation of sensitization to chromium usually is made by patch tests on the skin of subjects with a known or suspected chromium sensitivity. The concentrations of chromium that are employed in the patch tests range from 0.005% to as high as 2% (5).

Although chromium can produce sensitivity and contact dermatitis in humans (43, 44), virtually all the evidence is based on occupational exposure to high levels of dusts and fumes. Once an individual is sensitized, subsequent exposures are able to produce varying degrees of contact dermatitis. The levels of exposure used in patch tests to produce overt symptoms in sensitive individuals are much higher than the levels that are likely to occur in contaminated groundwater (45). Although comparisons of this type are speculative, there is no evidence that dermal sensitization can result from primary exposure to the levels that would be encountered in contaminated groundwater.

6   POTENTIAL EXPOSURE TO CONTAMINATED GROUNDWATER

The population that could be exposed to chromium included residents to the south of the large basin near the area where a private well was found to contain chromium at a concentration of 0.17 mg/L. A second group of residents to the southwest of the site also had the potential to be exposed to chromium above the level of the drinking water standard. This was indicated by the measurement of chromium at a concentration of 0.18 mg/L from a test well at the southwest corner of the industrial site. The total number of residents in the potentially exposed population was probably no more than 100 people.

Not all of the potentially exposed population would be expected to be exposed to equal levels of chromium because, like most plumes, there was a concentration gradient with distance from the basin. The highest chromium concentration measured in groundwater at the industrial site was 0.37 mg/L (adjacent to the basin). As a worst-case estimate it was assumed that the maximum concentration of chromium measured in a test well at the site (0.37 mg/L) was the level of exposure in the exposed population. This concentration was considered as a maximum average concentration in highly exposed individuals over their entire lifetime.

It was assumed that exposed individuals consume 2 L/day of drinking water (7) and that all the drinking water contained chromium, even though some drinking water will normally come from non-chromium-bearing sources (e.g., individuals who worked away from the home). It is not known whether this concentration is representative of past concentrations or of future concentrations. On the other hand, some extremely active individuals in the population may consume more than 2 L/day of water on a daily basis. Furthermore, this amount may increase in the summer months and decrease in the winter months, but as suggested by the National Academy of Sciences (7), 2 L/day is a reasonable composite figure for water consumption over a lifetime.

Thus, the chromium dose to the exposed population, assuming an average weight of 70 kg/person, would be

$$0.37\,mg/L \cdot lifetime \times 2\,L/day \times 1/70\,kg = 0.011\,mg/kg \cdot day \text{ over a lifetime.}$$

The dose was expressed in mg/kg·lifetime because it is the most commonly used scaling factor for equivalence between human and animal doses, especially for agents that are not metabolized to a toxic species.

In evaluating the risks that specific substances might present to humans, it is important to determine whether the exposed populations have any characteristics that render them particularly susceptible to certain health effects (46). Thus, as discussed in the section above concerning the fate of chromium in organisms, because chromium(VI) is absorbed to a greater degree when gastric juices are avoided, any persons with reduced gastric acidity or impaired gastric juices—including individuals with ulcers or other gastric disorders—may be more susceptible to increased absorption of chromium. Persons with pernicious anemia have reduced gastric acidity and may be a more susceptible population. Also, because fasting decreases the flow of gastric juices and gastric acidity, a person who fasts for extended periods may also be susceptible to increased absorption. Extended treatment with antacids or systemic medications may decrease stomach acidity. In the case of antacids, however, the question of susceptibility is complicated because sodium-based antacids tend to induce a hyperacidity response, whereas other antacids may do so to a far lesser extent (47). Potentially susceptible populations of these types were not accounted for in the risk assessment.

Finally, a number of groups may have a chromium deficiency. These include the elderly, children, pregnant women, diabetics, siblings and children of diabetics, and individuals on low-chromium diets. However, because the bioavailability of chromium(VI) is low, it is not clear whether ingestion of drinking water containing chromium would have beneficial effects on individuals with a chromium deficiency.

7 POTENTIAL HEALTH RISKS

The evaluation of the possible risks to health associated with ingestion of water containing chromium at the levels found is complex. Despite extensive laboratory and field measurements concerning chromium levels, and considerable experimental and human evidence on potential toxicity, the available data do not permit quantitative estimates to be made with a high degree of confidence. Much of the data are derived from inappropriate routes of exposure, are outdated, or have other limitations. Therefore, in order to assess potential risks, it has been necessary to make a number of reasonable assumptions. Insofar as possible, these assumptions are explicitly delineated.

To evaluate potential risks, the exposure of specific populations is combined with the data on the dose–response relations for each type of toxicity. This comparison allows a judgment to be made about the probability that a specific effects will be observed in an exposed population. Because no demonstrable adverse effect has been observed as a result of adequate studies in either humans or experimental animals from the ingestion of either chromium(VI) or chromium(III), it is difficult to evaluate the risks. For cancer, risk evaluations are usually based on extrapolations from doses that produced tumors to doses that are presumed to represent an acceptable risk. However, the data on the carcinogenicity of chromium following oral ingestion do not permit this approach, nor are they warranted, since they are all negative.

To evaluate noncarcinogenic risks, the traditional approach has been to select the lowest no-observed-effect level (NOEL) from either human or experimental animal exposure data and apply a safety (or uncertainty) factor to this dose to derive a "safe" level of exposure for humans. The safety factor is usually 10, 100, or 1000, depending on the degree of confidence in the animal data (7). In this assessment the safety factor (or margin of safety) was calculated from the lowest dose that produces a particular effect in an experimental animal compared with the anticipated exposure of humans from the drinking water.

7.1 Cancer

Chromium(III) compounds are mutagenic in in vitro mammalian test systems, but not in in vitro bacterial test systems (5). Mutagenicity often is correlated with carcinogenicity, but the definitive test of carcinogenicity is achieved through evaluating the results of lifetime studies in animals. Although the mutagenicity of chromium(III) suggests that chromium(III) may be carcinogenic, this possibility seems remote in light of the results of the chronic study by Ivankovic and Preussmann (23).

While the evidence for carcinogenicity of chromium(VI) by inhalation in humans is substantial, the data on the metabolism of chromium(VI) appear to explain the absence of carcinogenic effects by ingestion and the carcinogenicity of chromium(VI) by inhalation or administered to the lungs or injected into muscle (5, 9, 29).

Even if chromium(VI) were carcinogenic following oral exposure—and there is no evidence to support this—a sufficient quantity must reach a susceptible cell population in order to initiate the carcinogenic process. Chromium(III) is essentially not absorbed, and a large proportion of ingested chromium(VI) will be reduced to chromium(III) by gastric juices (10). Virtually all of the amount of chromium(VI) that is absorbed will be taken up by red blood cells and other plasma proteins (20). Chromium(VI) readily crosses the red blood cell membrane where most or all of it then is reduced to chromium(III) in the cell. Chromium(III) is bound to macromolecules in the cell and thus is unable to leave. In addition, chromium(III), but not chromium(VI), has a strong tendency to complex with organic ligands, including proteins, to form chemical complexes or insoluble polynuclear species with extracellular components (5, 40). This further reduces the amount of chromium(VI) available to other cells.

The small amount of chromium(VI) that is not tightly bound in blood will first pass through the liver, which contains microsomal enzymes that have been shown to be able to reduce chromium(VI) to chromium(III) (5, 48). Liver mitochondria have been shown to accumulate chromium(VI) rapidly with subsequent reduction to chromium(III) (22). This would leave even less chromium(VI) available to pass into the nucleus of susceptible cells to interact with DNA and related materials involved in mutagenicity and the possible induction of cancer.

In summary, although it cannot be proved conclusively that chromium(VI) or chromium(III) is not carcinogenic when ingested, there is no experimental evidence to suggest that chromium(III) or chromium(VI) is carcinogenic when ingested. Furthermore, the totality of the evidence concerning absorption and metabolism offers a plausible explanation for the absence of carcinogenic effects of chromium following ingestion.

7.2 Reproductive Impairment

Gross and Heller (28) have published the only study that presents even equivocal evidence of possible reproductive effects due to chromium exposure. Sterility was reported in rats following administration of a chromium(VI) compound at doses as low as 0.125% of the diet. As previously noted, neither the sex of the sterile animals nor the nature of the sterility was reported, although it was most likely secondary to starvation. While this is not a convincing study of reproductive impairment, a margin of safety between the lowest reported effective dose observed in this study and the highest anticipated residential exposure can be calculated.

At 0.125% of the diet over a lifetime, rats in the Gross and Heller study were consuming chromium(VI) at a daily rate of approximately

$$1.25 \times 10.3 \times 20 \, \text{g food/day} = 0.025 \, \text{g} \quad \text{or} \quad 25 \, \text{mg Cr(VI)/day.}$$

Considering the average weight of the rats was about 200 g, or 0.20 kg, their daily dose was

$$\frac{25 \, \text{mg/day}}{0.20 \, \text{kg}} = 125 \, \text{mg/kg·day.}$$

The equivalent dose for the potentially exposed residents was 0.011 mg/kd·day. The safety factor (or margin of safety) between the lowest effective dose that was reported to induce sterility in the animals and the highest potential exposure in residents is

$$\frac{125}{0.011} = 11,000 + .$$

This is a considerable margin of safety because the dose–response curves for reproductive hazards tend to be steep; that is, the effects, if observed, will tend to occur in a narrow range of doses (49). Even if there are specially susceptible individuals in the population, the margin of safety is more than adequate. While it is recognized that most evaluations of this type rely upon the no-observed-effect level (NOEL), this was not available. However, the margin of safety derived from the lowest-observed-effect level (LOEL) is so large that the probability of reproductive effects from exposure is virtually zero.

7.3 Other Toxicities

Because no chronic studies have demonstrated unequivocal target organ toxicities for chromium, it is difficult to estimate the margin of safety for such toxicity. However, the approach taken by the EPA in determining water quality criteria can be adapted for this purpose (9). It is the EPA's policy that chronic studies do not establish a no-effect-level for any type of target organ toxicity. Therefore, the EPA used the maximum tested doses to estimate the minimum effective doses. For chromium(VI), this dose was 2.5 mg/kg·day administered over a lifetime, based on the study by MacKenzie et al. (11) in which rats were administered chromium(VI) in drinking water at 25 ppm. The margin of safety between a *clearly nontoxic dose* and the maximum estimated exposure to contaminated groundwater can be calculated as

$$\frac{2.5 \, \text{mg/kg·day}}{0.011 \, \text{mg/kg·day}} = 220.$$

If the 2.5 mg/kg·day were associated with some toxicity, this margin of safety could arguably be considered insufficiently protective. However, because the dose used represents a clearly nontoxic one, it is more than adequate.

The Gross and Heller (28) study also may be used to identify a minimum effective dose. They administered potassium chromate in drinking water to rats to doses up to 500 ppm for a period of 10 months. Because chromium(VI) does not accumulate in the body, 500 ppm in drinking water for 10 months is approximately equivalent to a lifetime (24 months) dose approximately 200 ppm (e.g., 200 mg/L of potassium chromate in drinking water). The rats in this experiment weighed approximately 250 g and would be expected to drink approximately 25 mL/day. This corresponds to a lifetime average daily dose of

$$200 \, \text{mg/L} \times \frac{0.025 \, \text{L/day}}{0.25 \, \text{kg}} = 20 \, \text{mg/kg·day}.$$

The margin of safety is therefore

$$\frac{20 \, \text{mg/kg·day}}{0.011 \, \text{mg/kg·day}} = 1800.$$

This margin of safety appears to be a better descriptor of the true margin of safety than the 220 value. The highest safety factor that is usually applied to equivocal animal data when estimating a safe dose for humans is 1000 (7, 46).

7.4   Conclusions

A critical review and analysis of chromium toxicity revealed an insignificant degree of risk for adverse health effects associated with consumption of drinking water containing chromium at the highest detected level at this site. This analysis demonstrated that there was a sufficient margin of safety between the highest detected level and the levels that might be anticipated to produce adverse health effects.

Based on several negative feeding studies in addition to compelling biochemical, metabolic, and physiological considerations, chromium(III) or chromium(VI) does not appear to pose a cancer risk following ingestion. Consequently, no cancer risk estimates are needed or even possible. The EPA's Office of Drinking Water most recent evaluation of the available data reached a similar conclusion: "since chromium has not been shown to be carcinogenic through ingestion exposure, the compound will be regulated based upon chronic toxicity data" (4). The margins of safety calculated for reproductive and other toxic effects suggest a de minimus level of risk associated with the concentrations of chromium detected near the site. The insignificant risk associated with the degree of contamination was reflected in the EPA's recent decision to raise the recommended maximum contaminant level (RMCL) for chromium [total chromium(III) and chromium(VI)] in drinking water from 0.05 to 0.12 mg/L (4).

REFERENCES

1. J. W. Grishan (Ed.), *Health Aspects of the Disposal of Waste Chemicals.* Pergamon, Oxford, 1986.

2. S. M. Pier and K. M. Bang, The role of heavy metals in human health. In N. M. Trief, Ed., *Environment and Health.* Ann Arbor Sci. Publ., Ann Arbor, MI, 1980, Chap. 11.

3. F. M. Sunderman, Jr., Mechanisms of metal carcinogenesis. *Biol. Trace Elem. Res.* **1**, 63–86 (1979).

4. Environmental Protection Agency, National primary drinking water regulations; Synthetic organic chemicals, inorganic chemicals and microorganisms. Proposed rulemaking. *Fed. Regist.* 50(219), 46966–7 (1985).

5. U.S. Environmental Protection Agency, *Health Assessment Document for Chromium* (rev. draft). Environmental Criteria and Assessment Office, USEPA, Research Triangle Park, NC, 1983.

6. W. Mertz, Chromium occurrence and function in biological systems. *Physiol. Rev.* **49**, 163–239 (1969).

7. National Academy of Sciences, *Drinking Water and Health*, Vol. 1. NAS, Washington, DC, 1977.

8. National Academy of Sciences, *Drinking Water and Health*, Vol. 3. National Academy Press, Washington, DC, 1980.

9. U.S. Environmental Protection Agency, *Ambient Water Quality Criteria for Chromium*, NTIS No. PB81-117467. USEPA, Washington, DC. 1980.

10. R. M. Donaldson and R. F. Barreras, Intestinal absorption of trace quantities of chromium. *J. Lab. Clin. Med.* **68**, 484–493 (1966).

11. R. D. Mackenzie, R. U., Byerrum, C. F. Decker, C. A. Hoppert, and R. F. Langham, Chronic toxicity studies. II. Hexavalent and trivalent chromium administered in drinking water to rats. *AMA Arch. Ind. Health* **18**, 232–234 (1958).

12. Y. Sayato, K. Nakamuro, S. Matsui, and M. Ando, Metabolic fate of chromium compounds. I. Comparative behaviour of chromium in rat administered with Na_2CrO_4 and $CrCl_3$. *J. Pharm. Dyn.* **3**, 17–23 (1980).

13. R. D. Mackenzie, R. A. Anwar, R. U. Byerrum, and C. A. Hoppert, Absorption and distribution of Cr in the albino rat. *Arch. Biochem. Biophys.* **79**, 200–205 (1959).

14. M. H. Samitz and S. Gross, Effects of hexavalent and trivalent chromium compounds on the skin. *Arch. Dermatol.* **84**, 94–99 (1961).

15. B. B. Dutkiewicz, Absorption of hexavalent chromium by skin in man. *Arch. Toxicol.* **47**, 47–50 (1981).

16. J.E. Wahlberg and E. Skog, Percutaneous absorption of trivalent and hexavalent chromium. *Arch. Dermatol.* **92**, 315–318 (1965).

17. J. W. H. Mali, Some aspects of the behavior of chromium compounds in the skin. *J. Invest. Dermatol.* **41**, 111–122 (1963).

18. W. J. Visek, I. B. Whitney, U. S. G. Kuhn, III, and C. L. Comer, Metabolism of Cr-51 by animals as influenced by chemical state. *Proc. Soc. Exp. Biol. Med.* **84**, 610–615 (1953).

19. B. Dannielsson, E. Hassoun, and L. Dencker, Placental transport of chromium (Cr) and its effects on cartilage formation. *Teratology* **26**, 47 (abstr.) (1982).

20. J. Aaseth, J. Alexander, and T. Norseth, Uptake of (51) Cr-chromate by human erythrocytes— A role of glutathione. *Acta Pharmacol. Toxical.* **50**, 310–315 (1982).

21. F. L. Petrilli and S. DeFlora, Metabolic deactivation of hexavalent chromium mutagenicity. *Mutat. Res.* **54**, 139–147 (1978).

22. J. Alexander, J. Aaseth, and T. Norseth, Uptake of chromium by rat liver mitochondria. *Toxicology* **24**, 115–122 (1982).

23. S. Ivankovic and R. Preussmann, Absence of toxic and carcinogenic effects after administration of high doses of chromic oxide pigment in subacute and long-term feeding experiments in rats. *Food Cosmet. Toxicol.* **13**, 347–351 (1975).

24. R. A. Anwar, R. F. Langham. C. A. Hoppert, B. V. Alfredson, and R. U. Byerrum, Chronic toxicity studies. III. Chronic toxicity of cadmium and chromium in dogs. *Arch. Environ. Health* **3**, 92–96 (1961).

25. H. A. Schroeder and M. Mitchener, Scandium, chromium(VI), gallium, yttrium, rhodium, palladium, indium in mice: Effects on growth and life span. *J. Nutr.* **101**, 1431–1438 (1971).

26. P. B. Hammond and R. P. Beliles, Metals. In J. Doull, C. D. Klaassen, and M. O. Amdur, Eds., *Casarett and Doull's Toxicology: The Basic Science of Poisons*, 2nd ed. Macmillan, New York, 1980, Chap. 17.

27. M. Kanisawa and H. S. Schroeder, Life term studies on the effect of trace elements on spontaneous tumors in mice and rats. *Cancer Res.* **29**; 892–895 (1969).

28. W. G. Gross and V. G. Heller, Chromates in animal nutrition. *J. Ind. Hyg. Toxicol.* **28**, 52–56 (1945).

29. International Agency for Research on Cancer, *IARC Monographs on the Evaluation of Carcinogenic Risk of Chemicals to Man. Some Inorganic and Organometallic Compounds*, Vol. 2. IARC, Lyon, 1972.

30. International Agency for Research on Cancer, *IARC Monographs on the Evaluation of Carcinogenic Risk of Chemicals to Humans. Chemicals, Industrial Processes and Industries Associated with Cancer in Humans*, IARC Monogr., Vols 1–29, IARC Monogr. Suppl. 4. IARC, Lyon, 1982.

31. H. A. Schroeder, J. J. Balassa, and W. H. Vinton, Chromium, lead, cadmium, nickel and titanium in mice: Effect on mortality, tumors and tissue levels. *J. Nutr.* **83**, 239 (1964).

32. H. A. Schroeder, J. J. Balassa, and W. H. Vinton, Chromium, cadmium and lead in rates: Effects on lifespan, tumors and tissue levels. *J. Nutr.* **86**, 51 (1965).

33. G. Tamino, L. Peretta, and A. G. Levis, Effects of trivalent and hexavalent chromium on the physiochemical properties of mammalian cell nucleic acids and synthetic polynucleotides. *Chem. Biol. Interact.* **37**, 309–319 (1981).

34. M. Stella, A. Montaldi, R. Rossi, G. Rossi, and A. G. Levis, Clastogenic effects of chromium on human lymphocytes in vitro and in vivo. *Mutat. Res.* **101**, 151–164 (1982).

35. H. Tsuda and K. Kato, Chromosomal aberrations and morphological transformation in hamster embryonic cells treated with potassium dichromate in vitro. *Mutat. Res.* **46**, 87–94 (1977).

36. A. G. Levis and F. Majone, Cytotoxic and clastogenic effects of soluble chromium compounds on mammalian cell cultures. *Br. J. Cancer* **40**, 523–533 (1979).

37. M. A Sirova and L. A. Loeb, Infidelity of DNA synthesis *in vitro*: Screening for potential metal mutagens or carcinogens. *Science* **194**, 1434–1436 (1976).

38. A. G. Levis, V. Bianchi, G. Tamino, and B. Pegoraro, Effects of potassium dichromate on nucleic acid and protein synthesis and on precursor uptake in BHK fibroblasts. *Cancer Res.* **38**, 110–116 (1978).

39. A. Fradkin, A. Janoff, B. P. Lsane, and M. Kuschner, *In vitro* transformation of BHK 21 cells grown in the presence of calcium chromate. *Cancer Res.* **35**, 1058–1063 (1975).

40. J. M. Gentile, K. Hyde, and J. Schubert, Chromium genotoxicity as influenced by complexation and rate effects. *Toxicol. Lett.* **7**, 439–489 (1981).

41. W. Lofroth, The mutagenicity of hexavalent chromium is decreased by microsomal metabolism. *Naturwissenschaften* **65**, 207–208 (1978).

42. J. E. Gruber and K. W. Jennette, Metabolism of the carcinogen chromate by rat liver microsomes. *Biochem. Biophy. Res. Commun.* **82**, 700–706 (1978).

43. S. Fregert and H. Rorsman, Allergy to trivalent chromium. *Arch. Dermatol.* **90**, 4–6 (1961).

44. S. L. Husain, Contact dermatitis in the west of Scotland. *Contact Dermatitis* **3**, 327–332 (1977).

45. S. Fregert, N. Hjorth, B. Mannusson, H. J. Bandmann, C. D. Calnan, E. Cronin, K. Malten, C. L. Meneghini, V. Pirila, and D. S. Wilkinson, Epidemiology of contact dermatitis. *Trans. St. John's Hosp. Dermatol. Soc.* **55**, 17–35 (1969).

46. E. J. Calabrese, *Principles of Animal Extrapolation.* Wiley, New York, 1983.

47. S. C. Harvey, 1980. Gastric antacids and digestants. In A. E. Gilman, L. S. Goodman, and A. Gilman, Eds., *The Pharmacological Basis of Therapeutics*, 6th ed. Macmillan, New York, 1980, Chap. 42.

48. F. L. Petrilli and S. DeFlora, Toxicity and mutagenicity of hexavalent chromium on *Salmonella typhimurium. Appl. Environ. Microbiol.* **33**, 805–809 (1977).

49. I. C. T. Nisbet and N. J. Karch, *Chemical Hazards to Human Reproduction.* Noyes, Park Ridge, NJ, 1983.

D

ASSESSING AIR CONTAMINANTS

17

Formaldehyde Exposure and Risk in Mobile Homes

R. G. Gammage and C. C. Travis

Health and Safety Research Division, Oak Ridge National Laboratory, Oak Ridge, Tennessee*

1 INTRODUCTION

No one escapes exposure to formaldehyde, either in the air that is breathed or, in the final analysis, at the hands of the embalmer! Furthermore, formaldehyde is produced in the human body as an important intermediary; this endogenous formaldehyde, however, is present in bound form rather than as free formaldehyde. Anthropogenic formaldehyde vapor is ubiquitous to modern residential and nonindustrial, occupational indoor environments. This exogenous formaldehyde enters the body primarily through inhalation, with absorption being primarily in the upper respiratory tract.

During the 1960s there was a rapid rise in the manufacture of formaldehyde; output peaked in 1972 and has remained reasonably constant since that time. Domestic production of formaldehyde in 1987 is estimated at 6.1 billion pounds as a 37% solution (1); future formaldehyde output is forecast to be flat or only slightly up. About half of the total consumption of formaldehyde goes into production of urea, phenol, and melamine formaldehyde resins. Most of these resins are used to produce housing materials such as the pressed-wood products of indoor quality plywood and paneling, particleboard, and medium-density fiberboard that is used mainly for furniture.

Humans have long been exposed to formaldehyde. Formaldehyde was introduced as a disinfectant in 1888. Cigarette smoke contains as much as 40 ppm formaldehyde (2). One can be reasonably sure, however, that the concentrations of formaldehyde in indoor air are now considerably higher than they were prior to World War II; particleboard bonded with urea-formaldehyde (UF) resin was not invented until 1943 (3). It is the UF resins used as adhesives in pressed-wood products that are the major sources of formaldehyde vapor indoors (4). This is especially the case with mobile homes. Mobile homes have high loading factors, exceeding $1 \text{ m}^2/\text{m}^3$ (surface area of pressed-wood products containing UF resin/volume of indoor air). This type of housing tends also to

*Research sponsored by the U.S. Department of Energy, under contract DE-AC05-840R21400 with the Martin Marietta Energy Systems, Inc.

have minimal ventilation and to be more poorly insulated than conventional housing. All these factors contribute to mobile homes being the type of dwelling with the generally highest levels of indoor formaldehyde (5). Thus it is natural to focus health concerns of formaldehyde exposure on those who live in mobile homes.

Formaldehyde is a colorless, reactive gas with a strong, pungent odor. At 0.05 ppm in air some persons can sense formaldehyde (6). Most people can smell formaldehyde at 1 ppm and experience some irritation at a few ppm. At 10 ppm formaldehyde becomes unpleasant, extremely irritating, and adversely affects nearly everyone. Precise thresholds have not been established for the irritant effects of formaldehyde; nor is there information regarding threshold values for sensitization to formaldehyde as an inhaled allergen (7).

There is, however, an abundance of anecdotal evidence and litigation, linking a variety of largely subchronic illnesses with sometimes unsatisfactory indoor environments of mobile homes (8). Formaldehyde is usually the first offending agent to be suspected, either by itself or in concert with other indoor air agents (9). Except in cases where very high concentrations of formaldehyde are encountered, definitive evidence to implicate formaldehyde in building air sickness is usually inadequate. There are, however, rare exceptions (10). Aside from complaints of acute toxicity by mobile home occupants, formaldehyde has been classified by the Environmental Protection Agency (EPA) as a probable human carcinogen. It is principally on this score that formaldehyde exposures in mobile homes are being assessed for risk to human health. The EPA's estimates of the increased cancer risks associated with lifetime exposure are relatively small; about 1–3 in 100,000 for lifetime exposures to ambient exposure levels (11). It is our opinion that the overall seriousness of risks of subchronic toxicity to the sensitive or hypersensitive segment of the population probably outweighs any carcinogenic risk.

2   CONCENTRATIONS OF FORMALDEHYDE OUTDOORS

Indoor concentrations of formaldehyde must be evaluated in light of concentrations outdoors; ingressing air will carry the outdoor formaldehyde indoors.

The natural background of formaldehyde is believed to result from the degradation of methane and other organic compounds. Formaldehyde concentrations in clean maritime air are only a few tenths of a ppb; in rural continental areas, mean values of 1 or 2 ppb are typical (12). Urban ambient levels of formaldehyde have recently been reported for a number of cities in the United States (13). The average concentrations were in the range of 10–20 ppb during warmer weather with lower concentrations measured in colder weather; the highest single concentration of formaldehyde reported was 69 ppb in southern California.

Warm polluted air outdoors can be expected to contribute 10–20 ppb to the formaldehyde levels inside mobile homes located in urban centers. Higher contributions should be considered as exceptional. In rural locations the impact on the indoor air should normally be no greater than a few ppb.

3   CONCENTRATIONS IN PREVIOUSLY MANUFACTURED MOBILE HOMES

A summary of some reported formaldehyde levels in surveys of mobile homes is contained in Table 1. In mobile homes where occupants have complained, the highest concentrations

TABLE 1. Reported Levels of Formaldehyde Vapor in Mobile Homes

Location	Measurement Type/Date	No. Homes	CH$_2$O Concentration (ppm)		Reference
			Central Measures*	Range	
California, built 1981 or later	Passive, February/March, 1985	293	0.101 (AM) 0.090 (GM)	0.023–0.314	20a
California, built prior to 1981	Passive, February/March, 1985	222	0.077 (AM) 0.064 (GM)	0.017–0.306	20a
California, built 1981 or later	Passive, July/August, 1985	391	0.100 (AM) 0.080 (GM)	0.012–0.464	20a
California, built prior to 1981	Passive, July/August, 1985	266	0.078 (AM) 0.061 (GM)	<0.010–0.386	20a
Minnesota, median age 2 years	Chromotropic acid, 1979–81	397 Rm 1 390 Rm 2	0.43 (AM) 0.41 (AM)	0.02–2.96 0.02–3.69	20a
Wisconsin, median age 16.5 months	Chromotropic acid, 1978–79	65	0.47 (M)	<0.10–3.68	17
Washington, pre-1977	Chromotropic acid	74	0.49 (M)	0.03–2.54	8
Various locations (Never occupied)	Not listed	260	0.86 (AM)	—	20b
Wisconsin (Noncompliant) all ages from 0–9 years	Chromotropic acid average 6 consecutive monthly meas.	137	0.46 (AM) 0.39 (M) 0.37 (GM)	0.10–2.84	18
< 3 years		100	0.54 (AM)	0.10–2.84	
> 3 years		37	0.19 (AM)	0.10–2.84	
Texas 76% of homes ≥ 2 years of age when monitored	Mostly colorimetric detector tubes, April, 1979–May, 1982	443	≥ 2 ppm in 27% homes one year of age or less	<0.5–8.0	15

*Various measures of the centers of distribution including arithmetic mean (AM), geometric mean (GM), and median (M).
[a]The authors know of no more recently reported surveys that are illustrative of formaldehyde levels in today's stock of mobile homes.

of formaldehyde have been in the range of a few ppm (14). The highest reported formaldehyde concentration in a mobile home is 8 ppm (15).

A report published in 1982 gave the mean concentration of formaldehyde inside mobile homes as 0.38 ppm (16). A Wisconsin study of mobile homes, whose median age was 16 months, produced a median concentration of formaldehyde of 0.47 ppm (17). A more recent publication has given a median concentration of 0.39 ppm for 137 mobile homes in Wisconsin (18); mobile homes less than 3 years old had an average monthly concentration of 0.54 ppm while those older than 3 years averaged 0.19 ppm.

These data provide a clear message that persons living in mobile homes at the beginning of the decade were routinely being exposed to formaldehyde well in excess of the American Society for Heating, Refrigeration, and Air Conditioning Engineers's (ASHRAE) comfort guideline for indoor air of 0.1 ppm (19). Neither was it unusual, in those years, for concentrations to exceed the 0.4-ppm target subsequently established for mobile homes by the Department of Housing and Urban Development.

The age of the urea-formaldehyde-bearing resins in a mobile home, and hence the age of the mobile home, strongly influences the airborne levels of formaldehyde. The influence of mobile home age is clearly impacting the data in Table 1 (20–20b). The dependence of formaldehyde levels on the age of mobile homes is shown in Fig. 1. These data reported by Preuss et al. (21) indicate an exponential decrease in the emission of formaldehyde into the indoor air and a half-life of about 4–5 years. Aging in itself is thus a form of remedial action. Recently reported, week-long integrated measurements of formaldehyde in about 200 older mobile homes bear this out; measurements made in February–March 1985 inside mobile homes built before 1981 produced an arithmetic mean of 0.077 ppb and a maximum single value of 0.3 ppm (20ᵃ). This result indicates that after aging for 5 years or more, the formaldehyde levels in the older stock of mobile homes can, on average, meet the ASHRAE guideline of 0.1 ppm (19).

ORNL-DWG 88-10604

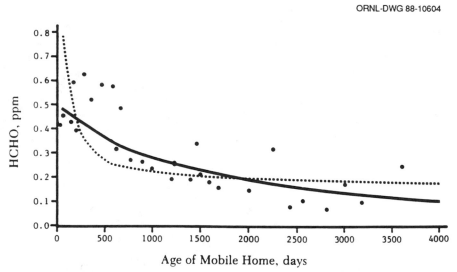

Figure 1. Dependency of formaldehyde levels on the ages of mobile homes; ●, actual data points; ---, power curve fit; —, exponential curve fit.

4   CONCENTRATIONS IN CONTEMPORARY MOBILE HOMES

What levels of formaldehyde are the occupants of newly manufactured mobile homes being exposed to? This is the question of most concern.

The Department of Housing and Urban Development (HUD) proposed a product standard for emissions of formaldehyde from particleboard and hardwood plywood paneling (22). The standard was published as rule No. 24 CFR Part 3280 in 1985 (23). HUD believes that enforcement of this product standard will prevent concentrations of formaldehyde in indoor ambient air from exceeding 0.4 ppm. The available medical and scientific evidence, in HUD's opinion, indicates that the majority of persons will not suffer adverse health effects if exposed to formaldehyde at levels of up to 0.4 ppm. It is acknowledged by HUD, however, that certain individuals may become sensitized to formaldehyde and even to the extent of reacting adversely to any measurable level of formaldehyde. Such persons benefit little from any standard. To alert these persons, HUD requires warning labels to be posted in manufactured homes.

Already in the spring of 1984 an estimated 53% of total U.S. plant capacity could meet the HUD standard (24). The situation appears to have improved considerably since that time; in presentations delivered to the National Particleboard Association in January 1987, 89 and 87% of domestically manufactured products for particleboard and hardwood plywood paneling, respectively, were meeting the HUD standard.

Industry has produced and still is working to produce new resin formulations and scavenger systems to minimize further the emissions of formaldehyde. In fact, it is claimed that the best state-of-the-art materials are capable of keeping indoor levels from exceeding 0.1 ppm at standard conditions and only 1 month after manufacture (25). These same authors showed a 10-fold variation between formaldehyde emissions from the best and worst currently produced medium-density fiberboard that they examined. It therefore seems likely that considerable differences exist between mobile homes from different manufacturers. The magnitude of these differences in levels of formaldehyde awaits the taking and publication of actual indoor measurements in the United States.

Recently published measurements for new mobile homes in the Federal Republic of Germany (FRG) indicate that even if construction is with the lowest emitting particleboards classified E1 ($\leqslant$ 10 mg formaldehyde content/100 g), the 0.1 ppm guideline is still not guaranteed. Formaldehyde levels of up to 0.2 ppm were encountered (26). The problem lay with air exchange rates of only 0.1–0.3 per hour, much lower than the 1 per hour used during the E1 classification test.

Some manufacturers of mobile homes have recently begun substituting gypsum and other non-formaldehyde-containing wallboard in the place of hardwood-plywood wall paneling. This measure will produce some further reductions in the indoor levels of formaldehyde. Prefabricated houses in the FRG that were new and unfurnished but constructed with boards made with phenolic resins, diisocyanates, or gypsum indeed had formaldehyde levels significantly below 0.1 ppm (26). There seems to be reasonable likelihood that in a growing fraction of new mobile homes the occupants have the good fortune not to be exposed to levels greater than 0.1 ppm.

5   FLUCTUATIONS IN FORMALDEHYDE LEVELS

The foregoing commentary in the previous sections has been confined to situations where environmental conditions of temperature and humidity were generally benign (e.g., 77°F and 50% relative humidity) and the ventilation rate adequate (e.g., 0.5 air changes per hour or more). The HUD product standard, for example, specifies testing under these moderate conditions of climate and ventilation.

It is important to appreciate that extremes of temperature and humidity can have a pronounced influence on the levels of formaldehyde that occupants experience. Short-term measurements over 1 or 2 hours may not adequately reflect the time-averaged daily 24-h or longer exposure of a house-bound occupant. Certainly the short-term measurement could miss peak exposures important for consideration of acute health effects.

The experimental effects of temperature on formaldehyde emission are now well known (27); a rise in temperature from 25 to 35°C, such as when the wall of a mobile home is heated by the sun, can triple the rate of release for formaldehyde. Five fold increases in levels of formaldehyde have been measured in a mobile home in Florida (28) as the wall temperatures increased from about 16 to 36°C.

Air humidity can affect airborne formaldehyde concentrations in complex ways. The effect of change in relative humidity from 70 to 30% in a new mobile home was reported recently to bring about a 40% reduction in formaldehyde levels (29). Persistent high humidity can slowly hydrolyze UF resin and increase the generating rate for formaldehyde. Moisture enhances the release of formaldehyde from resins.

Wood absorbs a considerable amount of moisture. Formaldehyde reversibly hydrolyzes in this wood moisture to become methylene glycol, otherwise known as formalin. A large amount of water, and therefore formaldehyde, can be bound up in the wood products of a mobile home; wood moisture varies from 6 to 27 wt.% at 30 and 96% relative humidity, respectively (30). In diurnal and seasonal cycles, sorbed moisture and its incipient formaldehyde can be desorbed into the occupants' immediate environment.

Knowledge about the fluctuations in levels of formaldehyde produced by environmental factors will certainly be important when considering any acute illness. Normally these fluctuations will be of lesser importance when considering any carcinogenic potential due to long-term exposure. A threshold concentration may exist, however, which is related to the concentration needed to penetrate the mucous fluids and react with underlying cellular material in respiratory passages. In such cases, a greater weighting would need to be assigned to the peak exposures than to a long-term average exposure.

6   CARCINOGENIC EFFECTS OF FORMALDEHYDE

Evidence of a causal relation between exposure to formaldehyde and human cancers is sparse and conflicting (7). Nevertheless, there are some epidemiological data that formaldehyde is a carcinogen in humans and strong evidence that it is a carcinogen in animals. On the basis of this evidence, the EPA has classified formaldehyde as a probable human carcinogen. We briefly review the evidence.

While over 28 epidemiological studies related to formaldehyde exposure have been conducted, there is little evidence of cancer deaths associated with formaldehyde exposure. The strongest evidence comes from three recent studies. Blair et al. (31, 32) observed significant excesses in lung and nasopharyngeal cancer among 26,000 workers occupationally exposed to formaldehyde. They conclude that there may be an association between formaldehyde exposure and nasopharyngeal cancer (32), but that there was little evidence of an association between lung cancer deaths and formaldehyde exposure since cancer risk did not increase consistently with either increasing intensity or cumulative formaldehyde exposure (31). The EPA believes that the lung cancer results are meaningful despite the lack of significant trends with exposure (33).

Stayner et al. (34) reported statistically significant excesses in buccal cavity tumors among garment workers exposed to formaldehyde. Risk was highest among workers with the longest duration of exposure and follow-up period. Vaughan et al. (35, 36) showed a significant association between nasopharyngeal cancer and having lived 10 years or more in mobile homes. Based primarily on these three studies, the EPA has concluded that there is limited evidence indicating that formaldehyde is a human carcinogen. (The EPA defines limited evidence as indicating that a causal relation is credible but that alternative explanations cannot be excluded.)

The principal studies showing that formaldehyde is an animal carcinogen are Kerns et al. (37), Albert et al. (38), and Tobe et al. (39). These studies have shown increases in malignant tumors (squamous cell carcinomas) in the nasal cavities of male and female rats and in male mice. Neither in these studies nor in other studies have effects been observed beyond the initial site of nasal contact. The EPA chose to use the Kerns et al. (35) data set in developing a quantitative risk assessment for formaldehyde.

The Albert et al. (38) study was not used because it contains only a single nonzero exposure level, while the Tobe et al. (39) study was not used because it obtained tumor response only at the highest dose level.

Additional evidence that formaldehyde might be a carcinogen includes the results of short-term tests designed to measure the effect of formaldehyde on DNA. Formaldehyde has been shown to be mutagenic in numerous tests involving bacteria, fungi, and insects (Drosophila). It can transform cells in culture and cause DNA cross-linking, sister chromatid exchanges, and chromosome aberrations. It has been shown to form DNA adducts and to interfere with DNA repair in human cells.

7   LOW-DOSE EXTRAPOLATION OF BIOASSAY DATA

Since risk at low exposure levels cannot be measured directly either in animal studies or in human epidemiological studies, mathematical models have been developed to extrapolate from high to low doses. Almost all extrapolation methods give a reasonable fit to observed data but lead to large differences in projected risk at low dose. Both OSTP (40) and EPA guidelines for carcinogen risk assessment (41) state that in selection of a low-dose extrapolation model, it is appropriate to consider the mechanism of action of the carcinogen. The biological evidence indicates that formaldehyde acts through both an initiation and promotional mechanism of action. Formaldehyde is known to be able to cause mutations and DNA damage, indicating that it can initiate the cancer process. At high doses, it is also known to cause increased DNA synthesis and increased cellular proliferation. However, currently accepted low-dose extrapolation models do not allow for the separation of the initiation properties of a carcinogen (which may occur over the whole dose range) from its promotional aspects (which may only occur in the high-dose range).

The relation between exposure and tumor response in rats is very nonlinear. In the Kerns et al. (37) study, no rats developed tumors at 2 ppm, 1% at 5.6 ppm, while 50% responded at 14.3 ppm. Formaldehyde's ability to increase cell proliferation and its ability to bind to DNA have been suggested as possible mechanisms for the steep dose–response curve.

Studies by Swenberg et al. (42) and Chang et al. (43) have shown formaldehyde exposure increases the cell turnover rate in the nasal cavity of rats and mice. However, the increase in squamous metaplasia is only twofold between 5.6 and 14.3 ppm, not the 50-fold increase seen in squamous cell carcinomas. Thus, increased cellular proliferation does not appear to be the total explanation for the observed linearity in the cancer bioassay.

Casanova-Schmitz et al. (44) reported a nonlinearity in the amount of covalent binding of formaldehyde to DNA of the respiratory mucosa. Covalent binding to mucosa DNA was 10.5 times higher at 6 ppm than at 2 ppm. Starr and Buck (45) have suggested that these data can be used as input to a quantitative risk assessment for formaldehyde. The EPA Science Advisory Board (SAB) (46), while praising the DNA adduct data as an important contribution, believes more study is necessary before such data can be used in quantitative risk assessment (33). Thus, while attempts have been made to consider the mechanism of action of formaldehyde, it is the general scientific consensus that insufficient data exist to justify deviation from use of the linearized multistage model for low-dose extrapolation.

8   QUANTITATIVE RISK ASSESSMENT

Given the limited evidence that formaldehyde is a human carcinogen, the EPA (33) based its estimates of human cancer risk from formaldehyde exposure on the Kerns et al. (37) study in rats. This study produced both squamous cell carcinomas (malignant tumors) and polypoid adenomas (benign tumors) in the rats. It is normal EPA procedure to combine benign and malignant tumor data in developing risk estimates (41). However, since squamous cell carcinomas and polypoid adenomas arise from different cell types, it was not considered appropriate to combine them (7, 33). Had the EPA used both benign and malignant tumor responses in the quantitative estimation of human cancer risk, the predicted human risk would have been about 10 times higher.

Besides a low-dose extrapolation model, human risk estimation based on animal data necessitates the choice of the proper interspecies scaling factor. The standard EPA practice is to use surface area. However, studies show that nonhuman primates and rats have similar carcinogenic responses to formaldehyde exposure. Consequently, humans were assumed to have the same response as rats at equivalent exposure levels and duration (7, 33). If nasal surface area had been used, the estimated human cancer risks would have been about 10 times higher.

Based on these assumptions, the EPA (33) estimates that the upper-bound excess lifetime risk of developing cancer is 2×10^{-4} for residents of mobile homes who are exposed for 10 years to an average formaldehyde level of 0.1 ppm. The actual risk of developing cancer may of course be zero. It should be pointed out that the excess cancer incidence observed in the human epidemiologic studies are consistent with projections based on the rat nasal carcinoma data (33).

9   SUMMARY

Mobile homes generally have higher levels of airborne formaldehyde than conventional housing because of higher loading factors for pressed-wood products and less ventilation. Because of previous complaints by residents of mobile homes claiming a variety of adverse acute health effects due to formaldehyde, manufacturers have taken public opinion into account; the particleboard industry now offers a wide range of products that are either formaldehyde free or have much lower emission rates than in the past. The sometimes excessively high airborne formaldehyde concentrations (several ppm) are undoubtedly a thing of the past. The Department of Housing and Urban Development (HUD) product standard published in 1985 is designed to prevent formaldehyde in the ambient indoor air of new mobile homes from exceeding 0.4 ppm, a level at which a majority of persons will not suffer adverse acute health effects. The majority of today's domestically manufactured particleboard and hardwood plywood paneling can meet the product standard. The American Society of Heating, Refrigeration, and Air Conditioning Engineers (ASHRAE) has established a comfort guideline for indoor air of 0.1 ppm formaldehyde, adequate to satisfy all but the most highly sensitive persons. The best state-of-the-art materials are claimed to be capable of keeping indoor levels from exceeding this 0.1 ppm guideline if the climatic conditions are moderate. Some limited data from the Federal Republic of Germany indicate that in new mobile homes, with the best available particleboard, up to 0.2 ppm occurs because of low air exchange rates. Formaldehyde-free product substitution in contemporary mobile homes, such as the use of gypsum wallboard instead of formaldehyde containing pressed-wood, is contributing further to reduced levels of formaldehyde in indoor air. In previously manufactured mobile homes, aging of ureaformaldehyde (UF) resins generally reduces the emission rate of formaldehyde. After aging for five years or more, formaldehyde levels in the older stock of mobile homes can, on the average, meet the ASHRAE guideline of 0.1 ppm. Thus the majority of persons today living in mobile homes, whether they be older or new homes, are being exposed to average concentrations near or below 0.1 ppm. Extremes of high temperature and humidity, however, can cause levels of formaldehyde to be elevated above the norm. In particular, the heating of mobile home walls by the sun can produce temporary, several-fold increases in airborne formaldehyde concentration. Such peak concentrations of a few tenths ppm are probably of more significance in establishing or triggering responses in persons predisposed or disposed to chemical sensitivity than for any carcinogenic potential.

REFERENCES

1. M. S. Reisch, Top 50 chemicals production turned back up in 1987. *Chem. Eng. News* **66**(15), 31 (1988).

2. Formaldehyde: Evidence of carcinogenicity. *NIOSH Bull.* **34** (1981).

3. F. Farni, Procède pour la fabrication des plaques artificielles en bois comprise. French Patent 81, 781 (1943).

4. R. M. Orheim, Letter to the Editor. Resin, not foam, is problem?, *Chem. Eng. News* **60**(17), 2 (1982).

5. B.Meyer, Formaldehyde exposure from building products. *Environ. Int.* **12**, 283–288 (1986).

6. R. Niemela and H. Vainis, Formaldehyde exposure in work and general environment. *Scand. J. Work Environ. Health* **7**, 95–100 (1981).

7. Report on the consensus workshop on formaldehyde. *Environ. Health Perspect.* **58**, 323–381 (1984).

8. P. A. Breysse, Formaldehyde in mobile and conventional homes. *Environ. Health Saf. News* **26**, 19 (1977).

9. R. Ahlstrom and B. Berglund, Formaldehyde odor and it's interaction with the air of a sick building. *Environ. Int.* **12**, 289–295 (1986).

10. W. T. Hanna and P. Painter, A syndrome resembling Henoch–Schonlein purpura and chloroderma in association with formaldehyde. University of Tennessee College of Medicine and Memorial Hospital. *JAMA, J. Am. Med. Assoc.* (submitted for publication).

11. EPA says formaldehyde likely a carcinogen. *Chem. Eng. News*, April 27, p. 18 (1987).

12. *Formaldehyde.* MMV Medizin Verlag, Muenchen, 1985, p. 21.

13. L. J. Salas and H. B. Singh, Measurements of formaldehyde and acetaldehyde in the urban ambient air. *Atmos. Environ.* **20**, 1301–1304 (1986).

14. R.B. Gammage and A. R. Hawthorne, Current status of measurement techniques and concentrations of formaldehyde in residences. *Adv. Chem. Ser.* **210**, 125 (1985).

15. S. W. Norsted, C. A. Kozinetz, and J. F. Annegers, Formaldehyde complaint investigations in mobile homes by the Texas Department of Health. *Environ. Res.* **37**, 93–100 (1985).

16. K. C. Gupta, A. G. Ulsamer, and P. W. Preuss, Formaldehyde in indoor air: Sources and toxicity. *Environ. Int.* **8**, 349–358 (1982).

17. K. A. Dally, L. P. Hanrahan, M. A. Woodbury, and M. S. Kanarek, Formaldehyde exposure in nonoccupational environments. *Arch. Environ. Health.* **36**, 277–284 (1984).

18. L. P. Hanrahan, H. A. Anderson, K. A. Dally, A. D. Eckmann, and M. S. Kanarek, Formaldehyde concentrations in Wisconsin mobile homes. *J. Air Pollut. Control Assoc.* **35**, 1164–1167 (1985).

19. American Society of Heating, Refrigerating, and Air-Conditioning Engineers, *ASHRAE STANDARDS: Ventilation for Acceptable Indoor Air Quality*, ANSI/ASHRAE 62-1981R. ASHRAE, New York, 1981.

20. K. Sexton, K. S. Liu, and M. X. Petreas, Formaldehyde concentrations inside private residences: A mail-out approach to indoor air monitoring. *J. Air Pollut. Control Assoc.* **36**, 698–704 (1986).

20a. I. M. Ritchie and R. G. Lehnen, An analysis of formaldehyde concentrations in mobile and conventional homes. *J. Environ. Health* **47**, (6), 300–305 (1985).

20b. Clayton Environmental Consultants, *Fed. Regist.* **48**, 37139 (1983).

21. P. W. Preuss, R. L. Dailey, and E. S. Lehman, Exposure to formaldehyde. *Adv. Chem. Ser.* **210**, 251–252 (1985).

22. *Federal Register*, **48**, No. 159, 37137 (1983).

23. *Federal Register, Manufactured Homes Construction and Safety Standards.* FR, Washington DC, 1985, pp. 31996–32013.

24. Heiden Associates, *Comparison of Costs Associated with In-Plant Techniques for Reducing Formaldehyde Emissions from Particleboard and Hardwood Plywood Paneling,* Report to the Formaldehyde Institute. Submitted to the Environmental Protection Agency, 1984.

25. B. Meyer and K. Hermanns. Formaldehyde release from pressed wood products. *Adv. Chem. Ser.* **210**, 113 (1985).

26. R. Marutzky, Formaldehyde injuries in prefabricated houses: Causes, prevention, and reduction. *Proc. Indoor Air* **2**, 690–694 (1987).

27. A. Berge, B. Mellegaard, P. Hanetho, and B. P. Ormstad, Formaldehyde release from particleboard—Evaluation of a mathematical model. *Holz Roh- Werkst.* **38**, 251 (1980).

28. B. Meyer and K. Hermanns, Diurnal variations of formaldehyde exposure in mobile homes. *J. Environ. Health*, **48**, 57–61 (1985).

29. T. Godish and J. Rouch, Mitigation of residential formaldehyde contamination by indoor climate control. *Am. Ind. Hyg. Assoc. J.* **47**(12), 972–797 (1986).

30. B. Meyer and K. Hermanns, Reducing indoor air formaldehyde concentrations. *J. Air Pollut. Control Assoc.* **35**, 816–821 (1985).

31. A. E. Blair, P. A. Stewart, M. O'Berg, W. Gaffey, J. Walrath, J. Ward, R. Bales, S. Kaplan, and D. A. Cubit, Mortality among industrial workers exposed to formaldehyde. *JNCI, J. Natl. Cancer Inst.* **76**, 1071–1084 (1986).

32. A. Blair, P. A. Stewart, R. N. Hoover, J. F. Fraumeni, Jr., J. Walrath, M. O'Berg, and W. Gaffey, Cancers of the nasopharynx and oropharynx and formaldehyde exposure. *JNCI, J. Natl. Cancer Inst.* **78**(1), 191 (1987).

33. Environmental Protection Agency, *Assessment of Health Risks to Garment Workers and Certain Home Residents from Exposure to Formaldehyde*. Office of Pesticides and Toxic Substances, April 1987.

34. L. Stayner, A. B. Smith, G. Reeve, L. Blade, L. Elliott, R. Keenlyside, and W. Halperin, Proportionate mortality study of workers exposed to formaldehyde in the garment industry. Presented at the Society for Epidemiologic Research 17th Annual Meeting, Houston, Texas. *Am. J. Epidemiol.* **120**, 458–459 (1984).

35. T. L. Vaughan, C. Strader, S. Davis, and J. R. Daling, Formaldehyde and cancers of the pharynx, sinus, and nasal cavity. I. Occupational exposures. *Int. J. Cancer* **38**(5), 677–683 (1986).

36. T. L. Vaughan, C. Strader, S. Davis, and J. R. Daling, Formaldehyde and cancers of the pharynx, sinus and nasal cavity. II. Residential exposures. *Int. J. Cancer* **38**(5), 685–688 (1986).

37. W. D. Kerns, K. L. Pavkov, D. J. Donofrio, E. J. Gralla, and J. A. Swenberg, Carcinogenicity of formaldehyde in rats and mice after long-term inhalation exposure. *Cancer Res.* **43**, 4382–4392 (1983).

38. R. E. Albert, A. R. Sellakumar, S. Laskin, M. Kuschner, N. Nelson, and D. A. Snyder, Gaseous formaldehyde and hydrogen chloride induction of nasal cancer in the rat. *JNCI, J. Natl. Cancer Inst.* **68**, 597–603 (1982).

39. M. Tobe, T. Kaneko, Y. Uchida, E. Kamata, Y. Ogawa, Y. Ikeda, and M. Saito, *Studies of the Inhalation Toxicity of Formaldehyde*. National Sanitary and Medical Laboratory Service, Japan, 1985.

40. Office of Science and Technology Policy, Executive Office of the President, Chemical carcinogens: A review of the science and its associated principles. *Fed Regist.* II. 10371–10442 (1985).

41. Environmental Protection Agency, proposed guidelines for carcinogen risk assessment. *Fed. Regst.* **49**, 46294 (1986).

42. J. A. Swenberg, C. S. Barrow, C. J. Boreiko, H. D'A. Heck, F. J. Levine, K. T. Morgan, and T. B. Starr, Nonlinear biological responses to formaldehyde and their implications for carcinogenic risk assessment. *Carcinogenesis (London)* **4**, 945–952 (1983).

43. J. C. F. Chang, E. A. Gross, J. A. Swenberg, and C. S. Barrow, Nasal cavity deposition histopathology and cell proliferation after single or repeated formaldehyde exposures in B6C3F1 mice and F344 rats. *Toxicol. Appl. Pharmacol.* **68**, 161–176 (1983).

44. M. Casanova-Schmitz, T. B. Starr, and H. D'A. Heck, Differentiation between metabolic incorporation and covalent binding in the labeling of macromolecules in the rat nasal mucosa and bone marrow by inhaled [14C]- and [³H] formaldehyde. *Toxicol. Appl. Pharmacol.* **76**, 26–44 (1984).

45. T. B. Starr and R. D. Buck, 'The importance of delivered dose in estimating low-dose cancer risk from inhalation exposure to formaldehyde. *Fundam, Appl. Toxicol.* **4**, 740–753 (1984).

46. Environmental Protection Agency, Science Advisory Board, and Environmental Health Committee, *Review of Draft Document—Preliminary Assessment of Health Risks to Garment Workers and Certain Home Residents from Exposures to Formaldehyde* (draft). Letter to Lee M. Thomas, October 1, 1985, from R. A. Griesemer and N. Nelson.

18

Environmental Lung Cancer Risk from Radon Daughter Exposure

Naomi H. Harley

Department of Environmental Medicine, New York University Medical Center, New York

1 INTRODUCTION

Radon is a naturally occurring radioactive gas. It is a member of the uranium series and its immediate parent is ^{226}Ra. In the earth's crust, the normal or average radioactivity of each element in the series is in equilibrium at about 1 pCi/g soil or rock (37 mBq/g). The entire uranium series decay chain is shown in Fig. 1. Near the soil surface, radon is not in equilibrium but, because it is a gas, it either diffuses or flows due to pressure gradients into the open volume. In outdoor air, the radon concentration is low (0.2 pCi/L, or 7 mBq/L) because of the large dilution capability of the atmosphere, but in an enclosed volume such as a mine, the gas and its immediate short-lived daughters can build up to much higher concentrations. If the rock in mines is uraniferous with consequently higher ^{226}Ra, radon can build up to thousands of pCi/L (2).

The risk of lung cancer from radon daughter exposure in underground mines has been known for 500 years. Agricola in 1597 (3) reported on deaths from respiratory illness in the Schneeburg and Joachimstahl mines in the Erzgebirge on the border of Saxony and Bohemia. Harting and Hesse in 1879 (4) recognized the disease as lung cancer in these same mines at the end of the 19th century but did not know the etiology of the disease. They stated that 75% of deaths in miners was due to lung cancer and that onset of the disease occurred after about 20 years work in the mines. Arnstein in 1913 (5) reported statistical data showing that, from 1875 to 1912, 276 of these miners had died from lung cancer, 64 from tuberculosis, and 206 from other causes. Lung cancer mortality was 40% for this study and this estimate of mortality is still regarded as valid (6). In 1921, Uhlig (7) published some of his histological findings and speculated that the etiology might be ionizing radiation. In 1924, Ludewig and Lorenser (8) were apparently the first to postulate that radon was the important factor in lung cancer in the Schneeburg miners.

Evans and Goodman in 1940 (9) were the first to propose occupational guidelines for radon based on a review of the human data from these mines and the radium dial-painter experience with bone cancer from ingested radium. They proposed that the high mortality from lung cancer was due to prolonged exposure at radon concentrations of about

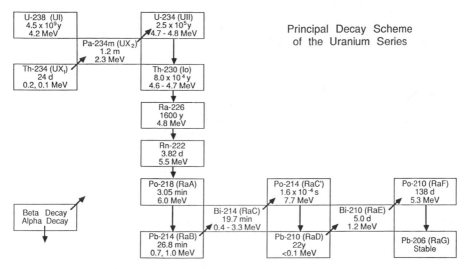

Figure 1. Principal decay scheme of the uranium series.

1000 pCi/L. They suggested a factor of 100 be applied to arrive at a permissible concentration for radon of 10 pCi/L in "plant, laboratory or office air."

In 1951, both Harley (10) and Bale (11) determined that the actual dose delivered to lung tissue was from the short-lived radon daughters rather than from radon gas itself. During the mid-1950s, the mines in the United States operated under the guideline set by the U.S. Public Health Service (12), which was 100 pCi/L of radon in equilibrium with its daughters. Because of the complication of the disequilibrium of the short-lived daughters with radon, the unit of working level (WL) equal to 1.3×10^5 MeV/L of potential alpha energy release with complete decay of the short-lived daughters in air was devised. The working level did not depend on daughter equilibrium and was an easy measurement to perform in the mines. It required a 5-min sampling of air on a filter followed by a single alpha count. In general, the daughter equilibrium in mines was such that 1 WL was equivalent to 300 pCi/L of radon. Total exposure was reported in units of WL multiplied by the time spent underground in units of the work month (an exposure to 1 WL for 1 working month of 170 h) is a cumulative exposure of 1 working level month or WLM). Thus, the occupational guideline was 12 WLM in a year during the years of most active uranium mining in the United States.

Unfortunately, many of the mines were not in compliance with the occupational guidelines and exposures many times the permitted 12 WLM/yr were reported. Miners in the United States worked underground for an average of 10 years and total exposures of 120 WLM should have been a maximum. Instead, individuals received up to 10,000 WLM in some of the mines (13).

In 1963, reports of excess lung cancer in U.S. miners began to emerge (14). A cohort of 3362 miners from the Colorado plateau was assembled for follow-up. Miners with at least 1 month underground experience between 1950 and 1963 were included in this group. It is the experience with this group and three similar cohorts in Czechoslovakia (the same mines as were reported on as far back as 1597), Canada, and Sweden that form the basis for all the occupational and environmental risk estimates (15–19).

The U.S. cohort of Colorado plateau miners showed a clear excess of lung cancer and in

1971 (20), based on preliminary data from the prospective study, the U.S. Department of Interior reduced the occupational standard to 4 WLM/yr with maximum air concentrations not to exceed 1 WL (21).

2   HAZARD IDENTIFICATION

Many studies from different countries have been published which show excess lung cancer in underground miners. Reports are available from British iron and tin miners, French iron miners, Newfoundland fluorspar miners, and Swedish lead and zinc miners. Added to these are the reports of the Czechoslovakian, Canadian, French, Swedish, and U.S. uranium miners already mentioned.

To date, the only cancer significantly in excess for the exposed groups is bronchogenic lung cancer. The excess lung cancer is consistent in that it is related to radon daughter concentration in many mining environments that varied widely in other atmospheric contaminants.

A standardized mortality ratio,

$$SMR = \frac{\text{observed deaths}}{\text{expected deaths}},$$

of greater than 1 was observed in the U.S. (22), Canadian (18), and Swedish (19) cohorts for stomach cancer but the SMR increase is not statistically significant. Since the effect is reported in three of the mining groups, stomach cancer is likely to be in excess for miners although at a low level (near expected) of risk.

The Canadian follow-up of Ontario miners is ongoing and is designed to investigate various contaminants in the air other than radon daughters. Among these are asbestiform materials, arsenic, blasting fumes, total dust, free silica, and diesel fumes. It is noteworthy in the Canadian Ontario miners that no significant excess lung cancer was observed in other types of mines such as nickel, copper, or iron mines. An excess risk of lung cancer was observed in Canadian gold miners (23) and an attempt was made to show a possible association with atmospheric contaminants, since gold mines do not have particularly high radon daughter concentrations. There was a positive association of lung cancer in gold miners exposed to high dust levels in combination with arsenic and asbestos fibers in the ore. Gold miners not exposed to high dust levels (giving a potential for asbestos, arsenic, etc.) still showed significantly increased lung cancer. Radon daughter levels were not well documented in the gold mines and so radon-daughter-related lung cancer is still a possibility.

In the Swedish iron mining cohort, Radford (19) showed that samples of the bedrock indicated no arsenic, chromium, or nickel and samples of mine air indicated no identifiable asbestos fibers. Diesel exhaust could be ruled out because 70% of the lung cancer cases had appeared before diesel equipment was introduced into the mines. A case control study was used with this group to show that the odds ratio (ratio of exposed to unexposed in the cases divided by this ratio in the controls) for the frequency of silicosis in cases versus controls did not differ significantly from unity. Obviously, iron oxide dust was present in these mines.

Based on the exposure–response data discussed in Section 3 and the studies performed with the existing cohorts, the primary risk factor for lung cancer appears to be the alpha dose to cells in the bronchial epithelium from radon daughters deposited on airway surfaces.

Other contaminants in the air may contribute somewhat to the excess lung cancer as suggested by the Canadian gold miners. The possibility exists that these substances account for the slight excess of stomach cancer in three of the mining groups and this could be chemical carcinogenesis. The alpha dose to the stomach from radon daughters cleared from the bronchial tree and swallowed would be vanishingly small compared with the lung dose and it is doubtful whether radiation could be involved.

3   EXPOSURE–RESPONSE RELATION (HAZARD EVALUATION)

The value of attributable risk per year per unit exposure is needed for projecting the observed lung cancer excess to whole life either from a single or short-term exposure as in mines or, as in the case of environmental exposure, for continuous exposure over whole life.

The published underground miner epidemiology has been reviewed by the National Council on Radiation Protection and Measurements (NCRP) (24) and Figs. 2 and 3 are taken from this report. The lung cancer risk for the various mining groups can be estimated over the various (short) time intervals of follow-up reported of from 10 to 20 years. It may be estimated as an excess or attributable lung cancer risk per year per WLM exposure.

Figure 2 shows the lung cancers attributable to radon daughter exposure for the various mining groups where data are available on excess mortality and exposure. Figure 3 shows the excess risk as of the date of last follow-up in terms of the total risk per person per unit exposure rather than risk per person per year.

At the time Fig. 2 was prepared, the updated Canadian data had not been published. Muller (18) extended the Ontario cohort data through 1981 and if these are added (excluding gold miners) the attributable risk is between 2 and 5 per person per year per WLM for each of their exposure categories from 4 to 350 WLM. Including the updated

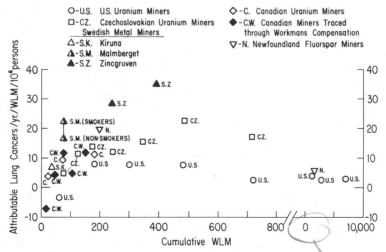

Figure 2. Attributable annual lung cancer mortality as a function of cumulative radon daughter exposure. (From Ref. 24).

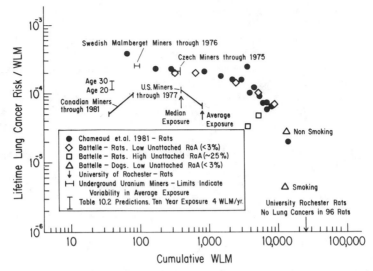

Figure 3. Lifetime lung cancer risk in humans and animals as a function of cumulative radon daughter exposure. (From Ref. 24).

Canadian data would not change the average attributable risk value determined from the data in Fig. 2 of $(12 \pm 2) \times 10^{-6}$ per person year per WLM.

Figure 3 (modified to include the updated Canadian data) expresses the risk for the four cohorts as total excess lung cancer risk to the time of follow-up of the study per WLM exposure. Included in this figure are the relevant experimental animal data that have been published. It can be seen that the excess attributable risks for the rat and beagle dog are similar to that for human underground miners.

At exposures greater than 1000 WLM, the response per WLM decreases. One explanation of this is that, at this high an exposure, each stem cell in the bronchial epithelium has been hit by an alpha particle about 10 times, on average, and it is likely that some cell death occurs (25).

The support for the lifetime human risk of about 2×10^{-4} per WLM by experimental animals is important since it allows other studies to be performed that cannot be resolved with the human data.

Other groups or individuals have published various risk estimates based on analysis of the same data used by NCRP. For example, BEIR III (26) selected the Newfoundland and Czechoslovakian groups to give a value of 19×10^{-6} per person year per WLM and developed an age-dependent risk (per million per year per WLM) of 10 for those 35–49 at time of diagnosis, 20 for those aged 50–65, and 50 for those over age 65.

4   EXPOSURE ASSESSMENT

The weakest part of the underground miner epidemiology is the estimate of actual exposure. In the U.S. study, 43,000 radon daughter measurements were made between 1951 and 1969. Approximately 2500 different mines were in existence during this time and measurements could not be made in each individual mine. Estimates of the mine atmospheres were made by interpolation. In the Czechoslovakian mines, 120,000 radon measurements were made but the daughter equilibrium was not measured. Measurements were not made in the Swedish iron mines until 1968 yet all miners were included in the study who worked underground for more than 1 calendar year between 1897 and 1976. Exposures in the past were estimated from a knowledge of the radon concentration dissolved in groundwater (the source of radon in these Swedish mines) and the ventilation rates, which were increased over the years as radon daughter hazards were recognized.

In all radiation-related epidemiological studies to date, <u>it appears that exposure (the independent variable) is the poorest known of the factors</u>.

For this reason, it is important to use all of the mining studies together rather than relying on a single study since the errors in exposure measurement and estimation should be minimized with this approach.

The Canadian epidemiologists were aware of this problem and chose to use a range of exposures, which they termed the special and standard exposures to denote what they believed to be the maximum and minimum values of exposure, respectively. The attributable or relative risk, which they estimate, is thought to be between the two values given by the exposure range.

For environmental exposures, measurements have been made for many years of the outdoor concentrations of radon. These average about 0.2 pCi/L for much of the world, not only the United States (27). Only recently have indoor measurements become available (1, 28, 29).

Cumulative exposure, which is the basic unit for risk estimation, is given in terms of WLM for the environment as well as the mines. The risk as determined in the epidemiological studies was related to the measured air concentration of radon daughters in WL multiplied by the time spent in the mine at that concentration in multiples of the working month (170 h). Currently, radon rather than radon daughters is the measurement of choice in homes while radon daughters are still measured in the U.S. mines. To convert radon concentration in pCi/L to WL, an equilibrium factor for the daughters is necessary. Based on existing data (27), an equilibrium factor of 0.7 is appropriate for outdoor air, 0.4–0.5 for indoor air, and 0.3 for mines.

$$\text{exposure in WL} = (\text{pCi }^{222}\text{Rn/L}) \times F/100, \tag{1}$$

where F is the equilibrium factor. The cumulative exposure is

$$\text{cumulative exposure in WLM} = (\text{WL}) \times (\text{hours exposed})/170. \tag{2}$$

An outdoor concentration of 0.2 pCi/L is therefore equal to an exposure of 0.0014 WL and, if this were the only exposure, would equal $\underline{0.0014 \times 50 = 0.07 \text{ WLM}}$ in 1 year. *Rounding*

The first indoor measurements of radon were made by Hultqvist (30) in Sweden and Glauberman (31) in New York City. They reported values of about 1 pCi/L as an average for indoor air, but Hultqvist had a few measurements of high radon levels in homes. Hultqvist's early data were generally ignored as simply odd or unusual because there were no numerical values of lung cancer risk available to place his data in context.

NCRP estimated the U.S. indoor average concentration in 1984 based on only 50 indoor measurements. Since that time many other data sets have been published with much larger number of homes surveyed. One problem with the recent data is that high radon concentrations in homes were observed beginning with the Watras family in Boyertown, Pennsylvania in 1984, where radon levels were equal to those measured in the

TABLE 1. Distribution of Radon Concentrations in Single-Family Dwellings

Group	Approximate Number of Dwellings	Number of States	pCi/L Air Mean	Median	GSD
NCRP (1)	50	3	1.0	0.66	2.5
Nero et al. (28)	800	17	1.5	0.9	2.8
Cohen (29)	450	42	1.5	1.0	2.4

Schneeburg and Joachimstahl mines of a few thousand pCi/L. For this reason many surveys seek to find "hot" homes to effect remedial action and the data being obtained are not representative of a national average. Some random survey data are available such as that reported by Cohen (29) and some measured for special purposes such as that reported by Nero (28). A summary of these data sets is shown in Table 1.

It appears at the present time that survey data of homes in the United States are distributed in a log–normal manner with an average of 1.5 pCi/L (median 1.0 and geometric standard deviation 2.5). Perhaps a few thousand very high homes in the United States exist which do not fall into this log–normal distribution but represent unusual and special circumstances. The Watras home is one such example but about 500 such homes have already been uncovered in surveys performed by the states of Pennsylvania, New Jersey, and New York, by the U.S. EPA, or by individuals, notably, Bernard Cohen at the University of Pittsburgh.

It has been demonstrated that the source of indoor radon is the soil beneath the building. Only in some cases, for example, in apartments on high floors, does building construction material contribute significantly to the indoor concentration (32). Apartments (high floors) tend to have about twice the outdoor concentration while the normal living areas in single-family homes have five times the outdoor levels (29). Radon dissolved in water (particularly deep well water) when used indoors for dishwashers, showers, and so on contributes to the total indoor concentration by a few percent (33). Only in very special cases does water contribute significantly to the total indoor concentration because the ratio of radon concentration in air to that in water is low (about 1:10,000).

The average indoor ^{222}Rn concentration used in this chapter for purposes of risk estimation is 1 pCi/L (rounded to one significant figure to indicate the uncertainty in the measured U.S. average).

5   RISK PROJECTION MODELS

The mining cohorts studied have not gone to completion so values of lifetime risk must be projected using a particular technique. One special problem when estimating risk of lung cancer following radon daughter exposure is that the epidemiology is based on an occupationally exposed group of male miners. The ubiquitous nature of radon and the recent finding that radon in some homes exceeds permissible occupational standards have made the risk from environmental exposure in the entire United States a national concern (1). Environmental exposure is continuous from birth and this requires a risk assessment model different from that for miners.

Two models are currently applied to the mining data to project lifetime risk. These are (i) the absolute risk model modified to accommodate the normal age appearance of lung cancer and the reduction in risk that appears to occur subsequent to a given exposure, and

TABLE 2. Comparison of Risk Estimates

Source	Risk/WLM for 10^6 person-yr	Period of Expression	Risk/WLM per 10^6 Persons during Expression Period	Relative Risk	Lifetime Risk for 1 WLM/yr
NCRP (24)	10	Remaining lifetime	200		0.9%
UNSCEAR (37)	5–10	40 yr	450		
ICRP (38)	5–15	30 yr	150–450		
NAS (26)	10–50[a]	Remaining lifetime	730[b]		
U.S. EPA (39)		Lifetime	300–700	1.2–2.8%	3.2–7.0%[c] 1.3–2.8[d]
				1–4%	1.3–5.0%[e]
Thomas et al. (40)	3–18		600[b]	2.3%	2.0%

[a] According to age.
[b] Calculated by U.S. EPA.
[c] U.S. EPA WLM.
[d] Standard WLM.
[e] From U.S. EPA *Citizens Guide to Radon.* Assumes 75% occupancy for 70 years.
Source: Reference 36. Printed with permission from Pergamon Press, Ltd, Copyright © 1986.

(ii) the relative risk model that increases the normal age-specific lung cancer risk in the population by a constant fraction per unit radon daughter exposure. It appears, as the miners are followed until death, that the correction for reduced effect subsequent to exposure is necessary in this model also (34).

The mining data lend themselves to development of either risk projection model. The modified absolute model follows the normal age appearance of cancer (above age 40) and risk is expressed for a unit exposure (of 1 WLM). Other factors such as smoking do not affect this model.

Relative risk can be derived from the same data and this model assumes that the risk following an individual exposure is a multiple of the baseline risk for the specific population per unit exposure. This model implies that radon daughter exposure is affected by other agents that make up the age-specific mortality for the particular group. If this is true, then the lung cancer effect of radon daughters in a group of smokers is higher than in a group of nonsmokers (13). Also, the risk for blacks would be considerably greater than for whites.

The Environmental Protection Agency (EPA) (35) issued guidelines in 1986 for radon remediation levels in homes. Their recommendations are based on a constant relative risk model with a range of risk coefficients of 0.01–0.04 per WLM. The risk coefficients and the risk per WLM from the various groups are shown for comparison in Table 2 (36–40).

One of the first published lifetime lung cancer risk estimates for environmental radon daughter exposure was performed by Harley (41) and later extended to both occupational and environmental lifetime risk estimates by NCRP (24).

Risk projection for environmental situations is possible, assuming the choice of a valid model. There are currently two approaches, as described previously—a modified absolute risk model and a relative risk model. In either case, it appears evident that the risk from radon daughter exposure decreases with time after cessation of exposure (34). This was also apparent in the published data from the Czechoslovakian studies, which showed a higher total risk for miners first exposed at older ages than could be explained by the age-specific mortality curves. It suggested that the risk from early exposures had decreased from first exposure as these miners aged.

The first model—the modified absolute risk model—is shown stylistically in Fig. 4. If an exposure (say a 1 year exposure) occurs before the minimum age for cancer appearance

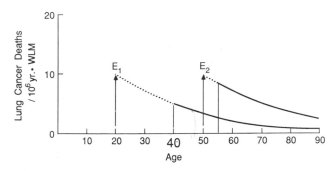

Figure 4. NCRP model for annual appearance of lung cancer attributable to a single exposure of radon daughters. Solid lines indicate the years during which risk is expressed. Risk from exposure at age 20 not expressed until the age at which lung cancer normally appears; risk from exposure at ages greater than 40 not expressed until after the minimum latent interval of 5 years. Risk coefficient reduced from time of exposure with 20-year half-life.

(age 40) there is a latent period from exposure to age 40 before the cancer risk is expressed. If exposure occurs after age 40, there is at least a 5-year interval before a frank cancer can be detected. This latter interval is known as the minimum latent period. Following each (year's) exposure there is an exponential reduction of risk with an empirically estimated 20-year half-time. The risk at age $t > 40$ from a single year's exposure at age t_0 can be expressed beginning at age 40 to end of life (taken as age 85) as

$$A(t|t_0) = (RC)(E)\exp[-K(t - t_0)]P_t/P_{t0}. \qquad (3)$$

$A(t|t_0)$ is the attributable annual lung cancer rate at age $t > 40$ due to a single exposure at age t_0. If exposure occurs after age 40, risk commences at age $t_0 + 5$; if exposure occurs before age 35, risk commences at age 40. RC is the risk coefficient taken as 10×10^{-6} (person year)$^{-1}$ WLM^{-1}. P_t/P_{t0} is the life table correction for death from other causes, where P_t is the probability that an individual will be alive at age t and P_{t0} is the probability that an individual will be alive at age t_0. E is the exposure in WLM/yr and K is the risk reduction factor $\ln(2)/20 \text{ yr}^{-1}$.

The lifetime risk from a single exposure at age t_0 is

$$LR(t_0) = \sum_{t}^{85} A(t|t_0), \qquad (4)$$

where

$$t = 40 \text{ to } 85 \quad \text{for } t_0 \leqslant 35;$$

$$t = t_0 + 5 \text{ to } 85 \quad \text{for } t_0 > 35.$$

For multiyear exposures such as from continuous environmental exposure, E per year, the lifetime risk is

$$LR = \sum_{t_0}^{t_n} LR(t). \qquad (5)$$

The lifetime risks for various exposure regimes may be calculated readily for the modified absolute model. These are shown in Table 3 for exposures of from 1-year duration to lifetime and for ages at first exposure of from birth to age 60. The table values are taken from the NCRP model (24).

Illustrative Example 1 (NCRP Model). An individual resides in a home with a measured annual average radon concentration of 4 pCi/L from birth until death at age 85. This is the maximum risk from radon daughter exposure that this home can pose. The annual exposure in WLM is, assuming 50% equilibrium for the daughters,

$$WLM/yr = \left(\frac{^{222}Rn \text{ pCi/L}}{200}\right)\left(\frac{8760 \text{ h/yr}}{170 \text{ h}}\right) = \left(\frac{4}{200}\right)\left(\frac{8760}{170}\right) = 1 \text{ WLM/yr}.$$

From Table 3, the lifetime risk of lung cancer is 0.0091 or about 1%. This is the additional risk from radon alone; other risks of lung cancer such as from smoking are not included in this value. The expected lung cancer risk for smokers is about 10% and to nonsmokers 1%.

TABLE 3. Lifetime Lung Cancer Risk as a Function of Age and Duration of Exposure under Environmental Conditions per WLM per Year[a]

Exposure Duration	Age at First Exposure								Lung Cancers in a Population of 10^5 Persons[b]
	1	10	20	30	40	50	60	70	
1 year	6.4×10^{-5}	9.1×10^{-5}	1.3×10^{-4}	1.8×10^{-4}	2.1×10^{-4}	1.7×10^{-4}	1.3×10^{-4}	7.0×10^{-5}	13
5 years	3.4×10^{-4}	5.0×10^{-4}	6.9×10^{-4}	9.8×10^{-4}	1.0×10^{-3}	8.4×10^{-4}	5.5×10^{-4}	2.8×10^{-4}	66
10 years	7.7×10^{-4}	1.1×10^{-3}	1.5×10^{-3}	2.1×10^{-3}	2.0×10^{-3}	1.4×10^{-3}	9.1×10^{-4}	3.8×10^{-4}	130
30 years	3.4×10^{-3}	4.8×10^{-3}	5.5×10^{-3}	5.5×10^{-3}	4.2×10^{-3}	2.5×10^{-3}	1.3×10^{-3}	3.8×10^{-4}	380
Life	9.1×10^{-3}	9.1×10^{-3}	7.7×10^{-3}	7.7×10^{-3}	4.5×10^{-3}	2.7×10^{-3}	1.3×10^{-3}	3.8×10^{-4}	560

[a]For radon daughters measured under environmental rather than underground mining conditions.
[b]For a population with age characteristics equal to that in the whole United States in 1975.
Printed with permission from the National Council on Radiation Protection and Measurements.

Illustrative Example 2 (NCRP Model). A person lives in two homes: the first from birth until age 30 with radon concentration of 10 pCi/L and then in home 2 with radon concentration of 1 pCi/L from age 30 until death at age 85. The homes are occupied 80% of the time by this person; the other 20% of the time is spent outdoors or in a working environment where the radon concentration is 0.2 pCi/L. For this example it is assumed that radon daughter equilibrium is 50% for both indoors and outdoors. Actually, outdoor equilibrium is usually somewhat higher with 70% being typical. The annual exposure in home 1 is

$$\text{WLM(1)} = [(10 \text{ pCi/L})(0.8) + (0.2 \text{ pCi/L})(0.2)](1/200)(51.5) = 2.07 \text{ WLM/yr}.$$

In home 2 the annual exposure is

$$\text{WLM(2)} = [(1 \text{ pCi/L})(0.8) + (0.2 \text{ pCi/L})(0.2)](1/200)(51.5) = 0.21 \text{ WLM/yr}.$$

From Table 3, the lifetime risk of lung cancer will be

$$\text{LR} = (2.07)(0.0034) + (0.21)(0.0077) = 0.0086$$

or about 0.9% lung cancer risk.

The relative risk model is shown stylistically in Fig. 5. Each years exposure increases the baseline age-specific mortality by a fraction, RC:

$$R(t) = (RC)(E)M(t)P_t/P_{t0}, \tag{6}$$

where $M(t)$ is the age-specific mortality rate at age t. The same minimum latent interval as in Eq. (3) applies. RC is the risk coefficient or fractional increase in mortality/WLM. Lifetime risk from this single year's exposure is

$$\text{LR}(t_0) = \sum_{t}^{85} R(t|t_0) \tag{7}$$

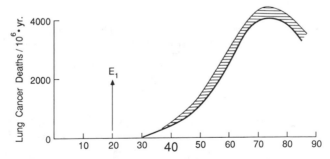

Figure 5. Stylistic representation of a constant relative risk model. Shaded area is the increased risk per WLM from exposure E_1. Risk is calculated as the constant fractional increase in the age-specific lung cancer mortality (solid line) for the group selected. For exposure after the age where lung cancer appears, there is a 5-year minimum latent interval before risk is expressed.

and lifetime risk from continuous exposure would be

$$LR = \sum_{t_0}^{t_n} LR(t). \tag{8}$$

Lifetime risks for various exposures where RC was taken as 0.01 per WLM are shown in Table 4. From Table 4 it can be seen that for the average exposure in the U.S. cohort of miners (800 WLM and 10-years duration) almost 50% mortality from lung cancer would be expected. This is not in agreement with observations of this group, which show that less than 10% mortality from lung cancer has occurred and that the total lung cancer mortality when all miners have died is not expected to double. Whittemore (13), in an analysis of the U.S. miner cohort, found that a relative risk coefficient of 0.0031 per WLM gave a best fit to the data.

Hornung (34) has reported that in the U.S. cohort it is apparent that a reduction in risk after cessation of exposure has occurred. He indicates that in a relative risk model the half-time for risk reduction is 10 years. Introducing this correction factor into the relative risk model yields

$$R(t|t_0) = (RC)(E)M(t)\exp[-c(t-t_0)]P_t/P_{t0}, \tag{9}$$

$$c = \ln 2/10 \, \text{yr}^{-1}.$$

A minimum latent interval of 5 years is always used, to agree with the observation that it requires at least this time for the appearance of lung cancer.

These calculations are shown in Table 5 for RC = 0.01 or a 1% relative risk coefficient.

It is of scientific interest to know which of the two models described, or whether perhaps another form of model, is most correct for human risk projection of lung cancer from radon daughter exposure. There is some evidence that the relative risk model is not entirely appropriate. Samet (42) in a study of Navajo uranium miners in New Mexico showed that the lower 95% confidence limit for the relative risk of lung cancer associated with uranium mining was 14.4. Unfortunately, radon daughter exposure was not accurately known. This high relative risk for primarily nonsmokers suggests that the risk in smoker and nonsmoker may be similar, pointing toward an absolute model. Radford (19) found a similar result in the Swedish iron miners with a relative risk coefficient of 0.107 per WLM for nonsmokers and 0.024 per WLM for smokers. This

TABLE 4. Calculated Lifetime Lung Cancer Mortality per Million Persons from Radon Daughter Exposure of 1 WLM/year as a Function of Age at First Exposure and Exposure Duration[a]

Exposure Duration	Age at First Exposure				
	Birth	10	20	30	50
1 year	670	680	680	700	650
10 years	6,800	6,800	6,900	7,000	6,000
20 years	14,000	14,000	14,000	14,000	10,000
30 years	20,000	21,000	21,000	20,000	12,000
Lifetime	46,000	39,000	32,000	25,000	12,000

[a]Constant relative risk model with 0.01 increased mortality per WLM; 5-year minimum latent interval.

TABLE 5. Calculated Lifetime Lung Cancer Mortality per Million Persons from Radon Daughter Exposure of 1 WLM/year as a Function of Age at First Exposure and Exposure Duration[a]

Exposure Duration	Age at First Exposure				
	Birth	10	20	30	50
1 year	8	17	34	69	200
10 years	120	240	480	940	2100
20 years	360	720	1400	2500	4000
30 years	840	1700	3000	4700	5000
Lifetime	7200	7100	6800	6500	5000

[a] Relative risk model with risk coefficient of 0.01 increased mortality per WLM reduced exponentially with 10-year half-time; 5-year minimum latent interval.

indicates a similar risk for smokers and nonsmokers. This same finding is documented by Blot for Japanese atomic bomb survivors exposed to external gamma-ray radiation, and it is accepted that lung cancer induced by gamma-ray radiation is best described by an absolute risk model (43).

6 BRONCHIAL ALPHA DOSIMETRY

The only justification for the use of mining epidemiology in environmental situations is by comparison of the alpha dose delivered to stem cells in bronchial epithelium from the activity on the airways that arises through deposition and clearance of material on the bronchial tree. Several calculations of the alpha dose have been performed since the original work of Altshuler (44) and Jacobi (45). The detailed alpha dose has been updated over the years as new information concerning the lung morphometry (46, 47), particle size of the attached and unattached radon daughters (48, 49), and deposition by turbulent diffusion (50, 51) appears. The most recent detailed alpha dose estimates published are those of Harley (52, 53) and James (54, 55). The calculations have shown that the dose delivered to men and women in the environment is the same per unit WLM exposure as that in mines even though the particle size, fraction of unattached daughters, and breathing rates are somewhat different. The 10 major factors that must be accounted for in the dosimetry tend to be compensating from one environment to the other. This means that the mining epidemiology can be used directly without any additional treatment to estimate or project environmental risks. The most recent dosimetry update includes experimental deposition studies by Cohen (51), using the particle sizes of interest in hollow casts of a human lung. The measurements show that the calculated airway activity is realistic and allows correction for the slightly enhanced deposition by turbulence in the upper few airways of the bronchial tree.

There is a short time interval at around 10 years of age where the calculated dose per unit exposure is almost a factor of 2 higher than for an adult. The significance of this is not likely to be great as a significant amount of lung cancer does not develop before about age 40 and there are data that confirm a reduction in the effect of exposure to radon daughters with time postexposure, presumably due to repair or stem cell death. Also, this increased dose per unit exposure in childhood lasts only for a few years and does not add substantially to the lifetime dose.

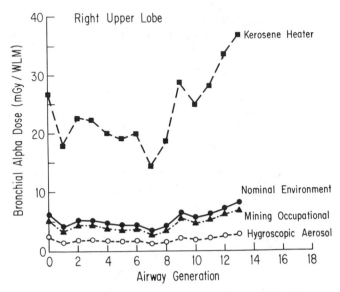

Figure 6. Bronchial alpha dose in mGy/WLM to cells in bronchial epithelium from radon daughters in the adult male. Alpha dose for four conditions: occupational underground mining, typical environmental, environmental with small aerosol size, and environmental with aerosol that will grow hygroscopically in the airways.

The dose per unit exposure as calculated by Harley (53) for the airways in the right upper lobe in a typical miner and for an environmentally exposed adult male are shown in Fig. 6. The dose is shown for airways in the upper right lobe of the human lung but is similar for all five lobes. The site of most lung cancer in the human is the first few airway branches or generations (generations 1–6 of the bronchial region) regardless of whether induction is from radiation exposure, cigarette smoking, or unknown etiology.

Also shown in Fig. 6 are the doses per unit exposure for two unusual conditions. Most radon daughters are attached to the ambient aerosol and the particle size of the aerosol determines the fractional deposition in the airway branches. In special circumstances, such as open flame burning (e.g., kerosene heaters), a very small aerosol is formed and deposition in the upper airways is more efficient. In this case a higher dose per unit exposure results. If the aerosol is hygroscopic, the particles will grow upon entry into the lung, because of the high moisture present, and reduced deposition in the upper airways occurs. These two extremes of dose are unusual and, in most circumstances, mining and environmental doses to the airways are the same.

Small fractions of the ^{218}Po and ^{214}Pb (which decays to the alpha emitter ^{214}Po on the bronchial airways) are not attached to the ambient aerosol. In mines about 4% of the ^{218}Po occurs in the "unattached form" and in environmental situation about 10%. The ratio of unattached ^{218}Po:^{214}Pb is approximately 10:1. There is some concern about the unattached fraction of the daughters because their small size (1–20 nm) ensures 100% deposition on the upper airways. The alpha dose received by the unattached daughters is disproportionally high because of their high deposition (100% versus a few percent for the attached daughters) but the alpha dose from them is generally less than 30% of the total alpha dose because of their low concentration in air.

7   ENVIRONMENTAL RISK EVALUATION

More data are needed to give an accurate description of the average exposure of the U.S. population to indoor radon and radon daughters. These are needed to provide a proper assessment of the lung cancer risk. As of the writing of this chapter, there are three published estimates of indoor radon in the United States which can be used to obtain the "average exposure." These data are shown in Table 1. Applying the best estimate of the average indoor equilibrium factor F of 0.4 for the radon daughters leads to

$$\text{average exposure in WLM} = (1 \text{ pCi/L})F \times \frac{8760 \text{ h exposed}}{170 \times 100}$$

$$= 0.2 \text{ WLM/yr}.$$

This calculation assumes full time spent indoors at the rounded average concentration of 1 pCi/L. Estimates are that about 80% of the time is spent indoors at some location, whether home or in a public or office building. Public buildings tend to be between the concentrations found in single-family homes and the outdoor concentration of about 0.2 pCi/L. Accurate measurements of radom samples taken in a large cross section of homes, offices, and public buildings is an obvious need.

From Tables 3 and 5, regardless of whether a modified absolute risk model or a modified relative risk model is used, the lifetime risk of lung cancer from exposure to average concentrations of indoor radon is about 0.2% or 2 cases per 1000 persons. For the population of the United States this would translate to about 10,000 lung cancer deaths per year due to average indoor radon daughter exposure.

One other possibility exists: that there is a threshold for very low exposures to radon daughters (an exposure below which no lung cancer risk exists). The Canadian mining epidemiology has recorded excess lung cancer at 50 WLM, and so a threshold, if one exists, is very near the average environmental exposures. Current radiobiological theory with support from animal exposure data at low exposures argues against a threshold.

Epidemiology on miners is for 10-year exposure, whereas environmental exposure is over the full lifetime (a possible dose rate effect). The modified absolute risk model accounts for this difference with the exponential reduction in risk for early exposure. It appears that the relative risk model also requires this exponential reduction factor.

8   CONCLUSIONS REGARDING THE MOST LIKELY RISK TO HUMANS

The chain of events leading to an estimate of the population risk from radon daughter exposure in the United States has both strong and weak points. Starting with the underground mining epidemiology, there is a clear excess of lung cancer that cannot be strongly causally related to any air contaminant other than radon daughters. The exposure estimates in these studies are poor, for the most part relying on reconstruction of ventilation changes and mining conditions and on assumptions about radon daughter equilibrium. Studies are underway where more frequent radon daughter measurements were made and where better individual exposure estimates are available for each miner. These studies should provide a stronger base for the numerical risk projections. Such a study is in progress at the University of New Mexico in a prospective follow-up of New

Mexico miners. Epidemiological studies now underway in the United States, Canada, and Sweden to detect excess lung cancer from environmental exposures should resolve the issue of a possible threshold for radon-daughter-induced lung cancer. From the results of the Canadian Ontario miner study, with average exposures of 50 WLM indicating excess lung cancer and with support from the experimental animal studies at even lower exposures, it seems highly improbable that a threshold exists.

Lifetime exposures of 50 WLM are currently experienced in the indoor environment in many homes; in fact, the current EPA guideline of 0.02 WL (4 pCi/L) leads to a lifetime exposure of just over 50 WLM.

The exact modeling technique that should be used to project lifetime risk is not known. As the mining studies go to completion, the appropriate model should emerge. At present, the conventional modeling techniques using reduction in risk with time postexposure yield similar values of lifetime risk and are in agreement with the miner epidemiology and with reasonable estimates of the lung cancer in the environment. It is important scientifically to know the temporal pattern of appearance of tumors for a better understanding of radon-daughter-induced carcinogenesis.

REFERENCES

1. National Council on Radiation Protection, Exposures from the uranium series with emphasis on radon and its daughters. *NCRP Rep.* **77** (1984).

2. D. A. Holaday, History of the exposure of miners to radon. *Health Phys.* **16**, 547–552 (1969).

3. G. Agricola, *De Re Metallica* translated by H. C. Hoover and L. H. Hoover). Dover, New York, 1950 (originally published in 1597).

4. F. H. Harting and W. Hesse, Der Lungenkrebs die Bergkrankheit in den Schneeberger Gruben. *Vierteljahresschr. Gerichtl. Med. Oeff. Sanitaetswes.*, pp. 296–309.

5. A. Arnstein, as cited by Hueper, in *Occupational Tumors and Allied Disease*. Thomas, Springfield, IL, 1942; *Wien. Klin. Wochenschr.* **26**, 748–752 (1913).

6. J. Muller, private communication (1986).

7. M. Uhlig, Ueber den Schneeberger Lungenkrebs. *Med. Clin. North Am.* **4**, 1811–1837 (1921).

8. P. Ludwig and E. Lorenser, as cited by Hueper, in *Occupational Tumors and Allied Disease*. Thomas, Springfield, IL, 1942; *Strahlentherapie* **17**, 428–435 (1924).

9. R. D. Evans and C. Goodman, Determination of the thoron content of air and its bearing on lung cancer hazards in industry. *J. Ind. Hyg. Toxicol.* **22**, 89 (1940).

10. J. H. Harley, A study of the airborne daughter products of radon and thoron. Thesis, Rensselaer Polytechnic Institute (RPI), Troy, NY, 1952.

11. W. F. Bale, Hazards associated with radon and thoron. Unpublished memorandum to the U.S. Atomic Energy Commission, reprinted in *Health Phys.* **38**, 1061 (1980).

12. D. A. Holaday, D. E. Rushing, R. D. Coleman, P. F. Woolrich, H. L. Kusnetz, and W. F. Bale, Control of radon and daughters in uranium mines and calculations on biologic effects. U.S. *Public Health Serv. Rep.* **494** (1957).

13. A. S. Whittemore and A. McMillan, Lung cancer mortality among U.S. uranium miners. *JNCI, J. Natl. Cancer Inst.* **71**, 489 (1983).

14. J. K. Wagoner, V. E. Archer, F. E. Lundin, D. A. Holaday, and J. W. Lloyd, Radiation as the cause of lung cancer among uranium miners. *N. Engl. J. Med.* **273**, 181–188 (1965).

15. J. Sevc, E. Kunz, and V. Placek, Lung cancer in uranium mines and long-term exposure to radon daughters. *Health Phys.* **30**, 433 (1976).

16. E. Kunz and J. Sevc, Lung cancer mortality among uranium miners (methodological aspects). *Health Phys.* **35**, 579 (1978).

17. E. Kunz, J. Sevc, V. Placek, and J. Horacek, Lung cancer in man in relation to different time distribution of radiation exposure. *Health Phys.* **36**, 699 (1979).

18. J. Muller, W. C. Wheeler, J. F. Gentleman, G. Suranyi, and R. A. Kusiak, *Study of Mortality of Ontario Miners.* Ministry of Labor, Toronto, Ontario, 1983.

19. E. P. Radford and K. G. S. Renard, Lung cancer in Swedish iron miners exposed to low doses of radon daughters. *N. Engl. J. Med.* **310**, 1485–1494 (1984).

20. F. E. Lundin, J. K. Wagoner, and V. E. Archer, *Radon Daughter Exposure and Respiratory Cancer: Quantitative and Temporal Aspects,* Jt. Monogr. National Institute for Occupational Safety and Health, and National Institute for Environmental Health Sciences, NTIS, Springfield, VA, 1971.

21. FR, *Federal Register,* Vol. 34, No. 576; Vol. 36, Nos. 101 and 9840 (1971).

22. R. J. Waxweiler, R. J. Roscoe, V. E. Archer, M. J. Thun, J. K. Wagoner, and F. E. Lundin, mortality follow-up through 1977 of the white underground miners cohort examined by the U.S. Public Health Service. In M. Gomez, Ed., *International Conference on Radiation Hazards in Mining, Golden, Corado.* Kingsport Press, Kingsport, TN, 1981, p. 823.

23. J. Muller, R. A. Kusiak, G. Suranyi, and A. C. Ritchie, *Study of Mortality of Ontario Gold Miners, 1955–1977.* Ministry of Labor, Toronto, Ontario, 1986.

24. National Council on Radiation Protection (NCRP), Evaluation of occupational and environmental exposures to radon and radon daughters in the United States. *NCRP Rep* **78** (1984).

25. N. H. Harley Interaction of alpha particles with bronchial cells. *Health Phys.* (1988) (in press).

26. National Academy of Sciences, *The Effects on Populations of Exposure to Low Levels of Ionizing Radiation,* Report, BEIR III. National Academy Press, Washington, DC, 1980.

27. National Council on Radiation Protection, Exposure of the populations in the United States and Canada to natural background radiation. *NCRP Rep.* **94** (1987).

28. A. V. Nero, M. B. Schwehr, W. W. Nazaroff, and K. L. Revzan, Distribution of airborne radon-222 concentrations in U.S. homes. *Science* **234**, 992–996 (1986).

29. B. L. Cohen, A national survey of Rn-222 in U.S. homes and correlating factors. *Health Phys.* **51**, 175 (1986).

30. B. Hultqvist, Studies on naturally occurring ionizing radiations. Thesis (in English). *K. Sven. Vetenkapsakad. Handl., Ser. 4* **3**, 6 (1956).

31. H. Glauberman and A. J. Breslin, *Environmental Radon Concentrations,* HASL NYO-4861. U.S. Atomic Energy Commission, Health and Safety Laboratory, New York, 1957.

32. N. H. Harley and T. Terilli, *Measurement and Apportionment of Radon Source Terms,* Final Report to USDOE. New York University, New York, 1986.

33. F. T. Cross, N. H. Harley, and W. Hofmann, Health effects and risks from Rn-222 in drinking water. *Health Phys.* **48**, 649 (1985).

34. R. W. Hornung and T. J. Meinhardt, *Quantitative Risk Assessment of Lung Cancer in U.S. Uranium Miners* National Institute for Occupational Safety and Health Report. Canters for Disease Control, Cincinnati, OH, 1986.

35. U.S. Environmental Protection Agency, *A Citizens Guide to Radon.* EPA, Washington, DC, 1986.

36. N. H. Harley and J. H. Harley, Risk assessment for environmental exposures to radon daughters. *Environ. Int.* **12**, 39–43 (1986).

37. *UNSCEAR Ionizing Radiation: Sources and Biological Effects.* United Nations, New York, 1982.

38. International Commission on Radiological Protection, *Limits for Inhalation of Radon Daughters by Workers,* ICRP Publ. 32. Pergamon, Oxford, 1981.

39. Environmental Protection Agency, *Draft Background Information Document: Proposed Standards for Radon-222 Emissions to Air from Underground Mines,* Rep. 520/1-85-010. USEPA, Washington, DC, 1985.

40. D. C. Thomas, K. G. McNeill, and C. Dougherty, Estimates of lifetime lung cancer risks resulting from radon progeny exposure. *Health Phys.* **49**, 825 (1985).

41. N. H. Harley and B. S. Pasternack, A model for predicting lung cancer risks induced by environmental levels of radon daughters. *Health Phys.* **40**, 307 (1981).

42. J. M. Samet, O. M. Kutvirt, R. J. Waxweiler, and C. R. Key, Uranium mining and lung cancer in Navaho men. *N. Engl. J. Med.* **310**, 1481–1484 (1984).

43. W. J. Blot, S. Akiba, and H. Kato, Ionizing radiation and lung cancer: A review, including preliminary results from a case control study among A-bomb survivors. In R. L. Prentice and D. J. Thompson, Eds., *Atomic Bomb Survivor Data, Utilization and Analysis.* SIAM, Philadelphia, PA, 1984.

44. B. Altshuler, N. Nelson, and M. Kuschner, Estimation of lung tissue dose from the inhalation of radon and daughters. *Health Phys.* **10**, 1137–1161 (1964).

45. W. Jacobi, The dose to the human respiratory tract by inhalation of short-lived Rn-222 and Rn-220 decay products. *Health Phys.* **10**, 1166 (1964).

46. E. R. Weibel, *Morphometry of the Human Lung.* Academic Press, New York, 1963.

47. H. C. Yeh and M. Schum, Models of human lung airways and their application to inhaled particle deposition. *Bull. Math. Biol.* **42**, 461 (1980).

48. A. C. George, E. O. Knutson, and K. W. Tu, Radon daughter plateout. I. Measurements. *Health Phys.* **45**, 439–444 (1983).

49. E. O. Knutson, A. C. George, R. H. Knuth, and B. R. Koh, Measurements of radon daughter particle size. *Radiat. Prot. Dosim.* **7**, 121 (1984).

50. D. Martin and W. Jacobi, Diffusion deposition of small sized particles in the bronchial tree. *Health Phys.* **23**, 23 (1972).

51. B. S. Cohen, Deposition of ultrafine particles in the human tracheobronchial tree: A determinant of the dose from radon daughters. *Proc. Am. Chem. Soc. Annu. Meet.,* ACS Symposium series 331, pp. 475–486 (1986).

52. N. H. Harley, Comparing radon daughter dose: Environmental versus underground exposure. *Radiat. Prot. Dosim.* **7**, 371 (1984).

53. N. H. Harley and B. S. Cohen, Updating radon daughter bronchial dosimetry. *Proc. Am. Chem. Soc. Annu. Meet., 1986* ACS Symposium series 331 pp. 419–429 (1986).

54. A. C. James, Dosimetric approaches to risk assessment for indoor exposure to radon daughters. *Radiat. Prot. Dosim.* **7**, 353 (1984).

55. A. C. James, A reconsideration of cells at risk and other key factors in radon daughter dosimetry. *Proc. Am. Chem. Soc. Annu. Meet.,* ACS Symposium series 331, pp. 400–418. (1986).

19

Assessment of Potential Health Hazards Associated with PCDD and PCDF Emissions from a Municipal Waste Combustor

David Lipsky
Environmental Risk Management Division, Dynamac Corporation, Fort Lee, New Jersey

1 INTRODUCTION

With many urban areas running out of space for traditional landfills for the disposal of solid and sanitary wastes, and because landfilling has become increasingly prohibitive due to costs, environmental risks, and stiff environmental regulations, the construction of municipal waste combustors (MWCs) to incinerate waste in modern waste-to-energy resource recovery facilities is becoming a favored mechanism to help manage the growing solid waste management problem. Currently, there are approximately 68 waste-to-energy municipal solid waste combustion facilities in the United States. By the year 2000, it is estimated that at least 200 additional plants will be constructed in the United States alone (1). However, construction of these facilities has frequently been delayed due to a number of concerns, the most prominent of which is the issue of toxic emissions and quite often the emissions of polychlorinated dibenzodioxins (PCDDs) and polychlorinated dibenzo-furans (PCDFs).

PCDDs and PCDFs are tricyclic organic compounds that exhibit similar physical and chemical properties. As shown in Fig. 1, PCDDs consist of two benzene rings connected by two oxygen atoms, while PCDFs consist of two benzene rings connected by only one oxygen atom. The isomers of each compound differ by the number and position of chlorine atoms attached to the benzene rings. Figure 1 describes some of the abbreviations and nomenclature used in discussions of PCDDs and PCDFs.

Concerns about dioxin emissions from MWCs were expressed in the late 1970s following the detection of dioxins in fly ash from incinerators in Europe and the detection of the highly toxic 2, 3, 7, 8-TCDD isomer in a stack sample from a Hempstead, Long Island Resource Recovery plant in 1980 (2–5). PCDDs, as well as PCDFs, were also discovered on fly ash from municipal waste combustors. Subsequent reports from Canada,

PCDFs

135 congeners*

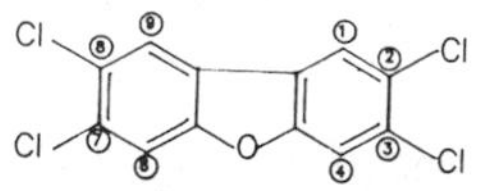

2,3,7,8-TETRACHLORODIBENZOFURAN

Lateral ring positions are 2,3,7 and 8

PCDDs

75 congeners*

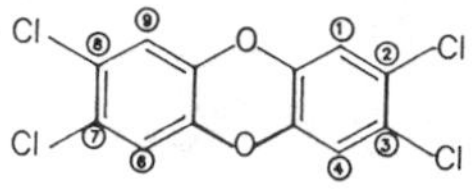

2,3,7,8-TETRACHLORODIBENZODIOXIN

Homologue*	Abbreviation	Number of* Isomers
Monochlorinated dibenzofuran	M_1CDF	4
Dichlorinated dibenzofuran	D_2CDF	16
Trichlorinated dibenzofuran	T_3CDF	28
Tetrachlorinated dibenzofuran	T_4CDF	38
Pentachlorinated dibenzofuran	P_5CDF	28
Hexachlorinated dibenzofuran	H_6CDF	16
Heptachlorinated dibenzofuran	H_7CDF	4
Octachlorinated dibenzofuran	O_8CDF	1
Monochlorinated dibenzo-p-dioxin	M_1CDD	2
Dichlorinated dibenzo-p-dioxin	D_2CDD	10
Trichlorinated dibenzo-p-dioxin	T_3CDD	14
Tetrachlorinated dibenzo-p-dioxin	T_4CDD	22
Pentachlorinated dibenzo-p-dioxin	P_5CDD	14
Hexachlorinated dibenzo-p-dioxin	H_6CDD	10
Heptachlorinated dibenzo-p-dioxin	H_7CDD	2
Octachlorinated dibenzo-p-dioxin	O_8CDD	1

Figure 1. Numbering and nomenclature system for chlorine atoms of the PCDF and PCDD congeners. (*Congener denotes any isomer of any homologue. Homologue defines a group of isomers with the same number of chlorine atoms. An isomer is defined by the arrangement of chlorine atoms within the homologue.)

Japan, France, and the United States confirmed the presence of PCDDs and PCDFs in combustion emission products (6–10).

Based on what was then known about the acute toxicity and suspected high carcinogenic potency of 2, 3, 7, 8-TCDD, the discovery of dioxins in MWC emissions prompted environmental regulatory agencies in Canada, Europe, Japan, and the United States to examine the potential health significance and extent of the dioxin emission problem from MWCs.

In response of these concerns, between 1981 and 1983 the EPA completed risk assessments on six municipal waste combustors (11, 12). These risk assessments were limited to the assessment of the potential carcinogenic risks associated with inhalation of dioxins emitted from the MWC's stacks and by the initial assumption that dioxin-related health risks were restricted to the 2, 3, 7, 8-TCDD isomer. These assessments focused on the 2, 3, 7, 8 isomer since it was the most toxic isomer and, although our understanding of 2, 3, 7, 8-TCDD is still not complete, it has become one of the most studied chemicals so that a good deal of data were available on which to evaluate the risks. As a conservative assumption in their risk assessments, the EPA also calculated carcinogenic risks assuming that all the tetrachlorinated dioxin isomers possessed equal carcinogenic potency as 2, 3, 7, 8-TCDD. In all six assessments, the EPA judged the risks to be insignificant even when extrapolated upper-bound increased carcinogenic risks were estimated in one case at up to 4.6×10^{-5}.

In recent years the above approach to risk assessment has been criticized as being too simplistic. Evaluation of other pollutants emitted from point source stack emissions, such as smelters, and/or from nonpoint sources have indicated that ingestion and dermal absorption of particulate emissions deposited on ground or living surfaces may also be significant exposure pathways (13–15). There is also evidence that indirect routes of exposure such as uptake of PCDDs and PCDFs in meat and milk via the food chain and subsequent human ingestion are also important exposure pathways in some situations (15, 16). Consequently, the traditional approach to risk assessment probably underestimated the degree of total exposure to chemicals released from stacks; although, the human health risks may not be significantly different from those previously predicted owing to the conservatism incorporated in them.

Of note, the EPA has released a new multiexposure pathway risk assessment methodology to account for multicomponent emissions products and to account for the potential risks associated with multiple pathways of exposure (e.g., ingestion, dermal contact, plant uptake, runoff to surface water, and infiltration to groundwater) (1). Furthermore, in the past 2 years several risk assessments for other resource recovery projects have been submitted to state regulatory agencies which evaluate the degrees of risk associated with multiple pathways of exposure (17–21). These assessments have concluded that predicted risks associated with multiple pathways of exposure are significant, in comparison with the risks predicted solely for the inhalation pathway.

In 1984, I co-authored a risk assessment that evaluated the potential risks associated with the release of PCDDs and PCDFs from the proposed Brooklyn Navy Yard Resource Recovery Facility (BNYRRF) in New York City (22). This risk assessment was one of the first to address some of the shortcomings of the EPA risk assessment procedures. Using highly conservative assumptions, we concluded that the upper-bound excess cancer risk for the maximally exposed individual (MEI), due to the complex mixture of PCDDs and PCDFs predicted to be emitted from the BNYRRF, was less than 5.9×10^{-6}. Because of the highly conservative assumptions used in the risk assessment, this level of risk was judged to be insignificant.

The purpose of this chapter is to present the results of the BNYRRF risk assessment and demonstrate some of the procedures used and the assumptions made in evaluating dioxin-related risks from MWCs. However, in this chapter, I have tried to incorporate as much as possible the substantial amount of new information that has become available concerning dioxin emissions from MWCs.

The BNYRRF is one of five waste-to-energy plants to be built in New York City. The New York City Department of Sanitation has generally advocated the construction of these facilities as a means of solid waste disposal and to extend the lifetime of the city's one remaining active sanitary landfill, the Fresh Kills Landfill in Staten Island. The Board of Estimate funded the initial study to address the concerns raised by many in New York City about the alleged potential dioxin-related health risks associated with resource recovery facilities.

The BNYRRF will be a 3000 ton per day (tpd) mass burn facility that will include four 750-tpd combustion units each sharing a 500-ft tall stack and will incorporate the Martin stoker system that has been used elsewhere in the United States, Europe, and Japan. The BNYRRF will have natural gas auxiliary burners located at the point where secondary air will be injected to maintain a minimum secondary combustion temperature of 980°C. Emission control systems that were evaluated in the risk assessment included a high-efficiency (greater than 99.5%) fabric filter to meet an outlet particulate emission loading of 0.015 gr/dscf at 12% O_2. Subsequent to completion of the risk assessment, a dry acid gas scrubber system was added to the pollution control ensemble (22).

The key parts of the risk assessment are as follows:

- Evaluation of physical, chemical, and biological properties of PCDDs and PCDFs.
- Identification of the estimated human cancer risk associated with given degrees of uptake of PCDDs and PCDFs.
- Estimation of the potential PCDD and PCDF emissions from the BNYRRF.
- Estimation of the dispersion and flux of the PCDD and PCDF emissions.
- Estimation of the resulting cancer risk.

2 PROPERTIES OF PCDDs AND PCDFs

2.1 Physical Properties

PCDDs and PCDFs are lipophilic compounds that are only very slightly soluble in water (23). The most studied isomer, 2, 3, 7, 8-TCDD has a high octanol–water partition coefficient and a sorption partition coefficient (k_{oc}) of approximately 10^6 (2, 24). As such, dioxins bind tightly to soils, sediments, and fly ash (2). The extent of this binding may be correlated with the percentage of carbon in the particle, the particle size, and the particle morphology (25). This affinity is demonstrated by the lengthy, difficult, and harsh sample preparation procedures used to extract dioxins and furans from fly ash. For example, Kooke et al. pretreated with hydrochloric acid to extract PCDDs from fly ash (26).

In general, dioxins are stable even when exposed to rigorous conditions including acids, bases, and heat (2, 27). They appear to be fairly resistant to thermal degradation (28). From kinetic and thermodynamic principles, Shaub and Tsang estimated that 99.99% destruction of TCDDs in the gas phase at 727°C may require about 15 min. At 977°C, however, the decomposition may require less than 1 s (28).

Dioxins can undergo photolytic degradation (27, 29, 30). According to a study by Crosby and Wong, 2, 3, 7, 8-TCDD will photolyze in sunlight in the presence of a hydrogen donor (31). Photolytic decomposition of large quantities of TCDD-contaminated soils has been demonstrated with a reported destruction efficiency of 99.94% over a period of several weeks (32). In Seveso, Italy, a hydrogen donor in an aqueous solution was applied to a heavily dioxin contaminated area of grassland in order to enhance photodegradation. After 9 days, 80–90% of the TCDD was destroyed (33, 34). Although an increase in chlorine content may tend to decrease photodegradation, the position of the chlorine atoms may be critical to this process (35, 36).

Laboratory experiments have documented photolytic degradation of PCDDs ranging from 0% for TCDD crystals on a glass plate exposed to sunlight for 14 days to up to 50% degradation of TCDD when irradiated in an isooctane and 1-octanol solution for 40 min with artificial sunlight (24). Vapor phase TCDD is predicted to photolyze rapidly in the atmosphere with a calculated upper-limit half-life of 58 min (29). Based on the above, photolysis may be a significant removal and destruction mechanism for PCDDs on fly ash although the extent to which this occurs is not known.

Very little is known concerning the environmental half-life of dioxins in other environmental matrices. The half-life of 2, 3, 7, 8-TCDD in soil has been reported to range from 6 months to 12 years (37–40). Almost certainly, the degradation of TCDD in soil is dependent on the type of soil, availability of the light to reach the TCDD (e.g., only the top $\frac{1}{2}$ cm would be affected), and the presence of other chemicals (41, 42). Freeman and Schroy have conducted modeling studies of soil sprayed with TCDD-contaminated soil at Times

Beach Missouri. They have predicted that over 67% of the TCDD should volatilize during the first summer from the top 1 cm of soil (43). However, field studies indicate that only approximately 20% of the TCDD actually has been lost from the top 1 cm (42).

The half-life of dioxins in the atmosphere, particularly when bound to fly ash from MWCs is not known; although a calculated upper-bound half-life (for summer sunlight at 40° latitude) of 58 min has been reported (29). However, in addition to removal from the atmosphere by wet and dry deposition processes, dioxins may volatilize from particles and surfaces despite their low vapor pressure (40, 44). Nash and Beall have demonstrated volatilization of TCDD from soil in both field and chamber studies (45). Theoretical calculations by Freeman and Schroy (43) and by Thibodeaux (46) also indicate that volatilization may be a significant removal pathway.

The primary removal mechanism for dioxin in water is through absorption by sediment or biota, although volatilization and photodegradation may occur to some extent (30, 48, 49). A calculated half-life of 6 days has been reported for TCDD in clean surface water (40° latitude under summer lighting conditions) (29). Microbial degradation in most systems is negligible compared to other chemicals.

2.2 Toxicology

2.2.1 Acute Toxicity. PCDDs possess high acute toxicity with an LD_{50} of 0.16 µg/kg for 2, 3, 7, 8-TCDD in male guinea pigs. While other congeners are somewhat less toxic, the LD_{50} values are still in the µg/kg range. As shown in Table 1, considerable variation in toxicity exists among different test species with an LD_{50} of up to 3000 µg/kg in dogs. The least sensitive species is the male hamster with an LD_{50} value of 5051 µg/kg (50). The Wistar rat has also been shown resistant to TCDD's acute toxicity (50). LD_{50} values are approximately 20–30 times higher in mice, monkeys, and rabbits compared to guinea pigs. Differences in the acute toxicity values for the different isomers of PCDD and PCDF are presented in Table 2. The most toxic congeners are those fully substituted in the 2, 3, 7, 8 position.

Some of this variability in acute toxicity probably results from variations in the abilities of different species to metabolize and eliminate PCDDs and PCDFs, whereas some may result from variations in the distribution of cytosolic receptor proteins and consequent activation of aryl hydrocarbon hydroxylase enzymes (AHHs). However, not all interspecies variability can be explained by these factors (51, 52). For example, guinea pigs are

TABLE 1. 2, 3, 7, 8-TCDD LD_{50} for Several Animal Species

Species	Sex	LD_{50} (µg/kg BW)
Guinea pig	Male	0.6–2.1
	Female	3
Rabbits	Mixed	115
Rat, Sherman	Male	22
	Female	45
Rat, Charles River	Mixed	100
Rat, Porton	Female	190
Mouse	Male	114
Dog	Mixed	300–3000
Monkey, rhesus	Female	70

Source: Reference 113.

TABLE 2. Biological Activity of Various PCDD Isomers

Materials	AHH Induction Relative to 2, 3, 4, 8-TCDD	Acute Lethality for Vertebrates LD_{50} (ng/g BW)[a]
2, 3, 7, 8-TCDD	1	0.6–5,000
1, 2, 3, 7, 8-P_5CDD	15	3–338
1, 2, 3, 4, 7, 8-H_6CDD	21	70–800
1, 2, 3, 6, 7, 8-H_6CDD	85	70–1,300
1, 2, 3, 7, 8, 9-H_6CDD	130	60–1,400
1, 3, 7, 8-TCDD	240	
1, 2, 3, 4, 6, 7, 8-H_7CDD	370	600
1, 2, 3, 8-TCDD	1,700	
2, 3, 7-T_3CDD	3,000	30,000
1, 2, 3, 4, 6, 7, 9-H_7CDD	10,000	
1, 2, 3, 4-TCDD	33,000	1,000,000
2, 8-DCDD	33,000	300,000
2, 7-DCDD	33,000	2,000,000
O_8CDD	53,000	1,000,000
1, 2, 3, 6, 7-P_5CDD	220,000	
1, 2, 4, 7, 8-P_5CDD	330,000	1,000–5,000

[a]Units are nanograms per gram of body weight (BW). The number preceding the dish (–) is for the guinea pig (the most sensitive of experimental animals) and the number after the dash is the highest LD_{50} for any vertebrate tested for acute toxicity to PCDDs.
Source: Reference 2.

much more sensitive to the acute lethal effects of PCDDs and PCDFs than are hamsters or rats, yet PCDDs do not induce AHH activity in guinea pigs, and guinea pigs metabolize and excrete PCDDs and PCDFs as rapidly as do rats. Susceptibility of mice to most of the toxic effects of PCDDs and PCDFs is genetically controlled and is associated with the AH locus (51). Table 2 also shows differences in AHH enzyme induction activity for several of the PCDD and PCDF isomers.

The principal effect observed in all species after acute exposure to 2, 3, 7, 8-TCDD is weight loss and thymic atrophy (53). The decrease in weight proceeds slowly even following exposure to a single high dose. Depending on the test animal, deaths occurred up to 45 days after exposure. During this interval, test animals exhibit a general wasting syndrome, associated with poor weight gain or loss of weight. The mean time to death is unaffected by increasing the dose of 2, 3, 7, 8-TCDD (50).

Some effects of 2, 3, 7, 8-TCDD are more species specific. Chloracne, a clinical marker of human dioxin exposure, also occurs in some mice, rhesus monkeys, and rabbits (50). It has not been observed in guinea pigs, hamsters, and some tester strains of mice (53). In rats, rabbits, and mice, 2, 3, 7, 8-TCDD produces an acute liver injury that is not observed in either monkeys, hamsters, or guinea pigs (50).

2.2.2 Chronic Noncarcinogenic Effects.

Several major feeding studies have been performed in order to assess the chronic effects of 2, 3, 7, 8-TCDD in test animals. Effects observed include reduced survival rates, toxic hepatitis, dermatitis, and immunotoxicity (54–59). Chronic toxicity data from these long-term studies have been used to derive a no observed effect level (NOEL) for noncarcinogenic effects for 2, 3, 7, 8-TCDD. Many regulatory agencies base their position regarding acceptable levels of human exposure on the rat feeding studies of Kociba et al. (55) or Murray et al. (59) in arriving at a NOEL of 0.001 μg/kg·day.

2.2.3   Carcinogenicity. Several major long-term animal studies have demonstrated that 2, 3, 7, 8-TCDD is carcinogenic in certain animal species (54–57). The study by Kociba et al. (55) in particular provides substantial evidence that 2, 3, 7, 8-TCDD is a carcinogen in rats, a result confirmed by NCI's investigations (56). 2, 3, 7, 8-TCDD has been classified as a B2 carcinogen using the EPA weight-of-evidence classification system (50). This means that it has been demonstrated to be a carcinogen in animal test models and is a probable human carcinogen. The only other dioxin isomer tested, a mixture of HCDD congeners, has also been tested in rats and been classified as a B2 carcinogen (50).

Although 2, 3, 7, 8-TCDD is carcinogenic to animals, it is not clear whether it can act both as an initiator and as a promoter of carcinogenesis; however, the weight of data indicates that it does not possess genotoxic activity (60, 61). One study showed that 2, 3, 7, 8-TCDD was a potent promoter of liver cancer after initiation with diethylnitrosamine (62). Another study confirmed this observation using 3-methyl chloranthrene (63). Other investigations have produced negative results (64, 65). This issue has been critically reviewed by Shu and co-workers (61). Recently, a special blue ribbon committee established by the EPA indicated that the available data do not suggest that 2, 3, 7, 8-TCDD is an initiator (60).

2.2.4   Human Epidemiology. Studies of the possible effects of TCDD in humans have involved groups reportedly exposed as a result of industrial accidents or through occupational exposure to phenoxy herbicides or chlorophenols (containing TCDD as a by-product) through residence near areas where phenoxy herbicides or chlorophenols were manufactured, or though exposure to areas where industrial wastes were disposed. These studies have been reviewed in several publications (50, 53, 66–69). The noncarcinogenic health effects observed in humans as a result of acute exposure to chemical mixtures containing TCDD have included chloracne, liver disorders, peripheral neuropathy, cardiovascular disease, neurasthenia, and other effects. Aside from chloracne and some reversible acute symptoms, major epidemiological studies have failed to find conclusively serious long-term adverse health effects (53, 60, 66–69). However, in no case was there any quantitative characterization of TCDD exposure and in most cases even qualitative characterization of exposure was incomplete. These factors severely limit the conclusions that can be drawn about the effects of TCDD in humans.

The most extensively studied incident resulting in widespread acute exposure to TCDD occurred in Seveso, Italy in 1976. This accident, caused by the release of a reaction vessel's contents into the atmosphere, exposed workers and residents of the area to 2, 3, 7, 8-TCDD, 2, 4, 5-TCP, and other halogenated compounds. A total of 447 people developed chloracne and some complained of nausea, vomiting, headache, and other symptoms (66, 70–72). Most of these symptoms were reported within several weeks. Although liver problems such as enlarged livers and some abnormal results for liver function tests were reported, when the overall results of these studies were evaluated, no severe systemic health effects were noted (73). Similarly, several follow-up studies of workers potentially exposed to TCDD due to a process accident in the manufacture of 2, 4, 5-T indicated the persistence of chloracne in over 50% of the workers exposed, even after a period of over 30 years (74, 75). Aside from chloracne, investigators failed to demonstrate significant adverse long-term health effects (53, 74, 75).

With respect to potential chronic low-dose exposure to TCDD, some sublethal and nonstatistically significant effects were alleged in residents living at sites contaminated with dioxin-contaminated waste oil (76); however, the results were later found to be incorrectly interpreted or the subclinical effects had subsided (77).

Epidemiological and human health studies have produced contradictory results with respect to TCDD carcinogenicity. These studies have focused primarily on the relation between phenoxy acid herbicides and chlorophenols. The link between these studies and TCDD is the presumptive presence of TCDD as an impurity in phenoxy acids or chlorophenols. As noted above, the inability to quantify actual exposure to TCDD has been a methodological shortcoming of these epidemiological studies.

Several Swedish epidemiological studies have reported an association between occupational exposure to phenoxy acid herbicides or chlorophenols and increased incidence of certain cancers including soft tissue sarcomas, non-Hodgkin's lymphomas, and nasopharyngeal cancers (78–81). However, a case control study of similar design in New Zealand failed to demonstrate a significantly increased risk of soft tissue sarcoma (82–84). There have been several case reports of soft tissue sarcomas among U.S. workers exposed to phenoxy acids and/or PCDDs (85–87). However, some of these reports may be based on erroneous pathological diagnoses (88). Exposure to TCDD-contaminated materials has also been linked to increased stomach cancer mortality rates (89, 90). These results are contradicted by studies that do not show increased stomach cancer rates (85, 86, 91, 92).

In summary, exposure to phenoxy herbicides and chlorophenols has been shown in some studies to be associated with soft tissue sarcoma, lymphoma, stomach cancer, and nasal cancer, but the results have been contradicted by other studies. As a result, no outcome has been conclusively established or rejected (67).

2.2.5 Developmental Effects.

2, 3, 7, 8-TCDD has been demonstrated to be teratogenic in mice and rats (93) and to be fetotoxic in rabbits (94) and monkeys (95, 96). However, the fetotoxicity has been attributed to severe maternal toxicity (53). A three-generation reproduction study showed that the reproductive capacity of rats was affected at TCDD levels of 0.01 and 0.1 μg/kg·day but not at 0.001 μg/kg·day (59).

Although there have been a number of studies attempting to correlate TCDD exposure (again using herbicide exposure as a surrogate for TCDD exposure) with birth defects and abortions in humans, the results of these studies have been conflicting and/or the study design was flawed. A study of birth defects and reproductive outcomes among the wives of military personnel involved with the spraying of herbicides in Vietnam (Operation Ranch Hand) found increases in spontaneous abortions and in birth defects (97). However, the data were obtained largely upon subjective self-reports that require medical record and birth cerfiticate verification (53). Moreover, quantification of exposure concentrations is lacking.

A CDC case–control study in the Atlanta area provided strong evidence that Vietnam veterans as a group had no greater risk for siring babies with serious birth defects (98) than a control population. However, there was a weak association noted between alleged Agent Orange exposure and specific types of birth defects. The AMA in its review of the data indicated that the evidence was weak and that the associations may be due to chance or the result of some unknown bias or uncontrolled confounding factor (53). One study of Australian veterans found no excess birth defects (67). However, none of the findings could be correlated with herbicide exposure because no specific dose–response effect could be shown.

In summary, no data indicate that TCDD has caused teratogenic effects in humans. Additional epidemiologic observations from well-designed studies are warranted before any conclusions can be reached concerning dioxins' ability to produce adverse reproductive effects in humans.

3   DETERMINATION OF "RISK"

Historically, there have been two approaches to estimating risk levels from exposure to toxic agents. One approach involves calculating an acceptable daily intake (ADI) by applying a safety factor to doses of the agent that did not produce an observed effect in laboratory animals (no observed effects level, NOEL). This approach is typically used for noncarcinogenic toxic effects (99). The second approach relies on the use of mathematical models to extrapolate experimental dose–response information obtained from animal exposure studies using high dosage levels to the low levels likely to be encountered by human populations. This latter approach is often used for carcinogens and generally assumes that there is no threshold for the response being extrapolated; that is, any dose, no matter how small, will pose some risk (100–102).

3.1   ADI/NOEL Approach

As discussed previously, 2, 3, 7, 8-TCDD has a variety of toxic effects on laboratory test animals, including embryotoxicity and teratogenicity. Effects have also been observed in various organs and systems including the thyroid, liver, and skin, as well as the immune system (50). Only the 2, 3, 7, 8-TCDD and a mixture of HCDD isomers have been demonstrated to be animal carcinogens. They are both ranked in the B2 category using the EPA's weight-of-evidence classification (50).

Normally, an ADI is not derived from a NOEL for compounds that have been found to be carcinogenic. However, 2, 3, 7, 8-TCDD has not been proved to be an initiator of neoplastic growth (2, 53, 60, 61). In light of this fact, several agencies have found it appropriate to use a NOEL to calculate a guideline or standard. For 2, 3, 7, 8-TCDD, a

TABLE 3. ADIs for 2, 3, 7, 8-TCDD Used by Various Regulating Agencies

Agency[a]	Basis	ADI
Canada	NOEL of 1 ng/kg·day, safety factor of 100	10 pg/kg·day
The Netherlands	NOEL of 1 ng/kg·day, safety factor of 250	4 pg/kg·day
Kimbrough (CDC)	LOEL of 1.8 ng/kg·day, safety factor of 1000	4 pg/kg·day
NYSDOH	NOEL of 1 ng/kg·day, safety factor of 500	2 pg/kg·day
West Germany	NOEL of 1 ng/kg·day, safety factor of 100–1000	1–10 pg/kg·day

[a]References: Canada (104):; The Netherlands (104a); Kimbrough (105); NYSDOH (106); West Germany (106a).

NOEL of 1 ng/kg of body weight per day in rats has been reported in both a three-generation reproduction study by Murray et al. (59) and a 2-year oncogenic study by Kociba (55). On the basis of these studies, regulatory agencies in Canada, The Netherlands, Germany, and elsewhere have developed guidelines or standards by applying safety factors ranging from 100 to 1000 to the NOEL (61). A NOEL of 0.18 μg/kg·day has been reported for a mixture of HCDDs tested in rats (103). NOELs have not been determined for other PCDD and PCDF isomers. A list of the guidelines established by regulatory agencies or published by various authors using the ADI/NOEL approach is provided in Table 3 (104–106a).

3.2 Extrapolating Carcinogenic Risks from High-Dosage Bioassays

For suspected carcinogens, the approach used to determine excess carcinogenic risk is to extrapolate dose–response (i.e., tumor count) data from high-dose animal studies to low-dose risk levels by application of various mathematical extrapolation models. [The true shape of the dose–response curve at low dosages is not known. From a mathematical point of view, determining the actual shape of the dose–response curve at low dosages through low-dose animal feeding studies is probably impossible because of the enormously large and costly number of animals that would be required (100)]. A conversion (and somewhat arbitrary) factor, based on surface area, is then applied to convert animal dosage to human dosage.

A number of mathematical models and assumptions can be applied to the dose–response extrapolation (102). The linearized multistage model has been adopted by the EPA as the primary basis for risk extrapolation in the low-dose region of the dose–response relation (101). The risk estimates resulting from this model should be regarded as conservative, representing a plausible, unlikely, upper limt of the risk; that is, the true risk is not likely to be higher than the estimate, but it could be dramatically lower. Depending on the approach used, the standard cancer models can predict risks of 1 in 1,000,000 at doses of 2, 3, 7, 8-TCDD as small as 6.4 fg/kg·day to as high as 140,000 fg/kg·day (Table 4) (107, 108).

The use of the linear nonthreshold model to extrapolate risk may be a particularly conservative assumption for TCDD since TCDD probably acts as a promoter rather than as an initiator in carcinogenesis (60, 61). The use of a linear extrapolation model is believed to produce an overestimate of risk for carcinogens that are primarily promoters. This argument, however, is open to challenge (100, 109).

TABLE 4. Extrapolated Human-Equivalent Dose–Response Data to Estimate an Upper Bound to Carcinogenic Risk

PCDD Isomer	Agency[a]	10^{-6} Cancer Risk
2, 3, 7, 8-TCDD	Canada	30–90 fg/kg·day
	U.S. EPA	6.4 fg/kg·day
	CDC	28–1428 fg/kg·day
	FDA	57 fg/kg·day
	California	8.0 fg/kg·day
	Sielken	140,000 fg/kg·day
HCDD[b]	U.S. EPA	161 fg/kg·day

[a]References: Canada (2); U.S. EPA (50); CDC (105); FDA (50); California (107); U.S. EPA–HCDD (50); Sielkin (108).
[b]Mixture of 1, 2, 3, 6, 7, 8 and 1, 2, 3, 7, 8, 9 isomers.

Several agencies, including the U.S. Environmental Protection Agency (U.S. EPA), the Centers for Disease Control (CDC), the California Department of Health Survey (CDHS), New York State Department of Health (NYSDOH), and the National Research Center of Canada (NRCC) have published excess carcinogenic risk estimates for 2, 3, 7, 8-TCDD (50, 104–107, 110). The basis for these risk estimates include the 2-year rat-feeding study published by Kociba et al. (55), with an independent pathology review performed by Squire (111) and an NCI study using rats and mice (56). A carcinogenic risk estimate for a mixture of HCDD isomers has also been published by the EPA, based on one NCI study in rats and mice (50, 103).

The carcinogenic risk estimates published by these agencies, using essentially the same data bases, vary over three orders of magnitude as shown in Table 4. The data are presented in terms of the estimated quantity of 2, 3, 7, 8-TCDD or HCDD in fg/kg of body weight which, if consumed each day over a 70-year lifetime, might produce 1 increased case of cancer for every 1,000,000 people exposed to that concentration. It is apparent from this table that the most conservative assessment—one that represents an upper bound to cancer risk—is the risk estimate published by the EPA. For perspective, a cancer risk estimate by Sielken (108) is included in the table to demonstrate that the extrapolated cancer risk may be substantially less than predicted by these regulatory agencies.

There are several factors that account for differences in the risk estimates. First, extrapolations from animals to humans can be done on the basis of either relative weights or surface areas. The latter approach may more closely approximate human pharmacological responses. It is not clear which of the two approaches is more appropriate for carcinogens. The use of extrapolation based on surface area rather than weight increases the unit risk estimates by a factor of 5.8 for rats and about 13 for mice (110). Second, extrapolations can be performed by using the most sensitive responders or by averaging responses. Similarly, these extrapolations can be performed by either grouping different lesion sites to average the risk or by fitting the tumor data from each lesion site. This last procedure can suggest the most sensitive risk levels and target organs (101). The CDC fitted separately the tumor data for each lesion site, thereby providing for a range of extrapolated risk estimates (105). Third, a correction for high early mortality of animals in the high-dose group was used by the EPA to provide an adequate fit of the data to the dose–response extrapolation.

Finally, several different extrapolation models can be used to provide a best fit for the data. Moreover, the method used to extrapolate and fit the dose–response data has a very strong impact in the calculated carcinogenic potencies (102, 108, 112). For example, Sielken has demonstrated that the procedure used to fit the dose–response data reported by Kociba to the linearized multistage model makes the slope of the curve unresponsive to the low experimental dose data and potentially significantly overestimates the carcinogenic potency 2, 3, 7, 8-TCDD (108).

3.3 Multiple Components in Incinerators

Toxicity data required to evaluate risks exist principally for the 2, 3, 7, 8-TCDD isomer, which represents only a small fraction of the PCDD emissions from MWCs. Total PCDD emissions, in turn, may be present in smaller amounts than PCDFs. Therefore, the overall toxicity of the complex mixture of PCDDs and PCDFs predicted in the emission products remains in question. Several approaches have been taken to deal with this uncertainty.

First, all isomers of TCDD can be regarded to be as toxic or carcinogenic as 2, 3, 7, 8-TCDD. This approach is likely to overestimate risks significantly, since the available data

TABLE 5. Weighting Factors Used to Calculated TCDD Toxic Equivalence[a]

Compound	EPA	NYSDOH	Swiss	Ontario[b]	California
2,3,7,8-TCDD	1	1	1	1	1
Other TCDDs	0.01	0	0.01	0.01	0
2,3,7,8-PeCDD	0.5	1	0.1	0.1	1
Other PeCdd	0.005	0	0.1	0.1	0
2,3,7,8-HxCDDs	0.04	0.033	0.1	0.1	0.03
Other HxCDDs	0.0004	0	0.1	0.1	0
2,3,7,8-HpCDD	0.001	0	0.01	0.01	0.03
Other HpCDDs	0.00001	0	0.01	0.01	0
OCDD	0	0	0	0.0001	0
2,3,7,8-TCDF	0.1	0.33	0.1	0.5	1
Other TCDFs	0.001	0	0.1	0.5	0
2,3,7,8-PeCDFs	0.1	0.33	0.1	0.5	1
Other PeCDFs	0.001	0	0.1	0.5	0
2,3,7,8-HxCDFs	0.01	0.011	0.1	0.1	0.03
Other HxPCDFs	0.0001	0	0.1	0.1	0
2,3,7,8-HpCDFs	0.001	0	0.01	0.01	0.03
Other HpCDFs	0.00001	0	0.01	0.01	0
OCDF	0	0	0	0.0001	0

[a]References: EPA (117); NYSDOH (116); Swiss (114); Ontario (104); California (107).
[b]The Ontario method also includes TEFs for mono-, di-, and tri-CDD/CDF.

suggest that substitution in three or four of the 2, 3, 7, 8 positions influences toxicity significantly (113).

A second approach is to use one of several methods for estimating a toxic equivalency factor (TEF) based on the biological activity of the individual isomers for the complex mixture. For example, the Swiss EPA developed a procedure for estimating a TEF by taking into account the relative ability of the various isomers to induce microsomal enzymes (114). A third approach uses bioassay systems to measure 2, 3, 7, 8-TCDD equivalency (115, 116).

Most recently, the Chlorinated Dioxins Technical Panel of the EPA Risk Assessment Forum published a peer-reviewed interim procedure for calculating TEFs from measured or predicted concentrations of PCDD and PCDF homologues. The procedure was based on the EPA's assessment of the literature concerning the biological activity of the various isomers and, in general, gives lower toxic equivalency values than other previously used procedures (117). Table 5 summarizes, for several of the more commonly used procedures, the different weighting factors used to calculate toxic equivalency. Using these various procedures with data on emissions predicted for the BNYRRF, the TEF calculations vary by two orders of magnitude (Table 6).

For the purposes of this risk assessment, two approaches were used to estimate a TEF. For conservatism, an approach similar to the one used by the Swiss EPA was used to calculate a TEF. However, a smaller TEF derived using the EPA weighting procedure was also used to estimate risks in our analysis of uncertainties. The Swiss method was modified somewhat because the Swiss EPA did not address the weighting factor of tri-CDDs or tri-CDFs. Based on limited experiments with 2, 3, 7-tri-CDD, however, the relative toxicity and enzyme induction capacity of the tri-CDDs are at least three orders of magnitude less than 2, 3, 7, 8-TCDD (2). Therefore, a weighting factor of 0.01 was applied as the appropriate weighting factor for the tri-CDDs and tri-CDFs. Based on predicted dioxin

TABLE 6. Calculation of Toxic Equivalency Factors Using Different TEF Estimation Procedures

Isomer/Homologue	Homologue (%)	BNYRRF Emission Rate[a]	EPA b	EPA c	NYSDOH b	NYSDOH c	California 1985 b	California 1985 c	Swiss b	Swiss c	Ontario b	Ontario c
2,3,7,8-TCDD	0.05	0.42	1.00	0.42	1.00	0.42	1.00	0.42	1.00	0.42	1.00	0.42
TCDD	0.95	5.82	0.01	0.06	0.00	0.00	0.00	0.00	0.01	0.06	0.01	0.06
2,3,7,8-PeCDD	0.07	0.76	0.50	0.38	1.00	0.76	1.00	0.76	0.10	0.08	0.10	0.08
PeCDD	0.93	9.94	0.01	0.05	0.00	0.00	0.00	0.00	0.10	0.99	0.10	0.99
2,3,7,8-HCDD	0.30	4.92	0.04	0.20	0.03	0.16	0.03	0.15	0.10	0.49	0.10	0.49
HCDD	0.70	11.48	0.00	0.00	0.00	0.00	0.00	0.00	0.10	1.15	0.10	1.15
2,3,7,8-HpCDD	0.50	3.90	0.00	0.00	0.00	0.00	0.03	0.12	0.01	0.04	0.01	0.04
HpCDD	0.50	3.90	0.00	0.00	0.00	0.00	0.00	0.00	0.01	0.04	0.01	0.04
OCDD	1.00	2.60	0.00	0.00	0.00	0.00	0.00	0.00	0.00	0.00	0.00	0.00
2,3,7,8 TCDF	0.03	2.43	0.10	0.24	0.33	0.80	1.00	2.43	0.10	0.24	0.50	1.21
TCDF	0.97	89.77	0.00	0.09	0.33	0.00	0.00	0.00	0.10	8.98	0.50	44.89
2,3,7,8 PeCDF	0.07	1.90	0.10	0.19	0.33	0.63	1.00	1.90	0.10	0.19	0.50	0.95
PeCDF	0.93	24.70	0.00	0.02	0.00	0.00	0.00	0.00	0.10	2.47	0.50	12.35
2,3,7,8 HxCDF	0.20	12.70	0.01	0.13	0.01	0.14	0.03	0.38	0.10	1.27	0.10	1.27
HxCDF	0.80	50.80	0.00	0.01	0.00	0.00	0.00	0.00	0.10	5.08	0.10	5.08
2,3,7,8 HpCDF	0.50	3.85	0.00	0.00	0.00	0.00	0.03	0.12	0.01	0.04	0.01	0.04
HpCDF	0.50	3.85	0.00	0.00	0.00	0.00	0.00	0.00	0.01	0.04	0.01	0.04
OCDF	1.00	0.60		0.00	0.00	0.00	0.00	0.00	0.00	0.00	0.00	0.00
Sum				1.80		2.91		6.27		21.57		69.09
TEF (sum/2,3,7,8-TCDD)				4.28		6.94		14.93		51.36		164.51

[a] Predicted BNYRRF emission rate (Table 7) for isomer or homologue class, assuming equal distribution of chlorines within each homologue (units ng/NM³).
[b] These columns provide the TEF weighting factors used by the different regulatory agencies.
[c] These columns represent the product of the BNYRRF emission rate times the respective column b.

TABLE 7. Calculation of Toxic Equivalents: Brooklyn Navy Yard Facility

	Concentration in Flue Gas[a] (ng/NM^3)	Relative Toxicity	Toxic Equivalent Concentration
Tri-CDF	307.4	0.01[b]	3.07
Tetra-CDF	92.2	0.10	9.22
Penta-CDF	26.6	0.10	2.67
Hexa-CDF	63.5	0.10	6.35
Hepta-CDF	7.7	0.01	0.08
Octa-CDF	0.6	0.00	0.00
Tri-CDD	13.3	0.01[b]	0.13
Tetra-CDD	6.5	0.01	0.06
Penta-CDD	10.7	0.10	1.07
Hexa-CDD	16.4	0.10	1.64
Hepta-CDD	7.8	0.01	0.08
Octa-CDD	2.6	0.00	0.00
2,3,7,8-TCDD	0.42	1.00	0.42
Total			24.79

$$\frac{\text{Total toxic equivalent}}{2,3,7,8\text{-TCDD}} = \frac{24.79}{0.42} = 59$$

[a]Based on data from the Chicago Northwest and Zurich-Josefstrasse facilities.
[b]Relative toxicity for tri-CDD and tri-CDF assumed based on 3000-fold difference in enzyme induction and 30,000-fold difference in acute toxicity (2).

emission rates from the BNYRRF (see Table 9), a TEF equal to 59 times the toxicity of the 2, 3, 7, 8-TCDD emitted from the BNYRRF was calculated as provided in Table 7. It is important to note that this approach is based on enzyme induction, which may have no relation to toxicity or carcinogenesis. A toxic equivalency of 59 is believed to be a conservative estimate of toxic equivalency on the basis of the limited experiments using fly ash or soot in animal feeding or enzyme bioassay experiments (115, 116, 118).

It should be stressed that the selection of a TEF is arbitrary. The data base is too limited to provide experimentally determined upper and lower limits to toxic equivalency for incinerator emissions. Furthermore, the degree to which a given model can accurately predict toxic equivalency level bioassays has not been fully evaluated. For example, in one feeding study, the use of the Swiss and NYSDOH TEFs overestimated the toxic equivalency of fly ash by a factor of 10–20 times (118).

4 METHODS

4.1 Predicting Emissions from Point Sources

Predicted dioxin emission rates for the BNYRRF were developed based on an analysis of the available literature. In selecting a data set to estimate dioxin emissions, the objective was to evaluate data from modern, well-operated MWCs with heat recovery units, similar in design, operations, and waste type to the proposed Brooklyn facility. Furthermore, the

TABLE 8. Compilation of pre-1984 PCDD Emission Data Used in BNYRRF Risk Assessment[a]

Incinerator	Location	Total Emissions (ng/Nm^3)	References
Chicago Northwest	Chicago	180	119
Zurich-Josefstrasse	Switzerland	202	113
Eskjo	Sweden	532	119[a]
Como	Italy	722	119[b]
Sweden	Sweden	1,436	119[c]
Sweden	Sweden	280	119[c]
Sweden	Sweden	28	119[c]
Hampton	Virginia	12,620	119[d]
Milan I	Italy	1,413	120
Milan II	Italy	204	120
Busto Arisio	Italy	79	120
Desio	Italy	143	120
Italy 1	Italy	537	120[a]
Italy 2	Italy	56,454	120[a]
Italy 3	Italy	8,952	120[a]
Italy 4	Italy	7,988	120[a]
Italy 5	Italy	1,502	120[a]
Italy 6	Italy	639	120[a]
Zaanstad	The Netherlands	2,713	120[b]

[a]Not all homologues quantified in all studies.

test data to be evaluated had to have been obtained using methods that were compatible with sampling, analytical, and quality assurance protocols of the U.S. EPA.

The emission data selected as the most representative of the BNYRRF was the data from the Chicago Northwest facility and the Zurich-Josefstrasse facility (114, 119). The latter facility was used to provide supplementary data on penta-CDD emission rates since the penta-CDDs were not speciated in the Chicago study.

Both facilities use a furnace design similar to that proposed for the BNYRRF. The Chicago facility is located in an urban area with a waste stream presumably similar to new York City's and was tested under the sponsorship of the U.S. EPA using sampling methods to capture both gaseous and particulate forms of PCDDs and PCDFs. In addition, stringent quality assurance controls were used in order to assure data representativeness. The Zurich-Josefstrasse facility was tested by the Swiss counterpart to the U.S. EPA using similarly rigorous sampling and analytical protocols. It is important to note that there continues to be disagreement on the selection of appropriate data sets to predict emissions from MWCs. First, dioxin emission rates from MWCs tested prior to 1984 have been shown to vary by two to three orders of magnitude. As shown in Table 8 (119a–120b), the Chicago Northwest facility had some of the lower dioxin emission rates. Therefore, it was suggested that the Chicago data set may be biased toward a "best-case" rather than the "average" or "worst-case" estimate of probable emissions from the BNYRRF. Second, the data indicate that while as a general trend emissions of dioxins appear to be inversely related to furnace temperature and good combustion efficiency, emissions are not related to furnace conditions alone. Rather, emissions probably depend on a number of complex variables related to the design and operation of the incineration process (including postcombustion formation phenomena outside the firebox) (1, 121). For example, three systems that were designed for resource recovery emitted PCDDs and PCDFs that were two to three orders of magnitude higher than Chicago. These are the two plants in Milan, Italy with Volund steam generation systems and the Hampton, Virginia refuse-fired steam boiler (5, 120). Similarly, a test of the ANSWERs RDF plant indicated that dioxin emissions were higher while using an auxiliary burner to maintain high secondary combustion temperatures than when the system was turned off (122). Accordingly, using one data set to make simple comparisons between incinerators of reasonably similar design may not be appropriate in estimating emissions.

A third source of disagreement is based on our still incomplete understanding of the rate-determining steps controlling dioxin emission rates. For example, Commoner and others have proposed that the rate-controlling step effecting dioxin emissions is not the destruction of dioxin and its precursors in the furnace of the MWC, rather it is the formation of dioxin as a postcombustion product through de novo synthesis between phenolic compounds produced when lignin (from the paper wastes) breaks down in the heat of the furnace and reacts with chlorine on fly ash surface (121). If this theory is correct, then selection of a data set on the basis of comparable MWC design and combustion parameters may not be a sufficient condition for ensuring comparable dioxin emission rates. This theory is supported by recent data from PEI and from the Westchester plant where higher concentrations of dioxins were detected in the stack downstream of the furnace (123, 124). Furthermore, Vogg has demonstrated that the reaction chemistry of fly ash supports the hypothesis of postcombustion formation of dioxins since simply heating fly ash obtained from an operating incinerator at 300–400°C results in significant dioxin formation on the fly ash caused by precursors present on the fly ash. Above 400°C dioxin volatilization and degradation of dioxins predominate (125). Similar evidence for catalytic synthesis of dioxins on fly ash has recently been reported by Karasek (126).

While the above indicates that there is incomplete knowledge concerning the factors regulating dioxin emission rates, recent tests from newly constructed MWCs with advanced combustion and air pollution control equipment support the use of the Chicago data set for the purpose of this risk assessment. As indicated in Table 9 (127–127c), dioxin emissions at these facilities (particularly facilities equipped with a dry scrubber and baghouse air pollution control equipment) were found to have emission levels similar to or lower than the levels measured in Chicago. Moreover, when the available emissions data from properly operated mass burn facilities with some form of heat recovery and excess air

TABLE 9. Dioxin Emission Test Results from Recently Constructed Waste-to-Energy Facilities

| Facility Name | Date Constructed | Air Pollution Control Equipment | Dioxin Emissions Data (ng/NM^3 at 12% CO_2) | | |
			Date	PCDDs	PCDFs	References
Chicago Northwest	1970[a]	ESP	1980	58	259	119
Zurich-Josefstrasse	1978	ESP	1981	171	134	113
Wurzburg	1984	Dry scrubber	1985	22.1	27.9	120[a]
Tulsa, OK	1986	ESP	1986	18.9	15.5	120[b]
Hogdalen, Sweden	1986	Dry scrubber Feb. filter	1986	6.4	12.7	127
Marion County, OR	1986	Dry scrubber Fab. filter	1986	1.1	0.4	127[a]
Westchester, NY	1985	ESP	1985	24	76	127[b]
North Andover	1985	ESP	1986	114	234	127[c]

[a]Includes estimated values for nonquantified isomers.

TABLE 10. Predicted PCDF and PCDF Emissions from BNYRRF[a]

	Concentration in Flue Gas[b] (ng/NM^3)	Mass Emission Rate (μg/s)
Tri-CDF	307.4	51.18
Tetra-CDF	92.2	15.35
Penta-CDF	26.6	4.33
Hexa-CDF	63.5	10.58
Hepta-CDF	7.7	1.28
Octa-CDF	0.6	0.10
Total CDF	498.0	82.92
Tri-CDD	13.3	2.22
Tetra-CDD	6.5	1.07
Penta-CDD	10.7	1.79
Hexa-CDD	16.4	2.73
Hepta-CDD	7.8	1.30
Octa-CDD	2.6	0.43
Total-CDD	57.3	9.54
2, 3, 7, 8-Tetra-CDD	0.42	0.07

[a]Assuming all emitted PCDDs and PCDFs are in gaseous form.
[b]Based on testing of the Chichago Northwest and Zurich-Josefstrasse facilities. Corrected to flue gas conditions projected for BNYRRF: that is, 10.5% CO_2 (dry basis) and 13.63% H_2O.

are examined, the Chicago emissions factor is above the median values (when measured as TCDD toxic equivalents) (120a). Thus, from the risk assessment perspective, the Chicago data set provides a reasonably conservative emission rate compared with recently tested facilities.

By using the Chicago Northwest and Zurich-Josefstrasse data, the estimated BNYRRF emissions corrected for the size of the BNYRRF and assuming a flue gas emission rate of 99,900 Nm^3/min are presented in Table 10.

4.2   Correcting Emission Rates for Fabric Filter Pollution Control

The Chicago and Zurich-Josefstrasse facilities utilized electrostatic precipitators (ESP) for pollution control, whereas the BNYRRF will utilize fabric filters designed to emit less than half the weight of fly ash emitted by an ESP comparable in efficiency to those used in Chicago. Therefore, since it was assumed that some of the dioxins were adsorbed to particulates, the dioxin emissions from the BNYRRF should be less than those observed for comparable facilities using an ESP.

Recent testing indicates that without appreciable cooling of the combustion gas, up to 75% of the dioxins will be in a gaseous state or attached to aerosol particles less than 0.1 μm in diameter (1). However, the data from individual facilities that have been tested vary widely so that the exact degree of partitioning is not known (127). In the absence of empirical data, the emissions from the BNYRRF were calculated in two ways: case 1 assuming all dioxins emitted from the test facilities were gaseous, and case 2 assuming that dioxin emissions were particulate bound. The true emission rates will fall between these two values.

A further refinement to the emission rates was developed based on an assumption that dioxin concentrations per unit mass of particles were inversely proportional to particle size. This assumption is based on the hypothesis that the adsorption and/or synthesis of dioxin on particulates takes place on surface reactive sites, by analogy with data on trace metal concentrations in fine particles emitted from incinerators and coal-fired power plants (128–130), and by studies on dioxin formation on fly ash residues (126). This hypothesis is also supported by several investigations, which have reported from 2 to 12 times higher concentrations of dioxins emitted on fly ash from incinerator stacks than on the larger fly ash particulates collected from the electrostatic precipitator hoppers (130–133). However, it should be noted that other investigators report inconclusive results (134). It has also been postulated that dioxin concentrations in fly ash may be impacted by adsorption primarily to a porous carbonaceous core covered by a constant-thickness outer layer such that the larger particles are enriched for dioxins rather than the smaller particles (17).

While the exact relation between fly ash particle size and dioxin concentrations is still being investigated, for the purpose of this risk assessment, and consistent with current EPA guidance (1), it has been assumed that an inverse relation between particle size and PCDD and PCDF concentrations exists.

The particle size distribution expected to be emitted from the BNYRRF's stack is not known with certainty since there is only a limited amount of test data from similarly designed mass burn facilities equipped with fabric filters and acid gas air pollution control systems (1). For this risk assessment, the particle size distribution of stack emitted particulates from the Braintree Municipal Incinerator (Table 11), which is a mass burn facility with an ESP, was used to estimate particle size distributions emitted from the BNYRRF (135). (Recently, data have been published for several other MWCs. However, the Braintree data set appears to be a reasonable data set to use at this time since it provides a mass median particle diameter that is the approximate average value of these facilities.)

TABLE 11. Particle Size Distribution in Resource Recovery Stack Emissions (Electrostatic Precipitator Outlet)

Geometric Mean Particle Diameter (μm)	Percentage of Total Weight[a] (%)	Percentage of Total Surface Area (%)
15.0	12.8	1.5
12.5	10.5	1.5
8.1	10.4	2.2
5.5	7.3	2.3
3.6	10.3	5.0
2.0	10.5	9.2
1.1	8.2	12.9
0.7	7.6	16.6
< 0.7	22.4	48.8

[a]From an average of six tests run at the resource recovery plant electrostatic precipitator outlet.
Source: Reference (135).

The emissions data from the Chicago and Zurich-Josefstrasse facilities (Table 10) and the particulate emissions data from Braintree (Table 11) were used in a series of calculations (numbered 1–4) to determine the PCDD and PCDF emission rates by particle size expected from the BNYRRF assuming the installation of a fabric filter pollution control system instead of the ESP that was used in the Chicago facility. These data in turn were used as input to the air dispersion models described in Section 5.

Example Calculation 1. Calculating the Surface Area to Weight Ratio of Each Particle Size Class

Given:

- Assume aerodynamically spherical particles.
- Specific surface area (S) of a spherical particle with radius r:

$$S = 4\pi r^2$$

- Volume (V) of spherical particle with radius r ($r = 7.5\,\mu\text{m}$ for 15-μm particle):

$$V = \tfrac{4}{3}\pi r^3.$$

Then

$$S/V = 4\pi r^2 / \tfrac{4}{3}\pi r^3 = 3/r \tag{1}$$

Example:

$$S/V = 3/7.5 = 0.4 \quad \text{(results for other size particles not shown)}.$$

Multiplying the ratio of the surface area to volume by the percent weight fraction of particles emitted in a given size category should approximate the amount of surface area available for adsorption in that particle size category. Dividing the surface area for each particle category by the total available surface area for all particles gives an estimation of the fraction of total area on any size particle. If the emission rate of a pollutant in grams per second is known, then the multiplication of the emission rate times the fraction of available surface area per particle size will determine the emission rate of the pollutant as a function of particle size. See the next calculation.

Example Calculation 2. Determining the Available Surface Area of Each Particle Size Class

Given:

- Particle density is constant and therefore the particle volume is proportional to the particle weight.
- S/V_i is the surface to volume (or weight) ratio of a given particle size class i [Eq. (1)].
- F_{wi} is the weight fraction of a given particle size class i (obtained from Braintree; see Table 11).
- SA_i is the relative proportion of total surface area for size class i.

Then:

$$SA_i = (S/V_i) \times F_{wi}. \tag{2}$$

Example:

$$S/V_i = 0.4.$$

$$F_{wi} = 12.8\% = 0.128 \quad \text{(Table 11)}.$$

$$SA_i = 0.0512 \quad \text{(other values not shown)}.$$

Example Calculation 3. Calculating the Percentage of the Total Surface Area Comprised of Particle Size Class i

Given:

- SA_i is the relative proportion of total surface area for size class i.
- $\sum SA$ is the sum of SA_i for all i ($\sum SA = 3.44$—not shown).
- F_{si} is the fraction of the total surface area comprised of size class i particles.

Then:

$$F_{si} = SA_i/\sum SA. \tag{3}$$

Example:

$$SA = 0.0512.$$

$$\sum SA = 3.44.$$

$$F_{si} = 0.0149 = 1.5\% \quad \text{(all other values for } F_{si} \text{ are given in Table 11)}.$$

Assuming that dioxins are adsorbed to particulates in proportion to available surface area, then 12.8% of the emitted fly ash weight and 1.5% of the particle surface area is comprised of 15-μm particles (Table 11). For particle size class i, the PCDD emission rate (μg/s) will equal the total PCDD emission rate (9.54 μg/s from Table 10) times the fraction of total surface area. (Note: The total PCDD emission rate of 9.54 μg/s is based on testing of the Chicago NW and Zurich–Josefstrasse facilities corrected to the conditions projected for the BNYRRF-correction calculations not shown.) The total fly ash emission rate for class i will equal the total fly ash emission rate (7.94 g/s—obtained from PDEIS) times the percentage weight of that size class. This information in turn was used in Example Calculation 4 to compute the PCDD emission rates per gram of fly ash emitted.

Example Calculation 4. Determining PCDD and PCDF Emission Rates per Gram of Fly Ash Emitted for Each Particle Size Category

Given:

- FA is the fly ash emission rate (obtained from PDEIS and equal to 7.94 g fly ash/s).

TABLE 12. Calculated Concentration of PCDF and PCDD in Fly Ash Emissions as a Function of Particle Size at the Outlet of an ESP

Mean Particle Diameter (μm)	PCDD Concentration (ng/g)	PCDF Concentration (ng/g)
15.0	141	1,224
12.5	172	1,492
8.1	254	2,209
5.5	379	3,291
3.5	583	5,070
2.0	1,053	9,150
1.1	1,890	16,429
0.7	2,624	22,812
<0.7	2,618	22,751

- DA is the total PCDD emitted (taken from Table 10 and equal to 9.54 μg PCDD/s).
- DA_i is the number of μg PCDD/g emitted fly ash for particle size class i.

Then:

$$DA_i = \frac{DA(\mu g/s) \times F_{si}}{FA(g/s) \times F_{wi}}. \tag{4}$$

Example:

$$DA_i = (9.54 \ \mu g/s \times 0.015)/(7.94 \ g/s \times 0.128)$$

$$= 0.141 \ \mu g \ PCDD/g \ fly \ ash \ P141 \ ng/g$$

(The values for other size class categories are provided in Table 12). For the case of a fabric filter instead of an ESP, the particle size distribution by weight and a total fly ash emission rate for a fabric filter system were provided by the contractor (Table 13). PCDD emission rates, assuming the use of fabric filter for various particle size categories, were calculated as described below.

Example Calculation 5. Calculating PCDD and PCDF Emission Rates if a Fabric Filter Rather Than an ESP Were Used in the BNYRRF

Given:

- FA_{ff} is the fly ash emission rate for a fabric filter pollution control system (equal to 3.97 g/s according to contractor).
- F_{wi} is the weight fraction of ith particle size class for a fabric filter system (data obtained from contractor and provided in Table 13).
- DA_i is the dioxin concentration on ith particle size class in ng PCDD/g of fly ash as determined in Table 12.
- DER_i is the dioxin emission rate (ng/s) for ith particle size class.

Then:

$$DER_i = FA_{ff} \times F_{wi} \times DA_i. \tag{5}$$

TABLE 13. Predicted PCDF and PCDD Emission Rates from BNYRRF as a Function of Particle Size at the Outlet of a Fabric Filter

Mean Particle Diameter (μm)	Weight Percent[a] (%)	Fly Ash Emission Rate (g/s)	PCDD Emission Rate (ng/s)	PCDF Emission Rate (ng/s)
15.0	24	0.953	134	1,166
12.5	11	0.437	75	652
8.1	7	0.278	71	614
5.5	5	0.199	75	655
3.5	7	0.278	162	1,409
2.0	7	0.278	293	2,544
1.1	14	0.556	1,051	9,135
0.7	10	0.397	1,042	9,056
< 0.7	15	0.596	1,560	13,560
Total	100	3.972	4,463	38,791

[a]Weight percent fractions for particle sizes were calculated from data contained in personal communication.

TABLE 14. Predicted PCDF and PCDD Emissions from BNYRRF[a]

	Fraction	Concentration on Fly Ash (ng/g)	Mass Emission Rate (μg/s)
Tri-CDF	0.6173	6029	23.946
Tetra-CDF	0.1851	1808	7.180
Penta-CDF	0.0534	521	2.071
Hexa-CDF	0.1275	1245	4.946
Hepta-CDF	0.0155	151	0.0601
Octa-CDF	0.0012	12	0.047
Total CDF	1.0000	9766	38.791
Tri-CDD	0.2321	261	1.036
Tetra-CDD	0.1135	127	0.0507
Penta-CDD	0.1867	210	0.833
Hexa-CDD	0.2862	322	1.277
Hepta-CDD	0.1361	153	0.607
Octa-CDD	0.0454	51	0.203
Total CDD	1.0000	1124	4.463
2, 3, 7, 8-Tetra-CDD	0.0073	8	0.0326

[a]Assumes that all emitted PCDFs and PCDDs are on particulates.

Example:

$$FA_{ff} = 3.97 \quad \text{(Table 13).}$$

$$F_{wi} = 0.24 \quad \text{(Table 12).}$$

$$DA_i = 141 \, ng/g \quad \text{(Table 12).}$$

$$DER_i = 134 \, ng/s \quad \text{(all other values for DER are provided in Table 13).}$$

Based on Example Calculation 5, the PCDD and PCDF emission rates are presented in the last two columns of Table 13; the total emission rates are 4463 ng/s for PCDD and 38,791 ng/s for PCDF. Assuming the ratios between homologues remains unchanged following collection by the fabric filter, the emissions of isomer groups from the fabric filter outlet are presented in Table. 14.

5   EXPOSURE ASSESSMENT

5.1   Air Quality Impacts

In order to assess the impact of the emissions from the proposed BNYRRF on the general population, computer modeling was performed on the emissions data to predict downwind dioxin concentrations in ambient air, soil, dust, and dirt. The prediction of ambient air concentrations of dioxins quantifies potential population exposure through the inhalation pathway, while the deposition analysis provides an estimation of potential human exposure through the ingestion of contaminated dirt and dust, as well as human exposure through dermal contact with these materials.

The model approved by the NYCDEP, as the one appropriate for analyzing air quality impacts resulting from the BNYRRF stack emissions, was the MPTERU model (136). This model is a modification of the MPTER model and uses dispersion coefficients determined empirically to be more suitable for urban areas. These coefficients are considered by the NYCDEP to be more appropriate for dispersion analyses of point sources in New York City.

The MPTERU program was used to determine normalized concentrations of pollutants at all potential receptor locations in the area of significant impact including ground-level receptors within 25 km of the Brooklyn Navy Yard, as well as elevated receptors in New York. Five years of historical meteorological data from the area of the incinerator were used to compute hour-by-hour impact concentrations at each receptor location. The hourly concentrations were then averaged to arrive at normalized ambient air concentrations.

The maximum ground-level receptor concentrations of PCDD and PCDF were determined by multiplying the maximum normalized concentrations (for the worst-case receptor location) times the emission rate for dioxin ($\mu g/s$) to obtain the ambient concentrations ($\mu g/m^3$). Ground-level and elevated receptor impacts were determined to be almost identical. If we assume as case 1 that all dioxins are emitted from the stack in a gaseous state, then application of the emission rates shown in Table 10 to the maximum normalized concentrations results in the maximum ambient air concentrations shown in the first column of Table 15. Application of the emission rates shown in Table 14 for case 2, assuming 100% adsorption to particulates, provides maximum ambient air concentrations of dioxins as shown in the second column of Table 15.

TABLE 15. Predicted Maximum Annual Average Exposure Concentrations of PCDFs and PCDDs Due to Emissions from the BNYRRF

	Case 1: PCDF and PCDD Emissions Are Gaseous	Case 2: All PCDF and PCDD Emissions Are Adsorbed on Particulates				
	Maximum Concentration in Air (pg/m^3)	Maximum Concentration in Air (pg/m^3)	Maximum Annual Deposition Rate (ng/m^2)	Concentrations in Soil After 1 year (fg/g) (a)	Concentrations in Street Dirt (pg/g) (b)	30-day Accumulation in House Dust (pg/m^2) (c)
Tri-CDF	1.2283	0.5747	4.790	299	64	100
Tetra-CDF	0.3684	0.1723	1.436	90	19	30
Penta-CDF	0.1063	0.0497	0.414	26	6	9
Hexa-CDF	0.2539	0.1187	0.990	62	13	21
Hepta-CDF	0.0307	0.0144	0.120	8	2	2.5
Octa-CDF	0.0024	0.0011	0.009	0.6	0.1	0.2
Total-CDF	1.9900	0.9309	7.759	486	104	163
Tri-CDD	0.0533	0.0249	0.208	13	3	4
Tetra-CDD	0.0257	0.0012	0.101	6	1	2
Penta-CDD	0.0430	0.0120	0.167	10	2	3.5
Hexa-CDD	0.0655	0.0306	0.256	16	3	5
Hepta-CDD	0.0312	0.0146	0.122	8	2	2.5
Octa-CDD	0.0103	0.0049	0.041	3	0.6	0.9
Total-CDD	0.2290	0.0882	0.895	56	12	18
2,3,7,8-TCDD	0.00168	0.000782	0.0065	0.41	0.088	0.135

[a] Calculated using Eq. (10).
[b] Calculated using Eq. (11).
[c] Maximum annual deposition rate × (30/365) × 25%.

To present a conservative analysis of the inhalation exposure for case 2, the particulates that deposit on the ground were also assumed to be available for inhalation. However, since the larger particles deposit and the smaller particles have the higher concentrations, these represent only 1–2% of the total dioxins emitted. Therefore, there is a slight double-count in the inhalation exposure. However, since this is a small amount, it was not subtracted, thus adding to the conservatism of the model.

5.2 Deposition Model

The pathway of ingestion and dermal exposure of particles emitted from the Brooklyn Navy Yard facility stack would originate with solid particulates that settle to the ground and are mixed with ambient dust, dirt, and soil.

The Industrial Source Complex (ISC) computer model developed under the sponsorship of the U.S. EPA by a private contractor was used to calculate particulate dispersion rates through dry deposition (137). The deposition algorithm was developed under contract to the U.S. Army (138). The model is not equipped to handle terrain features or elevated receptors when calculating deposition rates, and it is not able to account for any physical transformations or changes in particle size occurring in the atmosphere. Therefore, some inaccuracies may be introduced due to flow obstruction by buildings and by particle size changes. In addition, no losses due to wet deposition, photodegradation, runoff, or volatilization have been assumed, thus providing some conservatism to the model.

The long-term (ISCLT) model version was used to calculate annual deposition rates at ground-level receptors. The annual deposition rates were computed at 612 receptor points extending out to 12 km from the proposed site. The deposition rates were also calculated using meteorological conditions observed over a 5-year period from 1966 to 1970 at the LaGuardia Airport weather station. The emission rates from case 2 in Table 14, where all PCDFs and PCDDs were assumed to be adsorbed on fly ash, were used in this analysis. If only a portion of the PCDFs and PCDDs are adsorbed on fly ash, then the deposition rates will be less than those presented.

From the empirical relation established in the ISC model, the proportion of fly ash emitted from the BNYRRF that will ultimately settle to the ground is determined as shown in Table 16. This is computed from the reflection coefficients, that is, the fraction of fly ash in a particular particle size category that is reflected from the ground when the carrier (air) is reflected from the ground surface. This is also the fraction of fly ash that remains suspended in air and does not settle at all. The reflection coefficient is a function of the particle settling velocity, which is a function of particle size and density. For example, from Table 16, 20% by weight (100 minus a reflection coefficient of 80) of the particles with a mean diameter of 15 μm will deposit.

To calculate the quantity of PCDDs and PCDFs depositing on the ground per gram of deposited fly ash, Example Calculations 6–8 were performed.

Example Calculation 6. Calculating Fly Ash Deposition Rate for Particle Size Class i

Given:

- R_i is the reflection coefficient for ith particle size class (Table 16).
- F_{wi} is the weight fraction of ith particle size class (Table 13).

TABLE 16. PCDF and PCDD Concentrations in Deposited Fly Ash

Particle Diameter (μm)	Reflection Coefficient (dimensionless)	Fraction Depositing	Weight Fraction of Fly Ash Emitted	Fly Ash Deposited (g/s)	Fraction of Emission that Ultimately Deposits	PCDD Concentration (ng/g)	Contribution of PCDD in Deposited Fly Ash (ng/g)	PCDF Concentration (ng/g)	Contribution of PCDF in Deposited Fly Ash (ng/g)
15.0	0.80	0.20	0.24	0.191	0.552	141	77.8	1,224	675.7
12.5	0.82	0.18	0.11	0.079	0.228	172	39.2	1,492	340.2
8.1	0.85	0.15	0.07	0.042	0.121	254	30.7	2,209	267.3
5.5	0.90	0.10	0.05	0.020	0.058	379	22.0	3,291	190.9
3.6	0.95	0.05	0.07	0.014	0.041	583	23.9	5,070	207.9
2.0	1.0	0.00	0.07	0.000	0.000	1,053	0.0	9,150	0.0
1.1	1.0	0.00	0.14	0.000	0.000	1,890	0.0	16,429	0.0
0.7	1.0	0.00	0.10	0.000	0.000	2,624	0.0	22,812	0.0
<0.7	1.0	0.00	0.15	0.000	0.000	2,618	0.0	22,751	0.0
Total				0.346			193.6		1682.0

- FA_{ff} is the total fly ash emission rate from fabric filter (3.972 g/s; from Table 13).
- FAD_i is the fly ash deposition rate (g/s) for particle size class i.

Then:

$$FAD_i = (1 - R_i) \times F_{wi} \times FA_{ff}. \tag{6}$$

Example:

$$R_i = 0.8 \quad \text{(Table 16)}.$$
$$F_{wi} = 0.24 \quad \text{(Table 13)}.$$
$$FA_{ff} = 3.97 \text{ g/s} \quad \text{(Table 13)}.$$
$$FAD_i = 0.191 \text{ g/s} \quad \text{(see Table 16 for other values)}.$$

Summing the deposition rate for all size classes (see Table 16), only 0.346 g/s will settle, which constitutes 9% of the fly ash emitted from the stack. As indicated below, the 15-μm particle size class represents 55.2% of the total fly ash that ultimately deposits.

Example Calculation 7. Calculating the Fraction of Particles within the ith Size Class That Ultimately Deposits

Given:

- FAD_i is the fly ash deposition rate for ith particle size category.
- $\sum FAD$ is the total fly ash deposited for all i particle size classes.
- D_i is the fraction of emissions that ultimately deposits.

Then:

$$D_i = FAD_i/\sum FAD. \tag{7}$$

Example:

$$FAD = 0.191 \text{ g/s} \quad \text{(Table 16)}.$$
$$\sum FAD = 0.346 \text{ g/s} \quad \text{(Table 16)}.$$
$$D_i = 0.552 \quad \text{(Table 16)}.$$

The fraction of depositing particles in the 15-μm size class represents 55% by weight of all particles that settle, while the concentration of PCDD is 141 ng/g (Table 12). For each particle size category, the total quantity of PCDDs and PCDFs depositing per gram of fly ash was calculated using Example Calculation 8.

Example Calculation 8. Calculating the Total Quantity of PCDD and PCDF Depositing per Gram of Fly Ash

Given:

- D_i is the fraction of emissions that ultimately deposits for each particle size class.

- DA_i is the PCDD concentration per gram of emitted fly ash for the ith particle size class [Eq. (4)].
- CD_i is the PCDD concentration in deposited fly ash for the ith particle size class.
- $\sum CD$ is the PCDD concentration in deposited fly ash summed for all particle size classes.

Then

$$CD_i = D_i \times DA_i. \tag{8}$$

Example:

$D_i = 0.552$ (Table 16).

$DA_i = 141\,\text{ng/g}$ (Table 12).

$CD_i = 77.8\,\text{ng/g}$ PCDD in 15-μm particles that deposit on the ground.

$\sum CD = 193.6\,\text{ng/g}$ PCDD concentration in deposited fly ash.

The BNYRRF design parameters along with the projected fly ash and PCDD and PCDF emission rate data were used as input to the ISC model to determine fly ash deposition rates. Potential exposures for the maximally exposed individual were determined by multiplying the maximum annual fly ash deposition rate ($0.004613\,\text{g/m}^2\cdot\text{yr}$) determined by the ISC model by the concentration of PCDD and PCDF in the fly ash particles that deposit on the ground as shown below.

Example Calculation 9. Calculating the Annual Deposition Rate of PCDDs and PCDFs at the Point of Maximum Impact

Given:

- DEP_{fly} is the fly ash deposition rate at point of maximum potential impact.
- $\sum CD$ is the concentration of PCDD in deposited fly ash.
- DEP_{PCDD} is the annual deposition rate of PCDD at point of maximum potential exposure.

Then:

$$DEP_{PCDD} = \sum CD \times DEP_{fly}. \tag{9}$$

Example:

$DEP_{fly} = 0.004613\,\text{g/m}^2\cdot\text{yr}$ determined using MWC design

parameters and the ISC model (data not shown).

$\sum CD = 193.6\,\text{ng/g}$ fly ash for PCDD   (Table 16).

$DEP_{PCDD} = 0.8949\,\text{ng/m}^2\cdot\text{yr}$ (annual deposition rate for

PCDD at the point of maximum exposure).

In summary, the maximum deposition rate was calculated at $0.895 \, \text{ng/m}^2 \cdot \text{yr}$ for PCDDs and $7.759 \, \text{ng/m}^2 \cdot \text{yr}$ for PCDFs (Table 15).

5.3   Predicted Maximum Concentrations of PCDFs and PCDDs in Soil, Dirt, and Dust

Where the fly ash particles land on ambient soil, a conservative interpretation would be that the fly ash particles mix within the top centimeter of ambient soil or dust by mechanical means without resuspension, reentrainment, or degradation. A typical soil density is $1.6 \, \text{g/cm}^3$, and the concentrations of PCDF and PCDD compounds mixed in a layer of soil 1 cm thick are presented in Table 15 (column a) for accumulations after 1 year. Subsequent accumulations can be determined by multiplying these values by the number of accumulating years. These data were derived using Example Calculation 10.

Example Calculation 10. Determining the Concentrations of 2, 3, 7, 8-TCDD in Soil After One Year

Given:

- DEP_{2378} is the annual deposition rate ($\text{ng/m}^2 \cdot \text{yr}$ of $2, 3, 7, 8$-TCDD at point of maximum potential exposure (Table 15).
- ρ is the density of soil (g/cm^3).
- CF is the correction factor.
- CM is the thickness of mixing zone (cm).
- C_{soil} is the concentration of $2, 3, 7, 8$-TCDD (fg/g) in soil after 1 year.

Then:

$$C_{\text{soil}} = \frac{DEP_{2378}}{\rho \times CM \times CF}. \tag{10}$$

Example:

$$DEP_{2378} = 0.0065 \, \text{mg/m}^2 \cdot \text{yr} \quad \text{(Table 15)}.$$

$$\rho = 1.6 \, \text{g/cm}^3.$$

$$CM = 1 \, \text{cm} \quad \text{(see text)}.$$

$$CF = (10{,}000 \, \text{cm}^2/\text{m}^2) \times (10^{-6} \, \text{mg/fg}) = 0.01.$$

$$C_{\text{soil}} = 0.41 \, \text{fg/g soil}.$$

For this risk assessment, a conservative assumption was made that PCDDs do not gradually accumulate in the soil over time; rather, the receptor is assumed to be exposed over a 70-year period to the concentration of PCDD deposited as a slug (in year 1) in soil over a 20-year accumulation period. A 20-year accumulation period appears to be a reasonable approximation of the steady-state concentration assuming a half-life of PCDD in soil of 12 years.

Although it is consistent with EPA guidance (1), a mixing zone of 1 cm also seems highly conservative. At locations where there is the greatest potential for exposure such as playgrounds, gardens, and ballfields, the soil is likely to be disturbed so that surficial materials would be mixed to a depth greater than 1 cm. Other evidence that 1 cm is a conservative mixing zone value comes from known contamination areas such as Seveso, Italy, where vertical movement of dioxins to a depth of 15–30 cm has been reported (139, 140).

Particles depositing as dust on outdoor surfaces will settle at the rates presented in Table 15 along with total particulate from other sources. These particles, which would become associated with street dirt, would be subject to frequent washout due to deliberate washing and natural rains. Therefore, a long-term accumulation rate would not be appropriate. Instead, the fly ash particles are assumed to be diluted with settleable ambient particulates at all times.

This is a very conservative assumption that places an upper bound on the potential PCDD concentration expressed on a weight basis. It states that for every gram of settleable PCDD emitted from the stack, the PCDD will be diluted only by the settleable particulate present in the ambient air from all sources. As a first approximation, it was assumed that if the PCDD containing particulate is removed (e.g., by rain), then the non-PCDD particulate present will also be lost at the same rate. Therefore, the concentration of PCDD in dust will not change with time, nor will PCDD accumulate (since if the PCDD accumulates so does the non-PCDD containing particulate, at the same rate). The settleable particulate data have been provided by the City of New York Department of Environmental Protection as total dustfall data measured in Brooklyn. This was $0.62 \, mg/cm^2$ per month, or $74.4 \, g/m^2$ per year (141). The concentrations of PCDFs and PCDDs in settleable dust and street dirt are presented in Table 15 (column b) based on Example Calculation 11.

Example Calculation 11. Determining the Concentration of 2,3,7,8-TCDD on Settleable Dust and Street Dirt

Given:

- DEP_{2378} is the annual deposition rate ($ng/m^2 \cdot yr$) at point of maximum potential exposure.
- DEP_{dust} is the measured deposition rate of dust for New York City.
- C_{dust} is the concentration of 2,3,7,8-TCDD in settleable dust and dirt.

Then:

$$C_{dust} = DEP_{2378}/DEP_{dust}. \qquad (11)$$

Example:

$$DEP_{2378} = 0.0065 \, ng/m^2 \cdot yr \quad (Table \ 15).$$
$$DEP_{dust} = 74.4 \, g/m^2 \cdot yr \quad (Ref. \ 90).$$
$$C_{dust} = 8.8 \times 10^{-14} \, g/g \ dust = 0.088 \, pg/g.$$

On a weight basis, the TCDD concentration in home dust was assumed to be equal to the concentration in street dirt, an assumption that is used by CDC in its risk assessment and supported by some studies of lead contamination in indoor versus outdoor environments (142).

Estimated PCDD levels in home dust and street dirt on a surface area basis were also used to estimate risk. For outdoor deposition the accumulation period in urban streets is unknown. The Swiss EPA in their assessment of dioxin emissions from incinerators, used an estimated half-life equal to 14 days for rural environments (114). Consistent with the Swiss EPA Assessment, we have assumed 30 days as a reasonable period of accumulation. Therefore, the TCDD concentration on outdoor surfaces per square meter is equal to the maximum annual deposition rate times 30/365.

The maximum accumulation rate for indoor surfaces was estimated at 25% of the outdoor rate, also with a 30-day accumulation period as provided in Table 15 (column c).

There is some evidence to suggest that a 30-day accumulation period in homes is overly conservative. For example, the data provided by Solomon et al., if extrapolated, indicate that there is from 0.6 to 1 g dust/m^2 in single-family urban middle-class homes (gas heated) in Champagne–Urbana, Illinois. Their data, if applied to the PCDD and total particulate deposition rates, would indicate that steady-state conditions for dust buildup in homes would be reached in 3–5 days (143).

6   COMPUTATION OF AN UPPER BOUND TO THE LEVEL OF RISK ASSOCIATED WITH EMISSIONS FROM THE BNYRRF

In this section, an upper-bound limit of risk for each of three potential pathways (inhalation, ingestion, and dermal absorption) for PCDD and PCDF exposure is calculated for the maximally exposed individual (MEI). An upper-bound limit of risk is a predicted upper limit or maximum risk, using worst-case assumptions, at the point of maximum exposure, for the maximally exposed individual, for a period of a 70-year lifetime.

It is important to note that the use of a series of conservative assumptions carries the danger that the potential risks will be vastly overstated and unrealistic. For this risk assessment, the upper-bound risk calculated for the MEI represents a value that is almost certain to overestimate the actual risk by a great margin. Specifically, the upper-bound risk is based on a person that would live a 70-year lifetime at the point of maximum exposure and who has routine contact with the soil. For perspective, less conservative assumptions have been applied in the section on uncertainties to estimate risk for an average exposed individual.

It should be noted that recent risk assessments for MWCs have evaluated risks associated with other potential pathways of exposure including food chain uptake of PCDDs and subsequent ingestion of meat, fish, vegetables, and human breast milk. However, given the urban character of New York City, the relatively small quantity of locally grown produce, meat, fish, and poultry available for local consumption, and the large degree of uncertainty inherent in evaluating such risks, the analysis of these additional pathways was not considered in this risk assessment.

To calculate an upper-bound limit of risk, we have estimated a PCDD and PCDF daily intake for each of the three pathways, using the dispersion and deposition models for dioxin emissions presented in Section 5 and data regarding the uptake and bioavailability of PCDDs and PCDFs from air, soil, dust, and street dirt. The PCDD daily intake was then compared with existing ADIs and the cancer dose–response data to determine if there are any potential health impacts that might be associated with the predicted BNYRRF emissions.

Several general assumptions were used in the assessment.

1. The air dispersion and particulate deposition modeling of the stack emissions from the stack adequately represents the transport of the PCDD emissions to ground level.
2. The composition of emission products found at ground level is identical to the composition (but not the concentration) found in the stack.
3. We have assumed conservatively that the population is exposed to the maximum annual average ground-level concentration from the incinerator for 24 h/day throughout a 70-year lifetime.
4. We have assumed conservatively, that there is no loss of PCDDs through volatilization or photodegradation.

6.1 Inhalation Exposure

6.1.1 Calculation of a Daily Intake. To calculate a daily intake from inhalation (DI_{inh}), the maximum average ambient air concentration of 2, 3, 7, 8-TCDD (Table 15) was multiplied by the average amount of air exchanged per day, the particulate retention rate, and the bioavailability of the inhaled material as provided in Eq. (12).

In the absence of quantitative data, a conservative assumption has been applied, namely, that indoor ambient air contaminant concentrations equal outdoor concentrations. In fact, as reviewed by Yocum, this is not true for contaminants of outdoor origin (144). For contaminants attached to particulates, the long-term indoor versus outdoor concentration is reduced by the scrubbing of outdoor air as it penetrates the building shell. The degree of reduction is in turn dependent on the season of the year, with higher indoor concentrations reported during warm weather, when windows are kept open. For contaminants such as lead or nonmethane hydrocarbons, the indoor concentration may equal only 50–66% of the outdoor concentration. Since the average person spends at least $\frac{1}{3}$–$\frac{1}{2}$ of his or her life indoors, the assumption that the indoor and outdoor concentrations are equal may overestimate risk by at least 11–17%.

Reported air exchange volumes (averages for adult men and women combined) range from 13 to 20 m^3. For this assessment, the CDC estimate of 15 m^3/day was used since this represents a reasonable estimate for a population that includes children in addition to working adults (105).

Not all particulate matter inhaled into the lungs is retained by them. Thus, the amount of exposure depends on the particle size distribution. We used an EPA estimate that 75% of the inhaled particulates are retained (11). This estimate is based on studies done by the International Commission of Radiological Protection. It appears to be a conservative estimate in that 50% of the particles by weight are of the size category (less than 2 μm) expected to settle deeply into the lungs (145). The remaining 50% will be deposited in the upper respiratory tract and subsequently swallowed. Other investigators looking at the distribution of particles retained in the lungs as a function of particle size, who have made certain assumptions regarding the bioavailability of inhaled and ingested fly-ash-bound PCDDs and PCDFs, have concluded that only 30–50% of the inhaled dose is absorbed (145, 146). No data are available regarding the bioavailability of PCDDs and PCDFs in laboratory animals subjected to PCDD dosing through inhalation exposure. In the absence of such data, a conservative assumption has been used that all inhaled PCDDs and PCDFs retained in the lungs are bioavailabile. To derive an upper limit to DI_{inh}, we assumed a maximum annual average concentration of 2,3,7,8-TCDD for ground-level and elevated receptors equal to $0.00168 \, pg/m^3$. This concentration was obtained from Table 15 using the case 1 scenario, where it was assumed for the purpose of modeling that all PCDD emissions leave the stack in a gaseous state.

Based on the above discussion, the upper-bound maximum daily intake of 2,3,7,8-TCDD from the inhalation pathway, for the maximally exposed individual (MEI), was calculated as follows.

Example Calculation 12. Determining the Maximum Daily Intake of 2,3,7,8-TCDD Through Inhalation Assuming All PCDD Are Emitted from the Stack in a Gaseous State

Given:

- DI_{inh} is the daily intake of 2,3,7,8-TCDD through inhalation (g/day).
- C_1 is the maximum ambient air concentration (g/m^3) of 2,3,7,8-TCDD assuming case 1—that all dioxins are emitted in a gaseous state.
- V is the average ventilation rate (m^3/day).
- R is the percent particulate retention in lungs.
- B_{inh} is the percent bioavailability (inhalation).

Then:

$$DI_{inh} = C_1 \times V \times R \times B_{inh}. \tag{12}$$

Example:

$$C_1 = 0.00168 \, pg/m^3 \text{ (from Table 15)}$$
$$= 1.68 \times 10^{-15} \, g/m^3.$$
$$V = 15 \, m^3/day.$$
$$R = 75\% = 0.75.$$
$$B_{inh} = 100\% = 1.$$
$$DI_{inh} = 1.9 \times 10^{-14} \, g/day.$$

For case 2, the maximum ambient air concentration of 2,3,7,8-TCDD would equal $0.000782 \, pg/m^3$ and DI_{inh} would equal $8.8 \times 10^{-15} \, g/day$.

6.1.2 Comparison of Daily Intake from Inhalation with Acceptable Daily Intake Levels (ADIs).

Several regulatory agencies in this country and abroad have set 2,3,7,8-TCDD standards and criteria on the basis of an acceptable daily intake as presented in Table 3. These agencies felt that the ADI approach was a reasonable method for determining very safe dose levels, particularly for compounds that are believed to be promoters rather than initiators of carcinogenesis.

The upper-bound estimate of 2,3,7,8-TCDD intake through the inhalation pathway in comparison with these ADIs is presented in Table 17 and the impacts are shown to be negligible. For example, the maximum estimated intake of 2,3,7,8-TCDD through the

TABLE 17. Estimated Percentage of Acceptable Daily Intake (ADI) Attributable to Inhalation of PCDD and PCDF Emissions from the BNYRRF

Upper-Bound Daily Intake for Inhalation Pathway (pg/kg· day)	Acceptable Daily Intake (ADI)			
	Canada (10 pg/kg· day)	The Netherlands (4 pg/kg· day)	NYSDOH (2 pg/kg· day)	West Germany (1.0 pg/kg· day)
2,3,7,8-TCDD $(2.7 \times 10^{-4})^a$	0.0027%	0.007%	0.014%	0.027%
TCDD $(4.2 \times 10^{-3})^b$	0.042%	0.11%	0.21%	0.42%
TCDD toxic equivalency $(1.6 \times 10^{-2})^c$	0.16%	0.40%	0.80%	1.59%

$^a DI_{inh}$ (pg/kg·day) $= DI_{inh}$ (g/day)/70 kg $= (1.9 \times 10^{-2}$ pg/day)/(70 kg) $= 2.7 \times 10^{-4}$ pg/kg·day.
$^b DI_{inh}(TCDD) = DI_{inh}(2,3,7,8\text{-}TCDD) \times 15.5.$
$^c DI_{inh}(\text{toxic equivalents}) = DI_{inh}(2,3,7,8\text{-}TCDD) \times 59.$

inhalation pathway for a 70-kg human is only 0.027% of the most conservative published ADI of 1.0 pg/kg·day.

As an added safety factor, we compared the daily intake with published ADIs using two other conservative assumptions: first, that all TCDDs were as toxic as the 2,3,7,8-TCDD, and second, that the toxicity of the complex mixture of PCDDs and PCDFs was 59 times that of 2,3,7,8-TCDD alone, using the toxic equivalency approach. Using these assumptions, the maximum daily intake of TCDD toxic equivalents through inhalation of gaseous or particulate emissions from the BNYRRF ranged from 0.042 to 1.59% of the various ADIs. These levels are well below very safe dose levels suggested by these regulatory agencies. Consequently, the data indicate that risks associated with potential noncarcinogenic toxic effects due to inhalation of PCDD and PCDF emissions from the BNYRRF are not significant.

TABLE 18. Upper-Bound Estimated Increased Cancer Risk for Population of One Million People Exposed for a 70-year Period to the Maximum Daily Intake via the Inhalation Pathway^a

	Dose for 1×10^{-6} Excess Cancer Risk			
	Sielkin (140 pg/kg· day)	Kimbrough (1.4 pg/kg· day)	Kimbrough (0.028 pg/kg· day)	EPA (0.0064 pg/kg· day)
Daily Intake	Upper Bound Excess Risk for 70-kg Human			
1.9×10^{-2} pg/day (2,3,7,8-TCDD)	0.000019	0.0019	0.010	0.042
0.15 pg/day (1,2,3,6,7,8- and 1,2,3,7,8,9-HCDD)				0.013

6.1.3 Comparison of Daily Intake from the Inhalation Pathway with Cancer Risk Estimates.

The daily intake calculations for inhalation exposure have been compared in Table 18 with three different risk extrapolation models in order to estimate the excess cancer risk for the MEI resulting from the projected operations of the BNYRRF. This table provides an estimate of the increased cancer incidences per 1,000,000 people exposed (to the maximum concentrations) over a 70-year lifetime. It is important to reiterate that there is very little empirical evidence to support either the use of one dose–response extrapolation model over another, or to convert animal test data to human equivalent dosages. As a consequence, several other equally plausible dose–response extrapolations have been made that indicate that the estimated dose which would yield an added risk of 1 $\times 10^{-6}$ could be as high as 140 pg/kg·day. The excess cancer risk was calculated using Eq. 13.

Example Calculation 13. Calculating Excess Cancer Risk for Inhalation Pathway

Given:

- DI_{inh} is the daily intake (pg/day) of 2, 3, 7, 8-TCDD through inhalation [from Eq. (12)].
- BW is body weight (kg).
- VSD is the virtual safe dose corresponding to 1×10^{-6} risk (pg/kg·day) (Table 4).
- P is 1×10^{-6} risk.
- R is the excess individual cancer risk.

Then:

$$R = \frac{DI_{inh} \times P}{BW \times VSD}. \tag{13}$$

Example:

$$DI_{inh} = 1.9 \times 10^{-14} \text{ g/day} = 1.9 \times 10^{-2} \text{ pg/day} \quad [\text{Eq. (12)}].$$

$$BW = 70 \text{ kg}.$$

$$VSD = 0.0064 \text{ pg/kg·day}.$$

$$P = 1 \times 10^{-6}.$$

$$R = 0.042 \times 10^{-6}.$$

The EPA dose–response model predicts that the inhalation of 1.9×10^{-2} pg/day of 2, 3, 7, 8-TCDD results in an upper limit of risk for an individual equal to 0.042×10^{-6}, which is equivalent to less than 0.042 increased cancer cases for every 1,000,000 people exposed (Table 18) to the maximum concentration for a 70-year lifetime.

Two isomers of HCDD (1, 2, 3, 6, 7, 8 and 1, 2, 3, 7, 8, 9) have been tested as a mixture and have been shown to be carcinogenic in animal feeding studies. These two isomers make up only 20% of the total number of possible HCDD isomers. To estimate the risks associated with inhalation of HCDD isomers, we assumed equal distribution of the various HCDD isomers in particulate emissions. Therefore, the daily intake for the carcinogenic isomers of HCDD was calculated by multiplying the total HCDD intake [from Eq. (12)] by 20%. Consequently, $DI_{inh}(HCDD) = 0.15$ pg/day. Using Eq. (13) we found that this corresponds to an upper limit of risk equal to less than 0.013 increased cancer cases for every 1,000,000 people exposed.

As demonstrated in Table 18, using the most conservative model, the EPA risk model, and assuming that the excess risks from 2,3,7,8-TCDD and HCDD are additive, the projected levels of exposure through the inhalation pathway would not result in more than 0.06 new cases of cancer in a population of 1,000,000 exposed to the estimated maximum levels and assuming a maximum daily intake over a 70-year lifetime. In more common terminology, the excess cancer risk for a 70-year lifetime is less than 0.06×10^{-6} or 6 in 100,000,000. If the other dose extrapolations are more representative, it can be seen that the cancer risk levels are substantially less by one to five orders of magnitude.

6.2   Ingestion and Dermal Exposure

6.2.1   Discussion. Until recently, the standard practice for most regulatory agencies performing risk assessments was to consider inhalation of emission products as the only pathway of exposure. Studies performed on other pollutants emitted from point sources, such as smelters, or from nonpoint sources indicate that ingestion and dermal absorption of particulate emissions deposited on living area surfaces may also be exposure pathways (13, 14). These pathways are typically ignored since the data needed to characterize the environmental fate, transport, and biological uptake of toxic contaminants, in relation to ingestion and dermal exposure pathways, are not well documented. Nonetheless, as an additional safety factor, we tested the sensitivity of the risks derived for the inhalation pathway to the additive impacts of ingestion and dermal absorption of dioxin-contaminated dust, dirt, and soil.

For the purpose of calculating a maximum daily intake of PCDD through ingestion and dermal exposure, the case 2 scenario was used where it was assumed that all dioxins enter the baghouse attached to particulates.

6.2.2   Daily Intake through the Ingestion Pathway. A daily intake of 2,3,7,8-TCDD through ingestion (DI_{ing}) was estimated in two ways. First, DI_{ing} was determined based on an estimated rate of soil ingestion in grams per day, the 2,3,7,8-TCDD concentration (weight basis) in soil or dirt, and a percentage bioavailability. Using a different surface area approach, we also determined a concentration of TCDD in g/m^2 on home and street surfaces and calculated DI_{ing} based on an estimate of bioavailability and the surface contact area for hands, feet, and other exposed areas.

The issue of how much soil or dust a child or adult ingests is being widely debated in the risk assessment field. Several risk assessments, including the original BNYRRF assessment, utilized as a worst-case assumption the CDC risk assessment of dioxin-contaminated soils, which concluded that the average person ingests from 0.1 to 10 g soil/day depending on the age group. Using the CDC data, a weighted averaged ingestion rate for a 70-year lifetime would equal 0.41 g/day (105). However, the ingestion levels used by the CDC seem quite high and therefore too conservative when compared with other studies. For example, Duggan and Williams have summarized the literature on the amount of lead ingested through street dust (147). In their opinion, a quantity of 50 μg of lead is ingested daily by children. Assuming, on the high side, an average lead concentration in urban environments of 1000 ppm, this would indicate an ingestion of 50 mg/day of soil and dirt per day.

Lepow et al. (148), in an assessment of lead exposure in children caused by ingesting dirt and dust, estimated a rate of dirt ingestion equal to 100 mg/day (specifically 10 mg of dirt ingested 10 times a day). In a recent Dutch study, the amount on hands ranged from 4 to 12 μg (149). Assuming maximum lead concentrations of 500 μg/g (the levels were typically lower) and assuming the child ingested the entire contents adsorbed on his hand on 10 separate occasions, we calculate the amount of ingested dirt as equal to 240 mg. Thus, to eat 10 g soil/day, as suggested by the CDC, the child would have to place his hand in his mouth 410 times, a rate that seems improbable. Binder has estimated that children 1–3 years of age ingest about 180 mg/day of soil based on the quantity of silicon and aluminum found in the feces (150). In a more recent Dutch study, the amounts of aluminum, titanium, and acid-soluble residue in the feces of hospitalized and nursery school children aged 2–4 were determined. Based on the differences between the hospitalized children (presumably not exposed to soil while hospitalized) and the nursery school children, it was estimated that the nursery school children ingested approximately 56 mg of soil each day (151). The EPA in its lead criteria document assumed that a child ingested 50 mg/day of household dust, 40 mg/day of street dust, and 10 mg/day of dust derived from their parents' clothing for a total ingestion rate of 100 mg of soil and dust per day (13). The EPA in its risk assessment of dioxin-contaminated soil and in the *Superfund Public Health Evaluation Manual* estimates that adults ingest 100 mg/day (152, 153). In summary, the data indicate that children between the ages of 1 and 6 years of age are more likely to ingest, at most, 100 mg of soil or dirt per day rather than the 10 g/day used by the CDC.

Older children and adults are likely to ingest less than 100 mg/day of soil. Paustenbach has estimated that adults are unlikely to ingest more than 10–20 mg soil/day through indirect ingestion of soil attached to vegetation and food products and through poor personal hygiene (154). Although it is likely that adults ingest less soil than young children, for the purpose of this risk assessment, a lifetime ingestion rate of 100 mg of soil or dirt per day was used to assess the risks for the maximally exposed individual. Different assumptions will be utilized in our analysis of uncertainties.

Daily intake levels via the ingestion pathway were also calculated using a surface area approach. In their risk assessment of the Binghamton office fire, NYSDOH made the assumption that contaminants contained on 5–25% of the surface area of the hands were ingested. Based on the average hand surface area for females, the material contained on 0.0033–0.016 m^2 of surface would be ingested each day (106). For the purpose of this assessment, the maximum figure of 0.016 m^2/day will be used to estimate risks for the MEI.

Recent studies in several laboratories have shown that the bioavailability of PCDD from environmental samples can vary widely depending on, for example, the matrix, the age of the sample, and the presence of other compounds in the matrix (155). Studies of rats given TCDD in the diet reported 50–60% absorption (156). A mixture of TCDD in acetone and corn oil given to rats by gavage resulted in 86% absorption (157). A study reported by McConnell indicates high bioavailability in guinea pigs and rats fed dioxin-contaminated soil from Times Beach (158). Lucier reports a bioavailability of PCDD in soil that was dose dependent ranging from 24 to 50% (159). Umbreit recalculated the guinea pig data of McConnell and reported an oral bioavailability of 85% (160). However, the guinea pig data are believed to be flawed based on the almost 100% mortality of the animals at high dose (161).

In contrast to the high degree of bioavailability reported in Times Beach soil, Umbreit has demonstrated only a low degree of bioavailability (less than 0.5%) for TCDD-contaminated soil from a Neward 2, 4, 5-T manufacturing site and moderate (21%) bioavailability in a New Jersey metal salvage yard contaminated with dioxin from an outside source (160). These data suggest the importance of matrix effects on bioavailability since the Newark soils were harder to extract and appeared to bind TCDD more highly than Times Beach soils (160).

Recent experiments by Shu indicate a mean oral bioavailability of 43% for rats fed Missouri soil contaminated with TCDD in the early to mid-1970s (161). Based on McConnell's work, the CDC used a bioavailability of 30% in its risk assessment of dioxin-contaminated soils (105).

It should be noted that dioxin is believed to bind more tightly to fly ash than to most soils. Frequently, very difficult extraction techniques are required to desorb the material from fly ash. Feeding of fly ash containing PCDDs to rats over a 19-day period resulted in lower absorbed PCDD levels than for a similar PCDD concentration extracted from fly ash in toluene (162). For example, rats fed with fly ash stored PCDDs and PCDFs in their livers at concentrations that were at least three to five times lower than rats fed with a comparable amount of a fly ash extract. For penta-CDD, hexa-CDF, and hexa-CDD isomers, these concentrations were 10–20 times lower. A recent experiment by van den Berg demonstrated that the bioavailability of fly ash fed to rats is approximately 9% (163).

The data indicate that the bioavailability of dioxins bound to soils is somewhere in the range of 20–50%. The bioavailability of dioxins bound to fly ash is probably lower at approximately 10%. For this risk assessment, an oral bioavailability of 30% suggested by the CDC will be used to estimate the potential absorbed dose for the MEI.

To summarize, a determination of the daily intake due to ingestion was derived on the basis of several different assumptions concerning the patterns of exposure. These assumptions include:

- Ingestion of 100 mg of soil or dust per day and 30% bioavailability.
- Contact with surfaces at up to 0.016 m²/day and 30% bioavailability.

Each of these assumptions was tested further by assuming three different sources of

TABLE 19. Estimated Daily Intake of 2, 3, 7, 8-TCDD through the Ingestion Pathway

	Source of Exposure		
	Home Dust	Street Dirt	Soil
A. Weight Approach			
Concentration of 2, 3, 7, 8-TCDD[a]	8.8×10^{-14} g/g	8.8×10^{-14} g/g	8.2×10^{-15} g/g
DI_{ing}[b]	2.6×10^{-15} g/day	2.6×10^{-15} g/day	2.5×10^{-16} g/day
B. Surface Area Approach			
Concentration of 2, 3, 7, 8-TCDD[c]	1.35×10^{-13} g/m²	5.4×10^{-13} g/m²	
DI_{ing}[d]	6.5×10^{-16} g/day	2.6×10^{-15} g/day	

[a] Assumes a 20-year accumulation period for soil.
[b] Calculated using Eq. (14).
[c] Assumes a 30-day accumulation period for street dirt with home dust equal to 25% of outdoor accumulation.
[d] Calculated using Eq. (15).

exposure—home dust, street dirt, and soil. The estimated daily intake through the ingestion pathway calculated on a weight or surface area basis is presented in Table 19. Example calculations are provided below.

Example Calculation 14. Calculating the Maximum Daily Intake through Ingestion Using a Weight Approach

Given:

- C_s is the 2, 3, 7, 8-TCDD concentration in soil, dirt, or dust (g/g soil).
- Ing is the amount of soil, dust, or dirt ingested per day (g/day).
- B_{ing} is the bioavailability via ingestion.
- DI_{ing} is the daily intake of 2, 3, 7, 8-TCDD through ingestion (g/day).

Then:

$$DI_{ing} = C_s \times Ing \times B_{ing}. \tag{14}$$

Example:

$$C_s = 8.2 \times 10^{-3} \, pg/day = 8.2 \times 10^{-15} \, g/day \quad \text{(from Table 15)}.$$
$$Ing = 100 \, mg/day = 0.1 \, g/day.$$
$$B_{ing} = 30\% = 0.3.$$
$$DI_{ing} = 2.5 \times 10^{-16} \, g/day.$$

Example Calculation 15. Calculating the Maximum Daily Intake through Ingestion Using a Surface Area Approach

Given:

- C_{sa} is the 2, 3, 7, 8-TCDD concentration in dust or street dirt per unit surface area (g/m^2).
- SC is the surface area contacted by hands and other exposed areas (m^2/day).

Then:

$$DI_{ing} = C_{sa} \times SC \times B_{ing}. \tag{15}$$

Example:

$$C_{sa} = 0.135 \, pg/m^2 = 1.3 \times 10^{-13} \, g/day \quad \text{(from Table 15)}.$$
$$SC = 0.016 \, m^2/day \quad \text{(see text)}.$$
$$B_{ing} = 0.3.$$
$$DI_{ing} = 6.2 \times 10^{-16}.$$

The maximum estimated daily intake calculated by either method provides for slightly different results (Table 19). On a weight basis, the maximum estimated daily intake of

2, 3, 7, 8-TCDD ranged from 2.5×10^{-16} to 2.6×10^{-15} g/day. On a surface area basis, the daily intake ranged from 6.5×10^{-16} to 2.6×10^{-15} g/day.

6.2.3 Daily Intake from Dermal Absorption.

The daily intake via dermal absorption (DI_{derm}) is a function of the surface area of exposed skin, the frequency of contact between the exposed skin and contaminated surfaces, and the rates of dermal absorption for PCDDs and PCDFs bound tightly to soil, dust, and fly ash. Information to calculate these data are not well documented.

Based on their analysis of skin surface area, contact rates, and other considerations, the CDC in its risk assessment of dioxin-contaminated soils estimated that a person might be dermally exposed to up to 0.55 g soil/day over a 70-year lifetime (105).

By making different assumptions about surface area and frequency of contact in its risk assessment of the Binghamton office fire, NYSDOH used a surface area approach and assumed a transfer of surface materials proportional to the surface area of the hands and arms of female workers (106). The EPA has used still other assumptions for the surface area of exposed skin and the amount of soil accumulating on the skin to derive estimates of dermal absorption rates (1).

For the purpose of this assessment, we have used two methods to derive DI_{derm}. The first method shown in Example Calculation 16 was derived from the NYSDOH procedure (106). This method is referred to here as a *surface area approach* since the PCDD concentrations used as input to Example Calculation 16 are expressed in surface area units (mg/m^2). Transfer of dirt and dust on indoor or outdoor surfaces was assumed to be proportional to the surface area of the hands and arms of female workers. Contact between skin and living surfaces was estimated to occur over 10, 25, or 50% of the surface area of exposed hands and arms. This estimate resulted in the assumption that there was complete transfer to the hands and arms of the material contained on surfaces ranging in size from 0.028 to $0.14 \, m^2$ each day. For conservatism, the upper value of $0.14 \, m^2$ was used as the contact area for the MEI.

The second method shown in Example Calculation 17 is based on similar assumptions regarding the exposed surface area of skin in children and adults and the amount of soil accumulating on skin. However, it is referred to here as a *weight approach* since the PCDD concentrations used in Eq. (17) are expressed on a weight-to-weight basis.

The amount of soil accumulating on skin is considered by the EPA to have an upper limit of $1.5 \, mg/cm^2$ for children based on the reports of Lepow et al. (164) and Roels (165). For adults, Hawley has suggested that the soil coating on adults could be as great as $3.5 \, mg/cm^2$ (166). The exposed surface area for adults is estimated to be $2940 \, cm^2$ and for children it is $980 \, cm^2$ (150). These areas correspond to people wearing short sleeved, open-necked shirts, long pants and shoes, without gloves or a hat.

For this assessment an exposed surface area equal to $2940 \, cm^2$ and a lifetime average contact amount of $3.5 \, mg/cm^2$ will be used to calculate DI_{derm} for the MEI. Those values appear to be highly conservative. A contact amount of $3.5 \, mg/cm^2$ times an exposed surface area of $2940 \, cm^2$ means that up to 10 g of soil, dust, and dirt are sticking to skin surfaces each day. This is considerably more than the CDC estimate that up to 0.55 g of soil are contacted each day. A more realistic assumption for contact amount has been proposed by Paustenbach, who estimates an average contact amount of $0.5 \, mg/cm^2$ (154).

For the purpose of calculating exposure for the maximally exposed individual, contact time was assumed to be 12 h/day for the entire year. The assumption of a 12-h exposure seems to be a plausible but conservative assumption based on the fact that much of the day is taken up by activities that are unlikely to result in contact with dirt or dust (e.g., sleeping, eating). The assumption that exposure occurs throughout the year is implausible and conservative with respect to exposure to soil and street dirt, since exposure is not likely to occur for one-half of the year due to weather and other factors. The assumption is probably a conservative but plausible assumption for home dust.

The study by Poiger et al. (167) is one of two studies providing data on the absorption of TCDD through the skin. Application of TCDD in methanol or TCDD in a soil–water paste resulted in TCDD accumulation in the liver amounting to 2% of the administered dose. Application in an activated carbon–water paste completely eliminated absorption. Dermal application in polyethylene glycol resulted in 9.3% absorption compared with oral feeding of TCDD dissolved in ethanol. The data further suggest that dermal bioavailability decreases as TCDD concentration decreases. However, recent experiments by Shu et al. (168) using rats indicate that the dermal bioavailability of TCDD-contaminated soils is around 1.3%. Since rats have higher permeability skin compared to human skin, a bioavailability of 1% based on experiments with rats represents a probable upper-bound limit for humans.

In the absence of any other data on TCDD, regulatory agencies such as the CDC and the EPA have adopted 1 and 0.07–3%, respectively, as the dermal bioavailability of soil-bound TCDD. Since TCDD is expected to be bound tightly to fly ash, the amount absorbed from fly ash may be less than that for soil. For this risk assessment, a bioavailability of 1% will be used as a reasonably conservative estimate.

The daily intake due to dermal absorption was calculated in two ways using either Example Calculation 16 or 17.

Example Calculation 16. Calculating the Daily Intake of 2, 3, 7, 8-TCDD through Dermal Absorption Using a Surface Area Approach

Given:

- CA is the surface area contacted by exposed hands and feet (m^2/day).
- B_{derm} is the bioavailability through dermal contact.
- S_{sa} is the concentration of 2, 3, 7, 8-TCDD in dust or dirt calculated on a surface area basis (ng/m^2) (from Table 15).
- DI_{derm} is the daily intake of 2, 3, 7, 8-TCDD through dermal absorption.

Then:

$$DI_{derm} = CA \times B_{derm} \times S_{sa}. \qquad (16)$$

Example:

$$CA = 0.14 \, m^2/day \quad \text{(see text)}.$$

$$B_{derm} = 1\% = 0.01.$$

$$S_{sa} = 0.135 \, pg/m^2 \quad \text{(Table 15)}.$$

$$DI_{derm} = 1.9 \times 10^{-16} \, g/day.$$

Example Calculation 17. Calculation of the Daily Intake of 2, 3, 7, 8-TCDD throuh Dermal Absorption Using a Weight Approach

Given:

- DI_{derm} is daily intake through dermal absorption (g/day).

672   DAVID LIPSKY

- CT is the contact time (h).
- SA is the exposed surface area (cm^2).
- CA is the contact amount (g/cm^2).
- B_{derm} is the dermal bioavailability (%).
- S_{sol} is the concentration in soil, dirt, or dust (g/g).

Then:

$$DI_{derm} = (CT \times SA \times CA \times B_{derm} \times S \div 24\,h). \qquad (17)$$

Example:

$$CT = 12\,h.$$
$$SA = 2940\,cm^2.$$
$$CA = 3.5\,mg/cm^2 = 0.0035\,g/cm^2.$$
$$B_{derm} = 0.01.$$
$$S_{sol} = 8.8 \times 10^{-14}\,g/g \quad (from\ Table\ 15).$$
$$DI_{derm} = 4.5 \times 10^{-15}\,g/day.$$

Table 20 presents the DI_{derm} based on exposure to either soil, street dirt, outdoor dust, or home dust. Daily intake of 2, 3, 7, 8-TCDD ranges from 4.2×10^{-16} to 4.5×10^{-15} g/day using the weight approach, and from 1.9×10^{-16} to 7.6×10^{-16} g/day using the surface area approach.

TABLE 20. Estimated Daily Intake of 2, 3, 7, 8-TCDD from Dermal Absorption

	Source of Exposure		
	Home Dust	Street Dirt	Soil
A. Weight Approach			
Concentration of 2, 3, 7, 8-TCDD[a]	8.8×10^{-14} g/g	8.8×10^{-14} g/g	8.2×10^{-15} g/g
DI_{derm}[b]	4.5×10^{-15} g/day	4.5×10^{-15} g/day	4.2×10^{-16} g/day
B. Surface Area Approach			
Concentration of 2, 3, 7, 8-TCDD[c]	1.35×10^{-13} g/m^2	5.4×10^{-13} g/m^2	
DI_{derm}[d]	1.9×10^{-16} g/day	7.6×10^{-16} g/day	

[a] Assumes a 20-year accumulation period for soil.
[b] Calculated using Eq. (17).
[c] Assumes a 30-day accumulation period for street dirt with home dust equal to 25% of outdoor accumulation.
[d] Calculated using Eq. (16).

6.3   Impacts of Ingestion and Dermal Absorption Pathways on Risk Estimates

The sensitivity of the risk estimates derived for the inhalation pathway to the additional risks that might be attributable to the ingestion and dermal pathways was tested. These latter two pathways were not considered initially because of the high degree of uncertainty in the estimates of ingestion, absorption, and bioavailability rates and because of the difficulties in modeling PCDD concentrations in soil, dirt, and dust.

The data (Table 21) indicate that for the case 1 scenario, the only contribution to exposure is through the inhalation pathway. Under this scenario, the daily intake (DI) equals 1.9×10^{-14} g/day. For the case 2 scenario, assuming that the lowest values for DI_{derm} and DI_{ing} reported in Tables 19 and 20 are applicable, the daily intake (DI_{min}) for all pathways combined equals 9.3×10^{-15} g/day. Under this set of assumptions, the total daily intake is one-half the total daily intake estimated under the case 1 scenario, with the combined contribution of the ingestion and dermal pathways representing only approximately 5% of the total.

However, assuming some of the maximum estimates for intake through ingestion and dermal absorption are applicable, we find that the daily intake (DI_{max}) for all pathways combined equals 1.6×10^{-14} g/day. Under this set of assumptions, the total daily intake is approximately 85% of the daily intake estimated under the case 1 scenario, with the combined contribution of the ingestion and dermal pathways representing slightly less than one-half the total.

In summary, under all conditions tested, the primary source of exposure is due to the inhalation pathway. The daily intake calculated for the inhalation pathway (1.9×10^{-2} pg/day) under case 1 is not likely to be exceeded and may in fact be lowered if the ingestion and dermal exposure pathways are considered.

6.4   Additional Issues

6.4.1   Risks Associated with the Complex Mixture of PCDDs and PCDFs.   It can be argued that the procedures used to predict the increased cancer risk associated only with $2,3,7,8$-TCDD and HCDD exposure underestimate the cancer risk of the complex mixture of PCDDs and PCDFs emitted from the BNYRRF.

TABLE 21. Calculation of a Total Daily Intake of 2,3,7,8-TCDD for Inhalation, Ingestion, and Dermal Absorption Pathway

Case 1: PCDDs and PCDFs Enter Fabric Filter in Gaseous Phase

$DI = DI_{inh} + DI_{ing} + DI_{derm}$
$DI = 1.9 \times 10^{-14} + 0 + 0$
$DI = 1.9 \times 10^{-14}$ g/day

Case 2: PCDDs and PCDFs Enter Fabric Filter Attached to Particulates

$DI = DI_{inh} + DI_{ing} + DI_{derm}$
$DI_{min} = 8.8 \times 10^{-15} + 2.5 \times 10^{-16} + 1.9 \times 10^{-16}$
$DI_{max} = 8.8 \times 10^{-15} + 2.6 \times 10^{-15} + 4.5 \times 10^{-15}$
$DI_{min} = 9.3 \times 10^{-15}$ g/day
$DI_{max} = 1.6 \times 10^{-14}$ g/day

TABLE 22. Table of Uncertainties

1. Case 1 Scenario

A. Previous assumption
  - Maximum ambient air concentration of 2, 3, 7, 8-TCDD $0.00168\,\text{pg/m}^3$

  Changed assumption
  - AEI exposed to 75% of maximum $0.00126\,\text{pg/m}^3$

B. Previous assumption
  - Indoor air quality equals outdoor air quality $0.00168\,\text{pg/m}^3$

  Changed assumption
  - Indoor air quality = 60% of outdoor air quality; AEI spends 16 h/day indoors; change represents average 70-yr exposure $0.00123\,\text{pg/m}^3$

C. Previous assumption
  - 75% of inhaled particulates retained   0.75

  Changed assumption
  - 30% of inhaled particulates retained   0.30

2. Case 2 Scenario

A. Previous assumption
  - Maximum ambient air concentration of 2, 3, 7, 8-TCDD $7.8 \times 10^{-4}\,\text{pg/m}^3$

  Changed assumption
  - AEI exposed to 75% of maximum $5.9 \times 10^{-4}\,\text{pg/m}^3$

B. Previous assumption
  - DI_{inh} for MEI $8.8 \times 10^{-3}\,\text{pg/day}$

  Changed assumptions
  - Same changes made as in 1A and 1C $3.4 \times 10^{-3}\,\text{pg/day}$

C. Previous assumption
  - Maximum deposition rate of 2, 3, 7, 8-TCDD $6.5 \times 10^{-3}\,\text{ng/m}^2$

  Changed assumption
  - Average deposition rate 75% of maximum $4.9 \times 10^{-3}\,\text{ng/m}^2$

D. Previous assumption
  - Average lifetime ingestion rate   100 mg/day

  Change assumption
  - Average of MEI value and lower reported value of (10 mg)   55 mg/day

E. Previous assumption
  - Surface area contact $0.016\,\text{m}^2/\text{day}$

  Changed assumption
  - Average of MEI value and lower reported value (0.0033) $0.010\,\text{m}^2/\text{day}$

F. Previous assumption
  - Oral bioavailability   0.30

  Changed assumption
  - Average of MEI value and lower reported value (10%)   0.20

G. Previous assumption
  - Soil mixing zone   1 cm

  Changed assumption   10 cm

H. Previous assumption
  - Indoor dust accumulation period   30 days

  Changed assumption   15 days

I. Previous assumption
  - TCDD concentration in street dirt $8.8 \times 10^{-2}\,\text{pg/g}$

  Changed assumption
  - Deposition of particles diluted by equal weight of dirt, debris, soil, etc. $6.6 \times 10^{-2}\,\text{pg/g}$

674

TABLE 22. (*Continued*)

J. Previous assumption	
• Contact area	$0.14\,\mathrm{m}^2$
Changed assumption	
• Average value for MEI and lower value of 0.028	0.084
K. Previous assumption	
• Soil Accumulation on skin	$3.5\,\mathrm{mg/cm}^2$
Changed assumption	
• Average of MEI value and lower reported value of	
$0.5\,\mathrm{mg/cm}^2$	$2\,\mathrm{mg/cm}^2$
L. Previous assumption	
• Average annual exposure time	12 h/day
Changed assumption	8 h/day

3. General

A. Previous assumption	
• Swiss-based TEF	59
Changed assumption	
• EPA-based TEF	4.3
B. Previous assumption	
• EPA cancer potency	6.4 fg/kg BW/day
Changed assumption	
• CDC cancer potency	28 fg/kg BW/day

4. Summary—Case 1 Scenario

• DI for MEI—Case 1	1.9×10^{-2} pg/day
• DI for AEI—using assumptions 1A and 1C	7.4×10^{-3} pg/day
Cancer risk for MEI	4.2×10^{-8}
Cancer risk for MEI; TEF $= 59$	2.5×10^{-6}
Cancer risk for AEI	1.7×10^{-8}
Cancer risk for AEI; TEF $= 59$	9.7×10^{-7}
Cancer risk for AEI; TEF $= 4.3$	7.1×10^{-8}
Cancer risk for MEI using CDC cancer potency	
and TEF $= 4.3$	4.2×10^{-8}
Cancer risk for AEI using CDC cancer potency	
and TEF $= 4.3$	1.6×10^{-8}

5. Summary—Case 2 Scenario

• DI_{min} in for MEI	9.3×10^{-3} pg/day
• DI_{max} for MEI	1.6×10^{-2} pg/day
• DI_{min} for AEI	3.4×10^{-3} pg/day
• DI_{max} for AEI	4.5×10^{-3} pg/day
Cancer risk for AEI (assume DI_{max})	1.0×10^{-8}
Cancer risk for AEI; TEF $= 59$	5.9×10^{-7}
Cancer risk for AEI; TEF $= 4.3$	4.3×10^{-8}
Cancer risk for AEI using CDC cancer potency	
and TEF $= 4.3$	9.8×10^{-9}

It would be desirable to estimate the carcinogenic risk of this mixture for all other PCDD and PCDF isomers. However, dose–response data are lacking. Several regulatory agencies use the concept of toxic equivalency to evaluate toxicities of complex mixtures and there is experimental evidence to support this approach in dealing with noncarcinogenic risks. However, there is no data regarding the applicability of this method to the assessment of carcinogenic risks arising from the complex mixtures of PCDDs and PCDFs emitted from MWCs. In other words, it is not clearly established experimentally that toxic equivalency correlates with carcinogenic equivalency.

Assuming for the purposes of this assessment that toxic equivalency equals carcinogenic equivalency, we can calculate that the risk due to the carcinogenic potential of the complex mixture of PCDD and PCDF would equal 59 times the risk due to $2,3,7,8$-TCDD. Given the inherent uncertainty regarding the most appropriate model or procedure to use in estimating human equivalent dose–response for $2,3,7,8$-TCDD, multiplication of the most conservative $2,3,7,8$-TCDD dose–response extrapolation (EPA's) by 59 may significantly overestimate risk.

Based on the daily intake values shown in Table 21 and the EPA cancer risk extrapolation model, the increased cancer risk due to the predicted concentration of $2,3,7,8$-TCDD in BNYRRF emissions, for all three pathways of exposure, was estimated to range from 0.021 to 0.042×10^{-6}. Through use of the toxic equivalency method, the increased cancer risk due to the complex mixture of PCDDs and PCDFs present in the emissions was predicted to range from 1.2 to 2.5×10^{-6}. By using other equally plausible cancer potency models or TEFs, the predicted risks would be substantially lower.

6.4.2 Uncertainties. The multiplication of worst-case assumptions typically used in estimating the level of risk for the MEI potentially overestimates the risk substantially. Consequently, for perspective, Table 22 presents a list of plausible alternative assumptions that were used to calculate the increased cancer risk for an average exposed individual (AEI). The primary source of exposure for the AEI continues to be the inhalation pathway. Upper-bound excess cancer risks for the AEI (case 1), assuming a TEF equal to 59, equals 9.7×10^{-7} or 39% less than the upper-bound risk for the MEI.

More importantly, using a different but equally plausible set of assumptions concerning the cancer potency and the TEF, we find that the data in Table 22 demonstrate that the cancer risks for both the AEI and the MEI may be substantially lower than the upper-bound limits discussed in Section 6.4.1. For example, excess cancer risks were calculated causing a cancer potency of 28 fg/kg·day for the 1×10^{-6} risk and a TEF of 4.3. The former was selected as a reasonably conservative cancer potency estimate used by the CDC in some of their risk assessments. A TEF of 4.3 was calculated using the EPA TEF weighting scheme. While the upper-bound estimate of excess cancer risk for the MEI was found to equal 2.5×10^{-6}, by using equally plausible assumptions for cancer potency and TEFs, the excess cancer risk could be less than 9.7×10^{-8}.

7 SUMMARY AND CONCLUSIONS

A risk assessment was performed to estimate the risks associated with predicted rates of PCDD and PCDF emissions from the BNYRRF. The assessment compared the predicted ambient air concentrations and estimated daily intake levels for PCDDs and PCDFs with concentrations of PCDDs and PCDFs known or suspected to cause a toxic effect.

Several safety factors were incorporated into our assessment to ensure conservatism. They include the following:

- Assessment of three potential pathways of exposure: inhalation of gaseous or particulate emission, and ingestion or dermal absorption of particulates deposited on outdoor and indoor surfaces.

- Application of a toxic equivalency multiplier equal to 59. This equivalency factor was also used to estimate carcinogenic equivalency as a worst-case assumption although such an application is speculative.

- No losses of PCDDs were assumed through volatilization or degradation or through such actions as rainfall.

- Indoor ambient air quality was assumed to equal outdoor air quality.

- Risks were calculated based on continuous exposure over a 70-year lifetime at the point of maximum impact.

- The most conservative cancer risk extrapolation model was included to estimate an upper-bound limit to increased cancer risk.

- Conservative assumptions for bioavailability and rates of ingestion and dermal contact were included to estimate worst-case daily intakes of PCDDs.

The results of this risk assessment are summarized below. Risks associated with inhalation of PCDDs and PCDFs at the maximum ambient air concentrations were determined by comparing a predicted maximum daily intake through inhalation (DI_{inh}) with ADIs and cancer dose–response extrapolations. The maximum daily intake DI_{inh} of 2,3,7,8-TCDD, HCDD, and TCDD toxic equivalents are predicted to be well below (less than 1.6%) any ADI promulgated by any regulatory agency. These ADIs provide a margin of safety and they identify a very safe dose, below which risks are insignificant for noncarcinogenic toxic effects.

An upper bound to carcinogenicity risk was also determined by comparing DI_{inh} with three different cancer dose–response extrapolations. The upper-bound excess risk due to exposure to 2,3,7,8-TCDD and HCDD, at the point of maximum impact, ranges from less than 0.0019 to less than 0.055×10^{-6} or less than 5 cases per 100,000,000 people exposed to the maximum concentration over a 70-year lifetime.

The sensitivity of the risk estimate derived for the inhalation pathway to the additional risks that might be attributable to the ingestion and dermal pathways was tested. These two pathways were not considered initially because of the high degree of uncertainty in the estimates of ingestion, absorption, and bioavailability rates and because of the difficulties in modeling PCDD concentrations in soil, dirt, and dust. A range of daily intake estimates for the MEI was calculated for these pathways. Under all conditions tested, the upper-bound excess cancer risk predicted to be less than 0.055×10^{-6} for the case 1 scenario will not be exceeded if the contribution of the ingestion and dermal pathways are considered. For the case 2 scenario, the upper-bound excess cancer risk is predicted to be reduced in comparison to the case 1 scenario by from 15 to 50%. This result differs from our original estimate in which we concluded that the ingestion and dermal pathways might increase the total cancer risk by 2.4 times. The difference in these results are attributed to the use of more realistic but still conservative estimates of soil ingestion rates and bioavailability.

As an additional safety factor to our assessment, we examined the risks due to PCDD exposure assuming that carcinogenic equivalency equals toxic equivalency. For the MEI, using one of the most conservative TEFs (equal to 59) and the most conservative cancer potency estimates, the upper-bound increased cancer risk due to the complex mixture of PCDDs and PCDFs present in the emissions ranges from less than 1.1×10^{-7} (case 2) to an upper-bound limit less than 2.5×10^{-6} (case 1), again assuming a 70-year lifetime exposure, 24 h/day, to the maximum concentrations. Within the context of the assumptions used in the risk assessment, and by considering current regulatory practice regarding acceptable versus unacceptable table health risks, a worst-case upper-bound excess cancer risk less than 2.5×10^{-6} represents an insignificant risk. Using the same conservative numbers for cancer potency and TEFs, we find that the excess cancer risk for the average exposed individual will probably not exceed 1×10^{-6}. Using equally plausible but less conservative assumptions regarding either cancer potency or TEFs, we find that the excess cancer risk is predicted to be substantially less than 1×10^{-6}.

REFERENCES

1. D. Cleverly, L. Fradkin, R. Bruins, P. M. McGinnis, G. W. Dawson, and R. Bond, *Methodology for the Assessment of Health Risks Associated with Multiple Pathway Exposure to Municipal Waste Combustion Emissions.* Office of Air Quality Planning and Standards, USEPA, Washington, DC, 1986.

2. National Research Council of Canada, *Polychlorinated Dibenzo-p-dioxins: Criteria for Their Effects on Man and His Environment,* NRCC 18574, ISSN 0316-0114. NRCC, Ottawa, Canada, 1981.

3. J. W. Lustenhouwer, Chlorinated dibenzo-p-dioxins and related compounds in incinerator effluents. A review of measurements and mechanisms of formation. *Chemosphere* **9**, 501–522 (1980).

4. K. Olie et al., Chlorinated-p-dioxins and chlorodibenzofurans are trace components of fly ash and flue gas of some municipal incinerators in the Netherlands. *Chemosphere* **6**, 455–459 (1977).

5. T. O. Tiernan et al., Characterization of toxic components in the effluents from a refuse-fired incinerator. *Resour. Conserv.* **9**, 343–354 (1982).

6. G. A. Eicemen et al., Analysis of fly ash from municipal incinerators for trace organic compounds. *Anal. Chem.* **51**, 2343–2350 (1979).

7. G. A. Eicemen et al., Variations in concentrations of organic compounds including PCDDs and polynuclear aromatic hydrocarbons in fly ash from a municipal incinerator. *Anal. Chem.* **53**, 955–959 (1981).

8. F. W. Karasek, Dioxins from garbage: Previously unknown source of toxic compounds is being uncovered using advanced analytical instrumentation. *Cancer Res.* 1316 (1980).

9. R. R. Bumb et al., Trace chemistries of fire: A source of chlorinated dioxins. *Science* **210**, 385–390 (1980).

10. L. L. Lamparski and T. J. Nestrick, Determination of tetra, hexa, hepta, and octa chlorinated dioxin isomers in particulate samples at parts per trillion levels. *Anal. Chem.* **52**, 2045–2054 (1980).

11. U.S. Environmental Protection Agency, *Interim Evaluation of Health Risks Associated with Emissions of Tetrachlorinated Dioxins from Municipal Waste Resource Recovery Facilities.* Office of the Deputy Administrator, USEPA, Washington, DC, 1981.

12. U.S. Environmental Protection Agency, *Memo from Mike Cook on TCDD Emissions for Municipal Waste Combustors.* Office of Solid Waste and Emergency Response, USEPA, Washington, DC, 1983.

13. U.S. Environmental Protection Agency, *Air Quality Criteria for Lead,* EPA-600/8-77-017. Office of Research and Development, USEPA, Washington, DC, 1977.

14. U.S. Environmental Protection Agency, *Health Assessment Document for Inorganic Arsenic,* EPA-600/8-83-021F. Office of Health and Environmental Assessment, USEPA, Washington, DC, 1984.

15. G. A. Holton, C. C. Travis, E. L. Etnier et al., *Multiple-Pathways Screening-Level Assessment of a Hazardous Waste Incineration Facility,* Publ. ORNL/TM-8652. Oak Ridge Natl. Lab., Oak Ridge, TN, 1984.

16. G. F. Fries, *Assessment of Potential Residues in Foods Derived from Animals Exposed to TCDD-Contaminated Soils*. Presented at Dioxin 86, Fukuoka, Japan, 1986.

17. Radian Corp., *Stanislaus Waste-To-Energy Facility Health Risk Assessment*. Submitted to Stanislaus County (California) Air Pollution Control District, October 16, 1986.

18. A. Eschenroeder, P. Guldberg, D. Kellermeyer, A. Smith, and S. Wolff, *An Analysis of Health Risks from the Irwindale Resource Recovery Facility*. Submitted to the California Energy Commission, Sacramento, March 7, 1986.

19. Clement Assoc., *Risk Assessment for the Proposed Trash-To-Steam Municipal Solid Waste Incinerator at the U.S. Naval Base in Philadelphia, PA*. Submitted to the Philadelphia Public Health Advisory Commission, December 2, 1986.

20. Environ Corp., *Documentation of the Methodology and Assumptions Used in the Preliminary Risk Analysis for PCDDs and PCDFs at the Proposed Adirondack Resource Recovery Facility*. Prepared for Foster Wheeler USA Corp., August 14, 1986.

21. Camp Dresser and McKee, *Multimedia Risk Assessment*. Prepared for Lanchester County Solid Waste Management Authority, Lanchester, PA, 1987.

22. Fred C. Hart Associates, *Assessment of Potential Public Health Impacts Associated with Predicted Emissions of Polychlorinated Dibenzodioxins and Polychlorinated Dibenzofurans from the Brooklyn Navy Yard Resource Recovery Facility*. Submitted to New York City Dept. of Sanitation, August 17, 1984.

23. L. Marple, R. Brunck et al., Experimental and calculated physical constants for 2, 3, 7, 8-TCDD. In J. H. Exner, Ed., *Solving Hazardous Waste Problems—Learning from Dioxins*. American Chemical Society, Washington, DC, 1987.

24. M. P. Esposito, *Dioxins*. USEPA, Washington, DC, 1980.

25. D. G. Barnes, *Dioxin Production from Combustion of Biomass and Wastes*. Presented at the Institute of Gas Technology Symposium, Lake Buena Vista, FL, January 1983.

26. R. Kooke et al., Extraction efficiencies of PCDDs and PCDFs from fly ash. *Anal. Chem.* **53**, 461–463 (1981).

27. G. C. Miller and R. G. Zepp, 2, 3, 7, 8-TCDD: Environmental chemistry. In J. H. Exner, Ed., *Solving Hazardous Waste Problems—Learning from Dioxins*. American Chemical Society, Washington, DC, 1987.

28. W. M. Shaub and W. Tsang, Physical and chemical properties of dioxins in relation to their disposal. In R. Dullen et al., Ed., *Human and Environmental Risks of Chlorinated Dioxins and Related Compounds*, Plenum. NY (1983) pp. 731–748.

29. R. T. Podoll, H. M. Jaber, and T. Mill, Tetrachlorodibenzodioxin rates of volatilization and photolysis in the environment. *Environ. Sci. Technol.* **20**, 490–492 (1986).

30. D. Dullen, H. Drossman, and T. Mill, Products and quantum yields for photolysis of chloroaromatics in water. *Environ. Sci. Technol.* **20**, 72–77 (1986).

31. D. G. Crosby and A. S. Wong, Environmental degradation of 2, 3, 7, 8-TCDD. *Science* **195**, 1337–1338 (1977).

32. Chemical and Engineering News, Dioxin in report. *Chem. Eng. News* **61**, 20–64 (1983).

33. H. K. Wipf et al., Field trials of photodegradation of TCDD on vegetation after spraying with vegetable oil. In M. P. Esposito et al., Eds., *Dioxins*. USEPA, Washington, DC, 1980.

34. D. G. Crosby, Conquering the monster—The photochemical destruction of chlorodioxins. In M. P. Esposito et al., Eds., *Dioxins*. USEPA, Washington, DC, 1980.

35. T. J. Nestrick et al., Methodology and preliminary results for the isomer specific determination of TCDDs and higher chlorinated dioxins in chimney particulates from wood fueled furnaces located in the United States. *Environ. Sci. Res.* **26** (1983).

36. D. G. Crosby, Photodecomposition of chlorinated dibenzo-p-dioxins. *Science* **173**, 748–749 (1971).

37. P. C. Kearney et al., Persistence and metabolism of chlorodioxins in soils. *Environ. Sci. Technol.* **6**, 1017–1019 (1972).

38. International Agency for Research on Cancer, *IARC Monograph on the Evaluation of the Carcinogenic Risk of Chemicals to Man for Fumigants, Herbicides, Chlorinated Dioxins, and Miscelleneous Chemicals*, IARC Monogr., Vol. 15. IARC, Geneva, 1977.

39. A. L. Young, Long-term studies on the persistence and movement of TCDD in a natural ecosystem. *Environ. Sci. Res.* **26** (1983).

40. A. DiDomenico et al., Environmental persistence of 2, 3, 7, 8-TCDD at Seveso. In O. Hutzinger et al., Eds., *Chlorinated Dioxins and Related Compounds*. Pergamon, Oxford, 1980.

41. D. J. Paustenbach, Assessing the potential environmental and human health risks of contaminated soil. *Comments Toxicol.* (1987) (in press).

42. R. A. Freeman, F. Hileman, R. Noble, and J. Schroy, Experiments on the mobility of 2, 3, 7, 8-TCDD at Times Beach, Missouri. In J. H. Exner, Ed., *Solving Hazardous Waste Problems— Learning from Dioxins*. American Chemical Society, Washington, DC, 1987.

43. R. A. Freeman and J. M. Schroy, *Environmental Mobility of Dioxins*. Presented at the Eighth ASTM Aquatic Toxicology Symposium, Fort Mitchell, KY, April 15–17, 1984.

44. L. J. Thibodeaux, Off-site transport of 2, 3, 7, 8-TCDD from a production and disposal facility. In G. Choudhary et al., Eds., *Chlorinated Dioxins and Dibenzofurans in the Total Environment*. Butterworth, Woburn, MA, 1983.

45. R. G. Nash and M. L. Beall, Distribution of silvex, 2, 4,-D, and TCDD applied to turf in chamber and field plots. *J. Agric. Food Chem.* **28**, 614–623 (1980).

46. L. J. Thibodeaux and D. Lipsky, A fate and transport model for 2, 3, 7, 8-TCDD in fly ash on soil and urban surfaces. *Hazard. Waste Hazard. Mater.* **2**, 225–235 (1985).

47. F. Matsumura et al., Microbial degradation of TCDD in a model ecosystem. *Environ. Sci. Res.* **26** (1980).

48. C. T. Ward and F. Matsumura, Fate of 2, 3, 7, 8-TCDD in a model aquatic ecosystem. *Arch. Environ. Contam. Toxicol.* **7**, 349–357 (1978).

49. American Society of Mechanical Engineers, *Study of State-of-the-Art of Dioxin from Combustion Sources*, Res. Commun. Ind. Municipal Wastes, ASME, New York, 1981.

50. U.S. Environmental Protection Agency, *Health Assessment Document for PCDDs*, Final Report, EPA/600/8-84/014F. Office of Health and Environmental Assessment, USEPA, Washington, DC, 1985.

51. A. Poland and J. C. Knutson, 2, 3, 7, 8-TCDD and related halogenated hydrocarbons: Examination of the mechanism of toxicity. *Annu. Rev. Pharmacol. Toxicol.* **22**, 517–554 (1982).

52. R. A. Neal, T. Gasiewicz, L. Geiger, J. Olson, and T. Sawahata, Metabolism of 2, 3, 7, 8-TCDD in mammalian systems. *Banbury Rep.* **18**, 39–60 (1984).

53. American Medical Association, *The Health Effects of "Agent Orange" and Polychlorinated Dioxin Contaminants: An Update 1984*. AMA, Chicago, IL, 1984.

54. J. P. Van Miller et al., Increased incidence of neoplasms in rats exposed to low levels of 2, 3, 7, 8-TCDD. *Chemosphere* **6**, 537–544 (1977).

55. R. J. Kociba, D. G. Keyes, and J. E. Beyer, Results of a two year chronic toxicity and oncogenicity study of 2, 3, 7, 8-TCDD in rats. *Toxicol. Appl. Pharmacol.* **46**, 279–303 (1978).

56. National Toxicology Program, *A Bioassay of 2, 3, 7, 8-TCDD for Possible Carcinogenicity (Gavage Study)*, DHHS Publ. No. (NIH) 82–1765. NCI, NTP, Bethesda, MD, 1980.

57. K. S. Toth et al., Carcinogenicity testing of herbicide 2, 4, 5,-trichlorophenoxyethanol containing dioxin or of pure dioxin in Swiss mice. *Nature (London)* **278**, 548–549 (1979).

58. K. S. Toth et al., Carcinogenic bioassay of the herbicide 2, 4, 5,-trichlorophenoxyethanol with different 2, 3, 7, 8 TCDD content in Swiss mice. *Prog. Biochem. Pharmacol.* **14**, 82–93 (1978).

59. F. J. Murray et al., Three generation reproduction study of rats given 2, 3, 7, 8-TCDD in the diet. *Toxicol. Appl. Pharmacol.* **50**, 241–251 (1979).

60. Pitot Committee Report, Dioxin Update Committee, Office of Pesticides and Toxic Substances, EPA, Washington, DC, 1986.

61. H. P. Shu, D. J. Paustenbach, and F. J. Murray, A critical evaluation of the use of mutagenesis, carcinogenesis, and tumor promotion data in a cancer risk assessment of 2, 3, 7, 8-TCDD. *Regul. Toxicol. Pharmacol.* **7**, 57–88 (1987).

62. H. C. Pitot, T. Goldsworthy, and H. Poland, Promotion by 2, 3, 7, 8-TCDD of hepatocarcinogenesis from diethylnitrosamine. *Cancer Res.* **40**, 3616–3620 (1980).

63. R. E. Kouri et al., 2, 3, 7, 8-TCDD as co-carcinogen causing 3-methylcholanthrene initiated subcutaneous tumors in mice geneteically "nonresponsive" at the Ah locus. *Cancer Res.* **38**, 3777–3783 (1978).

64. National Toxicology Program, *Bioassay of 2, 3, 7, 8-TCDD for Possible Carcinogenicity (Dermal Study)*, DHHS Publ. No. (NIH) 80–1757. NCI, NIH, Bethesda, MD., 1980.

65. D. L. Berry, T. J. Slaga, J. Digiovanni, and J. R. Juchau, Studies with chlorinated dibenzodioxins, polybrominated biphenyls, and polychlorinated biphenyls in a two-stage system of mouse skin tumorigenesis. *Ann. N.Y. Acad. Sci.* **320**, 405–414 (1979).

66. G. Reggiani, An overview of the health effects of halogenated dioxins and related Compounds—the Yusho and Taiwan episodes. In F. Couston and F. Pocchiari, Eds., *Accidental Exposure to Dioxins: Human Health Aspects*. Academic Press, New York, 1983.

67. M. A. Fingerhut, M. H. Sweeney, W. E. Halperin, and T. M. Schnorr, Epidemiology of populations exposed to dioxins. In J. H. Exner, Ed., *Solving Hazardous Waste Problems—Learning from Dioxins*. American Chemical Society, Washington, DC, 1987.

68. R. D. Kimbrough and V. N. Houk, Effects of chlorinated dibenzodioxins. In J. H. Exner, Ed., *Solving Hazardous Waste Problems—Learning from Dioxins*. American Chemical Society, Washington, DC, 1987.

69. A. Blair, Review of the epidemiology data regarding dioxin and cancer. In Pitot Committee Report to EPA's Office of Pesticides and Toxic Substances, EPA, Washington, DC, 1986.

70. F. V. Pocchiari, V. Silano, and A. Zampieri, Human health effects from accidental release of TCDD at Seveso, Italy. *Ann. N.Y. Acad. Sci.* **320**, 311–320 (1979).

71. G. Reggiani, Acute human exposure to TCDD in Seveso, Italy. *J. Toxicol. Environ. Health* **6**, 27–43 (1980).

72. G. Reggiani, Medical problems raised by the TCDD contamination in Seveso, Italy. *Arch. Toxicol.* **40**, 161–168 (1978).

73. G. Reggiani, Toxicology of TCDD and related compounds: Observation in man. In O. Hutzinger, R. Frei, E. Merian, and F. Pocchiari, Eds., *Chlorinated Dioxins and Related Compounds: Impact on the Environment*. Pergamon, Oxford, 1982.

74. R. R. Suskind and V. S. Hertzberg, Human health effects of 2, 4, 5,-T and its toxic contaminants. *JAMA, J. Am. Med. Assoc.* **251**, 2372–2380 (1984).

75. M. Moses, R. Lilis, K. D. Crow et al., Health status of workers with past exposure to 2, 3, 7, 8-TCDD in the manufacture of 2, 4, 5-trichlorophenoxyacetic acid: Comparison of findings with and without chloracne. *Am. J. Ind. Med.* **5**, 161–182 (1984).

76. R. E. Hoffman, P. Stehr-Green et al., Health effects of long-term exposure to 2, 3, 7, 8-TCDD. *JAMA, J. Am. Med. Assoc.* **255**, 2031–2038 (1986).

77. J. H. Dean and R. D. Kimbrough, Immunotoxicity of the chlorinated dibenzodioxins and dibenzofurans. In Pitot Committee Report to Office of Pesticides and Toxic Substances, EPA, Washington, DC, 1986.

78. L. Hardell and A. Sandstrom, Case-control study: Soft-tissue sarcomas and exposure to phenoxyacetic acids or chlorophenols. *Br. J. Cancer* **39**, 711–717 (1979).

79. L. Hardell, Malignant lymphomas of the histiocytic type and exposure to phenoxyacetic acids as chlorophenols. *Lancet* **1**, 55–56 (1979).

80. M. Erikson, L. Hardell, D. O. Berg et al., Soft-tissue sarcomas and exposure to chemical substances: A case-reference study. *Br. J. Ind. Med.* **38**, 27–33 (1981).

81. L. Hardell, B. Johansson, and O. Axelson, Epidemiological study of nasal and naso-pharyngeal cancer and their relation to phenoxy acid or chlorophenol exposure. *Am. J. Ind. Med.* **3**, 247–257 (1982).

82. A. H. Smith, D. O. Fisher et al., Do agricultural chemicals cause soft-tissue sarcoma? Initial findings of a case-control study in New Zealand. *Community Health Stud.* **6**, 114–119 (1982).

83. A. H. Smith, D. O. Fisher et al., The New Zealand soft-tissue sarcoma case-control study: Interview findings concerning phenoxyacetic acid exposure. *Chemosphere* **12**, 565–571 (1983).

84. A. H. Smith, N. Pearce, D. O. Fisher et al., Soft-tissue sarcoma and exposure to phenoxy-herbicides and chlorphenols in New Zealand. *JNCI, J. Natl. Cancer Inst.* **75**, 1111–1114 (1984).

85. R. R. Cook et al., Mortality experience of employees exposed to 2, 3, 7, 8-tetrachloro-dibenzo-p-dioxin. *J. Occup. Med.* **22**, 530–532 (1980).

86. J. A. Zack, and R. R. Suskind, The mortality experience of workers exposed to tetrachloro-dibenzodioxin in a trichlorophenol process accident. *J. Occup. Med.* **22**, 11–14 (1980).

87. J. A. Zack and W. R. Gaffey, A mortality study of workers employed at the Monsanto Company plant in Nitro, West Virginia. In R. E. Tucker, A. L. Young, and A. P. Gray, Eds., *Human and Environmental Risks at Chlorinated and Related Compounds.* Plenum Press, New York, 1983, pp. 575–591.

88. Radian Corp., *Final Emissions Test Report.* North Andover Resource Recovery Facility, North Andover, MA. 1986.

89. O. Axelson, L. Sundell, K. Andersson et al., Herbicide exposure and tumor mortality. *Scand. J. Work Environ. Health* **6**, 73–79 (1980).

90. A. M. Thiess, R. Frentzel-Beyme, and R. Link, Mortality study of persons exposed to dioxin in a trichlorophenol-process accident in the BASEF AG. *Am. J. Ind. Med.* **3**, 179–189 (1982).

91. V. Riihimaki, S. Asp, and S. Hernberg, Mortality of 2, 4-dichlorophenoxyacetic acid and 2, 4, 5-trichlorophenoxyacetic acid herbicide applicators in Finland. *Scand. J. Work Environ. Health* **8**, 37–42 (1982).

92. M. G. Ott, B. B. Holder, and R. D. Olson, A mortality analysis of employees engaged in the manufacture of 2, 4, 5-trichlorophenoxyacetic acid. *J. Occup. Med.* **22**, 47–50 (1980).

93. K. D. Courtney and J. A. Moore, Teratology studies with 2, 4, 5-T and 2, 3, 7, 8-TCDD. *Toxicol. Appl. Pharmacol.* **20**, 396–403 (1971).

94. E. Giavini, M. Prati, and C. Vismara, Rabbit teratology study with 2, 3, 7, 8-TCDD. *Environ. Res.* **27**, 74–78 (1982).

95. J. R. Allen, D. A. Barsotti, L. Lambrecht, and J. P. Van Miller, Reproductive effects of halogenated aromatic hydrocarbons on nonhuman primates. *Ann. N.Y. Acad. Sci.* **320**, 419–425 (1979).

96. W. P. McNulty, Fetocidal and teratagenic actions of TCDD. In W. W. Lawrence, Ed., *Public Health Risks of the Dioxins.* William Kaufmann, Los Altos, CA, 1984, pp. 245–253.

97. G. D. Lathrop, W. H. Wolfe et al., *An Epidemiologic Investigation of Health Effects in Air Force Personnel Following Exposure to Herbicides: Baseline Morbidity Study Results.* U.S. Air Force School of Aerospace Medicine, Brooks Air Force Base, TX, 1984.

98. J. Erikson, J. McLinere et al. Vietnam veterans' risks for fathering babies with birth defects. *JAMA, J. Am. Med. Assoc.* **252**, 903–912 (1984).

99. M. L. Dourson and J. F. Stara, Regulatory history and experimental support of uncertainty (SAFETY) factors. *Regul. Toxicol. Pharmacol.* **3**, 224–238 (1983).

100. National Research Council, *Risk Assessment in the Federal Government*. National Academy Press, Washington, DC, 1983.

101. Environmental Protection Agency, Proposed guidelines for carcinogen risk assessment. *Fed. Regist.* **49**, 46294–46301 (1984).

102. F. C. Munro and D. Krewski, Risk assessment and regulatory decision making. *Food Cosmet. Toxicol.* **19**, 549–560 (1981).

103. National Toxicology Program, *Bioassay of 1, 2, 3, 6, 7, 8- and 1, 2, 3, 7, 8, 9-HCDD (Gavage) for Possible Carcinogenicity*, DHHS Publ. No. (NIH) 80–1754. NCI, NIH, Bethesda, MD, 1980.

104. Ontario Ministry of the Environment, *Scientific Criteria Document for Standard Development No. 4–84: PCDDs and PCDFs*. OME, Ontario, Canada, 1985.

104a. C. A. Vander Heijden, A. G. Knapp et al., *Evaluation of the Carcinogenicity and Mutagenicity of 2, 3, 7, 8-TCDD.....*, Rep. DOC/LCM 300/292. Bilthoven, Netherlands, 1982.

105. R. Kimbrough et al., Health implications of 2, 3, 7, 8-TCDD contamination of residential soil. *J. Toxicol. Environ. Health* **14**, 47–93 (1984).

106. N. Kim and J. Hawley, *Revised Risk Assessment, Binghamton State Office Building, Albany, NY*. New York State Dept. of Health, Bureau of Toxic Substance Assessment, January 17, 1984.

106a. Federal Environmental Agency, *Report on Dioxins*. FEA, Federal Republic of Germany, 1984.

107. California Department of Health Services, *Health Effects of 2, 3, 7, 8-TCDD and Related Compounds*. Epidemiological Studies Section, Berkeley, CDHS, CA, April 1985.

108. R. L. Sielken, Quantitative cancer risk assessment for TCDD. *Food Chem. Toxicol.* **25**, 257–267 (1987).

109. F. P. Perera, The genotoxic/epigenetic distinction; relevance to cancer policy. *Environ. Res.* **34**, 175–191 (1984).

110. U.S. Environmental Protection Agency, (USEPA), *Memo from S. Bayard to Interagency Meeting of Dioxin Working Group*. USEPA, Washington, DC, January 25, 1984.

111. R. A. Squire, *Pathologic Evaluations of Selected Tissues from the Dow Chemical TCDD and 2, 4, 5-T Rat Studies*, Contract 68-01-5092. Submitted to the Carcinogen Assessment Group, USEPA, Washington, DC, August 15, 1980.

112. C. J. Portier, D. G. Hoel, and J. Van Ryzin, Statistical analyses of the carcinogenesis bioassay data relating to the risk of exposure to 2, 3, 7, 8-TCDD. In W. Lawrence, Ed., *Public Health Risks of the Dioxins*. William Kaufmann Publ., Los Altos, CA, 1984.

113. D. H. Harding, *Chlorinated Dioxins and Dibenzofurans, Ambient Air Guideline*. Health Studies Service, Special Studies and Services Branch, Ministry of Labor, Ontario, Canada, 1982.

114. Swiss Federal Office for Environmental Protection, Environmental pollution due to dioxins and furans from communal rubbish incineration plans. *Schriftenr. Unweltschutz.* No. 5 (1982).

115. T. Sawyer et al., Bioanalysis of PCDF and PCDD mixtures in fly ash. *Chemosphere* **12**, 529 (1983).

116. G. Eadon, K. Aldous, G. Fienkel et al., *Comparison of Chemical and Biological Data on Soot Samples from the Binghamton State Office Building*. New York State Dept. of Health, Albany, March 1982.

117. U.S. Environmental Protection Agency, *Interim Procedures for Estimating Risks Associated with Exposure to Mixtures of Chlorinated Dibenzodioxins and Dibenzofurans*, EPA/625/3-87/012. USEPA, Washington, DC, March 1987.

118. M. Suter Hoffman and C. Schlatter, Toxicity of particulate emissions from a municipal incinerator: Critique of the concept of TCDD-equivalents. *Chemosphere* (1986).

119. D. Redford et al., *Emissions of PCDDs and PCDFs from Combustion Sources.* Presented at the International Symposium on Chlorinated Dioxins and Related Compounds, Arlington, Va, October 1985.

119a. C. Rappe et al., PCDDs, PCDFs and other polynuclear aromatics formed during incineration and polychlorinated biphenyl fires. In G. Choudary et al., Eds., *Chlorinated Dioxins and Dibenzofurans in the Total Environment.* Butterworth, Woburn, MA, 1983.

119b. F. Gizzi et al., PCDD and PCDF in emissions from an urban incinerator. *Chemosphere* **11**, 577–583 (1982).

119c. B. Ahling and A. Lindskog, Emissions of chlorinated organic substances from combustion. In O. Hutzinger et al., Eds., *Chlorinated Dioxins and Related Compounds—Impact on the Environment.* Pergamon, Oxford, 1982.

119d. T. O. Tiernan, Chlorodibenzodioxins, chlorodibenzofurans, and related compounds in the effluents from combustion processes. *Chemosphere* **12**, 595–606 (1983).

120. A. Cavallaro et al., Sampling, occurrence and evaluation of PCDDs and PCDFs from incinerated solid urban waste. *Chemosphere* **9**, 611–621 (1980).

120a. A. Cavallaro et al., Summary of results of PCDD analyses from incinerator effluents. *Chemosphere* **11**, (1982).

120b. K. Olie et al., PCDD and related compounds in incinerator effluents. In O. Hutzinger et al., Eds., *Chlorinated Dioxins and Related Compunds—Impact on the Environment.* Pergamon, Oxford, 1980.

121. B. Commoner et al., *Environmental and Economic Analysis of Alternative Municipal Solid Waste Disposal Technologies.* Center for the Biology of Natural Systems, Queens College, New York, December 1, 1984.

122. NYSDEC, *ANSWERS: Emission Source Test Report: Sheridan Avenue RDF Plant.* Bureau of Air Toxics, Division of Air Resources, NYSDEC, Albany, January 29, 1985.

123. Environment Canada, *Natural Incenerator Testing and Evaluation Program: Two-Stage Combustion, Prince Edward Island,* Rep. EPS 3/UP/. September, 1985.

124. A. J. Fossa, R. Kerr et al., *Air Emission Characterization of Municipal Waste Combustors in New York State.* Abstr. 87-57.5. Presented at the APCA Annual Meeting, New York City, 1987.

125. H. Vogg and L. Stiegler, Thermal behavior of PCDD/PCDF in fly ash from municipal incenerators. *Chemosphere* **15**, 9–12, 1986.

126. F. W. Karasek and L. C. Dickson, Model studies of PCDD formation during municipal refuse incineration. *Science* **237**, 754–756 (1987).

127. A. Smith, M. Smith et al., *Health Risk Assessment for the Brooklyn Navy Yard Resource Recovery Facility.* Health Risk Associates, 1987.

127a. P. Siebert, D. Alston et al., *Statistical Properties of Available Worldwide Combustion Dioxin/Furan Emissions,* Abstr. 87-94.1. Presented at the APCA Annual Meeting, New York City, 1987.

127b. J. L. Hahn, H. P. von dem Fange, R. Zurlinden et al., *Air Emissions Testing at the Wurzbug, West Germary Waste-To-Energy Facility.* Presented at the 1986 National Waste Processing Conference, Denver, CO, 1986.

127c. R. Zurlinden, H. von dem Fange, and J. L. Hahn, *Environmental Test Report—Executive Summary; Walter B. Hall, Resource Recovery Facility, Tulsa Oklahoma,* Rep. No. 102. Ogden Projects, Inc., Tulsa, OK, 1986.

128. S. L. Law and G. E. Gordon, Sources of metals in municipal incinerator emissions. *Environ. Sci. Technol.* **13**, 432 (1979).

129. D. F. Natusch et al., Toxic trace elements: Preferential concentrations in respirable particles. *Science* **183**, 202–204 (1974).

130. California Air Resources Board, *Air Pollution Control at Resource Recovery Facilities,* Preliminary Draft Report. CARB, Sacramento, CA, 1984.

131. M. L. Taylor et al., Assessment of incineration processes as sources of supertoxic chlorinated hydrocarbons..... In G. Choudhary et al., Eds., *Chlorinated Dioxins and Dibenzofurans in the Total Environment.* Butterworth, Woburn, MA, 1983.

132. K. Ballschmitter, Reported by C. C. Kemp, in *Notes on PCDDs and PCDFs in Connection with Waste-to-Energy Plants.* Browning-Ferris Industries, April 1983.

133. O. Hutzinger, personal communication (1984).

134. F. W. Karasek, Distribution of PCDDs and other toxic compounds generated on fly ash particulates in municipal incinerators. *J. Chromatogr.* **239**, 173–189 (1982).

135. M. Golembiewski et al., *Environmental Assessment of a Waste-to-Energy process*, USEPA Rep. No. 600/7-80-149, Midwest Research Institute, 1980.

136. T. E. Pierce and D. B. Turner, *User's Guide for MPTER*, EPA-600/8-80-016. USEPA, Washington, DC, 1980.

137. H. F. Cramer Co., Inc., *Industrial Source Complex (ISC) User's Guide*, Vol. 1, NTIS PB80-133044 1979.

138. R. K. Dumbauld et al., *Dispersion Deposition from Aerial Spray Releases*, Pre-print volume for the Third Symposium on Atmospheric Diffusion and Air Quality. American Meteorological Society, Boston, MA, 1976.

139. A. DiDomenico, V. Silano et al., Accidental release of 2, 3, 7, 8-TCDD in Seveso, Italy II. TCDD distribution in the soil surface layer. *Ecotoxicol. Environ. Saf.* **4**, 298–320 (1980).

140. A. DiDomenico, V. Silano et al., Accidental release of 2, 3, 7, 8-TCDD in Seveso, Italy IV. Vertical distribution of TCDD in soil. *Ecotoxicol. Environ. Saf.* **4**, 327–338 (1980).

141. H. Nudelman, New York City Department of Environmental Protection, Personal communication to Ben Miller, New York City Department of Sanitation, June 29, 1984.

142. R. M. Harrison, Toxic metals in street and household dusts. *Sci. Total Environ.* **11**, 89 (1979).

143. R. L. Solomon and K. A. Reinbold, *Environmental Contamination by Lead and Other Heavy Metals*, Publ. No. NSF/RA 770681-5, National Science Foundation, Washington, DC, 1977.

144. J. F. Yocum, Indoor-outdoor air quality relationships. *J. Air Pollut. Control Assoc.* **32**, 500 (1982).

145. H. Leung and D. J. Paustenbach, A proposed occupational exposure limit for 2, 3, 7, 8-TCDD (in press).

146. M. Lippman and R. B. Schlesinger, *Chemical Contamination in the Human Environment.* Oxford Univ. Press, London and New York, 1979.

147. M. J. Duggan and S. Williams, Lead in city streets. *Sci. Total. Environ.* **7**, 91–97 (1977).

148. M. L. Lepow et al., Role of environmental lead in increased body burdens of lead in Hartford children. *Environ. Health Perspect.* 99–101 (1974).

149. B. Brunekreff et al., Blood lead levels of Dutch city children and their relationship to lead in the environment. *J. Air. Pollut. Control Assoc.* **33**, 9 (1983).

150. S. Binder, D. Sokol, and D. Maughan, Estimating the amount of soil ingested by young children through tracer elements. *Arch. Environ. Health* **41**, 341–345 (1986).

151. P. Clausing, B. Brunekreff, and J. H. Van Wijnen, A method for estimating soil ingestion by young children. *Int. Arch. Occup. Environ. Health* **59**, 73–82 (1987).

152. J. Schaum, *Risk Analysis of TCDD Contaminated Soil.* Office of Health and Environmental Assessment, Office of Research and Development, USEPA, Washington, DC, 1984.

153. ICF Inc., *Superfund Public Health Evaluation Manual*, EPA Contract No. 68-01-7090, OSWER Directive 9285 4-1. ICF Inc., December 18, 1985.

154. D. J. Paustenbach, H. P. Shu, and F. J. Murray, A critical examination of assumptions used in risk assessments of dioxin contaminated soil. *Regul. Toxicol. Pharmacol.* **6**, 284–307 (1986).

155. M. Gallo, Bioavailability of dioxins from complex mixtures. In *Pitot Committee Report to EPA's Office of Pesticides and Toxic Substances.* EPA, Washington, DC, 1986.

156. G. F. Fries and G. S. Marrow, Retention and excretion of 2, 3, 7, 8-TCDD by rats. *J. Agric. Food Chem.* **23**, 265–269 (1975).

157. J. Q. Rose, The fate of 2, 3, 7, 8-TCDD following single and repeated doses to the rat. *Toxicol. Appl. Pharmacol.* **36**, 209–226 (1976).

158. E. McConnell, G. Lucier, G., Rumbaugh, et al., Dioxin in soil: Bio-availability after ingestion by rats and guinea pigs. *Science* **223**, 1077–1079 (1984).

159. G. W. Lucier, R. C. Rumbaugh et al., Ingestion of soil contaminated with 2, 3, 7, 8-TCDD alters heapatic enzyme activities. *Fundam. Appl. Toxicol.* **6**, 364–371 (1986).

160. T. H. Umbriet, E. J. Hess, and M. Gallo, Acute toxicity of TCDD contaminated soil from an industrial site. *Science* **232**, 497–499 (1986).

161. H. Shu, D. Paustenbach, J. Murray et al., Bioavailability of soil-bound TCDD: Oral bioavailability in the rat. *Fundam. Appl. Toxicol.* **10**, 648–654 (1988).

162. Van den Berg et al., Uptake and selective retention in rats of orally administered CDDs and CDFs from fly ash and fly ash extract. *Chemosphere* **12**, 537–544 (1983).

163. M. Van Den Berg, M. Greevenbroek et al., Bio-availability of PCDDs and PCDFs on fly ash after semi-chronic oral ingestion by the rat. *Chemosphere* **15**, 509–518 (1986).

164. M. L. Lepow, M. Gillette et al., Investigations into sources of lead in the environment of urban children. *Environ. Res.* **10**, 415–426 (1975).

165. H. A. Roels, J. P. Buchet, and R. R. Lauwerys, Exposure to lead by the oral and pulmonary routes of children living in the vicinity of a primary lead smelter. *Environ. Res.* **22**, 81–94 (1980).

166. J. K. Hawley, Assessment of health risk from exposure to contaminated soil. *Risk Anal.* **5**, 289–302 (1985).

167. H. Poiger and C. Schlatter, Influence of solvents and absorbents in dermal and intestinal absorption of TCDD. *Food Cosmet. Toxicol.* **18**, 477 (1980).

168. H. Shu, P. Teitelbaum, A. S. Webb et al., Bioavailability of soil-bound TCDD: Dermal bioavailability in the rat. *Fundam. Appl. Toxicol.* **10**, 335–343 (1988).

169. R. Zurlinden, H. von dem Fange, and J. L. Hahn, *Environmental Test Report—Executive Summary—Marion County Solid Waste-To-Energy Facility*, Rep. No. 108. Ogden Projects Inc., 1986.

170. NYSDEC, *Emission Source Test Report*, Preliminary report on Westchester Resco. NYSDEC, Albany, 1986.

E

ASSESSING OCCUPATIONAL HAZARDS

20

Assessing Health Risks in the Workplace: A Study of 2, 3, 7, 8-Tetrachlorodibenzo-*p*-dioxin

Hon-Wing Leung
Syntex Corporation, Palo Alto, California

Dennis J. Paustenbach
McLaren Environmental Engineering, ChemRisk Division, Alameda, California

INTRODUCTION

The principal goal in an occupational hygiene program is to protect the health of workers handling industrial chemicals. Since exposure to these chemicals cannot be totally eliminated, it becomes necessary to define some acceptable levels of exposure at which a worker's health will not be jeopardized. These health-based standard are often called occupational exposure limits (OELs). There are many types of OELs: some are in the form of voluntary, concensus standards and guidelines, while other are legal regulations.

HISTORY OF OCCUPATIONAL EXPOSURE LIMITS

Perceptions of what constitutes appropriate working conditions have changed over the years (Fig. 1). However, it has long been recognized that exposure to airborne dusts and chemicals could cause occupational illness and injury. The concentrations and lengths of exposure at which this might be expected to occur were unclear because of the lack of documentation. Beginning in 1937, a committee of the American Conference of Governmental Industrial Hygienists (ACGIH) was convened to assemble all the data that related the degree of exposure to a toxicant with the likelihood of producing an adverse effect. After 4 years of intensive research and documentation, the first set of values were released in 1941 (1).

Over the past 45 years, many organizations in numerous countries have proposed exposure limits for airborne contaminants. Presently in the United States at least six groups recommend exposure limits for the workplace. These include the threshold limit values (TLVs) of the ACGIH, the exposure limits recommended by the National Institute for Occupational Safety and Health of the U.S. Department of Health and Human

&. Notice &.
To Employees

1. Godliness, cleanliness and punctuality are the necessities of a good business.

2. This firm has reduced the hours of work, and the clerical staff will now only have to be present between the hours of 7 a.m. and 6 p.m. on weekdays.

3. Daily prayers will be held each morning in the main office. The clerical staff will be present.

4. Clothing must be of a sober nature. The clerical staff will not disport themselves in raiment of bright colours, nor will they wear hose, unless in good repair.

5. Overshoes and top-coats may not be worn in the office, but neck scarves and headwear may be worn in inclement weather.

6. A stove is provided for the benefit of the clerical staff. Coal and wood must be kept in the locker. It is recommended that each member of the clerical staff bring in 4 pounds of coal each day during cold weather.

7. No member of the clerical staff may leave the room without permission from Mr. Rogers. The calls of nature are permitted and the clerical staff may use the garden below the second gate. This area must be kept in good order.

8. No talking is allowed during business hours.

9. The craving for tobacco, wines or spirits is a human weakness and as such is forbidden to all members of the clerical staff.

10. Now that the hours of business have been so drastically reduced, the partaking of food is only allowed between 11:30 a.m. and noon, but work will not, on any account, cease.

11. Members of the clerical staff will provide their own pens. A new sharpener is available, on application to Mr. Rogers.

12. Mr. Rogers will nominate a senior clerk to be responsible for the cleanliness of the main office and the private office, and all boys and juniors will report to him 40 minutes before prayers, and will remain after closing hours for similar work. Brushes, brooms, scrubbers and soap are provided by the owners.

13. The new increased weekly wages are as hereunder detailed: Junior boys (up to eleven years) 1s.4d., Boys (to 14 years) 2s.1d., Juniors 4s.8d., Junior clerks 8s.7d., Clerks 10s.9d., Senior Clerks (after 15 years with owners) 21s.

The owners recognise the generosity of the new Labour Laws, but will expect a great rise in output of work to compensate for these near utopian conditions.

Figure 1. Office regulations posted in a Burnley cotton mill in 1852. It represents an interesting contrast to the working conditions found in the United States and Europe in the twentieth century.

Services, the workplace environmental exposure limits developed by the American Industrial Hygiene Association, standards for workplace air contaminants suggested by the Z37 Committee of the American National Standards Institute, and, lastly recommendations made by local, state, and regional governments. In addition to these, permissible exposure limits (PELs) that must be met in the workplace because they are law have been established by the Occupational Safety and Health Administration (OSHA) of the Department of Labor.

Outside the United States, as many as 50 other groups have established workplace exposure limits (2, 3). Many of these limits are nearly or exactly the same as the ACGIH TLVs developed in the United States. In some cases, such as in the Soviet Union, Japan, and other Soviet bloc countries, the limits are dramatically different from those in the United States (4). Differences among various limits recommended by other countries may be due to a number of factors:

1. Difference in the philosophical objective of the limits and the undesirable effects they are meant to minimize or eliminate.
2. Difference in the predominant age and sex of the workers.
3. The duration of the average workweek.
4. The economic state of affairs in that country.
5. The OELs serve simply as a guide because of a lack of enforcement.

RISK ASSESSMENT CONSIDERATIONS

Exposure limits for workplace air contaminants are based on the premise that, although all chemical substances are toxic at some concentration when experienced over a specific period of time, there exists a concentration at which no injurious effect should result no matter how often the exposure is repeated (5). This premise also applies to substances that cause irritation, nuisance, or other forms of stress as the primary biological effect.

It is important to recognize that OELs refer to airborne concentrations of substances to which nearly all workers may be repeatedly exposed day after day without adverse effect (6). They do not necessarily prevent discomfort or injury for everyone. Because of the wide range in individual susceptibility, a small percentage of workers may experience discomfort at concentrations at or below the exposure limit, and a smaller percentage may be affected more seriously by aggravation of a preexisting condition (7, 8). This limitation, although less than ideal, is a practical one since levels so low as to protect all hypersusceptible individuals would be infeasible due to either engineering or economic limitations.

OELs are based on the best available information from industrial experience and experimental human and animal studies. The rationale for each of the established values may differ from substance to substance. Protection against impairment of health may be a guiding factor for some, while reasonable freedom from irritation, narcosis, nuisance, or other forms of stress may form the basis for others (9). The age and completeness of the information available for establishing OELs also vary; consequently, the precision of each particular OEL is subject to variation (10).

OELs established both in the United States and elsewhere are derived from a wide number of sources. As shown in Table 1, the 1968 TLVs (those adopted by OSHA as federal regulations) were based largely on human experience. This indicates that an

TABLE 1. Distribution of Procedures Used to Develop ACGIH TLVs for 414 Substances through 1968

Procedure	Number	Percentage of Total
Industrial (human) exprience	157	38
Human volunteer experiments	45	11
Animal, inhalation—chronic	83	20
Animal, inhalation—acute	8	2
Animal, oral—chronic	18	4.5
Animal, oral—acute	2	0.5
Analogy	101	24

exposure limit was set after it had been found to have toxic, irritational, or other undesirable effects on humans. Many of the more recent exposure limits for systemic toxicants, especially those internal limits set by manufacturers, have been based primarily on animal toxicology tests prior to commercial production (11).

The criteria used to develop the TLVs may be classified into four groups: morphologic, functional, biochemical, and miscellaneous (nuisance, cosmetic) (12). About half of the TLVs have been derived from human data and 30% from animal data. Of the human data, most have been derived from the effects noted in workers who were exposed for many years. Consequently, most of the existing TLVs have been based on the results of workplace monitoring and qualitative and quantitative human responses (13). Recently, TLVs for new compounds have been based primarily on the results of animal studies rather than human experience. It is noteworthy that only about 50% of the TLVs are set to prevent systemic toxic effects, while 40% are based on irritation and about 1–2% are intended to prevent cancer (13).

By setting exposure limits, the ACGIH and its counterparts throughout the world acknowledge that chemical carcinogens are likely to have a threshold, or at least a practical threshold (14). The following was cited by ACGIH to support the concept of threshold for carcinogens:

- Evidence from epidemiologic studies and carcinogenic studies in animals (15).
- Biochemical, pharmacokinetic, and toxicologic evidence demonstrating inherent, built-in anticarcinogens and processes in our bodies (14).

Although the TLV committee and other groups that recommend exposure limits believe that there is likely to be a threshold for carcinogens, another equally credible school of thought is that there is little or no evidence for the existence of thresholds for chemicals that are genotoxic (16). In an attempt to take into account the philosophical postulate that chemical carcinogens do not have a threshold even though a no observed effect level is often observed in an animal experiment, modeling approaches for estimating the carcinogenic response at low doses have been developed (17, 18).

METHODS USED IN SETTING OCCUPATIONAL EXPOSURE LIMITS

Many approaches for deriving OELs from toxicological data have been proposed and put into use over the past 45 years (10, 19). Although there are many ways to set OELs, the quantitative relation between the extent of exposure to a chemical agent and the physiological response of the exposed population (dose–response relation) is fundamental to the development of exposure limits. Five common methods that have been used to establish OELs and selected examples to illustrate their application are presented below.

Safety Factors

In this widely used method, one tries to identify from the dose–response relation a dose at which none of the population shows any adverse effect, that is, no observed effect level (NOEL). Since most dose–response experimentation has been conducted in laboratory animals, one must predict the species differences in extrapolating data from animals to humans (20, 21).

In many cases, even when physiological differences are accounted for mathematically, the extrapolation of animal data to humans is not always predictable (22). Therefore, some arbitrary safety factor is used to account for the possibility that humans will be more sensitive than the species tested (23, 24).

The size of the safety factor used depends on the quality of the data determining the dose–response relation. In general, the more reliable the data, the smaller the size (25). A survey of the documentation of TLVs (26) suggests that even for chemical substances suspect of carcinogenic potential in humans, safety factors from 2 to 10 have been applied to the NOEL identified in animal studies to establish the TLV (Table 2).

Illustrative Example 1. Safety Factor Approach (Phenyl Ether)

Data. A repeated inhalation study exposed rats, rabbits, and dogs at mean concentrations of 5 and 10 ppm phenyl ether vapor for 7 h/day, 5 days/wk for a total of 20 exposures (27). No signs of toxicity or irritation were observed in animals exposed to 5 ppm.

Solution. Applying a safety factor of 5 on the NOEL, we obtain

$$\text{TLV} = \frac{\text{NOEL}}{\text{safety factor}} = \frac{5\,\text{ppm}}{5} = 1\,\text{ppm}.$$

The recommended TLV for phenyl ether is 1 ppm, as a time-weighted average (6).

Illustrative Example 2. Safety Factor Approach (Estradiol). A variation of the safety factor approach applies specifically to chemicals related to naturally occurring substances

TABLE 2. Implied Size of Safety Factor Used to Arrive at the Threshold Limit Values of Chemicals with an A2 Designation

Chemical	TLV	NOEL	Species	Safety Factor
Chloroform	10 ppm	30 ppm	Rat	3.0
Ethylene oxide	1 ppm	10 ppm	Rat	10.0
Formaldehyde	1 ppm	2 ppm	Rat	2.0
Hexachlorobutadiene	0.24 mg/m^3	0.2 mg/kg·day	Rat	5.8
2-Nitropropane	10 ppm	27 ppm	Rat and rabbit	2.7
Vinyl bromide	5 ppm	50 ppm	Rat	10.0

produced in the human body. In this method, a level of exposure equivalent to 1%
increase in body burden over the daily endogenous production rate is considered not
to pose any significant health effect. This is analogous to considering the daily endogenous
production rate as the NOEL and applying a safety factor of 100 to obtain the OEL.

Data. In human males, the endogenous production of estradiol is about $50 \, \mu g/day$ (28).
A typical worker is assumed to breathe $10 \, m^3$ of air in an 8-h workday.

Solution. The OEL for estradiol is therefore equal to 1% of the daily production rate
divided by the volume of air breathed:

$$\frac{50 \, \mu g/day \times 0.01}{10 \, m^3} = 0.05 \, \mu g/m^3.$$

Mathematical Models

This approach is most often used for genotoxic carcinogens. The rationale for a modeling
approach is that it is impossible to conduct toxicity studies at low doses near those
measured in the environment because the number of animals necessary to elicit a
statistically significant response at these doses in a laboratory experiment would be too
great (29). Consequently, results of animal studies conducted at high doses are
extrapolated by mathematical models to those levels found in the workplace or the
environment (30).

The most popular models for low-dose extrapolation are the one-hit, multistage,
Weibull, multihit, logit, and Probit (31). Since for genotoxic carcinogens it is presumed
that at any dose, no matter how small, a response could occur in a sufficiently large
population, an arbitrary risk level is usually selected as presenting an insignificant or de
minimus level of risk. The exposure level corresponding to this de minimus risk is the
virtually safe dose. Regulatory agencies may make judgments about the biologic and
economic feasibility and reasonableness of establishing a standard based on this virtually
safe dose (32). Often the use of models to extrapolate exposure to carcinogens from
high dose to low dose is erroneously called risk assessment. In practice, modeling is
only one part of the risk assessment process. A true risk assessment to determine
safe levels of occupational exposure actually requires exhaustive analysis of all the
information obtained from studies of mutagenicity, acute toxicity, subchronic toxicity,
chronic studies, pharmacokinetics, metabolism data, and epidemiology before a limit is
recommended (33, 34).

The modeling approach is conservative since it does not account for biological repair
or detoxification process; consequently, the exposures predicted by mathematical models
are sometimes too low to be economically or practically feasible. Another drawback in
the modeling approach is that different equally valid mathematical models may lead to
widely different risk estimates (35). Quantitative risk modeling can be useful in the overall
process of setting OELs for genotoxic carcinogens, but because of the above-mentioned
shortcomings, they should not be used as the sole basis for deriving these limits.

Illustrative Example 3. Mathematical Model Approach (Ethylene Oxide). Because there
is a paucity of human studies available on ethylene oxide, OSHA's risk assessment on
ethylene oxide (36) was derived from results of a 2-year inhalation study on rats. Using
the multistage model, OSHA predicted an excess lifetime risk for cancer from exposure

to ethylene oxide at 50 ppm to be 63–110 per 1000 workers, with 95% upper confidence limits on the excess risk of 101 to 152 deaths per 1000 workers. The risk estimated at 1 ppm was approximately 1.2–2.3 excess deaths per 1000, with 95% upper confidence limits of 2.1–3.3 excess deaths per 1000. To extrapolate from the animal carcinogenicity data in making risk predictions for humans, OSHA employed a milligram per kilogram body weight per day adjustment to scale the animal dose to equivalent human doses. The total volume of air that a worker would be expected to breathe in a normal working day was assumed to be 9.3 m^3, and the typical working lifetime was taken to be 8 h/day, 5 days/wk, 46 wk/yr for 45 years.

Illustrative Example 4. Mathematical Model Approach (Asbestos). Unlike most chemicals where only animal data are available, there are several human studies on asbestos. OSHA used a linear model to describe the relation between the excess relative risk of lung cancer and asbestos exposure (37):

$$R_L = R_E[1 + (K_L)(f)(d_{t-10})],$$

where R_L = lung cancer mortality resulting from the asbestos exposure

  R_E = expected mortality in the absence of exposure

  f = intensity of exposure in fibers/cm^3

  d = duration of exposure in years

  t = time from the onset of asbestos exposure in years (minus 10 years to allow for a minimum latent period)

  K_L = proportionality constant measuring the carcinogenic potency of asbestos exposure.

A best estimate of K_L was obtained from 11 epidemiologic studies. Using the equation above and a K_L value of 0.01, OSHA was able to predict a lifetime excess risk of total cancer for a lifetime exposure (45 years) to various asbestos fiber concentrations. Reduction in the PEL from 2 to 0.2 fibers/cm^3 reduces the calculated risk from lifetime exposure from 64 per 1000 to 6.7 per 1000.

Analogy

This method is most commonly applied to a series of analogous chemicals when there is no or very limited toxicological data on some of them. In this approach, an OEL for one of the chemicals in the series has been established based on toxicological data. Identical OELs are then adopted for other chemicals in the series which lack toxicity data. The limitation of the approach is that it is restricted to chemicals that relate closely with one another and produce identical biological endpoint. Another drawback is that it does not take into account the biological potency of the individual chemical.

Illustrative Example 5. Analogy Approach (Alkylamines). The TLVs for ethylamine, methylamine, diethylamine, dimethylamine, and trimethylamine are all 10 ppm, based primarily on analogy to prevent irritative effects (26).

Illustrative Example 6. Analogy Approach (Alkyl Ketones). The TLVs for methyl propyl ketone, methyl isopropyl ketone, and diethylketone are all 200 ppm, based primarily on analogy to prevent narcotic effects and significant irritation (26).

Correlation with Thermodynamic Properties

The rationale of this approach is based on the principle that biological effects can be induced by simple physical interactions between a chemical and receptive centers (38). If the effect of a series of chemicals is purely physical, then the thermodynamic properties can be used to provide a scale to express the potency of each member in a homologous series. The advantage of this approach over simple analogy to establish OEL is that the potency of the biological response is correlated quantitatively with a common thermodynamic parameter among the homologues.

Illustrative Example 7. Correlation Approach (Alkylbenzenes). Nielsen and Alarie (39) determined the median concentrations necessary to depress the respiratory rate of mice due to sensory irritation of the upper respiratory tract for a variety of alkylbenzenes. They found that the potency of the alkylbenzenes increased with chain length. However, the ratio of equipotent concentration/saturated vapor concentration for these alkylbenzenes varied very little. Knowing the vapor pressure enabled prediction of the sensory irritation potency and by extension the OELs for these alkylbenzenes. The quantitative relation for a series of 8 alkylbenzenes is

$$\text{OEL (ppm)} = 0.0054 \text{ vapor pressure (ppm)}.$$

The predicted values using this relation were in close agreement with established TLVs for toluene, ethylbenzene, isopropylbenzene, and butyltoluene. Acceptable OELs for *n*-propylbenzene, *n*-butylbenzene, *t*-butylbenzene, *n*-amylbenzene, and *n*-hexylbenzene, which currently have no established TLVs, were estimated to be 50, 20, 20, 10, and 5 ppm, respectively.

Illustrative Example 8. Correlation Approach (Organic Acids). Leung and Paustenbach (40) observed that there exists an association between the equilibrium proton dissociation constant (pK_a) and the OELs of organic acids that produce irritation as the primary adverse effects. The regression equation for a series of 10 organic acids is

$$\log \text{OEL} (\mu \text{mole/m}^3) = 0.43 pK_a + 0.53.$$

The OEL of a variety of organic acids can be predicted using this relation.

Physiologically Based Pharmacokinetic Model

This newest approach attempts to scale up a simulated physiological system derived from laboratory animal data to describe the behavior of a chemical in the human body (41, 42). Physiological modeling is used to describe the animal in terms of particular organs with the associated blood flows, volumes, and partition coefficients. This approach allows the extrapolation of data obtained in one species to another by accounting for differences in physiology and biochemistry between the tested and untested species. The approach models the movement of a chemical throughout the body by sets of mass-balance differential equations that account for the disposition of chemical entering the various compartments of the model. These models represent the mammalian system in terms of specific organs (or groups of tissues lumped together based on a common characteristic), all of which are defined. It is the coherent relation of the anatomical and physiological characteristics between different species that provide the basis for extrapolation of pharmacokinetic data from laboratory animals to humans. One shortcoming of this approach is that the mathematics are very complex and solutions are feasible only with the aid of a computer.

Illustrative Example 9. Physiological Pharmacokinetic Model Approach (Haloalkanes). For an example of how this method is applied to risk assessment, see Chapters 5 and 23.

A CASE STUDY OF OCCUPATIONAL RISK ASSESSMENT: 2, 3, 7, 8-TETRACHLORODIBENZO-*p*-DIOXIN

2, 3, 7, 8-Tetrachlorinated dibenzodioxins (TCDD) are contaminants produced during the manufacture of chlorophenols, hexachlorophene, and phenoxy herbicides. They may also be produced by the incineration of certain materials (43). Most human exposure to TCDD is believed to be associated with the use of Agent Orange in Vietnam, 2, 4, 5-T in agriculture, the manufacture of these agents and pentachlorophenol, and at incinerators where certain materials are burnt. TCDD is also present in the soil of numerous industrial sites, landfills, and residential communities due to the past disposal of TCDD-containing waste (44, 45). Many of these have been designated as Superfund hazardous waste sites. Remediation of these sites may involve soil excavation, which may present potential exposure to airborne dust containing the dioxin.

ANIMAL TOXICOLOGY

Among the 75 isomers of chlorinated dioxins, 2, 3, 7, 8-tetrachlorodibenzo-*p*-dioxin is the most toxic (46). Table 3 shows that there is a marked species difference in the acute toxicity of TCDD. Humans appear to be less sensitive than laboratory animals to the toxic effects of TCDD (47). Generally, the liver and adipose tissue are the major storage depots for TCDD in most species. There is also a large species difference in the whole body excretion half-life of TCDD, as shown in Table 3.

The toxicity of TCDD is characteristically delayed. Animals generally suffer a rapid weight loss and depletion of adipose tissue—wasting syndrome (48). TCDD is a potent inducer of aryl hydrocarbon hydroxylase and the cytochrome P_1-450 (P-448) enzymes (49). Thymic atrophy has been seen in many animal species and mucosal hyperplasia or metaplasia has been observed in the gastric, intestinal, and urinary tracts of primates and cattle exposed to TCDD, but not in the rat, mouse, and guinea pig. Chloracne, a

TABLE 3. Oral LD$_{50}$ and Whole-Body Excretion Half-Life of TCDD in Different Animal Species

Animal	LD$_{50}$ (μg/kg)	$t_{1/2}$ (days)
Guinea pig	1	30–94
Rat	22–45	31
Monkey	< 70	455
Rabbit	155	—
Mouse	144	15
Dog	> 300	—
Hamster	5000	15

similar hyperplastic epidermal change in the skin, is the most characteristic lesion observed in exposed human populations (50).

Mutagenicity

The mutagenicity data have been critically reviewed (51, 52). The *Salmonella*/Ames bacteria tests were all negative except two studies. The validity of these two positive studies had been questioned (52). The results with yeast and mammalian cell systems have been mixed, although predominantly negative. The cogency of the positive studies has also come under question (51, 52). In other studies, TCDD induced neither unscheduled DNA synthesis nor dominant lethal mutation. In addition, TCDD was inactive in the sex-linked recessive lethal test. Both the dominant lethal assay and the sex-linked recessive lethal test are in vivo tests and are regarded as more definitive than the in vitro bacterial and cell culture assays in predicting the mutagenic potential for humans.

The cytogenetic activity of TCDD has been evaluated in several test systems including humans. The available evidence indicates that TCDD is not clastogenic, that is, inactive in inducing chromosomal aberrations, sister chromatid exchange, or micronucleus formation.

The preponderance of the evidence supports the conclusion that TCDD is not mutagenic. The absence of significant chromosomal effects in human populations who were likely exposed to TCDD lends further credence to this conclusion (52).

Oncogenicity

An early study on TCDD found no tumorigenic activity on mouse skin (53) and another study found an inhibitory effect on skin tumors (54). In contrast, TCDD was carcinogenic in female Swiss–Webster mice by the dermal route (55). The fibrosarcomas induced were limited to the site of TCDD application and were preceded by necrosis and ulceration of the dermis, which could result in the material being applied directly to the underlying mesenchymal tissue. The authors concluded there was no evidence that TCDD was a systemic tumorigen, and they urged caution in attempting to interpret the increased incidence of localized fibrosarcoma in the female mice. Historical data have indicated that this type of fibrosarcoma can easily be induced in rodents with numerous innocuous materials.

There are two cancer bioassays widely used in assessing the cancer risk of TCDD (56, 57). In one study (56), Sprague–Dawley rats were fed a diet containing TCDD. A dose-related increase in the incidence of hepatocellular carcinoma was observed in female rats given 0.01 and 0.1 μg/kg·day. No increase in neoplastic lesions was seen in animals given 0.001 μg/kg·day. The other study (57) was a gavage study involving B6C3F1 mice and Osborne–Mendel rats. In the rat, a dose of 0.07 μg/kg·day produced an increased incidence of hepatocellular carcinoma and thyroid tumors. No increase in tumor incidence was observed in rats given a dose of 0.0014 μg/kg·day. In the mouse, a dose of 0.3 μg/kg·day elicited hepatocellular and thyroid tumors in the female animals, and a dose of 0.07 μg/kg·day induced hepatocellular tumors in the male animals. No increase in tumor incidence of any type was seen in either animal below a dose of 0.007 μg/kg·day. Thus, these two cancer bioassays (56, 57) identified a NOEL of 0.001 μg/kg·day for the carcinogenic response in rodents.

Since neither TCDD nor its metabolites form covalent adducts with DNA in vivo or in vitro (58), this suggests that TCDD acts as a promoter rather than as an initiator of carcinogenesis in rodents. This view is substantiated by several promotion studies (59, 60). These data and the fact that TCDD is not mutagenic indicate that TCDD induced tumors in rodents by an epigenetic rather than a genotoxic mechanism (52).

Developmental Toxicity

2, 4, 5-Trichlorophenoxyacetic acid containing 30 ppm of TCDD produced an increased incidence of cleft palate in mice and cystic kidney in the rat, while no teratogenesis was observed at 1 ppm (61). Doses of TCDD at 0.5 μg/kg·day during organogenesis caused developmental toxicity, but the effect was slight at 0.125 μg/kg·day (62).

Mice exposed to TCDD in utero had poorly developed lymphatic systems and hepatic fatty infiltrates (63). TCDD caused prenatal hydronephrosis, and renal function of the neonates was impaired, although lesions were not evident (64). A NOEL of 0.1 μg/kg·day for developmental effects in mice has been identified (65).

In another study, pregnant rabbits treated orally with 0.25 μg/kg of TCDD aborted, but not at 0.1 μg/kg (66). The high abortion rate was ascribed to severe maternal toxicity. Gross and histological examination of the fetuses did not reveal any signs of teratogenicity.

Pregnant rhesus monkeys treated with 0.2 μg/kg of TCDD had no increase in abortion or maternal toxicity. At 1.0 μg/kg, three of four monkeys aborted, and half of the dams had signs of toxicity (67).

A three-generation study showed that the reproductive capacity of rats was clearly affected at TCDD levels of 0.01 and 0.1 μg/kg·day, but not at 0.001 μg/kg·day (68).

HUMAN EXPERIENCE AND EPIDEMIOLOGY

Workers involved in the manufacture and use of trichlorophenol, hexachlorophene, and 2, 4, 5-trichlorophenoxyacetic acid represent the population most heavily exposed to TCDD. The following summarizes the medical findings in some of the major studies.

Monsanto Study

This incident involved a "runaway reaction" during the manufacture of 2, 4, 5-trichloro-phenoxyacetic acid. The most frequent symptom reported was acneform lesions. A cohort mortality study of persons with chloracne revealed lower mortality rates than expected. No apparent excess of deaths from malignant neoplasms or circulatory diseases was observed (69). A follow-up study showed that chloracne persisted in 53% of the expos-ed subjects, compared to none in the unexposed group (70). However, no significant differences in a variety of clinical parameters were detected between the exposed and nonexposed groups. A recent survey found that the mean duration for residual chloracne was 26 years (71).

Dow Study

A study of Dow Chemical workers who might have been exposed to TCDD revealed a comparable mortality rate as controls (72). Overall cancer deaths were elevated, but no particular tumor type predominated, and the difference was not statistically significant (73). Of these 61 workers, 49 developed chloracne. A study of wives of workers with exposure to TCDD revealed no statistically significant differences in adverse reproductive outcome compared to controls (74).

Ranch Hand Study

This study was organized to evaluate the long-term health effects from occupational exposure to Agent Orange during military service in Vietnam. The first phase, a mortality study, has shown no unusual findings attributable to the herbicide. The second phase, designed to determine morbidity incidence, has also shown no definitive clinical endpoints, such as soft tissue sarcoma, porphyria cutanea tarda, or chloracne (75).

Centers for Disease Control Study

This case–control study attempted to identify an association between Vietnam service and subsequent male parentage of congenitally malformed offspring. The results indicated that veterans were at no greater risk than other men for siring babies with all types of serious structural birth defects combined (76).

Swedish Studies

Exposure to phenoxyacetic acids or chlorophenols has been suggested to be associated with an increased risk of soft tissue sarcoma and malignant lymphoma (77–79). It was, however, not known from these investigations if the increased risk was attributed to the pure chemical substances, contamination with TCDD, or a combination of these materials. Hardell's works are not accepted by all scientists and these studies have been heavily criticized for their study design, interpretation, and on the basis of disease identification (80). A recent study on these cancer patients found no difference in TCDD level in their adipose tissue compared to the control population with no exposure to phenoxy acids (81).

PROPOSAL AND RATIONALE

Most potent carcinogens share common characteristics that should be qualitatively incorporated into the extrapolation of the response to low doses and the eventual setting of an exposure limit. For example, carcinogens such as aflatoxin and vinyl chloride are metabolized to proximate electrophilic intermediates that bind to DNA bases. Substances in this class usually are carcinogenic in more than one species and produce tumors at multiple sites; the latency period is often short and inversely dose related. Such chemicals usually induce a high proportion of malignant tumors as well as a spectrum of preneoplastic changes. Furthermore, these substances are active in short-term tests for mutagenicity and genotoxicity. For chemicals possessing these characteristics, a conservative approach to risk assessment similar to that provided by mathematical extrapolation models is warranted.

Conversely, for animal carcinogens such as estrogens, phenobarbital, saccharin, and PCBs, a less conservative approach to risk assessment is indicated. These substances are not metabolized to electrophiles, and they or their metabolites do not bind to cellular components. Often these substances produce tumors in only one species or only at doses high enough to induce extensive tissue necrosis and regeneration. These chemicals are generally inactive in mutagenicity tests and show little evidence of genotoxicity. The available data indicate that TCDD falls into this category (52). The International Agency for Research on Cancer (82) has confirmed that there is insufficient data to conclude that TCDD is a human carcinogen.

In light of TCDD's lack of genotoxicity, the safety factor approach is appropriate to establish safe levels of human exposure (18). This approach has been used to set virtually every OEL, including those dealing with carcinogens (24, 25).

Chronic (Time-Weighted Average OEL)

The subchronic and chronic developmental effects of TCDD in laboratory animals have been studied. In rats, TCDD below a dose of $0.125\,\mu g/kg \cdot day$ was not teratogenic, and no embryotoxic or fetotoxic effects were observed (63). In a three-generation reproductive study in rats, a NOEL of $0.001\,\mu g/kg \cdot day$ was identified (68). Two lifetime cancer bioassays in rodents suggested that the NOEL was also $0.001\,\mu g/kg \cdot day$ (56, 57).

The available evidence from epidemiological studies and industrial experience suggests that TCDD is not a human carcinogen. However, since it is carcinogenic in rodents, TCDD has been considered for regulatory purposes as a chemical substance suspect of carcinogenic potential in humans (83).

A time-weighted average OEL for TCDD can be estimated by applying a 100-fold safety factor to the animal NOEL of $0.001\,\mu g/kg \cdot day$. A typical worker is assumed to work 220 days/yr for 40 years per 70-year lifetime and breathe $10\,m^3$ of air in an 8-h workday.

$$\text{Time-weighted average OEL} = (\text{acceptable intake})(70/40)(365/220)(\text{body wt})/(\text{air breathed})$$

$$= (10\,pg/kg)(1.75)(1.66)(70\,kg)/(10\,m^3)$$

$$= 200\,pg/m^3.$$

A safety factor of 100 rather than the customary factor of 10 is used for TCDD (Table 2) because of the diverse species difference between animals and humans, the uncertainty regarding its mechanism of action, and its extremely long biological half-life in humans (84). An additional margin of safety is incorporated in this proposed limit since most workers are not likely to be involved in the remediation of TCDD-contaminated sites for much of their 40-year working lifetime.

The proposed OEL is based on free TCDD. However, TCDD encountered in ambient environment will most frequently be bound to soil or other particulates. To estimate the OEL for TCDD on dust, one must adjust the concentration with respect to several parameters, including particle size of the dust, location of deposition in the respiratory tract, and bioavailability. The characteristics of TCDD-contaminated dust have been discussed (85), and the bioavailability of soil-bound TCDD has been critically reviewed (86). An OEL for TCDD-contaminated soil can be calculated according to the following formula:

$$(\text{TCDD})(\text{IP})[(F_a)(B_a) + (F_u)(B_u)] = 200\,pg/m^3,$$

where F_a = fraction of particles deposited in the alveolar region = 0.3
F_u = fraction of particles deposited in upper airways = 0.6
(these particles are cleared by mucociliary apparatus and ultimately swallowed)

B_a = bioavailability of TCDD deposited in alveolar region = 100%
B_u = bioavailability of TCDD deposited in upper respiratory tract = 25%
TCDD = TCDD concentration on particles
IP = concentration of inhalable particles.

Illustrative Example 10. A hazardous waste site has been uniformly contaminated with 100 ppb TCDD, what is the acceptable level of total inhalable dust for that setting?

Solution. Applying the TCDD concentration on dust particles to the general equation, we obtain

$$(100\,\text{pg/mg})(\text{IP})[(0.30)(100\%) + (0.60)(25\%)] = 200\,\text{pg/m}^3$$

$$\text{IP} = 4.4\,\text{mg/m}^3.$$

If we assume that half of the particulates at this site are inhalable, then a concentration of 8.8 mg/m^3 total suspended particulates would be acceptable for dust containing 100 ppb TCDD.

Although various assumptions in the calculation will yield different acceptable levels of exposure depending on a particular site's characteristics, the above calculation illustrates that the levels of airborne dust containing TCDD will generally be acceptable at most hazardous waste sites.

Acute (Short-Term OEL)

Epidemiological studies have indicated that the most prominent acute adverse effect due to TCDD exposure is chloracne (50). In a study where TCDD was applied dermally, 8 of 10 human volunteers given a total dose of 16 mg over 6 weeks developed chloracne, but no other clinical symptoms. None of the other volunteers developed chloracne or other adverse effects. A NOEL for chloracne was 8 μg for this group of men (47). A short-term OEL for TCDD can be estimated:

$$\text{short term OEL} = (\text{NOEL})/(\text{air breathed in 15 min})(\text{safety factor})$$

$$= (8.0\,\mu\text{g})/(0.02\,\text{m}^3/\text{min} \times 15\,\text{min})(100)$$

$$= 0.27\,\mu\text{g/m}^3 = 270\,\text{ng/m}^3.$$

Although this short-term OEL is expected to prevent chloracne, the overall daily dose will exceed the time-weighted average OEL of 200 pg/m^3 following less than 1 min of exposure. Consequently, a short-term OEL does not seem prudent for TCDD. In short, exposures need only be controlled to limit uptake to 10 pg/kg·day, that is, 200 pg/m^3.

CANCER RISK ASSESSMENT

As previously discussed, the biological data on TCDD do not support the use of mathematical models for low-dose extrapolation. Nonetheless, for policy reasons, many regulatory agencies employ these models to estimate the theoretical upper bound of risk from exposure to all chemical carcinogens.

TABLE 4. Lifetime Risk of Death from Cancer Associated with Occupational Exposure at OSHA Permissible Exposure Limits for selected Substances

Substance	PEL	Risk/1000
Inorganic arsenic	$10\,\mu g/m^3$	8
Ethylene oxide	1 ppm	1–2
Ethylene dibromide	20 ppm	0.2–6
Benzene	1 ppm	5–16
Vinyl chloride	1 ppm	4
Dibromochloropropane	1 ppb	2
Asbestos	$0.2\,fiber/cm^3$	6.7
TCDD	$200\,pg/m^3$	0.357

Even assuming TCDD were genotoxic and applying the linear multistage model on the data of Kociba (56), exposure to TCDD at the proposed OEL of $200\,pg/m^3$ would have produced a theoretical cancer risk of 3×10^{-4}. This level of risk is still much less than that typically considered acceptable for occupational exposures. Historically, regulatory agencies have promulgated OELs with upper plausible risks of 10^{-3} rather than 10^{-6}, the risk level often referred to in environmental regulations (32). Furthermore, estimated risks in the range of 10^{-3}–10^{-4} have been considered acceptable for environmental contaminants when the exposed population is relatively small ($< 10^5$). Table 4 shows that the risk of TCDD exposure to the proposed OEL is much less than those from exposure to other chemicals at their respective PELs (87). The actual cancer risk is almost certainly much less than these estimates because of the conservatism of the risk models, and their inability to incorporate biologic protective mechanisms.

OELs have been established for over 1700 agents (3). Of these, about 30 TLVs have been set for animal carcinogens. The justification for setting OELs for nongenotoxic carcinogens with the safety factor approach has been discussed (24, 25). The proposed OEL for TCDD is based on an acceptable intake of $10\,pg/kg\cdot day$, which takes into account TCDD's lack of genotoxicity, the NOEL determined in two cancer bioassays and a three-generation reproduction study, and the favorable epidemiology data

TABLE 5. Acceptable Daily Intakes for TCDD Calculated by Various Regulatory Agencies

Agency[a]	Risk Analysis Approach	Allowable TCDD Intake (fg/kg·day)	Extrapolated OEL (pg/m³)	Reference
EPA	Linearized multistage	6.4	0.13	88
CDC	Linearized multistage	28–1,428	0.57–30	45
OME	Safety factor (100)	10,000	200	89
SINH	Safety factor (250)	4,000	80	90
FEA	Safety factor (100–1000)	1,000–10,000	20–200	91
FDA	Safety factor (77)	13,000	260	92
NYSDH	Safety factor (500)	2,000	35	93

[a]EPA, Environmental Protection Agency (U.S.); CDC, Centers for Disease Control (U.S.); OME, Ontario Ministry of Environment (Canada); SINH, State Institute of National Health (Netherlands); FEA, Federal Environmental Agency (Germany); FDA, Food and Drug Administration (U.S.); NYSDH, New York State Department of Health (U.S.).

704   H.-W. LEUNG AND D. J. PAUSTENBACH

regarding the lack of chronic health effects in workers who had exposures sufficient to cause chloracne. Table 5 shows that the proposed OEL for TCDD is in line with the majority of extrapolated OEL based on the acceptable TCDD intake suggested by a variety of governmental agencies (88–93).

STEADY-STATE ADIPOSE TISSUE LEVEL

Since TCDD is highly lipophilic and has a long biologic half-life in humans, it is expected to accumulate in adipose tissue with repeated daily exposure. TCDD levels in the adipose tissue of nonoccupationally exposed persons in the United States is about 7 ppt (94).

The steady-state level of TCDD in adipose tissue resulting from occupational exposure to 200 pg/m^3 can be estimated by

$$\frac{1.44(D_t)(t_{1/2})}{10.5 + (59.5/10)}$$

where D_t is the daily intake.

This calculation assumes that the TCDD concentration in the liver and other tissues is about $\frac{1}{10}$ that in adipose tissue (95), and the average human weighs 70 kg with 10.5 kg (15%) body fat.

If the half-life is assumed to be 4–8 years (84), the steady-state TCDD concentration in adipose tissue resulting from occupational exposure at the proposed OEL will be 89–179 ppt.

The health risks associated with these levels of TCDD in the adipose tissue are de minimus. The reasons are several-fold. First, the concentration of TCDD measured in the adipose tissue of rats exposed for 2 years to the NOEL of 0.001 μg/kg·day was 540 ppt. Since humans sequester more TCDD in adipose tissue than lower species, which is speculated by some scientists as a protective mechanism, a comparable level in human fat should yield a lesser risk than that suggested in rodent studies. Second, humans exposed to 16 mg TCDD had a theoretical peak adipose tissue level of about 1.3 ppm (16 mg/12.25 kg), yet they only developed chloracne, which resolved within 6 months

TABLE 6. Estimated Steady-State Adipose Tissue Level of Chemicals Following Chronic Exposure at the OEL

Chemical	OEL	$t_{1/2}$ (year)	Background[a]	Exposed	E/B[b]
DDT[c]	1 mg/m^3	1.5	6 ppm	480 ppm	80
Dieldrin	0.25 mg/m^3	1.0	0.29 ppm	80 ppm	276
PCB[d]	1 mg/m^3	1.5	1 ppm	800 ppm	800
TCDD	200 pg/m^3	4–8	7 ppt	89–179 ppt	13–26

Adipose Tissue Level spans Background, Exposed, E/B columns.

[a]Background levels referred to those in nonoccupationally exposed general population.
[b]E/B is the ratio of steady-state adipose tissue level in the occupationally exposed to that in the background.
[c]DDT, dichlorodiphenyl trichloroethane.
[d]PCB, polychlorinated biphenyl.

(47). None of those who received 8 μg TCDD developed chloracne, yet their peak adipose tissue levels were about 650 ppt (8 μg/12.25 kg).

Table 6 shows that the 26-fold increase over background (179/7) in the concentration of TCDD in adipose tissue among workers exposed for many years at the OEL is not unusual when compared with other industrial chemicals following workplace exposure at their corresponding TLVs. Third, and most importantly, the available toxicology and epidemiology data indicate that daily intake of TCDD at 100-fold below the animal NOEL for carcinogenicity (i.e., 10 pg/kg·day) poses no human health hazards.

COMPARISON OF EXPOSURE ESTIMATES WITH PROPOSED EXPOSURE LIMIT

Illustrative Example 11. Hexachlorophene Production Workers. Patterson et al. (96) measured the adipose tissue level of TCDD in 15 chemical workers in a hexachlorophene manufacturing facility in Verona, Missouri. A median TCDD concentration of 24.7 ppt was found (range: 3.5–750 ppt). These individuals had a history of last exposure to TCDD about 13 years prior to the determination of the fat level. Assuming a biological elimination half-life of 6 years (84) and a first-order process, one can estimate the median TCDD concentration in the adipose tissue of these individuals at the cessation of last exposure as follows:

$$C_0 = C/e^{-0.693(t)/t_{1/2}}$$

$$= 24.7/e^{-0.693(13)/6}$$

$$= 111 \text{ ppt},$$

where C_0 is the concentration at the end of exposure.

The adipose tissue level of 111 ppt TCDD suggests a probable occupational exposure about equal to that from exposure to the proposed OEL for TCDD, which would have been expected to produce a level of 89–179 ppt. The fact that no adverse medical symptoms have been reported in these workers is consistent with the estimation that occupational exposure had been close to the proposed OEL of 200 pg/m^3.

Illustrative Example 12. Ranch Hand Workers in Vietnam. In a study of 20 Vietnam veterans (97) who were engaged in the Ranch Hand operation where the herbicide Agent Orange, a 1:1 mixture of 2, 4, 5-trichlorophenoxyacetic acid and 2, 4-dichlorophenoxyacetic acid, was used for aerial defoliation, a median concentration of 5 ppt TCDD was found in the adipose tissue of these exposed subjects (range: nondetectable to 99 ppt). The time between last exposure and tissue analysis was about 13 years. Thus, the extrapolated median adipose tissue level at the end of exposure is about 30 ppt, which suggests that the probable exposure had been well below the OEL recommended here. It is interesting to note that while varied health complaints have been alleged, no consistent medical problems including chloracne have been documented in these individuals (75).

An alternative exposure estimate was discussed by Gough (98). The concentration of TCDD in the Agent Orange was estimated to be about 2 ppm, and the efficiency of TCDD transfer from the environment into an individual's body is assumed to be about 0.05% (99). The low efficiency of transfer results from clothing protecting most of the skin and from little of the TCDD being on the person's lips where it can be ingested. A soldier standing under Agent Orange spray in a jungle environment would have received an internal dose of 39 pg or 0.56 pg/kg. This estimated level of exposure is well below the acceptable daily intake of 10 pg/kg·day used in the setting of the proposed OEL.

CONCLUSION

The key to the success of OELs is that the setting of any goal gives a sense of purpose and direction to occupational health programs. It establishes an objective, which can be mutually pursued by the industrial hygienists, safety engineers, occupational physicians, and management. By way of illustrative examples and an in-depth case study of TCDD, we have demonstrated the application of the complex risk assessment process to evaluate health risk from exposure to chemicals in the occupational environment.

REFERENCES

1. H. E. Stokinger, Threshold limit values. In N. I. Sax, Ed., *Dangerous Properties of Industrial Materials Report*, vol. 1, No. 5, Van Norstrand Reinhold, New York, 1981, pp. 8–13.

2. H. E. Stokinger, International threshold limit values. *Am. Ind. Hyg. Assoc. J.* **24**, 469–474 (1963)

3. W. A. Cook, *A Compilation of World-Wide Occupational Exposure Limits.* American Industrial Hygiene Association, Akron, OH, 1987.

4. R. L. Zielhuis, Permissible limits for occupational exposure to toxic agents: A discussion on differences in approach between U.S. and USSR. *Int. Arch. Arbeitsmed.* **33**, 1–13 (1974).

5. J. H. Gaddum, The estimation of the safe dose. *Br. J. Pharmacol.* **11**, 156–160 (1956).

6. American Conference of Governmental Industrial Hygienists, *Threshold Limit Values and Biological Exposure Indices for 1986–1987.* ACGIH, Cincinnati, OH, 1986.

7. W. C. Cooper, Indicators of susceptibility to industrial chemicals. *J. Occup. Med.* **15**, 335–359 (1983).

8. G. S. Omenn, Predictive identification of hypersusceptible individuals. *J. Occup. Med.* **24**, 369–374 (1983).

9. D. J. Paustenbach, Occupational exposure limits, pharmacokinetics and unusual work schedules. In L. J. Cralley and L. V. Cralley, Ed., *Patty's Industrial Hygiene and Toxicology,* 2nd ed., Vol. 3A. Wiley, New York, 1985.

10. R. L. Zielhuis and W. R. F. Notten, Permissible levels for occupational exposure; basic concepts. *Int. Arch. Occup. Environ. Health* **42**, 269–281 (1979).

11. D. J. Paustenbach and R. Langner, Corporate exposure limits: The current state of affairs. *Am. Ind. Hyg. Assoc. J.* **47**, 809–818 (1986).

12. T. F. Hatch, Criteria for hazardous exposure limits. *Arch. Environ. Health* **27**, 231–235 (1973).

13. H. E. Stokinger, Criteria and procedures for assessing the toxic responses to industrial chemicals. In *Permissible Levels of Toxic Substances in the Working Environment.* International Labor Office Geneva, 1970.

14. H. E. Stokinger, The case for carcinogen TLV's continues strong. *Occup. Health Safety* **46**, 54–58 (1977).

15. C. Brown, Mathematical aspects of dose-response studies in carcinogenesis—the concept of thresholds. *Oncology* **33**, 62–65 (1976).

16. K. S. Crump, D. Hoel, C. Langley, and R. Peto, Fundamental carcinogenic processes and their implications for low dose risk assessment. *Cancer Res.* **36**, 2973–2979 (1976).

17. E. Crouch and R. Wilson, Calculating and comparing various acceptable levels of risk. *Risk Anal.* **1**, 42–51 (1981).

18. D. Krewski, C. Brown, and D. Murdock, Determining "safe" levels of exposure: Safety factors or mathematical models? *Fundam. Appl. Toxicol.* **4**, S383–S394 (1984).

19. E. J. Calabrese, *Methodological Approaches to Deriving Environmental and Occupational Health Standards.* Wiley, New York, 1978.

20. G. N. Krasovskii, Extrapolation of experimental data from animals to man. *Environ. Health Perspect.* **13**, 51–58 (1976).

21. E. J. Calabrese, *Principles of Animal Extrapolation.* Wiley, New York, 1983.

22. R. L. Dixon, Problems in extrapolating toxicity data for laboratory animals to man. *Environ. Health Perspect.* **13**, 43–50 (1976).

23. D. W. Gaylor, The use of safety factors for controlling risk. *J. Toxicol. Environ. Health* **11**, 329–336 (1983).

24. R. L. Zielhuis and F. Van Der Dreek, The use of a safety factor in setting health based permissible levels for occupational exposure. I. A Proposal. *Int. Arch. Occup. Environ. Health* **42**, 191–201 (1979).

25. M. Dourson and J. Stara, Regulatory history and experimental support of uncertainty (safety factors). *Regul. Toxicol. Pharmacol.* **3**, 224–238 (1983).

26. American Conference of Governmental Industrial Hygienists, *Documentation of Threshold Limit Values and Biological Exposure Indices*, 5th ed. ACGIH, Cincinnati, OH, 1986.

27. R. E. Hefner, Jr., B. K. J. Leong, R. J. Dociba, and P. J. Gehring, Repeated inhalation toxicity of diphenyl oxide in experimental animals. *Toxicol. Appl. Pharmacol.* **33**, 78–86 (1975).

28. C. Longcope, D. S. Layne, and J. F. Tait, Metabolic clearance rates and interconversion of estrone and 17ß-estradiol in normal males and females. *J. Clin. Invest.* **47**, 93–106 (1968).

29. D. Salsburg, The use of statistics when examining lifetime studies in rodents to detect carcinogenicity. *J. Toxicol. Environ. Health* **3**, 611–628 (1977).

30. Food Safety Council, *Proposed System for Food Safety Assessment.* FSC, Washington, DC, 1980.

31. M. F. Crammer, Extrapolation from long term low dose animal studies. I. Review. In G. G. Berg, Ed., *Measurement of Risks.* Plenum Press, New York, 1981.

32. C. C. Travis, S. A. Richter, E. A. C. Crouch, R. Wilson, and E. D. Klema, Cancer risk management: A review of 132 federal regulatory decisions. *Environ. Sci. Technol.* **21**, 415–420 (1987).

33. D. B. Clayson, D. Krewski, and I. Munro (Eds.), *Toxicological Risk Assessment*, Vol. 1. CRC Press, Boca Raton, FL, 1985.

34. Environmental Protection Agency, Guidelines for carcinogen risk assessment. *Fed. Regist.* **51**, 33992–34003 (1986).

35. N. Mantel and M. A. Schneiderman, Estimating "safe" levels, a hazardous undertaking. *Cancer Res.* **35**, 1379–1386 (1975).

36. Occupational Health and Safety Administration, Occupational exposure to ethylene oxide; quantitative risk assessment. *Fed. Regist.* **49**, 25755–25763 (1984).

37. Occupational Health and Safety Administration, Occupational exposure to asbestos; quantitative risk assessment. *Fed. Regist.* **51**, 22631–22644 (1986).

38. J. Ferguson, The use of chemical potentials as indices of toxicity. *Proc. R. Soc. London* **127**, 387–404 (1939).

39. G. D. Nielsen and Y. Alarie, Sensory irritation, pulmonary irritation, and respiratory stimulation by airborne benzene and alkylbenzenes: Prediction of safe industrial exposure levels and correlation with their thermodynamic properties. *Toxicol. Appl. Pharmacol.* **65**, 459–477 (1982).

40. H.W. Leung and D. J. Paustenbach, Setting occupational exposure limits for irritant organic acids and bases based on their equilibrium dissociation constants. *Appl. Ind. Hyg.* **3**, 115–118 (1988).

41. K. B. Bischoff, Current applications of physiological pharmacokinetics. *Fed. Proc., Fed. Am. Soc. Exp. Biol.* **39**, 2456–2459 (1980).

42. L. E. Gerlowski and R. K. Jain, Physiologically-based pharmacokinetic modelling: Principles and applications. *J. Pharm. Sci.* **72**, 1103–1127 (1983).

43. O. Hutzinger, M. J. Blumich, M.V.D. Berg, and K. Olie, Sources and fate of PCDDs and PCDFs: An overview. *Chemosphere* **14**, 581–600 (1985).

44. T. H. Umbreit, E. J. Hesse, and M. A. Gallo, Acute toxicity of TCDD contaminated Soil from an industrial site. *Science* **232**, 497–499 (1986).

45. R. Kimbrough, H. Falk, P. Stehr, and G. Fries, Health Implications of 2, 3, 7, 8-tetrachloro-dibenzo-p-dioxin (TCDD) contamination of residential soil. *J. Toxicol. Environ. Health* **14**, 47–93 (1983).

46. A. Poland and J. C. Knutson, 2, 3, 7, 8-Tetrachlorodibenzo-p-dioxin and related halogenated aromatic hydrocarbons: Examination of the mechanism of toxicity. *Annu. Rev. Pharmacol. Toxicol.* **22**, 517–544 (1982).

47. F. H. Tschirley, Dioxin, *Sci. Am.* **254**, 29–35 (1986).

48. B. A. Schwetz, J. M. Norris, G. L. Sparschu, V. K. Rowe, P. J. Gehring, J. L. Emerson, and C. G. Gerbit, Toxicology of chlorinated dibenzo-p-dioxins. *Environ. Health Perspect.* **5**, 87–99 (1973).

49. J. B. Greig and F. DeMatteis. Effects of TCDD on drug metabolism and hepatic microsomes in rats and mice. *Environ. Health Perspect.* **5**, 211–219 (1973).

50. R. R. Suskind, Chloracne: The hallmark of dioxin intoxication. *Scand. J. Work Environ. Health* **11**, 165–171 (1985).

51. J. S. Wassom, A review of the genetic toxicology of chlorinated dibenzo-p-dioxins. *Mutat. Res.* **47**, 141–160 (1977).

52. H. P. Shu, D. J. Paustenbach, and F. J. Murray, A critical evaluation of the use of mutagenesis, carcinogenesis and tumor promotion data in a cancer risk assessment of 2, 3, 7, 8-TCDD. *Regul. Toxicol. Pharmacol.* **7**, 57–88 (1987).

53. J. A. DiGiovanni, A. Viaje, and D. L. Berry, Tumor initiating ability of 2, 3, 7, 8-TCDD and arochlor 1254 in a two stage system of mouse skin carcinogenesis. *Bull. Environ. Contam. Toxicol.* **18**, 522–527 (1977).

54. D. L. Berry, J. DiGiovanni, M. R. Juchau, W. M. Bracken, G. L. Gleason, and T. J. Slaga, Lack of tumor-promoting ability of certain environmental chemicals in a two-stage mouse skin tumorigenesis assay. *Res. Commun. Chem. Pathol. Pharmacol.* **20**, 101–108 (1978).

55. National Toxicology Program, *Carcinogenesis Bioassay of 2, 3, 7, 8-TCDD in Swiss–Webster Mice (Dermal Study)*, Tech. Rep. No. 121, NIH Publ. No. 82-1757. Research Triangle Park, NC, 1982.

56. R. J. Kociba, D. G. Keys, J. E. Beyer, R. M. Carreson, C. E. Wade, D. A. Dittenber, P. O. Kalmins, L. F. Franson, P. N. Park, S. D. Barnard, P. A. Hummel, and C. G. Humiston, Results of a two-year chronic toxicity and oncogenicity study of 2, 3, 7, 8-TCDD in rats. *Toxicol. Appl. Pharmacol.* **46**, 279–303 (1978).

57. National Toxicology Program, *Carcinogenesis Bioassay of 2, 3, 7, 8-TCDD in Osborne–Mendel Rats and B6C3F1 Mice (gavage study)*, DHHS Publ. No. (NIH) 82–1765. Research Triangle Park, NC, 1980.

58. A. Poland and E. Glover, An estimate of the maximum in vivo convalent binding of 2, 3, 7, 8-tetrachlorodibenzo-p-dioxin to rat liver protein, ribosomal RNA and DNA. *Cancer Res.* **39**, 3341–3344 (1979).

59. A. Poland, D. Palen, and E. Glover, Tumor promotion by TCDD in skin of HRS/J hairless mice. *Nature (London)* **300**, 271–273 (1982).

60. H. C. Pitot, T. Goldsworthy, H. A. Campbell, and A. Poland, Quantitative evaluation of the promotion by 2, 3, 7, 8-tetrachlorodibenzo-p-dioxin in hepatocarcinogenesis from diethylnitrosamine. *Cancer Res.* **40**, 3616–3620 (1980)

61. K. D. Courtney, D. W. Gaylor, M. D. Hogan, and H. L. Falk, Teratogenic evaluation of 2, 4, 5-T. *Science* **168**, 864–866 (1970).

62. G. L. Sparschu, F. L. Dunn, and V. K. Rowe, Study of tetratogenicity of 2, 3, 7, 8-TCDD. *Food Cosmet. Toxicol.* **9**, 405–412 (1976).

63. D. Neubert, P. Zens, A. Rothenwallner, and H. J. Merker, A survey of the embryotoxic effects of TCDD in mamalian species. *Environ. Health Perspect.* **5**, 233–240 (1973).

64. J. E. Gibson, Perinatal nephropathies. *Environ. Health Perspect.* **15**, 121–130 (1976).

65. F. A. Smith, B. A. Schwetz, and K. D. Nitsche, Teratogenicity of 2, 3, 7, 8-TCDD in CF-1 mice. *Toxicol. Appl. Pharmocol.* **38**, 517–523 (1976).

66. E. Giavini, M. Prati, and C. Vismara, Rabbit teratology study with 2, 3, 7, 8-TCDD. *Environ. Res.* **27**, 74–78 (1982).

67. W. P. McNulty, Teratogenicity and fetotoxicity. In W. W. Lowrance, Ed., *Symposium on Public Health Risk of Dioxins.* Rockefeller University, Kaufman Publ., Los Altos, CA, 1984, pp. 245–254.

68. F. J. Murray, F. A. Smith, K. D. Nitschke, C. G. Humiston, R. J. Kociba, and B. A. Schwitz, Three generation reproduction study of rats given 2, 3, 7, 8-tetrachlorodibenzo-p-dioxin (TCDD) in the diet. *Toxicol. Appl. Pharmacol.* **50**, 241–252 (1979).

69. J. A. Zack, and W. R. Gaffey, A mortality study of workers employed at the Monsanto plant in Nitro, West Virginia. In R. E. Tucker, A. L. Young, and A. P. Gray, Eds., *Human and Environmental Risks of Chlorinated Dioxins and Related Compounds.* Plenum Press, New York, 1983, pp. 575–591.

70. R. R. Suskind, and V. S. Hertzberg, Human health effects of 2, 4, 5-T and its toxic contaminants. *JAMA, J. Am. Med. Assoc.* **251**, 2372–2380 (1984).

71. M. Moses, R. Lilis, K. K. Crow, J. Thornton, A. Fischbein, H. A. Anderson, and I. J. Selikoff, Health status of workers with past exposure to 2, 3, 7, 8-tetrachlorodibenzo-p-dioxin in the manufacture of 2, 4, 5-trichlorophenoxyacetic acid; Comparison of findings with and without chloracne. *Am. J. Ind. Med.* **5**, 161–182 (1984).

72. R. R. Cook, G. G. Bond, R. A. Olson, M. G. Ott, and M. R. Gondek, Evaluation of the mortality experience of workers exposed to the chlorinated dioxins. *Chemosphere* **15**, 1769–1776 (1986).

73. G. G. Bond, M. G. Ott, and F. E. Brenner, Medical and morbidity surveillance findings among employees potentially exposed to TCDD. *Br. J. Ind. Med.* **40**, 318–324 (1983).

74. J. C. Townsend, K. M. Bodner, P. F. D. Van Peenen, R. D. Olsen, and R. R. Cook, Survey of reproductive events of Wives of Employees Exposed to chlorinated dioxins. *Am. J. Epidemiol.* **115**, 695–713 (1982).

75. G. D. Lathrop, W. D. Wolfe, R. A. Albanese, and P. M. Moynahan, An epidemiologic investigation of health effects in Air Force personnel following exposure to Herbicides, executive summary baseline morbidity study. *Banbury Rep.* **18**, 471–474 (1984).

76. J. D. Erickson, J. Mulinare, and P. W. McClain, Vietnam veterans' risks for fathering babies with birth defects. *JAMA, J. Am. Med. Assoc.* **252**, 903–912 (1984).

77 L. Hardell and A Sanstrom, Case control study: Soft-tissue sarcomas and exposure to phenoxyacetic acids or chloropenols. *Br. J. Cancer* **39**, 711–717 (1979).

78. M. Eriksson, L. Hardell, N. O. Berg, T. Moller, and O. Axelson, Soft-tissue sarcomas and exposure to chemical substances: A case-referent study. *Br. J. Ind. Med.* **38**, 27–33 (1981).

79. L. Hardell, M. Eriksson, P. Lennier, and E. Lundgren, Malignant lymphoma and exposure to chemicals, especially organic solvents, chlorophenols and phenoxy acids: A case-control study. *Br. J. Cancer* **43**, 169–176 (1981).

80. National Research Council of Canada, 2, 4-D: *Some Current Issues*, NRCC Publ. No. 20647. NRCC, Ottawa, Ontario, 1983, pp. 60–64.

81. L. Hardell, L. Domellof, M. Nygren, M. Hansson, and C. Rappe, *Levels of Polychlorinated Dibenzodioxins and Dibenzofurans in Adipose Tissue of Patients with Soft-tissue Sarcoma and Malignant Lymphoma Exposed to Phenoxy Acids and of Unexposed Controls.* American Chemical Society, Miami, FL, 1985 pp. 167–168.

82. International Agency for Research in Cancer, *Some Fumigants, the Herbicides 2, 4-D and 2, 4, 4-T Chlorinated Dibenzodioxins and Miscellaneous Industrial Chemicals,* Vol. 15. World Health Organization, Lyon, France, 1977, pp. 41–102.

83. Natural Toxocology Program, *Fourth Annual Report on Carcinogens,* NTP 85–002. U.S. Department of Health and Human Services, Washington DC, 1985 p. 185.

84. H. Poiger and C. Schlatter, Pharmacokinetics of 2, 3, 7, 8-TCDD in man. *Chemosphere* **15**, 1489–194 (1986).

85. J. Schaum, *Risk Analysis of TCDD Contaminated Soil.* Office of Health and Environmental Assessment, U.S. Environmental Protection Agency, Washington, D.C. 1984.

86. D. J. Paustenbach, H. P. Shu, and F. J. Murray, A critical examination of assumptions used in risk assessments of dioxin contaminated soil. *Regul. Toxicol. Pharmacol.* **6**, 284–307 (1986).

87. J. V. Rodricks, S. M. Brett, and G. C. Wrenn, Significant risk decisions in federal regulatory agencies, *Regul. Toxicol. Pharmacol.* **1**, 307–320 (1987).

88. Environmental Protection Agency, *Health Assessment Document for Polychlorinated Dibenzo-p-dioxins,* Final Report, EPA-600/8-84-014F. Office of Environmental Assessment, Cincinnati, OH, 1985.

89. Ontario Ministry of the Environment, *Scientific Criteria Document for Standard Development No. 4-84: Polychlorinated Dibenzo-p-dioxins (PCDD's) and Polychlorinated Dibenzofurans (PCDF's)* OME, Ontario, Canada, 1985.

90. C. A. Van Der Heijden, A. G. A. C. Knapp, P. G. N. Kramers, and M. J. Van Logten, *Evaluation of the Carcinogenicity and Mutagenicity of 2, 3, 7, 8-Tetrachlorodibenzo-1, 4-Dioxin (TCDD): Classification and No-Effect Level,* Rep. DOC/LCM 300/292. State Institute of National Health, Bilthoven, The Netherlands, 1982.

91. Federal Environmental Agency, *Report on Dioxins.* Erich Schmidt, Verlag. Berlin, 1984.

92. F. Cordle, The use of epidemiology in the regulation of dioxins in the food supply. *Regul. Toxicol. Pharmacol.* **1**, 379–387 (1981).

93. M. K. Kim and J. Hawley, *Revised Risk Assessment Binghamton State Office Building* (draft). New York State Department of Health, Albany, 1983.

94. D. G. Patterson, Jr., J. S. Holler, S. J. Smith, J. A. Liddle, E. J. Sampson, and L. L. Needham, Human adipose tissue data for 2, 3, 7, 8-TCDD in certain U.S. samples. *Chemosphere* **15**, 2055–2060 (1986).

95. J. J. Ryan, A. Schecter, R. Lizotte, W. F. Sun, and L. Miller, Tissue distribution of dioxins and furans in humans from the general population. *Chemosphere* **14**, 929–932 (1985).

96. D. G. Patterson, Jr., R. E. Hoffmann, L. L. Needham, J. R. Bagby, D. W. Roberts, J. L. Pirkle, H. Falk, E. J. Sampson, and V. N. Hauk, Levels of 2, 3, 7, 8-tetrachlorodibenzo-p-dioxin in adipose tissue of exposed and control persons in Missouri, *JAMA, J. Am. Med. Assoc.* **256**, 2683–2686 (1986).

97. M. L. Gross, J. O. Lay, P. A. Lyon, D. Lippstreu, N. Kangas, R. L. Harless, S. E. Taylor, and A. E. Dupuy, Jr., 2, 3, 7, 8-tetrachlorodibenzo-p-dioxin levels in adipose tissue of Vietnam veterans. *Environ. Res.* **33**, 261–268 (1984).

98. M. Gough, *Dioxin, Agent Orange, The Facts.* Plenum Press, New York, (1986).

99. K. M. Stevens, Agent Orange toxicity: A quantitative perspective. *Hum. Toxicol.* **1**, 31–39 (1981).

21

A Case Study of Developmental Toxicity Risk Estimation Based on Animal Data: The Drug Bendectin

E. Marshall Johnson

Jefferson Medical College, Philadelphia, Pennsylvania

1 INTRODUCTION: MAGNITUDE OF THE PROBLEM

Recent years have witnessed a marked upturn in the attention paid to problems of in utero development, particularly the effects that exogenous agents may have on this development. There is no basis for suggesting that the incidence of congenital malformations is increasing. In fact, their occurrence seems to be about the same today as they have been throughout the years for which some quantified data are available. What has changed is that some other problems of childhood have been overcome to some significant extent. This increases the visibility of developmental problems and their recognition as major problems because so many others of childhood have been eliminated. For example, not too long ago infectious diseases such as bacterial infections were major and oftentimes overwhelming problems for the newborn. As these have been overcome to some significant extent, developmental problems increase in relative importance. Coupled with this are two additional considerations. There is a marked awareness of environmental contamination in contemporary society and family size is decreasing. As couples choose to have fewer children, there are greater efforts to have better children. Congenital problems of development continue as a major health problem, and more than one million people are hospitalized each year due to developmental problems (1).

Depending on the level of examination, the congenital malformation rate in the human population is approximately 3% of live-born (2). This is a general estimate considered to include only those problems that have clinical significance and to exclude developmental variants that perturb neither the quality nor the quantity of the individual's life. By the time a population reaches puberty, the number of developmental problems is approximately doubled (3). That as many as 6% of the live newborns may have developmentally relatable problems seems large and is of itself a significant health problem. Actually, it may be only the tip of the iceberg. Over 40% of the preimplantation embryos are considered to be abnormal (4), and Nishimura (5) has provided data indicating that the incidence of abnormal offspring increases with increasing gestational

711

age up to a maximum and thereafter declines through term. Lastly, there is a significant malformation rate in the 15–20% of recognized human pregnancies that abort spontaneously. However, even with these losses of concepti that bear developmental defects, some abnormal offspring are delivered and live.

Even though the rate of developmental defects does not appear to be increasing, the amount of attention and concern that is focused on this aspect of human experience has increased and shows every sign of continuing to do so for the foreseeable future. With these thoughts in mind, and in view of the fact that a certain undefined proportion of human developmental problems may be due to exogenous agents, a discussion of developmental toxicity risk estimation is warranted.

2   IDENTIFICATION OF HAZARDS

It is a generally accepted dogma that approximately 25% of human congenital malformations have an associated genetic basis (6) but the cause of the unfavorable genetic constitution tends to escape analysis. How many of these, in the final analysis, may be due to an effect of an exogenous agent on the genome is undetermined. Environmental and pharmacologic agents are not known to be directly responsible for a large number of human congenital malformations (6). Therefore, since the majority of congenital malformations are due to unknown causes, the question emerges about the origin of the stimulus that causes so many human embryos to develop abnormally. The obvious and facile answer to this question is that it is a multifactorial problem entailing interactions between the genetics of the mother and child as the foundation of developmental potentialities on which various types, sequences, and severities of exogenous drugs or other chemicals exert their influence.

It is axiomatic that a potential developmental toxicant's effect will be modulated to a larger or lesser extent by the genetics of both the mother and her conceptus (7). There may, however, be some noteworthy exceptions to this generalization. One is thalidomide, which although it did not cause congenital malformations in all the women exposed, it did so in a high percentage of those exposed between the 20th and 35th days of gestation (8). This may be due to the fact that thalidomide has a marked prediction for disrupting some aspect of embryonic development in the absence of any acute signs of toxicity in the mothers. The exact developmental phenomenon perturbed by thalidomide is not established, but whatever it is, it apparently is common to all embryos. Another kind of exception is a compound such as a folic acid antagonist, which again, at least in experimental animals, seems to produce a high percentage of malformations somewhat independent of the genetics of the population exposed or treated. In this instance the vulnerability of embryos of different genetic composition to the adverse effects of the agent may be due to the fact that its action is at the level of interference with cell division (9) on which in utero development is dependent is every species.

3   HAZARD EVALUATION

Shephard et al. (10) provided an excellent pictorial of the testing methods currently available to protect the human embryo from the adverse effects of in utero exposure to exogenous agents. In this he considered that animal tests were the initial means by which one could detect an agent that was hazardous to the human embryo. The most commonly applied animal test of developmental effects is made in animals treated by a somewhat standard experimental procedure. The most comprehensive statement of this developmental effects test, which is conducted in at least two animal species, was prepared by the Environmental Protection Agency (11). As this document clearly outlines, the Segment II type of test (12) is considered to be a powerful test of in utero effects and to provide data relevant for extrapolation of effect levels to humans.

The Segment II test is termed a developmental toxicity evaluation because it is not merely a test for teratogenicity, as strictly defined. This is because a mammalian embryo that has been exposed to a toxicant above its threshold to regulate its own development and safely deal with the challenge or repair the damage may (i) die, (ii) become structurally abnormal but live (terata), (iii) suffer a developmental delay, or (iv) have a decrement of anticipated postnatal function. In fact, if one sought to restrict developmental toxicity evaluations to teratogenicity alone, the Segment II type of evaluation would not be the proper test to use (13). The Segment II protocol is a vigorous and broad test and causes developmental effects at lower treatment levels than do short pulses of treatment, which are more likely to produce live abnormal offspring. It is by far the most commonly executed developmental toxicity test. Importantly, in this test, chemicals known from epidemiologic studies to affect human development adversely also produce effects in laboratory animals.

In the Segment II evaluation, rats and rabbits are the experimental animals most commonly used. Groups of pregnant animals are exposed to the test agent at three treatment levels. The lowest must produce no adverse effect on either the mothers or the offspring; the third or highest treatment level generally should produce no more than 10% maternal deaths but must show some signs of maternal effect (11); and the second or intermediate dose can be positioned between these two, based on a variety of arithmetic and/or biologic considerations. The study requires a concurrent control group treated with any carrier or vehicle used for the test compound. The endpoint assays of maternal toxicity are maternal death, a decrement of maternal weight gain during gestation (often linked with measurement of food and water consumption, which may or may not correlate with maternal body weight change), and clinical signs, that is, daily cage-side observations of animal status. Treatment of the pregnant animals begins just after the embryos have implanted into the uterus and generally ceases at the end of the second third of gestation, when major organogenesis largely is completed. The fetuses are obtained by cesarean section the day before anticipated delivery and examined externally, weighed, and then evaluated for both soft and osseous tissue status by a series of somewhat standardized manipulations and examination techniques (14).

There are test protocols, as well as endpoint assays of effects, other than the Segment II that also can be used to test for developmental effects of exogenous agents. For example, in utero exposure may result in subtle functional (15) or behavioral (16) effects that are not examined in the Segment-II-type test. The effects of prenatal exposure on postnatal behavior have been an area of particular attention for some years. It is sometimes reported that behavioral effects are produced at exposure or treatment levels below those capable of producing structural abnormalities or other signs of developmental toxicity. However, consistent and clear examples are not available to establish that altered behavior is produced at exposure levels below those that would produce other manifestations of altered development in a Segment II or similar evaluation and more standardized endpoint assays of effects (17). Behavioral tests are valuable for detecting the type of effects that may be produced by an agent applied too late in gestation to produce more obvious types of developmental effects, but they are not an effective means to define the developmental toxicity no-observed-effect level (NOEL).

Also relevant to considerations of developmental toxicity test sensitivity are the topics of treatment severity and duration. A treatment period shorter than that of the Segment II protocol produces effects different from the more protracted exposure period of the Segment II evaluation (18). When one varies the period during gestation that a short treatment is applied, this too alters the pattern and incidence of developmental effects produced (19). More routinely recognized is the fact that the severity of maternal exposure also markedly affects the nature of the developmental outcome. This was used effectively at the Sloan–Kettering Institute (20) as the basis for an early teratogen screening system. In this technique, pregnant animals were treated with the acute single dose LD_{50} amount of a test agent. If developmental effects were produced, the chemical was administered for several gestational days at lower treatment levels in an attempt to detect stage-specific types of developmental effects. The key point here is that, as the duration of treatment during the initial period of embryogenesis increases, the pattern of effects changes and the treatment level required to cause developmental effects decreases.

Failure to understand this type of confounder of developmental toxicity studies (21) can lead to disproportionate concern about the developmental hazard potential of specific chemicals (22). For example, ethylene glycol monomethyl ether was given by gavage to pregnant ICR mice (21) on either a single day or for 2–3 days during the critical stages of embryogenesis. It was considered by the authors to be uniquely hazardous to the embryo because the brief treatment period did not produce Segment-II-type toxicity in the mothers at term. No data were available on the status of the mothers during treatment. This study demonstrated that a single dose of 500 mg/kg administered during organogenesis produced developmental effects, but when treatment extended over 2 or 3 days, only 250 mg/kg were needed to produce developmental effects. The crucial point is that when the same chemical was tested in ICR mice by the more protracted treatment period of a Segment-II-type protocol (23), developmental effects in the offspring were evident when the mothers were treated with 31.25 mg/kg·day, which was also the maternal-effect level. In other words, if exposure is controlled below the NOEL of a Segment II evaluation, the much higher level needed to elicit effects with a short pulse will also be avoided. On the other hand, a Segment II is not invariably the optimal developmental toxicity test for NOEL determination. It may be inadequate for a compound that very slowly bioaccumulates, that is, has a long biologic half-life. For these chemicals a multigenerational type of experiment is recommended (24).

Animal tests for identifying developmental effects tend to produce effects remarkably similar to those detected in humans (manuscript in preparation). In the past there has been some confusion on this point, but increasingly it has become evident that the embryos of animals are not markedly different from the embryos of humans in their basic developmental processes or their vulnerability and response to a noxious stimulus. A good example of this consistency between species was provided some time ago by the drug chlorambucil, which was demonstrated to result in renal agenesis both in the rat (25) and in the human (26). More recent examples are also available. Ethanol is reported to have produced developmental effects in the rat (27) which have come to be considered remarkably similar to the human fetal alcohol syndrome. At the present time excess vitamin A, a well-known developmental toxicant in experimental animals (28, 29) that causes a particular variety or pattern of malformations, is reported to produce the same general types of effects in human embryos from mothers treated with high levels of retinoid congeners (30).

Not only are the animal and human developmental toxicity data comparable qualitatively, they also are similar quantitatively. The Council on Environmental Quality (31) compared animal and human exposure levels and found that, in general, human embryos were not markedly more susceptible than animal embryos, that is, human embryos do not necessarily undergo abnormal development at markedly lower exposure levels than do animal embryos.

The two outcomes of the Segment II evaluation discussed above—that is, pattern of effect and dose level at which no effects will be produced—are two of the outcomes of Segment-II-type testing. A third is the slope of the dose–response curve. Most developmental toxicity occurs over a narrow span of doses. This very steep dose–response curve is somewhat unusual in toxicologic studies and does not occur invariably in studies of developmental toxicants. A good case in point is ethyl alcohol, which has a somewhat less steep dose–response curve, so that the NOEL is best identified in studies employing larger numbers of exposed animals.

The fourth and more recently recognized but potentially very useful Segment II outcome is the relation between the exposure level necessary to produce a Segment-II-type maternal effect and the treatment level necessary to affect the embryo adversely. The adult (A) NOEL and the developmental (D) NOEL can be formed into a ratio based on the protocol and endpoint assays from the data of contemporary Segment II protocols made according to the EPA guidelines (11). The larger the A/D ratio, the greater is the propensity of a test compound to affect embryogenesis adversely in the absence of maternal toxicity. Conversely, an agent with a very low A/D ratio may still be capable of producing developmental effects but tends to do so only at, or very near to, maternally toxic exposure levels (32). In these latter cases it can be difficult to determine whether the adverse effects in the fetus are due to a direct action of the agent on development or a secondary effect of altered maternal homeostasis. In either case it is not highly relevant to safety evaluations and risk estimation, because as long as the exposure level is held below the NOEL for both the mother and the conceptus, neither would be considered to be at risk. Agents with larger A/D ratios are the primary developmental toxicants (33). For them, exposure of the pregnant animal must be kept below the developmental NOEL if developmental effects are to be precluded. In so doing, the maternal animal has an automatic, if you will, level of protection.

If an agent is shown in a Segment II protocol to have a very low A/D ratio, that does not mean it cannot adversely affect human embryos. For example, thalidomide has an A/D ratio that is very large (larger than 30). Excess vitamin A has an A/D ratio in the neighborhood of 2. The difference between these two agents, both of which are known animal and human teratogens, is that thalidomide has a large A/D ratio and had the ability to affect development adversely even though it was not used at acute maternally toxic treatment levels. In the case of excess vitamin A, the treatment, and certainly the therapeutic level in some instances, is also the maternally acutely toxic level. The mother may tolerate or recover from the toxicity of the vitamin and in fact may actually benefit from the high exposure. However, the embryo can become diverted into a pattern of abnormal development from which it is unable to escape. A definition of a human teratogen, then, is that it is either an agent with a large A/D ratio or, if it has a lower A/D ratio, one that is experienced at, or very near to, the maternally toxic exposure level.

In the context of risk assessment of developmental toxins, considerations such as those listed above are necessary to make an accurate evaluation of the analytical data that are the basis for the process. The hazard identification step in the risk assessment of developmental toxicants is perhaps somewhat more clear than it is for some other types of toxicologic effects. Hazard identification is the process whereby one determines whether a test agent has the ability to cause a particular kind of adverse effect. In developmental toxicology the degree of hazard posed by specific agents can be quantified by use of the A/D ratio derived from the endpoint assays of the Segment II evaluation. The regulatory framework most relevant to developmental toxicity must be based on the no-effect level and a prudent safety factor, because developmental toxicity is a threshold-type phenomenon (27, 34, 35). If something can adversely affect the embryo, this does not necessitate its proscription. In fact, we know that many if not most chemicals, when a sufficiently high dose is administered to the mother, will produce adverse effects in the offspring.

The basis for most of the discrepancy between the number of animal and human teratogens is simply a matter of exposure severity. Many agents have been demonstrated to alter development in animals but few are known to have interfered with human development because experimental animals are treated with high exposure levels seldom encountered by pregnant humans. In Segment II tests, it is essential to use very high treatment levels to ensure that agents are tested vigorously. The way to assure vigorous tests is to require that treatment levels high enough to affect the mother adversely be used for the high-dose group of the Segment II protocol. In those rare instances where this cannot be attained because the test agent is unable to produce maternal effects, a limit test of 1 g/kg is used. The overwhelming majority of the animal "teratogens" produce their effects only at maternally toxic exposure levels and such severe exposure tends to be avoided by humans. The animal tests are not inadequate; rather, the evaluation and interpretation of the data are incorrect. Failure to appreciate this leads to the erroneous cliche that animal tests are not relevant to human safety.

In general, developmental toxicity evaluations made by the regulatory agencies, or de facto by society through the courts and usage, are consistent with the scientific facts and productive of human well-being. This is not invariably the case, however, and there are some notable exceptions or inconsistencies between science and the use of some substances (36). An excellent example of this is the no-longer-available pharmacologic Bendectin.

Bendectin was a mixture of the antihistamine doxylamine and vitamin B_6 and was an effective antiemetic, particularly applicable during the first trimester of pregnancy. It is no longer available commercially because manufacturing and marketing were halted in the face of extensive litigation. Bendectin is one of the more thoroughly animal-tested chemicals to which humans have ever been exposed deliberately. One of the experiments is particularly powerful and can serve to illustrate many of the points that one expects to find in a well-designed and well-executed developmental toxicity safety evaluation. Such studies are powerful tests for both developmental toxicity hazard identification and risk estimation.

4   BENDECTIN: HAZARD IDENTIFICATION

Between October 1982 and March 1983, Bendectin was studied in rats for the National Center for Toxicologic Research using a standard Segment II protocol (37). In this study, rats were treated by oral gavage from days 6 through 15 of gestation and killed on day 20, at which time their fetuses were removed and evaluated by the standard means for detection for both soft and osseous tissue effects.

A pilot or range-finding study was conducted with eight pregnant animals in each group before the definitive study was begun (37). The groups treated received either 0, 200, 400, 600, 800, or 1000 mg/kg·day between days 6 and 15 of gestation. Severe maternal toxicity was evident in the high-dose group, as evidenced by the death of four females.

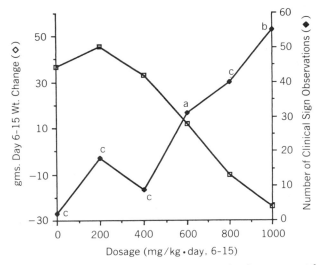

Figure 1. Maternal effects. a = seven pregnant females at term; b = four pregnant females at term; c = eight pregnant females at term. $*p \leqslant 0.05$.

There was one death in the 600-mg/kg·day group. None died at any other treatment level.

The other two endpoint assays of maternal effects recorded in this range-finding study are shown in Fig. 1. Pregnant rats at the 1000-, 800-, and 600-mg/kg·day dosage levels clearly had a dosage-related reduction in weight gain during treatment. Those treated with 400 mg/kg·day, while still on the same dose–response curve, could not be clearly identified as having been affected. When clinical signs were evaluated on an incidence basis, the findings were similar to the maternal weight gain data. The three groups receiving the higher treatment levels clearly were affected severely. In this preliminary study, even though females of the two lower-dose groups had slightly elevated incidences of clinical sign reports, they were not in a strict dose–response relation. One is not able to determine whether this parameter of toxicity showed an effect on the dams treated with 200 or 400 mg/kg·day.

Figure 2 is a depiction of the fetal effects seen in the offspring of the dams. At treatment levels of 400, 600, 800, and 1000 mg/kg, fetal weight was reduced. Again, one cannot be certain that treatment levels of 200 or 400 mg/kg resulted in a compound-related reduction. Another very useful fetal-effects parameter is the percentage of implantations resorbed, but there was no marked effect on resorptions, except perhaps at the two higher treatment levels. When the fetuses were examined for gross anatomical malformations, some were found (Fig. 3) in the two higher treatment groups. No pattern of malformations was evident, perhaps indicating there was not a selective effect on embryogenesis but that effects on development were secondary to altered maternal homeostasis.

On the basis of the preliminary study, the definitive experiment was begun at dose levels of 200, 500, and 800 mg/kg (37). This was an unusually powerful study in that, instead of the usual 15–20 animals, 30–37 female rats were exposed to each of three treatment levels and to distilled water, which was the vehicle for the test material. Maternal effects were evident at each treatment level, as indicated by the curve of female weight gain during treatment (Fig. 4), as well as by the incidence of the clinical

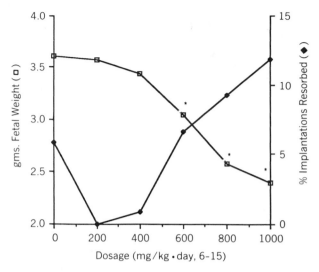

Figure 2. Fetal effects. *$p \leqslant 0.05$.

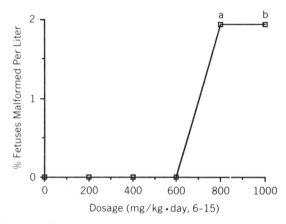

Figure 3. External fetal malformations. a = one with agnathia, one with agnathia plus cleft palate; b = one with single-digit bilateral microdactyly.

sign—piloerection between days 7 and 17. The erection of the guard hairs, often associated with a humpback-type posture, is a rather common sign of maternal perturbation in rats. These indications of maternal effects were consistent with the intake of feed during treatment, which was depressed at each dosage level. Feed intake at 500 and 800 mg/kg was statistically significantly different from the controls (Fig. 5). As frequently occurs for both maternal weight gain (not evident in this study) and also for maternal feed intake, there was a rebound phenomenon at the cessation of treatment. The upper line of Fig. 5 indicates increased feed intake by the severely affected dams of the 500- and 800-mg/kg groups.

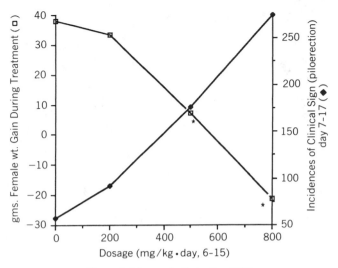

Figure 4. Maternal effects. *$p \leqslant 0.05$.

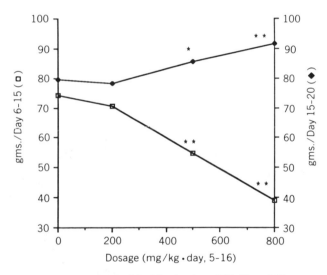

Figure 5. Maternal feed intake. *$p \leqslant 0.05$; **$p \leqslant 0.01$.

In Fig. 6 data regarding embryonic survival are presented. Preimplantation loss was higher in all treated groups than it was in controls. This is not considered as an agent effect and serves as an excellent example of data that can be interpreted incorrectly. Note that a clear dose–response relation is lacking and the rate and range of loss were what one expects in pregnant rats. Furthermore, and even more importantly, preimplantation loss could not have been affected by this treatment period. Implantation begins on day 6 in rats and treatment did not begin until implantation had already begun.

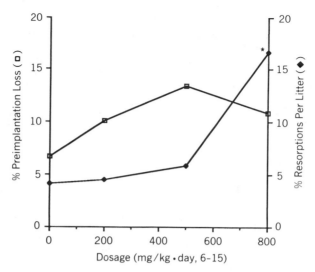

Figure 6. Embryonic survival. *$p \leqslant 0.05$.

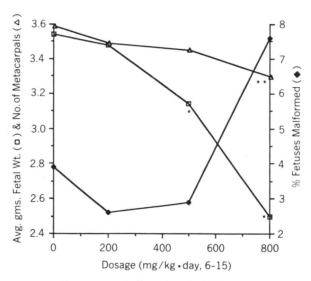

Figure 7. Fetal effects. *$p \leqslant 0.05$; **$p \leqslant 0.01$.

The percentage of resorptions per litter was severely increased for the 800-mg/kg group but was within normal range in the 200- and 500-mg/kg groups. Fetal weights were depressed at each treatment level (Fig. 7), which was associated with a dose-related decrease in the number of metacarpals ossified. Ossification of the fetal and postnatal skeletal elements is a rather rigid sequence by which one can generally age-date a young individual with some accuracy. This developmental delay of ossification in offspring of experimental animals is not unusual. It generally is expected and even pathognomonic of altered maternal status in experimental rats. The percentage of fetuses malformed and the percentage of resorption did not increase except at the highest treatment level of 800 mg/kg·day.

5   BENDECTIN: HAZARD EVALUATION

From these data the preliminary or range-finding experiment seemed to indicate that a treatment level of 400 mg/kg was a no-effect level for maternal weight gain during treatment. Clearly, 600 was an effect level. Actually, one cannot be certain that 400 was not also. The standard errors of measurement of the data points for maternal weight change during treatment were 2.61, 1.63, 2.84, 4.07, 5.13, and 6.75 for the control through 1000-mg/kg groups, respectively. The experience of developmental toxicologists is that, as maternal parameters change due to a toxic effect, the standard error of measurement or standard deviation tends to increase. The standard deviation at 400 mg/kg was not different from those at lower doses and was as one would expect in untreated animals. On this basis, one would lean tentatively toward the view that 400 mg/kg·day measured by this parameter in this experiment was a maternal no-effect level. The issue would be resolved in the definitive study that used larger group sizes.

In the definitive study, it becomes evident that the level of 200 mg/kg is a maternal effect level based on the dose–response curve alone. This is corroborated by the incidence of piloerection in the pregnant rats, which was markedly increased in a directly dose-related manner at each treatment level. (Other clinical signs of maternal perturbation showed similar increases, but the sign plotted here is piloerection, simply because it was the most frequently reported sign.) Maternal weight gain during treatment at 200 mg/kg·day was not retarded to a statistically significant extent, but the direct dose relation is difficult to ignore. One must allow that this parameter, in conjunction with clinical signs, showed an adverse maternal effect. Less clear, yet consistent with there being a marginal effect on maternal status at 200 mg/kg·day, is the fact that feed intake during treatment, although not statistically significant, was slightly lower than in the controls. This parameter was statistically significantly depressed in a dose-related manner at the two higher treatment levels.

In summary, maternal effects were evident in at least two of the standard endpoint assays of maternal toxicity at a treatment level of 200 mg/kg·day. They also might have been evident, not to a statistically significant but possibly to a dose-related extent, in one other assay, that is, maternal weight gain and its associated maternal feed intake during treatment.

Fetal effects were less evident than were maternal effects in this study. At the severely maternally toxic treatment level of 800 mg/kg·day there was a statistically significant increase in the incidence of resorptions per litter. The percentage of fetuses malformed was also higher than that of any of the other groups. The most sensitive parameter of fetal effect was fetal weight at cesarean delivery. It was statistically significantly depressed at a dosage of 500 mg/kg. At 200 mg/kg there were no clearly compound-related effects evident in the fetuses. The metacarpal developmental stage as well as fetal weights tended to be smaller than concurrent controls. However, in view of the possible suppression of maternal weight gain at this time and the clearly evident increase in maternal perturbation as evidenced by the clinical signs, minor skeletal maturational delay at this dosage is more reasonably attributable to altered maternal homeostasis than to Bendectin.

The adult toxicity level is therefore 200 mg/kg·day and developmental toxicity is evident at 500 mg/kg·day. Thus, the data suggest that the developmental hazard index (A/D ratio) for Bendectin is less than 1, indicating that this test compound produced no developmental toxicity except at treatment levels high enough to produce obvious signs of altered maternal homeostasis. Bendectin did not evidence any selective ability to disrupt the conceptus in this study. One could hold that the fetal parameters of day-20 weight and skeletal ossification, similar to maternal effects, were directly attributable to Bendectin. Groups treated with 100 mg/kg could have been used but actually this was not necessary, since the data indicate no fetal malformations in the presence of even the severe maternal perturbation produced at the dose of 500 mg/kg·day.

6   BENDECTIN: ASSESSMENT OF DEVELOPMENTAL RISK

By this standard evaluative technique, Bendectin has been found to have a developmental toxicity NOEL of 200 mg/kg·day during the most sensitive period of in utero development. Humans were given two 10-mg tablets per day during this same gestational stage. A standard means for establishing permissible human exposure levels is to determine the margin of safety (MOS). As an initial rule-of-thumb, a MOS above 100 is considered desirable. When based on adequate data, this size margin of uncertainty is more than adequate to prevent risk to human pregnancies. Actually, many margins of safety for industrial chemicals are well below 100, yet evidence of human birth defects are not found even in such carefully monitored populations. One of the more widely used drugs is aspirin, which has a margin of safety rather significantly below 100 and, based on use, actually may merit reevaluation. The margin of safety of Bendectin from this study is calculated as

$$\frac{200 \, mg/kg \, (animal \; NOEL)}{0.36 \, mg/kg \, (20 \, mg/55 \, kg \; woman)} = 555 \, (MOS).$$

Based on this excellent study in rats and similar type studies made in other species (38), Bendectin does not appear to pose a hazard to human in utero development. The margin of safety clearly indicates that the risk of humans ingesting sufficient Bendectin to affect development adversely does not exist. The absence of risk from Bendectin has been confirmed by epidemiologic studies (39). Bendectin was ingested by millions of pregnant women and the evidence is that no birth defects were produced by it. In addition, cessation of its use some years ago has not been associated with a recognized reduction in the incidence of human birth defects. In developmental toxicology as well as other assays of adverse effects, it is important to avoid situations where useful substances that can be safely used are avoided at the price of perpetuating circumstances of unknown, but probably significant (40), hazard potential.

Not only is Bendectin not a hazard, if Bendectin reduces maternal nausea, it could be associated with a better nutritional status and lower catecholamine levels—two factors with margins of safety that are much smaller than that for Bendectin.

7   CONCLUSION

Developmental toxicity is a threshold phenomenon and the threshold can be identified by careful examination of data derived from standardized testing in pregnant laboratory animals. A margin of safety can be established to allow for uncertainties in the data base and differences in susceptibilities of different populations.

Bendectin is an example of a situation where withdrawal of a substance incorrectly perceived as hazardous is probably hazardous to human well-being. It is unfortunate that there is not a means to redress an issue such as this after it is demonstrated that the substance is not uniquely hazardous to development and is used by humans with an adequate margin of safety. Developmental toxicity data should be used to control those agents that are hazardous and make available those that are beneficial as well as nonhazardous.

REFERENCES

1. March of Dimes Birth Defects Foundation, *Facts/1985*. MDBDF, White Plains, NY, 1985.

2. M. E. Davis and E. L. Potter, Congenital malformations and obstetrics. *Pediatrics* **19**, 719–724 (1957).

3. T. H. Shepard, J. R. Miller, and M. Marois, *Methods for Detection of Environmental Agents that Produce Congenital Defects*. Am. Elsevier, New York, 1975.

4. D. H. Carr, Detection and evaluation of pregnancy wastage. In J. G. Wilson and F. C. Fraser, Eds., *Handbook of Teratology*, Vol. 1. Plenum Press, New York, 1977, pp. 189–213.

5. H. Nishimura and N. Okamoto, *Sequential Atlas of Human Congenital Malformations*. University Park Press, Baltimore and London Igaku Shoin Ltd., Tokyo, 1976.

6. J. G. Wilson, *Environment and Birth Defects*. Academic Press, New York, 1973,

7. F. C. Fraser, The multifactorial/threshold concept: Uses and misuses. *Teratology* **14**, 267–280 (1976).

8. W. Lenz, in M. Fishbein, Ed., *Congenital Malformations*. Int. Med. Congr., New York, 1964, pp. 263–276.

9. E. M. Johnson, Effects of maternal folic acid deficiency on cytologic phenomena in the rat embryo. *Anat. Rec.* **149**, 49–56 (1964).

10. T. H. Shephard, J. R. Miller, and M. Marois, Eds., *Methods for Detection of Environmental Agents that Produce Congenital Defects*. Am. Elsevier, New York, 1975.

11. Environmental Protection Agency, Guidelines for the health assessment of suspect developmental toxicants. *Federal Register* **51**, 34028–34040 (1986).

12. E. M. Johnson and B. E. C. Gabel, An artificial embryo for detection of abnormal developmental biology. *Fundam. Appl. Toxicol.* **3**, 243–249 (1983).

13. E. M. Johnson and M. S. Christian, When is a teratology study not an evaluation of teratogenicity? *J. Am. Coll. Toxicol.* **3**, 431–434 (1984).

14. J. G. Wilson, Embryological considerations in teratology. In J. G. Wilson and J. Warkang, Eds., *Teratology: Principles and Techniques*. Univ. of Chicago Press, Chicago, IL, 1964.

15. L. M. Newman and E. M. Johnson, Effect of prenatal excess vitamin A on lung morphology and oxygen consumption in the newborn rat. *Teratology* **27**, 66A (1983).

16. D. E. Hutchings, Behavioral Teratology: A new frontier in neurobehavioral research. In E. M. Johnson and D. M. Kochhar, Eds., *Teratogenesis and Reproductive Toxicology*, Vol. 65. Springer-Verlag, Berlin and New York, 1983.

17. E. M. Johnson, The utility of behavioral tests for in utero developmental toxicity NOEL determinations (in preparation).

18. M. M. Nelson, Teratogenic effects of pteroylglutamic acid deficiency in the rat. In *Ciba Foundation Symposium on Congenital Malformations*. Little, Brown, Boston, MA, 1960, pp. 134–151.

19. C. D. C. Baird, M. M. Nelson, I. W. Monie, and H. M. Evans. Congenital cardiovascular anomalies induced by pteroylglutamic acid deficiency during gestation in the rat. *Circ. Res.* **2**(6), 544–554 (1954).

20. M. L. Murphy, Factors influencing teratogenic response to drugs. In J. G. Wilson and J. Warkany, Eds., *Teratology: Principles and Techniques.* Univ. of Chicago Press, Chicago, IL, 1964, pp. 145–184.

21. V. L. Horton, R. B. Sleet, J. A. John-Greene, and F. Welsch, Developmental phase-specific and dose-related teratogenic effects of ethylene glycol monomethyl ether in CD-1 mice. *Toxicol. Appl. Pharmacol.* **80**, 108–118 (1985).

22. F. Welsch, The applicability of in vitro methods to teratogenicity testing and to studies on the mechanisms of action of chemical teratogens. *Chem. Ind. Inst. Toxicol. Act.* **6**(10), 1, 3–8 (1986).

23. K. Nagano, E. Nakayama, H. Oobayashi, T. Nishizawa, O. Hirokazu, and Y. Kazunori, Experimental studies on toxicity of ethylene glycol alkyl ethers in Japan. *Environ. Health Perspect.* **57**, 75–84 (1984).

24. E. M. Johnson, *J. Am. Coll. Toxicol.* **5**, 197–201 (1986).

25. I. W. Monie, Chlorambucil induced abnormalities of the urogenital system of rat fetuses. *Anat. Rec.* **139**, 145 (1961).

26. D. Shotton and I. W. Monie, Possible teratogenic effect of chlorambucil on a human fetus. *JAMA. J. Am. Med. Assoc.* **186**, 74 (1963).

27. S. Sandor and D. Amels, Action of ethanol on the prenatal development of albino rat. *Rev. Roum. Embryol. Cytol., Ser. Embryol.* **8**, 105–118 (1971).

28. S. Q. Cohlan, Excessive intake of vitamin A as a cause of congenital anomalies in the rat. *Science* **117**, 535—536 (1953).

29. S. Q. Cohlan, Congenital anomalies in the rat produced by excessive intake of vitamin A during pregnancy. *Pediatrics* **13**, 556–557 (1954).

30. F. W. Rosa, A. L. Wilk, and F. O. Kelsey, Vitamin A congeners. In J. L. Seaver and R. L. Brent, Eds., *Teratogen Update Environmentally Induced Birth Defect Risks.* Liss, New York, 1986, pp. 61–70.

31. Clement Associates, Inc., *Chemical Hazards to Human Reproduction*, Council on Environmental Quality, 1981.

32. E. M. Johnson, A tier system for developmental toxicity evaluations based on considerations of exposure and effect relationships. *Teratology* **35**, 405–427.

33. E. M. Johnson, A prioritization and biologic decision tree for developmental toxicity safety evaluations. *J. Am. Coll. Toxicol.* **3**, 141–147 (1983).

34. J. G. Wilson, *Environment and Birth Defects.* Academic Press, New York, 1973.

35. E. M. Johnson, Cross-species extrapolations and the basis for safety factor determinations in developmental toxicology. *Reg. Jot. Pharm.* **8**, 22–36 (1988).

36. E. M. Johnson, Perspectives on reproductive and developmental toxicity. *Toxicol. Ind. Health* **2**, 453–482 (1986).

37. National Center for Toxicologic Research, *Teratologic Evaluation of Bendectin®* (*CAS No. 8064-77-5) in CD Rats*, NCTR Contract No. 222-80-2031(c). NCTR, Washington, DC, 1984.

38. J. P. Gibson, R. E. Staples, E. J. Larson, W. L. Kuhn, D. E. Holtkamp, and J. W. Newberne, Teratology and reproductive studies with an antinauseant. *Toxicol. Appl. Pharmacol.* **13**, 439–447 (1968).

39. L. B. Holmes, Bendectin. In J. L. Seaver and R. L. Brent, Eds., *Teratogen Update Environmentally Induced Birth Defect Risks.* Liss, New York, 1986, pp. 53–59.

40. N. Chernoff, D. B. Miller, and M. B. Rosen, Developmental effects induced in the CD-1 mice by maternal stress: Effects of a single 12 hr stress on varying days during organogenesis. *Teratology* **35**, 38A (1987).

22

Risk Assessment Methodologies for Developmental and Reproductive Toxicants: A Study of the Glycol Ethers*

Dennis J. Paustenbach

McLaren Environmental Engineering, ChemRisk Division, Alameda, California

INTRODUCTION

In recent years, the public has expressed an increasing concern for those chemicals used in the workplace and the home which may adversely affect offspring or impair reproductive function (1, 2). Once known as teratology tests, these toxicological studies have been more appropriately defined as tests for developmental toxicity (2–5). Such tests attempt to identify those chemicals that can cause growth retardation, reduced viability, malformations, and functional impairment in the offspring of exposed animals (3, 6, 7). Tests which evaluate a substance's capacity to adversely effect oogenesis, spermatogenesis, and fertilization are part of the reproductive toxicology test battery. Following the identification of those substances that could alter development or reproduction, the hazard posed by the various proposed uses should be evaluated, human exposure measured, control measures considered, and risk management decisions reached (8).

Although the risk assessment process has frequently been used to evaluate carcinogenic substances (9–12), few human health assessments of chemicals that produce developmental or reproductive effects in animals have been published in the open literature (5). In 1986, the U.S. Environmental Protection Agency (EPA) published risk assessment guidelines for developmental toxicants and these represent good criteria on which to develop such analyses (3). The EPA document concluded that it is currently assumed that a threshold exists for developmental toxicants "because the embryo is known to have some capacity for repair of the damage or insult, that most developmental deviations are probably multifactorial in nature." Accordingly, the EPA indicated that safety factors are

*The majority of this text was published in the *Journal of Toxicology and Environmental Health*, vol. 23, pp. 29–75 (1988) and is reproduced with the permission of Hemisphere Publishing Corporation.

generally acceptable to evaluate human risk since there are no theoretical grounds for adopting mathematical models which are currently used to assess genotoxic carcinogens (3). The safety factor approach has been previously recommended (4, 5, 13–16).

The simple evaluation of whether a chemical has the capacity to affect the offspring of humans or their reproductive capacity based on animal data has been termed a *qualitative assessment* (17). More recently, the qualitative assessment has been called the hazard identification phase of a complete health risk assessment (8). The objective of this process is to determine whether a chemical *could* pose a particular hazard to humans. In contrast, a *quantitative assessment* is the process by which the likelihood of an adverse effect (e.g., a developmental effect) at a given dose is evaluated (17). Risk assessments should contain both qualitative and quantitative discussions. They should also incorporate all available data regarding the chemical and physical properties of the substance, its potency, magnitude of the exposure, timing of the exposure, mechanism of action, and its pharmacokinetic behavior. Interestingly, risk assessments of developmental agents, unlike the assessment of carcinogens, are further complicated because the timing of the exposure, as well as the type and severity of the untoward response, must also be considered. Furthermore, the chemical's dose–response curves for both the mother and the offspring should be understood (3). For reproductive toxicants, it is necessary to study not only the reproductive viability of the parents but also the first and perhaps second generations.

The EPA guidelines (3) noted that approaches to ranking agents for their selective developmental toxicity have been proposed and these have been reviewed (18, 19). Of current interest are those that develop ratios relating an adult toxic dose with the dose that affects fetal development (3, 20–25). Ratios near unity indicate the developmental toxicity occurs only at doses producing maternal toxicity; as the ratio increases, there is a greater likelihood of developmental effects occurring without maternal toxicity. The latter phenomena are known as developmental phase-specific effects (26). Although further validation is necessary (27), such approaches should ultimately help identify those agents that are likely to pose the greatest threat to the health of human offspring and help establish priorities for regulatory agencies and risk managers (3, 23).

In spite of the numerous uncertainties associated with any risk assessment, especially those dealing with agents that may effect offspring or reproductive function, the application of safety factors to the NOELs obtained in Segment II or three-generation reproduction studies represents the best available approach for objectively, and quantitatively, evaluating the likelihood of adverse health effects following a certain level of exposure to a xenobiotic. The benefits of using risk assessments to address difficult environmental issues have been demonstrated on numerous occasions (28–30). Since it is now known that virtually any chemical or drug—when a proper dose is administered at the proper stage of development to embryos of the proper species—will be effective in producing adverse developmental effects on the fetus (known as Karnofsky's law), the risk assessment process is particularly relevant to developmental toxins (30). Such assessments are important since they bring together the results of all pertinent toxicology tests, metabolism studies, and exposure assessments and then integrate them into a cohesive document from which a risk management decision can be reached (29, 31). From such assessments, managers and scientists within federal or state agencies, industry, and the public can make informed decisions. Assessments can also identify those areas where more scientific data are needed.

The public and scientific interest in the glycol ethers—especially 2-methoxyethanol (2-ME), 2-methoxyethanol acetate (2-MEA), 2-ethoxyethanol (2-EE), and 2-ethoxyethanol acetate (2-EEA)—has been to a large extent brought about by toxicology research, which has indicated that these chemicals can cause developmental effects in the offspring of exposed animals (26, 32–43) and, perhaps, reproductive toxicity (99–100, 110–114). Broadscale interest in these compounds has been spurred by the EPA's risk assessment of 2-methoxyethanol, 2-ethoxyethanol, and their acetates (42) and the interest of the Occupational Safety and Health Administration (OSHA)(43). Their acute toxicity in animals and humans has been recognized for a number of years (44–55).

A number of clinical reports describing the acute toxic effects of fairly heavy exposure to the glycol ethers were published about 50 years ago (50–54). Although these studies showed that the glycol ethers could cause depression of the central nervous system and hematopoietic effects, the available data suggested that exposure to airborne concentrations less than 25 ppm for 8 h/day would not be expected to produce acute adverse effects. Reports by Zavon (56) and Ohi and Wegman (57) described toxicity from 2-ME following exposure when it was used as a printing and ink solvent. Both studies suggested that dermal uptake was an important route of entry. Cohen (58) has observed that inhalation exposures of about 35 ppm of 2-ME, coupled with dermal uptake, can produce adverse effects on the hematopoietic system.

Recently, it was alleged that 2-ME had produced testicular cancer in a painter but a review of the data indicated that there was no scientific basis for this claim (59). In a case report of males exposed to above 25 ppm of 2-EE, in the manufacture of castings, a decrease in the average sperm count was reported (61). Another report involving workers exposed to 2-ME and 2-EE suggested that semen quality had been affected (62). Epidemiological studies of the reproductive outcome of workers exposed to low levels of the glycol ethers have not demonstrated an adverse effect (65, 66). Some firms, concerned about the animal toxicity data, have considered limiting the duties of women of childbearing age in jobs where exposure to certain glycol ethers is possible (67).

This chapter evaluates the developmental and reproductive hazards posed by the four most commonly used glycol ethers in the semiconductor industry. Concern has been expressed over the 20,000 persons who are potentially exposed to these chemicals within this industry (68–72). As is customary in developing a risk assessment, the available toxicity data, human data, industrial hygiene sampling results from this industry, and exposure assessment were used to evaluate the likelihood that these exposures could produce adverse effects in these workers or their offspring. Wherever appropriate, the terminology and methodologies for assessing risk which have been proposed by the EPA (3) have been used.

THE GLYCOL ETHERS

Characteristics and Use

The ethylene glycol ethers are a family of chemicals derived from ethylene oxide. The glycol ethers possess numerous physical properties that are different from the more commonly used ethylene glycol, known as antifreeze. Of the glycol ethers, 2-methoxyethanol (2-ME) is the most common and approximately 90 million pounds of 2-ME were sold in 1981 in the United States alone (73). The importance and use of glycol ethers and glycol ether esters in the coatings and semiconductor industries have been reviewed by Smith (74).

Glycol ether solvents were first introduced as commercial products in the late 1920s. Because *n*-butyl acetate was the primary solvent used in coatings, the introduction of the glycol ether solvents represented a major improvement for the coatings industry. Of the

TABLE 1. Evaporation Rate of Ethylene Oxide-based Glycol Ethers

Solvents	Relative Evaporation Rate[a] (n-Butyl Acetate = 1)	Flash Point[b] TCC (°F)
Ethylene glycol	0.0001	232
Ethylene glycol monomethyl ether (EGME or 2-ME)	0.5	120
Ethylene glycol monoethyl ether (EGEE or 2-EE)	0.3	115
Ethylene glycol monopropyl ether (EGPE or 2-PE)	0.2	125
Ethylene glycol monobutyl ether (EGBE or 2-BE)	0.07	165
Ethylene glycol monomethyl ether acetate (EGMEA or 2-MEA)	0.3	140
Ethylene glycol monoethyl ether acetate (EGEEA or 2-EEA)	0.2	150

[a]From Smith (74) or Rowe and Wolfe (73).
[b]From Rowe and Wolfe (73) or Olishifski (75).

commercially available ethylene oxide based glycol ethers and glycol ether ester solvents, ethylene glycol monomethyl ether or 2-methoxyethanol (EGME or 2-ME), ethylene glycol monoethyl ether or 2-ethoxyethanol (EGEE or 2-EE), ethylene glycol monopropyl ether or 2-propyl ether (EGPE or 2-PE), ethylene glycol monobutyl ether or 2-butoxyethanol (EGBE or 2-BE), ethylene glycol monomethyl ether acetate or 2-methoxy ethyl acetate (EGMEA or 2-MEA), and ethylene glycol monoethyl ether acetate or 2-ethoxyethyl acetate (EGEEA or 2-EEA) all have evaporation rates between 0.5 and 0.07 (see Table 1). The use of 2-ME and 2-MEA is generally limited to specialty appliances in the coatings and the semiconductor industries, but the other products (EGEE, EGPE, EGBE, and EGEEA) all have a broad range of uses in the coatings industry (74). As determined by the tag closed cup (TCC) technique (Table 1), the flash points vary between 115 and 232°F (75).

Within the semiconductor industry, the glycol ethers are primarily used in the photolithographic portion of the wafer manufacturing process (76). One of several different types of glycol ethers, used in positive photoresist, is applied to a wafer using either a spray coater or a spin coating device. In either case, the spray coater places a uniform film of the photoresist on a silicon wafer. A spin coater then deposits a metered amount of resist (e.g., a glycol ether) via a closed transport system onto a 3- or 4-in. wafer, which is then spun for a specific time period to achieve a uniform 0.3–2-μm layer across the surface of the wafer. These operations are performed in a clean room, usually under a laminar flow hood.

The basic function of a photoresist substance is to enable the manufacturer to transfer a pattern for a circuit or other element of a semiconductor device from a mask—a glass with the pattern to be etched on the smiconductor device printed on the glass—to the semiconductor device. Ultraviolet light is directed through the mask, exposing a layer of photoresist on a silicon wafer to the pattern on the mask. The wafer is then developed and subsequent baking, etching, and stripping processes are used to create a part of the circuit contained on the silicon wafer. A detailed description of the photoresist process has been presented by Gise and Blanchard (77).

Glycol ether solvents based on propylene oxide have also been available for many years and are generally mixtures of two components. The major component contains a secondary hydroxyl, while the minor component has a primary hydroxyl group but a branch structure. In contrast, the ethylene oxide based products have a linear structure with a primary hydroxyl. The ethylene oxide based products are generally better solvents and consequently they have dominated the coatings market (74). For example, when comparing the properties of 2-ME with the properties of propylene glycol monomethyl ether, the evaporation rate of the propylene oxide based product is about twice that of the ethylene oxide based product; the flash point is much lower, and the solution viscosity with coatings resins is very similar (74).

It is not always possible to match both solvent activity and the evaporation rate of an ethylene oxide based glycol ether with a propylene oxide based product. This is one of the reasons it is sometimes difficult to substitute ethylene oxide based solvents in coatings systems with propylene oxide based products. In most coating systems, ethylene oxide based products have better solvent activity, better coupling ability, and give better solvent release from a coating than the propylene oxide based products (74). Manufacturers are currently trying to develop other types of less hazardous but effective glycol ethers (78, 79).

Exposure Hazard Rating

Unlike so many of the common solvents used in industry, the glycol ethers enjoy a rather low vapor pressure. As shown in Table 2, the vapor pressure for the four glycol ethers discussed in this chapter range in value from 1 to 10 mm Hg at 25°C (room temperature). These are markedly lower than common solvents like toluene and acetone, which have

TABLE 2. Vapor Pressures, Vapor Hazard Indices (VHI), and Occupational Exposure Limits for Select Glycol Ethers and Several Other Common Industrial Solvents

Chemical	Vapor Pressure at 25°C (mm Hg)	OSHA PEL[a] (ppm)	ACGIH TLV[b] (ppm)	Vapor Hazard Index (PEL)[c]	(TLV)[d]
2-Methoxyethanol	10	25	5	0.40	2.00
2-Methoxyethanol acetate	5	25	5	0.20	1.00
2-Ethoxyethanol	5.3	200	5	0.03	1.00
2-Ethoxyethanol acetate	2	100	5	0.02	0.40
Acetone	227	1000	750	0.23	0.30
Methylene chloride	390	500	100	0.80	3.90
Perchloroethylene	19	100	50	0.20	0.38
Toluene	30	200	100	0.15	0.30

[a]OSHA permissible exposure limit (PEL). Based on CFR 1910.1000 (1970).
[b]ACGIH threshold limit values (TLV), 1985–1986 values.
[c]Vapor hazard index (VHI) is defined as the vapor pressure (mm Hg) at 25°C divided by the occupational exposure limit. This index is useful for identifying which chemical, among a group used in a similar manner, is likely to be the most difficult to control to acceptable airborne levels. The higher the index, the greater the likelihood that the concentration will approach the exposure limit. In this column, the VHI is based on the OHSA permissible exposure limit (PEL).
[d]Vapor hazard index based on 1985–1986 TLVs.

vapor pressures of 30 and 227 mm Hg, respectively, at the same temperature. The low vapor pressure of the glycol ethers, coupled with the conditions under which they are used, explains the low levels of airborne exposure which have been observed in the industrial hygiene surveys of the chip (wafer) manufacturing industry (81).

In an effort to predict which chemicals are most likely to be a concern in workplace air, industrial hygienists and ventilation engineers have found it useful to calculate the vapor hazard index (VHI) for the various chemicals used in a given process. The VHI is the vapor pressure (VP) at 25°C divided by the occupational exposure limit (VHI = VP/TLV) for that chemical (82). Although the VHI concept was devised in the 1940s, it remains a useful tool for identifying those chemicals that are likely to pose the greatest hazard in the workplace since it accounts for both volatility and toxicity/undesirability. One shortcoming is that for the VHIs to be comparable, it is assumed that the various chemicals are used within similar pieces of equipment and under similar use conditions. In short, a chemical with a high vapor pressure and a low TLV would have a high VHI and therefore would require special effort to ensure that the airborne concentrations would not reach excessive levels. On the other hand, chemicals that have VHIs less than 1 are generally easy to control. The VHI can be based on either OSHA PELs or ACGIH TLVs. For the glycol ethers, VHIs derived from the TLVs are particularly useful since the rationale for these limits considered their developmental toxicity and reproductive hazard (83).

Based solely on the volatility of these four glycol ethers, 2-methoxyethanol and 2-methoxyethanol acetate should be most difficult to control. 2-Ethoxyethanol acetate, on the other hand, should be found at the lowest airborne concentrations in the workplace, assuming that all other factors are equal (Table 2). As discussed later, the air sampling data confirm that volatility is a reasonably accurate predictor of the relative airborne concentrations for these chemicals.

Potential for Workplace Exposure

Relatively small quantities of the glycol ethers are used within a workroom at any given time during chip manufacturing. About 1–2 mL are applied to a 3- or 4-in. wafer (chip) during the spinning step. One-half- to 2-gal bottles of photoresist are normally placed in cabinets below the equipment in which they will be used. Generally, local exhaust ventilation is used to remove any vapor that is produced. The bottles of photoresist are changed as required and the technicians involved in the change-out procedure wear appropriate protective gloves and an apron to prevent skin contact. The procedure involves removing the aspirator delivery tube from the spent bottle of resist and installing a fresh bottle.

The spinner heads on the coaters are cleaned periodically to remove photoresist that has adhered to the assembly over time and this presents an opportunity for exposure. Typically, the clean-up requires the use of some type of solvent such as acetone or xylene to remove hardened resist. Cleaning operations are conducted in a cleaning station, which is equipped with a local exhaust system and drains that remove excess waste solvent. The technician involved in the cleaning operation wears appropriate protective equipment (gloves and apron) to prevent skin contact.

Personal Protective Equipment

In most semiconductor operations, personal protective equipment is required of all persons who handle the glycol ethers. Gloves are the primary protective device. On rare

TABLE 3. Time to Break-through and Permeation Rates for Various Gloves and Solvents[a,b]

	Sol-Vex Nitrile	Neoprene Unsupported	Neox Supported Neoprene	PVA Supported Polyvinyl Alcohol	Natural Rubber
Acetonitrile	30 min (F)	30 min (VG)	1.5 h (E)	1 h (E)	4 min (VG)
2-Methoxyethanol (2-ME)	1.5 h (VG)	1.5 h (VG)	ND (E)	10 min (G)	45 min (G)
2-Ethoxyethanol (2-EE)	3.5 h (G)	45 min (E)	4 h (E)	1.25 h (G)	45 min (G)
2-Ethoxyethanol acetate (2-EEA)	1.5 h (G)	25 min (G)	1.25 h (VG)	40 min (VG)	11 min (G)
Diacetone alcohol	4 h (E)	5 h (E)	ND (E)	2 h (VG)	20 min (VG)
2-Methoxyethanol (2-ME)	11 min (G)	25 min (G)	70 min (VG)	6 min (G)	4 min (VG)
Pyridine	—	—	—	50 min (G)	5 min (F)
1,1,1-Trichloro-ethene	1.5 h (P)	—	—	1 h (E)	—

[a] Based on Loreti and Nohrden (84). From Edmont Research and Development (84a).
[b] The first number represents the permeation breakthrough time followed by a permeation rating that corresponds to the following: ND, none detected during a 6-h test (equivalent to excellent); E, Excellent, permeation rate of less than $0.15 \, mg/m^2 \cdot s$; VG, very good, permeation rate of less than $1.5 \, mg/m^2 \cdot s$; G, good, permeation rate of less than $15 \, mg/m^2 \cdot s$; F, fair permeation rate of less than $150 \, mg/m^2 \cdot s$; P, poor, permeation rate of less than $1500 \, mg/m^2 \cdot s$; NR, not recommended, permeation rate of greater than $1500 \, mg/m^2 \cdot s$.

occasions, when concentrations are potentially in excess of 5 ppm, respirators are used. In 1981–1982, tests to evaluate the permeability of the glycol ethers through various glove materials in common use in the semiconductor industry were performed (84). These tests showed that gloves made of nitrile and butyl rubber or neoprene provided the best protection (Table 3) (84, 84a). These types of gloves are now the ones most frequently used in this industry.

Three kinds of respirators for preventing inhalation exposure to the glycol ethers are available for use; however, because of the low concentrations encountered, they are rarely necessary. One-half masks equipped with carbon canisters are the most common type. These are used in situations where exposures are not likely to exceed five times the TLV since these respirators usually only provide a protection factor of 10. Supplied-air respirators are occasionally worn by maintenance workers engaged in work or clean-up operations. When used, $15 \, ft^3$ of air per minute is supplied to full-face masks and this should provide a protection factor of at least 2000.

DEVELOPMENTAL TOXICOLOGY: TERMINOLOGY AND DEFINITIONS

The fields of reproductive biology and developmental toxicology have been rapidly evolving ones. The bulk of the research activity has occurred over the past 15 years and, even as late as 1985, there was some confusion over the terms to be used. This risk assessment, as much as possible, uses the following definitions, which were adopted by the EPA in their final risk assessment guidelines for developmental toxicants (3):

Developmental Toxicology—The study of adverse effects on the developing organism that may result from exposure prior to conception (either parent), during prenatal development, or postnatally to the time of sexual maturation. Adverse developmental effects may be detected at any point in the life span of the organism. The manifestations of developmental toxicity include: [1] death of the developing organism, [2] structural abnormality (teratogenicity), [3] altered growth, and [4] functional deficiency.

Embryotoxicity and Fetotoxicity—Any toxic effect on the conceptus as a result of prenatal exposure; the distinguishing feature between the two terms is the stage of development during which the injury occurred. The terms, as used here, include malformations and variations, altered growth, and in utero death.

Altered Growth—An alteration in offspring organ or body weight or size. Changes in body weight may or may not be accompanied by a change in crown–rump length and/or in skeletal ossification. Altered growth can be induced at any stage of development, may be reversible, or may result in a permanent change.

Functional Teratology—The study of the causes, mechanisms, and manifestations of alterations or delays in functional competence of the organism or organ system following exposure to an agent during critical periods of development either pre- and/or postnatally.

Malformations and Variations—A malfunction is usually defined as a permanent structural change that may adversely affect survival, development, or function. The term teratogenicity which is used to describe these types of structural abnormalities will be used to refer only to structural defects. A variation is used to indicate a divergence beyond the usual range of structural constitution that may not adversely affect survival or health. Distinguishing between variations and malformations is difficult since there exists a continuum of responses from the normal to the extreme deviant. There is no generally accepted classification of malformations and variations. Other terminology that is often used, but no better defined, includes anomalies, deformations, and aberrations.

Depending on dose, several of the developmental effects discussed above have, in at least one of the tests, been observed in animals exposed to these glycol ethers.

DEVELOPMENTAL TOXICOLOGY: BACKGROUND

Segment II studies are designed to evaluate the teratogenic potential of a test agent and they are the most common tests to evaluate prenatal toxicity. FDA Segment II evaluations are performed in both a rodent and a nonrodent species; most frequently the rat and rabbit. Males used for breeding are not administered the test agent. Typically, day 0 of presumed gestation is the day spermatozoa, a vaginal plug (rats, mice), or insemination (rabbits) occurs. Animals are treated during the period of major organogenesis and cesarean-sectioned 1 or 2 days prior to the expected time of natural delivery. Treatment periods for commonly used species are: rat, days 6–15 (C-section on day 20); mouse, days 6–15 (C-section on day 18); rabbit, days 6–18 (C-section on days 28–30); and hamster, days 6–14 (C-section on day 15). The Segment II test protocol is a rigorous one since the pregnant animal is exposed to the toxicant throughout the critical portions of the pregnancy (85).

There are four ways in which altered in utero development can be demonstrated: (i) death of the conceptus, (ii) gross structural abnormality, (iii) in utero growth retardation, or (iv) decrement of anticipated postnatal functional capabilities. These can arise from a variety of causes (3, 13). Currently, there is no internationally accepted congenital abnormality classification system, although the one developed by the World Health Organization (WHO) is quite good (25, 86). These classes of effects, however, as well as the mechanisms that cause them, have little influence on the risk assessment process.

Three terms are often used to describe the results of developmental toxicity tests. For purposes of risk assessment, *teratogenic* should describe those chemicals that have been shown to produce structural abnormalities. Embryotoxic and fetotoxic appear to be the most ill-defined terms. Several papers have used embryotoxic as the sum of all possible toxic actions affecting the embryo, including teratogenic, embryolethal, and other effects. Black and Marks (87) have proposed that *embryotoxicity* should describe the loss of an embryo and the term *fetotoxicity* should be reserved for less severe effects. Fetotoxicity has also been used to describe the toxic or degenerative effect on fetal tissues and organs after organogenesis (3, 88, 89). Some authors have suggested that fetotoxic effects are usually transient and that bones and organs would be expected to continue to develop to their normal appearance and function (88). However, there are examples of fetotoxicity (in humans and animals) where the adverse effects persist throughout growth and development, for example, phenylketonuria. Perhaps for this reason the EPA guidelines (1986) note that fetotoxic effects include malformations and variations, altered growth, and in utero development.

To predict the dose at which no health hazard should exist in humans, identification of a NOEL (no observed effect level) or a NOAEL (no observed adverse effect level) in developmental toxicity studies is usually necessary. As presented in Table 4, from studies of substances that are known to affect humans adversely and for which there is some knowledge of the level of human exposure, it is possible to evaluate the accuracy of animal data to predict the no-effect level in humans (2). From these historical data, it is evident that the application of a rather modest safety factor to the animal NOEL (no larger than 100) has usually been sufficient to protect humans from adverse developmental effects.

It is reassuring that all human teratogens, except possibly one, have been detected in animals (3, 27, 85, 90–93). Whether they were all prospectively detected is a different consideration, although this did occur with several chemicals such as the androgens (23, 24). This issue has been clouded, at least in part, because of the fact that thalidomide was not detected in animal tests before its effects were seen in humans. However, it is important to remember that thalidomide was the driving force behind development of the contemporary safety evaluation studies that replaced the old two-litter test, which

TABLE 4. Comparison of Human and Animal Developmental Toxicity Tests

Agent	Human Effect Level	Animal Species and Effect Level
Alcohol	0.4–0.8 g/kg·day	Rat 1.5
Aminopterin	50 μg/kg·day	Rat 100
Diphenylhydantoin	2 mg/kg·day	Mouse 50
DES	20–80 mg/kg·day	Rhesus 200
Methotrexate	42 μg/kg·day	Rat 200
Methylmercury	0.5 μg/kg·day	Rat 250
PCBs	70 μg/kg·day	Rhesus 125
Thalidomide	0.5–1.0 mg/kg·day	Rabbit 2.5

Source: CEQ (1981) and Nisbet and Karch (2).

probably would not have detected the adverse effects of thalidomide. Nevertheless, accusations that thalidomide would not be identified under the currently used Segment II test battery do not appear supportable. Johnson and Christian (7) have noted that the current Segment II tests would almost certainly have detected a variety of structural abnormalities in rabbits and, in all likelihood, rats would have shown greater resorptions rather than an increased incidence of abnormalities; either would have been sufficient to prevent its approval. Furthermore, the A/D ratio for thalidomide is about 20—a figure that would certainly have demanded special attention.

REPRODUCTIVE TOXICOLOGY: BACKGROUND

In general, reproductive function is evaluated through the use of rodents in a multigeneration study. These are designed to determine if the test substance produces abnormalities in parental activities (from mating through lactation), in the pregnancy itself, or in the growth and development of offspring (from conception through maturity). Unlike the Segment II developmental toxicity test, a reproductive toxicity study involves lifetime exposure to a chemical and is designed to assess subtle effects on reproduction such as decreased fertility, premature delivery, and smaller offspring (88a).

As discussed by Dixon (89a), multigeneration studies are intended to provide data on gonadal function, estrus cycle, mating behavior, conception, implantation, abortion, fetal and embryonic development, parturition, postnatal survival, lactation, maternal behavior, and postpartum growth. The advantage of a multigeneration test is that it evaluates a wide variety of reproductive processes, and adverse genetic and behavioral effects may be observed as well.

To date, no single test or test battery for assessing reproductive toxicity has been accepted by the Environmental Protection Agency (EPA), Food and Drug Administration (FDA), Consumer Product Safety Commission (CPSC), and Occupational Safety and Health Administration (OSHA). Each continues to develop protocols for specific chemicals or concerns on an as-needed basis, although it is likely a uniform test will be established in the next few years. The traditional three-generation study involves two litters in each generation, because the first litter produced by adolescent mothers often has a great deal of variation (88a). One reason that three generations have been popular is that they were also used to detect genetic abnormalities. More recently, EPA has suggested that two-generation tests, coupled with the results of a battery of mutagenicity tests, would be equally sensitive as the standard three-generation test. The other reason that three-generation tests have been used is that it was believed that cumulative effects would be better detected.

In the EPA multigeneration test, at least three dose levels, in addition to the control, are used. The highest dose should produce an observable toxic effect but not cause more than 10% fatalities. The lowest dose should produce no adverse effects. The test substance should be administered via the route most like that to which humans will be exposed. The substance should be administered to two generations of animals, and a third generation should be exposed in utero and through nursing (88a). Dosing of the animals in the first generation, F_0, begins as soon as possible (about 6 weeks) and is continued each day. Dosing continues until all F_1 generation animals have been weaned. Dosing of the animals selected from the F_1 generation for breeding begins as soon as the animal are weaned. The test substance is administered daily to these animals with dosing continuing until 30 days after all F_2 animals have been weaned. After the F_0 generation animals have received the substance for at least 100 days, they are bred to produce the F_1 generation. After random selection from the different litters of the F_1 generation, these animals are administered the substance for at least 120 days and then bred to produce the F_2 generation. The F_2 generation is not dosed.

A fairly large number of observations are made in this test. The weight of each weanling is recorded weekly until maturity, dates of delivery are kept, observations of the mother and offspring are recorded, and measurements of spermatogenesis of all males are made. In addition, the following parameters are recorded: litter size, number of stillborn, number of live births, pup weights, and physical as well as behavioral abnormalities. Importantly, the fertility, gestation, viability, and lactation indices are calculated from the multigeneration test results (88a). Numerous other tests are available for evaluating reproductive capacity but the multigeneration test has the benefit of yielding much information in a limited amount of time. Of course, if adverse effects are observed, other more specific tests which evaluate specific portions of the male or female reproductive system would probably be needed. There are at least 40 different parameters which could be evaluated in the male reproductive system and perhaps as many as 60 can be considered for study in females (89a). The complexity of the reproductive process makes the unraveling of the mechanism by which adverse effects occur a difficult and often time-consuming investigation.

HAZARD ASSESSMENT

A good deal of the confusion in developmental and reproductive toxicology has been caused by the lack of distinction between toxicity, hazard, and risk estimation. Toxicity is a property of a chemical like its flammability. In contrast, hazard is the ability of the test chemical under a given set of conditions to cause a specific kind of adverse effect (i.e., developmental toxicity, neurotoxicity, cardiotoxicity). Tests for developmental toxicity identify those chemicals that might pose a hazard to the developing fetus. On the other hand, the risk posed by a chemical is the probability or likelihood that an adverse outcome will occur in a group that is exposed to a particular concentration or dose. Risk is therefore generally a function of exposure.

One parameter in the hazard assessment of development toxicants is the relation between the lowest dose that produces signs of overt toxicity in adults (A) and the lowest dose that produces any one of the three signs of developmental toxicity in the offspring (D). Fabro et al. (5) suggested that the ratio of the LD_{05} in the mother compared to the dose that did not affect embryonal development, which they called the "relative teratogenic index," might be a useful index for identifying chemicals likely to be hazardous to humans. Regrettably, this approach has been found to have numerous shortcoming and has therefore received limited attention.

The usefulness of the A/D relation is illustrated in Fig. 1. Most agents tend to affect both the mother and the conceptus at approximately the same general dosage level (24, 25). These are known as coaffective agents; that is, they have a low hazard index, and they tend not to exhibit developmental selectivity (A/D < 1). For these chemicals, there is risk of developmental toxicity only if maternally toxic doses are approached or exceeded—situations that should not occur if occupational exposure limits such as TLVs are met (4, 24, 25). On the other hand, some agents can alter some aspect of development at a small fraction of the adult toxic dose, and these can present a genuine developmental hazard (A/D > 1). For these, there is a genuine risk of adverse effects on development at exposure levels that are innocuous to adults.

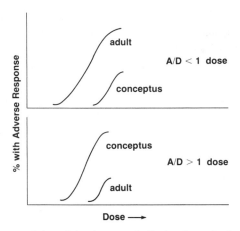

Figure 1. Relation between adult and developmental affective doses. In the plot where A/D is less than 1, toxic effects are seen in the pregnant animal at doses lower than those that adversely affect the conceptus. In contrast, where the A/D ratio is greater than 1, the conceptus is much more sensitive to the effects of the chemical than the mother (based on Johnson, 1986).

The A/D relationship is only one of many considerations when assessing the developmental hazard. For example, consideration must be given to those chemicals where the A/D ratio varies between species. In such situations, the species likely to be most similar to humans (metabolically and physiologically) should be given greater weight and, perhaps, the importance of the A/D ratio should be less emphasized. One shortcoming of the A/D ratio is that it is unable to reflect the differences in the severity of the adverse effects observed in the mother (e.g., weight loss) versus that observed in the offspring (e.g., gross deformity). The slope of the dose–response curve is also not reflected in this approach. Nonetheless, our experience to date suggests that the A/D ratio is generally informative and that chemicals likely to pose a significant risk to pregnant workers will usually meet two criteria. First, human exposure will be greater than $\frac{1}{100}$th the animal NOEL. Second, the adverse effect on development produced by the substance can occur at doses that do not elicit clear signs of toxicity in the adult; they have a high A/D ratio (4, 23).

Comparative Metabolism

When assessing the developmental effects of any chemical, it is useful to understand its metabolism in animals and, if possible, in humans. In 1983, Miller et al. (92) noted that little was known about the metabolism of 2-ME or the other glycol ethers except that ethylene glycol monobutyl ether (2-BE), a structural homologue of 2-ME, was apparently oxidized to n-butoxyacetic acid in the rat, rabbit, guinea pig, dog, monkey, and human (48). Jonsson and Steen (93) confirmed that n-butoxyacetic acid was a urinary metabolite of 2-BE in rats. Hutson and Pickering (94) have studied the metabolism of another structural homologue of 2-ME, ethylene glycol isopropyl ether (EGiPE) in rats. They showed that following an ip injection of [^{14}C]EGiPE, the major routes of excretion were urine (73%) and expired air (14%). Isopropoxyacetic acid and its glycine conjugate were identified as the two major urinary metabolites of EGiPE.

Based on results obtained with these close structural homologues of 2-ME, together

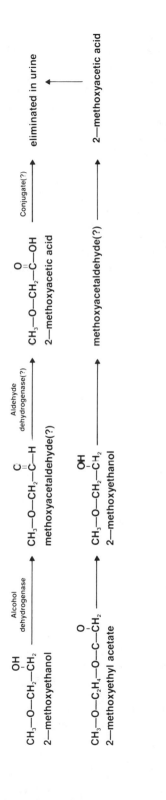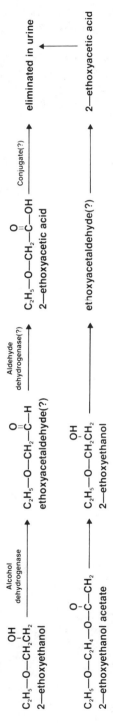

Figure 2. The likely metabolism of 2-ME, 2-MEA, 2-EE, and 2-EEA. The formation of methoxyacetaldehyde and ethoxyacetaldehyde, with subsequent conversion to methoxyacetic acid and ethoxyacetic acid, respectively, has been suggested but the evidence is not convincing. The methoxyacetic acid (MAA) and ethoxyacetic acid (EEA) are generally considered the chemicals responsible for causing the developmental effects.

737

with the fact that 2-ME is a substrate for human and equine alcohol dehydrogenase in vitro (92, 95–98), it was expected that 2-ME might be oxidized to methoxyacetaldehyde via alcohol dehydrogenase (ADH) and then further oxidized to methoxyacetic acid via aldehyde dehydrogenase (Fig. 2). In the study by Miller and co-workers (92), male Fischer 344 rats were given a single po dose of approximately 1 or 8.7 mmole/kg of [^{14}C]EGME (ethylene glycol monomethyl ether or 2-ME). Approximately 50–60% of the administered ^{14}C was excreted in urine, and about 12% was eliminated as $^{14}CO_2$ within 48 h after a single po dose of [^{14}C]EGME. Methoxyacetic acid was identified as the primary urinary metabolite of 2-ME, which accounted for 80–90% of the total ^{14}C in urine. Since methoxyacetic acid has been shown to produce the same spectrum of toxicity as 2-ME in male rats, it is likely that the adverse effects of 2-ME are the result of its in vivo bioactivation to methoxyacetic acid. Hence, Miller and co-workers (97) concluded that the differences of metabolites appeared to the underlying basis for the remarkably different toxicologic properties of 2-ME and propylene glycol monomethyl ether, PGME. Foster et al. (99) have suggested that methoxyacetaldehyde might be formed prior to the methoxyacetic acid and that the former could be the toxic species (Fig. 1). However, other studies have not indicated that the acetaldehyde is the proximate teratogen. Work by Brown and co-workers (32) and Ritter and co-workers (38) confirmed that methoxyacetic acid is the likely proximate teratogen for both 2-ME and di(2-methoxyethyl)phthalate (DMEP). Yonemoto et al. (100) also showed adverse effects of 2-methoxyacetic acid on rat embryos in culture.

The metabolism of 2-ME appears to be similar among several species. For example, a close structural homologue of 2-ME, ethylene glycol monobutyl ether (2-BE) is oxidized to n-butoxyacetic acid in a variety of species: rat, rabbit, guinea pig, dog, monkey, and human (48). In addition, this has been confirmed in rats by Jonsson and Steen (93). Their evidence plus studies by Miller et al. (92) provides confidence regarding cross-species consistency of metabolism (i.e., there are likely to be few major differences in the metabolism of this type of compound across several species). Recent work by NIOSH indicates that ethoxyacetic acid in the urine of workers exposed to 2-EE might be an appropriate indicator of exposure (64).

By analogy, it is likely that the acetates of 2-methoxyethanol and 2-ethoxyethanol are metabolized via hydrolysis to the parent molecules, 2-ME and 2-EE, respectively (83). In support of this postulate, it has been noted that on an equimolar basis, the respective acetate esters were about as potent as 2-ME and 2-EE in producing testicular effects and leukopenia in exposed animals (4, 96, 97). The available data strongly suggest that 2-ME and 2-EE are metabolized to methoxyacetic acid and ethoxyacetic acid, respectively (Fig. 1).

Mutagenicity

McGregor and co-workers (101, 102) subjected 2-ME to the following assays for genetic toxicity: Ames test, unscheduled DNA synthesis (UDS) assay in human embryo fibroblasts, sex-linked recessive lethal (SLRL) test in *Drosophila*, dominant lethal test in male rats, bone marrow metaphase analysis in male and female rats, and the sperm abnormality test in mice. In vivo test animals were exposed to atmospheric concentrations of 25 or 500 ppm 2-ME. Point mutations in the Ames test and UDS in fibroblasts were not increased while the SLRL test gave ambiguous results, which the authors believed to warrant further investigation. Chromosomal aberration frequencies were not increased in rat bone marrow, but there was evidence from the dominant lethal tests that 2-ME had profound effects on male rat fertility during the meiotic phase. Pregnancy frequency was greatly reduced and preimplantation losses were large. There was also evidence of postimplantation losses. Sperm abnormalities were slightly increased in the mice. These effects on male reproductive cells were seen only at 500 ppm. The likely teratogen, the 2-methoxyacetic acid metabolite of 2-ME, was not tested for mutagenicity and its formation is unlikely even in the activated portion of the Ames test battery. The author concluded that 2-ME lacked genotoxic potential but that due particularly to its effects on fertility, all data needed to be considered in any safety evaluation of this chemical.

DEVELOPMENTAL AND REPRODUCTIVE TOXICOLOGY TESTS

2-Methoxyethanol (2-ME)

2-ME has been studied in numerous animal species (rats, rabbits, and mice) in recent years (26, 105–108). Standard Segment II developmental toxicity studies were conducted via inhalation, the typical route of human exposure in industry. These data should provide a sufficient understanding of the dose–response relation and the no observed effect level (NOEL) for predicting the hazard and risk to exposed humans.

Hanley et al. (105) exposed pregnant CF1 mice to 2-ME for 6 h/day from days 6 to 15 of gestation at concentrations of 0, 10, and 50 ppm (see Table 5). The pregnant dams were autopsied on day 18 according to the standard Segment II protocol. At the highest dose level (50 ppm), there was a minimal depression of maternal weight gain during the treatment period along with some minimal changes in white blood cell and platelet counts.

TABLE 5. Summary of Developmental Toxicity Data on Selected Glycol Ethers

Chemical	Maternal NOEL[a] (A)	Developmental NOEL (D)	A/D[b]	Reference
2-Methoxyethanol	50 ppm (mice)	10 ppm	5	105
(2-ME)	50 ppm (rats)	10 ppm	5	106
	10 ppm (rabbits)	10 ppm	1	106
	31.25 mg/kg·day (mice)	ND[c]	—	109
2-Methoxyethanol		Considered analogous		
acetate (2-MEA)		to 2-ME		
2-Ethoxyethanol	250 ppm (rats)	50 ppm	5	116
(2-EE)	202 ppm (rats)	ND	—	117
	160 ppm (rabbits)	ND	—	117
	175 ppm (rabbits)	50 ppm	3.5	118
2-Ethoxyethanol	594 ppm (rats)	130 ppm	4	35
acetate (2-EEA)	100 ppm (rabbits)	25 ppm	4	126
	50 ppm (rats)	50 ppm (rats)	1	41
	50 ppm (rabbits)	50 ppm (rabbits)	1	41

[a]NOEL = no observed effect level (dose to which animals were exposed that does not elicit an adverse effect).
[b]A/D = the ratio of the dose at which no toxic effects were seen in the adult mother divided by the dose at which no developmental effects were seen in the offspring (D). The larger the ratio, the greater hazard to offspring. The A/D ratio can also be based on the lowest doses capable of producing overt toxicity in the adults and the lowest dose capable of producing any one of the three signs of developmental toxicity observed in a Segment II evaluation.
[c]ND = none determined.

Consequently, slight toxicity was observed in the mother at 50 ppm. At this same high dose, but not at 10 ppm, there were adverse effects on prenatal development. The number of fetuses per litter was reduced significantly at 50 ppm, and the number of resorbed implantation sites was increased as was the percentage of litters with resorptions. The skeletal variations, both in sternebrae as well as in incidence of lumbar ribs, were increased also at 50 ppm. Unilateral testicular hypoplasia and hemorrhage in the male fetuses were also reported at this dose level (4). In this and some of the other studies of the ethylene glycol ethers, the apparent difference in maternal body weight gain might have been lost if maternal weight had been corrected for the weight of uterine contents.

Nagano et al. (109) reported a Segment II study performed in pregnant ICR mice treated by intragastric intubation of 2-ME (see Table 5). Doses were 0, 31.25, 62.5, 125, 250, 500, and 1000 mg/kg of maternal body weight. Maternal body weight gain was depressed at doses of 125 mg/kg·day and above. This may have been due to the reduction in litter size. At both this dose and 31.25 mg/kg·day, there was a slight increase in the number of skeletal variations but there were no frank malformations. Syndactally, polydactally, and so on did not occur at an elevated rate below the dose also capable of interfering with maternal weight gain (125 mg/kg·day). No clear NOEL was identified in this study.

Hanley and co-workers (106) exposed pregnant rats to 0, 3, 10, and 50 ppm 2-ME (see Table 5). Exposure to 50 ppm reduced maternal weight gain very slightly at the onset of treatment and depressed a series of hematologic parameters in a concentration-related manner. The conceptus also showed delayed ossification patterns and rib spurs at 50 ppm. When rabbits were exposed to the same doses (0, 3, 10, and 50 ppm), the high-dose group had markedly depressed maternal weight gain from day 6 through 14 and significantly increased absolute liver weight. Examination of the fetal rabbits showed that resorptions were increased at the high dose whereas fetal body weight and skeletal maturation were both reduced. In addition, frank structural abnormalities were seen at the high dose in association with a marked effect on maternal weight gain (4). Rabbits exposed to 10 ppm had a statistically significant increase in the percentage of implantations undergoing resorption when compared to concurrent controls; but, as discussed by Johnson (4), this result was not biologically significant, as the study authors concluded, because the statistics are more a function of the low incidence of resorptions in the concurrent controls, that is, 4% on a per implantation basis. The resorption rate observed in the 10-ppm exposed groups was well within the historic control range for rabbits in this laboratory. This interpretation has been questioned since concurrent controls usually carry more weight than historical controls, especially if the animals were randomly selected (42).

In a complex study conducted by Miller et al. (108), adult rats and rabbits were exposed via inhalation for 13 weeks to 2-ME at concentrations of 0, 30, 100, and 300 ppm. In each test species, both absolute and relative testes weights were reduced at the high dose. In the rabbits, there was a reduction of testes weight at the 100-ppm level, while at both the 100- and 300-ppm levels reduced body weight gain were evident in both rats and rabbits. It should be noted, however, that rabbit weights can fluctuate randomly irrespective of treatment effects. Also observed was a concentration-related reduction in the numbers of platelets. When the 13-week inhalation study was repeated with just male rabbits at doses of 0, 3, 10, and 30 ppm, there were no adverse effects due to treatment (108). From these studies, an experimental NOEL of 30 ppm for testicular effects was clearly identified for both species (4).

Horton et al. (26) have evaluated the phase-specific and dose-related teratogenic effects of 2-ME in CD1 mice following oral administration. They showed that 2-ME (EGME) was not toxic to the adult female after multiple doses of 250 mg/kg or a single administration of

500 mg/kg; however, 2-ME produced fetal weight loss and increased resorptions at 500 mg/kg. The malformations were specifically related to the development stage at the time of exposure. The no observed effect dose for the induction of digit malformations after a single administration of 2-ME was 100 mg/kg. At 175 mg/kg, digit anomalies were induced without any concurrent reduction in fetal body weights (4). Horton et al. (26) suggested that the A/D ratio for the mouse may be at least 6.0. However, as discussed by Johnson (24), the A/D in this study would almost certainly have been less than 5 had the animals been dosed throughout their pregnancy since their test protocol did not give the mothers adequate time to illicit the toxic effects.

Reproductive Toxicity of 2-ME

A number of studies to evaluate the reproductive hazard of 2-ME have been conducted (see Table 6). Nagano et al. (109) orally dosed JCL-ICR mice with 2-ME at levels of 62.5, 125, 250, 500, 1000, 2000 and 4000 mg/kg·day for 5 days/wk for 5 weeks and evaluated them for testicular atrophy. The no-effect level for testis weight was 125 mg/kg·day.

In a less comprehensive study, Samuels et al. (110) exposed rats to a single saturated vapor of 2-ME and subsequently studied the effects on the testis. There were marked reductions in testicular weight 14 days after exposure to 2-ME. In a follow-up study, designed to establish the effect of a single exposure to 2-ME, mature male albino rats were exposed to various concentrations for a single 4-h period and sacrificed 14 days later. Following this single exposure, an exposure-related decrease in testis weight was observed in rats exposed to 5000, 2500, or 1250 ppm. Histopathological examination revealed disordered spermatogenesis and tubular atrophy in these animals. Minimal degenerative changes were seen in the testis of rats exposed to 625 ppm 2-ME. Testicular weights were reduced in rats examined 2 days after exposure to 2500 and 1000 ppm 2-ME and remained depressed when compared with control values for up to 19 days following exposure. Histopathological examination of the testis revealed disordered spermatogenesis in these animals.

Perhaps the most elaborate evaluation of the reproductive toxicity of 2-ME has been conducted by Rao et al. (111). They conducted a dominant lethal study in rats where either the adult males or adult females were treated by the inhalation route for 13 weeks at vapor

TABLE 6. Summary of Reproductive Toxicology Data on 2-Methoxyethanol

Species	Lowest Dose That Affected Reproductive System	NOEL for Reproductive Effects	Adverse Effect Observed	Reference
Mice	250 mg/kg·day	125 mg/kg·day	Testicular atrophy	114
Rabbits	100 ppm	30 ppm	Reproduction	126a
Rats	100 ppm	30 ppm	Reproduction	126a
Rats	300 ppm	100 ppm	Dominant lethal	111
Rats	1000 ppm	< 625 ppm	Altered spermatogenesis	110
Rats	500 mg/kg	250 mg/kg	Damages spermatocytes	112
Rats	100 mg/kg·day	50 mg/kg·day	Dominant lethal and sperm	113

concentrations of 0, 30, 100, and 300 ppm and were then bred to untreated partners. At the highest exposure level, male fertility was depressed, but no effect on this parameter was seen at 100 ppm. Parental hemotology and testes weight were affected at 300 ppm even 11 weeks postexposure. In marked contrast, there were no effects at 11 weeks following exposures of 30 and 100 ppm.

In a similar study, Foster et al. (112) dosed rats po with 50–500 mg/kg·day of 2-ME and 250–1000 mg/kg·day of 2-EE for 11 days. Testicular damage following 2-ME treatment was observed 24 h after a single dose of 100 mg/kg. At 16 h after a single dose of 500 mg/kg, mitochondrial damage in the spermatocytes was one of the first subcellular changes to be demonstrated. Animals treated with 2-EE developed a similar lesion to that produced by 2-ME; however, to obtain damage of equivalent severity, a larger dosage for a longer period was required. In limited studies with 2-methoxyacetic acid and 2-ethoxyacetic acid using equimolar doses to their parent compounds (500 mg/kg of 2-ME or 2-EE for 4 or 11 days, respectively) produced lesions of equivalent severity to the corresponding glycol ether. These data represent good evidence that 2-methoxyacetic acid and 2-ethoxyacetic acid are the likely metabolites and that they are responsible for the toxic effects. Following administration of 500 mg/kg·day of 2-ME for 4 days, the testes recovered weight, and the majority of tubules recovered their spermatogenic potential within one full maturation cycle. No effect levels for the 11-day treatment period were 50 and 250 mg/kg·day for 2-ME and 2-EE, respectively.

Chapin and Lamb (113) studied the histologic effects of 2-ME on the spermatocytes of Fischer 344 rats. Adult male Fischer 344 rats of proven fertility were dosed po with 0, 50, 100, and 200 mg/kg·day of 2-ME for 5 days. Each male was then mated with two females per week for 8 weeks. They found that the fertility of males treated with 200 mg/kg·day declined at week 4 and remained low for the rest of the study. There was a modest but significant increase in the number of resorption sites at week 5 and 6 in the high-dose group. A decrease in the number of litters observed at week 5 after dosing in the 100-mg/kg·day group was also observed. There were time- and dose-related decreases in sperm concentrations and motility, primarily in the 100- and 200-mg/kg·day groups, as well as concurrent elevations in the number of abnormal sperm forms in the epididymis. These studies showed that 2-ME was a very weak inducer of dominant-lethal mutations and produced effects on late-stage spermatids and spermatogonia.

The bulk of the data on the reproductive toxicology of 2-ME indicate that, in rats and rabbits, the adult NOEL is greater than 10 ppm and the NOEL for developmental effects on the embryo is virtually the same. In addition, mice treated by the most likely route of human exposure, inhalation, had NOELs similar to those in rats and rabbits. Based on these data, a NOEL of 10 ppm will, in calculations associated with this assessment, be considered the dose at which no adverse effects (NOEL) have been seen in animal tests.

2-Methoxyethanol Acetate (2-MEA)

The developmental toxicities of the acetates of the methoxy and ethoxy glycol ethers have not been evaluated as thoroughly as 2-ME and 2-EE, primarily because the apparent metabolic pathway for 2-MEA and 2-EEA has been expected to form the parent molecules then the proximate teratogen. As a result, the acetates are expected to present a developmental hazard similar to the parent molecules.

Nagano et al. (114) studied 2-MEA to evaluate its testicular toxicity and to assess whether the effects and potency were similar to 2-ME. In this study, groups of mice were dosed orally 5 days/wk for 5 weeks with 500 mg/kg of 2-ME, 500 mg/kg of 2-MEA,

2000 mg/kg of 2-EE, and 4000 mg/kg of 2-EEA. Approximately equal degrees of atrophy were produced from exposure to these doses, and each produced leukopenia. On an equimolar basis, the respective acetate esters were about as potent as 2-methoxyethanol and 2-ethoxyethanol in producing testicular effects and leukopenia (83, 114).

Based on the reported testicular effects and the likely hydrolysis of 2-MEA to 2-ME, the NOEL for developmental effects for 2-ME seems to be an appropriate estimate of the NOEL for 2-MEA. Both chemicals should be considered developmental and reproductive toxicants in animals. Since a NOEL of 10 ppm has been identified for 2-ME, a NOEL of 10 ppm for 2-MEA seems appropriate for risk assessment calculations. Based on the available data, the ACGIH TLV committee proposed that the TLV for 2-MEA be lowered from 25 to 5 ppm and this was formally accepted in 1984. This figure provides only a twofold margin of safety below the animal NOEL.

2-Ethoxyethanol (2-EE)

Ethylene glycol monoethyl ether (2-EE) has also been studied according to the standard Segment II developmental toxicity protocols via inhalation. Tinston et al. (116) exposed Wistar rats to 2-EE vapor for 6 h/day on days 6–15 of gestation at levels of 0, 10, 50, and 250 ppm. In this study, which was reviewed by Johnson (4), an unusually large number of endpoint assays were conducted. For instance, patterns and degrees of ossification were reported not just for vertebrae but for vertebrae at specific vertebral levels analyzed for portions of individual vertebrae, that is, centrum, arch (pedicle and lamina), and transverse processes (both left and right). Johnson noted that when so many parameters are examined, it can be expected that there will be instances of statistical differences occurring between groups that may not be biologically significant. Careful examination of the data regarding all endpoints (e.g., implantations, resorptions, litters, external viscera, and hard tissue status) showed marked effects at 250 ppm. In addition, at this dose there were slight effects on the maternal animal evidenced as a reduction in hemoglobin (g/dL) and on hematocrit. The conceptus tended to be smaller and have increased numbers of skeletal variations. No adverse effects on any aspect of maternal or developmental biology were observed at 50 ppm or below.

According to Johnson (4), the incidence of preimplantation loss at 10 and 50 ppm observed by Tinston and co-workers (116) should not be considered treatment related. Two reasons support this conclusion. First, no consistent dose–response relation was found (2.4% in controls, and 9.7, 14.3, and 6.2% in 10-, 50-, and 250-ppm groups, respectively). Second, concurrent control incidence was well below the historical control rate in this laboratory where implantation loss in controls in 10 other studies ranged from about 4 to 13% (4).

An elaborate study of 2-EE has been conducted in both rats and rabbits by Andrews et al. (117). Rats were exposed to 765 or 202 ppm of 2-EE vapor for 3 weeks before mating and then from day 1 through 19 of pregnancy. No significant effects were produced in the adult rats at 202 ppm, although marked toxicity was evident at 765 ppm. At 202 ppm, suppressed pup weight and an increased incidence of a variety of skeletal variations and developmental delays were observed. The same study was repeated in rabbits in which they were exposed from days 1 through 19 of pregnancy at levels of 0, 160, and 617 ppm, 7 days/wk and 7 h/day. The high dose of 617 ppm was severely toxic to the dams and markedly depressed maternal weight gain during pregnancy. At 160 ppm, this effect was less obvious but may be dose related. From these studies, the researchers did not identify a NOEL for either rats or rabbits.

In an attempt to identify a NOEL to rabbits (Dutch belted), Tinston et al. (118; see also 119, 120) conducted a standard Segment II study. Pregnant females were exposed to 2-EE by inhalation at levels of 0, 10, 50, and 175 ppm from days 6 to 18 of pregnancy for 6 h/day. The highest dose of 175 ppm increased the number of skeletal variations and minor abnormalities in the concepti but did not adversely affect maternal body weight or a variety of other adult toxicity endpoint parameters. At both 10 and 50 ppm, 2-EE did not adversely affect implantation, resorption, or soft or hard tissue when measured in these rabbit fetuses (4).

The studies by Tinston et al (116, 118) and Andrews et al. (117) of 2-EE suggest that 50 ppm is a likely NOEL for the fetus. It appears that 50 ppm is a no-effect level for developmental toxicity in two species (rat and rabbit) exposed by the route most relevant to humans. Comparing the available studies, it is clear that 2-EE is less potent than is 2-ME with respect to its developmental toxicity. In view of the consistency between studies and species, the criteria usually applied in selecting the size of a safety factor (121–125), and considering the results of testing involving similar glycol ethers (2-ME and 2-MEA), a safety factor less than 100 can be applied to this NOEL to estimate acceptable limits of exposure for humans (4, 121). In light of its favorable use in industry and these data, in 1982 the ACGIH TLV committee (83) set the TLV for 2-EE at 5 ppm (about 10-fold less than the animal NOEL).

2-Ethoxyethyl Acetate (2-EEA)

The National Institute for Occupational Safety and Health (NIOSH) has conducted some developmental toxicology studies on 2-EEA. Sprague–Dawley rats were exposed to 2-EEA by inhalation for 7 h/day from days 7 through 15 of gestation using a Segment II protocol (35). The maternal animal data are not available for analysis but the authors stated that maternal animals showed no overt toxicity. At concentrations of 594, 390, and 130 ppm, no adverse effects were noted in the mother; however, at 594 and 390 ppm, there were adverse effects on the embryo. The incidence of adverse effects was only minimally elevated at 130 ppm, indicating that this dose was at, or very near, the developmental NOEL for rats (4).

A state-of-the-art teratology study of 2-EEA has also been reported by Tinston et al. (126). Pregnant Dutch belted rabbits were exposed to 0, 25, 100, and 400 ppm 2-EEA for 6 h/day on days 6–18 of pregnancy and sacrificed on day 29, at which point fetal evaluations were conducted. In addition to the usual toxicologic endpoint assays characteristic of a Segment II type of developmental toxicity test, numerous maternal hematologic assays were also reported (4). Toxicity in the adult rabbits was observed at 400 ppm. Both maternal food intake and weight gain during treatment were significantly reduced. Similarly, hemoglobin (g/dL) in maternal blood was significantly reduced in the 400-ppm group. Exposure to 100 or 25 ppm did not affect pregnant females beyond body weight effects during days 6–18—effects that are possibly associated with reduced feed intake (4). The rabbit fetuses from mothers exposed to the maternally toxic concentration of 400 ppm showed significantly increased incidences of developmental variations as well as major and minor defects of both soft and hard tissues. In some assays, for example, fetal weights and skeletal development, offspring whose mothers were exposed to 100 ppm may also have been adversely affected to a minor extent. Exposure to 25 ppm produced no adverse effect of any type on embryonic or fetal development. Therefore, for this study a NOEL of 25 ppm was identified in rabbits.

Recently, Tyl et al. (41) studied 2-EEA and found that inhalation exposure of pregnant

New Zealand white rabbits during organogenesis resulted in maternal toxicity at 100–300 ppm, embryotoxicity at 200 and 300 ppm, and fetotoxicity at 100–300 ppm. Significant increases in malformations were observed at 200 and 300 ppm. Exposure of pregnant Fischer 344 rats to 2-EEA during organogenesis resulted in maternal toxicity at 100–300 ppm, embryotoxicity at 300 ppm, and fetotoxicity at 100–300 ppm. Significant increases in malformations were seen at 200 and 300 ppm. Importantly, they noted that exposure concentrations which produced embryofetal toxicity (including teratogenicity) also resulted in maternal toxicity in both species; thus, the A/D ratio was close to unity (23). Exposure of rabbits and rats to 50 ppm resulted in no maternal, embryonic, or fetal toxicity and no increased incidence of malformations or variations; that is, 50 ppm is the no observable effect level (NOEL).

In light of the results of these three studies, a NOEL of 100 ppm has been identified for the adult rabbits (A) and exposures of 25 ppm produced no adverse effects on the offspring (D), for example, A/D of 4. Based on these data, the developmental toxicity of 2-EEA is somewhat less than that of the parent molecule (2-EE). This was acknowledged by the ACGIH TLV committee (83) for 2-ME and 2-EE when it was noted that "on an equimolar basis, the respective acetate esters were about as potent as 2-methoxyethanol and 2-ethoxyethanol in producing testicular effects and leukopenia." This observation is consistent with the likely metabolism of the acetates and the results of toxicity tests of 2-MEA and 2-EEA.

Adequacy of the TLVs

Table 5 summarizes the developmental toxicity data that have been gathered on these glycol ethers and presents the A/D ratios. Johnson (23, 24) has observed that, in general, most chemicals that have been tested have A/D ratios near unity.

The studies of Hanley et al. (105, 106) indicate that 2-ME presents a moderate developmental hazard to humans since it has an A/D ratio of 1 in rabbits and no greater than 5 in mice and rats. As noted previously, the data of Horton et al. (26) indicated that the A/D ratio for 2-ME in the mouse was about 6.0; however, the A/D ratio would almost certainly have been less than 5 had the animals been dosed throughout their pregnancy. This example is important since it illustrates that for the A/D ratio to be useful, the conditions of the Segment II study must be used or the results will not be comparable between studies (24). Since 2-MEA is metabolized to 2-ME (in vivo), it will be assumed that the A/D for 2-MEA is also between 1 and 5. Based on the available data, the current TLV of 5 ppm for 2-ME and 2-MEA appears to contain a relatively small margin of safety against developmental effects since it is only two fold lower than its NOEL for developmental effects. A TLV in the range of 1–2 ppm, about 5–10 fold lower than the animal NOEL, would be more appropriate.

Table 6 lists the results of tests that evaluated the reproductive potential of 2-ME. The data indicate that the NOEL for adverse reproductive outcome for 2-ME is about 30 ppm in the three species tested. In light of the sixfold margin of safety, it can be expected that as long as exposures are controlled to levels below the current ACGIH TLV (5 ppm), no adverse effects on reproductive potential would be expected to occur in workers. However, in light of its potential effect on semen, the larger margin of safety afforded by a TLV of 1 or 2 ppm seems advisable.

Tinston et al. (116, 118) and Andrews (117) identified a maternal NOEL of 200 ppm for 2-EE while the NOEL for developmental effects in offspring was 50 ppm. The resulting A/D ratio of 4 categories 2-EE as a chemical posing a moderate developmental hazard to humans (23). Since the current TLV of 5 ppm for 2-EE is 10-fold less than the NOEL for developmental effects in test animals, this uncertainty factor appears to be minimal especially since dermal uptake must be negligible if this margin of safety is to be realized.

The hazard posed by exposure to 2-EEA is similar in magnitude to that of 2-EE. Although it is not stated explicitly, Nelson et al. (35) apparently found no toxicity in female rats exposed to concentrations up to 594 ppm. Based on information in their study and the study by Tinston et al. (126), it appears that no effects on development were observed in offspring following exposures to 100 ppm. Thus, the data suggest that 2-EEA has an A/D ratio of about 5. The current TLV of 5 ppm is 20-fold less than the animal NOEL; consequently, even though it has a moderate A/D ratio, the TLV seems appropriate.

Occupational Exposure

The Semiconductor Industry Association (SIA), a trade organization, conducted an industry-wide survey of industrial hygiene air sampling data during 1984–1985 in an attempt to describe the typical levels of exposure to several of the glycol ethers and their derivatives (Fig. 3). A total of 277 samples of workplace air were provided by seven member companies. It was estimated that these data represent about 60% of all the industrial hygiene data (personal samples) on these chemicals which had been collected by member firms up to 1984. Based on discussions with industrial hygienists from member companies, these sampling data appear to be representative of the industry. The National Institute for Occupational Safety and Health (NIOSH) also conducted a study of the semiconductor industry in 1982 and the results of their 92 industrial hygiene samples, collected as part of their Health Hazard Evaluation Program, were found to be comparable to those collected by the firms and are included in this assessment (81). In short, the data used to estimate employee exposure to these glycol ethers (both personal and area sampling) were based on a total of almost 400 air samples and appear to be representative of the industry.

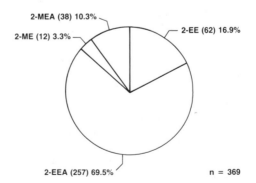

Figure 3. Distribution of industrial hygiene air sampling data collected among seven different firms in the semiconductor industry (1982–1985). Samples were assayed for 2-methoxyethanol (2-ME), 2-methoxyethanol acetate (2-MEA), 2-ethoxyethanol (2-EE), and 2-ethoxyethanol acetate (2-EEA).

Sampling and Analytical Methods

In workplace air monitoring studies of this industry, NIOSH Methods S361 and S79 were used to collect and identify 2-ME/2-MEA and 2-EE/2-EEA, respectively (127). The methodology involves drawing air through a charcoal tube (100 mg/50 mg) at a flow rate of 0.1–0.2 L/min. The glycol ethers were absorbed on coconut-based activated charcoal granules. Following collection, the glycol ethers were eluted (desorbed) with a solution of 5% methanol in methylene chloride. Samples are allowed to sit for 30 min prior to removal of an aliquot for subsequent analysis. The desorption efficiency was about 90% A 5-μL sample was injected into a gas chromatograph equipped with a flame ionization detecter. A variety of chromatographic columns are suitable for this analysis. A 10-ft stainless steel column $\frac{1}{8}$-in. ID containing 10% FFAP on 80/100 mesh, acid washed DMCS Chromosorb W, or a 20-ft stainless steel column containing 10% FFAP on 100/120 mesh Supelcoport have been recommended. The limit of detection for most of the analyses in this study was generally 0.05 ppm. The range for the analysis was 44–160 mg/m^3.

Discussion of Workplace Exposure Data

Figure 3 illustrates the distribution of industrial hygiene air sampling data for the four glycol ethers. Of the 369 samples, 70% were for 2-ethoxyethanol acetate (2-EEA). Only 20% of the samples contained detectable levels of the glycol ethers (limit of detection was 0.5 ppm). Of the 74 samples containing detectable amounts, only 4 (5.4%) were in excess of 1 ppm. The four samples in excess of 1 ppm contained 2-EEA. Occupational exposure data such as these are best described by the log–normal distribution; accordingly, the statistical analysis of these data were handled in this manner (128). It is important to note that throughout the statistical analysis of the exposure data, the limit of detection of the assay (rather than zero) was used in those instances when no detectable quantity was measured. As a result, the calculated margins of safety are actually greater than shown.

Table 7 provides details concerning the type of air samples collected. Of the 69 total samples, 194 (53%) were either area samples or other than personal samples. The remaining 175 (47%) were personal samples of the breathing zone (BZ) of operators (140 samples) or technicians (35 samples). In the semiconductor industry, the term *operator* applies to persons operating production equipment involved on the line in the fabrication

TABLE 7. Distribution of Industrial Hygiene Samples by Chemical and Type of Sampling Scheme

Chemical	Number of BZ[a] Samples		Number of "Other" Area Samples	Total
	Operators	Technicians		
2-EE	30	5	27	62
2-EEA	90	26	141	257
2-ME	6	1	5	12
2-MEA	14	3	21	38
Total	140	35	194	369

[a]BZ, breathing zone.

area (manufacturing). The term *technician* applies to persons whose primary job function is either the maintenance, adjustment, or profiling a production equipment or delivery/removal of chemical used in or on the equipment.

Exposure to 2-Ethoxyethanol (2-EE)

As shown in Table 8, a sufficient number (32) of time-weighted average (TWA) personal samples were collected for persons working with 2-EE to describe typical exposure. The average concentration in air was 0.55 ppm, which is about $\frac{1}{400}$th the current OSHA PEL (200 ppm) and about $\frac{1}{10}$th the ACGIH TLV established in 1984 (5 ppm). More importantly, the geometric mean (GM) for these data is 0.36 ppm—about 30% smaller than the mean. This indicates that, as expected, the typical concentration to which this group was exposed is less than that suggested by the arithmetic mean. The geometric standard deviation (GSD) was 3.65 for this data set, suggesting that there is a fairly broad range over which the data are distributed.

The short-term personal samples averaged 0.56 ppm and had a geometric mean of 0.16 ppm. The lesser geometric mean suggests that the bulk of the samples were close to the limit of detection of the assay and that several high results skewed the mean. These results, however, are consistent with the TWA sampling results and are lower than might be expected since short-term samples are generally collected in an effort to identify those jobs or tasks that are expected to pose the greatest exposure potential.

A total of 24 area samples were collected and these had an arithmetic mean of 0.99 ppm with a geometric mean of 0.97 ppm and GSD of 1.26. Like the short-term personal samples, area samples are generally used to identify those tasks where the concentration of the air contaminant is likely to be highest. The good agreement between the mean and geometric means and the very small GSD suggest that, in the vast majority of situations, the maximum anticipated personal breathing zone concentrations (time-weighted average) of 2-EE in the semiconductor industry are well below 1.0 ppm. Although the number of short-term area samples is too small to be significant, the arithmetic mean and geometric mean are consistent with other sampling data.

Even though GSDs in the range of 3–5 are larger than that frequently reported in the literature (129), they are not unusual and perhaps are typical of those observed in firms who have industrial hygiene programs. There are several reasons why relatively large GSDs can be expected in this study. First, whenever the arithmetic mean and geometric mean are close to the limit of detection of the assay, even samples as low as 1 ppm can markedly affect the GSD. Second, the studies that have been published by universities and NIOSH, which suggest that GSDs in the range of 2.0 are more typical of a

TABLE 8. Summary and Statistical Analysis of Industrial Hygiene Air Sampling Data for 2-Ethoxyethanol (2-EE)

Sampling Data[a]	N	Range	Mean ± SD	Geometric Mean ± GSD
Personal (TWA)	32	0.03–0.7	0.554 ± 0.280	0.357 ± 3.651
Personal (short-term)	4	0.3–2.0	0.563 ± 0.959	0.164 ± 5.917
Area (TWA)	24	0.05–1.1	0.992 ± 0.195	0.969 ± 1.263
Area (short-term)	20	0.06–2.0	1.03 ± 1.372	0.346 ± 11.935

[a]All concentrations are in ppm (v/v).

well-controlled workplace, were obtained in settings much different from those addressed in surveys within industry. For example, the university studies are generally obtained in a relatively small population of workers, involve one company, often involve one or two production areas (often within the same building), usually are collected over only 1 or 2 weeks of time, and usually are collected during only one season of the year. In short, these studies often describe employee exposure over a relatively "narrow" window in time and for only one kind of process or job description.

In contrast to studies involving rather narrowly defined workplaces, these data sets were gathered from seven different firms. Samples were obtained from numerous semiconductor manufacturing processes, from buildings containing various kinds of local exhaust and general ventilation systems, differing sampling times, as well as other differences. Consequently, the GSD observed in this study, although greater than desired, is not suprising.

Exposure to 2-Ethoxyethanol Acetate (2-EEA)

Table 9 summarizes the results of 357 samples of 2-EEA, a robust sampling. Personal samples were collected on 98 different occasions for periods of about 6–8 h with certain samples collected over periods of 12 h. The arithmetic mean for these samples was 0.05 ppm, the geometric mean was 0.02 ppm, and the GSD was 4.8. The data range in value from the limit of detection of 0.001 ppm to a maximum of 0.5 ppm. These results indicate that persons in the wafer manufacturing process are generally exposed to levels less than 0.05 ppm.

The results of short-term personal sampling, which wre collected for periods of about 15 min, indicate that the average level of exposure was about 2.8 ppm and that the geometric mean was about 0.10 ppm with a GSD of 33. Based on these data and the enormous GSD, one cannot describe the likely range of short-term exposures. However, in light of the ample number of personal samples and a peak concentration of 18 ppm, it is unlikely that short-term samples would rarely exceed 20 ppm.

The 128 area samples, which represent a much more sturdy data set than the short-term personal samples, indicate that exposures in those manufacturing areas which were thought to have the highest concentration of 2-EEA are very low. Specifically, the arithmetic mean was 0.05 ppm and the geometric mean was 0.01 ppm with a GSD of 6. The short-term area samples indicate that when samples were collected during the tasks believed to produce the highest levels, the airborne concentrations were in the range of 1.0–2.0 ppm.

TABLE 9. Summary and Statistical Analysis of Industrial Hygiene Air Sampling Data for 2-Ethoxyethanol Acetate (2-EEA)

Sampling Data[a]	N	Range	Mean ± SD	Geometric Mean ± GSD
Personal (TWA)	98	0.001–0.5	0.05 ± 0.08	0.02 ± 4.82
Personal (short-term)	21	0.001–18.0	2.82 ± 5.41	0.09 ± 32.77
Area (TWA)	128	0.001–1.8	0.05 ± 0.16	0.01 ± 6.08
Area (short-term)	10	0.005–15.0	1.56 ± 4.72	0.06 ± 10.66

[a]All concentrations are in ppm.

Exposure to 2-Methoxyethanol (2-ME)

As shown in Table 10, fewer personal and area samples were collected for 2-ME than for the other glycol ethers. Six personal TWA samples were collected and they ranged in value from the limit of detection of 0.03 ppm to 0.80 ppm. The arithmetic mean of these samples was 0.22 ppm and the geometric mean was 0.095 ppm with a GSD of 3.3. These data suggest that the bulk of the TWA samples were in the vicinity of 0.10 ppm.

Only one short-term personal sample was collected and one short-term area sample was collected. These data are virtually uninformative. Only four area samples were collected and these showed an average concentration of 0.23 ppm with a geometric mean of 0.08 ppm and a GSD of 4.7. This high GSD is not uncommon in light of the few number of samples collected.

Exposure to 2-Methoxyethanol Acetate (2-MEA)

2-MEA was studied more thoroughly than 2-ME and the results are summarized in Table 11. Sixteen personal samples were collected and these indicated that the average airborne concentration of 2-MEA was 0.01 ppm and that the geometric mean was 0.01 ppm with a GSD of 1.0. As suggested by the GSD, none of the samples contained levels in excess of the limit of detection of the analytical method (0.01 ppm). Only one short-term personal sample was collected and only one short-term area sample was collected; consequently, no conclusions can be reached about these exposures.

TABLE 10. Summary and Statistical Analysis of Industrial Hygiene Air Sampling Data for 2-Methoxyethanol (2-ME)

Sampling Data[a]	N	Range	Mean ± SD	Geometric Mean ± GSD
Personal (TWA)	6	0.04–1.0	0.22 ± 0.38	0.09 ± 3.30
Personal (short-term)	1	NA[b]	26.0 ± 0.0	NA
Area (TWA)	4	0.03–0.8	0.23 ± 0.38	0.08 ± 4.72
Area (short-term)	1	NA[b]	26 ± 0.0	NA

[a]All concentrations are in ppm (v/v).
[b]NA means not applicable.

TABLE 11. Summary and Statistical Analysis of Industrial Hygiene Sampling Data for 2-Methoxyethanol Acetate (2-MEA)

Sampling Data[a]	N	Range	Mean ± SD	Geometric Mean ± SD
Personal (TWA)	16	0.01	0.01 ± 0.00	0.010 ± 1.00
Personal (short-term)	1	NA[b]	17.0 ± 0.0	NA
Area (TWA)	20	0.01	0.01 ± 0.00	0.010 ± 1.00
Area (short-term)	1	NA	18.0 ± 0.0	NA

[a]All concentrations are in ppm (v/v).
[b]NA means not applicable.

None of the 20 area samples, which represent a substantial data set, showed vapor concentrations in excess of the limit of detection (0.01 ppm). As a result of the GSD of 1.0 (which indicates that there was no variability in the data set) one can, with reasonable confidence, infer that concentrations of 2-MEA in the workplace will usually be lower than 0.01 ppm.

RISK ASSESSMENT

The EPAs guidelines for assessing the risk posed by developmental toxicants state that

> At present, there are no mathematical models that are generally accepted for estimating developmental toxicity responses below the applied dose range. This is due primarily to the lack of understanding of the biological mechanisms underlying developmental toxicity, intra/ interspecies differences in the type of developmental events, the influence of maternal effects on the dose–response curve, and whether or not a threshold exists below which no effect will be produced by an agent. Many developmental toxicologists assume a threshold for most developmental effects; this assumption is based largely on the biological rationale that the embryo is known to have some capacity for repair of the damage or insult and that most developmental deviations are probably multifactorial in nature. The existence of a no-effect level (NOEL) in an animal study does not prove or disprove the essence or level of a true threshold; it only defines the highest level of exposure under the conditions of the test that are not associated with a significant increase in effect. The use of NOELs and uncertainty factors or margins of safety are attempts to ensure that the allowable levels are below those that will provide a significant increase in developmental effects (EPA, 1986).

The *uncertainty factor* approach to setting limits of exposure is conceptually a simple one. The no observed effect level (NOEL) is identified from studies (generally involving laboratory animals, but occasionally involving humans) that have been appropriately designed and conducted to assess the toxicological endpoint of interest. Uncertainty factors are arithmetic factors of varying magnitude (10, 50, 100, or 1000), which are applied to the NOEL to account for biological variances so that experimentally derived data can be extrapolated for setting limits of human exposure. In general, safety factors have been identified for most forms of chemical toxicity, except perhaps cancer and heritable mutations. For example, it has been customary to add a 2000-fold safety factor to the 90-day NOEL for neurotoxic agents when establishing a tolerance (based on acceptable daily intake) for pesticides that might be present in foods. A 100-fold safety factor has often been applied to the NOEL obtained in a chronic toxicity study to estimate the acceptable daily intake of food additives (130, 131). This was based on the assumption that rats were usually 10-fold less sensitive than humans to adverse toxic effects and the most susceptable human was 10-fold more sensitive than the typical human. Numerous developmental biologists, toxicologists, and physicians have indicated that the safety factor approach should also be appropriate for establishing safe levels of exposure to developmental or reproductive toxicants.

For many years, the *margin of safety approach* has been used by regulatory agencies both here and abroad to assess the risk associated with particular exposure scenarios (4, 122–125, 130–141). Usually, a margin of safety (MOS) is the ratio of the no observed effect level noted in animals (in this case, effects on offspring or reproductive function) and the dose to which persons are expected to be routinely exposed. The greater the difference between the animal NOEL and the anticipated human uptake, the greater is the margin of safety, and therefore, the greater the degree of protection. Margins of safety can also be defined as the difference between an acceptable level of exposure—such as an acceptable daily intake (ADI) or an occupational exposure limit, for example, TLV—and the level of human exposure. One advantage is that it provides a quantitative framework by which scientists, regulators, and the public can easily assess the degree of risk, or conversely, the freedom from harm, when a chemical is used in a particular way.

The following comments from a recent paper (135) represents a good review of the philosophical bases for thresholds:

> The prediction of thresholds for biological effects elicited by physical and chemical agents arises mainly from two broad categories of knowledge: (1) normal mammalian physiology (at all levels of organization); and (2) the response characteristics of the whole organism faced with exposures to exogenous substances.
>
> Investigations into the organismic, cellular, and subcellular functions of human and non-human mammalian organisms have revealed many important characteristics about the processes that protect the organism from the deleterious effects of outside influences. For example, it is known that, within limits, the body can protect itself from variations of external temperature, with some organs (e.g., the cardio-vascular system) having substantial versatility. For exposures to exogenous chemicals (i.e., zenobiotics), the body protects itself by: 1) controlling active absorption to limit the concentration in body fluids (Klassen, 1980; Schanker, 1971); 2) altering the distribution of a compound to modify concentrations at critical target sites (Klassen, 1980, Butler, 1971); 3) binding active chemical species (e.g., with sulfhydryl groups) and rendering a compound relatively innocuous (World Health Organization, 1978); 4) catalyzing the conversions of a chemical to a less toxic and more easily excretable form (Williams, 1949; Mandel, 1971) and at times increasing the catalytic rate (Gelboin, 1971); 5) redistributing an agent to body compartments far less susceptible to toxic influences—e.g., body fat—(Klassen, 1980); 6) requiring a minimum number of activated receptors to elicit an adverse response (Claus et al., 1974); 7) excreting a substance (Klassen, 1980; Cafrung, 1971); and 8) repairing damaged molecules and tissues (Robbins, 1964). For any given zenobiotic, all of these processes act in concert, each to a greater or lesser degree for an individual substances.

Overview of Risk Calculations

The data shown in Table 12 are the basic ones used in this assessment. For this analysis, the margin of safety (MOS) was defined as the ratio of the TLV (e.g., safe level

TABLE 12. The A/D Ratios for Selected Glycol Ethers and the Associated Risks for Workers Studies in the Semiconductor Industry (based on margins of safety)

Chemical	Hazard (A/D ratio)	Margin of Safety (TLV/exposure)[a]
2-Ethoxyethanol (ethylene glycol monoethyl ether or cellosolve) (2-EE)	1–5	14
2-Methoxyethanol (ethylene glycol monomethyl ether or methyl cellosolve) (2-ME)	3–5	53
2-Ethoxyethanol acetate (ethylene glycol monoethyl ether acetate) (2-EEA)	3–5	250
2-Methoxyethanol acetate) (ethylene glycol monomethyl ether acetate) (2-MEA)	4	500

[a]Margin of safety is defined as the current TLV devided by the geometric mean exposure of employees.

of exposure) and the geometric mean workplace air concentration. This appears to be the best available method for estimating the risk associated with developmental toxicants. For those chemicals where the TLV was not established to prevent adverse effects on development, the NOEL for developmental effects in a Segment II study divided by a factor of 100 could be used as a "preliminary exposure limit" (since this would represent the estimated human dose considered safe) if the A/D ratio was about 5 or less. When assessing the hazard posed by developmental toxicants, professional judgement needs to be exercised in selecting the appropriate safety factor for establishing acceptable levels of exposure since it should be influenced by the A/D ratio, severity of adverse effects, similarity of results between species, metabolic differences between species, and human experience. The margins of safety calculated in this analysis were probably greater than the actual value since the limit of detection for the air samples, rather than zero, was used in calculating the geometric mean exposure level.

Tests for developmental toxicity indicated that maternal exposure to 2-ME produced no adverse effects of pregnant adult rats and mice exposed to 10 ppm. Adverse effects on offspring were observed in mice exposed to about 50 ppm. In a 13-week experiment wherein rats and rabbits were exposed, a NOEL of 30 ppm was clearly identified. Based on all the available data, a NOEL of 10 ppm (in animals) seems to be a reasonable one on which to develop a quantitative evaluation of 2-ME.

Based on typical exposures in the semiconductor industry and the most appropriate occupational exposure limit—the TLV—the estimated MOS is 53 (Table 12). This MOS suggests that the risk of adverse effects on the offspring of exposed parents is insignificant for those employees who minimize or prevent dermal contact. Assuming that the TLV has been set at a level that was intended to protect the fetus, a margin of safety of one indicates that persons can, in general, be exposed to this hazard, yet not be at significant risk or injury.

Tests conducted by Andrews et al. (117) and Tinston et al. (116) indicate that adult pregnant rats exposed to 200 ppm of 2-EE were not adversely affected and no effects on development were observed in the offspring of mothers exposed to 50 ppm. It is noteworthy that there is a 10-fold difference between the 1986 TLV (5 ppm) and the inhalation dose that caused no adverse effects in animals. The 53-fold margin of safety between the TLV and the typical workplace air concentration suggests that this chemical is well controlled and that the offspring of pregnant workers should not be at an increased risk of adverse effects, assuming that dermal exposure is minimal.

The teratogenic potency of 2-EEA is roughly the same as the parent chemical, 2-EE. There is a fourfold difference between the dose that produced adverse effects on pregnant rabbits (100 ppm) and the dose at which no adverse effects were noted in offspring (25 ppm) (Table 5). The results of workplace air monitoring indicate that in the semiconductor industry, the airborne concentrations are quite low (0.02 ppm), thus providing a margin of safety sufficiently large that the offspring of pregnant workers should not be at increased risk as long as dermal exposure is minimized.

Pregnant adult animals and their offspring do not show adverse effects when exposed to 25 ppm of EEA. As shown in Table 12, the developmental toxicity of 2-MEA is approximately that of 2-EEA. The data indicate that there is a significant difference between the dose (vapor concentration × time) that produced adverse effects in the mother compared to the fetus (fourfold). Assuming that these data represent the typical workplace, the airborne concentrations are almost 5000-fold lower than the NOEL for offspring observed in animal studies. Consequently, assuming that skin contact is prevented or minimized, the offspring of pregnant workers in this industry should be at virtually no adverse risk of developmental effects.

SKIN ABSORPTION

During much of the past 40 years, the quantitative uptake of solvents through the skin of workers has been poorly understood and consequently often neglected by occupational health professionals. Recently, however, a number of toxicologists have developed tests to estimate the rate of dermal uptake using test animals and/or the skin of human cadavers. Jepson et al. (143) and McDougal et al (144) have developed some of the most sophisticated and accurate tests for estimating dermal uptake of vapors and liquids by animals. Dugard et al (1945) and Guest et al. (146) have specifically evaluated the dermal uptake of the glycol ethers. One shortcoming of animal tests is that human skin has generally been shown for a diverse class of chemicals to be less permeable to zenobiotics than the skin of rabbits and rats (147-148).

Dugard and co-workers (145) studied human skin (in vitro) and found that of the eight glycol ethers studied, 2-methoxyethanol (2-ME) was most readily absorbed (mean steady rate $2.82\,mg/cm^2 \cdot h$). For the monoethylene glycol ethers, they observed a reduction in the rate of absorption with increasing molecular weight or decreasing volatility (2-EE, $2.82\,mg/cm^2 \cdot h$; 2-ethoxyethanol, 2-EE, $0.796\,mg/cm^2 \cdot h$; 2-butoxyethanol, 2-BE, $0.198\,mg/cm^2 \cdot h$) and also within the diethylene glycol series: 2-(2-methoxyethoxy) ethanol (DM, $0.206\,mg/cm^2 \cdot h$); 2-(2-ethoxyethoxy) ethanol (DE, $0.125\,mg/cm^2 \cdot h$), and 2-(2-butoxyethoxy) ethanol (DB, $0.035\,mg/cm^2 \cdot h$). The rate of absorption of 2-ethoxyethyl acetate (2-EEA) was similar to that of the parent glycol ether, 2-EE. The absorption rates of diethylene glycol ethers were slower than their corresponding monoethylene glycol equivalents.

These authors noted that the results of their studies employing undiluted glycol ethers should not be extrapolated directly to solvent mixtures on a "rate proportional to concentration" basis, because components of the mixture may have a variety of effects on the absorption process. Based on their work, however, approximate absorption rates can be calculated for the most common glycol ethers.

Guest and co-workers (146) studied the rate of absorption of 2-EEA and 2-propoxyethyl accetate (2-PEA) in the beagle dog. Male beagle dogs were exposed to 50 ppm PEA or EEA for 5 h, and breath samples were collected during the exposure and a 3-h recovery period. Both compounds were rapidly absorbed through the lungs. After 10 min of exposure, the concentrations of the parent compounds in the expired breath were 5–10 ppm (80–90% absorption) and reached plateau values at about 3 h or 13 ppm for PEA (74% absorption) and 16 ppm for EEA (68% absorption). For studies of percutaneous absorption, $[^{14}C]PEA$ or $[^{14}C]EEA$ was added to undiluted compound and applied in a glass cell to a shaved area on a dog's thorax for 30 or 60 min. Blood and expired air were collected for 8 h and urine for 24 h. The pattern of urinary elimination for each compound was similar to that seen after intravenous dosing, with $[^{14}C]PEA$ being excreted more rapidly than $[^{14}C]EEA$. Although the excretion rates for the two compounds were markedly different, the absorption rates were similar. Estimated over a 60-min period, the percutaneous absorption rate was $110\,nmole/cm^2 \cdot min$ for EEA. This value is similar to those for other lipid-soluble compounds.

Although only about 30–60 chemicals have been studied in human skin (in vivo and in vitro), it appears that these four glycol ethers penetrate the skin at a rate similar to other solvents. For example, Piotrowski (149) determined that the dermal uptake of benzene, aniline, and toluene in humans (in vivo) was 0.4, 0.5, and $0.5\,mg/cm^2 \cdot h$, respectively. Dugard et al. (145) noted that compared with other solvents that have been measured using human epidermis, 2-ME has a very high dermal absorption rate.

Specifically, 2-ME penetrated the skin over 3 times more efficiently than 2-EE and 2-EEA, and about 10 times more efficiently than 2-butoxyethanol. Furthermore, 2-ME penetrates skin 4 times more efficiently than ethanol and 40 times more efficiently than n-butanol. Dugard and co-workers (145) have noted that the rapid absorption through human skin is in agreement with the clinical observations and results of pharmacokinetic studies by others who have studied 2-ME.

The following calculation illustrates the potential importance of skin absorption as a route of entry for the glycol ethers. In this example, it is assumed that a glove is heavily contaminated with 2-ME.

Scenario 1: Most of the glycol ethers have skin designations accompanying their TLVs, as do common solvents such as benzene, aniline, and trichloroethylene. Experimental data in animals (in vivo) and in humans (in vitro) indicate that the glycol ethers pass through the skin much like these solvents. For the sake of illustration, one can estimate how much 2-ME could possibly be absorbed (on an mg/kg basis) if a person has a heavily contaminated glove on one hand for about 30 minutes.

1. Surface area of the hands: $400 \, \text{cm}^2$ (Snyder, 1975)
2. Exposure time: 30 min
3. Rate of absorption: $28 \, \text{mg/cm}^2 \cdot \text{h}$

Uptake:

$$(400 \, \text{cm}^2)(2.8 \, \text{mg/cm}^2 \cdot \text{h})(0.5 \, \text{h})(\text{person}/70 \, \text{kg}) = 8 \, \text{mg/kg} \cdot \text{d}$$

Scenario 2: By comparison, how much 2-ME will be taken up by a 70-kg employee who is exposed for 8 h/d at the TLV of 5 ppm ($16 \, \text{mg/m}^3$), assuming an 80% uptake efficiency?

Uptake:

$$(16 \, \text{mg/m}^3)(10 \, \text{m}^3/8 \, \text{h workday})(0.8 \, \text{uptake})(\text{person}/70 \, \text{kg}) = 1.8 \, \text{mg/kg} \cdot \text{d}.$$

The calculations indicate that the uptake could be as much as $8 \, \text{mg/kg} \cdot \text{day}$ following 30 min of exposure. This dose is about four times greater than the predicted uptake of 2-ME when a person works for 8 h in an environment containing 2-ME at the TLV concentration. From this example, it is clear that the dermal route of entry can significantly contribute to the total absorbed dose.

Based on these data, a worker who is reasonably careless with respect to personal hygiene could easily take up more of the glycol ethers through skin contact than that taken up by inhalation of vapors at the TLV. Since the airborne concentrations of these glycol ethers in the semiconductor industry are a fraction of the current TLV, dermal uptake could easily be more important than inhalation.

DISCUSSION

The available toxicology data on these glycol ethers indicate that they can produce phase-specific developmental effects on offspring of pregnant animals. As noted by

Johnson (24), the A/D ratio for these chemicals is typically in the range of 1–5. Although the A/D concept is a relatively new one and additional data would be useful to confirm its merits, these values for A/D are sufficiently high to suggest that their potential hazard to humans should not be underestimated. Situations where dermal exposures are not well controlled could pose a significant hazard not only to adults but also to the fetus. Biological monitoring is very useful for estimating uptake of these kinds of chemicals, which can easily be absorbed through the skin. It appears that such methods are currently available for these four glycol ethers (64).

The results of the developmental toxicity tests, coupled with the workplace exposure data, indicate that workers in the semiconductor industry are exposed to levels of these glycol ethers which should not place them or their offspring at risk of adverse effects. The human hazard posed by these chemicals (A/D of approximately 5) is moderate. For comparison, the A/D ratio for thalidomide was about 20 in the four species tested. Among the four chemicals studied, the margin of safety for 2-EE is the smallest (14) while 2-MEA has the largest (500) (Table 12).

Some scientists have speculated that, in general, humans are less susceptible to developmental toxicants than rodents since there has been no apparent increase in other-than-normal births during the past 40 years even though there appears to have been a dramatic increase in human exposure to chemicals that are developmental toxicants. It has also been suggested that humans may have a more complex biological system for recognizing other-than-normal developing embryos and this may account for the high spontaneous abortion rate in humans. Others have postulated that the human embryo may have a more sophisticated detoxification and repair mechanism than lesser species, thus lessening the risks of adverse effects of exposure to xenobiotics. Physiological pharmacokinetic differences—that is, those differences between species such as average heart rate, surface area to weight ratios, ventilation rate, biochemical constants (e.g., V_{max} and K_m), and percentage of body fat—suggest that where the metabolite is the toxic moiety, for a given dose, animals are likely to be at greater risk of adverse developmental effects. Although no published papers have specifically addressed this phenomenon with respect to developmental toxins, some insight may be obtained from recent publications, which discuss techniques for estimating the toxic and carcinogenic response in humans based on the quantitative scale-up of animal data using biologically based disposition models (12, 150).

There are a number of uncertainties inherent in any risk assessment of a developmental or reproductive toxicant. Although our current understanding of reproductive biology and toxicology suggests that the approach used here should accurately describe the human health hazard, some assumptions and uncertainties should be recognized. First, metabolic differences between animals and humans are not uncommon and these are difficult to predict (150–152, 156). Such differences can result in greater or lesser production of toxic or nontoxic metabolites by humans when compared with lower species (rat or rabbit). In the case of the glycol ethers, such differences appear small given the similarity of the metabolic products between the four species exposed to 2-butoxyethanol (48). Miller et al. (126a) have demonstrated that 2-ME is likely to be metabolized by humans and rodents in a similar fashion.

Second, the possibility of delayed developmental effects in offspring also introduces some uncertainty into the risk assessment process. The field of behavioral teratology, which was been of considerable interest in recent years, has not yet developed "rules of thumb" that give much insight whether the offspring of humans are likely to be more or less susceptible to a given agent than the offspring of rodents. The purpose of a

Segment II test is not to identify those chemicals that might produce subtle adverse effects on the intellectual capabilities of offspring, and tests that clearly assess this hazard have yet to be fully developed. Third, the greatest uncertainty and concern is the possibility that the test species will underestimate the human hazard due simply to a difference in susceptibility.

Even though there are a number of uncertainties in assessing the human developmental hazard using animal studies, the historical experience of the 1970s and 1980s suggests that Segment II studies are an accurate and sensitive identifier of chemicals that might produce adverse effects on developing offspring. Since in these tests pregnant mothers are exposed to fairly significant levels of the test substances on each day following conception through early differentiation, proliferation, early growth, and organogenesis, we can feel confident that the tests aggressively challenge both the mother and the offspring during the most critical periods in the pregnancy.

More sophisticated techniques for estimating acceptable or safe levels of exposure from animal data are needed for both developmental and reproductive toxicants. Major advances in how best to scale-up data from rodents to humans should soon be realized when physiologically based pharmacokinetic models are used to predict the delivered dose to the embryo at various doses. At least in the near future, as noted by the EPA in their guidelines (3), the uncertainty factor approach needs to be used to estimate safe doses for humans. It results in a calculated exposure level believed to be unlikely to cause any developmental response in humans.

> The size of the uncertainty factor will vary from agent to agent and will require the exercise of scientific judgment, taking into account interspecies differences, the nature and extent of human exposure, the slope of the dose–response curve, the type of developmental effects observed and the relative dose levels for maternal and developmental toxicity in the test species.... Currently, there is no one laboratory animal species that can be considered most appropriate for predicting risk to humans (3).

Based on our understanding of the biological mechanisms surrounding developmental effects, and the susceptibility of rodents and rabbits, numerous scientific bodies and regulatory agencies have concluded that a threshold dose exists below which no adverse effects on offspring should exist. The exact nature of the developmental effects produced by a chemical may not always be identified in humans and experimental animals, but the concentrations (doses) at which developmental effects are produced tend to be very similar and only rather modest safety factors (2, 23, 24) are needed to allow the tests on these animal surrogates to provide a high level of protection for the human embryo. Specifically, if human exposures are maintained at levels about $\frac{1}{100}$th the NOEL observed in animal studies, experience suggests that the offspring of exposed persons should not be at risk of adverse effects. Uncertainty factors as low as 10 may be appropriate where ample experimental data are available or the human experience is favorable. Historically, the size of the uncertainty factor used to set acceptable limits of exposure for environmental contaminants has been much higher than those used in the occupational setting, justified primarily by the lesser number of exposed persons in the workplace and the concept of voluntary risk. The size of the safety factor can arguably be the responsibility of the risk assessor or the risk manager (3).

The available data on the reproductive and developmental toxicology of these glycol ethers should be sufficient to give a good indication of their qualitative and quantitative potential to affect adversely the offspring of exposed workers. By applying the concepts that have been discussed, and by using the inhalation exposure data that have been collected within the semiconductor industry, it can be concluded that workers and their offspring should not be at increased risk of adverse effects due to exposure to these glycol ethers, as long as airborne concentrations are maintained at current levels and dermal contact is avoided.

REFERENCES

1. J. Adler, Every parent's nightmare. *Newsweek*, March 16, pp. 57–66 (1987).

2. I. C. T. Nisbit and N. J. Karch, *Chemical Hazards to Human Reproduction*. Noyes Data Corp., Part Ridge, NJ, 1983.

3. Environmental Protection Agency (EPA). Guidelines for the health assessment of suspect developmental toxicants. *Fed. Regist.* **51** (185), 34028–34040 (1986).

4. E. M. Johnson, *A Synopsis and Critique of the Glycol Ethers Developmental and Reproductive Toxicology Data Bases*. Report to the CMA, 1984.

5. S. Fabro, On predicting environmentally-induced human reproductive hazards: An overall and historical perspective. *Fundam. Appl. Toxicol.* **5**, 609–614 (1985).

6. J. G. Wilson, *Environment and Birth Defects*. Academic Press, New York, 1973.

7. E. M. Johnson and M. S. Christian, When is a teratology study not an evaluation of teratogenicity. *J. Am. Coll. Toxicol.* **3**(6), 431–434 (1984).

8. National Research Council, *Risk Assessment in the Federal Government: Managing the Process*. National Academy Press, Washington, DC, 1983.

9. P. J. Gehring, P. G. Watanabe, and C. N. Park, Resolution of dose-response toxicity data for chemicals requiring metabolic activation: Example—vinyl chloride. *Toxicol. Appl. Pharmacol.* **44**, 581–591 (1978).

10. T. B. Starr and R. D. Buck, The importance of delivered dose in estimating low-dose cancer risk from inhalation exposure to formaldehyde. *Fundam. Appl. Toxicol.* **4**, 740–753 (1984).

11. D. Turnbull and J. Rodricks, Assessment of possible carcinogenic risk to humans resulting from exposure to Di(2-ethylhexyl)pathalate (DEHP). *J. Am. Coll. Toxicol.* **4**, 111–145 (1985).

12. M. E. Andersen, H. J. Clewell, M. L. Gargas, F. A. Smith, and R. H. Reitz, Physiologically-based pharmacokinetics and the risk assessment process for methylene chloride. *Toxicol. Appl. Pharmacol.* **87**, 185–205 (1987).

13. J. G. Wilson, In M. S. Christian, W. M. Galbraith, P. Voytek, and M. A. Mehlman, Eds., *Assessment of Reproductive and Tetratogenic Hazards*. Princeton Univ. Press, Princeton, NJ, 1983.

14. American Conference of Governmental Industrial Hygienists, *Threshold Limit Value for Chemical Substances and Physical Agents in the Workroom Environment with Intended Changes for 1985–6*. ACGIH, Cincinnati, OH, 1985.

15. W. L. Hart, R. L. Reynolds, W. J. Krasavage, T. S. Ely, R. H. Bell, and R. L. Raleigh. Evaluation of developmental toxicity data: A discussion of some pertinent factors. *Risk Anal.* **8**, 59–70 (1988).

16. M. D. Hogan and D. G. Hoel, Extrapolation to man. In A. W. Hayes, Ed., *Principles and Methods of Toxicology*. Raven Press, New York, 1982.

17. Food Safety Council, *A Proposed System for Food Safety Assessment: Final report of the Scientific Committee*. Nutrition Foundation, Washington, DC, 1982.

18. J. L. Schardein, Teratogenic risk assessment. In H. Kalter, Ed., *Issues and Reviews of Toxicology*, Vol. 1. Plenum Press, New York, 1983, pp. 181–214.

19. J. L. Schardein, B. A. Schwetz, and M. F. Kenel, Species sensitivities and prediction of teratogenic potential. *Environ. Health Perspect.* **61**, 55–67 (1985).

20. E. M. Johnson, Screening for teratogenic hazards: Nature of the problem. *Annu. Rev. Pharmacol. Toxicol.* **21**, 417–429 (1981).

21. S. Fabro, G. Schull, and N. A. Brown, The relative teratogenic index and teratogenic potency: Proposed components of developmental toxicity risk assessment. *Teratogen., Carcinogen, Mutagen.* **2**, 61–76 (1982).

22. E. M. Johnson, B. E. G. Gabel, and J. Larson, Developmental toxicity and structure/activity correlates of glycols and glycol ethers. *Environ. Health Perspect.* **57**, 135–140 (1984).

23. E. M. Johnson, A tier system for developmental toxicity evaluations based on considerations of exposure and effect relationships. *Teratology* (in press) (1988).

24. E. M. Johnson, A case study of developmental toxicity risk estimation based on animal data: The drug bendectin. Chap. 21.

25. E. M. Johnson and M. S. Christian, An overview of considerations basic to the extrapolation, evaluation and interpretation of developmental toxicity safety evaluation data: A short course. *Ann. Meet. Soc. Toxicol.* (1986).

26. V. L. Horton, R. B. Sleet, J. A. John-Greene, and F. Welsch, Developmental phase-specific and dose related teratogenic effects of ethylene glycol monomethyl ether in CD-1 mice. *Toxicol. Appl. Pharmacol.* **80**, 108–118 (1985).

27. J. F. Holson, C. Kimmel, C. Hogue, and G. Carlo, Data presented at the Toxicology Forum, Annual Meeting, Arlington, VA, 1981.

28. J. Rodricks and M. R. Taylor, Application of risk assessment to good safety decision making. *Regul. Toxicol. Pharmacol.* **3**, 275–307 (1983).

29. W. D. Ruckelshaus, *Risk Assessment and Management: Framework for Decision Making*, EPA Publ. No. 60019-85-002. USEPA, Washington, DC, 1984.

30. D. A. Karnofsky, in J. G. Wilson and J. Warkany, Eds., *Teratology: Principles and Techniques.* Univ. of Chicago Press, Chicago, IL, 1965, Chap. 8.

31. L. Lave, *Quantitative Risk Assessment in Regulation.* The Brookings Institution, Washington, DC, 1982.

32. N. A. Brown, D. Holt, and M. Webb, The teratogenicity of methoxyacetic acid in the rat. *Toxicol. Lett.* **22**, 93–100 (1984).

33. B. D. Hardin, R. W. Niemeier, R. J. Smith, M. H. Kuczuk, P. R. Mathenos, and T. E. Weaver, *Teratogenicity of 2-Ethoxyethanol by Dermal Application.* National Institute for Occupational Safety and Health, Cincinnati, OH, 1982.

34. C. C. Brown, High-to-low-dose extrapolation in animals. *ACS Symp. Ser.* **239**, 57–79 (1984).

35. B. K. Nelson, J. V. Setzer, S. Brightwell, P. M. Mathinos, M. H. Kuczuk, and T. E. Weaver, Comparative inhalation teratogenicity of four industrial glycol ether solvents in rats. *Teratology* **25**, 64A (1982).

36. B. K. Nelson and W. S. Brightwell, Behavioral teratology of ethylene glycol monomethyl and monoethyl ethers. *Environ. Health Perspect.* **57**, 43–46 (1984).

37. B. K. Nelson, W. S. Brightwell, J. V. K. Setzer, and T. L. O'Donohue, Reproductive toxicity of the industrial solvent 2-ethoxyethanol in rats and interactive effects of ethanol. *Environ Health Perspect.* **57**, 255–260 (1984).

38. E. J. Ritter, W. J. Scott, Jr., J. L. Randall, and J. M. Ritter, Teratogenicity of dimethoxyethyl phthalate and its metabolites methoxyethanol and methoxyacetic acid in the rat. *Teratology* **32**, 25–31 (1985).

39. B. K. Nelson, J. V. Setzer, W. S. Brightwell, P. R. Mathinds, M. H. Kuczek, T. E. Weaver, and P. T. Goad, Comparative inhalation teratogenicity of four glycol ether solvents and an amino derivative in rats. *Environ. Health Perspect.* **57**, 261–272 (1984).

40. R. W. Tyl, G. Millicovsky, D. E. Dodd, I. M. Pritts, K. A. France, and L. C. Fisher, Teratologic evaluation of ethylene glycol monobutyl ether in Fischer 344 rats and New Zealand White rabbits following inhalation exposure. *Environ Health Perspect.* **57**, 47–68 (1984).

41. R. W. Tyl, I. M. Pritts, K. A. France, L. C. Fisher, and T. R. Tyler, Developmental toxicity evaluation of inhaled 2-ethoxyethanol acetate in Fischer 344 rats and New Zealand white rabbits. *Fundam. Appl. Toxicol.* **10**, 20–39 (1988).

42. Environmental Protection Agency, *Preregulatory Assessment of 2-ME, 2-EE and Their Acetates.* Issued by G. Grindstaff, B. Cook and C. Scott, Exposure Evaluation Division, USEPA, Washington, DC, 1984.

43. Chemical Regulation Reporter, *Glycol Ethers: EPA Refers Regulatory Control to OSHA Based on Widespread Workplace Exposures*, May 23, Vol. 10. Bureau of National Affairs, Washington, DC, pp. 229–230, 1986.

44. H. W. Werner, J. W. Mitchell, and W. F. von Oettingen, The acute toxicity of vapors of several monoalkyl ethers of ethylene glycol. *J. Ind. Hyg. Toxicol.* **25**, 157–163 (1943).

45. H. W. Werner, C. Z. Nawrocki, J. W. Mitchell, and W. F. von Oettingen, Effects of repeated exposures to rats to vapors of monoalkyl ethylene glycol ethers. *J. Ind. Hyg. Toxicol.* **25**, 374–379 (1943).

46. C. P. Carpenter and H. F. Smyth. Jr., Chemical burns of the rabbit cornea. *Am. J. Ophthalmol.* **29**, 1363–1366 (1946).

47. H. W. Werner, J. W. Mitchell, and W. F. von Oettingen, Effects of repeated exposure of dogs to monoalkyl ethylene glycol ether vapors. *J. Ind. Hyg. Toxicol.* **25**, 409–414 (1943).

48. C. P. Carpenter, V. C. Pozzani, C. S. Weil, J. H. Nair, III, G. A. Keck, and H. F. Smyth, Jr., The toxicity of butyl cellosolve solvent. *AMA Arch. Ind. Health* **14**, 114–131 (1956).

49. F. Flury and W. Wirth, *Arch. Gewerbepathol. Gewerbehyg.* **5**, 52 (1933–1934), cited in *Toxicology and Hygiene of Industrial Solvents*, Williams & Wilkins, Baltimore, MD, 1943, p. 289.

50. C. E. Parsons and M. E. M. Parsons, Toxic encephalopathy and "granulopenic anemia" due to volatile solvents in industry: Report of two cases. *J. Ind. Hyg. Toxicol.* **20**, 124–133 (1938).

51. L. Greenburg, M. R. Mayers, L. J. Goldwater, W. J. Burke, and S. Moskowitz, Health hazards in the manufacture of "fused collars." I. Exposure to ethylene glycol monomethyl ether. *J. Ind. Hyg. Toxicol.* **20**, 134–147 (1937).

52. L. Greenburg, M. R. Mayers, L. J. Goldwater, and W. J. Burke, Health hazards in the manufacture of "fused collars." II. Exposure to acetone-methanol. *J. Ind. Hyg. Toxicol.* **20**, 148–154 (1937).

53. L. Greenburg, Toxic concentrations of ethylene glycol monomethyl ether. *Ind. Bull., N. Y. State Dep. Labor* **17**(6), 1–4 (1937).

54. E. Gross, in K. B. Lehmann and F. Flury, Eds., *Toxicology and Hygiene of Industrial Solvents.* Williams & Wilkins, Baltimore, MD, 1943, p. 287.

55. E. G. Young and L. B. Wooner, A case of fatal poisoning from 2-methoxyethanol. *J. Ind. Hyg. Toxicol.* **28**, 267–268 (1946).

56. M. R. Zavon, Methyl cellosolve intoxication. *Am. Ind. Hyg. Assoc. J.* **24**, 36–41 (1963).

57. G. Ohi and D. H. Wegman, Transcutaneous ethylene glycol monomethyl ether poisoning in the work setting. *J. Occup. Med.* **20**, 675–676 (1978).

58. R. Cohen, Reversible subacute ethylene glycol monomethyl ether toxicity associated with microfilm production: A case report. *Am. J. Ind. Med.* **6**, 441–446 (1984).

59. Chemical Regulation Reporter, *Testicular Cancer Direct Result of Spray Paint Operation, OSHA Told*, May 15, Vol. 11. Bureau of National Affairs, Washington, DC, 1987, pp. 439–440.

60. C. A. Kimmel and D. W. Gaylor, Issues in qualitative and quantitative risk analysis for developmental toxicology. *Risk Anal.* **8**, 15–20 (1988).

61. M. L. Meistrich, Estimation of human reproductive risk from animal studies: Determination of interspecies extrapolation factors for steroid hormones effects on the male. *Risk Anal.* **8**, 27–34 (1988).

62. National Institute for Occupational Safety and Health, *Health Hazard Evaluation Report*, HETA 84-115-1688. Precision Cast Parts Corp., Dept. of Health and Human Services, NIOSH, Washington, DC, 1986.

63. L. S. Welch, S. M. Schrader, T. W. Turner, and M. R. Cullen, Effects of exposure to ethylene glycol ethers on shipyard painters. I. Male reproduction. *Arch Environ. Health* (1988).

64. A. W. Smallwood, K. Kebord, J. Burg, C. Moseley, and L. Lowry, Determination of urinary 2-ethoxyacetic acid as an indicator of occupational exposure to 2-ethoxyethanol. *Appl. Ind. Hyg.* (1988).

65. R. R. Cook, K. M. Bodner, R. C. Kolesar, C. S. Uhlmann, P. F. Van Peenen, G. S. Dickson, and K. Flanasan, A cross-sectional study of ethylene glycol monomethyl ether process employees. *Arch. Environ. Health* **36**(6), 346–351 (1982).

66. H. Pastides, et al. A preliminary case-control study of reproductive outcome in a semiconductor manufacturing facility. *J. Iocc. Med.* (accepted for publication).

67. Anonymous, AT&T shifts pregnant women from semiconductor lines. *Occup. Health Saf. Lett.*, January 22, p. 4 (1987).

68. J. LaDou, The not-so-clean business of making chips. *Technol. Rev.*, May/June, pp. 24–31 (1984).

69. S. Harper, Unknown variables: Assessing risks in the semiconductor industry. *Occup. Health Saf.* **55**, 28–38 (1986).

70. J. LaDou, *Occupational Medicine: The Microelectronics Industry*. Hanley Belfus, Philadelphia, PA, 1985.

71. Chemical Regulation Reporter, *IBM Will Study Safety of Workers in Company's Semiconductor Operations*, May 29. Bureau of National Affairs, Washington, DC, 1987.

72. San Jose Mercury News, *Semiconductor Industry Appoints Scientific Panel to Evaluate Chemicals*, June 12, 1987.

73. V. K. Rowe and M. A. Wolf, Derivatives of glycols. In G. D. Clayton and F. E. Clayton, Eds., *Patty's Industrial Hygiene and Toxicology*, 3rd rev. ed., Vol. 2C, Wiley (Interscience), New York, 1982, pp. 3909–4052.

74. R. L. Smith, Review of glycol ether and glycol ether ester solvents used in the coating industry. *Environ. Health Perspect.* **57**, 1–4 (1984).

75. J. B. Olishifski, *Fundamentals of Industrial Hygiene*, 3rd ed. National Safety Council, Chicago, IL, 1987.

76. P. H. Wald and J. R. Jones, Semiconductor manufacturing: An introduction to processes and hazards. *Am. J. Ind. Med.* **11**, 203–221 (1987).

77. P. Gise and R. Blanchard, *Semiconductor and Integrated Circuit Fabrication Techniques*, 2nd ed. Reston Pub., Sunnyvale, CA, 1986.

78. J. D. Cox, Industrial health hazard update of glycol ethers. *Annu. Meet. Electrochem. Soc.*, Abstr. No. 294 (1985).

79. V. L. Horton and R. A. Owens, The use of cyclic ketones in the formation of positive photoresists for IC applications. *Annu. Meet. Electrochem. Soc.*, Abstr. No. 293 (1985).

80. American Conference of Governmental Industrial Hygienists, *Industrial Ventilation*, 22nd ed. Committee on Industrial Ventilation, ACGIH, Cincinnati, OH, 1986.

81. National Institute for Occupational Safety and Health, *Health Hazard Evaluation of the Semiconductor Industry*. NIOSH, Cincinnati, OH, 1982.

82. R. Wade, R. Williams, T. Mitchell, J. Wong, and B. Tuse, *Semiconductor Industry Study*. Publication of the State of California, Dept. of Industrial Relations, Sacramento, 1981.

83. American Conference of Governmental Industrial Hygienists, *Documentation of the Threshold Limit Values and Biological Exposure Indices*, 5th ed. ACGIH, Cincinnati, OH, 1986.

84. C. P. Loreti and J. C. Nohrden, *Permeation of Protective Gloves by Glycol Ether Solvents*, IBM Report, IBM, San Jose, CA, 1983.

84a. Edmont Research and Development, *Chemical Resistance Guide Containing Permeation and Degradation Data*, 3rd ed. Becton Dickinson, NJ, 1986.

85. M. S. Christian, Assessment of reproductive toxicology—state-of-the-art. In M. S. Christian, W. M. Galbraith, P. Voytek, and M. A. Mehlmann, Eds., *Assessment of Reproductive and Teratogenic Hazards*. [Princeton Univ. Press, Princeton, NJ, 1983.]

86. World Health Organization, *Principles and Methods for Evaluating the Toxicity of Chemicals*, Part 1. WHO, Geneva, 1978.

87. D. L. Black and T. A. Marks, Inconsistent use of terminology in animal developmental toxicology studies: A discussion. *Teratology* **33**, 333–338 (1986).

88. K. S. Rao, B. A. Schwetz, and C. N. Park, Reproductive toxicity risk assessment of chemicals. *Vet. Hum. Toxicol.* **23**, 167–175 (1981).

88a. R. L. Dixon and J. L. Hall. Reproductive toxicology. In A. W. Hayes, Ed., *Principles and Methods in Toxicology*, Raven Press, New York, 1982.

89. K. S. Rao and B. A. Schwetz, Protecting the unborn. *Occup. Health Saf.*, March, pp. 53–61 (1981).

89a. R. L. Dixon. Toxic responses of the reproductive system. In C. D. Klassen, M. O. Amdur, and J. Doull, Eds., *Casarett and Doull's Toxicology: The Basic Science of Poisons*, 3rd ed. Macmillan, New York, 1986.

90. O. P. Heinonen, D. Sloan, and S. Shapiro, *Birth Defects and Drugs in Pregnancy*. Publishing Sciences Group, Littleton, MA, 1977.

91. K. Hemminki and P. Vinels, Extrapolation of the evidence on teratogenicity of chemicals between humans and experimental animals: Chemicals other than drugs. *Teratogen., Carcinogen. Mutagen.* **5**, 251–318 (1985).

92. R. R. Miller, E. A. Hermann, P. W. Langvarot, M. J. McKenna, and B. A. Schwerz, Comparative metabolism and disposition of ethylene glycol monomethyl ether and propylene glycol monomethyl ether in male rats. *Toxicol. Appl. Pharmacol.* **67**, 229–237 (1983).

93. A. K. Jonsson and G. Steen, n-Butoxyacetic acid, a urinary metabolite from inhales n-butoxyethanol (butyl cellosolve). *Acta Pharmacol. Toxicol.* **42**, 356–356 (1978).

94. D. H. Hutson and B. A. Pickering, The metabolism of isopropyl oxitol in rat and dog. *Xenobiotica* **1**, 105–119 (1971).

95. C. S. Tsai, Relative reactivities of primary alcohols as substances of liver alcohol dehydrogenase. *Can. J. Biochem.* **46**, 381–385 (1968).

96. A. H. Blair and B. L. Vallee, Some catalytic properties of human liver alcohol dehydrogenase. *Biochemistry* **5**, 2026–2034 (1966).

97. R. R. Miller, E. A. Herman, L. L. Calhoun, P. E. Kastl, and D. Zakett, Metabolism and disposition of dipropylene glycol monomethyl ether (DPGME) in male rats. *Fundam. Appl. Toxicol.* **5**, 721–726 (1985).

98. R. R. Miller, E. A. Hermann, J. T. Young, T. D. Landry and L. L. Calhoun, Ethylene glycol monomethyl ether and propylene glycol monomethyl ethers: Metabolism, dispositon and subchronic inhalation toxicity studies. *Environ. Health Perspect.* **57**, 233–239 (1984).

99. P. M. D. Foster, D. M. Creasy, J. R. Foster, and T. J. B. Gray, Testicular toxicity produced by ethylene glycol monomethyl and monoethyl ethers in the rat. *Environ. Health Perspect.* **57**, 207–218 (1984).

100. J. Yonemoto, N. A. Brown, and M. Webb, Effects of Dimethoxyethyl phthalate, monomethoxy-ethyl phthalate, 2-methoxyethanol, and methoxyacetic acid on post-implantation rat embryos in culture. *Toxicol. Lett.* **21**, 97–102 (1984).

101. D. B. McGregor, Genotoxicity of glycol ethers. *Environ. Health Perspect.* **57**, 97–104 (1984).

102. D. B. McGregor, M. J. Willins, P. McDonald, M. Holmstrom, D. McDonald, and R. W. Niemeier, Genetic effects of 2-methoxyethanol and bis (2-methoxyethyl) ether. *Toxicol. Appl. Pharmacol.* **70**, 303–316 (1983).

103. M. R. Plasterer, W. S. Bradshaw, G. M. Booth, M. W. Carter, R. L. Schuler, and B. D. Hardin, Developmental toxicity of nine selected compounds following prenatal exposure in the mouse: Naphthalene, p-nitrophenol, sodium selenite, dimethyl phthalate, ethylenethiourea, and four glycol ether derivatives. *J. Toxicol Environ. Health* **15**(1), 25–38 (1985).

104. P. T. Goad and J. M. Cranmer, Gestation period sensitivity of ethylene glycol monoethyl ether in rats. *Toxicologist* **4**(345), 87 (1984).

105. T. R. Hanley, Jr., B. L. Yano, D. Nitochke, and J. A. John, *Ethylene Glycol Monomethyl Ether: Inhalation Teratology Study in Mice*, Contract No. 6-20-Ter-Ih/Dow. Chemical Manufacturers Association, Washington, DC, 1982.

106. T. R. Hanley, Jr., B. L. Yano, D. Nitochke, and J. A. John, *Ethylene Glycol Monomethyl Ethers: Inhalation Teratology Study in Rats and Rabbits*, Contract No. 6-20-Ter-Ih/-Dow. Chemical Manufacturers Association, Washington, DC, 1982.

107. R. R. Miller, L. L. Calhoun, and B. L. Yano, *Ethylene Glycol Monomethyl Ether: 13-week Vapor Inhalation Study with Male Rabbits*. Dow Chemical, 1982 (unpublished report).

108. R. R. Miller, J. A. Ayres, J. T. Young, and M. J. McKenna, Ethylene glycol monomethyl ether. I. Subchronic vapor inhalation study with rats and rabbits. *Fundam. Appl. Toxicol.* **3**, 49–54 (1983).

109. K. Nagano, E. Nakayama, J. Oobayashi, T. Yamada et al., Embryonic effects of ethylene glycol monomethyl ether in mice. *Toxicology* **20**, 335–343 (1981).

110. D. M. Samuels, J. E. Doe, and D. J. Tinston, The effects on the rat testis of single inhalation exposures to ethylene glycol monoalkyl ethers, in particular ethylene glycol monomethyl ether. *Arch. Toxicol., Suppl.* **7**, 167–170 (1984).

111. K. S. Rao, S. R. Cobel-Geard, J. T. Young, T. R. Hanley, W. L. Hayes, J. A. John, and R. R. Miller, Ethylene glycol monomethyl ether. II. Inhalation, reproduction and dominant lethal studies in rats. *Fundam. Appl. Toxicol.* **3**, 80–84 (1983).

112. P. M. Foster, D. M. Creasy, J. R. Foster, L. V. Thomas, M. W. Cook, and S. D. Gangolli, Testicular toxicity of ethylene glycol monomethyl and monoethyl ethers in the rat. *Toxicol. Appl. Pharmacol.* **69**, 385–399 (1983).

113. R. E. Chapin and J. C. Lamb. IV, Effects of ethylene glycol monomethyl ether or various parameters of testicular function in the F344 rat. *Environ. Health Perspect.* **57**, 219–224 (1984).

114. K. Nagano, E. Nakayama, M. Koyano, H. Oobayashi, H. Adachi, and T. Yamada, Testicular atrophy of mice induced by ethylene glycol monoalkyl ethers. *Jpn. J. Ind. Health* **21**(1), 29–35 (1979).

115. D. W. Hobson, A. P. D'Addario, R. H. Bruner, and D. E. Uddin, Subchronic dermal exposure study of diethylene glycol monomethyl ether and ethylene glycol monomethyl ether in the male guinea pig. *Fundam. Appl. Toxicol.* **6**, 339–348 (1986).

116. D. J. Tinston, J. E. Doe, M. J. Godlay, L. K. Head, M. Killick, M. H. Lutchfield, and G. A. Wiekramaratne, *Ethylene Glycol Monoethyl Ether (2-EE): Teratogenicity Study in Rats*, Rep. No. CTL/P/761. Imperial Chemical Industries PLC, England, 1983.

117. F. D. Andrews et al., *Teratologic Assessment of Ethylbenzene and 2-Ethoxyethanol*, NIOSH Contract. Batelle Pacific Northwest Laboratories, Washington, 1981.

118. D. J. Tinston, J. E. Doe, M. Thomas, and G. A. Wiekramaratne, *Ethylene Glycol Monoethyl Ether (2-EE): Inhalation Teratogenicity Study in Rabbits*, Rep. No. CTL/P776. Imperial Chemical Industries PLC, England, 1983.

119. J. E. Doe, Comparative aspects of the reproductive toxicology in rats of ethylene glycol

monomethyl ether and propylene glycol monomethyl ether. *Toxicol. Appl. Pharmacol.* **43**, 69–75 (1983).

120. J. E. Doe, Ethylene glycol monoethyl ether and ethylene glycol monoethyl ether acetate teratology studies. *Environ. Health Perspect.* **57**, 33–41 (1984).

121. E. M. Johnson, Current status of, and considerations for, estimation of risk to the human conceptus from environmental chemicals. In M. S. Christian, W. M. Galbraith, P. Voytek, and M. A. Mehlman, Eds., *Assessment of Reproductive and Teratogencic Hazards*, Sect. II. Princeton Univ. Press, Princeton, NJ, 1983, pp. 99–116.

122. C. S. Weil, Statistics versus safety factors and scientific judgement in the evaluation of safety for man. *Toxicol. Appl. Pharmacol.* **21**, 454–463 (1972).

123. M. Dourson and J. Stara, Regulatory history and experimental support of uncertainty (safety) factors. *Regul. Toxicol. Pharmacol.* **3**, 224–238 (1983).

124. M. Dourson, New approaches in the derivation of acceptable daily intakes (ADI). *Comments Toxicol.* **1**, 35–48 (1986).

125. E. J. Calabrese, *Methodological Approaches to Deriving Environmental and Occupational Health Standards*. Wiley, New York, 1978.

126. D. J. Tinston et al., *Ethylene Glycol Monoethyl Acetate (2-EEA) Teratogenicity Study in Rabbits*. Report prepared for the Chemical Manufacturers Association, Washington, DC, 1983.

126a. R. R. Miller, R. E. Carreon, J. T. Young, and M. J. McKenna, Toxicity of methoxyacetic acid in rats. *Fundam. Appl. Toxicol.* **2**, 158–160 (1982).

127. National Institute for Occupational Safety and Health (NIOSH), *NIOSH Sampling and Analytical Methods*, Vols. 2 and 4. NIOSH, Cincinnati, OH, 1984.

128. S. M. Rappaport and J. Selvin, A method for evaluating the mean exposure from a log-normal distribution. *Am. Ind. Hyg. Assoc. J.* **48**, 374–379 (1987).

128a. R. L. Sielken, Statistical evaluations reflecting skewness in the distribution of TCDD levels in human adipose tissue. *Chemosphere* **16**(8–9), 2135–2140 (1987).

129. K. A. Busch and N. A. Leidel, Statistical design and data analysis requirements. In L. J. Cralley and L. V. Cralley, Eds., *Patty's Industrial Hygiene and Toxicology*, 2nd ed., Vol. 3A. Wiley, New York, 1985, pp. 395–508.

130. A. Lehman and O. G. Fitzhugh, 100-Fold margin of safety. *Q. Bull.—Assoc. Food Drug Off. V.S.* **18**, 33–35 (1954).

131. C. S. Weil, Selection of number of the valid sampling units and a consideration of their combination in toxicological studies involving reproduction, teratogenesis or carcinogenesis. *Food Cosmet. Toxicol.* **8**, 177–182 (1970).

132. D. W. Gaylor, The use of safety factors for controlling risk. *J. Toxicol. Environ. Health* **22**, 329–336 (1983).

133. National Research Council, *Drinking Water and Health*, Vol. I. National Academy Press, Washington, DC, 1977.

134. M. E. LaNier, *Threshold Limit Values: Discussion and 35 Year Index with Recommendations (TLVs, 1946-81)*. American Conference of Governmental Industrial Hygienists, Cincinnati, OH, 1984.

135. J. Rodricks, R. Tardiff, and D. Turnbull, *Review of Risk Assessments Contained in EPA's Preregulatory Assessment of 2-ME, 2-EE and Their Acetates*. Environ Corp., Washington, DC, March 23, 1984. (Prepared for the Chemical Manufacturers Association, Washington, DC.)

136. R. L. Zielhuis and F. W. van der Kreek, The use of a safety factor in setting health based permissible levels for occupational exposure. Part I. A proposal. *Int. Arch. Occup. Environ. Health* **42**, 191–201 (1979).

137. R. L. Zielhuis and F. W. van der Kreek, Calculation of a safety factor in setting health

based permissible levels for occupational exposure. Part II. Comparison of extrapolated and published permissible levels. *Int. Arch. Occup. Environ. Health* **42**, 203–215 (1979).

138. J. A. John, D. J. Wroblewski, and B. A. Schwetz, Teratogencity of experimental and occupational exposure to industrial chemicals. *Issues Rev. Teratol.* **2**, 267–324 (1984).

139. E. J. Calabrese, *Principles of Animal Extrapolation*, Wiley, New York, 1983.

140. D. J. Paustenbach, Occupational exposure limits, pharmacokinetics and unusual work schedules. In L. J. Cralley and L. V. Cralley, Eds., *Patty's Industrial Hygiene and Toxicology*, 2nd ed., Vol. 3A. Wiley, New York, 1985, pp. 111–277.

141. K. S. Rao and B. A. Schwetz, Protecting the unborn: Dow's experience. *Occup. Health Saf.*, March, pp. 53–61 (1981).

142. J. L. Schardein, *Drugs as Teratogens*. CRC Press, Cleveland, OH, 1976.

143. G. W. Jepson, J. N. McDougal, and M. E. Andersen, Dermal absorption kinetics of liquid bromochloroethane in rats. *Toxicologist*, Abstr. 256 (1985).

144. J. N. McDougal, G. W. Jepson, H. J. Clewell, III, M. G. MacNaughton, and M. E. Andersen, A physiological pharmacokinetic model for dermal absorption of vapors in the rat. *Toxicol. Appl. Pharmacol.* **85**, 286–294 (1986).

145. P. H. Dugard, M. Walker, S. J. Mawdsley, and R. C. Scott, Absorption of some glycol ethers through human skin in vitro. *Environ Health Perspect.* **57**, 193–198 (1984).

146. D. Guest, M. L. Hamilton, P. J. Diesinger, and G. D. DiVincenzo, Pulmonary and percutaneous absorption of 2-propoxyethyl acetate and 2-ethoxyethyl acetate in beagle dogs. *Environ Health Perspect.* **57**, 177–183 (1984).

147. R. C. Webster and P. K. Noonan, Relevance of animal models for percutaneous absorption. *Int. J. Pharm.* **7**, 99–110 (1980).

148. M. J. Bartek and J. A. LaBudde, Percutaneous absorption, in vitro. In H. Maibach, Ed., *Animal Models in Dermatology*. Churchill-Livingstone, New York, 1975, pp. 103–120.

149. J. L. Piotrowski, *Exposure Tests for Organic Compounds in Industry*. National Institute of Occupational Safety and Health, Cincinnati, OH, 1973, pp. 77–144.

150. J. R. Ramsey and M. E. Andersen, A physiologically-based description of the inhalation pharmacokinetcis of styrene in rats and humans. *Toxicol. Appl. Pharmacol.* **73**, 159–175 (1984).

151. T. Butler, The distribution of drugs. In B. LaDu, H. G. Mandel, and E. L. Way, Eds., *Fundamentals of Drug Metabolism and Drug Disposition*. Williams Wilkins, Baltimore, MD, 1971, pp. 44–62.

152. E. Cafrung, Renal excretion of drugs. In B. LaDu, H. G. Mandel, and E. L. Way, Eds., *Fundamentals of Drug Metabolism and drug Disposition*. Williams Wilkins, Baltimore, MD, 1971, pp. 119–130.

153. H. G. Mandel, Pathways of drug biotransformation: Biochemical conjugation. In B. LaDu, H. G. Mandel, and E. L. Way, Eds., *Fundamentals of Drug Metabolism and Drug Disposition*. Williams Wilkins, Baltimore, MD, 1971, pp. 44–62.

154. C. D. Klaassen, Absorption, distribution and excretion of toxicants. In C. D. Klaassen, M. O. Amdur, and J. Doull, Eds., *Casarett and Doull's Toxicology*, 3rd ed. Macmillan, New York, 1986, pp. 33–64.

155. E. M. Johnson, Cross-species extrapolation and the biologic basis for safety factor determinations in developmental toxicology. *Regul. Toxicol. Pharm.* **8**, 22–36 (1988).

156. W. Slikker, The role of metabolism in the testing of developmental toxicants. *Regul. Toxicol. Pharm.* **7**, 390–413 (1987).

157. B. D. Hardin and C. J. Eisenmann, Relative potency of four ethylene glycol ethers for induction of paw malformations in CD-1 mouse. *Teratology* **35**, 321–328 (1987).

GENERAL REFERENCES

Altman, P. L., and Dittmer, D. S. (Eds.) (1979). *Biology Data Book*, 2nd ed., Vol. 2. Fed. Am. Soc. Exp. Biol., Bethesda, MD.

Baker, H. J., Lindsey, J. R., and Weisbroth, S. H. (Eds.) (1980). *The Laboratory Rat*, Vol. 2, Appendix 1. Academic Press, New York.

Beck, F. (1976). Comparative placental morphology and function. *Environ. Health Perspect.* **18**, 5–12.

Beckman, D. A., and Brent, R. L. (1984). Mechanisms of teratogenesis. *Annu. Rev. Pharmacol. Toxicol.* **24**, 483–500.

Buelke-Sam, J., Kimmel, C. A., and Adams, J., Eds. (1985). Design considerations in screening for behavioral teratogens: Results of the Collaborative Behavioral Teratology Study. *Neurobehav. Toxicol. Teratology* **7**(6), 537–789.

Butcher, R. E., Wootten, V., and Vorhees, C. V. (1980). Standards in behavioral teratology testing: Test variability and sensitivity. *Teratogenesis Carcinog. Mutagen.* **1**, 49–61.

Chemical Manufacturers Association (1984). *Comments on EPA's Advance Notice of Proposed Rulemaking and Preregulatory Assessment for 2-ME, 2-EE and their acetates.* CMA, Washington, DC.

Claus, G., Krisko, I., and Bolander, K. (1974). Chemical carcinogens in the environment and the human diet: Can a threshold be established? *Food Cosmet. Toxicol.* **12**, 737–746.

Collins, T. F. X (1978a). Reproduction and teratology guidelines: Review of the deliberations by the NTP. *J. Environ. Path. Toxicol.* **2**, 141–147.

Collins, T. F. X. (1978b). Multigeneration studies of reproduction. In J. G. Wilson and F. L. Fraser, Eds., *Handbook of Teratology Research Procedures and Data Analysis*, Vol. 4. Plenum, New York.

Crouch, E. C., and Wilson, R. (1979). Interspecies comparison of carcinogenic potency. *J. Toxicol. Environ. Health* **5**, 1095–1118.

Davies, J. (1978). Developmental aspects of the male reproductive system. *Environ. Health Perspect.* **24**, 45–50.

Donlett, D. E. (1936). Toxic encephalopathy and volatile solvents in industry: Report of a case. *J. Ind. Hyg. Toxicol.* **18**, 571–577.

Environmental Protection Agency (1980). *Assessment of Risks to Reproduction and the Development of the Human Conceptus from Exposure to Environmental Substances.* EPA, Washington, DC.

Environmental Protection Agency (1980). Water quality criteria documents; availability. Appendix C. Guidelines and methodology used in the preparation of health effect assessment chapters of the consent decree for water criteria documents. *Fed. Regist.* **45**, 79347–79357.

Food and Drug Administration (FDA) (1980). Caffeine; deletion of GRAS status, proposed declaration that no prior sanction exists, and use on an interim basis pending additional study. *Fed. Regist.* **45**, 69817–69837.

Gaylor, D. W., and Kodell, R. L. (1980). Linear interpolation algorithm for low dose risk assessment of toxic substances. *J. Environ. Pathol. Toxicol.* **4**, 305–312.

Gehring, P. J., Watanabe, P. G., and Blau, G. E. (1979). Risk assessment of environmental carcinogens utilizing pharmacokinetic parameters. *Ann. N.Y. Acad. Sci.* **329**, 137–152.

Gelboin, H. (1971). Mechanisms of induction of drug metabolism enzymes. In B. LaDu, H. G. Mandel, and E. L. Way, Eds., *Fundamentals of Drug Metabolism and Drug Disposition.* Williams Wilkins, Baltimore, MD, pp. 253–278.

Guyton, A. C. (1947). Measurement of the respiratory volumes of laboratory animals. *Am. J. Physiol.* **150**, 70–77.

Hardin, B. D., Bond, G. P., Sikov, M. R., Andrew, F. D., Beliles, R. P., and Niemeier, R. W. (1981). Testing of selected workplace chemicals for teratogenic potential. *Scand. J. Environ. Health* **4**, 66–75.

Interagency Regulatory Liaison Group (1979). Scientific bases for identification of potential carcinogens and estimation of risks. *JNCI, J. Natl. Cancer Inst.* **63**, 244–268.

Interagency Regulatory Liaison Group (1981). *Report of the Subcommittee on Teratology Endpoints*, Workshop on Reproductive Toxicology Risk Assessment. IRLG, Rockville, MD, Sept. 21–23.

Jackson, B. A. (1980). Safety assessment of drug residues. *J. Am. Vet. Med. Assoc.* **176**, 1141–1144.

Johnson, E. M. (1983). *Quantitative Assessments of Reproductive Outcomes*. Prepared for ICAIR Systems Division, Cleveland, Ohio, under Work Assignment 23 (D-507-23-1), July 6.

Johnson, E. M. (1980). Screening for teratogenic potential: Are we asking the proper question? *Teratology* **21**, 259.

Johnson, E. M., and Gabel, B. E. G. (1983). An artificial embryo for detection of abnormal developmental biology. *Fundam. Appl. Toxicol.* **3**, 243–249.

Johnson, E. M., Newman, L. M., and Schmidt, R. R. (1988). Postnatal effects of prenatal insult. *Risk Anal.* **8**, 35–44.

Kavlock, R. J., and Gray, J. A. (1983). Morphometrics, biochemical, and physiological assessment of perinatally induced renal dysfunction. *J. Toxicol. Environ. Health* **11**, 1–13.

Khera, K. S. (1981). Common fetal aberrations and their teratologic significance: A review. *Fund. Appl. Toxicol.* **1**, 13–18.

Kimmel, G. L. (1985). *In vitro* tests in screening teratogens: Considerations to aid the validation process. In M. Marois, Ed., *Prevention of Physical and Mental Congenital Defects*, Part C. Alan R. Liss, New York, pp. 259–263.

Kimmel, C. A., Kimmel, G. L., and Frankos, V. (1986). Interagency Regulatory Liaison Group workshop on reproductive toxicity risk assessment. *Environ. Health Perspect.* **66**, 193–221.

Kolata, G. (1986). Blindness of prematurity unexplained. *Science* **231**, 20–22.

Lamb, J. C., Gulati, D. K., IV, Russell, V. S., Hommel, L., and Sabharwal, P. S. (1984). Reproductive toxicity of ethylene glycol monoethyl ether tested by continuous breeding of CD-1 mice. *Environ Health Perspect.* **57**, 85–91.

Lee, I. P., and Dixon, R. L. (1978). Factors influencing reproduction and genetic toxic effects on male gonads. *Environ. Health Perspect.* **24**, 117–127.

Manson, J. (1986). Teratogens. In J. Doull, C. D. Klaussen, and M. O. Andur, Eds., *Casarett and Doull's Toxicology*, 3rd ed. Macmillan, New York.

Meistrich, M. L., and Brown, C. C. (1983). Estimation of the increased risk of human infertility from alterations in semen characteristics. *Fertil. Steril.* **40**, 220–230.

Monie, I. W. (1976). Comparative development of the nervous, respiratory, and cardiovascular systems. *Environ. Health Perspect.* **18**, 55–60.

Murphy, L. M. (1965). Factors influencing teratogenic response to drugs. In J. G. Wilson and J. Warkany, Eds., *Teratology: Principles and Techniques*. Univ. of Chicago Press, Chicago, IL, p. 147.

National Institute for Occupational Safety and Health (1983). Glycol ethers: 2-methoxyethanol and 2-ethoxyethanol. *Curr. Intell. Bull., No. 39.*

National Research Council (1977). *Principles and Procedures for Evaluating the Toxicity of Household Substances.* Report of the Committee for Revision of Principles and Procedures for Evaluating the Toxicity of Household Substances. National Academy Press, Washington, DC.

National Research Council (1980). *Drinking Water and Health*, Vol. 3. National Academy Press, Washington, DC.

Nelson, G. O., and Harder, C. A. (1974). Respirator cartridge efficiency studies. Part V. Effect of solvent vapor. *Am. Ind. Hyg. Assoc. J.* **35**, 391–399.

Nelson, M. M. (1957). Production of congenital anomalies in mammals by maternal dietary deficiencies. *Pediatrics* **19**, 764–76.

Neubert, D., Barrach, H. J., and Merker, H. J. (1980). Drug-induced damage to the embryo or fetus. In E. Grundmann, Ed., *Drug-Induced Pathology*. Springer–Verlag, New York, pp. 241–331.

768   D. J. PAUSTENBACH

Occupational Safety and Health Standards (1976). Occupational Safety and Health Administration, Title 29, Code of Federal Regulations, Part 1910.

Office of Technology Assessment (1981). *Assessment of Technologies for Determining Cancer Risks From the Environment.* OTA, Washington, DC.

Oudix, D. J., Zenick, H., Niewenhuis, R. J. and McGinnis, P. M. (1984). Male reproductivity toxicity and recovery associated with acute ethoxyethanol exposure in rats. *J. Toxocol. Environ. Health* **13**(4–6), 763–775.

Palmer, A. K. (1981). Regulatory requirements for reproductive toxicicology: Theory and practice. In C. A. Kimmel and J. Buelke-Sam, Eds., *Developmental Toxicology.* Raven Press, New York, pp. 259–287.

Paull, J. M. (1984). Origin and basis of the threshold limit values. *Am. J. Ind. Med.* **5**, 227–238.

Robbins, S. L. (1964). *Textbook of Pathology with Clinical Applications.* Saunders, Philadelphia, PA. pp. 81–89.

Schanker, L. (1971). Drug absorption. In *Fundamentals of Drug Metabolism and Drug Disposition.* Williams & Wilkins, Baltimore, MD, pp. 22–43.

Scortichini, B. H. John-Greene, J. A., Quast, J. F., and Rao, K. S. (1986). Tetratologic evaluation of dermally applied diethylene glycol monomethyl ether in rabbits. *Fundam. Appl. Toxicol.* **7**, 68–75B.

Seleyan, S. G. and Lemasters, G. K. (1987). The dose-response fallacy in human reproductive studies of toxic exposures. *J. Occ. Med.* **29**, 451–454.

Sever, L. E. and Hessol, N. A. (1984). Overall design considerations in male and female occupational reproductive studies. In J. E. Lockey, G. K. Lemasters, and W. R. Keye, Eds., *Reproduction: The New Frontier in Occupational and Environmental Research.* Alan R. Liss, New York, pp. 15–48.

Shepard, T. H. (1983). *Catalog of Teratogenic Agents,* 4th ed. Johns Hopkins Univ. Press, Baltimore, MD.

Sleet, R. B., Gohn-Greene, J. A., and Welsch, F. (1985). Paw dymsmorphogenesis in CD-1 mice treated with 2-ME and 2-MEA in combination with ethanol. *Teratology* **31**, 48A.

Sleet, R. B., John-Greene, J. A. and Welsch, F. (1986). Localization of Radioactivity from 2-methoxy [1, 2^{14}C] ethanol in maternal and conceptus compartments of CD-1 mice. *Toxicol. Appl. Pharmacol.* **84**, 25–35.

Smalley, H. E., Curtis, J. M., and Earl, F. L. (1968). Teratogenic action of carbaryl in beagle dogs. *Toxicol. Appl. Pharmacol.* **13**, 392–403.

Smyth, H. F., Jr., Seaton, J., and Fischer, L. (1941). *J. Ind. Hyg. Toxicol.* **23**, 259–264.

Snyder, W. S. (1975). *Report of the Task Group on Reference Man.* Pergamon, Oxford.

Truhaut, R., Dutertre-Catella, N., Phu-Lich, N., and Huyen, V. N. (1979). Comparative toxicology study of ethylglycol acetate and Butylglycol acetate. *Toxicol. Appl. Pharmacol.* **51**, 117–128.

Tuchmann-Duplessis, H. (1983). The teratogenic risk. *Am. J. Ind. Med.* **4**, 245–258.

Wang, G. M. and Schwerz, B. A. (1987). An evaluation system for ranking chemicals with teratogenic potential. *Teratogenesis, Carcinog. Mutagen.* **7**, 133–139.

Weil, C. S., and McCollister, D. C. (1963). Safety evaluation of chemicals. Relationship between short- and long-term feeding studies in designing an effective toxicity test. *Agric. Food Chem.* **11**, 486–491.

Williams, R. T. (1949). *Detoxication Mechanisms.* Wiley, New York.

Wilson, J. G. (1973). Present status of drugs as teratogens in man. *Teratology* **7**, 3–16.

World Health Organization (1980) *Occupational Exposure Limits for Airborne Toxic Substances,* 2nd ed., Occup. Saf. Health Ser. No. 37. Int. Labor Office, WHO, Geneva.

Zenick, H., Oudiz, D., and Niewenhuis, R. J. (1984). Spermatotoxicity associated with acute and subchronic ethoxyethanol treatment. *Environ. Health Perspect.* **57**, 255–232.

23

A Physiologically Based Pharmacokinetic Approach for Assessing the Cancer Risk of Tetrachloroethylene

Curtis C. Travis, Robin K. White, and Angela D. Arms

Health and Safety Research Division, Oak Ridge National Laboratory,* Oak Ridge, Tennessee

1 INTRODUCTION

Risk assessment is a procedure that synthesizes all available data and the best scientific judgment to estimate the risks associated with human exposure to chemicals (1). Because of gaps in our current scientific understanding of the cancer-causing process, human risk assessment for chemicals that have demonstrated carcinogenicity in rodents requires the use of a series of judgmental decisions on numerous unresolved scientific issues. Major assumptions are based on the necessity to extrapolate experimental results (i) across species from mice or rats to humans, (ii) from the high-dose regions to which animals are exposed in the laboratory to the low-dose regions to which humans are exposed in the environment, and (iii) across routes of administration. Recently, physiologically based pharmacokinetic (PB-PK) models have been used to reduce uncertainties associated with these three aspects of extrapolation (2–8).

The purpose of this chapter is to present a PB-PK model that is capable of describing the pharmacokinetics of tetrachloroethylene (perchloroethylene; PCE) in mice, rats, and humans (6). Model predictions are compared with empirical data to demonstrate that the model can be used to describe the time course of PCE concentrations in mice, rats, and humans. Lastly, the PB-PK model is applied to long-term animal cancer bioassay data for PCE to provide biologically based estimates of the carcinogenic risk associated with human exposure to PCE.

*Operated by Martin Marietta Energy Systems, Inc. for the U.S. Department of Energy under Contract No. DE-AC05-840R21400.

2 TETRACHLOROETHYLENE

Tetrachloroethylene (perchloroethylene, perc, PCE), a moderately volatile chlorinated hydrocarbon, is a colorless, nonflammable liquid that has a chloroform-like odor. PCE has a molecular weight of 165.8 and is relatively insoluble in water (150 mg/L at 25°C) (9). It is used extensively as a dry cleaning solvent and as a degreaser in the fabrication of metal parts. Annual domestic production of PCE is approximately 300×10^6 kg (10).

PCE is ubiquitous in the environment. Although there are no known natural sources of emissions, 90% of total PCE produced is expected to be released into the atmosphere (approximately 250×10^6 kg/yr). Ambient air concentrations vary from trace amounts in rural areas to 10 parts per billion (ppb) or 0.068 mg/m^3 in some large urban areas (10, 11). Because of its low solubility, PCE is rarely detected in surface and drinking water; when it is, concentrations are generally low—between 1 and 2 ppb (10).

PCE has been detected in foods including dairy products (0.3–13 μg/kg), meat (0.9–5 μg/kg), fruits and vegetables (0.7–2 μg/kg), fresh bread (1 μg/kg), and oils and fats (0.01–7 μg/kg) (12). PCE levels of 0.5–29.2 μg/kg (wet tissue) have been detected in postmortem human tissue (12).

With the molecular structure $Cl_2C = CCl_2$, PCE is similar to the suspected carcinogens trichloroethylene ($ClCH = CCl_2$) and vinylidene chloride ($CH_2 = CCl_2$). PCE has been shown to produce a statistically significant increase in hepatocellular carcinomas in mice following both inhalation and gavage exposures (13, 14), but not in rats. Based primarily on the animal bioassay data, the EPA's Carcinogenic Assessment Group has classified PCE as a Group B2 compound, a probable human carcinogen. The International Agency for Research on Cancer (IARC) and the American Conference of Government and Industrial Hygienists (ACGIH), however, have not classified PCE as to its carcinogenicity (15). Because of PCE's widespread use and frequent detection in the environment, it is important to determine the potential carcinogenic risk to humans exposed to environmental and occupational levels.

3 PHARMACOKINETIC MODELING

Pharmacokinetics is the study of the absorption, distribution, metabolism, and elimination of chemicals in humans and animals (16). Predictive PB-PK models provide an effective approach for interpreting empirical data relating to pharmacokinetics (2, 3, 6, 17). These models use actual physiological parameters of the experimental animals such as breathing rates, blood flow rates, and tissue volumes to describe the metabolic process. These models can often quantitatively relate exposure concentrations (in air, water, or food) to concentrations of parent compound or metabolite in various tissues of the body, allowing the prediction of the relation between applied dose of a chemical and effective dose at the target tissue(s) (8, 18). A chief advantage of the PB-PK model is that by simply using the appropriate physiological, biochemical, and metabolic parameters, the same model can describe the dynamics of chemical transport and metabolism in mice, rats, and humans. The ability of PB-PK models to extrapolate between species significantly improves the risk assessment process for estimating human cancer risks from animal cancer bioassays.

A pharmacokinetic model divides the body into physiologically realistic compartments connected by the arterial and venous blood flow pathways. The PB-PK model for PCE

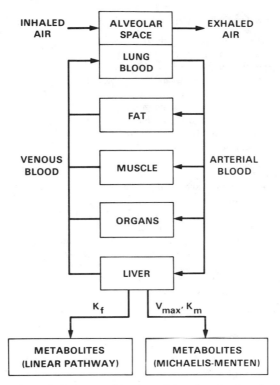

Figure 1. Diagram of a typical pharmacokinetic model used to simulate the behavior of PCE.

(Fig. 1 and Table 1) was patterned after the model developed by Ramsey and Andersen (2) and is described in detail in Ward et al. (6).

Tissue groups used in the model include (i) organs such as brain, kidney, and viscera; (ii) muscle; (iii) fat; and (iv) metabolic organs (principally the liver). The model is described mathematically by a set of differential equations that calculate the rate of change of the amount of chemical in each compartment (see the appendix). Metabolism, which in this model occurs only in the liver, is described using both a linear metabolic component and a Michaelis–Menten component describing saturable metabolism. Thus, there are three kinetic constants describing metabolism: the linear metabolic constant K_f (h^{-1}) and the two Michaelis–Menten metabolic constants V_{max} (mg/h) and K_m (mg/L blood).

The physiological and chemical parameters used to describe the pharmacokinetics of PCE are presented in Table 2. The parameters used in the model can be divided into three classes: physiological, chemical, and metabolic. The physiological parameters (such as breathing rates, blood flow rates, and tissue volumes) are well defined for mice, rats, and humans (19) and are fixed a priori before using the model. The chemical parameters describe the partitioning of a given chemical between air and blood and blood and tissues. These parameters can be determined in the laboratory using a vial equilibration technique (20), which allows for quantification of the blood–air and tissue–air partition coefficients. The tissue–blood partition coefficients are obtained by dividing the tissue–air partition coefficients by the blood–air partition coefficients.

TABLE 1. Nomenclature Used in Describing Physiologically Based Pharmacokinetic Model

Q_{alv}	Alveolar ventilation rate (L air/h)
C_{inh}	Concentration in inhaled air (mg/L air)
C_{alv}	Concentration in alveolar air (mg/L air)
λ_b	Blood–air partition coefficient (L air/L blood)
Q_b	Cardiac output (L blood/h)
C_{art}	Concentration in arterial blood (mg/L blood)
C_{ven}	Concentration in mixed venous blood (mg/L blood)
V_{max}	Michaelis–Menten metabolism rate (mg/h)
K_m	Michaelis constant (mg/L blood)
K_f	Linear metabolism rate (h^{-1})
A_m	Amount metabolized in the liver (mg)
Q_i	Blood flow rate to tissue group i (L blood/h)[a]
V_i	Volume of tissue group i (L)
C_i	Concentration in tissue group i (mg/L)
A_i	Amount in tissue group i (mg)
C_{vi}	Concentration in venous blood leaving tissue group i (mg/L blood)
λ_i	Tissue–blood partition coefficient for tissue i (L blood/L i)
$\lambda_{i/a}$	Tissue–air partition coefficient for tissue i (L air/L i)
k	Gavage or oral rate constant (h^{-1})
D_o	Total quantity of PCE absorbed via gavage route (mg)

[a]Subscripts: i for tissue groups or compartments; l, liver (metabolizing tissue group); f, fat; o, organs; and m, muscle.

TABLE 2. Physiological and Chemical Parameters Used in Describing the Behavior of Tetrachloroethylene in the PB-PK Model

	Parameter	Mouse	Rat	Human
Body weight (kg)	BW	0.024[a]	0.25	70.0[b]
Alveolar ventilation coefficient (L/h)	Q_{alvc}	21	22.2	15.2
Alveolar ventilation (L/h)	Q_{alv}	1.33	7.96	352.5
Cardiac output coefficient (L/h)	Q_{bc}	21	14.4	16.0
Blood flow fractions				
Total blood flow rate (L/h)	Q_b	1.33	5.16	371.1
Blood flow fraction in the liver	Q_l/Q_b	0.25	0.25	0.25
Blood flow fraction in the fat	Q_f/Q_b	0.09	0.09	0.05
Blood flow fraction in the organs	Q_o/Q_b	0.51	0.51	0.51
Blood flow fraction in muscle	Q_m/Q_b	0.15	0.15	0.19
Tissue group volume fractions				
Volume fractions in the liver	V_l/BW	0.06	0.04	0.04
Volume fractions in fat	V_f/BW	0.10	0.07	0.20
Volume fractions in the organs	V_o/BW	0.05	0.05	0.05
Volume fractions in muscle	V_m/BW	0.72	0.75	0.62
Blood–air partition coefficient	λ_b	16.9	18.9	10.3
Tissue–air partition coefficients				
Liver–air partition coefficient	$\lambda_{l/a}$	70.3	70.3	70.3
Fat–air partition coefficient	$\lambda_{f/a}$	2060	2300	1638
Organ–air partition coefficient	$\lambda_{o/a}$	70.3	70.3	70.3
Muscle–air partition coefficient	$\lambda_{m/a}$	20.0	20.0	80.0
Gastric absorption constant (h^{-1})	k	0.6	—	—

[a]With the exception of Buben and O'Flaherty (25) (0.04 kg).
[b]With the exception of Fernandez et al. (29) (83 kg).

TABLE 3. Metabolic Parameters for Tetrachloroethylene

Parameter	Mouse	Rat	Human
Body weight (kg)	0.024	0.25	70.0
V_{max} (mg/h)	0.11	0.068	3.5
K_m (mg/L blood)	0.4	0.3	0.3
K_f (h^{-1})	1.84	2.73	0.0

The metabolic parameters for a particular volatile compound can be determined either through closed chamber studies (21–23) or through optimization techniques to determine the best metabolic parameters consistent with empirical data.

Ward et al. (6) determined the metabolic parameters for PCE by fitting model predictions to species-specific empirical data. These parameters are given in Table 3. Comparison of model results with independent empirical data on inhalation and gavage exposures in mice, rats, and humans demonstrates that the pharmacokinetic model can be used to determine the time course of PCE in these species.

4   COMPARISON OF MODEL RESULTS WITH EMPIRICAL DATA

4.1   Mice

The metabolism of PCE in mice (B6C3F$_1$) was investigated by Schumann et al. (24). Mice were exposed for 6 h by inhalation to 10 ppm (67.8 mg/m^3) ^{14}C-labeled PCE and to a single oral dose of 500 mg ^{14}C-labeled PCE/kg body weight. Following inhalation of 10 ppm ^{14}C-labeled PCE, total metabolites were found to account for 88% of total radioactivity recovered, while unchanged PCE in expired air accounted for 12%. The reverse situation was observed after a single oral dose of 500 mg/kg. Approximately 83% was detected unchanged in expired air, while 17% appeared as metabolites. This shift in the major route of elimination is a result of saturation of the oxidative metabolic pathway; that is, metabolism could not rapidly reduce the high blood concentrations resulting from the gavage exposure, and therefore most of the PCE was expired.

Buben and O'Flaherty (25) also studied the metabolism of PCE in mice. Male Swiss–Cox mice were given PCE in corn oil by gavage five times a week for 6 weeks in doses of 20, 100, 200, 500, 1000, 1500, and 2000 mg/kg·day. Urinary metabolites were quantified to estimate the extent of metabolism. The fraction of each dose metabolized decreased with increasing dose, a result consistent with a saturable metabolic pathway. At low doses, about 25% of PCE was detected as urinary metabolites, while at high doses, only 5% of the administered dose was metabolized.

Since empirical values of the metabolic parameters for mice are not available, Ward et al. (6) determined values for these parameters (see Table 3) which produced the best fits with both the inhalation and gavage data from Schumann et al. (24) and the gavage data from Buden and O'Flaherty (25). Table 4 contains the experimental results of Schumann et al. (24) and the model predictions. In Fig. 2, model predictions (shown as a solid line) are compared with in empirical data (shown as vertical bars) from Buben and O'Flaherty (25). The graph shows the relation between PCE metabolism (amount of urinary metabolites in mg/kg excreted in 24 h) and dose. The model provides a good fit to both the inhalation data from Schumann et al. (24) and the gavage data from Schumann et al. (24) and Buben

TABLE 4. Schumann et al. (24) Data Versus Model Predictions for Mice[a]

Quantity	Data	Model Predictions
Inhalation of 10 ppm PCE for 6 h		
Total amount (mg)		
Metabolized + expired	0.4	0.37
Metabolized (%)	88.0 ± 2.3	88.3
Expired (%)	12.0 ± 2.2	11.7
Percentage expired over intervals		
360–540 (min)	7.70 ± 0.51	6.3
540–720	2.26 ± 0.95	2.8
720–1080	1.45 ± 0.53	2.0
1080–1800	0.41 ± 0.17	0.57
Gavage (500 mg/kg)		
Total amount (mg)		
Metabolized + expired	10.77 ± 0.51	12.0
Metabolized (%)	17.40 ± 3.9	18.6
Expired (%)	82.6 ± 4.6	81.4
Percentage expired over intervals		
0–180 (min)	32.3 ± 7.2	41.0
180–360	20.1 ± 3.6	20.0
360–720	26.9 ± 4.2	15.7
720–1440	3.14 ± 2.53	4.5
1440–2160	0.12 ± 0.03	0.17

[a] Body weight = 0.024 kg.

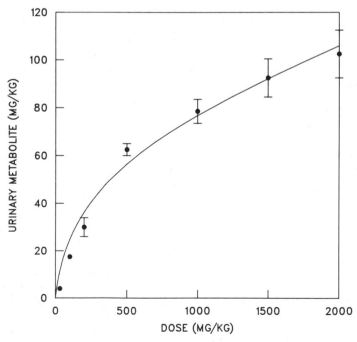

Figure 2. Model predictions of urinary metabolites of PCE as a function of dose. Based on the experimental data of Buben and O'Flaherty (25).

and O'Flaherty (25), substantiating the model's ability to perform correctly over a wide dose range for both inhalation and gavage routes of administration.

4.2   Rats

Adult male Sprague–Dawley rats weighing 250 g were exposed to ^{14}C-labeled PCE by inhalation for a duration of 6 h in experiments conducted by Pegg et al. (26). In the 72 h following exposure to 10 ppm, metabolism accounted for 20% of total radioactivity recovered, while unchanged PCE in expired air accounted for 70%. Pulmonary elimination of PCE in these rats had a half-life of about 7 h.

The biological parameters and partition coefficients used by Ward et al. (6) to model the empirical data of Pegg et al. (26) are presented in Table 2. In Fig. 3, model predictions (shown as solid points) are compared with the empirical data (shown as vertical bars) of Peggs et al. (26). The figure shows the percentage of PCE recovered in expired air in rats (for a number of different time intervals) following an exposure to 10 ppm PCE for 6 h. The vertical bars represent the range of the empirical data. The predictions and empirical data are integrated from the beginning of each time interval to the time at which the points and bars are drawn. Note that the length of the time intervals vary, causing the data points to be nonmonotonic. The model predicted that 68% of the body burden of PCE would be recovered in expired air during the 72 h after exposure, in good agreement with the experimentally determined value of 70%.

Adult male Sprague–Dawley rats weighing 250 g were given ^{14}C-labeled PCE orally in

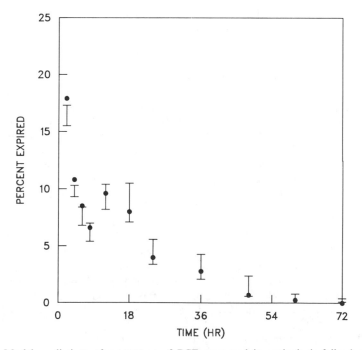

Figure 3. Model predictions of percentage of PCE recovered in expired air following 10-ppm inhalation exposure of rats for 6 h. Empirical data from Pegg et al. (26).

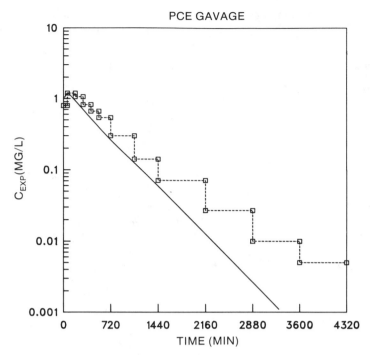

Figure 4. Model predictions of percentage of PCE recovered in expired air following oral administration of 500 mg/kg to rats. Empirical data from Pegg et al. (26).

corn oil in experiments conducted by Pegg et al. (26). In the 72 h following exposure to 500 mg/kg, metabolism accounted for 5% of total radioactivity recovered while unchanged PCE in expired air accounted for 90%. There was no significant difference in elimination half-life (approximately 7 h) with dose or route of administration.

In Fig. 4, model predictions of expired air concentrations (solid line) are compared with the empirical data of Pegg et al. (26). The model, based on parameters obtained from the inhalation study, slightly overpredicted the rate of elimination of PCE, which might be attributable to the effects of corn oil as a carrier. Withey et al. (27) and Angelo et al. (28) have shown that an oil carrier can affect the elimination pattern of volatile organic compounds like PCE.

4.3 Humans

Fernandez et al. (29) exposed 24 subjects to concentrations of 100 ppm of PCE for 1–8 h. During the first hours after exposure, the concentration of PCE in alveolar air decreased rapidly; however, Fernandez and his associates reported that more than 2 weeks were required to eliminate most (> 99%) of PCE retained following an 8-h exposure to 100 ppm.

The biological parameters and partition coefficients used to model the data of Fernandez et al. (29) are also presented in Table 2. Figure 5 shows the alveolar concentrations resulting from a 100-ppm exposure for various exposure durations

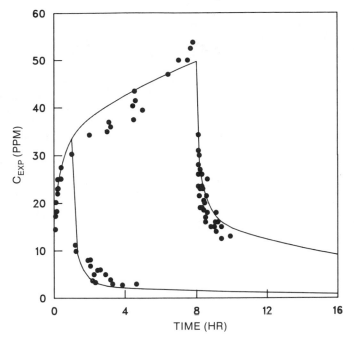

Figure 5. Model predictions of concentrations of PCE in human alveolar air following 100-ppm exposure. The exposure was 1 h for the data on the left and 8 h for the data on the right. Empirical data from Fernandez et al. (29).

reported by Fernandez et al. (29). The model results, calculated assuming 19% adipose tissue in humans, are shown as solid lines and are in good agreement with the empirical values.

5 ANIMAL BIOASSAYS

Several long-term bioassays have been carried out to study the carcinogenicity of PCE administered through either gavage or inhalation (13, 14, 30, 31). Because the dose–response data from Rampy et al. (30) and the original NTP (14) studies are ambiguous, only the NCI (13) and the final NTP (14) studies are discussed here. The National Cancer Institute (NCI) studied the response of mice and rats exposed to PCE through gavage (10, 13). B6C3F$_1$ mice were divided into two treatment groups for each sex, 50 animals per group. The male mice treatment groups received doses of 1072 and 536 mg/kg body weight per day; the two female groups received doses of 772 and 386 mg/kg body weight per day (10, 13). Osborne–Mendel rats were divided into similar treatment and control groups. Male rats received doses of 941 and 471 mg/kg body weight per day, respectively; females received 949 and 474 mg/kg body weight per day, respectively. The animals received PCE in corn oil through gastric intubation once a day, 5 days/week, for 78 weeks.

Results of the NCI study showed PCE to be carcinogenic in mice, inducing highly statistically significant increases in hepatocellular carcinomas in both sexes of mice when

TABLE 5. Incidence of Hepatocellular Carcinomas in B6C3F₁ Mice Fed PCE

	Dose (mg/kg·day)	Number of Animals	TBA[a]	Incidence (%)
Males	0	17	2	12
	Vehicle-control	20	2	10
	536	49	32	65
	1072	48	27	56
Females	0	20	2	10
	Vehicle-control	20	0	0
	386	48	19	40
	772	48	19	40

[a]Tumor-bearing animals.
Source: Ref. 13.

TABLE 6. Incidence of Hepatocellular Carcinomas in B6C3F₁ Mice Exposed to PCE Inhalation

	Dose (ppm)	Number of Animals	TBA[a]	Incidence (%)
Males	0	49	7	14
	100	49	25	51
	200	50	26	52
Female	0	48	1	2
	100	50	13	26
	200	50	36	72

[a]Tumor-bearing animals.
Source: Ref. 14.

compared to the incidence of tumors in either the vehicle-control or untreated control groups (10). In male mice, PCE-treated animals showed increased incidence over controls of 53 and 44%. Both treatment groups of female mice displayed increased incidence over controls of 30% (Table 5). Because of the low survival rates in rats, no conclusions could be drawn from this study about PCE's carcinogenicity in rats.

A second long-term animal study by the National Toxicology Program (NTP) examined the effects on B6C3F₁ mice and F344/N rats exposed to PCE through inhalaton 6 h/day, 5 days/week, for 2 years. Exposure concentrations used were 100 and 200 ppm in mice and 200 and 400 ppm in rats (32). In mice, PCE produced a statistically significant increase in the incidence of heptatocellular carcinomas at both treatment concentrations. In males, after the background rate of the control group was deducted, incidence rates were 37 and 38% for the respective exposure levels. In females, the effective incidence rates were 24 and 70% (Table 6).

In rats, PCE produced no increase in the incidence of hepatocellular carcinomas in the females and a slight increase in the males (14). In the males after deduction of the background rates, there was a 6% increase at the 200-ppm dose level and a 2% increase at the 400-ppm dose level (Table 7). These increases were not statistically significant.

TABLE 7. Incidence of Hepatocellular Carcinomas in F344/N Male Rats Exposed to PCE Inhalation

Dose (ppm)	Number of Animals	TBA[a]	Incidence (%)
0	50	4	8
200	50	7	14
400	49	5	10

[a]Tumor-bearing animals.
Source: Ref. 14.

6   ANALYSIS OF BIOASSAY DATA

The PB-PK model for PCE of Ward et al. (6) can be adapted to analyze the data from the animal bioassays. Using the exposure rate, exposure time, and route of administration from each of the bioassays (the gavage study from NCI and the inhalation study from NTP), total metabolite production under each of the animal bioassay protocols (33) can be evaluated.

The metabolic pathways of PCE are still speculative, but there is convincing evidence that the principal site of metabolism is the hepatic microsomal cytochrome P-450 system. The first product of this system is thought to be a highly reactive, epoxide intermediate, 1, 1, 2, 2-tetrachloroethylene oxide (34–36), which then rearranges to form PCE's most prominent metabolite, trichloroacetic acid (TCA) (10, 37–39). The epoxide intermediate has been shown to bind in vitro and in vivo to cellular macromolecules (24, 26, 32, 39). Both the epoxide and the ultimate metabolite, TCA, have been indicated as putative carcinogenic moieties (10, 37).

In addition to this primary TCA pathway, PCE is believed to be metabolized also by secondary pathways that produce other principal metabolites, oxalic acid and CO_2. The results of Yllner (40), Dmitrieva (41), Pegg et al. (26), and Schumann et al. (24) are consistent with the existence of secondary pathways of PCE metabolism, but these pathways have not yet been identified.

For purposes of this study, we assume that PCE is metabolized by two pathways. The first is a nonlinear pathway that acts by mixed function oxidative (MFO) reactions to produce PCE oxide and TCA. The second is a linear pathway (LP) that acts by as yet unidentified mechanisms to produce other metabolites. Our initial approach is to compare cancer incidence with total applied dose and with the amount of metabolite produced by the linear pathway and the amount of metabolite formed in the nonlinear mixed function oxidase pathway.

Figure 6 presents cancer incidence versus applied dose for both the NCI and NTP bioassays. For the gavage study, applied dose was given in mg/kg. For the inhalation studies, we computed applied dose (mg/kg) as exposure concentration (mg/m^3) times alveolar ventilation rate (m^3/h) times duration of exposure (h), divided by body weight. The dose–response curve was obtained as a least squares fit to the data using the equation $Y = 1 - \exp(-q_1 d - q_2 d^2)$. The dose–response curve in this figure represents the classical approach to risk assessment in which risks (probability of cancer) are expressed in terms of applied dose. Note that cancer incidence decreases in mice at high doses. In the classical approach (no consideration of pharmacokinetics), this decrease is explained in terms of cellular toxicity at high doses and subsequent cell death. Also, note that the cancer

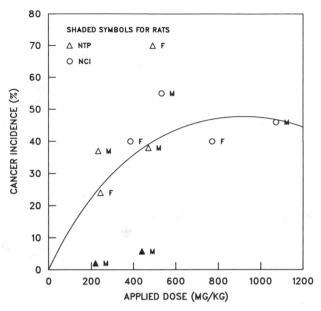

Figure 6. Cancer incidence for mice and rats from NCI gavage (13) and NTP (14) inhalation studies plotted as a function of applied dose (mg/kg·day).

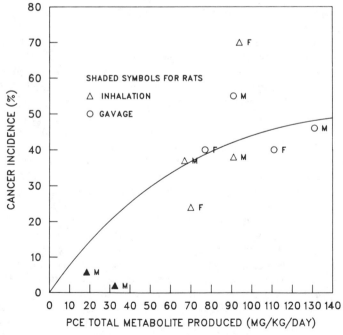

Figure 7. Cancer incidence for mice and rats from NCI gavage (13) and NTP (14) inhalation studies plotted as a function of total metabolites produced (mg/kg·day).

incidence obtained in rats is inconsistent with that of the mice. In the classical approach, this is taken to mean that PCE does not appear to be carcinogenic in rats (10, 13, 14). We now attempt to use pharmacokinetics to analyze the animal bioassay data.

Figure 7 shows cancer incidence versus total metabolite production for both the NCI and the NTP bioassays. The incidence rate is not well linearized when plotted against total metabolite production. However, the dose–response curve is increasing (i.e., it does not decrease at high doses) and the cancer incidence for rats is more consistent with that for the mice. We now split the total metabolite dose into that produced by the linear and nonlinear pathways.

Figure 8 displays cancer incidence versus metabolite production along the linear pathway. Again, the incidence rate is not well linearized. In fact, cancer incidence appears to be independent of dose. This suggests that the metabolite produced via the linear pathway is not carcinogenic. That is, there does not appear to be a relation between the amount of metabolite produced via the linear pathway and the cancer incidence in the animal bioassays. Figure 9 shows cancer incidence versus metabolite production along the nonlinear MFO pathway and presents a much better correlation between cancer incidence rates and metabolite production. The dose–response curve was obtained as a least squares fit to the data using the equation $Y = 1 - \exp(-q_1 d - q_2 d^2)$. The dose–response function is now nearly linear and the cancer incidence in rats is consistent with that in mice.

These results indicate that the tumor incidence rates in the NCI and NTP bioassays are more clearly correlated with the amount of the intermediate, reactant metabolite produced by the nonlinear metabolic pathway of PCE than with either the exposure or

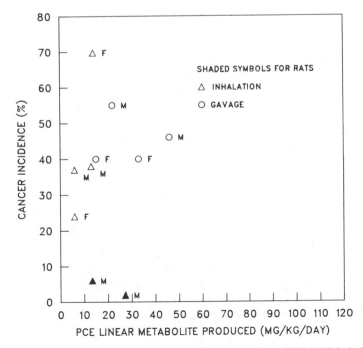

Figure 8. Cancer incidence for mice and rats from NCI gavage (13) and NTP (14) inhalation studies plotted as a function of PCE metabolites produced along the linear pathway (mg/kg·day).

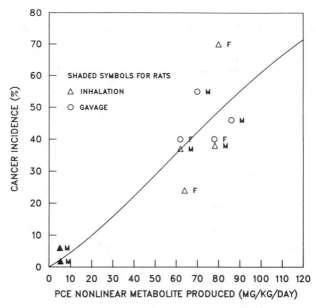

Figure 9. Cancer incidence for mice and rats from NCI gavage (13) and NTP (14) inhalation studies plotted as a function of PCE metabolite produced along the nonlinear pathway (mg/kg·day).

applied dose of the parent compound or the metabolite produced via the linear pathway. In summary, we can conclude the following:

1. The carcinogenic metabolite is produced via the nonlinear metabolic pathway.
2. The decrease in the classical dose–response curve at high doses is a result of saturation of the carcinogenic nonlinear metabolic pathway and not cell death.
3. PCE may be carcinogenic in *both* rats and mice. (The reason rats did not develop cancer in the NTP study was that the metabolized doses were too small).

7   CLASSICAL RISK ASSESSMENT METHODOLOGY

Traditionally, human risk from exposure to hazardous compounds has been estimated on the basis of administered dose. An outline of the administered dose approach used by federal regulatory agencies is as follows:

- It is *assumed* that if administered dose is measured in the proper units, cancer response will be approximately the same in all species.
- The proper units for equivalent dose are *assumed* to be either mg/kg body weight per day or mg/m² surface area per day.
- Carcinogenic response at low doses is *assumed* to be linear.
- The relation between administered dose (in the proper units) and cancer incidence in animals is determined on the basis of animal bioassays.
- The dose–response relation in humans is *assumed* to be the same as for animals.

This approach assumes that risks are a function of the dose taken into the body. It treats the body as a whole unit and assumes that rodent and human anatomy, physiology, and biochemistry are similar. The approach has several weaknesses:

- It does not account for metabolic differences between species.
- It does not account for differences in metabolic rates at high and low doses.
- It does not differentiate between parent compound and metabolites as the carcinogenic moiety.

However, when species-specific pharmacokinetic data are lacking, it is generally agreed that the administered dose approach is reasonable (1). The administered dose approach to estimating risk from PCE exposure is outlined in the following sections.

7.1 Interspecies Extrapolation

The first step in the classical risk assessment approach is the choice of an appropriate measure of equivalent carcinogenic dose in mice and humans. Equivalent dose can be expressed in terms of a concentration per medium or quantity per animal body weight. Effective doses measured as concentration per medium (e.g., mg/g food consumed, ppm, mg/m^3 in air) are most useful for describing situations involving direct contact between the medium and the receptor tissue (42). In most situations, however, equivalent dose is best described in terms of mg/kg body weight or mg/m^2 surface area.

The U.S. Food and Drug Administration (FDA) uses mg/kg body weight as a unit of dose on the assumption that the volumes of body fluids throughout which the carcinogen is distributed are proportional to body weight. The EPA uses surface area as the measure of equivalent dose. Because of the difficulty in empirically determining surface area, body weight to the 2/3 power is used as a surrogate measure of surface area. Surface area extrapolation is justified by the belief that metabolic rates (which influence concentrations of parent compound and by-products in the body) are proportional to body surface area. This assumption is supported by the classic Freireich et al. (43) analysis of 18 anticancer agents in mice, rats, dogs, monkeys, and humans. Freireich et al. (43) concluded that surface area provided the best measure of equivalent dose across species.

7.2 Dose–Response Relation in Animals

In its *Guidelines for Carcinogen Risk Assessment* (44), the EPA suggests that the cancer incidence at the most statistically sensitive tumor site in the most sensitive animal species and strain should be used as the basis for estimations of human risk. Thus, for tetrachloroethylene, the EPA (10) indicates that risk estimates should be based on dose–response data for hepatocellular carcinomas in female $B6C3F_1$ mice resulting from inhalation exposure.

Because the doses used in experimental studies are generally higher than those involved in most environmental exposures, a mathematical model must be applied to the experimental data to compute the dose–response curve in the low-dose range. In accordance with the assumption that there is no threshold of carcinogenic response and that dose–response is linear in the low-dose range, the EPA uses a linearized, multistage model to compute the dose–response curve. While the EPA recognizes that other dose–response models might fit the experimental data equally well, the *Guidelines for Carcinogen Risk Assessment* (44) state that "in the absence of adequate information to the contrary, the linearized multistage procedure will be employed." To determine the dose–response relation for tetrachloroethylene, the GLOBAL83 version of the linearized, multistage model (45) is applied to the incidence exhibited in female mice. GLOBAL83 calculates the dose–response relation for carcinogens by the formula

$$P(d) = 1 - \exp(-q_0 - q_1 d - q_2 d^2). \tag{1}$$

Thus, incremental cancer risk can be defined as

$$F(d) = \frac{P(d) - P(0)}{1 - P(0)} = 1 - \exp(-q_1 d - q_2 d^2). \tag{2}$$

From this, the model derives q_u, the 95% upper bound estimate of the linear slope, q_l. At low doses, the upper bound risk R can be predicted by $q_u d$, where d is the measure of dose. In their administered dose approach to estimating risk from PCE exposure, the EPA used the bioassay data from the female mouse inhalation study. The first step in the process is to estimate the administered doses in the NTP inhalation study.

Mice in the NTP study were exposed to 100 and 200 ppm, 6 h/day, 5 days/week, for 104 weeks. Exposure concentrations can be converted to administered dose by the following formula. First, exposure concentration in ppm is converted to mg/L and multiplied by the alveolar ventilation rate (L/min) and the duration of exposure (min) to yield administered dose in mg/day. This product is then divided by the animal body weight to obtain administered dose in mg/kg·day. For a 100-ppm exposure, the administered dose in females is calculated as

$$\frac{100\,\text{ppm}}{\text{L}} \times \frac{165.8\,\text{g/mol}}{24.45\,\text{L/mol}} \times \frac{1\,\text{g}}{1000\,\text{mg}} \times \frac{0.0315\,\text{L}}{\text{min}} \times 360\,\text{min} \times \frac{1}{0.032\,\text{kg}} \tag{3}$$

$$= 240.31\,\text{mg/kg·day}$$

When experimental exposure conditions are not continuous over the lifetime of the animal, the EPA risk estimates are based on a lifetime average exposure (LAE) which is calculated as (10):

$$240.31\,\text{mg/kg·day} \times \frac{5\,\text{days}}{7\,\text{days}} \times \frac{104\,\text{weeks}}{112\,\text{weeks}} = 159.4\,\text{mg/kg·day LAE}. \tag{4}$$

A similar computation for a 200-ppm exposure yields a LAE administered dose of 318.8 mg/kg·day.

TABLE 8. 95% Upper Bound Potency Estimates in Humans Based on Administered Dose to Mice in Inhalation Bioassay

	Body Weight Extrapolation	Surface Area Extrapolation
Male mice	3.3×10^{-3}	4.1×10^{-2}
Female mice	2.7×10^{-3}	3.6×10^{-2}

Source: Ref. 14.

Table 8 presents the q_u (95% upper bound estimate of the potency slope) for the doses administered to male and female mice. The q_u values in column 1 are calculated assuming mg/kg BW provides the best measure of equivalent dose; column 2 of Table 8 presents the calculation of q_u assuming surface area provides the best measure of equivalent dose.

7.3   Calculation of Administered Dose in Humans

In assessing the risk to humans exposed to a particular compound, regulators calculate the human risk that results from exposure to a standard unit of concentration, 1 μg of compound inhaled per m³ of air breathed in. Use of this standard unit of exposure concentration allows comparison of risk from one compound with the risks produced by exposure to other compounds. The risk due to human exposure to 1 μg of a compound per m³ of air is known as the *unit risk*.

In order to calculate the unit risk of PCE, we must begin by calculating the administered dose to humans (in units of mg/kg·day) that results from exposure to the unit concentration of 1 μg/m³. The administered dose to humans that results from exposure to 1 μg/m³ can be estimated as the product of the exposure concentration and daily air intake divided by human body weight. Since not all inhaled air is available for gas exchange in the lungs, the alveolar ventilation rate is used instead of the total ventilation rate. The estimated administered dose associated with human exposure to 1 μg/m³ of PCE in air is

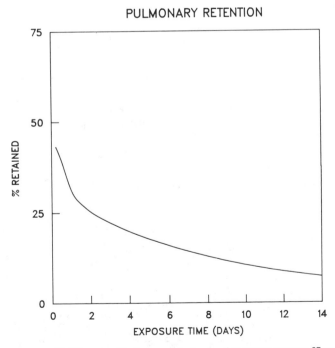

Figure 10. Percentage of PCE retained in the lungs during continuous exposure to 57 ppm of PCE for 14 days. Based on the data of Bolanowska and Golacka (46).

$$D = (1 \, \mu g/m^3)(13.4 \, m^3/day)(1/70 \, kg)(1 \times 10^{-3} \, mg/\mu g)$$
$$= 1.9 \times 10^{-4} \, mg/kg \cdot day$$

where $13.4 \, m^3/day$ is the daily alveolar ventilation rate of a 70-kg person based on a daily air intake of $20 \, m^3/day$. This calculation also assumes 100% absorption of the compound. In actual situations, the percentage of compound absorbed would decrease with length of exposure due to saturation of the blood's ability to take up additional chemical (Fig. 10) (46). As a result, this method of dose calculation overestimates actual human exposure. PB-PK models can account for this phenomena in a more realistic fashion. (This will be discussed in section 8.3.)

7.4 Classical Calculation of Human Risk

This estimation of administered dose can now be used with the potencies (q_u's) in Table 9 to compute human risk due to exposure to $1 \, \mu g/m^3$ of PCE in air. At low doses the upper bound risk R equals the product of the 95% upper bound of the linear slope (q_u) and dose (d). When mg/kg body weight is considered to produce equivalent dose across species, the risk to humans associated with $1 \, \mu g/m^3$ of PCE in air is

$$R = (2.7 \times 10^{-3})(1.9 \times 10^{-4}) = 5.1 \times 10^{-7}.$$

The EPA risk estimates assume that extrapolations based on surface area ($BW^{0.67}$) provide the best estimate of equivalent dose across species. Using surface area extrapolation, the risk to humans associated with $1 \, \mu g/m^3$ of PCE in air is

$$R = (3.6 \times 10^{-2})(1.9 \times 10^{-4}) = 6.8 \times 10^{-6}.$$

8 PHARMACOKINETIC RISK ASSESSMENT METHODOLOGY

The cancer process can be separated into a pharmacokinetic phase and a pharmacodynamic phase. The former relates applied dose to effective dose at target tissue, while the latter relates effective dose with biological effect.

TABLE 9. Dose–Response Data and 95% Upper Bound Potency Slope Estimates for B6C3F$_1$ Mice Exposed to PCE by Inhalation

	Administered Dose LAE (mg/kg·day)	Number of Animals	TBA[a]	95% Upper Bound Potency Estimates (q_u)
Males	0	49	7	
	152.4	49	25	3.3×10^{-3}
	304.8	50	26	
Females	0	48	1	
	158.4	50	13	2.7×10^{-3}
	318.8	50	36	

[a]Tumor-bearing animals.
Source: Ref. 14.

Federal regulatory agencies (47) have recently begun to use pharmacokinetic information in the risk assessment process. An outline of the pharmacokinetic approach used by federal agencies is as follows:

- A pharmacokinetic model is used to obtain the relation between administered dose and dose to target tissue.
- It is *assumed* if dose to target tissue is measured in the proper units, cancer pharmacodynamics will be the same in all species.
- The proper units for equivalent effective dose to target tissue are *assumed* to be either mg/kg body weight per day or mg/m^2 surface area per day.
- Cancer pharmacodynamics at low effective dose to target tissue is *assumed* to be linear.
- The relation between effective dose (in the proper units) and cancer incidence in animals (i.e., the pharmacodynamic relation) is determined on the basis of animal bioassays.
- The pharmacodynamic relation in humans is *assumed* to be the same as for animals.

While this approach is an improvement over the classical "administered dose approach" in that it accounts for species differences in pharmacokinetics, it still contains several weaknesses:

- It does not account for pharmacodynamic differences between species.
- It does not account for possible differences in pharmacodynamics at high and low doses.
- It does not differentiate between chemicals that cause cancer through direct interaction with genetic material and those that act indirectly through affecting cellular dynamics.

Nevertheless, the pharmacokinetic approach represents a significant step in the direction of making risk assessments more biologically based. The pharmacokinetic approach to estimating risk from PCE exposure is outlined in the following sections.

8.1 Interspecies Extrapolation

In the classical (administered dose) approach to risk assessment, it is assumed that when administered dose is expressed in the proper units (body weight basis or surface area basis), cancer incidence will be the same in all species. Thus the equivalent metric dose is assumed to account for interspecies differences in both the pharmacokinetic and pharmacodynamic phases for the cancer process. In the pharmacokinetic approach to risk assessment, the PB-PK model accounts for interspecies differences in pharmacokinetics. Thus, the PB-PK model provides the proper species-specific relation between exposure and effective dose to target tissue. However, it is still not known if a unit of toxin per unit of mouse tissue results in the same reponse as an equal unit of toxin per unit of human tissue. That is, the question arises as to the proper measure of effective dose to target tissue so that pharmacodynamic response is the same in all species. Again, possible choices are mg metabolite/kg weight of target tissue per day or mg metabolite/m^2 surface area target tissue per day. Since organ sizes scale approximately with body weight across species, equivalent metabolized dose at target tissue can be expressed in units of mg/kg body weight per day or mg/m^2 surface area per day.

8.2   Dose–Response Relation in Mice

The classical method of estimating risk assumes that the biological effects of a particular compound are directly related to the administered dose. Pharmacokinetic estimation of risk assumes that biological effect is related to the quantity of parent chemical that actually reaches the target tissue, the liver. In the case of PCE, the dose of concern appears to be the amount of metabolite produced along the nonlinear MFO pathway since this metabolite correlates best with hepatocellular carcinoma incidence in the female mice (see Fig. 11). Thus, in order to determine the dose–response curve for the nonlinear metabolite, the PB-PK model for PCE must be used to determine the amount of nonlinear metabolite in the liver which results from a known administered dose.

By using Eq. (4), the nonlinear metabolized doses calculated by the PB-PK model at 100 and 200 ppm are converted to lifetime average doses for the females of 42.1 and 52.9 mg/kg·day, respectively. The potency of PCE in mice, q_u, can now be determined by applying the multistage model to the lifetime average metabolized dose in the liver and the incidence of hepatocellular carcinomas in the females. At low doses the upper bound risk R equals the product of potency q_u and effective dose d. This formula is equivalent to assuming that at low effective doses to the liver, the pharmacodynamic relation is linear.

As with exposure of administered dose, the appropriate measure of equivalent metabolized dose in mice and humans must be determined. Table 10 presents q_u based on the effective dose of PCE (nonlinear metabolite in the liver) in male and female mice. The

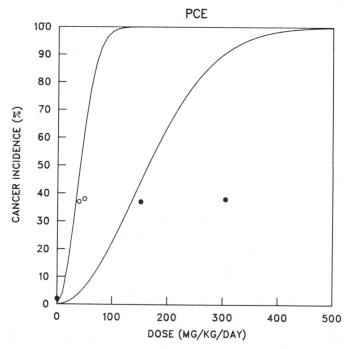

Figure 11. The multistage model maximum-likelihood estimates for PCE-induced hepatocellular carcinomas in female mice. Open circles represent metabolized dose versus incidence; solid circles represent administered dose versus incidence.

TABLE 10. 95% Upper Bound Potency Estimates in Humans Based on Effective Dose to Mice in Inhalation Bioassay

	Body Weight Extrapolation	Surface Area Extrapolation
Male mice	1.7×10^{-2}	2.2×10^{-1}
Female mice	1.0×10^{-2}	1.3×10^{-1}

Source: Ref. 14.

q_u values in column 1 are computed on the basis of body weight extrapolation; the q_u values in column 2 are computed on the basis of surface area extrapolation.

8.3   Calculation of Effective Dose in Humans

The potencies presented in Table 10 may now be used with pharmacokinetically derived metabolized dose to estimate human risk resulting from continuous exposure to 1 $\mu g/m^3$ of PCE in air. In the classical approach to risk assessment, the dose to humans is based on the effective dose, the PB-PK model estimate of the amount of PCE nonlinear metabolite that reaches the liver. PB-PK model simulation of PCE transport in humans estimates that a continuous exposure to 1 $\mu g/m^3$ of PCE in air results in an effective dose to the liver of 3.1×10^{-5} mg/kg·day.

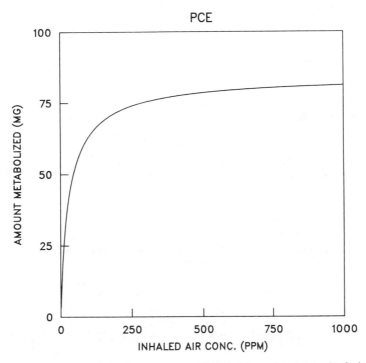

Figure 12. Effect of pathway saturation on amount of metabolite produced per unit of administered dose.

TABLE 11. Dose–Response Data and 95% Upper Bound Potency Slope Estimates for B6C3F$_1$ Mice Exposed to PCE by Inhalation

	Effective Dose LAE (mg/kg·day)	Number of Animals	TBA^a	95% Upper Bound Potency Estimates (q_u)
Males	0	49	7	
	42.1	49	25	1.7×10^{-2}
	51.7	50	26	
Females	0	48	1	
	42.4	50	13	1.0×10^{-2}
	53.0	50	36	

^{a}Tumor-bearing animals.
Source: Ref. 14.

Furthermore, application of the PB-PK model shows that metabolized dose to the liver does not increase linearly with exposure dose absorbed through the lungs, but rather reaches a maximum level and remains constant. Figure 12 shows that exposure to 1 ppm of PCE produces 3.3 mg of PCE metabolite, which increases to 22.8 mg metabolite at 10 ppm and 63.3 mg metabolite at 100 ppm. However, because of saturation of the nonlinear pathway, at 1000 ppm only 81.1 mg metabolite are produced. Thus, unlike the classical method, which assumes that effective dose increases linearly with exposure dose, use of the PB-PK model assumes that at higher dose levels, the amount of active compound reaching the liver does not increase. This phenomenon is a direct result of saturation of the nonlinear metabolic pathway and implies that carcinogenic risk to humans does not continue to increase with administered dose of PCE.

8.4 Pharmacokinetic Calculation of Human Risk

The potencies presented in Table 11 and the PB-PK model estimation of metabolized dose to the liver may be used to calculate a pharmacokinetically derived estimate of human risk due to continuous exposure of 1 μg/m^3 of PCE in air. At low doses the product of the 95% upper bound of the linear slope (q_u) and dose (d) represents the upper bound risk R. Thus, when mg/kg body weight is considered to be the appropriate measure of equivalent dose, the risk to humans associated with 1 μg/m^3 of PCE in air is

$$R = (1.0 \times 10^{-2})(3.1 \times 10^{-5}) = 3.1 \times 10^{-7}.$$

Using the EPA's assumption that surface area (mg/kg$^{0.67}$·day) provides the best measure of equivalent dose, the unit risk for humans is

$$R = (1.4 \times 10^{-1})(3.1 \times 10^{-5}) = 4.3 \times 10^{-6}.$$

9   COMPARISON OF HUMAN RISK ESTIMATES

Table 12 presents a comparison of human liver cancer risk estimates associated with 1 μg/m^3 of PCE in air calculated with and without the use of the PB-PK model. Potencies

TABLE 12. Risk of Human Exposure to 1 µg/m³ of PCE in Air

Method	Body Weight Extrapolation	Surface Area Extrapolation
Classical Method	5.1×10^{-7}	6.8×10^{-6}
PB-PK model	3.1×10^{-7}	4.3×10^{-6}

have been extrapolated between species using both mg/kg·day (body weight extrapolation) and mg/kg$^{0.67}$·day (surface area extrapolation). Our calculations assume that a female mouse weighs 0.032 kg and inhales 0.067 m³ of air per day and that a person weighs 70 kg and inhales 20 m³ of air per day. Table 12 shows that regardless of the method of extrapolation, at low exposures, incorporation of pharmacokinetics into the risk assessment for PCE exposure lowers the risk estimates by a factor of about 1.6.

As the nonlinear pathway saturates and the amount of metabolite reaching the liver stabilizes, however, incorporation of pharmacokinetics into the risk assessment greatly reduces the estimation of human risk. Figure 13 shows that at small administered doses (1 µg/m³ to 1 ppm) the reduction in risk gained from use of the PB-PK model remains

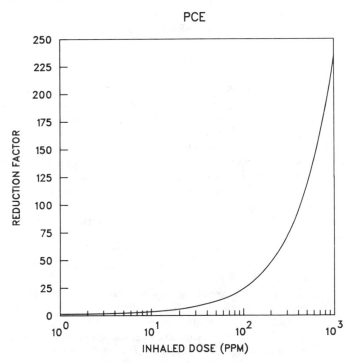

Figure 13. Reduction in risk estimates gained from use of PB-PK model in risk assessment. Increasing inhaled dose is plotted against the ratio of risk estimate without PB-PK modeling to risk estimate with PB-PK modeling.

constant at a factor of 1.6. As administered dose increases, the resulting reduction in risk also increases linearly with dose. At an exposure concentration of 100 ppm, for example, use of the PB-PK model reduces the risk estimate by about a factor of 24; at an exposure concentration of 500 ppm, use of pharmacokinetics reduces the risk estimate by about 118 times.

10 DISCUSSION

The classical method of estimating risk from exposure to a volatile organic assumes that the biological effect of a compound is directly related to the dose absorbed via the lungs. Pharmacokinetics allows the risk estimate to be based on the quantity of toxic substance that actually reaches the target tissue. The expected dose to target tissue can be obtained through computer solution of a set of equations describing the distribution and metabolism of the compound in the human body. This set of equations is termed a pharmacokinetic model. PB-PK models utilize three types of data: the anatomical and physiological structure of the animal, the partitioning of chemicals in various tissues, and metabolic parameters in various organs. For animals, all these parameters can be easily obtained from the literature or from laboratory experiments. For humans, the physiological and partitioning parameters are available, but the metabolic parameters must be indirectly inferred.

In this chapter, we have compared the classical and pharmacokinetic approaches to estimation of cancer risk from tetrachloroethylene. In the classical approach, carcinogenic response is assumed to be related to administered dose because of a lack of human data. The relation between administered dose and carcinogenic response is generally determined using animal data. Response in humans is assumed to be the same as for animals if dose is expressed in the proper units.

In the pharmacokinetic approach, the cancer process is separated into a pharmacokinetic and a pharmacodynamic phase. A pharmacokinetic model is used to determine the relation between administered dose and dose to target tissue. The relation between effective dose to target tissue and carcinogenic response in humans is then determined using animal data.

Since the carcinogenic metabolite is produced along the nonlinear metabolic pathway and since the nonlinear pathway saturates, incorporation of pharmacokinetics into the risk assessment for PCE can greatly reduce the estimate of human risk. A continuous lifetime exposure at 1 ppm would be expected to present a human cancer risk no greater than 4.3×10^{-6}. The lifetime risks associated with continuous 100- and 500-ppm exposures are 2.8×10^{-5} and 2.9×10^{-5}.

To date, a pharmacokinetic approach to cancer risk assessment has only been used for a few compounds (3, 47). Nevertheless, since this approach incorporates more realistic biological data, it promises to improve the risk assessment process. The PCE example illustrated in this chapter shows the usefulness of pharmacokinetic models in formulating a hypothesis for the mechanism of tumorigenicity of a compound. It also illustrates the use of pharmacokinetic models in extrapolating pharmacokinetic responses across species and across routes of administration. Pharmacokinetic models provide a tool to evaluate quantitatively and improve assumptions currently used in the risk assessment process. Because of these attributes, their use in risk assessment will undoubtedly increase in the near future.

APPENDIX

The physiologically based pharmacokinetic model for PCE is fully characterized by Ward et al. (6). Explanation of the nomenclature used in the model is found in Table 1. Parameters used are presented in Table 2. The following presents the mathematical equations describing the model.

Gas Exchange Compartment

$$Q_{alv}C_{inh}dt + Q_bC_{ven}dt = Q_{alv}C_{alv}dt + Q_bC_{art}dt$$

or

$$Q_{alv}(C_{inh} - C_{alv}) = Q_b(C_{art} - C_{ven}). \qquad (A.1)$$

$$C_{art} = \lambda_b C_{alv}. \qquad (A.2)$$

Tissue–Blood Exchanges

$$Q_i C_{art}dt = dA_i + Q_i C_{vi}dt$$

or

$$\frac{dA_i}{dt} = Q_i(C_{art} - C_{vi}). \qquad (A.3)$$

$$C_{vi} = C_i/\lambda_i. \qquad (A.4)$$

$$C_i = \frac{A_i}{V_i}. \qquad (A.5)$$

Metabolism

$$\frac{dA_m}{dt} = \frac{V_{max}C_{vl}}{K_m + C_{vl}} + K_f V_l C_{vl}. \qquad (A.6)$$

$$\frac{dA_l}{dt} = Q_l(C_{art} - C_{vl}) - \frac{dA_m}{dt}. \qquad (A.7)$$

Mixed Venous Blood

$$C_{ven} = \frac{1}{Q_b}\left(\sum_i Q_i C_{vi}\right). \qquad (A.8)$$

Arterial Blood

$$C_{art} = \frac{Q_{alv}C_{inh} + Q_bC_{ven}}{Q_b + Q_{alv}/\lambda_b}. \qquad (A.9)$$

Gavage—Absorption from the Gut

$$\frac{dA_l}{dt} = Q_l(C_{art} - C_{vl}) - \frac{dA_m}{dt} + KD_o e^{-kt}. \tag{A.10}$$

REFERENCES

1. Office of Science and Technology Policy, Executive Office of the President (OSTP), Chemical carcinogens: A review of the science and its associated principles, February, 1985. *Fed. Regist.* **2**, 10371–10442 (1985).

2. J. C. Ramsey and M. E. Andersen, A physiologically based description of the inhalation pharmacokinetics of styrene in rats and humans. *Toxicol. Appl. Pharmacol.* **73**, 159–175 (1984).

3. M. E. Andersen, H. J. Clewell III, M. L. Gargas, F. A. Smith, and R. H. Reitz, Physiologically based pharmacokinetics and the risk assessment process for methylene chloride. *Toxicol. Appl. Pharmacol.* **87**, 185–205 (1987).

4. M. E. Andersen, M. G. MacNaughton, H. J. Clewell III, and D. J. Paustenbach. Adjusting exposure limits for long and short exposure periods using a physiological pharmacokinetic model. *Am. Ind. Hyg. Assoc. J.* **48**, 335–343.

5. R. H. Reitz, R. J. Nolan, and A. M. Schumann, Organohalides. In *Proceedings of the National Academy of Science Workshop on Pharmacokinetics.* Safe Drinking Water Committee, Subcommittee on Pharmacokinetics, Board on Environmental Studies and Toxicology, National Research Council, Washington, DC, 1987.

6. R. C. Ward, C. C. Travis, D. M. Hetrick, M. E. Andersen, and M. L. Gargas, Pharmacokinetics of tetrachloroethylene. *Toxicol. Appl. Pharmacol.* **93**, 108–117 (1988).

7. D. J. Paustenbach, M. E. Andersen, H. J. Clewell, III, and M. L. Gargas, A physiologically-based pharmacokinetic model for inhaled carbon tetrachloride in the rat. *Toxicol. Appl. Pharmacol* (1988) (in press).

8. C. C. Travis, Interspecies and dose-route extrapolations. In *Proceedings of the National Pharmacokinetics and Risk Assessment: Drinking Water and Health* (Vol. VIII). Safe Drinking Water Committee, Subcommittee on Pharmacokinetics, Board on Environmental Studies and Toxicology, National Research Council, Washington, DC, 1987.

9. International Agency for Research on Cancer, *IARC Monogr. Eval. Carcinog. Risk Chem. Man* **20**, 491–494 (1979).

10. U.S. Environmental Protection Agency, *Health Assessment Document for Tetrachloroethylene (Perchloroethylene)*, Publ. No. EPA/600/8-82/005F. Office of Research and Development, Office of Health and Environmental Assessment, Environmental Criteria and Assessment Office, USEPA, Washington, DC, 1985.

11. B. B. Fuller, *Air Pollution Assessment of Tetrachloroethylene*, Rep. No. MTR-7143. Mitre Corp., McLean, VA (available from National Technical Information Service), Springfield, VA, 1976.

12. G. McConnell, D. M. Ferguson, and C. R. Pearson, Chlorinated hydrocarbons and the environment. *Endeavour* **34**, 13–18 (1975).

13. National Cancer Institute, *Bioassay of Tetrachloroethylene for Possible Carcinogenicity*, Publ. No. (NIH) 77–813. U.S. Department of Health, Education, and Welfare, Public Health Service, National Institutes of Health, NCI, Washington, DC, 1977.

14. National Toxicology Program, *NTP Technical Report on the Toxicology and Carcinogenesis of Tetrachloroethylene (Perchloroethylene), CAS 127-18-4, in F344/N Rats and B6C3F1 Mice (Inhalation Studies)*, NTP TR 311, NIH Publ. No. 85–2567. U.S. Department of Health and Human Services, Public Health Service, National Institutes of Health, NTP, Washington, DC, 1985.

15. American Conference of Governmental Industrial Hygienists, *Threshold Limit Values and Biological Exposure Indices for 1986–1987.* ACGIH, Cincinnati, OH, 1987 (ISBN: 0-936712-69-4).

16. M. Gibaldi and D. Perrier, *Pharmacokinetics.* Dekker, New York, 1975.

17. L. E. Gerlowski and R. K. Jain, Physiologically based pharmacokinetic modeling: Principles and applications. *J. Pharm. Sci.* **72**, 1103–1126 (1983).

18. M. E. Andersen, Tissue dosimetry in risk assessment, or What's the problem here anyway? In *Proceedings of the National Academy of Science Workshop on Pharmacokinetics. Pharmacokinetics in Risk Assessment*, Volume 8, *Drinking Water and Health*, National Academy Press. Washington, DC, 1987.

19. A. D. Arms and C. C. Travis, *Reference Physiological Parameters in Pharmacokinetic Modeling* U.S. EPA Final Report. EPA No. 600/6-88/004. NTIS order No. PB 88-196019, April 1988.

20. A. Sato and T. Nakajima, Partition coefficients of some aromatic hydrocarbons and ketones in water, blood, and oil. *Br. J. Ind. Med.* **36**, 231–234 (1979).

21. M. E. Andersen, M. L. Gargas, R. A. Jones, and L. J. Jenkins, Determination of the kinetic constants for metabolism of inhaled toxicants *in vivo* using gas uptake measurements. *Toxicol. Appl. Pharmacol.* **54**, 100–116 (1980).

22. J. G. Filser and H. M. Bolt, Pharmacokinetics of halogenated ethylenes in rats. *Arch. Toxicol.* **3**, 201–210 (1979).

23. M. L. Gargas, H. J. Clewell, III, and M. E. Andersen, Metabolism of inhaled dihalomethanes *in vivo*: Differentiation of kinetic constants for two independent pathways. *Toxicol. Appl. Pharmacol.* **82**, 211–223 (1986).

24. A. M. Schumann, J. F. Quast, and P. G. Watanabe, The pharmacokinetics and macromolecular interactions of perchloroethylene in mice and rats as related to oncogenicity. *Toxicol. Appl. Pharmacol.* **55**, 207–219 (1980).

25. J. A. Buben and E. J. O'Flaherty, Delineation of the role of metabolism in the hepatotoxicity of trichloroethylene and perchloroethylene: A dose-effect study. *Toxicol. Appl. Pharmacol.* **78**, 105–122 (1985).

26. D. G. Pegg, J. A. Zempel, W. H. Braun, and P. G. Watanabe, Disposition of tetrachloro(^{14}C)ethylene following oral and inhalation exposure in rats. *Toxicol. Appl. Pharmacol.* **51**, 465–474 (1979).

27. J. R. Withey, B. T. Collins, and P. G. Collins, Effect of vehicle on the pharmacokinetics and uptake of four halogenated hydrocarbons from the gastrointestinal tract of the rat. *J. Appl. Toxicol.* **3**(5), 249–253 (1983).

28. M. J. Angelo, A. B. Pritchard, D. R. Hawkins, A. R. Waller, and A. Roberts, The pharmacokinetics of dichloromethane I: Disposition in B6C3F1 mice following intravenous and oral administrations. *Food Chem. Toxicol.* **24**(9), 965–974 (1986).

29. J. Fernandez, E. Guberan, and J. Caperos, Experimental human exposures to tetrachloroethylene vapor and elimination in breath after inhalation. *Am. Ind. Hyg. Assoc. J.* **37**, 143–150 (1976).

30. L. W. Rampy, J. F. Quast, M. F. Balmer, B. K. J. Leong, and P. J. Gehring, *Results of a Long-Term Inhalation Toxicity Study: Perchloroethylene in Rats.* Toxicology Research Laboratory, Health and Environmental Research, Dow Chemical Co., Midland, MI, 1978 (unpublished).

31. National Toxicology Program, *Bioassay of Tetrachloroethylene in Female B6C3F1 Mice* (draft, not peer reviewed). U.S. Department of Health and Human Services, Public Health Service, National Institutes of Health, NTP, Washington, DC, 1983.

32. U.S. Environmental Protection Agency, *Addendum to the Health Assessment Document for Tetrachloroethylene (Perchloroethylene)* (draft, not peer reviewed), Publ. No. EPA/600/8-82/005FA. Office of Research and Development, Office of Health and Environmental Assessment, USEPA, Washington, DC, 1986.

33. C. C. Travis, R. K. White, and J. L. Quillen, Cancer risk of human exposure to tetrachloroethylene (draft) (1987).

34. G. Bonse, T. H. Urban, D. Reichert, and D. Henschler, Chemical reactivity, metabolic oxiraine formation and biological reactivity of chlorinated ethylenes in the isolated perfused rat liver preparation. *Biochem. Pharmacol.* **24**, 1829–1834 (1975).

35. S. A. Kline, J. J. Solomon, and B. L. Van Duuren, Synthesis and reactions of chloroalkene epoxides. *J. Org. Chem.* **43**, 3596–3600 (1978).

36. N. Sakamoto, Metabolism of tetrachloroethylene in guinea pigs. *Jpn. J. Ind. Health.* **18**, 11–16 (1976).

37. H. M. Bolt, R. J. Laib, and J. G. Filser, Reactive metabolites and carcinogenicity of halogenated ethylenes. *Biochem. Pharmacol.* **31**, 1–4 (1982).

38. O. Pelkonen and H. Vaino, Spectral interactions of a series of chlorinated hydrocarbons with cytochrome P-450 of liver microsomes from variously treated rats. *FEBS Lett.* **51**, 11 (1975).

39. A. K. Costa and K. M. Ivanetich, Tetrachloroethylene metabolism by the hepatic microsomal cytochrome P-450 system. *Biochem. Pharmacol.* **29**, 2863–2869 (1980).

40. S. Yllner, Urinary metabolites of C^{14}-tetrachloroethylene in mice. *Nature (London)* **191**, 820–821 (1961).

41. N. V. Dmitrieva, Contribution to the metabolism of tetrachloroethylene. *Gig. Tr. Prof. Zabol.* **11**, 54–56 (1967) (Engl. Transl.).

42. Midwest Research Institute, *Risk Assessment Methodology for Hazardous Waste Management.* Office of Policy Planning and Evaluation, MRI, U.S. Environmental Protection Agency, Washington, DC, 1986.

43. E. J. Freireich, E. A. Gehan, D. P. Rall, L. H. Schmidt, and H. E. Skipper, Quantitative comparison of toxicity of anticancer agents in the mouse, rat, hamster, dog, monkey, and man. *Cancer Chemother. Rep.* **50**(4), 219–244 (1966).

44. Federal Register, Guidelines for carcinogen risk assessment. *Fed. Regist.* **51**, 33992–34003 (1986).

45. R. B. Howe, *GLOBAL3: An Experimental Program Developed for the U.S. Environmental Protection Agency as an Update to GLOBAL 82: A Computer to Extrapolate Quantal Animal Toxicity Data to Low Doses.* K. S. Crump & Co., Inc., Ruston, LA, 1983 (unpublished).

46. W. Bolanowska and J. Golacka, Absorption and elimination of tetrachloroethylene in humans under experimental conditions. *Med. Pr.* **23**(2), 109–119 (1972). (Eng. Transl.).

47. U.S. Environmental Protection Agency, *Update to the Health Assessment Document and Addendum for Dichloromethane (Methylene chloride): Pharmacokinetics, Mechanisms of Action and Epidemiology,* Publ. No. EPA/600/8-87/030A. Office of Health and Environmental Assessment, USEPA, Washington, DC, 1987.

24

The Worker Hazard Posed by Re-entry into Pesticide-Treated Foliage: Development of Safe Reentry Times, with Emphasis on Chlorthiophos and Carbosulfan

J. B. Knaak
California Department of Health Services, Sacramento, California

Yutaka Iwata
ICI Americas Inc., Richmond, California

K. T. Maddy
California Department of Food and Agriculture, Sacramento, California

1 INTRODUCTION

The introduction of organic pesticides into modern agriculture has increased production and provided consumers worldwide with high-quality fruits and vegetables. The continuous use of these materials, however, has resulted in contamination of water, soil, and air. The chlorinated hydrocarbons, principally DDT, were the first class of compounds to be recognized as toxic environmental pollutants. DDT was replaced in the 1950s by an ever-growing number of biodegradable but dermally toxic organophosphorus and N-methylcarbamate insecticides. The use of these pesticides, principally ethyl parathion, on citrus in California resulted in a series of serious poisoning incidents among workers reentering treated groves to harvest fruit.

Established preharvest intervals (time between the last application of pesticide) varying from several days to several weeks were originally considered to be adequate to protect the health of workers "entering" or "reentering" a sprayed crop to harvest fruit or vegetables. Workers entering treated crops for activities other than harvesting (e.g., thinning, pruning) were not protected by the preharvest interval. On an annual basis in California there are over 300,000 field workers involved in handling crops treated at sometime with

TABLE 1. Chemical Identification of Pesticides Mentioned in Text

Pesticide	Chemical Designation
Acephate	O, S-Dimethyl acetylphosphoroamidothioate
Aldicarb	2-Methyl-2(methylthio) propionaldehyde O-(methyl carbamoyl) oxime
Azinphosmethyl	O, O-Dimethyl S-(4-oxo-1, 2, 3-benzotriazin-3($4H$)-yl) methyl phosphorodithioate
Carbaryl	1-Naphthyl methylcarbamate
Carbofuran	2, 3-Dihydro-2, 2-dimethyl-7-benzofuranyl methylcarbamate
Carbosulfan	2, 3-Dihydro-2, 2-dimethyl-7-benzofuranyl-[(di-n-butylamino)thio] methylcarbamate
Chlorobenzilate	Ethyl-4, 4′-dichlorobenzilate
Chlorthiophos	O-[2, 5-Dichloro-4-(methylthio)phenyl] O, O-diethyl phosphorothioate
Dialifor	S-[2-Chloro-1-(1, 3-dihydro-1, 3-dioxo-$2H$-isoindol-2-yl)ethyl] O, O-diethyl phosphorodithioate
Dimethoate	O, O-Dimethyl S-(N-methyl carbamoylmethyl) phosphorodithioate
Dioxathion	S, S'-(1, 4-dioxane-2, 3-diyl) bis(O, O-diethyl phosphorodithioate)
Ethion	O, O, O', O'-Tetraethyl S, S-methylene diphosphorodithioate
Malathion	O, O-Dimethyl S-[1, 2-di(ethoxycarbonyl) ethyl] phosphorodithioate
Methamidophos	O, S-Dimethyl phosphoramidothioate
Methidathion	S-[(5-Methoxy-2-oxo-1, 3, 4-thiadiazol-3($2H$)-yl)methyl] O, O-dimethyl phosphorodithioate
Methomyl	S-Methyl-N-[(methylcarbamoyl)oxy] thioacetimidate
Mevinphos	2-Methoxycarbonyl-1-methylvinyl dimethyl phosphate
Monocrotophos	Dimethyl 1-methyl-2-(methylcarbamoyl) vinyl phosphate
Oxamyl	S-Methyl N', N'-dimethyl-N-[(methylcarbamoyl)oxy-1-thiooxamimidate]
Paraoxon	O, O-Diethyl O-(4-nitrophenyl) phosphate
Parathion	O, O-Diethyl O-(4-nitrophenyl) phosphorodithioate
Phosphamidon	2-Chloro-2-diethylcarbamoyl-1-methyl vinyl dimethyl phosphate
Thiodicarb	Dimethyl N, N' [thio-bis(methylimino) carbamoyloxy thioacetimidate]

pesticide chemicals. The large number of workers, crops (e.g., 692,000 acres of grapes, 175,000 acres of citrus), and organophosphorus and N-methylcarbamate pesticides used ($< 1,500,000$ lb annually) on foliage on these two crops provide an insight into the potential magnitude of the field reentry problem as it exists in California alone.

This chapter presents poisoning cases reported in California agriculture, field management of these poisoning cases, federal and state regulatory responses, and the development of research procedures for characterizing dislodgeable foliar residues, their transfer to skin and clothing, their percutaneous absorption, and their effect on red cell cholinesterase activity. Currently acceptable procedures for calculating "safe foliar residues" and "safe reentry intervals" based on reentry research are provided using a number of pesticides employed in agriculture. Chemical designations of pesticides mentioned in the text are listed in Table 1.

2   HISTORICAL BACKGROUND

2.1   Poisoning Incidents

Poisoning incidences among workers who reentered pesticide-treated groves and vineyards were first reported in California in 1949 after the registration of ethyl parathion,

TABLE 2. Incidence of Multiple Case Systemic Illnesses of Agricultural Field Workers from Exposure to Residues of Organophosphorus Pesticides in California, 1949–1986

Date	Location	Number Ill	Probable Number Exposed	Crop and Activity[a]	Pesticides Implicated	AIA[b]	Worker Entry Time[c]	Previous Applications of Other Organophosphates the Same Season	
								Pesticide Used	Interval[d]
7/8/49	Marysville	20–25	56	Pears	Parathion	2.50	12	—[e]	—
6/27/51	Delano	16	24	Grapes	Parathion	1.87	33	—	—
8/27/52	Riverside	11	30	Oranges	Parathion	2.00	16	—	19
7/6/53	Riverside	7	—	Oranges	Parathion	—	17	—	—
7//53	Riverside	—	—	Citrus	Parathion	—	34	—	—
7//53	Bryn Mawr	—	—	Citrus	Parathion	—	33	—	—
//59	Entire state	275	—	Citrus	Parathion	—	—	—	—
10/5/61	Terra Bella	10	—	Lemons	Parathion	3.00	17	Parathion	97
8/9/63	Hughson	94	—	Peaches	Parathion	2.00	14–38	Parathion	36–110
6/29/66	Terra Bella	9	15	Oranges	Parathion	1.87	15	—	—
7/8/66	Porterville	6	11	Oranges	Parathion	1.33	32	—	—
7/21/66	Lindsay	3	30	Oranges	Parathion	2.00	13	—	—
8/2/66	Navelencia	11	22	Oranges	Parathion and malathion	13.50	28	—	—
						—	28		
8/11/66	Terra Bella	9	28	Oranges	Parathion and ethion	3.75	46	—	—
						—	46		
9/2–23/67	Hughson	23	—	Peaches	Azinphosmethyl and ethion	1.50	30+	TEPP	15–30
						200	38–47		
9/17–18/67	Ballico	3	—	Peaches	Azinphosmethyl	1.75	66	None	None
5//68	Lindsay	19	—	Oranges	Parathion	3.75	38–47	None	—
5/5/70	Porterville	3	30	Lemons, pruning	Dioxathion and naled	6.00	1	—	—
						1.00	1		
5/25/70	Lindsay	2	22	Oranges	Parathion and ethion	7.50	14	Parathion	17
						6.75	14		
5/27–28/70	Terra Bella	8–11	—	Oranges	Azinphosmethyl and ethion	12.00	8	Azinphosmethyl	10–12
						4.00	11		

TABLE 2 (*Continued*)

Date	Location	Number Ill	Probable Number Exposed	Crop and Activity[a]	Pesticides Implicated	AIA[b]	Worker Entry Time[c]	Pesticide Used	Interval[d]
								Previous Applications of Other Organophosphates the Same Season	
9/14–17/70	McFarland	35	35	Oranges	Parathion	9.00	34–37	Dioxathion	120
10/1/70	Orosi	11	55	Oranges	Parathion and malathion	3.00 / —	31 / 31	Azinphosmethyl	180
8/16–24/71	Orange Cove	8	9	Olives, pruning	Parathion	6.00	31	—	—
5/6/72	Lind Cove	3	—	Oranges	Parathion	2.50	21	—	—
9/15/72	Exeter	9	22	Oranges	Parathion	5.00	12	—	—
9/9/72	Huron	4	31	Lettuce, weeding	Parathion	2.50	1	Parathion	4–25
8/30/73	Fowler	27	32	Grapes	Dialifor	1.00	39	Phosalone / Phosmet / Ethion	41 / 57 / 57
9/3/74	Kerman	2	5	Grapes	Azinphosmethyl	1.00	28	Phosalone	67–68
6/12/75	Lemon Cove	16	20	Oranges	Parathion	2.00	16–20	None	None
6/76	Fresno	4	4	Lettuce, thinning	Mevinphos	—	14 h	—	—
9/8–10/76	Madera	118	120	Grapes	Dialifor	1.00	10	Phosalone	93
7/16/77	Orange Cove	39	39	Oranges	Parathion	5.00	22	—	—
6/10/78	Tulare	7	—	Grapes	Ethion	—	16	—	—
8/14–15/80	Ballico	6	24	Peaches	Azinphosmethyl	1.50	32+	Phosalone	—
7/11/80	Salinas	22	22	Cauliflower, banding	Mevinphos and phosphamidon	1.00	3 h	—	—

Date			Location	Crop	Pesticide	Pounds per acre[b]	Days	Pesticide	
4/23/81	41	80	King City	Lettuce	Mevinphos	1.00	2h	—	—
8/3/82	17	32	Strathmore	Oranges	Parathion	7.50	35	Parathion	—
9/18/82	35	35	Salinas	Cauliflower, banding	Mevinphos	1.00	1	Oxydemeton-methyl	1
4/16/82	17	27	Salinas	Cauliflower, weeding	Oxydemeton-methyl	0.50	1	Dimethoate	1
6/17/83	2	2	San Juan, Bautista	Irrigating	Azinphosmethyl	—	<1	—	—
5/22/84	2	2	Firebaugh	Cotton, irrigating	Chlorpyrifos and acephate	1.00 / 0.75	6h	—	—
7/15/85	4	15	Ducor	Grapefruit	Parathion	8.00	48	—	—
6/13/86	2	9	Watsonville	Strawberries, weeding	Malathion	2.00	21h	—	—
7/2/85	25	32	Five Points	Cotton, weeding	Methamidophos	0.50	2h	—	—
7/31/86	3	40+	Three Rocks	Cotton, running from border patrol	Methamidophos	0.80	1h	—	—

[a]Unless otherwise indicated in Crop column, workers are engaged in picking operation.
[b]Active ingredient expressed in pounds per acre.
[c]Days postapplication (unless otherwise stated).
[d]Days elapsed between exposure date and the most recent previous application.
[e]Dash means unknown.
Source: California Department of Food and Agriculture.

as shown in Table 2. The poisonings were characterized by sweating, vomiting, dizziness, and general body weakness. Red blood cell cholinesterase was depressed in most cases more than 20%. This and the poisoning incidents described later indicated to state and federal regulatory officials that "reentry intervals or times" separate and distinct from preharvest intervals were necessary to protect the health of workers. At this time California is the only state establishing and enforcing its own reentry intervals. Reentry intervals, however, have been established by the EPA for the other states.

From 1949 through 1958, six multiple case poisoning incidents occurred in California involving at least 79 persons entering groves treated with ethyl parathion (Table 2). In 1959, 275 workers were poisoned in six separate citrus groves throughout the state (Table 2). An additional 87 workers were poisoned during the years 1961–1969. Two incidents involved azinphosmethyl and ethion, while the remaining illnesses were attributed to the use of ethyl parathion.

Quinby and Lemmon (1) studied these early poisoning episodes. They documented 11 episodes, 6 in the state of Washington and the balance in California. Dermal exposure was determined to be the likely route of exposure. In California, Milby et al. (2) studied the effects of organophosphorus pesticide residues on 186 peach orchard workers; percutaneous absorption of the oxidation products (oxons) of the organophosphorus esters was identified as the likely cause of the poisonings. From 1970 to 1972 there were nine episodes involving 86 persons poisoned with ethyl parathion in citrus groves in California.

This group of episodes led to the passage of legislation in California in 1972 establishing a Workers Health and Safety (WHS) group in the California Department of Food and Agriculture (CDFA) and the adoption of Worker Safety Regulations (3) involving reentry into crops treated with organophosphorus pesticides in cooperation with the California Department of Health Services (CDHS). The adoption of regulations and the formation of the Worker Health and Safety group provided the CDFA with the legal means to investigate illnesses, establish reentry intervals, and prosecute violators. At this time other states have not passed similar regulations or established enforcement agencies.

Since 1964, each poisoning incident in California has been investigated by the CDFA to determine the reasons for the occurrence and to identify ways to prevent such illnesses (Table 2). For example, the use of a new chemical, dialifor, on grapes in 1973–1974 resulted in illnesses among workers harvesting the grapes. A thorough investigation by the CDFA staff resulted in the establishment of a 75-day reentry interval and the eventual deregistration of dialifor in California (4–6). It was shown that the formation and percutaneous absorption of foliar residues of dialifor oxon were the principal reasons for the illnesses observed in the workers. Compliance with legally designated reentry intervals kept workers out of fields where excessive leaf residues were present.

Incidents of ethyl parathion poisonings in citrus groves during 1977, 1982, and 1985 were determined to be caused by the presence of high levels of paraoxon in soil dust underneath trees (7). Soil dust served as a vehicle for transferring paraoxon to the hands, arms, legs, and feet of workers harvesting fruit (8). Parathion and paraoxon residues on foliage were at levels considered to be safe for reentry as a result of compliance with long reentry intervals (3).

Immediately following the dialifor and several of the parathion illness incidents, harvesting was stopped, and large acreages of ripe fruit remained to be harvested. Analyses of residues in soil and on foliage were performed to identify treated fields safe to harvest. The guidelines used for determining a "safe" field residue are covered later in this chapter. Workers with normal red blood cell cholinesterase activity were placed under medical supervision and allowed to harvest these fields. Fields considered unsafe for harvest were quarantined until they were safe to reenter and harvest the crop (9).

Whorten and Obrinsky (10) studied a reentry poisoning incident involving mevinphos- and phosphamidon-treated row crops. Poisoning was induced by the parent compounds when reentry occurred illegally within 1–24 h after application. In order to protect workers, their blood cholinesterase levels were followed until values returned to normal and the workers could return to work. In some cases, a period of 3 months was needed before values return to normal levels. This illustrates the degree of interpersonel variability encountered with respect to exposure, percutaneous absorption, and cholinesterase inhibition.

N-methylcarbamates can cause cholinesterase inhibition when inhaled or ingested (11). In a few instances, dermal exposure to foliage, within 1 or 2 days after application, has resulted in the poisoning of field workers. The incident that involved the most injury to date occurred in Indiana in August 1974. Seventy-four young men and women of a work crew of 150 became ill while detasseling corn within 24 h of a foliar application of carbofuran (12). Sufficient carbofuran was absorbed through the skin of the hands and arms to produce the effects observed in these workers. Occasionally, other smaller scale incidents have been reported with N-methyl carbamates. For example, in the summer of 1981, 4 out of 12 workers in a California grape vineyard were poisoned by methomyl applied to foliage less than 24 h prior to reentry. The workers recovered from their illnesses within a period of 4 or 5 h.

In addition to the foliar residue problem with carbofuran and methomyl, poisoning occasionally occurs in California when uninformed persons enter a field or grove to drink water from irrigation equipment containing pesticides. Several persons have been seriously poisoned from ingesting oxamyl; reentry restrictions are now required on the oxamyl label to prevent such occurrences.

2.2 Field Reentry Studies

During the 1970s, several incidents with organophosphorus pesticides prompted a number of agricultural chemical companies to conduct medically supervised reentry studies. Tobin (13) conducted a study with workers harvesting fruit from a citrus grove treated with ethion 1 day prior to reentry. A reduction in red blood cell cholinesterase activity occurred. Reentry studies with workers reentering a peach orchard treated 1 week before with azinphosmethyl were conducted (14, 15). Here again, a reduction in red blood cell cholinesterase activity occurred in the workers. Studies involving workers and reentry into cotton previously treated separately with ethyl and methyl parathion (16) and monocrotophos and ethyl and methyl parathion (17, 18) were conducted. Workers reentered treated cotton fields 12–72 h after application of the pesticides. Red blood cell cholinesterase depression was detected in the workers.

Spear et al. (19) conducted an ethyl parathion field reentry study in citrus groves involving several application rates and reentry intervals. Cholinesterase activity was depressed by 35% in workers entering as late as 25 days postapplication. The dose–response information obtained in this study has been of considerable value in establishing reentry periods for a number of organophosphorus pesticides in California coupled with the results of the reentry studies conducted by Kilgore (20) involving azinphosmethyl on peaches. A reentry period of up to 90 days was established for parathion and a 14-day reentry interval for azinphosmethyl. The procedure for setting the reentry intervals is discussed in Section 6, which deals with the mathematics of setting safe levels on foliage.

2.3   Federal Reentry Standards

The Occupational Safety and Health Administration (OSHA) was the first federal agency to propose pesticide reentry standards to protect the health of farm workers (21). The first standards, adopted on May 1, 1973, included 21 organophosphorus insecticides and five crops (citrus, peaches, grapes, tobacco, and apples) in wet and dry areas. These standards were replaced 6 weeks later with less stringent standards covering only nine organophosphorus insecticides with intervals ranging from 1 to 3 days for wet areas and 14 days for dry areas (22).

During the summer of 1973, a jurisdictional dispute between the U.S. Environmental Protection Agency (EPA) and OSHA over which agency would set and administer reentry standards occurred and was finally resolved in Federal Court in favor of the EPA. A year later the Federal Working Group on Pest Management appointed T. H. Milby to chair a Task Group on Occupational Exposure to Pesticides (23). The Task Group recommended that registrants should be required to (i) submit data to the EPA for establishing reentry intervals and (ii) pay attention to geographical differences and that (iii) the Federal Government should support research into the fundamental factors that influence reentry intervals with respect to farm worker safety.

In the *Federal Register* on March 11, 1974 (24), the EPA published 48-h reentry standards for 11 organophosphorus insecticides, endrin, and endosulfan. The regulations also recognized state responsibility and authority to set additional restrictions to meet local problems as carried out by the California Department of Food and Agriculture. In order to develop reentry intervals, the CDFA put into place monitoring requirements based on the recommendations of the California Department of Health Services (25). These monitoring studies utilized changes in field worker blood cholinesterase levels to determine if dislodgeable residues were at a "safe level." Since these requirements included the use of human subjects (i.e., field workers), the studies were to be conducted in a manner conforming to ethical requirements involving medical supervision and the safeguarding of the individual subject's safety and dignity.

Several well-controlled reentry studies were conducted by Knaak et al. (26) and Popendorf et al. (27), respectively, with phosalone on citrus and peaches in California. The study by Knaak and co-workers followed conventional field workers while the study by Popendorf followed college students working as fruit pickers. The results of these studies provided useful information for establishing reentry intervals for phosalone. None of the workers entering groves after the application of phosalone developed cholinesterase poisoning symptoms or a decrease in red blood cell cholinesterase activity.

The monitoring requirements were later modified in 1975 to exclude the use of farm workers as subjects in monitoring studies. This policy was based on the contentions that under the current conditions in California agriculture, truly informed and voluntary consent, free from any duress, could not be obtained from farm field workers. In a meeting of CDFA and EPA officials held in San Francisco in 1977, the Federal Government took the position that California's approach to establishing reentry intervals used human subjects in a manner inconsistent with the current views of the Federal Agency concerning informed consent as covered in the Guidelines for Protection of Human Subjects (28) promulgated by the U.S. Department of Health, Education, and Welfare. The use of animal models was recommended as a means for obtaining the necessary data for setting reentry intervals.

In 1980, the EPA presented a new set of methodologies for setting reentry intervals (21). Three types of data were determined to be necessary to calculate a reentry interval:

(i) dose–response data, (ii) estimates of a relation between surface residues and total body exposure and (iii) time versus residue data. In this procedure an allowable exposure level (AEL) was determined. In 1984 the EPA published the methodologies in detail in *Pesticide Assessment Guidelines, Subdivision K, Exposure: Reentry Protection* (12). The reentry study involving chlorthiophos presented in Section 6 of this chapter is referenced in this document.

3   HAZARD EVALUATION

A chapter on the pesticide field reentry problem would not be complete without a brief discussion of the toxic properties of the organophosphorus and *N*-methylcarbamate pesticides, their action on acetylcholinesterase, bioassay procedures used to determine their effects on circulating red blood cell cholinesterase, procedures for measuring dermal dose–ChE response, and percutaneous absorption in model animals. The automated cholinesterase procedure described in Section 3.2 was used to detect these pesticides in field workers and in model animals. These procedures play an important role in determining safe level for organophosphorus esters and *N*-methylcarbamates on foliage.

3.1   Properties of Toxic Organophosphorus and Carbamate Esters

The organophosphorus pesticides inhibit acetylcholinesterase in the nervous system and in red blood cells of humans and animals by reacting with the active site of this enzyme. Organophosphorus insecticides vary in their affinity for the enzyme and in their ability to irreversibly phosphorylate the enzyme (29). Six types of organophosphorus insecticides are produced and used in the United States and are represented by phosphates, phosphorothioates, phosphorothiolates, phosphorodithioates, phosphoroamidates, and phosphonates. The phosphorothioates (parathion) and phosphorodithioates (azinphosmethyl, dialifor, methidathion, dimethoate, and phosalone) are oxidized on foliage to produce more toxic products called oxons (phosphates and phosphorothioates). The oxons are better inhibitors of acetylcholinesterase and their formation on plant foliage is the principal reason for the reentry poisoning in California (23).

The insecticidal carbamates, esters of *N*-methylcarbamic acid, are also inhibitors of acetylcholinesterase. They vary in their affinity for the enzyme. The enzyme–inhibitor complex is unstable, resulting in the release of the intact carbamate and enzyme (11).

The poisoning symptoms observed in workers exposed to organophosphorus and carbamate esters were caused by the inhibition of acetyleholinesterase in the nervous system. Red blood cell cholinesterase activity measurements in workers and experimental animals are routinely used to estimate indirectly the in vivo effects of these pesticides on nervous system cholinesterase. According to studies in the rat, administration of AChE inhibitiors produces an almost immediate decrease in both red blood cell and brain cholinesterase activity.

Recovery of AChE activity, inhibited by organophosphorus esters, occurs by direct synthesis of new enzyme, dissociation of the enzyme–inhibitor complex and reactivation of the phosphorylated enzyme, or in the case of the carbamates mainly by reactivation of the carbamylated enzyme. Poisoning and the treatment of poisoning were recently reviewed by Hirschberg and Lerman (30) and Lerman et al. (31).

Blood cholinesterase activity assays are the principal procedures used to determine worker exposure to cholinesterase inhibitors and to examine the dermal dose–ChE response relation in animal models. The blood cholinesterase assay is discussed in Section 3.2 of this chapter.

Technical organophosphorus (OPs) and N-methylcarbamate insecticides respectively, are supplied by manufacturers as viscous liquids and crystalline solids to be formulated with organic solvents, detergents, and water as emulsifiable concentrates or as water–soluble powders for dilution in water for application (32). Most of these materials are strongly lipophilic. Exceptions, however, exist as a number of the OPs and N-methylcarbamates are quite water soluble. Acephate is a white solid material, soluble to 65% w/v in water and to only 10% w/v in acetone–ethanol and 5% w/v in aromatic solvents. Its hydrolysis product, methamidophos, is even more water soluble than acephate and less soluble in organic solvents. Methomyl, a white crystalline N-methylcarbamate used extensively in agriculture, is soluble in water to the extent of 5.8% w/v in water and 100% w/v in methanol. Oxamyl, closely related in structure to methomyl, is even more soluble in water, 28% w/v, and methanol, 144% w/v.

The organophosphorus insecticides vary in their acute oral toxicity from less than 1.0 mg/kg of body weight for the most toxic oxons such as paraoxon to well over 1500 mg/kg for the less toxic OPs (e.g. malathion). The N-methylcarbamates also vary widely in their acute oral toxicities, which range from a low of 8.0 mg/kg (aldicarb) to several hundred mg/kg (i.e., carbaryl).

Field workers, however, are dermally exposed to residues of organophosphorus and carbamate insecticides on foliage. The EPA regulations (33) currently group pesticide products into three toxicity categories based on the results of dermal LD_{50} studies in the rabbit. Category I materials have a dermal LD_{50} of < 200 mg/kg, category II materials a dermal LD_{50} of 200–1000 mg/kg, and category III materials a dermal LD_{50} of > 1000 mg/kg. The oxons formed from the phosphorothioates and phosphorodithoates have a dermal LD_{50} of < 200 mg/kg. Reentry intervals may be required by EPA (12) and the California Department of Food and Agriculture (34) for pesticide products assigned to categories I and II. The relation between a dermal dose of an organophosphorus or carbamate ester and its effect on blood cholinesterase activity is discussed in Section 3.3 and used in Section 6 of this chapter to set reentry intervals.

3.2 Blood Cholinesterase Assay

The Milby report (23) recommended the use of the Michel (35), pH-Stat (Nabb and Whitfield, (36) or colorimetric method (Ellman et al., 37) for measuring blood cholinesterase activity of field workers. The pH-Stat and colorimetric methods are suitable for measuring the inhibitory action of organophosphorus and carbamate esters, while the Michel method was found suitable only for organophosphorus esters. Long incubation periods at high pH resulted in the reactivation of cholinesterase. All three methods were manual methods requiring a substantial amount of time and effort to obtain reproducible results. The automated Ellman method of Humiston and Wright (38) was modified by Knaak et al. (39) to run on the Technicon Auto Analyzer II system. This two-channel system uses in one channel whole blood (intact red cells) or plasma as enzyme, acetylthiocholine as substrate, and a dialyzer system to separate the enzyme from the hydrolysis product, thiocholine, prior to reacting DTNB [5,5-dithiobis(2-nitrobenzoic acid)] with thiocholine to produce a yellow color. The second channel blanks out color resulting from nonenzymatic hydrolysis of acetylthiocholine.

The cholinesterase activity of the red blood cells is obtained by substracting the activity of the plasma from the activity of whole blood using the sample's hematocrit in Eq. (1):

$$RBC = \frac{\text{whole blood activity} - \left(\dfrac{1 - \text{hematocrit}}{100}\right)(\text{plasma activity})}{\text{hematocrit}/100}. \qquad (1)$$

The activity of whole blood, RBCs, and plasma are reported in terms of micromoles of
—SH released per minute per milliliter of sample. Plasma from Sigma Chemical
Company, St. Louis, Missouri is used as the enzyme standard and reduced glutathione as
the instrument standard. In field worker studies involving human blood, whole blood was
diluted 1:6 with pH 7.7 buffer and plasma was diluted 1:3 with buffer, while in the dermal
dose–ChE response studies discussed in Section 3.3 whole blood from the rat was diluted
1:3.5 with buffer, while plasma was used without dilution. The results with enzyme
standards are reproducible from run to run. After 10 years of field and laboratory use, the
method is being considered by the California Department of Health Services as an official
clinical laboratory method.

3.3 Dermal Dose–ChE Response

The field reentry studies involving farm field workers were conducted to determine the
relation between foliar pesticide residues in $\mu g/cm^2$ and cholinesterase depression in order
to set safe reentry intervals. These studies were costly and often provided little information

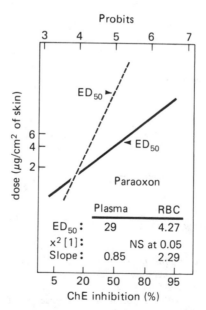

Figure 1. Dermal dose–ChE response curves obtained for paraoxon in the rat. Paraoxon was applied
to the clipped backs (25 cm²) of 220–240-g male Sprague–Dawley rats. Blood ChE activity was
determined after 72 h of exposure. Figure taken from Knaak et al. (42). ----Plasma ChE activity; —
RBC ChE activity. (Reprinted with permission from Springer-Verlag, *Bulletin of Environmental
Contamination and Toxicology*.)

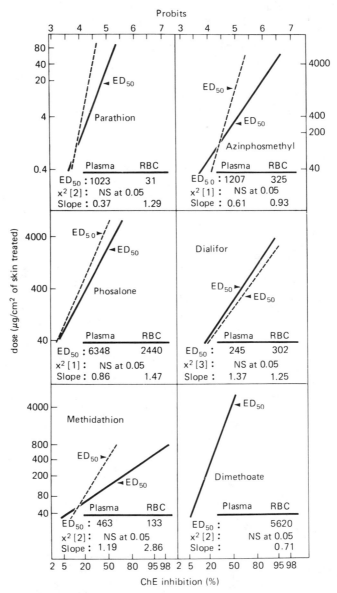

Figure 2. Dermal dose–ChE response curves for six organophosphorus pesticides. Male Sprague–Dawley rats weighing 220–240 g were used. A 25-cm² area of back skin was treated. Blood ChE activity was determined after 72 h of exposure. - - -, Plasma ChE; —, RBC ChE. Figure taken from Knaak et al. (42). (Reprinted with permission from Springer-Verlag, *Bulletin of Environmental Contamination and Toxicology*.)

relating foliar residue data to cholinesterase inhibition, because exposure times and foliar residue levels were not sufficient in magnitude to produce a dose-related effect in workers.

Gaines (40, 41) was the first to develop extensive acute dermal toxicity (LD_{50}) data in mg/kg of body weight on organophosphorus pesticides in the rat. As good as the mortality data were, it could not readily be used to relate residue levels or dermal dose in $\mu g/cm^2$ to cholinesterase inhibition. Knaak et al. (42) were the first to develop dermal dose–response curves (ED_{50}) in the rat relating dose in $\mu g/cm^2$ of skin surface to cholinesterase inhibition for a number of the organophosphorus pesticides of interest. Figures 1 and 2 give the dermal dose–response curves obtained by Knaak et al. (42) for paraoxon, parathion, dialifor, phosalone, azinphosmethyl, dimethoate, and methidathion. The dose (ED_{50}) resulting in 50% red blood cell and plasma cholinesterase inhibition after 72 h of exposure is given along with the slopes of the log–probit regression lines. The 72-h exposure period simulated a 3-day harvesting period. The results of these studies were used by Knaak et al. (42, 43) to establish safe levels on tree foliage (in $\mu g/cm^2$). Popendorf and Leffingwell (44) used these cholinesterase inhibition data to develop their "unified field model."

This work was extended by Knaak et al. (45) to include several important *N*-methyl carbamates, used extensively in California agriculture, for the purpose of establishing safe foliar levels and reentry intervals as described for organophosphates in Section 6.1. The dermal dose–ChE response curves for methomyl, thiodicarb, methiocarb, and methiocarb sulfoxide are given in Figs. 3 and 4.

The dose–response curve for methomyl is included with the curve for thiodicarb,

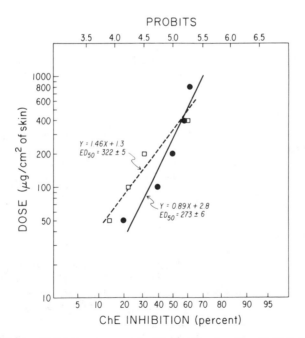

Figure 3. Dermal dose–ChE response curves for thiodicarb and methomyl. Male Sprague–Dawley rats weighing 220–240 g were used. A 25-cm² area of back skin was treated. RBC blood ChE activity was determined after 24 h of exposure. – – –, Thiodicarb; —, methomyl. Figure taken from Knaak et al. (45). (Reprinted with permission from American Chemical Society book publications.)

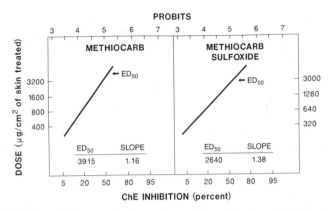

Figure 4. Dermal dose–ChE response curves for methiocarb and methiocarb sulfoxide. Male Sprague–Dawley rats weighing 220–240 g were used. A 25-cm² area of back skin was treated. Red cell ChE activity was determined after 24 h of exposure. Figure taken from Knaak et al. (45). (Reprinted with permission from American Chemical Society book publications.)

because of their structural similarities. Thiodicarb may be described as a molecule of methomyl linked to a second molecule of methomyl via an N–S–N bridge. In the rat, thiodicarb is metabolized to methomyl. The dermal dose–ChE response curves indicate that these two pesticides are similar in their ability to produce cholinesterase inhibition when topically applied. This is surprising, because they possess different physical properties. Methomyl is soluble in water to the extent of 5.8% w/v, while thiodicarb is virtually insoluble in water and organic solvents. Safe levels were determined for both methomyl and thiodicarb using the procedure of Knaak et al. (42).

3.4 Percutaneous Absorption

A number of dermatopharmacokinetic studies were conducted using radiolabeled organophosphorus and carbamate pesticides (46, 47) to determine the fate of pesticides. A few of these studies were conducted in conjunction with dermal dose–cholinesterase response studies to provide kinetic as well as cholinesterase inhibition data.

The fate, absorption kinetics, and dermal dose–ChE response of topically applied [ring-U-^{14}C]parathion, [ring-U-^{14}C]carbaryl, and [acetyl-1-^{14}C]thiodicarb were studied by Knaak et al. (46, 47). According to these studies, a 40-μg/cm² dose of parathion is absorbed at the rate of 0.5 μg/h·cm². The retention time on skin, $t_{1/2} = 24.3$–28.6 h, was less than its half-life, 28.5–39.5 h, in plasma.

Carbaryl was not absorbed as readily as parathion. The retention half-life for a 40-μg/cm² topical dose was 40 h, while the $t_{1/2}$ for elimination from plasma was 67 h. Thiodicarb dissipated at an initial rate (0–24 h; $t_{1/2}$, alpha phase) of 40 h from the skin of adult female rats and at a final rate (24–167 h; $t_{1/2}$, beta phase) of 254 h. Thiodicarb equivalents were at plateau levels in plasma during the study. The time–concentration curves for the absorption and elimination of [^{14}C]parathion and [^{14}C]carbaryl in select-ed tissues are given in Figs. 5 and 6. The time-course recoveries of dermally applied ^{14}C-labeled parathion, carbaryl, and thiodicarb are shown in Fig. 7. The model given in Fig. 8 describes the overall absorption and elimination of a topically applied dose. Maibach

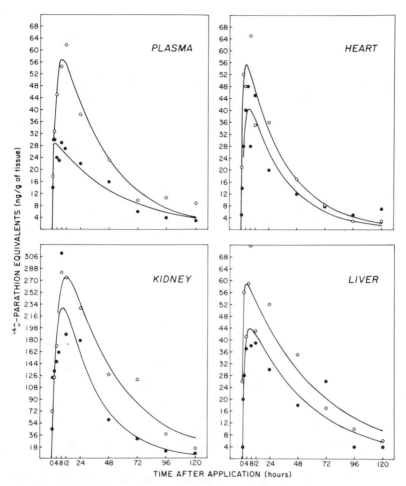

Figure 5. Time–concentration curves for the simultaneous absorption and elimination of [^{14}C]parathion equivalents in plasma, heart, kidney, and liver. ●, Adult males; ○, adult females. The mean coefficient of variation for the tissue values at each time interval was 37%. Figure taken from Knaak et al. (46). (Reprinted with permission from Academic Press, *Toxicology and Applied Pharmacology*.)

et al. (48) studied the absorption of [^{14}C]parathion and [^{14}C]carbaryl in human volunteers. A 5-day period was required to achieve a completely absorbed and eliminated topically applied dose. The studies indicated that carbaryl was more readily absorbed than parathion.

The results of parathion dermal dose–ChE response studies in male and female rats of variable age are given in Table 3. Blood samples were taken and analyzed for red blood cell cholinesterase activity 72 h after the application of the dose. Parathion was more toxic to females of varying ages than to males, and less toxic to young animals, on a weight basis. On a surface area basis, parathion was more toxic to females than males, equally toxic to young and adult males, but less toxic to young females, than adult females. Carbaryl at

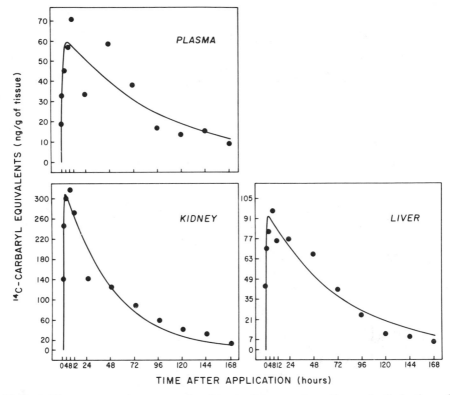

Figure 6. Time–concentration curves for the simultaneous absorption and elimination of [^{14}C]carbaryl equivalents in plasma, kidney, and liver of adult male rats. The mean coefficient of variation for the tissue values at each time interval was 27%. Figure taken from Knaak et al. (46). (Reprinted with permission from Academic Press, *Toxicology and Applied Pharmacology.*)

dose levels as high as 4000 μg/cm^2 of skin did not inhibit red blood cell ChE activity 24 h after the application of the dose even though it was absorbed through skin. According to these absorption studies, the nature of the chemical, the nature of the skin and skin site, the size of the exposure area, the concentration on skin (in μg/cm^2), and the time are the major factors governing the amount of pesticide absorbed.

4   EXPOSURE ASSESSMENT

The development of the dislodgeable residue methodology and procedures for measuring the transfer of pesticide foliar residues to workers provided the environmental data for estimating dermal dose.

4.1   Dislodgeable Leaf Residue Methodology

4.1.1   Application of Pesticides to Small Plots. The maximum hazard that a worker might encounter in a treated field is typically estimated by applying the maximum

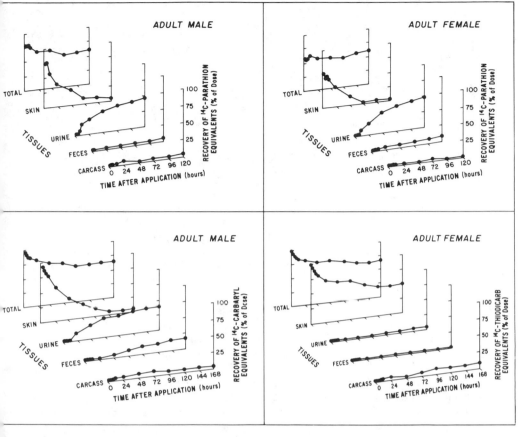

Figure 7. Time-course recovery of topically applied ^{14}C-labeled parathion, carbaryl, and thiodicarb equivalents in percentage of dose in feces, urine, carcasses, and skin (surface and penetrated residues) after application. Figure taken from Knaak and Wilson (47). (Reprinted with permission from American Chemical Society book publications.)

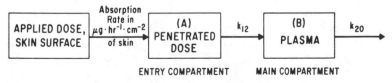

Figure 8. Two-compartment model with a central compartment (B) and an entry compartment (A) which takes up the topically applied dose. Figure taken from Knaak and Wilson (47). (Reprinted with permission from American Chemical Society book publications.)

TABLE 3. Parathion: Dermal Dose–Red Cell ChE Response in Male and Female Rats of Variable Age[a]

Sex, Age, Weight[b]	Slopes	$ED_{50}(\mu g/cm^2$ of treated area)[c]	$ED_{50}(\mu g/cm^2$ of total body surface)[c]	$ED_{50}(mg/kg$ of body weight
M, 10 weeks, 296 g	1.7	24.3 ± 3.7	1.7 ± 0.3	2.4
M, 5 weeks, 145 g	1.3	22.7 ± 4.2	1.6 ± 0.3	2.9
F, 13 weeks, 279 g	1.9	14.0 ± 3.7	1.0 ± 0.3	1.4
F, 5 weeks, 147 g	1.5	19.0 ± 4.1	1.3 ± 0.3	1.8

[a]Total area treated (7% of body surface).
[b]Sprague–Dawley rats, Simmonsen, Gilroy, CA.
[c]Values given with 95% confidence limits.
Source: Knaak et al. (46).

registered or proposed label rate, even though the normal use rate may be lower. The equipment used for the pesticide application should be typical of that used by the growers. The method of application should be selected such that the maximum foliar residue results. For example, the maximum label rate can often be applied to citrus trees by using either an oscillating boom sprayer or an airblast sprayer. Because the amount of water used with an oscillating boom sprayer may be on the order of 1500 gal/acre while that for an airblast sprayer is about 100 gal/acre, the amount of pesticide deposited on the outer foliage is different for the two applications. Airblast applications deposit more pesticide than boom applications.

The selection of the size of the test plot should be based on the ability to simulate an actual pesticide application made by a commercial operator. Ideally, the plot should be part of a larger field of the same crop so that the environmental conditions are representative of the crop. An isolated row of citrus, for example, would experience different climatic conditions than a row of citrus located within a grove of similar trees. If climatic factors, such as low humidity and high solar radiation, are believed to produce additional toxic residues such as organothiophosphate oxygen analogues (oxons), pesticide applications should be made in typically hot geographic regions and months of the year. However, the geographic region and time of year should not be atypical for the treated crop or the pesticide used, so as to produce atypical results of pesticide residues.

4.1.2 Development of the Leaf-Punch Sampler.

Pesticide residue data are generally expressed in terms of weight of pesticide per unit weight of matrix, such as micrograms per gram of soil, or weight of pesticide per unit volume of matrix, such as micrograms per liter of water. In both cases, one is interested only in the ratio of the amount of pesticide to the amount of matrix. When attempting to assess the hazards of reentry, it was recognized that only that portion of the total residue which was transferable to the worker was of concern. Pesticide residues inside plant tissues or surface waxes are not available to the agricultural worker, except through ingestion of the plant part, and therefore need not be considered. Conversely, pesticide residues on the plant surfaces are clearly the chief concern.

Residues may also be present as a liquid or solid pesticide deposit on the leaf surface, or they can be present in dust particles or clay particles, especially when they are used as formulation carriers. In general, surface residues require a surface area measurement so that the amount of pesticide can be reported on a per unit area basis, such as micrograms per square centimeter. Because foliage was initially suspected as the primary source of pesticide exposure, a technique to measure contamination was needed. An estimation of leaf area was possible using templates, but it was impractical. However, Gunther and co-workers (50) recognized that leaves, analogous to sheets of paper, could be punched in standard sizes. By knowing the aperture of the leaf punch and the number of leaf disks collected, the total area represented by the sample can readily be calculated. Thus, the leaf-punch sampler was developed as the tool of choice for collecting samples of foliage for residue analysis (50).

Two different apertures were initially used. A 2.5-cm (1-in.) aperture was used for sampling citrus leaves. A 1.8-cm aperture was used for peach leaves to accommodate the thinner nature of these leaves compared to citrus and grape leaves for excising purposes and the narrower nature of peach leaves. The punch had a concave surface to avoid disturbance of the surface residues. Unlike later leaf punches, the earlier models were designed so that the punch rotated one-eighth of a turn during the downward stroke to shear the leaf tissue and enhance the excision process. The first leaf punch was based on the

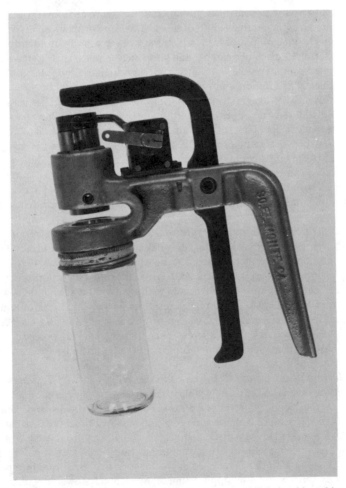

Figure 9. Punch for obtaining leaf disks for analysis of dislodgeable residues.

basic design of Smith and Little (51) and was privately manufactured by Norman Willett. Currently, leaf-punch samplers are available from Birkestrand Company (2563 Loma Avenue, South El Monte, CA 91733). A photograph of the leaf-punch sampler is shown in Fig. 9.

The simplicity of this sample collection procedure allowed the collection of a large number of leaf disks per treated field. Both statistically adequate sample size and appropriate field representation can easily be achieved. A collection jar for the sample simply screws onto the sampler and is replaced with a clean jar after each batch sample has been collected (Fig. 9). The jar containing the sample is simply capped and returned to the laboratory. An 8-oz jar is recommended to reduce the likelihood that the leaf disks will remain clumped together during the dislodgeable residue removal step.

4.1.3   Collection with the Leaf-Punch Sampler.   Leaf-disk samples are collected such that representative samples are obtained. In the case of tree crops, leaf disks are collected such that leaves from each octant around the tree are sampled equally by using eight or more trees. For row crops such as grapes, random samples from various heights are collected from a representative length of a field row. The primary objective is to collect samples from the type of foliage from which the worker will obtain the most contact or residues. A set of 40 disks per sample and three field replicates is deemed adequate. A stroke-activated counter on the leaf-punch sampler is used to keep track of the number of leaf disks collected. Variation among field replicates averages about 15%.

Field experience has demonstrated that the cutting edge needs to be cleaned after each batch sample with a tissue paper or a cotton swab moistened with water or acetone to remove plant juices, to maintain easy operation of the punch and to prevent cross-contamination between samples. It is best not to rely solely on the stroke-activated counter but to keep track mentally of the number of leaves sampled. The leaves should be free of excess moisture at the time of sampling; moisture resulting from a spray application, rain, overhead sprinkler irrigation, or morning dew should be allowed to evaporate before sampling is undertaken. Sample storage has been addressed by Gunther et al. (52).

4.1.4   Removal of Dislodgeable Residues.   The dislodgeable residue procedure involves the removal of surface residues by shaking the leaf disks with a dilute aqueous surfactant solution. The surfactant used was the American Cyanamid Company's Sur-Ten consisting of sodium dioctylsulfosuccinate. The first published procedure gave instructions that the leaf-disk sample be first shaken with 50 mL of the surfactant solution for 1 h and then with 50 mL of fresh solution for 30 min, and finally with 25 mL of solution for 5 s. The three wash solutions were combined in a separatory funnel and extracted with an organic solvent to recover the pesticide. This residue removal procedure with some variations has become a standard method for recovering dislodgeable residues (53).

4.1.5   Plotting Results and Determining the Half-Life of Residues.   Following application, the dissipation of dislodgeable residues from foliage is a complex process. It is dependent on the chemical and physical properties of the pesticides and their alteration products. If the logarithm of the residue is plotted against time, the dissipation process appears to have as many as three distinct parts. During the initial 1–3 days after application, residues may decline at a very rapid rate. Pesticides may be lost through volatilization along with the water used as a diluent or may penetrate into plant tissues. Between 1 day and 3 weeks after application, there is a much slower loss of residues. Then finally, after 3–4 weeks after application there is a very slow loss of residues. The entire

dissipation process is influenced by the presence of water, surfactants, emulsifiers, hydrocarbons, clays, and other materials present in the formulations.

4.2   Examples of Dislodgeable Residue Dissipation Curves

Dissipation curves for foliar applications of parathion, azinphosmethyl, and methidathion are given, respectively, in Figs. 10, 11, and 12. Paraoxon was formed on citrus foliage from parathion within the first 3 days postapplication (Gunther et al., 54). Whereas parathion residues continued to decline, paraoxon residues appeared to remain stable on the foliage. This high persistence of a very toxic compound was the main reason for the poisoning episodes associated with this pesticide. Azinphosmethyl dissipated more slowly on citrus with the formation of its oxygen analogue at the 6-1b AI/acre application rate (Kvalvag et al., 55). At lower rates of application, the oxon of azinphosmethyl was not detected. The oxygen analogue of methidathion was formed from the parent compound shortly after its application to citrus foliage (56). As the level of parent insecticide declines, the amount of oxon lost matched the amount formed and led to a "steady-state" residue level. When the parent insecticide reached lower levels, oxon dissipation was not offset by any additional oxon being formed and the oxon level declined.

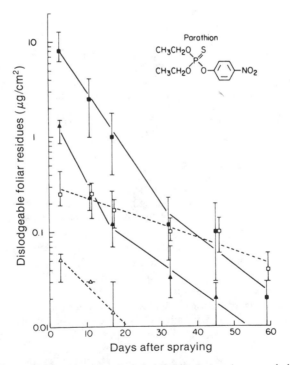

Figure 10.   Dissipation of parathion (closed symbols) and paraoxon (open symbols) on orange trees by gas chromatography. ■, and □, 10 lb AI parathion/100 gal per acre; ▲ and △, 10 lb AI parathion/1600 gal per acre. Figure taken from Knaak and Iwata (71). (Reprinted with permission from American Chemical Society book publications.)

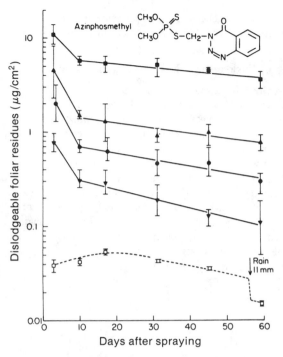

Figure 11. Dissipation curves for dislodgeable foliar residues of azinphosmethyl after a Guthion 2EC application to orange trees at 6 lb AI/100 gal (■) and at 6 lb AI/1200 gal (▲) per acre and at 2 (●) and 1 (▼) lb AI/500 gal per acre. Azinphosmethyl oxon (□) was determined only at the 6-lb AI/100 gal per acre treatment rate. Vertical lines give the range of values for six field sample replicates analyzed for azinphosmethyl and two field sample replicates analyzed for oxon. Data from Gunther et al. (54) and Kvalvag et al. (55). (Reprinted with permission from American Chemical Society book publications.)

4.3 Transfer of Foliar Residues to Workers

Investigative studies dealing with the hazards to workers contacting foliar residues of organophosphorus pesticides (OPs) principally involve ethyl parathion (Spear et al., 19), dioxathion (57), and phosalone (27) in California. Milby et al. (2) and Westlake et al. (57) estimated dermal exposure by washing unabsorbed residues from skin and measuring the residues in the washings by gas chromatography or by estimating the dermal dose indirectly from the amount of dust removed by scrubbing and rinsing skin, assuming that the pesticide concentration on skin was equal to the concentration in foliar dust.

The present and currently most acceptable method for measuring the dermal dose makes use of a multilayered cloth patch attached to skin or clothing to collect residues. The method was first used by Durham and Wolfe (58) in their investigations. Exposure patches consisted of 10.2 cm × 10.2 cm (4 in. × 4 in.) glassine weighing paper backing, a 4 in. × 4 in. alpha-cellulose center, and a 10-ply 4 in. × 4 in. surgical sponge outer dust collection medium. The patches are attached on the inside or outside of clothing, on both shoulders, chest, back, both forearms, and both upper arms, thighs, and shins. Residues on the hands are collected by washing the hands with soap and water or using alcohol.

Popendorf and Leffingwell (44) published the first quantitative model that relates field

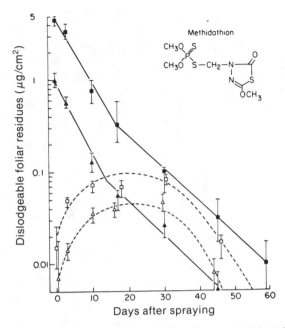

Figure 12. Dissipation curves for dislodgeable foliar residues of methidathion (closed symbols) and methidathion oxon (open symbols) after a Supracide 2E application to orange trees at 5.6 lb AI/100 gal (■, □) and 5.6 lb AI/2250 gal (▲, △) per acre. Vertical lines give the range of values obtained for six field sample replicates. Data from Iwata et al. (56). (Reprinted with permission from American Chemical Society book publications.)

worker exposure to foliar pesticide residues. The data used in this model were obtained from a series of field reentry studies conducted in California with dioxathion, ethyl parathion, and methidathion on grapes, citrus, and peaches. Each pesticide was applied by commercial equipment according to the instructions on the label. Workers equipped with dermal patches were allowed to reenter and harvest fruit on a daily basis from 1 to 3 days after application. Patches were removed after the end of the workday or some fraction of the day and analyzed for pesticide residues according to worker, day, and anatomical site. During each workday, leaf-punch samples were taken in the area of the vineyard or grove being harvested. The leaf samples were collected and analyzed according to the method of Gunther et al. (50).

The procedures used by Popendorf and Leffingwell (44) for calculating the rate of exposure (total body exposure in μg/h) from dermally collected (patches) and extracted residues are described by Davis (59) and Popendorf (60). These procedures extrapolate the dose rate on the patch to that on the skin surrounding each patch. Data were adjusted (61) based on the mensuration formula characteristic of each location and anatomic dimensions of the 50th percentile man (62, 63). Figure 13 presents key skin areas as a percentage of the total surface area (SA). Log–log regression analysis of the data showed that the relation between residues and dose is essentially linear as indicated in Fig. 14. Popendorf and Leffingwell (44) defined the dose to the worker by

$$D' = k_d tR, \tag{2}$$

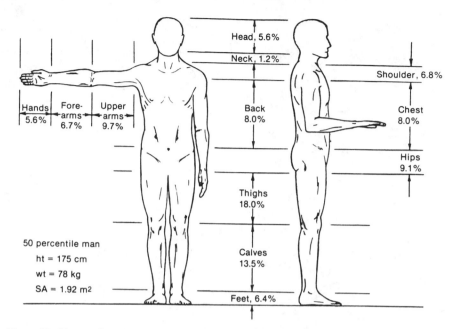

Figure 13. Human dermal surface area model derived from mensuration formula and anatomic dimensions. Each percentage corresponds to the proportion of the total surface area (SA) for each location. Figure taken from Popendorf and Leffingwell (44). (Reprinted with permission from Springer-Verlag, *Residue Reviews.*)

where D' is the dose (in mg), R is the measured residue (in ng/cm^2), t is the occupational exposure time (in h), and k_d is a crop or/and work practice-specific coefficient. The slope of the line (cm^2/h) of k_d value relates a foliar residue (ng/cm^2) to dose rate ($\mu g/h$) by simply multiplying a foliar residue level in ng/cm^2 by the k_d value in cm^2/h to give the dose rate in $\mu g/h$ for a one-sided leaf residue as shown in Fig. 14. To convert to a two-sided residue all residue values must be divided by 2. A k_d value of 5.1 was the transfer coefficient ($\mu g/h$ versus ng/cm^2) most often used by investigators involved in estimating pesticide exposure to workers reentering treated citrus. A k_d value of 5100 is used to relate a dose in $\mu g/h$ to a foliar residue in $\mu g/cm^2$.

The use of the model developed by Popendorf and Leffingwell (44) to predict harvester exposure to foliar residues in states such as Florida was questioned by Nigg et al. (64) who suggested that differences in California–Florida foliar and soil particulate matter might lead to a 10-fold greater California harvester exposure. This concern prompted these researchers (64) to develop a Florida model for predicting harvester exposure. Chlorobenzilate was applied to a mature block of Valencia oranges. Ten field workers wearing patches entered the grove 2, 3, and 4 days after the pesticide was applied to harvest fruit. Patches were collected at the end of the workday for analysis. All patch data were used in estimating total or partial body exposure ($\mu g/cm^2 \cdot h$). Good correlations were obtained for upper body exposure (excluding hands) versus leaf residues, $R = 0.70$; hand versus leaf residue, $R = 0.97$; lower body versus leaf residue, $R = 0.98$; and total body exposure versus leaf residue, $R = 0.98$.

The predictive equation was Y (estimated total body exposure, $\mu g/h) = (10652$

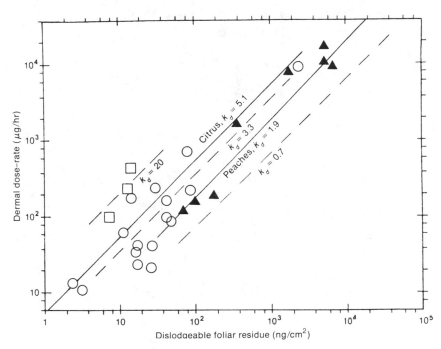

Figure 14. Composite dislodgeable residue versus dermal dose relations from Spear et al. (19), Popendorf et al. (27), and Popendorf (60): ○, citrus, multiple pesticides; □, citrus, superoxon; ▲, peaches, multiple pesticides. Figure taken from Popendorf and Leffingwell (44). (Reprinted with permission from Springer-Verlag, *Residue Reviews*.)

$\pm 2393 \, cm^2/h)X + (-74 \pm 430 \, \mu g/h)$, where X is the residue on the leaf surface in $\mu g/cm^2$. No log–log transformations were required as used in the California model. A reanalysis of the unmodified Popendorf and Leffingwell (44) data by Nigg et al. (64) yielded smaller errors in estimating the dose from the regression line than transformed data. Since Popendorf and Leffingwell (44) used one-sided leaf data in $\mu g/cm^2$, their data were divided by 2. The results indicated that there was no significant difference between the California and Florida models.

Nigg et al. (64) suggested that the two models for citrus fruit harvesters be averaged. The Y intercept values are small and should be canceled, leaving a simple equation for estimating total body exposure from foliar residues. This results in the following equation for a two-sided residue: exposure ($\mu g/h$) = 10^4 times residue (in $\mu g/cm^2$), where 10^4 is the slope of the regression line or transfer coefficient in cm^2/h.

This discussion shows that there are obvious differences in the data base. The Florida model is based on chlorobenzilate, an organochlorine miticide, while the California model is based on several experiments involving organophosphates, different workers, and different work conditions. The results, however, suggest that the differences in the work environment have been overemphasized between California and Florida. This also provides some assurances that estimation procedures used to estimate the uptake of chemicals by environmentally exposed persons are reasonably sturdy and not very sensitive to many of these factors.

5 EARLY AND CONCURRENT PROCEDURES FOR CALCULATING A REENTRY INTERVAL

Simple mathematical equations relating toxic foliar residues and cholinesterase inhibition were desired by regulatory officials to determine reentry intervals. A discussion of the early and concurrent procedures are given in this section.

5.1 Early Procedures

A mathematical procedure was proposed by Serat (65) to utilize organophosphorus pesticide foliar residue and cholinesterase depression data in workers exposed to these residues for estimating reentry times. The dissipation of the organophosphorus pesticide (in $\mu g/cm^2$ or ppm) was determined from leaf-punch samples taken at 2, 4, 8, and 28 days after a 7-lb/acre application. Ten workers were allowed to enter the field 3 days after application to harvest oranges for a period of 5 days. Cholinesterase activity was determined in the blood of these workers prior to and during the 5-day work period. Plasma activity was depressed. The residue data taken on each working day reflected the cumulative exposure of the workers. A semilogarithmic plot of ChE activity against cumulative insecticide exposure gave a straight-line relation. If a 10% decrease of ChE is acceptable, the residue producing this effect may be obtained from the curve. A plot of the residue data against time was then used to determine the reentry time.

Serat and Bailey (66) introduced the toxicological potential concept as the ratio between the pesticide residue level on foliage and the dermal LD_{50} value. In a latter study Serat et al. (67) suggested that worker reentry times could be estimated without exposing human beings to pesticide residues. The model combined the toxicological potential (66) concept with the earlier method for calculating safe reentry times (65), but the model neglected the effect of crop on the level of exposure and the toxicity of oxons in the dislodgeable residue.

In an unpublished paper by Spear (68) entitled "The Reentry Problem: Perspectives on the Regulatory Implications of Recent Research," the concept of setting safe pesticide levels on foliage in conjunction with safe reentry intervals was discussed in relation to the presence of ethion and the mono- and dioxons of ethion. The combined hazard of these materials is proportional to the sum of the amounts present weighted by the toxicity of each compound. According to Spear, the difficulties of indirectly estimating the relations between foliar residues, the residues transported to skin (dermal dose), and the absorbed dose leading to a toxic response led the Milby Committee (23) to conclude that "there is no substitute for basing worker safety re-entry intervals on carefully designed studies involving human beings, at least until a sufficient data base and experience permit similar latitude of design of reentry experiments."

Since the time of the report by the Milby Committee and the unpublished report by Spear (68), the relation between exposure, absorption, and the toxic effect has been defined using the results of field studies and animal dermal dose–ChE effect studies. The results of these studies and their usefulness in establishing safe levels and safe reentry times are presented in Sections 5.2 and 6.

5.2 Concurrent Procedures

Popendorf and Leffingwell (44) developed a "uniform field model' for evaluating foliar residue hazards and setting reentry intervals for organophosphorus pesticides. This model takes into consideration the residue initially deposited on foliage (R_0), the residue at reentry (R), the dose (mg) deposited on worker's skin (D'), the absorbed dose (D), and the response (change in AChE). The model is presented in the form of Eq. (3)–(6):

$$R = R_0 \exp(-k_r T) \tag{3}$$

$$D' = k_d t R, \tag{4}$$

$$D = \frac{k_a D'}{m}, \tag{5}$$

$$\Delta\text{AChE} = 1 - \exp\left(\frac{-k_e D}{\text{LD}_{50}}\right), \tag{6}$$

where k_r = pesticide specific residue decay coefficient
T = reentry interval (days)
k_d = residue transfer coefficient (cm^2/h)
t = exposure period (h)
k_a = absorption coefficient for fraction absorbed
m = body mass (nominal 70 kg)
ΔAChE = fraction of RBC cholinesterase inhibited
k_e = enzyme coefficient (use 6.0 for a topical dose and $k_a = 1$)
LD_{50} = dermal dose required to kill half the population.

In applying this model, the fractional change in acetylcholinesterase activity is estimated using eq. (3)–(6) or by combining them into Eq. (7):

$$\Delta\text{AChE} = 1 \exp\left[\frac{-k_e k_a\left(\dfrac{k_d t R_0 \exp(-k_r T)}{m}\right)}{\text{LD}_{50}}\right]. \tag{7}$$

This equation may be simplified further to Eq. (8) for citrus, where $R_0 = 1\ \mu g/cm^2$ (one-sided residue), $T = 0$, $k_d = 5.0\ cm^2/h$, and $t = 8.0\ h$:

$$\Delta\text{AChE} = 1 - \exp\left(\frac{-3.43}{\text{LD}_{50}}\right). \tag{8}$$

On the basis of Eq. (8), the fractional change in cholinesterase activity is dependent on the dermal LD_{50} of the organophosphorus insecticide under investigation. Equation (7) may be rearranged to determine a reentry interval T for an organophosphorus insecticide as shown in Eq. (9):

$$T = k_r^{-1} \ln\frac{-\text{LD}_{50} \ln(1 - \Delta\text{AChE})}{3.43}. \tag{9}$$

The uniform field model as described above has not been used to set reentry intervals for new pesticides such as chlorthiophos or carbosulfan as carried out in Sections 6.3 and 6.4.

Popendorf and Leffingwell (44) have used this model for calculation reentry intervals for parathion during high oxon production and high-oxon slow-decay conditions. Under conditions of high oxon production, a 35-day reentry interval was calculated for a 2% change in AChE activity. Under conditions of high oxon production and slow-decay rates, a 53-day reentry interval was determined for this change. This model was adjusted by Popendorf and Leffingwell (44) to take into consideration the combined toxicity of the parent pesticides (LD_{50}), their alteration products, and their rates of formation and dissipation (k_r). If the rate of absorption is significantly different for each of the products formed on the surface of the leaf, individual absorption rates may need to the determined for the pesticide and each alteration product. The Popendorf and Leffingwell (44) unified field model is conceptually sound but requires the development of enzyme, absorption, residue transfer, and residue decay coefficients in conjunction with dermal toxicity data and residue data to set reentry intervals. In the development of this model many of the parameters were estimated from a number of studies conducted with organophosphorus pesticides.

6   MATHEMATICS OF SETTING SAFE LEVELS ON FOLIAGE

Current mathematical procedures developed in California and used by the California Department of Food and Agriculture are described in this section along with procedures recommended by the U.S. Environmental Protection Agency (12).

6.1   Dermal Dose–ChE Response Studies and Field Worker Observations

The results of dermal dose–ChE response studies were used in conjunction with the results of field worker studies for estimating safe foliar residue levels for a number of

TABLE 4. Dermal Dose–ChE Response Expressed in Terms of Total Body Surface, Body Weight, and Safety Index

Pesticides	ED_{50} (μg/cm^2) of body surface[a]	ED_{50} (mg/kg)[b]	Dermal LD_{50} (mg/kg)	Safety Index LD_{50}/ED_{50} (mg/kg)
Paraoxon	0.33 ± 0.2	0.5	2.0^c	4.0
Parathion	2.4 ± 0.3	3.4	21.0^d	6.2
Methidathion	10.0 ± 0.3	15.0	150.0^e	10.0
Dialifor	23.0 ± 0.3	33.0	—	—
Azinphosmethyl	25.0 ± 0.5	35.0	220.0^d	6.3
Phosalone	188.0 ± 0.4	265.0	1450.0^f	5.5
Dimethoate	432.0 ± 2	611.0	1420.0^g	2.3

[a]Pesticides were individually applied in 1.0 mL of acetone to the clipped backs (25 cm^2) of 220–240-g male rats. Blood was taken 72 h after application for ChE determination. Response expressed in terms of total body surface (325 cm^2) from dermal dose–ChE response curves in Figs. 2 and 3. Values are given with 95% confidence limits.
[b]Values determined from dermal dose–ChE response curves.
[c]Estimated.
[d]Gaines (40).
[e]CIBA-GEIGY *Toxicology Data Bulletin.*
[f]Mazuret (49).
[g]Gaines (41).
Source: Knaak et al. (42).

TABLE 5. Establishment of Safe Levels ($\mu g/cm^2$) on Tree Foliage Using Results of Dermal Dose–ChE Response Studies in Male Rats and Field Reentry Studies

Pesticides[a]	Slopes	ED_{50} ($\mu g/cm^2$ of body surface)	Relative Toxicity[b]	Safe Level on Foliage ($\mu g/cm^2$)[c]
Paraoxon	2.3	0.33	1.0	0.02[d]
Methidathion	2.9	10.00	30.0	0.60
Azinphosmethyloxon	2.0	0.82	1.0	0.05[e]
Methidathionoxon	1.8	2.2	3.0	0.15
Dialifor	1.3	23.0	0.12	0.8
Parathion	1.3	2.4	0.013	0.09
Phosalone	1.5	188.0	1.0	7.0[f]
Azinphosmethyl	0.9	25.0	1.0	3.1[g]
Dimethoate	0.7	432.0	17.0	53.0

[a]Pesticide standard in italic.
[b]ED_{50} of pesticide under investigation divided by ED_{50} of pesticide standard.
[c]Relative toxicity multiplied by safe level of standard.
[d]Spear et al. (69).
[e]Estimated.
[f]Popendorf et al. (27).
[g]Richards et al. (70).
Source: Table is composite of data from Knaak et al. (42) and Knaak and Iwata (71).

organophosphorus and carbamate pesticides. Table 4 gives the dermal dose–ChE response data (ED_{50}) in terms of body weight and total body surface, and the dermal LD_{50} in terms of body weight. On the basis of total body surface, the quantities producing 50% red blood cell inhibition were 0.33, 2.4, 10.0, 23.0, 25.0, 188.0, and 432.0 $\mu g/cm^2$ of skin, respectively, for paraoxon, parathion, methidathion, dialifor, azinphosmethyl, phosalone, and dimethoate. In Table 5, these values and the results of studies conducted by Spear et al. (69), Richards et al. (70), and Popendorf et al. (27) were used by Knaak et al. (42, 43, 71) to estimate safe levels on foliage. The field exposure studies established safe levels for azinphosmethyl, azinphosmethyl oxon, phosalone, and paraoxon of 3.1, 0.05, 7.0, and 0.02 $\mu g/cm^2$, respectively. These pesticides and their safe foliar levels were used as standards for establishing additional safe levels on foliage for methidathion, methidathion oxon, dialifor, parathion, and dimethoate using their relative toxicities as shown in Table 4. In practice this was accomplished by grouping the pesticides under investigation and the pesticide standards according to their slopes, and determining a safe level for the pesticide under investigation using Eq. (10):

safe level ($\mu g/cm^2$) for pesticide under investigation

$$= \text{safe level of standard} \times ED_{50}\ (\mu g/cm^2)\ \text{of pesticide} \div ED_{50}\ \text{of standard.} \quad (10)$$

6.2   Reentry Intervals for Thions and Oxons

The oxidative conversion of methidathion, azinphosmethyl, and parathion on leaf surfaces to oxons necessitated the development of a procedure for establishing safe levels on foliage for the combined hazard posed by thion and oxon residues. This was accomplished for methidathion, azinphosmethyl, and parathion (71) by allowing the oxon to be present at a

TABLE 6. Procedure for Establishing Safe Levels (μg/cm²) for Thions + Oxons on Tree Foliage

Application to Citrus[a]	Days Elapsed[a]	Thion[a]	Oxon[a,b]	Thion + Oxon	Thion + Oxon × RT[c]	$\dfrac{\text{Thion} + \text{Oxon}}{\text{Thion} + \text{Oxon} \times \text{RT}} \times$ SL[d] for Thion
Parathion						
10 lb AI/1600 gal per acre	10	0.35	0.02	0.37	0.49	0.07
	20	0.09	0.01	0.10	0.16	0.06[e]
Methidathion						
5.6 lb AI/100 gal per acre	10	1.0	0.08	1.08	1.38	0.4
	20	0.25	0.1	0.35	0.73	0.3
	30	0.11	0.08	0.19	0.50	0.2[e]
Azinphosmethyl						
6.0 lb AI/1200 gal per acre	10	1.5	0.05	1.55	2.91	1.7
	20	1.3	0.05	1.35	2.86	1.6[e]
	30	1.1	0.05	1.15	2.51	1.5

[a]Taken from Fig. 10, 11, and 12.
[b]Oxons must be at safe level indicated in Table 2. Method assumes oxons will be at a safe level when safe level for thion + oxon is reached.
[c]RT = relative toxicity from Table 2 (ED_{50} of thion ÷ ED_{50} of oxon).
[d]SL = safe levels for thions from Table 2.
[e]Safe levels for thion + oxon.
Source: Knaak and Iwata (71).

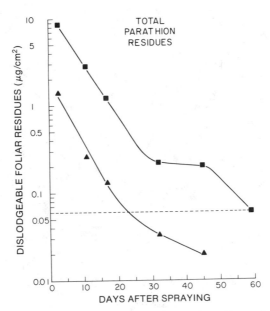

Figure 15. Dissipation of combined residues (thion + oxon) of parathion and paraoxon on orange trees. $-\blacksquare-$, 10 lb AI parathion/100 gal per acre; $-\blacktriangle-$, 10 lb AI parathion/1600 gal per acre. Dashed line is safe level for thion + oxon. Curves are drawn from Fig. 10. Figure taken from Knaak and Iwata (71). (Reprinted with permission from American Chemical Society book publications.)

safe level and by reducing the combined residue of oxon and thion to 0.06, 0.02, and 1.6 μg/cm^2, respectively, for parathion, methidathion, and azinphosmethyl; see Table 6. A safe level for the mixture may also be estimated by determining the toxicity (ED$_{50}$) of the oxon and thion mixture using the method of Finney (72) in Eq. (11):

$$ \text{ED}_{50}\ (\text{mixture, } \mu\text{g/cm}^2) = \left[\frac{P_1}{\text{ED}_{50,1}} + \frac{P_2}{\text{ED}_{50,2}} + \cdots + \frac{P_N}{\text{ED}_{50,N}} \right]^{-1}, \tag{11} $$

where P_1 and P_2 are the proportions of oxon and thion, respectively, on foliage after 10, 20, or 30 days as shown in Table 6. In the case of parathion–paraoxon at 10 days, the ED$_{50}$ of the mixture was 23.4 μg/cm^2, while the safe level for the mixture was 0.067 μg/cm^2 as determined by Eq. (12). This value is equivalent to the one given in Table 5 for parathion–paraoxon, 10 days after application.

$$ \text{SL, mixture}\ (\mu\text{g/cm}^2) = \frac{\text{ED}_{50},\ \text{thion} + \text{oxon}}{\text{ED}_{50},\ \text{phosalone}} \times \text{SL, phosalone}. \tag{12} $$

The relation between total parathion–paraoxon residues, their rate of dissipation, and the safe level for total thion and oxon is shown in Fig. 15. The dashed line is the safe level.

6.3 Reentry Interval for Chlorthiophos

These studies by Knaak et al. (42) and Knaak and Iwata (71) provided a method for determining a reentry interval for a new pesticide, chlorthiophos, on citrus. Figure 16

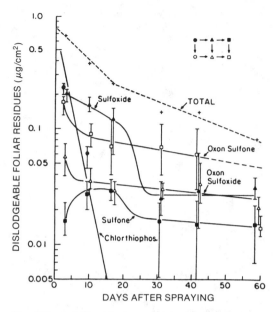

Figure 16. Dislodgeable residues of chlorthiophos and its oxidation products on orange foliage after application of Celathion 40WP at a rate of 9.5 lb AI/1900 gal per acre. Vertical lines indicate the range of values found for six replicate field samples. Figure taken from Iwata et al. (73). (Reprinted with permission from American Chemical Society, *Journal of Agriculture, Food and Chemistry.*)

Chlorthiophos

Chlorthiophos sulfoxide

Chlorthiophos sulfone

Chlorthiophos oxon

Chlorthiophos oxon sulfoxide

Chlorthiophos oxon sulfone

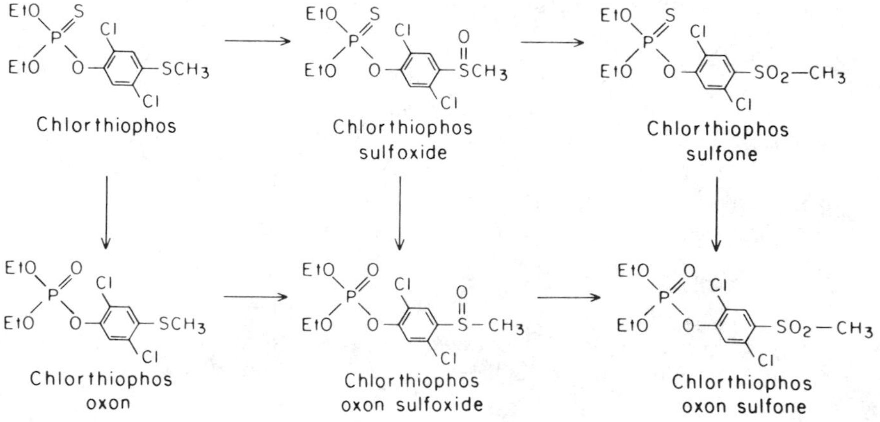

Figure 17. Chemical structure of chlorthiophos and five ChE-inhibition oxidation products. Figure taken from Iwata et al. (73). (Reprinted with permission from American Chemical Society, *Journal of Agriculture, Food and Chemistry.*)

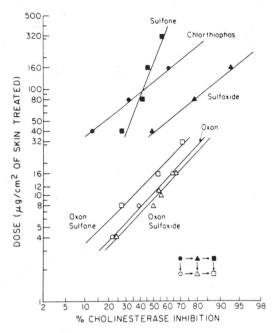

Figure 18. Percentage of red blood cell ChE inhibition in rats sacrificed 72 h after treatment of nature of skin surface with chlorithiophos or one of its five oxidation products. Figure taken from Iwata et al. (73). (Reprinted with permission from American Chemical Society, *Journal of Agriculture, Food and Chemistry*.)

(Iwata et al., 73) shows the dislodgeable residue data obtained when a commercial formulation of chlorthiophos, Celathion 40 W, is applied to citrus at a rate of 9.5 lb AI/1900 gal per acre. The chemical structures of the dislodgeable residues are given in Fig. 17. Chlorthiophos and five toxic oxidation products were found. Dermal dose–ChE response studies in the rat were performed on each toxicant to determine its ED_{50} value as shown in Fig. 18. The oxons were similar in their toxicity, while chlorthiophos, chlorthiophos sulfoxide, and chlorthiophos sulfone were less toxic. Safe levels on foliage were determined for each toxicant using the procedure of Knaak et al. (42). Paraoxon, parathion, and azinphosmethyl were used as pesticide standards (Table 7).

Two procedures were used to calculate safe reentry levels for chlorthiophos and its oxidation products on citrus. The first method used the procedure of Knaak and Iwata (71) for the combined thion and oxon residues as shown in Table 8. This method may be simplified using Eq. (11) and (12). Equation (11) first determines the ED_{50} of the mixture (thions and oxons). The value (15.1 $\mu g/cm^2$, 20 days after spraying) was used in Eq. 12, where it was divided by the ED_{50} of the oxon sulfoxide (40.3 $\mu g/cm^2$) and multiplied by the safe level (SL) for chlorthiophos sulfoxide (0.19 $\mu g/cm^2$) to give 0.07 $\mu g/cm^2$ as the safe level for the combined foliar residues in Table 8.

The second procedure (Iwata et al., 73) used to determine a safe reentry level was a modification of one proposed by the U.S. Environmental Protection Agency (12); see Table 9. A no observable effect level (NOEL) was determined (ED_{10}) for the combined residues of chlorthiophos sulfone and sulfoxide, and chlorthiophos oxon sulfoxide and

TABLE 7. Establishment of Safe Residue Levels (μg/cm²) on Citrus Tree Foliage Using Results of Dermal Dose–ChE Response Curves and Field Reentry Studies according to Knaak et al. (42)

Insecticide or Alteration Product[a]	Slope of Dose–Response Curve[b]	ED_{50} (μg/cm²) of total body surface)[c]	Relative Toxicity[d]	Safe Level on Foliage, (μg/cm²)[e]
Chlorthiophos sulfoxide	2.5	3.1	9.4	0.19
Chlorthiophos	2.4	8.8	27	0.54
Paraoxon	2.3	0.33	1	0.02[f]
Chlorthiophos oxon sulfone	2.0	1.2	3.6	0.07
Chlorthiophos oxon sulfoxide	1.9	0.69	0.29	0.03
Parathion	1.3	2.4	1	0.09[f]
Azinphosmethyl	0.9	25	1	3.0[g]
Chlorthiophos sulfone	0.8	13	0.53	1.6

[a]Reference compound is in italics; this compound is one for which actual field safety information is available.
[b]Slopes derived from Fig. 18 for chlorthiophos and its alteration products. Data used to construct the figure were statistically analyzed according to the log–probit analysis procedure of Finney (72).
[c]ED_{50} in μg/cm² multiplied by 25 cm² (treated area) and divided by 325 cm² (total surface area of the rat).
[d]ED_{50} of the compound under investigation divided by the ED_{50} of the reference compound.
[e]Relative toxicity multiplied by the established safe level of the reference as determined by actual reentry studies.
[f]Spear et al. (69).
[g]Richards et al. (70).
Source: Iwata et al. (73).

TABLE 8. Procedure for Establishing Safe Levels (μg/cm²) of Total Thions Plus Oxons of Chlorthiophos on Citrus Tree Foliage According to Knaak and Iwata (71)

Days After Spraying	Residues (μg/cm²)			Thion + Oxon × RT[c]	(Thion + Oxon)/ (Thion + Oxon × RT) × SL for Thion[d] (μg/cm²)
	Thion[a]	Oxon[b]	Thion + Oxon		
20	0.12	0.11	0.23	0.60	0.07
40	0.04	0.09	0.13	0.43	0.06
60	0.04	0.07	0.11	0.37	0.06

[a]Since no chlorthiophos is present at or after 20 days, thion residues are the sum of chlorthiophos sulfoxide and sulfone. Values were obtained from Fig. 16.
[b]Since no chlorthiophos oxon is present at or after 20 days, oxon residues are the sum of chlorthiophos oxon sulfoxide and sulfone. Values were obtained from Fig. 16.
[c]RT (relative toxicity) is the ED_{50} of the chlorthiophos sulfoxide divided by the ED_{50} of the oxon sulfoxide. This RT differs in definition from that in Table 7.
[d]SL (safe level) for the thion is 0.19 μg/cm² as given in Table 7 for the most toxic thion, chlorthiophos sulfoxide.
Source: Iwata et al. (73).

TABLE 9. Calculation of Reentry Intervals According to U.S. EPA Guidelines (12) with Slight Modifications[a]

Day	Compound Ratio[b]	NOEL[c] (μg/kg·day)	AEL[d] (μg/kg·day)	Total Dose[e] (μg/h)	Reentry Level[f] (μg/cm^2)
20	4:1:1:3	391	39.1	342	0.08
40	2:1:2:4	304	30.4	266	0.06
60	2:1:2:3	309	30.9	270	0.06

[a]The modification involves taking into account all toxic residues present on the foliage and using a total toxic residue level curve.
[b]This is the ratio of sulfoxide:sulfone:oxon sulfoxide:oxon sulfone present on foliage as shown in Fig. 16.
[c]No effect level (NOEL) calculated from data from dermal dose–ChE response curve. NOEL = ED_{10} $(25 \, cm^2)/(0.23 \, kg/day)$. Predicted $ED_{10} = [P_1/ED_{10,1} + P_2/ED_{10,2} + \cdots + P_N/ED_{10,N}]^{-1}$, where P = proportion of component in mixture (Finney, 72). ED_{10} values were extrapolated from Fig. 18. ED_{10} for chlorthiophos, its sulfoxide, its sulfone, its oxon, its oxon sulfoxide, and its oxon sulfone were 35, 12, 4, 2, 2, and 3.5 μg/cm^2, respectively.
[d]Allowable exposure level (AEL) = NOEL/SF. Safety factor (SF) = 10.
[e]Total dose = (AEL)(body weight, 70 kg)/(duration, 8 h/day).
[f]From total dose determine reentry level from graph of whole-body dermal dose (μg/h) versus dislodgeable foliar residues (ng/cm^2) from data of Popendorf (60) as abbreviated by U.S. Environmental Protection Agency (12).
Source: Iwata et al. (73).

sulfone on foliage, 20, 40, and 60 days after spraying. The ED_{10} values from the dermal dose–ChE response curves (Fig. 18) were used. The ED_{10} value for the mixture was determined using Eq. (13). The NOEL was calculated using the ED_{10} value for the mixture in Eq. (14), while an acceptable exposure level (AEL) was determined by Eq. (15).

$$ED_{10}(\text{mixture}, \mu g/cm^2) = \left[\frac{P_1}{ED_{10,1}} + \frac{P_2}{ED_{10,2}} + \cdots + \frac{P_N}{ED_{10,N}} \right]^{-1}, \tag{13}$$

$$NOEL\,(\mu g/kg \cdot day) = \frac{ED_{10}\,(25\,cm^2)}{0.23\,kg/day}, \tag{14}$$

$$AEL\,(\mu g/kg \cdot day) = \frac{NOEL}{SF}, \tag{15}$$

$$\text{total dose} = (AEL)(\text{body weight, 70 kg})(\text{duration, 8 h/day}). \tag{16}$$

A total dose was calculated using the AEL value in Eq. (16). Finally, in Eq. (17), a reentry level was determined by dividing the total dose by a transfer coefficient $k_d = 5.1$, determined graphically by Popendorf and Leffingwell (44) relating whole body dermal dose (μg/h) to dislodgeable foliar residues (ng/cm^2):

$$\text{reentry level (ng/cm}^2) = \frac{\text{total dose } (\mu g/h)}{k_d = 5.1\,cm^2/h}. \tag{17}$$

The reentry or safe levels determined by these two procedures gave almost equivalent values because the same dislodgeable residue and toxicological data base were used. Differences, however, exist in the manner in which these two methods used exposure data. In the first method, results of worker exposure studies were used to estimate safe residue levels for certain pesticides in the field using dislodgeable residue data and red blood cell cholinesterase measurements in the worker. The safe level for the pesticide was then used as a field standard in conjunction with relative animal potency data to relate the safe level of the standard to a pesticide under investigation. The second procedure did not use cholinesterase values from exposed workers, but rather developed a graph relating foliar residues (μg/cm^2) to dose (μg/h) for workers harvesting crops. Animal dermal dose–ChE response data were used to determine an acceptable AEL, total dose, and safe level from the graph.

Either method is acceptable for setting reentry intervals for organophosphorus pesticides. However, the Knaak and Iwata (71) method required field observations relating residue on foliage to changes in field worker cholinesterase values for the pesticide standard. Blood cholinesterase measurements in field workers are not required by the modification of the U.S. EPA procedure (12). In either case, workers should be monitored for AChE inhibition after a reentry interval is established on a new organophosphorus pesticide. On the basis of the calculated safe reentry levels determined for chlorthiophos, a 70-day reentry interval was proposed by Iwata et al. (73). Because of this long reentry interval and the marginal efficacy of this organophosphate, Celathion 40 W has not been registered in California.

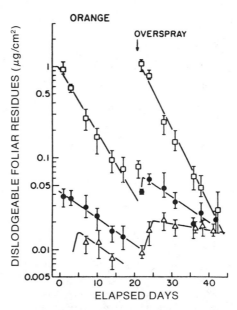

Figure 19. Dislodgeable foliar residues of carbosulfan ($\square$), carbofuran ($\bullet$), and 3-hydroxycar-bofuran ($\triangle$) after treatment of orange trees with Advantage 2.5EC insecticide formulation at 1.5 lb AI/200 gal per acre. Each datum point is the mean value obtained from six replicate field samples, and the vertical lines show the range of values found. Figure taken from Iwata et al. (74). (Reprinted with permission from American Chemical Society, *Journal of Agriculture, Food and Chemistry*.)

6.4   Reentry Interval for Carbosulfan

The procedure used to determine a safe level and reentry period for chlorthiophos was recently used by Iwata et al. (74) to establish a reentry interval for Advantage 2.5EC, a new insecticide containing carbosulfan as the active ingredient. This insecticide was applied to mature orange trees at a rate of 1.5 lb AI/200 gal per acre. Foliar dislodgeable residue data given in Fig. 19 were obtained over a period of 45 days. Carbosulfan is degraded on foliage to carbofuran and a metabolite, 3-hydroxycarbofuran. A safe reentry level was determined by Iwata et al. (74) for total residues of carbosulfan on oranges using the procedure used for chlorthiophos in Section 6.3.

Figure 20 gives the dermal dose–ChE response curves obtained for these products in the rat. Safe levels were determined using parathion as the reference standard for which actual field information was available. Carbosulfan, carbofuran, and 3-hydroxycarbofuran were all found to be less dermally toxic than parathion, as shown in Table 10. Safe levels varied from 0.3 to 1.3 μg/cm^2 with carbosulfan and carbofuran being equally toxic via the dermal route. In Table 11 the procedure of Knaak and Iwata (71) was used to determine safe levels for the the total carbamate residues of carbofuran on citrus foliage.

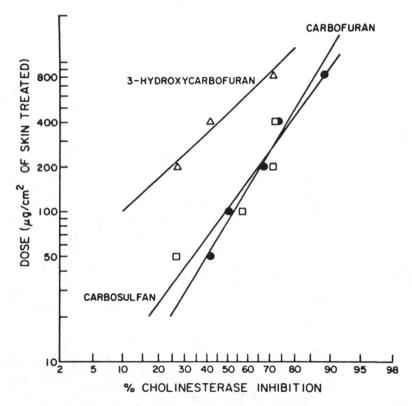

Figure 20.   Percentage of red blood cell ChE inhibition in rats sacrificed 24 h after treatment of 25 cm^2 of skin surface with carbosulfan, carbofuran, or 3-hydroxycarbofuran. Figure taken from Iwata et al. (74). (Reprinted with permission from American Chemical Society, *Journal of Agriculture, Food and Chemistry.*)

TABLE 10. Calculation of Safe Residue Levels ($\mu g/cm^2$) on Citrus Tree Foliage Using Results of Dermal Dose–ChE Response Curves and Field Reentry Studies According to Knaak et al. (42)

Insecticide or Alteration Product	Slope of Dose–Response Curve[a]	ED_{50} ($\mu g/cm^2$ of total body surface)[b]	Relative Toxicity[c]	Safe Level on Foliage ($\mu g/cm^2$)[d]
Carbofuran	1.12	6.6 ± 0.4	2.8	0.3
Carbosulfan	1.35	7.8 ± 0.4	3.3	0.3
3-Hydroxy carbofuran	1.95	34.4 ± 0.3	14.3	1.3
Parathion	1.3	2.4 ± 0.3	1.0	0.09^e

[a]Values for the three carbamate compounds were calculated from the data used to construct Fig. 19. Data were subjected to the log–probit analysis procedure of Finney (72).
[b]ED_{50} in $\mu g/cm^2$ multiplied by 25 cm^2 (treated area) and divided by 325 cm^2 (total surface area of the rat).
[c]ED_{50} of the compound under investigation divided by the ED_{50} of parathion, a reference compound for which actual field safety information is available.
[d]Relative toxicity multiplied by the established safe level of parathion, which was determined by actual reentry studies.
[e]Spear et al. (69).
Source: Iwata et al. (74).

Equations (11) and (12) may also be used to calculate a safe level for the mixture (total carbamates). In Eq. (12), the ED_{50} of the mixture (1, 3, 7, and 10 days after spraying) was divided by the ED_{50} of parathion and multiplied by the safe level determined in Table 10 for carbofuran (0.3 $\mu g/cm^2$). The small differences in the dermal ED_{50} values of carbosulfan (101 $\mu g/cm^2$) and carbofuran (86 $\mu g/cm^2$) and the small quantities of 3-hydroxycarbofuran formed on foliage resulted in safe levels for the mixture equivalent to carbosulfan or carbofuran.

Somewhat lower reentry levels were obtained in Table 12 when the reentry levels were calculated using the modified U.S. Environmental Protection Agency guidelines (12) as described in Section 6.3 for chlorthiophos. The lower values are probably a result of using the ED_{10} values in place of the ED_{50} values for the mixture of carbamates and the transfer coefficient of 5.1 (k_d for citrus). On the basis of these results and the dislodgeable residue data, a 7-day reentry time was selected as being sufficient to protect the health of workers.

Nigg et al. (75) conducted a similar study in Florida using carbosulfan. In experiment 1, Advantage 2.5EC was applied twice during the summer at the rate of 4 lb AI/750gal per acre to mature Valencia oranges. A similar spray program, experiment 2, was conducted by Nigg et al. (75) in Florida using a 1-lb rate. Carbofuran was the principal metabolite present on foliage.

Reentry intervals for the 4- and 1-lb AI/acre application rates in experiments 1 and 2 were calculated according to each of the two procedures used by Iwata et al. (74). The ED_{10} and ED_{50} values determined by Iwata et al. (74) for carbosulfan and carbofuran from dermal dose–ChE response studies were used in conjunction with dislodgeable residue data from experiments 1 and 2 to determine a safe reentry period for total carbamate residues using the procedure of Knaak and Iwata (71) in Table 13 and the modified U.S. Environmental Protection Agency method (12) in Table 14. This table indicates that safe reentry levels are reached in these experiments on days 2 and 3. The California–Florida citrus studies (Iwata et al., 74; Nigg et al., 75) with carbofuran were the first studies to

TABLE 11. Calculation of Safe Levels ($\mu g/cm^2$) Based on Total Carbamate Residues of Carbosulfan on Citrus Tree Foliage

Days After Spraying	Dislodgeable Foliar Residues ($\mu g/cm^2$)[a]				Toxic Equivalents, $(CS + CF) + (HCF \times RT)$[b] ($B$)	Safe Level for CS + CF + HCF Mixture, $(A/B) \times$ SL for CF ($\mu g/cm^2$)[c]
	Carbosulfan (CS)	Carbofuran (CF)	3-Hydroxycarbofuran (HCF)	Total Carbamate (A)		
1	0.94	0.038	<0.01	0.99	0.98	0.30
3	0.58	0.036	<0.01	0.63	0.62	0.30
7	0.27	0.029	0.012	0.31	0.30	0.31
10	0.17	0.023	0.012	0.21	0.19	0.32

[a]Values are those used to construct Fig. 19.
[b]RT (relative toxicity) is the ED_{50} of CS divided by the ED_{50} of HCF. This RT differs in definition from that given in Table 10.
[c]SL (safe level) is 0.3 $\mu g/cm^2$ as found for CF (Table 10), the most dermally toxic of the three carbamate compounds.
Source: Iwata et al. (74).

TABLE 12. Calculation of Reentry Intervals According to U.S. Environmental Protection Agency (12) Guidelines with Slight Modification[a]

Days After Spraying	Compound Ratio[b] CS:CF:HCF	NOEL[c] (μg/kg·day)	AEL[d] (μg/kg·day)	Total Dose[e] (μg/h)	Reentry Level[f] (μg/cm^2)
1	94:3.8:1	1224	122	1068	0.21
3	58:3.6:1	1209	121	1059	0.21
7	22.5:2.4:1	1197	120	1050	0.21
10	14.2:1.9:1	1200	120	1050	0.21

[a]Modification involves taking into account all toxic residues present on the foliage and using a total toxic residue curve.

[b]Ratios calculated from values used to construct Fig. 19.

[c]No effect level (NOEL) calculated from data from dermal dose–ChE response curve. NOEL = $ED_{10}(25\ cm^2)/(0.23\ kg/day)$. Predicted $ED_{10} = [P_1/ED_{10,1} + P_2/ED_{10,2} + \cdots + P_N/ED_{10,N}]^{-1}$, where P = proportion of component in mixture (Finney, 72). ED_{10} values were extrapolated from Fig. 19. ED_{10} values for CS, CF, and HCF were 11.5, 6.24, and 98.8 μg/cm^2, respectively.

[d]Allowable exposure level (AEL) = NOEL/SF. Safety factor (SF) = 10.

[e]Total dose = (AEL)(body weight, 70 kg)/(duration, 8 h/day).

[f]From total dose, reentry level was determined from the graph of whole-body dermal dose (μg/h) versus dislodgeable foliar residues (ng/cm^2) from the data of Popendorf and Leffingwell (44). Total dose was divided by 5.1, the k_d for citrus; derivation was based on the area of only one side of the leaf.

Source: Iwata et al. (74).

TABLE 13. Reentry Levels and Intervals for Total Carbamate Residues on Leaves

Days After Spraying	Dislodgeable Foliar Residues (μg/cm^2)[a] Carbosulfan (CS)	Carbofuran (CF)	Total Carbamates (CS + CF)	Reentry Level (μg/cm^2 total carbamates)[b]
	Experiment 1			
1	0.782	0.042	0.824	0.3
2	0.288	0.041	0.329	0.3
3	0.194	0.029	0.223	0.3[c]
	Experiment 2			
1	0.243	0.013	0.256	0.3[c]
2	0.165	0.025	0.190	0.3
3	0.157	0.034	0.191	0.3

[a]Values from dislodgeable residue tables.

[b]Safe reentry level is 0.3 μg/cm^2 for CS, CF, and total carbamates (CS + CF) according to Iwata et al. (74).

[c]Reentry interval is 3 days for experiment 1 and 1 day for experiment 2.

Source: Nigg et al. (75).

TABLE 14. Calculation of Reentry Intervals According to U.S. Environmental Protection Agency (12) Guidlines[a]

Days After Spraying	Compound Ratio[b] CS:CF	NOEL[c] (μg/kg·day)	AEL[d] (μg/kg·day)	Total Allowable CS + CF Dose[e] (μg/h)	CS + CF Reentry Level[f] (μg/cm^2)
		Experiment 1			
1	18.6:1	1198	120	1050	0.21
2	7.0:1	1131	113	989	0.19
3[g]	6.7:1	1127	113	989	0.19
		Experiment 2			
1	18.7:1	1199	120	1050	0.21
2[g]	6.6:1	1125	113	989	0.19
3	4.6:1	1087	109	954	0.19

[a] A slight modification of these guidelines is introduced here, which takes into account all toxic residues present on the foliage.
[b] Ratios calculated from dislodgeable residue tables.
[c] No effect level (NOEL) calculated from data from dermal dose–ChE response curve (Iwata et al., 74). NOEL = $ED_{10}(25\,\text{cm}^2)/(0.23\,\text{kg})$. Effective ED_{10} for mixture from $1/ED_{10} = P_1/ED_{10.2} + \cdots + P_N/ED_{10,N}$, where P_i = proportion of component i in the mixture (Finney, 72). $ED_{10,i}$ values were extrapolated from Fig. 19 Iwata et al. (74), and found to be 11.5 and 6.24 μg/cm^2·day for CS and CF, respectively.
[d] Allowable exposure level (AEL) = NOEL/SF. Safety factor (SF) = 10. [e] Total allowable dose = (AEL)(body weight, 70 kg)/(duration, 8 h/day).
[f] From total dose the reentry level is determined from a graph of whole-body dermal dose (μg/h) versus dislodgeable foliar residues (μg/cm^2) from the data of Popendorf and Leffingwell (44). Total dose divided by 5100 cm^2/h is k_d for citrus for a one-sided dislodgeable residue.
[g] Reentry interval (total carbamates from Table 13) is about 3 days for experiment 1 and 2 days for experiment 2.
Source: Nigg et al. (75).

provide dislodgeable residue data and estimate reentry intervals in these states for the same toxic organophosphate or methylcarbamate insecticide.

The transfer coefficient ($k_d = 5.1$) developed by Popendorf and Leffingwell in California was used by Iwata et al. (73, 74) and Nigg et al. (75) to estimate exposure. A repeat worker exposure study carried out by Nigg et al. (64) and discussed in Section 4.2 of this chapter yielded a k_d value of 5.3 cm^2/h, in close agreement with the California k_d of 5.1 cm^2/h. Popendorf and Leffingwell (44) developed their graphs using one-sided dislodgeable residue data. They assumed that all the residue was present on the top side of the leaf. Iwata et al. (73, 74) and Nigg et al. (75) reported their dislodgeable residue data in terms of a two-sided residue. Popendorf and Leffingwell (44) suggest that the two-sided residue data be divided by 2 to obtain one-sided data. If this procedure is carried out, unnecessarily long reentry intervals would be required by the modified U.S. Environmental Protection Agency procedure (12) when compared to the method used by Knaak and Iwata (71).

7 DISCUSSION

The large number of variables associated with the reentry problem prevented researchers from coming up with an easy and quick solution to the problem. However, by dividing the problem up into three distinct parts—(i) dissipation of the foliar residue, (ii) transfer of the residue to the skin and clothing of workers, and (iii) percutaneous absorption/dermal dose–ChE response—the reentry problem was resolved. A substantially large number of studies were conducted dealing with the dissipation of the foliar residues. These studies involved such factors as air temperature, humidity, ozone concentrations in air, rain, dust, season of the year, and a variety of other factors. The studies indicated that all these factors played a role in the conversion of foliar residues to toxic products, such as oxons, and in the dissipation of these residues. Several simple equations were written by California Department of Food and Agriculture scientists in the early 1970s in an attempt to describe the overall process. The equations did not adequately describe the process and the problem was finally solved as indicated in this chapter.

The overall dissipation process is still best described by a dissipation curve on a graph for the parent pesticide and each of the alteration products. Additional transfer studies are being conducted to relate foliar residues to residues on skin and clothing of workers. In a number of these new and unpublished studies conducted in Florida, the transfer coefficients are somewhat different from those described in this chapter. The reason for the discrepancy between the old and new data is unknown, but the results suggest that additional studies may be needed to understand fully the transfer process and the multitude of variables involved.

The recognition that a safe level on foliage exists for each pesticide, and that the safe level of one pesticide is related to that of another pesticide by their ability to inhibit cholinesterase when applied to skin, provided a practical procedure for establishing safe levels for new pesticides when a foliar safe level was known for an old pesticide. Dermal dose–ChE response studies in the rat provided a simple and inexpensive way of relating

TABLE 15. California Reentry Intervals

			Crop			All Other Crops
Pesticide	Apples	Citrus	Corn	Grapes	Peaches and Nectarines	
Anilazine (Dyrene)	2	2	2	2	2	2
Azinphosmethyl (Guthion)	14	30	—	21	14	—
Carbophenothion (Trithion)	2	14	2	14	14	2
Chlorpyrifos (Lorsban, Dursban)	—	2	—	—	—	—
Demeton (Systox)	2	5	2	7	7	2
Diazinon	—	5	—	5	5	—
Dicrotophos (Bidrin)	2	2	2	2	2	2
Dimecron (Phosphamidon)	2	14	2	2	2	2
Dimethoate (Cygon)	—	2	—	2	—	—
Dioxathion (Delnav)	—	30	—	30	30	—
Disulfoton (Di-syston)	2	2	2	2	2	2

TABLE 15 (*Continued*)

Pesticide	Apples	Citrus	Corn	Grapes	Peaches and Nectarines	All Other Crops
Endosulfan (Thiodan)	2	2	2	2	2	2
EPN	14	14	h	14	14	h
Endrin	2	2	2	2	2	2
Ethion	2	30	2	14	14	2
Malathion	—	1	—	1	1	—
Methamidophos (Monitor)	2	2	2	2	2	2
Methiocarb (Mesurol)	—	—	—	—	7	—
Methidathion (Supracide)	2	30	2	2	2	2
Methomyl (Lannate, Nudrin)	2	2	2	2	2	—
Mevinphos (Phosdrin)	2	4	2	4	4	2
Monocrotophos (Azodrin)	2	2	2	2	2	2
Naled (Dibrom)	—	1	—	1	1	—
Oxamyl (Vydate)	2	2	—	—	2	—
Onydemeton-methyl (Metasystox-R)	2	2	2	2	2	2
Parathion-ethyl	14	30[a,d] 45[b,d] 60[c,d]	14[e]	21	21	14[e]
Parathion-methyl	14	14[g]	14[g]	14[f]	21	14[g]
Parathion-methyl (encapsulated)	2	2	2	2	2	2
Phorate (Thimet)	2	2	2	2	2	2
Phosalone (Zolone)	—	7	—	7	7	—
Phosmet (Imidan)	—	—	—	5	5	—
Propargite (Omite)	—	14	—	14	—	—
Sulfur	—	1	—	1[i]	1	—
TEPP	2	4	2	2	4	2
All category 1 pesticides	1	1	1	1	1	1

[a] For all applications with spray mixtures containing 2 lb or less of parathion-ethyl per 100 gal, with rates of 8 lb or less per acre, and a total of no more than 10 lb/acre in the previous 12 months.

[b] For all applications with spray mixtures containing 2 lb or less of parathion-ethyl per 100 gal, with rates of more than 8 lb/acre, or more than 10 lb/acre in the previous 12 months.

[c] For all applications with spray mixtures containing more than 2 lb of parathion-ethyl per 100 gal.

[d] Any reentry interval for parathion-ethyl still in effect on May 15 in the counties of Fresno, Kern, Madera, and Tulare is extended to 90 days from the application date. All applications made after May 15 shall have a 90-day reentry interval except for any reentry interval still in effect on September 15, which is reduced to 30, 45, or 60 days, respectively, from the date of application, in accord with footnotes a, b, and c.

[e] For applications of 0.5–1.0 lb/acre of parathion-ethyl, there is a 7-day reentry interval. For applications of less than 0.5 lb/acre, the reentry interval is 2 days.

[f] The reentry interval for nonencapsulated parathion-ethyl on grapes in Monterey County is 6 days.

[g] When 1 lb or less per acre of parathion-methyl is applied there is a 2 day reentry interval.

[h] When more than 1 lb/acre of EPN is applied there is a 14-day reentry interval.

[i] For applications of sulfur in Riverside Country during March and April, and in San Joaquin, Stanislaus, Merced, Madera, Fresno, Kings, Tulare, and Kern Counties from May 15 through harvest, there is a 3-day reentry interval.

one pesticide to another in terms of potency or ability to inhibit cholinesterase. This procedure simplified the process, because a transfer coefficient and an acceptable exposure level (AEL) were not required.

The conversion of the parent pesticide to one or more highly toxic alteration products increased the complexity of the process by requiring ChE potency data for each product and potency data for the mixture present on foliage during the dissipation process. The toxicity of the mixture (ED_{10} or ED_{50}) was easily obtained using a simple equation.

California used the information obtained in these studies to establish reentry intervals for a number of organophosphorus and carbamate pesticides. Monitoring studies were conducted after the reentry intervals were established to determine if they were adequate to protect the health of field workers. Dislodgeable foliar residues were found to be below the calculated safe levels and no worker illnesses were associated with these levels. California has developed the most comprehensive regulatory response to prevent exposure during reentry. The current California reentry intervals specified in State Regulations are provided in Table 15.

REFERENCES

1. G. E. Quinby and A. B. Lemon, *JAMA, J. Am. Med. Assoc.* **166**, 740 (1985).

2. T. H. Milby, F. Ottoboni, and H. W. Mitchell, *JAMA, J. Am. Med. Assoc.* **189**, 351 (1964).

3. Title 3, Article 23 (Group 2) Section 2480, California Administrative Code. California Department of Food and Agriculture, Sacramento, 1974.

4. K. T. Maddy, *Residue Rev.* **62**, 21 (1975).

5. S. A. Peoples and K. T. Maddy, *West. J. Med.* **129**, 273 (1978).

6. J. B. Knaak, S. A. Peoples, T. Jackson, A. S. Frederickson, R. Enos, K. T. Maddy, J. Bailey, M. E. Dusch, F. A. Gunther, and W. L. Winterlin, *Arch. Environ. Contam. Toxicol.* **7**, 465 (1978).

7. F. A. Gunther, G. E. Carman, and Y. Iwata, *Worker Reentry Safety in Citrus Groves*, Contract No. 4288 with California Department of Food and Agriculture. Department of Entomology, University of California, Riverside, 1976.

8. Y. Iwata, *Residue Rev.* **75**, 127 (1980).

9. S. A. Peoples and K. T. Maddy. *West. J. Med.* **129**, 273 (1978).

10. M. D. Whorten and D. L. Obrinsky, *J. Toxicol. Environ. Health* **11**, 347 (1983).

11. J. E. Casida, Mode of action of carbamates. *Annu. Rev. Entomol.* **8**, 39 (1963).

12. U.S. Environmental Protection Agency, *Pesticide Assessment Guidelines, Subdivision K, Exposure: Reentry Protection.* USEPA, Washington, DC, 1984.

13. J. S. Tobin, *Citrus Pickers Working in Trees Treated with Ethion Formulations, July 24 to July 31, 1970, FMC Corporation Oct 8, 1970*, Public report to Hearing Record for Emergency Regulations adopted June 22, 1970. Submitted Oct 8, 1970 by the California Department of Agriculture.

14. T. B. Waggoner, C. A. Anderson, and D. L. Nelson, *Determination of the Hazards to Workers Picking Citrus Treated with Guthion Wettable Powder Formulation, Chemagro Corporation*, Public report to Hearing Record for Emergency Regulations adopted June 22, 1970. Submitted Oct 8, 1970 by the California Department of Agriculture.

15. T. B. Waggoner, C. A. Anderson, and D. L. Nelson, *Determination of the Hazards to Workers Picking Citrus Treated with Guthion Spray Concentrate Formulations, Chemagro Corporation*, Public report to Hearing Record for Emergency Regulations adopted June 22, 1970. Submitted Oct 8, 1970 by the California Department of Agriculture.

16. G. W. Ware, D. P. Morgan, B. J. Estesen, W. P. Cahill, and D. M. Whitacre, *Arch. Environ. Contam. Toxicol.* **1**, 48 (1973).

17. G. W. Ware, D. P. Morgan, B. J. Estesen, and W. P. Cahill, *Arch. Environ. Contam. Toxicol.* **2**, 117 (1974).

18. G. W. Ware and D. P. Morgan, *Arch. Environ. Contam. Toxicol.* **3**, 289 (1975).

19. R. C. Spear, W. J. Popendorf, J. T. Leffingwell, T. H. Milby, J. E. Davies, and W. F. Spencer, *J. Occup. Med.* **19**, 406 (1977).

20. W. W. Kilgore, *Human Physiological Effects of Organophosphate Pesticides in a Normal Agricultural Field Labor Population.* Food Protection and Toxicology Center, University of California, Davis, June 1977.

21. G. Zweig, J. D. Adams, and J. Blondell, Minimizing occupational exposure to pesticides: Federal reentry standards for farm workers (present and proposed). *Residue Rev.* **75**, 103–112 (1980).

22. U. S. Department of Labor, Occupational Safety and Health Administration: Emergency temporary standard for exposure to organophosphorous pesticides. *Fed. Regist.* **38**(83), 10715 (1973).

23. T. R. Milby, Report of the Task Group on Occupational Exposure to Pesticides to the Federal Working Group on Pest Management, Washington, D.C., January 1974.

24. U.S. Environmental Protection Agency, Farm-workers dealing with pesticides. Proposed health-safety standards. *Fed. Regist.* **39**(48), 9457 (1974).

25. E. Kahn, *Residue Rev.* **79**, 27 (1979).

26. J. B. Knaak, K. T. Maddy, M. A. Gallo, D. T. Lillie, E. M. Craine, and W. F. Serat, *Toxicol. Appl. Pharmacol.* **46**, 363 (1978).

27. W. J. Popendorf, R. C. Spear, J. T. Leffingwell, J. Yager, and E. Kahn, *J. Occup. Med.* **21**, 189 (1979).

28. U.S. Department of Health, Education, and Welfare, *Guidelines for Protection of Human Subjects*, 45 CFR 46. USDHEW, Washington, DC, 1981.

29. R. D. O'Brien, *Toxic Phosphorus Esters: Chemistry, Metabolism, and Biological Effect.* Academic Press, New York, 1960.

30. A. Hirschberg, and Y. Lerman, *Fundam. Appl. Toxicol.* **4**, 529 (1984).

31. Y. Lerman, A. Hirshberg, and Z. Shteger, *Am. J. Ind. Med.* **6**, 17 (1984).

32. *Farm Chemical Handbook.* Meister Publishing Co., Willoughby, OH, 1984.

33. 40 Code of Federal Regulations 162.10, July 1, 1983.

34. Title 3, Food and Agriculture, Chapter 6, Pesticides and Control Operations, Group 3, Article 3, Section 6770 of the California Administrative Code, September 16, 1986.

35. H. O. Michel, *J. Lab. Clin. Med.* **34**, 1564 (1949).

36. D. P. Nabb and F. Whitfield, *Arch. Environ. Health* **15**, 147 (1967).

37. G. L. Ellman, K. D. Courtney, V. Andres, Jr., and R. M. Featherstone, *Biochem. Pharmacol.* **7**, 85 (1961).

38. C. G. Humiston and G. J. Wright, *Toxicol. Appl. Pharmacol.* **10**, 467 (1967).

39. J. B. Knaak, K. T. Maddy, T. Jackson, A. S. Fredrickson, S. A. Peoples, and R. Love, *Toxicol. Appl. Pharmacol.* **45**, 755 (1978).

40. T. B. Gaines, *Toxicol. Appl. Pharmacol.* **2**, 88 (1960).

41. T. B. Gaines, *Toxicol. Appl. Pharmacol.* **14**, 515 (1969).

42. J. B. Knaak, P. Schlocker, C. R. Ackerman, and J. N. Seiber, *Bull. Environ. Contam. Toxicol.* **24**, 796 (1980).

43. J. B. Knaak, *Residue Rev.* **75**, 81 (1980).

44. W. J. Popendorf and J. T. Leffingwell, *Residue Rev.* **82**, 125 (1982).

45. J. B. Knaak, C. R. Ackerman, K. Yee, and P. Lee, *Reentry Research: Dermal Dose Red Cell Cholinesterase Response Curves for Methomyl, Thiodicarb, Methiocarb and Methiocarb Sulfoxide*, unpublished report. California Department of Food and Agriculture, 1982.

46. J. B. Knaak, K. Yee, C. R. Ackerman, G. Zweig, D. M. Fry, and B. W. Wilson, *Toxicol. Appl. Pharmacol.* **76**, 252 (1984).

47. J. B. Knaak and B. W. Wilson, Dermal dose—cholinesterase response and percutaneous absorption studies with several cholinesterase inhibitors. *ACS Symp. Ser.* **273** (1985).

48. H. I. Maibach, R. J. Feldmann, T. H. Milby, and W. F. Serat, *Arch. Environ. Health* **23**, 208 (1971).

49. L. J. Mazuret, *Phosalone, Methyl-Azinphos and Parathion, Acute Percutaneous Toxicity in the Rat,* unpublished report, 1971.

50. F. A. Gunther, W. E. Westlake, J. H. Barkley, W. Winterlin, L. Langbehn, *Bull. Environ. Contam. Toxicol.* **9**, 243 (1973).

51. G. L. Smith and D. E. Little, *Calif. Agric.,* June, p. 13 (1954).

52. F. A. Gunther, J. H. Barkeley, and W. E. Westlake, Worker environmental research. II. Sampling and processing techniques for determining dislodgeable pesticide residues on leaf surfaces. *Bull. Environ. Contam. Toxicol.* **12**, 641–644 (1974).

53. Y. Iwata, J. B. Knaak, R. C. Spear, and R. J. Foster, *Bull. Environ. Contam. Toxicol.* **18**, 649 (1977).

54. F. A. Gunther, Y. Iwata, G. E. Carman, and C. A. Smith, *Residue Rev.* **67**, 1 (1977).

55. J. Kvalvag, D. E. Ott, and F. A. Gunther, *J. Assoc. Off. Anal. Chem.* **60**, 911 (1977).

56. Y. Iwata, G. E. Carman, and F. A. Gunther, *J. Agric. Food Chem.* **27**, 119 (1979).

57. W. E. Westlake, F. A. Gunther, and G. E. Carman, *Arch. Environ. Contam. Toxicol.* **1**, 60 (1973).

58. W. F. Durham and H. R. Wolfe, *Bull. W.H.O.* **26**, 75 (1962).

59. J. E. Davis, *Residue Rev.* **75**, 33 (1980).

60. W. F. Popendorf, *Am. Ind. Hyg. Assoc. J.* **41**, 652 (1980).

61. W. J. Popendorf, An industrial hygiene investigation into the occupational hazards of parathion residues to citrus harvesters. Ph.D. Thesis, University of California, Berkeley (1976).

62. National Aeronautics and Space Administration, *NASA Life Sciences Data Book,* 1st ed. U.S. Government Printing Office, Washington, DC, 1962.

63. N. Diffrient, A. R. Tilley, and J. C. Bardagjy, *Human Scale 1/2/3.* MIT Press, Cambridge, MA, 1974.

64. H. N. Nigg, J. H. Stamper, and R. M. Queen, *Am Ind. Hyg. Assoc. J.* **45**, 182 (1982).

65. W. F. Serat, *Arch. Environ. Contam. Toxicol.* **1**, 170 (1973).

66. W. F. Serat and J. B. Bailey, *Bull. Environ. Contam. Toxicol.* **12**, 682 (1974).

67. W. F. Serat, D. C. Mengle, H. P. Anderson, and E. Kahn, *Bull. Environ. Contam. Toxicol.* **13**, 506 (1975).

68. R. C. Spear, *The Reentry Problem: Perspectives on the Regulatory Implications of Recent Research,* unpublished paper. University of California, Berkeley, 1977.

69. R. C. Spear, W. J. Popendorf, W. F. Spencer, and T. H. Milby, *J. Occup. Med.* **19**, 411 (1977).

70. D. M. Richards, J. F. Kraus, P. Kurtz, and N. O. Borhani, *J. Environ. Pathol. Toxicol.* **2**, 493 (1978).

71. J. B. Knaak and Y. Iwata, The safe level concept and the rapid field method: A new approach to solving the reentry problem. *ACS Symp. Ser.* **182**, 23 (1982).

72. D. J. Finney, *Probit Analysis,* 3rd ed. Cambridge Univ. Press, New York, 1972.

73. Y. Iwata, J. B. Knaak, G. E. Carman, M. E. Dusch, and F. A. Gunther, *J. Agric. Food Chem.* **30**, 215 (1982).

74. Y. Iwata, J. B. Knaak, M. E. Dusch, J. R. O'Neal, and J. L. Pappas, *J. Agric. Food Chem.* **31**, 1131 (1983).

75. H. N. Nigg, J. H. Stamper, and J. B. Knaak, *J. Agric. Food Chem.* **32**, 80 (1984).

F

ASSESSING POTENTIAL HAZARDS TO CONSUMERS

25

Methylmercury in Fish: Assessment of Risk for U.S. Consumers

Linda Tollefson

Epidemiology and Clinical Toxicology Unit, Center for Food Safety and Applied Nutrition, U.S. Food and Drug Administration, Washington, DC

1 INTRODUCTION

Public health officials have long been concerned about the hazards associated with methylmercury ingestion that occur from the consumption of contaminated fish (1). These hazards consist primarily of damage to the central nervous system, specifically cerebral and cerebellar lesions, and deleterious effects on the developing fetus. Paresthesia is usually the first clinical symptom noted, a numbness and tingling sensation around the mouth, lips, fingers, and toes. Also, Burbacher et al. (2) have reported reproductive failures in female primates associated with methylmercury exposure, including nonconception and early spontaneous abortions. Methylmercury compounds pass easily through the blood–brain barrier, the blood–testes barrier, and the placenta, causing damage both postnatally and prenatally. Methylmercury poisoning may be the cause of subtle neurological impairments even at low to moderate levels. Furthermore, parental life and early childhood may be especially vulnerable to low body burdens of methylmercury, because of the sensitivity of the developing nervous system.

All forms of mercury entering the aquatic environment, either as a result of human activities or from natural geologic sources, may be converted to methylmercury, which can be concentrated by fish and other aquatic species (3) Swedish investigators discovered that organisms present in aquatic sediments were able to methylate inorganic mercury (4). The form of mercury in edible fish muscle is almost entirely methylmercury (5), which is more likely to produce chronic effects than the nonalkyl forms of mercury.

Fish may concentrate methylmercury either directly through the water or through components of the food chain. Methylmercury has a very long half-life in fish—approximately 2 years (6). This is two to five times the half-life of inorganic mercury, and much longer than most of the chlorinated solvents. The distribution and elimination appear to occur in two stages: first, methylmercury is distributed throughout the tissues, primarily to muscle, over a period of a few weeks, and then it is discharged from the established binding sites very slowly. This extremely slow loss is one of the reasons why fish are a major source of mercury for humans. Furthermore, fish are continuously supplied with

845

methylmercury from the water, providing a mechanism for the continuous increase of residues in all tissues. Few other foodstuffs are known to contain appreciable quantities of methylmercury. Of all the substances analyzed by the FDA in a survey of 10 basic foods and in the food commodity class of the FDA total diet study, fish was the only potential source of hazardous levels of mercury (7).

Recently, data have become available indicating that the bioavailability of methylmercury to fish may be increased in an acidic environment. This has implications in regard to environmental pollution and the formation of acid rain, which can lower the pH of inland waters (8). It was originally thought that acidification enhanced methylation, but the newest evidence indicates that net methylation is actually inhibited with decreasing pH (9). Possible mechanisms by which the mercury burden is increased in fish in an acidic environment include increased gill premeability, decreased trophic state of the lake or river, and decreased growth rate of the fish (8, 9).

The hazardous nature of methylmercury residues in fish has been emphasized by the Minamata Bay (1953–1960) and Niigata (1965) poisoning episodes in Japan (10). A severe neurological disorder was first noted in the population in the vicinity of Minamata Bay, Japan, late in 1953. The disease was subsequently linked to consumption of seafood from the bay, which was contaminated by large levels of mercury as a result of an effluent from a chemical manufacturing plant. By 1978, the number of victims recognized by Japan for relief measures was 1303 with an additional 200 deaths (10). Levels of mercury as low as 10 ppm in hair and 30 ng/mL in blood were associated with toxic symptoms (11). However, there was a considerable time lapse between onset of symptoms and monitoring of blood and hair levels for mercury, so that the recorded levels cannot be reliably associated with the observed neurological symptoms.

In 1965, outbreaks of methylmercury poisoning occurred among persons living in villages near the mouth of the Agano River, in Niigata, Japan. This catastrophe was also due to industrial contamination of the Agano River. As a result, 6669 victims were recognized for relief measures by 1978 and there were 55 deaths (10). The first victims had high levels of mercury in their hair, ranging from 60 to 600 ppm. Through active monitoring, a number of asymptomatic subjects were discovered with hair mercury levels greater than 150 ppm; most of these later developed symptoms of methylmercury poisoning (12).

It has not been clearly established at what level methylmercury is toxic for aquatic organisms. There is some evidence that concentrations of mercury as low as 5 ppb in the water can have a detrimental effect (3). Before the onset of Minamata disease, it was believed that fish that accumulated methylmercury became moribound, but the contaminated fish and shellfish in Minamata did not behave abnormally (10).

A more recent poisoning episode occurred in the fall and winter of 1971–1972 in Iraq as a result of ingestion of home made bread prepared from wheat seed that had been treated with alkylmercury fungicide and intended for planting. As a result of this episode, 6530 cases were admitted to hospitals throughout the country, with 459 deaths (13). Blood samples collected 65 days (the approximate half-life of methylmercury in humans) after the poisoning episode from victims showing early signs of toxicity contained approximately 240 ng/mL (ppb) mercury.

Acute poisoning episodes of populations by methylmercury result in very dramatic effects. However, subclinical effects of methylmercury on some subgroups of the population are also of public health importance and constitute a threat that is more difficult to evaluate. Concern that low levels of methylmercury may have subtle neurological effects is the stimulus for continuing research efforts (14). Populations whose main protein source is fish constitute another group of consumers at increased risk to the dangers associated with methylmercury ingestion.

To determine if a hazard exists among fish consumers in the United States, data on fish consumption and mercury residues in fish in the United States are evaluated in this assessment. Fish consumption data were obtained from a study conducted in 1973–1974 commissioned by the Tuna Research Foundation (TRF). This is the latest fish-specific survey available. The most recent survey of mercury in U.S. fish was performed during the 1979 fiscal year by the Food and Drug Administration (FDA). These exposure data and also National Marine Fisheries Service (NMFS) residues data from 1974 are sufficiently thorough and valid to ensure a high degree of certainty in the results of this assessment.

The estimated exposure levels experienced by the vicims of the methylmercury poisoning epidemics and the pharmacokinetics of methylmercury in humans were used to estimate body levels. The best indices of exposure to methylmercury are levels of mercury in hair and blood. Whole body burdens can easily be related to blood and hair levels that have been associated with various toxic effects. To assess the risk of methylmercury to U.S. fish consumers, a safety factor of 10 was incorporated in the minimum level currently known to be associated with adverse effects. The risk to especially sensitive groups such as infants and prenatal life, as well as those populations known to consume large quantities of fish, was also evaluated. The approach to this assessment of risk for U.S. consumers from the ingestion of methylmercury in fish is consistent with that advocated by the National Research Council (15).

2 HAZARD IDENTIFICATION

The mercury contaminating the aquatic environment comes from two principal sources: leaching or volatilization from natural geological sources and human activities (1). Approximately 10,000 tons of mercury were produced in 1973 (16), and human activities cause an additional 10,000 tons of mercury to be released into the environment each year (16). Mercury compounds discharged into the environment from commercial sources consist primarily of the following (4):

1. Metallic mercury, Hg^0 (chloralkali and instrument plants).
2. Inorganic divalent mercury, Hg^{2+} (chloralkali plants).
3. Phenylmercury, $C_6H_5Hg^+$ (paints, pulp, and paper plants).
4. Methylmercury, CH_3Hg^+ (agriculture).
5. Methoxyethylmercury, $CH_3OCH_2CH_2Hg^+$ (agriculture).

Mercury has a biological cycle and any of its forms are potentially exchangeable among the air, land, and water phases (3) as indicated in Fig. 1. River and lake sediments as well as decomposing fish contain microorganisms that can form methylmercury and dimethylmercury from inorganic mercury even under anaerobic conditions (4). Both methylmercury and dimethylmercury are rapidly taken up and accumulated by fish. When dimethylmercury reaches the atmosphere, it is converted to inorganic mercury vapor plus methane and ethane (3).

Once methylmercury is formed in the sediment or suspended sediments in water, it is rapidly and efficiently taken up by aquatic organisms (17). Accumulation in bottom

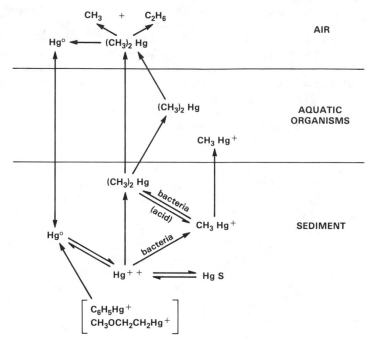

Figure 1. Biological cycle of methylmercury.

fauna is followed by accumulation in fish species. For the overall food chain, uptake through the gills is the key process; however, as the tropic level of the fish increases, the intake from food becomes more important (17). Large carnivorous fish at the end of a food chain such as tuna and swordfish can thus be expected to accumulate large amounts of mercury.

Approximately 95% of methylmercury is absorbed from the gastrointestinal tract in humans (17). Methylmercury becomes associated with the red blood cells rather than the plasma (13). It is uncertain how methylmercury accumulates in tissue but there is evidence that in humans a methylmercury–glutathione complex is important (18). Methylmercury is lipid soluble, can diffuse through cell membranes, and can attain appreciable concentrations in the brain (19). In primates it appears that the brain contains approximately 5% of the total amount of methylmercury in the body (20). However, at high blood-mercury concentrations brain concentration appears to be disproportionately increased (21). In humans, there is evidence that approximately 10% of the body burden of methylmercury accumulates in the brain, 5% in the blood, and the rest evenly distributed throughout the other tissues (16). Methylmercury also accumulates in hair as it is formed. The concentration of mercury in hair is proportional to the concentration in blood at the time of incorporation. At steady state, hair and blood concentrations have a ratio of 250:1 (17).

Methylmercury readily crosses the human placenta and enters the fetus (19). The mercury concentration in fetal red blood cells is 30% higher than in those of the mother; this may be due to the accumulation of methylmercury in cord erythrocytes (22, 23), or alternatively, it may be due to the different chemical structure of fetal and adult hemoglobin (16). Methylmercury distributes to all tissues in the fetus, including the brain, which is the principal target organ for prenatal toxicity.

The half-life of methylmercury in the adult human has been shown to be approximately 70 days (24). A small amount undergoes biotransformation to inorganic mercury by demethylation in the body (16). Inorganic mercury has been found in kidney, liver, feces, bile, and urine in primates after administration of methylmercury (16). The majority of the absorbed methylmercury in humans is eliminated by means of the liver into the bile and then feces, and to a lesser extent through the urine (17). Much of the methylmercury excreted in the bile is reabsorbed through an enterohepatic circulation (16), contributing to marked retention by the body. Methylmercury is also excreted into breast milk, the concentration being approximately 5% of the blood concentration (17, 25).

The clinical effects of methylmercury poisoning are primarily due to damage to the central nervous system. Paresthesia, a numbness and tingling sensation around the mouth, lips, fingers, and toes, is usually the first clinical symptom noted (12, 17). Ataxia—a stumbling gait and difficulty in articulating words—is the next progressive symptom, along with dysarthria—a constriction of the visual fields ultimately leading to tunnel vision—and impairment of hearing (10, 11). Neurasthenia—a generalized muscle weakness—fatigue, headache, irritability, and inability to concentrate often occur. In severe cases, myoclonic tremors or jerks are present, which frequently lead to coma and death (26).

Takeuchi and Eto (11) described distinct groups in the Minamata poisoning episode which differed in severity of symptoms:

1. The most serious outcome was death or permanent disability from severe mental abnormalities.
2. Those who were moderately poisoned but had advanced lesions showed paresthesia, ataxia, dysarthria, tremor, and hearing and vision problems.
3. Less advanced cases suffered from ataxia, dysarthria, and constriction of the visual field.
4. Those with less specific symptoms that were believed but not proved to be due to methylmercury poisoning suffered from fatigue, memory impairment, headaches, numbness, slight mental disorders, and tremors of the lips and fingers.

Takeuchi and Eto (11) made the disturbing observation that a prolonged period of 10 years or more could occur between exposure to methylmercury and appearance of symptoms. This latency period appears to be inversely related to blood concentrations (12). There is also evidence from the Minamata epidemic that the clinical symptoms associated with methylmercury toxicity had actually progressed over time, after exposure had ceased (27). Studies from the Niigata poisoning incident (28) support the finding that the clinical course of methylmercury poisoning, particularly the neurological symptoms, can progress over a period of years after exposure is discontinued.

Takeuchi (29) has described the neuropathological lesions from methylmercury that are found in the cerebral cortex and the granular layer of the cerebellum. Cerebral edema occurs acutely, with focal necrosis of neurons and replacement with glial cells. As the neurons are continually destroyed, cerebral atrophy occurs. The cerebral lesions occur mainly in the visual areas of the occipital cortex.

Many species of laboratory animals have shown similar effects as humans to methylmercury poisoning. Ataxia, lethargy, depressed peripheral sensation, and blindness have all been found (12). Peripheral nerve damage has been found in rats and guinea pigs but the evidence for this symptom has been equivocal in primates. Brain lesions in primates have been similar to those found in humans (30).

Prenatal life and infancy are the life stages most vulnerable to methylmercury because of the sensitivity of the developing nervous system. Prenatal poisoning cases resemble cerebral palsy; the children can be spastic, blind, deaf, and have severe mental impairment. Even at relatively low exposure levels, children may be affected with developmental retardation and mild neurological abnormalities (31).

Like the adult, pathological changes from methylmercury exposure in the fetus consist of cortical damage, particularly in the visual areas of the occipital cortex and the granular layer of the cerebellum since methylmercury tends to concentrate in these areas (29). However, infant brains show not only the focal neuronal changes as did the adults, but also developmental deficiencies in actual brain structure, such as hypoplasia and malformations (32). In Minamata, fetal brain lesions appeared more diffuse than in the adult (19). and in Iraq, abnormal neuronal migration in the cerebellum and cerebrum was evident (32).

There is evidence that methylmercury exposure affected reproductive outcome in female monkeys. Burbacher et al. (2) found an association between infertility and abortion and blood-mercury concentration. Rats have shown decreased fetal weight with lower, nonlethal exposure levels (33). Decreased survival of the offspring and decreased weight gain to weaning have also been noted (33). Spyker (34) found that mice exposed prenatally to methylmercury exhibit neuromuscular deficiencies later in life.

There is no evidence for mutagenic activity by methylmercury, but teratogenic effects are seen in many species of animals other than primates. Malformations may be correlated with high peak levels of blood methylmercury (12). As in the adult, the brain is the organ most susceptible to prenatal methylmercury toxicity. Learning deficits have been noticed in rats who were prenatally exposed at low doses and there is evidence that the deficits may develop with time (35).

The human epidemiology data available on the reproductive effects of methylmercury come primarily from epidemics that resulted in disastrous outcomes such as stillbirths, prenatal mortality, and severe infant neurological disabilities. Reproductive effects such as infertility, early spontaneous abortions, and malformations have not been specifically studied for methylmercury, although the reproductive effects of inorganic mercury are fairly well documented (36).

Similarly, occupational exposures to elemental mercury vapor have frequently been studied, particularly in the chloralkali industry, the manufacture of thermometers and graduated scientific glassware, the repair of electrical meters, the mining and milling of mercury, the manufacture of artificial jewelry, and the felt hat industry (17). However, occupational exposure to methylmercury has been limited to a few individuals and situations such as accidents among laboratory personnel, workers in pulp and saw mills, and workers involved in either the production of alkylmercury fungicides or their application to cereal seed (17). Exposure in these cases is by inhalation of the dust or absorption of liquid fungicide preparations through the skin (17). These reports of occupational exposures to methylmercury have contributed to the description of the signs and symptoms of poisoning but have contributed essentially nothing to an understanding of dose–response relations. Goldwater (37) reviewed occupational exposures to phenylmercury and methoxyethylmercury compounds, but these industrial hazards appear to be of minor public health importance.

A number of important studies have been published on the effect of selenium on the toxicity of methylmercury to experimental animals (38–40). These studies have established that although selenium exerts some protective effect, it does not eliminate the toxicity of methylmercury. Since 1974, when the above-referenced studies were published, other information on the selenium–methylmercury relation has become available. A workshop was jointly sponsored by the FDA and NMFS in 1977 to review recent research on the effects of selenium on methylmercury toxicity. (A copy of the report of the workshop is on file in the office of the Hearing Clerk, FDA.) The consensus of the workshop participants was that the findings are inconclusive and that any protective effect of selenium should be considered as a means of maintaining an adequate margin of safety.

3 HAZARD EVALUATION

The best indices of exposure to methylmercury are levels of mercury in hair and blood. Detailed studies of the victims of poisoning episodes, particularly those supplying information on mercury levels in blood, hair, and in some cases brain, have provided valuable information for estimating acceptable levels for exposure of humans to methylmercury. Additional information has also been provided by (i) studies in Scandinavia on the metabolism of trace amounts of ^{203}Hg-labeled methylmercury by humans, which allowed calculation of the half-life in humans (about 70 days) and also the relative concentration of mercury in the various parts of the body (24), and (ii) the relation between ingestion of methylmercury from contaminated fish and mercury levels in blood and hair.

The hair/blood ratio in humans has been consistently measured at approximately 250 (17). Mercury levels in hair can be used to assess past exposures and maternal exposure after the birth of an affected infant. Also, transient increases would become apparent from measurement of mercury levels in hair, whereas they would not become apparent from similar measurements of mercury levels in blood.

Apparently, the appearance of toxic symptoms from methylmercury exposure depends on both the blood level of methylmercury and the amount of time the blood levels are increased (12). If the duration of exposure has a significant effect, dose–response information obtained from acute poisoning epidemics such as occurred in Japan and Iraq may have little relevance to the effects of chronic low-level exposure such as occurs among most populations of fish consumers. A certain amount of methylmercury given acutely may produce toxic effects, whereas the same amount distributed over time may not result in mercury poisoning since excretion is continually occurring. Alternatively, an acute dose of methylmercury may not result in toxic effects, whereas the same dose given chronically may produce signs of poisoning due to accumulation to toxic levels.

For adults, inorganic mercury appears to be the most toxic form of mercury when given acutely, and methylmercury appears to be most toxic for chronic exposure (19). In the fetus, it is not known for certain which form of mercury is most acutely toxic. Methylmercury is by far the most hazardous form of mercury for chronic exposure to the fetus because of its ability to cross the placenta and accumulate in fetal tissues (19).

The majority of the human epidemiology evidence suggests that duration of exposure to methylmercury is extremely important to the development of toxic effects in both the adult and fetus (11). However, studies of populations exposed to methylmercury from consuming large amounts of fish for many years indicate otherwise (41, 42). Although there is disagreement as to how much emphasis should be placed on the duration of exposure to methylmercury, and how to incorporate such information into extrapolation models to estimate threshold levels, a regulatory agency such as the FDA will use the possibility of chronic exposure to justify decreasing the acceptable daily intake of methylmercury as a matter of safety to public health (1).

The inhabitants of Minamata Bay, Japan, were exposed to methylmercury from 1953 to 1960 by consuming fish from the bay that were contaminated by large amounts of mercury (10). Kurland et al. (43) summarized the clinical features seen during this poisoning epidemic. The onset of symptoms was characterized by progressive numbness of the distal parts of the extremities and the lips and tongue. Usually, ataxia appeared next, along with dysarthria, dysphagia, deafness, and blurring of vision due to constriction of the visual fields. Spasticity and rigidity were often present, and hypersesthesia was sometimes noted. Insomnia, agitation, and psychological disturbances frequently occurred. Among the severely affected patients, intellectual impairment and generalized muscle wasting could be expected.

In 1965, another outbreak of methylmercury poisoning occurred from the consumption of fish from an industrially contaminated river in Niigata, Japan (10). Most of the victims were discovered by active monitoring and search rather than by the spontaneous reporting of cases (12). The reported symptoms were similar to those described for the Minamata episode, but the Niigata incident represented a less severe epidemic (12).

Investigators have found evidence that victims in the Niigata area suffered nonspecific, milder symptoms such as headaches, fatigue, and dizziness at hair levels of 30–40 ppm, whereas the more severe symptoms were associated with levels in excess of 150 ppm (28). Evidence was also found of cases with delayed onset of symptoms and deterioration with time. Seven patients with hair-mercury levels greater than 200 ppm had the following sequence of symptoms over a 5-year period (28):

1. First symptom noted was sensory disturbance of extremities. This symptom become prevalent after 3 years.
2. Sensory disturbances around the mouth began 1 year after exposure and became prevalent after 4–5 years.
3. Ataxia began 1 year after exposure and became prevalent after 4–5 years.
4. Constriction of the visual field was noted after a delay of 4 years and become prevalent 1 year later.

Takeuchi and Eto (11) also reported on the delayed onset of symptoms from methylmercury poisoning, noting that the signs could occur 10 years after exposure. There is more evidence for the existence of a delayed syndrome among the prenatally exposed in Iraq (44) than in Japan. However, in general, the Japanese prenatally exposed victims were first examined at an older age than those in Iraq (45).

Studies of the victims of the Japanese poisoning epidemics continue, and information on the apparent recovery of some of the adult poisoning cases has been reported. Tokuomi (46) followed 26 victims of methylmercury poisoning for 10 years after first diagnosis. Ataxia in writing and walking remained but was improved slightly; incidence of finger tremor decreased from 75 to 54% of the 26 victims. Hearing impairment became less pronounced in some of the victims, but those who were deaf as the result of methylmercury did not regain their hearing. Some victims who suffered constriction of the visual field experienced widening. Superficial sensation disturbances, although still present in 80% of the victims, showed some improvement. However, almost all victims were still unable to live ordinary lives. Unfortunately, little information is available on the exposure dose these victims received.

A Swedish expert group evaluated data on human methylmercury toxicity derived from cases that occurred in Minamata and Niigata. The Swedish group determined (by extrapolation) that the lowest blood-mercury level associated with toxic effects was 200 ppb (ng/mL) and the lowest hair-mercury level associated with toxic effects was 50 ppm (47). There have been reports that evidence of methylmercury poisoning is present in Minamata victims with hair levels as low as 10 ppm (11, 28). Although the threshold may have been lowered by factors such as malnutrition, it appears most likely that these low levels are merely artifacts of the long time lapse between the onset of symptoms and the analysis of hair for methylmercury.

The Iraqi outbreak of methylmercury poisoning has been extensively studied by many investigators (13, 25, 31, 44, 48). In the autumn of 1971, after several years of low crop yields in Iraq, seed grain was imported for planting. The grain had been treated with mercury compounds to prevent fungal growth. Poisoning resulted from the ingestion of bread made from the methylmercury-treated seed grain intended for planting (25). Signs of poisoning were confined to the CNS, with an insidious and progressive onset, and consisted of symptoms similar to those identified during the Minamata and Niigata episodes (48). Those mildly affected showed symptoms such as irritability, headache, fatigue, and paresthesia circumorally and in the distal parts of the extremities. Those moderately affected also showed cerebellar signs such as ataxia, dysarthria, tremor, and hyperreflexia. Those severely affected also had visual and hearing impairments, some being completely blind and deaf.

On a group basis, the categories of symptomatology severity were related to the blood concentration of mercury (44, 48). Severe cases had blood levels greater than 2000 ppb (ng/mL), and those mildly affected had lower levels, but the relation was not consistent for individual symptoms (48). The level of mercury in whole blood at which symptoms of toxicity were first detected was approximately 240 ppb (ng/mL) (13). This calculation was made on samples collected 65 days after the end of exposure, which is the approximate half-life of methylmercury in humans (24). Since the actual clearance times from the blood were not known, the level may lie between 240 and 480 ppb. These values are for adult exposures only.

As in the Japanese epidemics, it was observed that improvement took place among the mild and moderately affected adults in Iraq (49). The symptom that disappeared earliest was paresthesia, which generally was one of the first signs to appear. Some improvement was also noticed among severe cases and appeared to be inversely proportional to the amount of damage (48). However, exacerbation of the symptoms of methylmercury poisoning over time, particularly among these exposed prenatally, was more marked in the Iraq epidemic than in Japan. It has been postulated that this may be due to the difference in the duration of exposure; the Iraqi patients were exposed acutely for a period of 1–2 months, while the Japanese patients were exposed for years (48). Many of the Japanese victims were not recognized until their symptoms were marked, and it was generally not possible to determine when their exposure had begun.

3.1   Prenatal Exposure

The first reports of fetal methylmercury toxicity came from Minamata, where approximately 6% of the children born between 1955 and 1959 developed cerebral palsy (19). The mothers generally had no overt symptoms of methylmercury poisoning during pregnancy or at the birth of their children, although some experienced mild paresthesia (50). No decrease in birth weight of the infants or changes in the duration of gestation were noticed (50). Malformations in the infants were rare, but microcephaly was observed in 60% of congenital Minamata disease cases (50).

Beginning in the sixth month after birth, the affected infants began to show instability of the neck, convulsion, and failure of the eyes to follow an object (50). Common symptoms included intellectual impairment, appearance of primitive reflexes, dysarthria, hyperkinesia, and hypersalivation. Such clinical signs occur with cerebral palsy in general, but these cases of congenital methylmercury poisoning exhibited a more marked degree of impairment of intelligence and cerebellar symptoms (50). No mercury levels in any body tissue were available for either the mothers or the infants (17). However, 2–5 years after exposure had ceased, high levels of hair mercury were found in both patients and their parents (50).

In the Iraqi cases, cerebral palsy was associated with very high maternal hair-mercury levels, in the range of 400–500 ppm (33, 44). Death in early infancy or childhood was associated with maternal mercury levels of 200–600 ppm in hair. There appears to be a very wide range of sensitivity for various effects in the fetus (44).

In a study of infant–mother pairs exposed to methylmercury during pregnancy during the Iraqi outbreak in early 1972, it was found that the infants' blood-mercury levels were higher than their mothers' levels for over 4 months after birth (45). In contrast to the Minamata experience, in only one infant–mother pair was the infant affected while the mother was not. The blood-mercury levels in the breast-fed infants were maintained by the passage of methylmercury via maternal milk. In this study the lowest measured blood-mercury level associated with methylmercury toxicity in an infant was 564 ppb. Also, six infants had blood-mercury levels of 200 ppb with no signs of poisoning. However, the investigators emphasized that these children should be followed prospectively in order to assess whether or not the toxic effects of methylmercury may become manifest in later years. In Japan, patients who had been prenatally exposed to methylmercury poisoning were examined at ages 1–7 years, whereas in this study the infants were 6–7 months old. Therefore, brain damage may have had time to become apparent in the Japanese population and may help to explain why so many more cases were found in which the infant was affected but the mother had no or minimal symptomatology. Also, the Japanese infants were continually exposed over a long period through contaminated fish, whereas the Iraqi infants were exposed during a single outbreak, by consuming bread made with contaminated wheat (45, 48). In any event, the study by Amin-Zaki et al. (45) demonstrated that infant blood-mercury levels remain higher than those of their mothers after birth, and therefore infants may be at higher risk of methylmercury poisoning than their mothers.

Magos et al. (51) studied the effect of lactation on excretion of methylmercury in Porton Wistar rats. Lactation did increase the elimination of mercury from the whole body but had no effect on the elimination of mercury from the brain. Both control and lactating animals had the same amount of brain histologic abnormalities. Greenwood et al. (52) studied blood-mercury clearance half-times of lactating and nonlactating females exposed during the Iraqi epidemic. Lactating females had a mean half-life of 42 days whereas nonlactating females and males had a mean half-life of 75 days. This may not be relevant in light of the fact that there was no difference in elimination of methylmercury from the brain—the target tissue—between lactating and nonlactating rats.

Magos et al. (53) studied the sensitivity of virgin and pregnant rats to methylmercury. Clinical signs as well as brain concentration and elimination parameters were identical in pregnant and virgin rats. Therefore, pregnant or lactating females are probably no more sensitive to methylmercury poisoning than those in other physiological states. The explanation for increased effects on the fetus must be due to the fetal dose–response relation.

In an attempt to characterize the dose–response relation for human fetal exposure to methylmercury, peak maternal hair-mercury concentrations were found to be related to neurological effects in infants involved in the Iraqi epidemic (54). Minimal symptoms were reported for both mothers and infants when peak maternal hair-mercury levels were less than 68 ppm. In another study (55), a few children of mothers with peak hair-mercury concentrations of less than 25 ppm were found to have symptoms such as delayed speech, mental retardation, and microcephaly.

Amin-Zaki et al. (44) conducted a follow-up study of 32 infants poisoned prenatally during the Iraqi epidemic. The most important finding was that many of the infants initially noted as being free of symptoms when first examined had neurological signs and delays in psychomotor development. At least half the children had a history of delayed development. Since there was no case-matched control group of infant–mother pairs, the abnormalities could not be conclusively attributed to methylmercury poisoning in utero. The authors reported that whereas adults and older children experienced some recovery from the effects of methylmercury poisoning, those prenatally exposed suffered permanent damage. They attributed this difference to the fact that the developing fetal and infant brain is more susceptible to the toxic effects of methylmercury.

Later, Amin-Zaki et al. (56) followed for 5 years 29 children who were exposed at the ages of 1–10 months, primarily through breast milk. Neurological signs became more evident as the children aged. Hyperreflexia, presence of Babinski's sign, and delayed motor development increased in incidence after examinations at 2 and 5 years postexposure. The authors attributed the neurological damage partially to the long period of exposure through breast milk. However, in children exposed at the age of 2–16 years, a high rate of improvement was noted (49), which was related inversely to the severity of the initial symptoms. No improvement was found in those with very severe damage, and the time for recovery or improvement was inversely related to the amount of damage. Since there is evidence for improvement with time since exposure (49), as well as for deterioration (44, 56), the age at exposure may play a major role.

4 EXPOSURE ASSESSMENT

Consumption of fish and shellfish is the most important source of methylmercury for the majority of individuals. It has been established that the form of mercury in edible fish muscle is almost completely methylmercury (5, 57). Only limited data are available on the form of mercury in shellfish, which indicate that the mercury in shrimp and lobster is mostly methylmercury (1). As discussed previously, food sources other than fish and shellfish contribute an insignificant amount to the total methylmercury intake of humans (7).

4.1 High Fish Consumers

Several populations exposed to methylmercury through high fish consumption have been studied epidemiologically. From Sweden there are reports of families consuming fish containing 0.3–7 mg Hg/kg (ppm) or up to 5 µg Hg/kg body weight of the consumer, resulting in blood-mercury levels up to 60 ppb with no signs or symptoms of poisoning (58).

Turner et al. (41) described a Peruvian population that was chronically exposed to methylmercury because of its long-term and heavy consumption of ocean fish. Approximately 70% of this population's dietary protein came from fish. Although the mean blood-methylmercury concentration was 82 ppb, no individual could be identified as having symptoms of methylmercury poisoning. There was a high prevalence of paresthesias in the population but the condition was no more frequent than in a neighboring control group with a mean blood-methylmercury concentration of 9.9 ppb. Hair analyses for methylmercury indicated that the mercury levels were constant over long periods, confirming the suggestion that this population had been chronically exposed to methylmercury for many years.

A group of fishermen in American Samoa who were at sea for periods up to 22 months and ate up to 9 oz of fish per day were studied. The average blood-methylmercury concentration of this group was 64 ppb. None of the fishermen showed any evidence of methylmercury poisoning (59).

In these studies, many normal individuals had blood-methylmercury levels that were higher than the lowest estimated level reported from Niigata that was associated with overt symptoms. Perhaps acute exposure to high levels of methylmercury results in disproportionately large amounts of mercury accumulating in the brain, whereas chronic exposure to lower quantities of methylmercury does not result in such marked brain insult. No specific attempt was made to search for the more subtle effects of methylmercury poisoning in these populations, such as behavioral problems and learning disabilities.

4.2   U.S. Consumers

To determine the intake of fish and shellfish in the United States, a consumption study was conducted in 1973–1974 by the National Purchase Diary Panel, Inc. (NPD). NPD is a marketing research and consulting firm that specializes in the analysis of consumer purchasing behavior as recorded in monthly diaries by families over time. This study was commissioned by the Tuna Research Foundation (TRF) to provide a representative and projectable sample of seafood consumption patterns among the continental U.S. population. It is the most recent fish-specific national survey available. Later surveys of general food intake exist, but these are not considered to be as valid as a fish-specific survey for determining U.S. fish consumption. The objective of the survey was to provide data on seafood consumption patterns (i) by species, (ii) by individuals within a family, (iii) by young children (10 years or less), and (iv) by pregnant women.

NPD maintains two national panels of over 6500 families in addition to panels in 35 local test markets. Members of one national panel plus 2000 families from local market panels were asked to participate in this project. Panelists recorded their seafood consumption by family member in a diary for a 1-month period. Data from one-twelfth of the sample population were recorded each month for 1 year, from September 1973 to August 1974. Total sample counts (returns) were: number of families, 7662; number of individuals, 25,165; number of young children, 4952; and number of pregnant women, 10. Because of the small number of pregnant women, no data on them are presented in the report (60).

The NPD panel is balanced nationally with regard to a number of major demographic characteristics. However, because diary panels nearly always gain better cooperation among some groups than others, NPD projects its data to total U.S. households. Because of small geographic and demographic panel imbalances, each panel family is simultaneously weighted upward or downward from this average, depending on whether they are over-represented or under-representated in the panel. Demographics controlled in this stage are (i) census region, (ii) inside/outside standard metropolitan statistical areas (SMSA), (iii) family size (iv) age of housewife, and (v) income.

On the basis of consumption data from the NPD survey, residue data provided by NMFS, and the assumption that the sampling methods are valid and the diary recording is reasonably accurate, it appears likely that the probability of a systematic exposure to substantial intakes of methylmercury in fish and shellfish by the average consumer is low. Some examples of the variables to be considered for a variety of the important species of fish and shellfish are presented in Table 1.

Approximately 93% of the individuals sampled consume seafood; tuna is the most usual seafood eaten, with 61.5% of all the individuals sampled eating tuna. The average consumption of total seafood per individual was 18.58 oz/month. This corresponds closely to the report of Newberne and Stillings (61), which estimated the national average fish consumption in the United States during the past 50 years to be approximately 16 oz/month.

The NPD survey provides information on the "average" U.S. fish consumer. However, sports fishermen may consume much more fish than the average U.S. consumer, and also fish consumption may vary dramatically among the regions of the United States. To determine if consumption patterns do actually differ among these groups, we abstracted data from the NPD survey for eight Great Lakes states. Table 2 contains data on fish consumption for Illinois, Indiana, Michigan, Minnesota, New York, Ohio, Pennsylvania, and Wisconsin. Although consumption is not given for fishermen specifically, many of these states are important areas for recreational fishing, and therefore consumption by fishermen should be reflected in the data.

TABLE 1. Consumption Patterns and Methylmercury Residues in Seafood[a]

Fish Species	Projected Number of Persons Consuming Fish	Monthly Consumption (g)		Mercury Level (ppm)	
		Mean ± SD	Range	Mean ± SD	Range
Tuna	132,025,000	166.4 ± 125.8	24.4–3728.3		
Albacore				0.156 ± 0.057	0.04–0.25
Yellowfin				0.324 ± 0.252	0.04–0.87
Skypjack				0.199 ± 0.083	0.03–0.39
Lobster	13,240,000	232.6 ± 173.8	18.2–1605.2	0.175 ± 0.148	0.07–0.28
Salmon	19,834,000	206.3 ± 319.5	23.9–3479.9		
Pink				0.018 ± 0.015	0.01–0.04
Coho				0.056 ± 0.055	0.02–0.21
Sockeye				0.059 ± 0.085	0.01–0.21
Halibut	5,140,000	216.4 ± 142.0	25.0–766.8	0.179 ± 0.123	0.01–0.38
Shrimp	47,081,000	224.4 ± 177.8	25.6–1439.9	0.113 ± 0.179	0.10–0.56
Swordfish	409,000	196.0 ± 74.9	99.4– 511.2	—[b]	

[a] Consumption data from ref. (60); residue data provided by NMFS
[b] No data provided.

TABLE 2. Consumption Patterns for Eight Great Lakes States[a]

| State | Fish Species | Monthly Consumption (g) | |
		Mean ± SD	Range
All	All	607.2 ± 567.9	9.0–6041.1
	Pike	312.6 ± 428.1	18.9–4806.9
	Salmon	148.8 ± 129.6	3.0–1764.0
Illinois	All	657.9 ± 552.0	24.0–5169.9
	Pike	336.9 ± 294.6	78.9–1332.0
	Salmon	129.9 ± 99.6	3.0– 585.9
Indiana	All	491.4 ± 393.3	9.0–2769.0
	Pike	266.1 ± 173.7	150.0– 609.0
	Salmon	168.3 ± 119.1	24.0– 680.1
Michigan	All	515.1 ± 391.5	38.1–1827.0
	Pike	274.2 ± 205.8	78.9– 780.0
	Salmon	153.9 − 135.3	17.1– 690.0
Minnesota	All	540.0 ± 528.3	29.1–3455.1
	Pike	303.0 ± 406.5	18.9–2640.0
	Salmon	123.6 ± 98.4	13.5– 488.1
New York	All	732.9 ± 656.1	9.9–5199.0
	Pike	255.3 ± 179.1	24.0– 810.0
	Salmon	157.8 ± 160.5	6.9–1764.0
Ohio	All	588.6 ± 720.9	16.5–6041.1
	Pike	487.5 ± 905.7	108.9–4806.9
	Salmon	142.8 ± 118.2	16.5– 888.0
Pennsylvania	All	567.3 ± 506.7	31.5–3464.1
	Pike	207.6 ± 142.5	24.0– 570.0
	Salmon	152.1 ± 119.7	20.7– 567.9
Wisconsin	All	591.9 ± 485.7	33.0–3312.0
	Pike	312.9 ± 333.9	36.0–2079.0
	Salmon	120.6 ± 78.0	30.9– 459.9

[a]Data from Tuna Research Foundation (TRF) (60).

The average consumption of all fish for all eight Great Lakes states was 21.38 oz/month compared to 18.58 oz for the average U.S. consumer. The amount of all fish species consumed monthly by state ranged from a low of 17.30 oz in Indiana to a high of 35.81 oz in New York. The mean consumption of salmon for all the eight Great Lakes states surveyed was 148.8 g/months, ranging from 120.6 for Wisconsin consumers to 168.3 for Indiana consumers. The mean consumption of salmon for all U.S. consumers is 206.32 g/month. These data give some assurance that regional fish consumption is not drastically different from the U.S. average, at least for the eight Great Lakes states discussed here.

NMFS attempted to determine if the persons eating more than 90 oz of seafood per month (1.4% of the sample survey) continued to consume seafood at this rate over a long period. These individuals kept an additional diary for an extra month in November 1974. The average consumption recorded for the first diary month was 124.2 oz per individual and the average consumption for the second diary month was 45 oz. This is a net change in consumption of − 64%. The highest mean consumption recorded in the two diaries was 197.5 oz/month. Therefore, few if any persons in the United States maintain a steady total seafood consumption of more than 200 oz/month.

4.3   FDA Data on Mercury Concentration in Fish on the U.S. Market

Fish from Minamata Bay in the 1950s had a median total mercury level of 11 mg/kg (ppm) fresh weight. Fish from the Agano River in Niigata caught during the epidemic had a median total mercury level of less than 10 mg/kg (ppm) fresh weight (17). Methylmercury accounts for practically all the mercury found in most species of marine or freshwater fish. The mean methylmercury content of the contaminated wheat in the Iraqi outbreak was found to be 7.9 mg/kg (ppm) (17).

Table 3 contains FDA data showing the mercury levels that existed in samples of domestic fish during the fiscal year 1979 (57). The maximum level of mercury rarely

TABLE 3. Mean Mercury Levels in FDA Fiscal Year 1979 Survey[a]

Species	Mean (ppm)	Maximum Level (ppm)
Bass, fresh water	0.19	0.62
Bass, salt water	0.07	0.25
Bluefish	0.19	0.81
Carp	0.11	0.37
Catfish	0.10	0.74
Cod	0.15	0.83
Halibut	0.27	0.51
Perch, fresh water	0.13	0.30
Perch, salt water	0.17	0.44
Pike, walleye	0.26	0.75
Pollack	0.05	0.14
Swordfish	0.83	1.82
Trout, fresh water	0.13	1.01
Trout, sea	0.09	0.24
White fish	0.06	0.24

[a]Data from FDA (57).

TABLE 4. Mean Mercury Levels in Selected Great Lakes Fish: FDA 1970 Survey[a]

Great Lake	Species	Mean ± Standard Deviation (ppm)
Lake Erie	Walleye	0.58 ± 0.26
	Perch	0.24 ± 0.14
	White bass	0.49 ± 0.31
	Smallmouth bass	0.51 ± 0.19
Lake St. Clair	Perch	0.88 ± 0.75
	All others	0.48 ± 0.32
Lake Michigan	All types	0.11 ± 0.11
Lake Ontario	All types	0.30 ± 0.30
Lake Huron	All types	0.19 ± 0.11
Lake Superior	All types	0.13 ± 0.11

[a]Data from Simpson et al. (7).

reached above 1.0 ppm, and with the exception of swordfish, the mean levels are well below 0.5 ppm. As can be seen in Table 1, even the species with the highest expected levels of mercury, those at the top of the food chain, have mean values well below 0.5 ppm.

Table 4 contains data reported by Simpson et al. (7) on mercury levels in freshwater fish from the Great Lakes, an area suspected of having a large amount of mercury from environmental contamination. Again, these data indicate that the average levels of methylmercury in most fish are well below the present 1.0-ppm FDA guideline.

5   RISK EVALUATION

Any chemical can be toxic to humans if enough is ingested. Therefore, most governments have tried to place a limit on the daily intake of various naturally occurring and industrial substances for the protection of the public health. The acceptable daily intake (ADI) is the amount of a food additive or residue that, in the opinion of a regulatory agency, can be consumed daily over a long time without risk (62). It is expressed in terms of milligrams of residue per kilogram of body weight of the consumer.

The concept of an ADI may not be applicable to trace contaminants because for the most part the level in food is unpredictable and uncontrollable, and consequently the daily intake is highly variable. In addition, the susceptibilities of the fetus, infant, and child to many substances are presently unknown and subclinical effects have not been adequately described. Moreover, in the case of methylmercury and many other contaminants that are cumulative, the individual daily exposure may only make a small contribution to the body burden. Hence, it would be reasonable to specify an average limiting weekly or monthly intake rather than daily.

A Joint Food and Agriculture Organization/World Health Organization (FAO/WHO) Expert Committee on Food Additives (63) established a provisional tolerable weekly intake of 0.3 mg of total mercury per person, of which no more than 0.2 mg should be present as methylmercury. These amounts are equivalent to 5 and 3.3 μg, respectively, per kilogram of body weight. If the value for methylmercury is used, the tolerable level corresponds to approximately 230 μg/wk for a 70-kg person, or 33 μg/day.

The estimate of tolerable weekly or daily intakes of methylmercury was based on information developed primarily by Swedish studies of Japanese individuals poisoned in the episode of Niigata, which resulted from consumption of contaminated fish and shellfish. Data on mercury levels in blood and hair provided a basis for establishing methylmercury levels at which toxic effects were observed. The blood level at the time of onset of symptoms was estimated by extrapolation and it was concluded that the lowest blood level for the appearance of signs and symptoms of methylmercury poisoning was 200 ppb (0.2 ppm) (47).

Pharmacokinetic studies in Finland and Sweden on the movement of methylmercury through the human system made it possible to relate blood-mercury levels to daily intake. By using trace amounts of radiolabeled methylmercury, it was shown that methylmercury is completely (more than 95%) absorbed from food and is distributed rapidly throughout the body, and that its estimated average biological half-life is about 70 days (24). This information was used to calculate the theoretical total body burden of mercury as a function of time when a constant dose of methylmercury is ingested. This calculated body burden becomes essentially steady after about 1 year (five times the biological half-life). At steady state, a conservative estimate of the total amount of methylmercury in the body is about 100 times the daily intake. At steady state, the blood-mercury level expressed in ng/mL (ppb) is approximately equal to the daily intake expressed in μg/day for a 70-kg person (26).

These relations have been found to hold true in a study of consumers of large quantities of fish in Sweden (58). A linear relation was found between daily ingested methylmercury and the level of methylmercury in blood, and the data indicated that a steady daily intake of approximately 300 μg Hg as methylmercury for a 70-kg person would result in a blood-mercury concentration of roughly 200 ppb at steady state (58). This is a somewhat lower body burden than that calculated by Clarkson's model (26), which is recognized to be conservative.

The more recent poisoning episode (1971–1972) in Iraq, caused by the ingestion of contaminated bread prepared from wheat seed that had been treated with alkylmercury fungicide and intended for planting, has provided additional data relating exposure to toxic effects. By using the kinetic data developed in Scandinavia, the body burden of methylmercury in these patients was calculated and related to the frequency and signs and symptoms in the population. The results of this study indicate that the effects of methylmercury can be noted at a body burden of approximately 25 mg Hg for a 70-kg person (25).

Clarkson et al. (64) reviewed the Iraqi data and determined that the lowest toxic body burden of methylmercury was approximately 50 mg for a 70-kg person. This is the level at which an increase over the background frequency of paresthesia could be detected.

Based on the available data, a threshold value at which symptoms of toxicity associated with methylmercury are first noticeable has been estimated at 50 ppm for hair and 200 ppb for whole blood, which would be reached with a minimum daily intake of 300 μg mercury present as methylmercury in the diet. Dose–response relations below this range of intake are not known.

There is continued concern about the relative sensitivity of the developing fetus. In this respect, it should also be noted that the studies in Iraq clearly demonstrated a wide variation in individual sensitivity to methylmercury as well as wide variations in the rate of excretion of methylmercury. The effect of the interaction of other chemical factors such as selenium on the toxicity of methylmercury has not been demonstrated conclusively at this time, but it may need to be considered when more information is developed. There is also evidence that ethanol can potentiate methylmercury toxicity in rats (65).

The following limitations to this approach were recognized: (i) it was not known to what extent particular individuals are more or less sensitive to mercury than others; (ii) the estimates were based on the lowest level that caused an effect rather than the normal procedure of using a no-effect dose level; (iii) paresthesia is usually the first symptom of methylmercury toxicity noted but is not sufficient to diagnose poisoning because it can be caused by many other factors (66); (iv) questions about dose–response relations in human fetuses and newborn infants were unanswered; and (v) there is a possibility of subclinical effects arising from exposure to very low levels of methylmercury.

Paresthesia continues to be the first symptom ascribed to methylmercury poisoning, but this effect occurs relatively late in the progression of toxic changes. Therefore, it would be desirable to find an earlier indicator of toxicity, or, ideally, of pretoxicity. Woods and Fowler (67) found that rats chronically exposed to methylmercury hydroxide had increased levels of urinary uroporphyrin and coproporphyrin as a result of changes in the renal heme biosynthetic pathway enzyme activities. No discernible organ damage was found at the dosage levels used in their experiment, suggesting the clinical utility of urinary porphyrin levels as a sentinel of pretoxic exposure to methylmercury. In this regard it is noteworthy that Minamata patients were observed to have porphyrinuria

(46). However, other investigators have indicated that renal damage in humans after exposure to methylmercury is very rare and is usually due to the inorganic ion (3, 17).

In the Woods and Fowler experiment (67), rats were divided into four groups receiving drinking water with 0, 3, 5, or 10 ppm methylmercury hydroxide for 6 months. Changes in activities of renal heme biosynthetic pathway enzymes were accompanied by increases in urinary heme precursors. There was a 5–12.5-fold increase in urinary uroporphyrin and a 14–21-fold increase in urinary coproporphyrin. Initial porphyrinuria occurred between 1 and 2 weeks following commencement of exposure. Later, Woods et al. (68) found that rats acutely treated with inorganic mercury did not have significant increases in urinary uroporphyrin levels. The authors suggested that further studies are needed to explain fully the porphyrinogenic response induced by chronic mercury exposure.

As discussed in Section 3 on hazard evaluation, there are indications that the duration of exposure should be considered when establishing safety limits for methylmercury exposure. The threshold for effects from long-term, low-level exposure may be lower than that for acute effects from poisoning epidemics. There is evidence (11) that the length of exposure to methylmercury results in clinical adverse effects regardless of the levels of mercury in blood and hair. Therefore, incorporation of a time factor for chronic exposure may lower the level at which toxicity symptoms first appear (12).

Similarly, we know that the fetus is much more sensitive to the effects of methylmercury (28, 31), and therefore it would be prudent to lower the minimum daily intake of methylmercury for pregnant women. This hypersusceptibility of the fetus, and possibly infant, to the toxic effects of methylmercury has not been quantified in any rigorous manner. During the methylmercury poisoning epidemic in Minamata, it was noted that an unusually large number of children were born who developed symptoms similar to cerebral palsy approximately 6 months after birth (19). It was soon determined that the affected infants were victims of congenital Minamata disease (50). However, their mothers, almost without exception, exhibited no signs of methylmercury toxicity either during pregnancy or at the birth of their affected children (50).

This phenomenon of severe effects in the fetus associated with no or minimal symptoms in the mother was not repeated during the Iraqi outbreak of methylmercury poisoning. However, in Iraq, the infants' blood-mercury levels exceeded that of their mothers' (45), and therefore the infants may have been at higher risk for the toxic effects of methylmercury. In addition, there does not appear to be any evidence for recovery from the symptoms of methylmercury poisoning when the exposure occurs in utero. This is attributed to the hypersusceptibility of the developing fetal and infant brains to methylmercury (44). Children exposed to methylmercury at ages from 1 to 10 months also did not show improvement in their neurological symptoms compared with children exposed at ages from 2 to 16 years (49), further suggesting that the age at exposure may play a significant role in the toxic effects of methylmercury.

Because of these areas of uncertainty, a factor of 10 has been used to provide a sufficient margin of safety. Such a safety factor, although not technically elegant or based in theory, has been shown to be satisfactory over many years of use (1). The legal basis of the FDA's use of safety factors can be found in the 1958 Food Additive Amendments to the Federal Food, Drung and Cosmetic Act [21 U.S.C. 348 (c)(5)(C)]. Thus a maximum tolerable level for all humans is estimated to be 30 μg methylmercury daily in the diet, resulting in 20 ppb of methylmercury in blood and 5 ppm in hair. Based on current knowledge, this should adequately protect prenatal life and populations chronically exposed to methylmercury.

6   DISCUSSION

Data from the TRF survey have indicated that the average consumption of all fish among the fish-eating population of the United States is 18.58 oz/month or approximately 18 g/day. Daily consumption of species containing relatively high levels of methylmercury such as tuna, swordfish, or halibut would be considerably less. For example, the mean daily consumption of halibut is 7.2 g with two standard deviations increasing the total to 16.6 g. This would include some 97.5% of all consumers of halibut. The consumption of 16.6 g of halibut with 0.179 ppm Hg would provide a daily methylmercury intake of approximately 2.9 μg.

The mean daily consumption of swordfish is 6.53 g with a standard deviation of 2.5 g. If 11.53 g of swordfish with a mercury level of 1.5 ppm were consumed each day, and this would include over 95% of all swordfish eaters, the daily mercury intake would be 17.3 μg, still below the ADI of 30 μg.

At the highest level of swordfish consumption shown by the TRF survey—that is, 511 g/month or 17 g/day, with a mercury residue of 1.5 ppm—the daily mercury intake would be 25.5 μg, still below the ADI of 30 μg. If in addition to the highest level of consumption of swordfish in the NMFS—that is, 17 g/day with a mercury residue of 1.5 ppm—the same individual consumed the average daily amounts of tuna, halibut, and salmon at the present average residue levels of mercury for each of the three species, then the the total daily intake of mercury from all four species would average 29.0 μg, still below the ADI:

$$(17.0 \text{ g swordfish} \times 1.5 \,\mu\text{g/g Hg}) + (5.5 \text{ g tuna} \times 0.324 \,\mu\text{g/g Hg})$$

$$+ (6.9 \text{ g salmon} \times 0.059 \,\mu\text{g/g Hg}) + (7.2 \text{ g halibut} \times 0.179 \,\mu\text{g/g Hg}) = 29.0 \,\mu\text{g Hg}.$$

Such consumption seems very unlikely, particularly since the cost of swordfish, halibut, and salmon is prohibitively high. Certainly the small number of persons who would conceivably consume such amounts does not justify the imposition of a lower regulatory action level for mercury in seafood than the current 1.0 ppm.

Additional data developed on the biological half-life of methylmercury in humans, however, indicate a need to take into account the problem of variations among individuals. In the Iraqi episode, 90% of the individuals studied had a biological half-life of methylmercury that was between 60 and 70 days, but 10% showed values of 110–120 days (69). This variability did not appear to be related to age or diet. Individuals having a long biological half-life would accumulate much higher steady-state levels than those having short biological half-lives and consequently might be at greater risk from the same level of methylmercury intake.

In addition, information has been developed on the so-called late onset of symptoms associated with methylmercury poisoning. Specifically, by 1973, in the Agano area of Niigata, Japan, new cases of methylmercury poisoning were detected years after the consumption of contaminated fish had ceased (70). Further evidence for latent effects was found among poisoning victims who experienced delayed onset of certain symptoms and, as discussed previously, deterioration of their initial symptoms (11, 28). These findings indicate that there may be some damage that is not diagnosed under current procedures, and it introduces further uncertainty into the determination of the lowest effect level used to estimate tolerable intakes. Further concern has been generated by the follow-up studies of Iraqi infants by Amin-Zaki et al. (44) in which the investigators found neurological and developmental dysfunctions in infants initially thought to be free of the toxic effects of methylmercury. Unfortunately, little information is available relating these latent effects to a specific dose of methylmercury or to levels of mercury in hair or blood.

The data currently available for quantitatively evaluating the association of neurological symptoms of toxicity with exposure to methylmercury are sparse and inconsistent. Additional studies are being carried out on the prenatal effects of methylmercury to determine that this lifestage continues to be protected by the FDA's 1.0-ppm regulatory level for mercury in seafood. However, even with the above-outlined uncertainties concerning the results of exposure in Japan and Iraq, where exposures were considerably higher than anything experienced in other countries, U.S. fish consumption data do not indicate any cause for concern of methylmercury poisoning for the average American. The majority of fish consumers in the United States could easily double their intake and still remain below the mercury ADI. The current 1.0-ppm regulatory level for all marine species provides more than adequate protection at the current average fish consumption levels in the United States. In addition, the enforced limit of 1.0 ppm mercury in marine fish provides a sufficient margin of safety for young children and for significant numbers of consumers exceeding the acceptable daily intake.

REFERENCES

1. U. S. Food and Drug Administration, Action level for mercury in fish and shellfish. Notice of proposed rule making, Fed. Regist. **39**, 42738 (1974).

2. T. M. Burbacher, C. Monnett, K. S. Grant, and N. K. Motter, Methylmercury exposure and reproductive dysfunction in the nonhuman primate, Toxicol. Appl. Pharmacol. **75**, 18–24 (1984).

3. R. A. Wallace, W. Fulkerson, W. D. Shults, and W. S. Lyon, Mercury in the Environment: The Human Element, ONRL-NSF Environ. Program. Oak Ridge National Laboratory, Oak Ridge, TN, 1971, pp. 15–20.

4. A. Jernelov, Conversion of mercury compounds. In M. W. Miller and G. G. Berg, Eds., Chemical Fallout: Current Research on Persistent Pesticides. Thomas, Springfield, IL, 1968, pp. 68–74.

5. G. Westoo, Determination of methyl mercury compounds in foodstuffs, I. Methyl mercury compounds in fish, identification and determination. Acta Chem. Scand. **20**, 2131–2137 (1966).

6. W. Stopford and L. J. Goldwater, Methylmercury in the environment: A review of current understanding. Environ. Health Perspect. **12**, 115–118 (1975).

7. R. E. Simpson, W. Horwitz, and C. A. Roy, Residues in food and feed. Pestic. Monit. J. **7**, 127–138 (1974).

8. A. Jernalov, The effects of acidity on the uptake of mercury in fish. In T. Y. Toribara, M. W. Miller, and P. E. Morrow, Eds., Polluted Rain. Plenum Press, New York, 1980, pp. 221–222.

9. S. O. Quinn and N. Bloomfield, Eds., Acidic Deposition, Trace Contaminants and Their Indirect Human Health Effects: Research Needs. Workshop Proceedings. Covallis Environmental Research Laboratory, Corvallis, OR, 1985, pp. 13–16.

10. Y. Takizawa, Epidemiology of mercury poisoning. In J. Nriagu, Ed., The Biogeochemistry of Mercury in the Environmental. Elsevier/North-Holland and Biomedical Press, Amsterdam, 1979, pp. 325–365.

11. T. Takeuchi and K. Eto, Minamata disease. Chronic occurrence from pathological viewpoints. In T. Tsubaki, Ed., Studies on the Health Effects of Alkylmercury in Japan. Environment Agency, Tokyo, Japan, 1975, pp. 28–62.

12. M. J. Inskip and J. K. Piotrowski, Review of the helath effects of methylmercury. *J. Appl. Toxicol.* **5**, 113–133 (1985).

13. T. W. Clarkson, L. Amin-Zaki, and S. K. Al-Tikriti, An outbreak of methylmercury poisoning due to consumption of contaminated grain. *Fed. Proc., Fed, Am. Soc. Exp. Biol.* **35**, 2395–2399 (1976).

14. G. D. Langolf, D. B. Chaffin, R. Henderson, and H. P. Whittle, Evaluation of workers exposed to elemental mercury using quantitative tests of tremor and neuromuscular functions. *Am. Ind. Hyg. Assoc. J.* **39**, 976–984 (1978).

15. National Research Council, *Risk Assessment in the Federal Government: Managing the Process.* National Academy Press, Washington, DC, 1983, pp. 1–50.

16. L. Friberg, G. F. Nordberg, and V. B. Vouk, Eds., *Handbook on the Toxicology of Metals.* Elseview/North-Holland Biomedical Press, Amsterdam, 1979, pp. 503–530.

17. World Health Organization, *Environmental Health Criteria 1. Mercury.* Environment Programme and the World Health Organization, Geneva, 1976, pp. 5–131.

18. A. Naganuma, Y. Koyama, and N. Imura, Behavior of methylmercury in mammalian erythrocytes. *Toxicol. Appl. Pharmacol.* **54**, 405–410 (1980).

19. S. Kitamura, K. Sumino, K. Hayakawa, and T. Shibata, Mercury content in 'normal' human tissues. In T. Tsubaki, Ed., *Studies on the Health Effects of Alkylmercury in Japan.* Environment Agency, Tokyo, Japan, 1975, pp. 20–27.

20. M. Berlin, J. Carlson, and T. Norseth, Dose-dependence of methylmercury metabolism. *Arch. Environ. Health* **30**, 307–313 (1975).

21. B. J. Koos and L. D. Longo, Mercury toxicity in the pregnant woman, fetus, and newborn infant. *Am. J. Obstet. Gynecol.* **126**, 390–409 (1976).

22. P. M. Kuhnert, B. R. Kuhnert, and P. Erhard, Comparison of mercury levels in maternal blood, fetal cord blood, and placental tissues. *Am. J. Obstet. Gynecol.* **139**, 209–213 (1981).

23. H. Tsuchiya, K. Mitani, K. Kodama, and T. Nakata, Placental transfer of heavy metals in normal pregnant Japanese women. *Arch. Environ. Health* **39**, 11–17 (1984).

24. J. K. Miettinen, Absorption and elimination of dietary mercury (2 +) ion and methylmercury in man. In M. W. Miller and T. W. Clarkson, Eds., *Mercury, Mercurials, and Mercaptans.* Plenum Press, New York, 1973, pp. 233–243.

25. F. Bakir, S. Al-Damluji, L. Amin-Zaki, M. Murtadha, A. Khalidi, N. Al-Rawi, S. Tiktiti, H. Dhahn, T. Clarkson, J. Smith, and R. Doherty, Methylmercury poisoning in Iraq. An interuniversity report. *Science* **181**, 230–240 (1973).

26. T. W. Clarkson, Mercury poisoning. *Dev. Toxicol. Environ. Sci.* **1**, 189–200 (1977).

27. A. Igata, K. Niina, R. Hamada, and Y. Ohkatsu, The late onset of organic mercury intoxication after exposure. In T. Tsubaki, Ed., *Studies on the Health Effects of Alkylmercury in Japan.* Environment Agency, Tokyo, Japan, 1975, pp. 178–179.

28. T. Tsubaki and K. Irukayama, Eds., *Minamata Disease: Methylmercury Poisoning in Minamata and Niigata, Japan.* Elsevier, Oxford, UK, and Kodansha, Tokyo, 1977, pp. 57–267.

29. T. Takeuchi, Pathogenesis of Minamater disease. In M. Kutsuma, Ed., *Minamata Disease.* Kumamoto Univ. Press, Kumamoto, Japan, 1968, pp. 141–228.

30. C. M. Shaw, N. K. Motter, E. S. Luschei, and D. F. Finocchio, Cerebrovascular lesions in experimental methylmercurial encephalopathy. *Neurotoxicology* **1**, 57–74 (1979).

31. D. O. Marsh, G. J. Myers, T. W. Clarkson, L. Amin-Zaki, S. Tikriti, and M. A. Majeed, Fetal methylmercury poisoning: Clinical and toxicological data on 29 cases. *Ann. Neurol.* **7**, 348 (1980).

32. B. B. Choi, L. W. Lapham, L. Amin-Zaki, and T. Saleem, Abnormal neuronal migration, deranged cerebral cortical organization, and diffuse white matter astrocytosis of human fetal brain. A major effect of methylmercury poisoning in utero. *J. Neuropathol. Exp. Neurol.* **37**, 719–733 (1978).

33. W. J. Chen, R. L. Body, and N. K. Mottet, Some effects of continuous low-dose congenital exposure to methylmercury on organ growth in the rat fetus. *Teratology* **20**, 31–36 (1979).

34. J. M. Spyker, Subtle and long-term consequences of parental exposure to methylmercury. In B. Weiss and V. G. Laties, Eds., *Behavioral Toxicology*. Plenum Press, New York, 1975, pp. 320–349.

35. H. R. Musch, M. Bornhausen, and H. Greim, Operant behavior performance changes in rats after prenatal methylmercury exposure. *Toxicol. Appl. Pharmacol.* **56**, 305–311 (1980).

36. National Research Council, *An Assessment of Mercury in the Environment*, A report prepared by the Panel on Mercury of the Coordinating Committee for Scientific and Technical Assessments of Environmental Pollutants. National Academy of Sciences, Washington, DC, 1978, pp. 97–105.

37. L. J. Goldwater, Aryl and alkoxyalloyl mercurials. In M. W. Miller and T. W. Clarkson, Eds., *Mercury, Mercurials, and Mercaptans*. Plenum Press, New York, 1973, p. 56.

38. H. E. Ganther and M. L. Sunde, Effect of tuna fish and selenium on the toxicity of methylmercury: A progress report. *J. Food Sci.* **39**, 1–5 (1974).

39. B. R. Stillings, H. Lagally, P. Bauersfeld, and J. Soares, Effect of cystine, selenium, and fish protein on the toxicity and metabolism of methylmercury in rats. *Toxicol. Appl. Pharmacol.* **30**, 243–254 (1974).

40. G. S. Stoewsand, C. A. Bache, and D. J. Liske, Dietary selenium protection of methylmercury intoxication of Japanese quail. *Bull. Environ. Contam. Toxicol.* **11**, 152–156 (1974).

41. M. D. Turner, D. O. Marsh, J. C. Smith, J. B. Inglis, T. W. Clarkson, C. E. Rubio, J. Chiriboga, and C. C. Chiriboga, Methylmercury in populations eating large quantities of maine fish. *Arch. Environ. Health* **35**, 367–378 (1980).

42. U. S. Food and Drug Administration, Action level for mercury in fish, shellfish, crustaceans, and other aquatic animals. Withdrawal of proposed rulemaking and termination of rulemaking proceeding. *Fed. Regist.* **44**, CF3990 (1979).

43. L. T. Kurland, S. N. Faro, and H. Siedler, Minamata disease. The outbreak of a neurologic disorder in Minamata, Japan, and its relationship to the ingestion of seafood contaminated by mercuric compounds. *World Neurol.* **5**, 370–391 (1960).

44. L. Amin-Zaki, M. A. Majeed, S. B. Elhassani, T. W. Clarkson, M. R. Greenwood, and R. A. Doherty, Prenatal methylmercury poisoning. Clinical observations over five years. *Am. J. Dis. Child.* **133**, 172–177 (1979).

45. L. Amin-Zaki, S. Elhassani, M. A. Majeed, T. W. Clarkson, R. A. Doherty, and M. R. Greenwood, Intra-uterine methylmercury poisoning in Iraq. *Pediatrics* **54**, 587–595 (1974).

46. H. Tokuomi, Minamata disease in human adults. In M. Kutsuma, Ed., *Minamata Disease*, Kumamoto Univ. Press, Kumamoto. Japan, 1968, pp. 37–72.

47. F. Berglund, M. Berlin, G. Birke, U. von Euler, L. Friberg, B. Holmstedt, E. Jonsson, C. Ramel, S. Skerfving, A. Swensson, and S. Tejning, Methylmercury in fish: A toxicology-epidemiologic evaluation of risks. Report from an expert group. *Nord. Hyg. Tidskr., Suppl.* **4**, 19–290 (1971).

48. F. Bakir, H. Rustam, S. Tikriti, S. F. Al-Damluji, and H. Shihristani, Clinical and epidemiological aspects of methylmercury poisoning. *Postgrad. Med. J.* **56**, 1–10 (1980).

49. L. Amin-Zaki, M. A. Majeed, T. W. Clarkson, and M. R. Greenwood, Methylmercury poisoning in Iraqi children. *Br. Med. J.* **1**, 613–616 (1978).

50. M. Harada, Congenital Minamata disease: Intrauterine methylmercury poisoning. *Teratology* **18**, 285–288 (1978).

51. L. Magos, G. C. Peristianis, T. W. Clarkson, and R. T. Snowden, The effect of lactation on methylmercury intoxication. *Arch. Toxicol.* **45**, 143–148 (1980).

52. M. R. Greenwood, T. W. Clarkson, R. A. Doherty, A. H. Gates, L. Amin-Zaki, S. Elhassani, and M. A. Majeed, Blood clearance half-times in lactating and nonlactating members of a population exposed to methylmercury. *Environ. Res.* **16**, 48–54 (1978).

53. L. Magos, G. C. Peristianis, T. W. Clarkson, R. T. Snowden, and M. A. Majeed, Comparative study of the sensitivity of virgin and pregnant rats to methylmercury. *Arch. Toxicol.* **43**, 283–291 (1980).

54. D. O. Marsh, G. J. Myers, T. W. Clarkson, L. Amin-Zaki, S. Tikriti, M. A. Majeed, and A. R. Dabbagh, Dose–response relationship for human fetal exposure to methylmercury. *Clin. Toxicol.* **18**, 1311–1318 (1981).

55. D. O. Marsh, G. J. Myers, T. W. Clarkson, L. Amin-Zaki, and S. Tikriti, Fetal methylmercury poisoning: New data on clinical and toxicological aspects. *Trans. Am. Neurol. Assoc.* **102**, 69–71 (1977).

56. L. Amin-Zaki, M. A. Majeed, M. R. Greenwood, S. B. Elhassani, T. W. Clarkson, and R. A. Doherty, Methylmercury poisoning in the Iraqi suckling infant: A longitudinal study over five years. *J. Appl. Toxicol.* **1**, 210–214 (1981).

57. U. S. Food and Drug Administration, in *Compliance Program Report of Findings. FY79 Pesticides and Metals in Fish Program.* U.S. Department of Health and Human Services, Public Health Service, Bureau of Foods, FDA, Washington, DC, 1982.

58. S. Skerfving, Methylmercury exposure, mercury levels in blood and hair, and health status in Swedes consuming contaminated fish. *Toxicology* **2**, 3–23 (1974).

59. D. O. Marsh, M. D. Turner, J. C. Smith, J. W. Choe, and T. W. Clarkson, Methylmercury in human populations eating large quantities of marine fish. I. Northern Peru. *Proc. 1st Int. Mercury Congr., Barcelona, 1974.*

60. Tuna Research Foundation (TRF), *Seafood Consumption Study.* National Purchase Diary Panel, Inc., Schaumberg, IL, 1975.

61. P. M. Newberne and E. R. Stillings, Mercury in fish: A literature review. *CRC Crit. Rev. Food Technol.* **4**, 311–335 (1974).

62. S. Margolin, Mercury in marine seafood: The scientific medical margin of safety as a guide to the potential risk to public health. *World Rev. Nutr. Diet.* **34**, 182–265 (1980).

63. Joint FAO/WHO Expert Committee on Food Additives, *Evaluation of Certain Food Additives and of the Contaminants Mercury, Lead, and Cadmium,* FAO Nutr. Meet. Rep. Ser. No. 51. FAO/WHO, Rome, 1972, pp. 9–16.

64. T. W. Clarkson, J. C. Smith, D. O. Marsh, and M. D. Turner, A review of dose-response relationships resulting from human exposure to methylmercury compounds. In T. W. Clarkson, Ed., *Heavy Metals in the Aquatic Environment.* Vanderbilt University, Nashville, TN, 1973.

65. C. J. Turner, M. K. Bhatnagar, and S. Yamashiro, Ethanol potentiation of methyl mercury toxicity: A preliminary report. *J. Toxicol. Environ. Health* **7**, 665–668 (1981).

66. T. W. Clarkson, B. Weiss, and C. Cox, Public health consequences of heavy metals in dump sites. *Environ. Health Perspect.* **48**, 113–127 (1983).

67. J. S. Woods and B. A. Fowler, Renal porphyrinuria during chronic methyl mercury exposure. *J. Lab. Clin. Med.* **90**, 266–272 (1977).

68. J. S. Woods, D. L. Eaton, and C. B. Lukens, Studies on porphyrin metabolism in the kidney. Effects of trace metals and glutathione on renal uroporphyrinogen decarboxylase. *Mol. Pharmacol.* **26**, 336–341 (1984).

69. H. Shahristani and K. Shihab, Variation of biological half-life of methylmercury in man. *Arch. Environ. Health* **28**, 342–344 (1974).

70. T. Tsubaki, K. Hirota, K. Shirakawa, K. Kondo, and T. Sato, Clinical, epidemiological and toxicological studies on methylmercury poisoning. In G. L. Plaa and W. A. M. Duncan, Eds., *Proceedings of the First International Congress on Toxicology: Toxicology as a Predictive Science.* Academic Press, New York, 1978, pp. 339–357.

26

A Comprehensive Risk Assessment of DEHP as a Component of Baby Pacifiers, Teethers, and Toys

Duncan Turnbull and Joseph V. Rodricks

Environ Corporation, Washington, DC

1 INTRODUCTION

Di-2-ethylhexyl phthalate (DEHP) (1) is a commercially important chemical whose major use (more than 300,000,000 lb in 1980) is as a plasticizer in polyvinyl chloride (PVC) plastics (1). PVC containing DEHP is widely used in consumer products, such as imitation leather, wallpaper, lawn furniture, swimming pool liners, flooring, footwear, rainwear, containers and tubing for transfusion of blood and blood products, other medical devices, and children's toys (1). The DEHP is not chemically bound within the polymer, and it can diffuse through and out of the PVC, giving the opportunity for human exposure.

Di-2-ethylhexyl phthalate (DEHP)

(1)

The ability of DEHP to migrate from blood bags into stored blood raised concern almost 20 years ago (2, 3). Since then, its use in these products has been reduced, but not eliminated. More recently, this concern was increased with the publication of a report from the National Toxicology Program (NTP) that showed that high dietary concentrations of DEHP caused an increased incidence of liver cancer in rats and mice (4). This finding encouraged the Consumer Products Safety Commission (CPSC) to investigate the possible risk to humans from DEHP in PVC plastics (5). CPSC's main objective was to

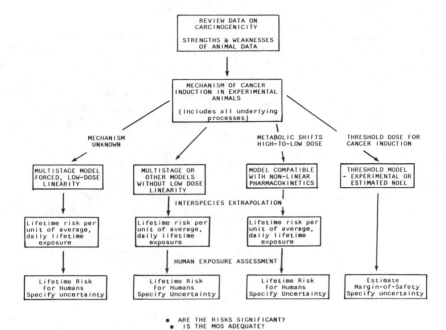

Figure 1. Broad outline of carcinogenesis risk assessment.

examine possible risks to children from DEHP in children's PVC toys, pacifiers, teethers, and so on.

Most soft plastic toys, teethers, and pacifiers are composed of PVC plastic containing a high concentration of DEHP, as high as 40% in the most flexible types. As noted above, the DEHP is free to diffuse within the PVC polymer and can move out of the polymer. This movement is governed by simple physical principles controlling chemical equilibria. As a result, when a DEHP-containing pacifier is sucked or chewed, some of the DEHP can move from the pacifier into the child's saliva. The rate of movement is affected by factors such as the relative solubility of DEHP in the PVC polymer and in saliva, the temperature, the thickness of the polymer, and any physical forces acting on the polymer (e.g., chewing).

This assessment examines four alternative approaches to risk assessment of DEHP and investigates the degree to which each is supported by the available data. A broad outline of this process is presented in Fig. 1. It follows the four-step process for risk assessment outlined by the National Academy of Sciences (6).

2 HAZARD IDENTIFICATION

The focus of this investigation was to evaluate the carcinogenic potential of DEHP in humans at exposure levels that they may currently receive. Although DEHP has other toxic effects in animals at very high exposure levels, notably testicular effects (7, 8), these other effects are not discussed in this chapter, except as they relate to its carcinogenic potential. The available data suggest that maintaining exposure at or below levels that would present no cancer hazard would also protect against those other potential adverse effects.

2.1   Evidence for Carcinogenicity

There are few studies in the published literature that examine the possible adverse effects of chronic exposure of humans to DEHP (9–11), and none specifically examines its possible carcinogenicity.

Prior to the NTP bioassay (4), several animal studies had shown no evidence of carcinogenicity of DEHP (12–15). Those studies, however, were probably insufficiently sensitive, because they used small numbers of animals or were of short duration, to have detected a weak carcinogenic effect similar in magnitude to that seen in the NTP study.

2.1.1   *NTP Bioassay.*   In the NTP bioassay (4), groups of 50 B6C3F$_1$ mice and 50 F-344 rats of each sex were given diets containing DEHP at 0, 3000, or 6000 ppm (mice) and 0, 6000, or 12,000 ppm (rats). In rats, survival was not affected by DEHP, but body weight gain was reduced in males at both dose levels and in high-dose females. Food consumption was reduced slightly in both sexes at both dose levels. In mice, there was a significant reduction in survival in low-dose females, but not in high-dose females or in males. There was, however, a dose-related reduction in body weight gain in females.

Both mice and rats showed significant increases in the incidence of liver tumors, as shown in Table 1. The liver was the only organ in which there was a significant increase in tumor incidence (4).

Although it has been suggested (16) that the maximum tolerated dose (MTD) was exceeded in the NTP bioassay, because body weight gain was depressed by more than 10% in low- and high-dose female mice, low- and high-dose male rats, and high-dose female rats, the NTP (4) has noted that the 10% weight-loss criterion for defining an MTD is only a guideline. The primary reason for not exceeding a theoretical MTD in chronic bioassays, according to NTP, is to avoid excess early deaths and pathological changes that might lead to tumor development by a secondary mechanism. NTP concluded that both these

TABLE 1. Incidence of Liver Tumors in Rats and Mice Fed DEHP in NTP Bioassay

	Control		Low Dose		High Dose	
	Male	Female	Male	Female	Male	Female
Rats						
Hepatocellular carcinoma	1/50	0/50	1/49	2/49	5/49	8/50[a]
Neoplastic nodules	2/50	0/50	5/49	4/49	7/49	5/50[a]
Combined	3/50	0/50	6/49	6/49[a]	12/49[a]	13/50[a]
Mice						
Hepatocellular carcinoma	9/50	0/50	14/48	7/50[a]	19/50[a]	17/50[a]
Hepatocellular adenoma	6/50	1/50	11/48	5/50	10/50	1/50[a]
Combined	14/50	1/50	25/48[a]	12/50[a]	29/50[a]	18/50[a]

[a]Significantly greater than corresponding control by Fisher's exact test ($p < 0.05$).
Source: Ref. 4.

reasons had been met in the case of DEHP. Many scientists and expert groups have pointed out that many chemicals at or above their MTD induce biological changes or are handled by the body's metabolic systems differently than at low dose levels, and these changes may influence cancer development in some cases. The question of a secondary mechanism of tumor production with DEHP, which would occur only at doses near the MTD, is discussed later.

2.2   Genotoxicity

DEHP has been studied in a wide variety of test systems for genotoxic activity. These include 11 studies of mutagenicity in bacterial mutation assays (9, 17–26), four studies of mutagenicity in mammalian cells in vitro (23, 27–29), six cytogenetic studies in vitro (30–35), four cytogenetic studies in vivo (23, 24, 36, 37), three dominant lethal mutation assays in mice (38–40), two studies of cell transformation in vitro (23, 24), and three studies examining binding of radiolabeled DEHP to DNA in vivo (41–43). In addition, a large number of studies have examined the genotoxicity of DEHP's major metabolites, mono-2-ethylhexyl phthalate (MEHP) and 2-ethylhexanol (18–20, 23–26, 28, 34, 37, 40, 44).

Evaluation of the genotoxicity of a chemical that has demonstrated an ability to increase the incidence of tumors in an experimental bioassay is important. As discussed in more detail in Section 3, there is reason to believe that the production of a genetic change at a critical target in the DNA, perhaps the activation of an oncogene, represents an early step in the development of cancer (45–47). Since such genetic changes are essentially irreversible once they are fixed in the genome, and since, in theory, a single molecule of genotoxic chemical could produce such an irreversible change, the genotoxicity of many carcinogens is often cited as evidence for the absence of thresholds for carcinogens.

Some chemicals that do not appear to possess genotoxic activity can also affect tumor incidence, but for those chemicals, prolonged exposure to high-dose levels appears to be necessary to produce their effect; and it is likely that a threshold exists for their tumorigenic activity (48).

Although a number of individual studies of the genotoxicity of DEHP have indicated apparent positive responses (24, 38, 39), these have generally not been confirmed by other studies, and the overall weight of the evidence is that DEHP is not genotoxic. There remains some uncertainty in the case of MEHP in light of several studies that suggest it possesses cytogenetic activity (23, 24, 34). If the proposed mechanism of carcinogenicity of DEHP in rodents (see Section 3.1) is correct, however, some genetic damage might be expected in assay systems containing peroxisomes.

3   DOSE–RESPONSE EVALUATION

3.1   Mechanism of Carcinogenicity

The exact details of the mechanism of action are not known for any carcinogen. It is clear, from the differences in the biological effects of different carcinogens, however, that more than one mechanism may produce an increase in tumor incidence (45). For the so-called genotoxic carcinogens, the mechanism of action seems to involve interaction, either directly or after metabolic activation to an electrophilic form, with DNA (45–47). Other chemicals appear to increase tumor incidences without interacting with DNA. These include tumor promoters and cocarcinogens, some hormones, immunosuppressive drugs, and various other nongenotoxic carcinogens (45). Because, as described in Section 2.2, DEHP appears to be devoid of genotoxic activity, it belongs in the general class of nongenotoxic carcinogens. Less is known about the details of how these chemicals influence the incidence of tumors than is the case for genotoxic carcinogens.

In the case of DEHP, there is considerable support for the hypothesis that it belongs to a diverse class of nongenotoxic carcinogens whose mechanism of action involves the proliferation of the cell cytoplasmic organelles, the peroxisomes (22, 49, 50). In this section, we examine the support for this hypothesis and its implications for risk at low-dose levels. We also examine another aspect of the biology of DEHP that may affect low-dose risk, that of its pharmacokinetics and metabolism.

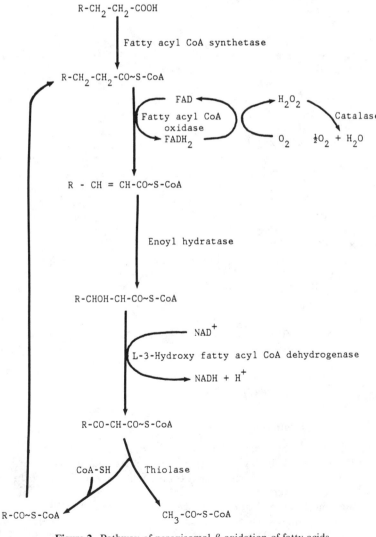

Figure 2. Pathway of peroxisomal β-oxidation of fatty acids.

3.1.1 Peroxisome Proliferation Hypothesis. Peroxisomes are small (0.2–1.5 mm) cytoplasmic organelles characterized by their morphology and enzyme activities (51–53). Peroxisomes are found throughout the plant and animal kingdoms. In mammals, they are most common in liver and kidney. Among the enzymes found in peroxisomes are catalase, which breaks down hydrogen peroxide to water (53), and several enzymes that generate hydrogen peroxide as a by-product (51). In particular, the peroxisomes contain a system of enzymes involved in β-oxidation of fatty acids, the first step of which generates hydrogen peroxide (54). This pathway is illustrated in Fig. 2.

Reddy et al. (49) proposed that there was a relation between peroxisome proliferation and liver carcinogenesis in rodents on the basis of their finding that a structurally diverse group of chemicals caused a reduction in serum lipid (particularly triglyceride) levels, liver enlargement without necrosis, proliferation of liver peroxisomes, and hepatocellular carcinoma in mice or rats, but were not mutagenic. Several other chemicals have since been shown to share these properties (50). Reddy et al. (22, 50, 55) have suggested that increased production of hydrogen peroxide by the peroxisomes may be responsible for the carcinogenic effect. Evidence supporting this hypothesis includes the following:

1. Enzymes involved in β-oxidation of fatty acids that generate hydrogen peroxide are increased in activity to a greater extent than is catalase, which inactivates hydrogen peroxide in animals fed chemicals, including DEHP, causing peroxisome proliferation (50, 56–60).
2. There is evidence of increased intracellular levels of hydrogen peroxide in animals fed some peroxisome proliferators (61–63) including DEHP (64).
3. Rats fed carcinogenic levels of several peroxisome proliferators show increased levels of lipofuscin, which is probably a product of lipid peroxidation (65).
4. Hydrogen peroxide or its products (66) can cause DNA and chromosome damage (67–75), is mutagenic (76), and appears to have tumor-promoting or cocarcinogenic activity (77–80).

There are limitations in this hypothesis, however. Some weak peroxisome proliferators, such as acetylsalicylic acid (aspirin) and fenofibrate do not appear to be carcinogenic (50, 81), but this may simply indicate that there is a threshold for this mechanism of carcinogenicity. Also, although a relation between increased hydrogen peroxide production and cancer development is plausible, there is no clear evidence that hydrogen peroxide itself can cause cancer.

3.2 Dose-Dependent Pharmacokinetics of DEHP

Following oral administration, the first step in the metabolism of DEHP is hydrolysis by a nonspecific lipase in the gut to yield mono-2-ethylhexyl phthalate (MEHP) and 2-ethylhexanol (2-EH). In rodents, MEHP subsequently undergoes ω- and $(\omega - 1)$-oxidation to yield the major metabolites shown in Fig. 3. The pathways illustrated there are inferred from knowledge of the structure of the urinary metabolites, based on the work of Albro et al. (41, 82, 83). Metabolites are numbered according to Albro's convention. Of particular interest here is the β-oxidation step going from metabolite V to metabolite I (see Fig. 3). Recall that peroxisomes contain the enzymes involved in β-oxidation of fatty acids and may therefore be involved in this step of the metabolism of DEHP in rodents, generating hydrogen peroxide. In humans, however, metabolite I has not been found, and

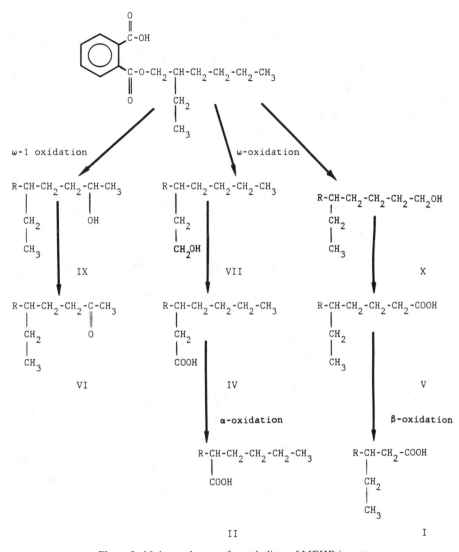

Figure 3. Major pathways of metabolism of MEHP in rats.

it is only a minor metabolite in nonhuman primates (41, 84). Peroxisome proliferation is much less extensive in primates than in rodents given DEHP (85). Hence, if peroxisomal β-oxidation is important in forming metabolite I, the finding (33, 41) of lower levels of metabolite I in primates would be expected, because of the lesser degree of peroxisome proliferation.

In addition to those interspecies differences in the production of metabolite I, a recent study (86) has demonstrated that there are dose-related changes in the proportions of the various metabolites of DEHP. Of particular interest, there is a dose-related increase in the proportion of the dose administered to rats that is excreted in the urine as metabolite I. In male F-344 rats fed DEHP for 20 days at 1000, 6000, or 12,000 ppm (the last two doses being equivalent to those fed in the NTP bioassay), the percentage of the daily dose excreted as metabolite I increased from 11% at 1000 ppm to 26% at 6000 ppm and 31% at 12,000 ppm. The immediate precursor (metabolite V) declined from 11% at 1000 ppm to 8% at 6000 ppm and 7% at 12,000 ppm. In addition, there was a decline in the percentage of the dose excreted via the feces, particularly as metabolite IX (see Fig. 3).

The dose-related changes in metabolism suggest that there is an increase with increasing dose in β-oxidation, since metabolite I is formed from metabolite V by β-oxidation (see Fig. 3) (83). Since the peroxisome proliferation that occurs at these dose levels in rats is accompanied by increases in peroxisomal β-oxidation activity, it is interesting to speculate that these dose-related changes in metabolism reflect concurrent peroxosome proliferation. It is not known, however, whether the β-oxidation step of DEHP metabolism occurs in the peroxisomes or in another cellular location (mitochondria or endoplasmic reticulum), but if it does occur in the peroxisomes, hydrogen peroxide would be generated, also in a nonlinear fashion. Furthermore, if the hypothesis that hydrogen peroxide generation is responsible for the carcinogenic effect of DEHP and other peroxisome proliferators is correct, a nonlinear relation between DEHP dose and tumor induction would be expected at low-dose levels (see Section 3.3).

3.3 Low-Dose Extrapolation

3.3.1 Extrapolation Models.
To estimate the carcinogenic risk to humans posed by xenobiotics shown to be carcinogenic in animals, two forms of extrapolation are generally needed—low-dose extrapolation and interspecies extrapolation. Low-dose extrapolation uses mathematical models together with information on the relation between dose of the chemical and carcinogenic response to predict the probability of an effect at dose levels in the range to which humans may be exposed. Interspecies extrapolation involves inferring risks to humans on the basis of the available data regarding metabolism, pharmacokinetics, and epidemiology, together with low-dose extrapolation.

For low-dose extrapolation, a number of different mathematical models have been developed (87, 88). Which of these models is most appropriate to use in any particular situation is one of the more controversial aspects of risk assessment. Wide differences in estimates of low-dose risk can arise through using different low-dose extrapolation models. Because of this uncertainty, we have used several different models, each with some degree of support, to examine their implications for low-dose human risk.

The multistage model is based, in part, on theories of cancer causation (89, 90), which suggest that a cell can give rise to a tumor only after it has undergone a certain number of heritable changes (stages). It is favored by regulatory agencies (5, 91) because it has some theoretical basis, and because it is conservative; that is, it yields higher estimates of risk than many other models. It has the mathematical form

$$P_D = 1 - \exp\left[-(q_0 + q_1 d + q_2 d^2 + \cdots + q_k d^k)\right]$$

where P_D = probability of a tumor at dose D

$q_0, q_1, \ldots, q_k$ = nonnegative parameters whose values are estimated based on the dose–response data

k = number of stages in the model.

As used by regulatory agencies, a 95th percentile upper confidence limit is calculated on the value of the linear parameter (q_1) in the model. This upper confidence limit, designated q_1^*, defines the excess risk at low-dose levels D: risk $= q_1^* D$. A computer model (GLOBAL 82) has been developed (92) to calculate the results of this co-called linearized multistage model.

The Mantel–Bryan log–probit model (93, 94) was the first mathematical model introduced specifically for carcinogen risk assessment. It represents a mathematical description of the distribution of tolerances, or thresholds, for a toxic effect in a population and has the form

$$P_D = P_0 + [1 - P_0 \Phi(a + b \log_{10} D)]$$

where P_D = probability of an effect at dose D
P_0 = probability of an effect in the absence of exposure
Φ = standard normal distribution function
a, b = parameters.

As proposed by Mantel and Bryan, the parameter b is fixed equal to 1 to ensure that the extrapolation is conservative. The parameter a is estimated from the experimental data. This procedure is less widely used than during the 1960s and 1970s because it has no basis in current theories of carcinogenesis. We use it here to give an idea of the possible range of uncertainty in the low-dose risk estimates. Also, since it is a description of the distribution of thresholds, it may be more appropriate than the multistage model if our proposed mechanism of carcinogenicity of DEHP is correct, because a threshold for DEHP would be expected at a dose level below that causing peroxisome proliferation.

If the proposed hypothesis that peroxisome proliferation is necessary for carcinogenesis by DEHP is correct, a threshold would be anticipated; at dose levels that do not induce peroxisome proliferation, no increase in tumor incidence would be expected. If this is true, then a safe exposure level should be identifiable by the same procedure that is used to identify safe levels of chemicals causing toxic effects other than cancer. This is the NOEL/safety factor approach. In this procedure, the highest dose level at which no adverse effects are produced is identified—the no observed effect level (NOEL)—and this dose level is divided by a safety factor, or uncertainty factor, to define a safe dose (95, 96). The magnitude of the safety factor used is governed by the quality and perceived relevance to the situation of human exposure of interest of the available toxicity data. Thus, for example, if high-quality human data are available, a safety factor of just 10-fold is often used to account for possible sensitive subgroups in the general population; if data from only a subchronic animal study are available, a safety factor of 1000 will often be used if a safe chronic human exposure level is desired (97). This safety factor covers both intraspecies and interspecies variability in sensitivity together with a factor to account for the differences in exposure duration (subchronic to chronic) (95, 97).

3.3.2 Units of Dose Measurement.
The most commonly used measure of dose in toxicological assessment is the applied dose measured in mg/kg body weight per day. However, in determining how risk varies with dose, a more relevant measure of dose would be the dose of the ultimate carcinogen at the target site. This latter dose, the target-site dose, will be a function of both the administered dose and the pharmacokinetics of the chemical (its absorption, distribution, biotransformation to active or inactive forms, and elimination). Provided all the pharmacokinetic parameters for a chemical are linear in

dose, the target-site dose will simply be proportional to the administered dose. It is becoming increasingly clear, however, that in many cases the pharmacokinetic parameters are not linear in dose throughout the dose range, and this can significantly affect estimates of risk at low dose levels (98–101).

Gehring et al. (98), for example, showed that the biotransformation of vinyl chloride to an active form was saturated at high doses, and this explained the flattening of the dose–response curve at high dose levels.

In the case of DEHP, we have only indirect information on the relation between applied dose and target-site dose with which to work. If the hypothesis for the mechanism of action of DEHP proposed in Section 3.1.1 is correct, the target-site dose of interest is the dose of hydrogen peroxide generated by the peroxisomes. Only an indirect measure of this dose is available at this time. It is based on the assumption that the production of DEHP metabolite I (Fig. 3) is a function of peroxisomal β-oxidation. If this assumption is correct, then because one molecule of hydrogen peroxide is generated for each β-oxidation cycle, the production of DEHP metabolite I might be an indirect measure of the production of hydrogen peroxide.

There is uncertainty in using metabolite I as a surrogate for target-site dose. We do not know whether metabolite I is formed in the peroxisomes or in the mitochondria (or another cellular compartment). Obviously, production of metabolite I in the mitochondria would not be an indicator of peroxisomal activity and would not involve peroxide generation; thus, the use of metabolite I production would overestimate peroxisomal activity and peroxide generation to the extent that mitochondrial β-oxidation is involved in metabolite I production. Peroxisomal production of metabolite I is supported by the results of recent studies by Lhuguenot et al. (102–104) who examined the effects of dose and time on the metabolism of MEHP using Wistar rats in vivo and rat hepatocytes in vitro. They found that both in vivo and in vitro production of metabolite I increased in parallel with increases in cyanide-insensitive peroxisomal β-oxidation activity. Also, the change in the rate of production of metabolite I from metabolite V with time of the hepatocytes in culture mirrored the change in the activity of cyanide-insensitive palmitoyl CoA oxidation in the hepatocytes (104).

In the past, pharmacokinetic data have been used to estimate target-site doses of genotoxic carcinogens, and these dose estimates have been used in place of measures of applied dose in risk extrapolation (98, 99). In assessing the risks of DEHP, use may be made of our knowledge of the nonlinear relation between applied dose of DEHP and urinary excretion of metabolite I to provide a surrogate to estimate the presumed nonlinear relation between applied dose of DEHP and peroxisome activity, which is in turn an indicator of the target-site dose of peroxide or other active oxygen species. To do this it is necessary to examine the quantitative relation between daily dose of DEHP and excretion of metabolite I under conditions approximating those of the NTP bioassay. Data describing the relation between DEHP dose and metabolite formation are derived from a study of the metabolism of DEHP in which male rats were fed DEHP at 1000, 6000, and 12,000 ppm in the diet for 20 days prior to receiving ^{14}C-labeled DEHP at the same dietary levels (86). These data are presented in Table 2.

The relation between daily dose of DEHP and daily excretion of metabolite I was fit to a power curve with the equation $I = 0.0187D^{1.43}$, where I is the daily excretion of metabolite I and D is the daily dose of DEHP. This curve was chosen as best fitting the data ($r = 0.9996$). This equation can be used to adjust the doses in the NTP bioassay to give doses that are surrogates for the target-site dose before fitting extrapolation models to the bioassay dose–response data. This adjustment is used with both the multistage model and

TABLE 2. Relation between Daily Dose of DEHP and Excretion of Metabolite I in Male Rats Fed DEHP for 20 Days

Dietary Concentration of DEHP (ppm)	Equivalent Daily Dose (mg/kg·day)[a]	Fraction of Dose Excreted in Urine as Metabolite I	Amount of Metabolite I Excreted per Day (mg/kg·day)[b]
1,000	54.97	0.11	7.15
6,000	370.81	0.25	92.76
12,000	769.64	0.31	238.59

[a]Based on consumption of food containing ^{14}C-labeled DEHP and terminal body weight (86).
[b]Amount excreted = daily dose of DEHP × fraction excreted as metabolite I.

the Mantel–Bryan model. Because of the uncertainties outlined above, this adjustment must be considered only semiquantitative. A superior approach would be the development of a physiologically based pharmacokinetic model.

3.3.3   Modeling of Rodent Carcinogenicity Data.

In order to estimate the low-dose risk to rodents, in an attempt to provide a conservative estimate of human risk, the combined incidences of hepatocellular carcinoma and adenoma/neoplastic nodules from the NTP bioassay (4) were used. To provide a better estimate of the background tumor incidence, pooled data from control groups were used, combining data from the four bioassays (DEHP, butyl benzyl phthalate, guar gum, and di-2-ethylhexyl adipate) that were performed in the same room of the same laboratory at the same time as the DEHP bioassay. The dose levels in mg/kg·day estimated by NTP (4) on the basis of food consumption were used. The four data sets used for risk extrapolation are presented in Table 3. Included are the estimates of the surrogate target-site doses based on the expected urinary levels of metabolite I for rats. These are derived as described in Section 3.3.2 using data from the multidose metabolism study (86). Since this metabolism study involved only

TABLE 3. Data Sets Used for Low-Dose Risk Extrapolation

Species	Sex	Dose (mg/kg·day) of DEHP (Metabolite I)	Incidence of Hepatocellular Tumors
Rat	Male	0	8/149
Rat	Male	322 (71.6)[a]	6/49
Rat	Male	674 (205.6)	12/49
Rat	Female	0	3/197
Rat	Female	394 (95.5)	6/49
Rat	Female	774 (250.5)	13/50
Mouse	Male	0	56/200
Mouse	Male	672	25/48
Mouse	Male	1325	29/50
Mouse	Female	0	10/200
Mouse	Female	799	12/50
Mouse	Female	1821	18/50

[a]Numbers in parentheses are estimated surrogate target-site dose levels calculated as described in the text.

TABLE 4. Multistage Model Dose Coefficients Based on DEHP Doses in NTP Bioassay[a]

	q_1 (mg/kg·day)$^{-1}$	q_2 (mg/kg·day)$^{-2}$	q_1^* (mg/kg·day)$^{-1}$
Male rats	1.42×10^{-4}	2.86×10^{-7}	4.88×10^{-4}
Female rats	2.13×10^{-4}	2.07×10^{-7}	4.96×10^{-4}
Male mice	4.59×10^{-4}	0	6.70×10^{-4}
Female mice	2.35×10^{-4}	0	3.29×10^{-4}

[a]The figures tabulated are the dose coefficients q_1 and q_2 in the multistage model: $P(d) = 1 - \exp[-(q_0 + q_1 d + q_2 d^2)]$, where $P(d)$ is the probability of developing a tumor after lifetime exposure to a dose of d mg/kg·day. For small values of d, the excess risk of developing a tumor closely approximates $q_1 d + q_2 d^2$. Also tabulated is q_1^*, the upper 95th percentile confidence limit on q_1.

TABLE 5. Multistage Model Dose Coefficients Based on Surrogate Target-Site Doses (Estimated Levels of Metabolite I) in NTP Bioassay[a]

	q_1 (mg/kg·day)$^{-1}$	q_2 (mg/kg·day)$^{-2}$	q_1^* (mg/kg·day)$^{-1}$
Male rats	1.03×10^{-3}	3.31×10^{-7}	1.77×10^{-3}
Female rats[b]	1.16×10^{-3}	0	1.70×10^{-3}

[a]The figures tabulated are the dose coefficients q_1 and q_2 in the multistage model: $P(d) = 1 - \exp[-(q_0 + q_1 d + q_2 d^2)]$, where $P(d)$ is the probability of developing a tumor after lifetime exposure to a dose of d mg/kg·day. For small values of d, the excess risk of developing a tumor closely approximates $q_1 d + q_2 d^2$. Also tabulated is q_1^*, the upper 95th percentile confidence limit on q_1.
[b]Although the data on metabolite I levels were derived from studies in male rats only, they are applied to females for purposes of conservative risk assessment since the female data predict slightly higher risks, recognizing the uncertainty of applying metabolic data derived from one sex to the other.

male rats, the adjustment, strictly, is applicable to male rats, but we have applied the same data to females also.

Dose-related metabolism data are not available for mice. Therefore, no such adjustments are made for the doses administered to mice, although a similar nonlinear relation between the applied dose of DEHP and the target-site dose probably also occurs in mice.

The results of applying the multistage model to all four data sets in Table 3 are presented in Table 4, which presents the dose coefficients q_1 and q_2 from the multistage model that best fit the data using the daily doses of DEHP. Also included are the values of q_1^*, the upper 95th percentile confidence limit on q_1. At low-dose levels, the excess risk above background to rodents is closely approximated by $P(d) = q_1 d + q_2 d^2$, where $P(d)$ is the risk at dose level d and q_1 and q_2 are the estimated dose coefficients. The upper confidence limit on low-dose risk is closely approximated by $P(d) = q_1^* d$.

Table 5 lists the corresponding values of q_1, q_2, and q_1^* derived using the surrogate target-site dose values. To derive the risk estimate for a given dose d of DEHP using these values, it is first necessary to convert the DEHP dose to the corresponding surrogate dose I using the equation $I = 0.0187 d^{1.43}$. The risk is then derived using the dose coefficients as described above (risk $= q_1 I + q_2 I^2$, or, upper 95th percentile confidence limit on risk $= q_1^* I$).

Table 6 lists the values of virtually safe dose corresponding to a risk of 10^{-6} and 10^{-8} predicted by the Mantel–Bryan probit procedure applied to the data on female rats and male mice.

TABLE 6. Virtually Safe Doses of DEHP Corresponding to Risks of 10^{-6} and 10^{-8} from Mantel-Bryan Model for Female Rats and Male Mice Based on DEHP Dose and on Surrogate Dose

	Virtually Safe DEHP Dose (μg/kg·day)			
	Based on DEHP Dose		Based on Surrogate Dose[a]	
	Risk = 10^{-6}	Risk = 10^{-8}	Risk = 10^{-6}	Risk = 10^{-8}
Female rats	46.8	6.5	791	198
Male mice	11.9	1.6	—	—

[a]Although the data on metabolite I levels were derived from studies in male rats only, they are applied to females for purposes of conservative risk assessment since the female data predict slightly higher risks, recognizing the uncertainty of applying metabolic data derived from one sex to the other.

3.4 Interspecies Extrapolation

Several factors strongly suggest that humans are likely to be much less sensitive to the carcinogenic effects of DEHP than are rats and mice. These are discussed below.

3.4.1 Interspecies Differences in Target-Site Susceptibility. In rats and mice exposed to very-high-dose levels of DEHP, the only site affected was the liver. The liver in rodents appears to be more susceptible to carcinogenesis than in humans. Various strains of mice show a high and variable incidence of spontaneous liver tumors that can be influenced markedly by factors such as stress and diet (105, 106). In rats, the liver appears to contain a high proportion of preneoplastic cells that can be stimulated to generate tumors by promoting agents (107–109). Furthermore, a high proportion of animal carcinogens are active in the rodent liver (110, 111), while few chemicals are known to cause liver cancer in humans (112). For example, of 98 chemicals reviewed by Griesemer and Cueto (111) which showed sufficient evidence of carcinogenicity in NCI bioassays, almost 60% produced hepatocellular tumors in mice or rats. Of the 98, 26 were significantly active only in the liver, and another 31 were active in the liver plus one or more other sites. By contrast, of the seven industrial processes and occupational exposures:

Auramine manufacture
Boot and shoe manufacture and repair (certain occupations)
Furniture manufacture
Isopropyl alcohol manufacture (strong-acid process)
Nickel refining
Rubber industry (certain occupations)
Underground hematite mining (with exposure to radon)

and 23 chemicals and groups of chemicals:

4-Aminobiphenyl
Analgesic mixtures containing phenacetin
Arsenic and arsenic compounds
Asbestos
Azathioprine

Benzene
Benizidine
N, N-Bis(2-chloroethyl)-2-naphthylamine (chlornaphazine)
Bis(chloromethyl) ether and technical-grade chloromethyl methyl ether
1, 4-Butanediol dimethanesulfonate (Myleran)
Certain combined chemotherapies for lymphomas (including MOPP)
Chlorambucil
Chromium and certain chromium compounds
Conjugated estrogens
Cyclophosphamide
Diethylstilbestrol
Melphalan
Methoxsalen with ultraviolet A therapy (PUVA)
Mustard gas
2-Naphthylamine
Soots, tars, and oils
Treosulfan
Vinyl chloride

that are considered by IARC (112) to be causally related to cancer in humans, only three (azathioprine, conjugated estrogens, and vinyl chloride) are associated with liver cancer. Of these three, only estrogens are associated with hepatocellular tumors like those commonly seen in rodents. Azathioprine is associated with hepatobiliary tumors, and vinyl chloride with liver angiosarcoma, which are of quite different histologic origins.

TABLE 7. Distribution of Urinary Metabolites of DEHP in Various Species

Metabolite[a]	Rat	Mouse	Green Monkey	Human
Residual DEHP	—	0.5	2.2	—
MEPH	Trace	18.6	28.9	18.3
I	17.2	16.8	0.1	—
II	2.0	1.0	—	1.8
III	1.2	0.4	—	—
IV	3.3	0.8	—	1.2
V	51.3	1.1	4.2	5.3
VI	2.6	14.9	5.9	12.1
VII	2.6	7.2	7.0	11.9
VIII	—	—	5.7	8.1
IX	13.3	12.3	38.2	36.2
X	0.6	2.2	0.1	0.1
A, B, C	4.1	8.1	7.6	4.9
Phthalic acid	1.8	12.4	0.1	0.1

[a]Metabolites are numbered according to the convention of P. W. Albro.
Source: Albro et al. (41).

Of specific relevance to DEHP, humans (and other primates) are less susceptible to peroxisome proliferation than are rats and mice (50, 113). These interspecies differences are likely to result in overestimates of human risk if the data from rodents are applied directly to humans.

3.4.2   Interspecies Differences in Metabolism of DEHP.   Previously, the potential importance of the production of DEHP metabolite I by β-oxidation as a possible indicator of peroxisomal β-oxidation activity was discussed. The production of metabolite I is one aspect of the metabolism of DEHP that clearly distinguishes humans and other primates from both rats and mice (see Tables 7 and 8). Not indicated in these tables is the fact that as much as 80% of the urinary metabolites in humans and other primates are excreted as glucuronide conjugates, while little if any conjugates are produced by the rat. Albro et al. (41) have noted that the differences in the metabolism of DEHP occurring in rats and primates would result in the overall demand on the oxidation potential in the liver being in opposite directions in rats and primates receiving high doses of DEHP. Albro et al. (41) further concluded that to the extent that the metabolism of DEHP is involved in its biological activity, one must question seriously whether rats are an appropriate model for humans.

TABLE 8. Urinary Metabolites of DEHP Expressed as Percentages of Total Urinary Radioactivity Excreted in First 24 h after Dosing

Metabolite[a]	Monkey	Rat	Mouse[b]
MEHP	11	—[c]	17
Phthalic acid	2	2	13
I	0.5	11	13
II	—	0.9	0.8
III	0.5	—	0.8
IV	0.5	4	3
V	25	29	1
VI	1	11	12
VII	7	3	6
IX	18	18	11
X	9	4	2
XII	2	6	5
XIII	6	6	7
Uncertain	15	1	5
XIV	2	1	2
Uncertain	1	1	1

[a]Metabolites are numbered according to the convention of P. W. Albro.
[b]The mouse urine extract analyzed by HPLC contained only 79% of the radioactivity excreted in 0–24 h. The remainder of the radioactivity was eluted from the SAC-2 resin in the acidic aqueous wash and probably contained some of the more polar metabolites, perhaps including glucuronides.
[c]Radioactivity in the sample was less than twice background for the system.
Source: Moran et al. (84)

The data shown in Table 7 were obtained under a variety of different conditions of exposure. The major differences in metabolism are confirmed, however, by the data shown in Table 8, which were obtained under comparable conditions of exposure. Importantly, if the hypothesis that production of metabolite I is an indicator of peroxisomal β-oxidation, and hence of hydrogen peroxide production, these data also suggest that humans would be less susceptible than rats or mice to the carcinogenic effect of DEHP.

3.4.3   Overview on DEHP's Carcinogenicity.   If the biological and metabolic data are indicators of relative carcinogenic activity, there is strong support for the contention that direct application to humans of low-dose extrapolation of the DEHP carcinogenicity data from rodents would overestimate human risk. Although direct evidence supporting this contention is lacking, the peroxisome-proliferation theory of carcinogenesis provides sufficient support to justify selecting an alternative to the more typical risk assessment approaches.

Having noted that the DEHP carcinogenicity data from rodents are probably not applicable to humans, we have nevertheless made use of these data to examine what the potential human risk might be, in the worst case, if the data were applicable to humans. In doing this, we have used all the low-dose extrapolation models described in Section 3.3.

4   EXPOSURE ASSESSMENT

A comprehensive and accurate assessment of human exposure to DEHP is critically important to the conduct of an adequate risk assessment. Unfortunately, studies that evaluate the degree of human exposure are few. In this assessment, the exposure of children to DEHP as a result of their contact with vinyl products containing the plasticizer is evaluated. The most useful source of information on children's exposure to DEHP comes from empirical measurements of migration of DEHP under conditions intended to simulate use (chewing and sucking pacifiers and teethers, and skin contact with other products) that were performed for CPSC by the Inhalation Toxicology Research Institute (114). Estimates of DEHP from plastics have also been made based on physicochemical factors (e.g., migration rates, partition coefficients, surface areas, temperature) (1).

4.1   Exposure Estimates Based on Laboratory Studies of DEHP Migration

The Inhalation Toxicology Research Institute (ITRI) (114) conducted tests for CPSC to estimate the extent of migration of DEHP from various consumer products, particularly children's products, in 1983. ITRI examined both oral and dermal exposure, but for this chapter we consider only the data relating to oral exposure. ITRI examined leaching of DEHP from pacifiers, teethers, and plastic toys into simulated saliva (phosphate-buffered saline solution containing 0.16% mucin) under various conditions, including conditions in which the objects were squeezed to simulate chewing.

Initial trials with human saliva demonstrated considerable variability in leaching rates (114). When two samples of a teether were immersed in different samples of human saliva at 37°C with shaking 30 times per minute over a 22-h period, the rate of DEHP leaching into saliva was 0.074 μg/h·cm^2 of teether in one sample, and in the other was 0.014 μg/h·cm^2. A comparable study using a similar teether and the simulated saliva showed a leaching rate of 0.032 μg/h·cm^2. It was assumed by ITRI that the leaching rate observed for the saliva simulant approximates that with human saliva.

Further trials by ITRI indicated that mechanical manipulation of a pacifier by squeezing it with a brass plunger while it was immersed in the saliva simulant substantially increased the rate of leaching. Since such squeezing was thought to mimic the chewing and sucking of items such as pacifiers, teethers, and, to a lesser extent, children's toys, this procedure was used in further studies by ITRI (114). However, since the entire product was immersed in saliva simulant during these studies, while only a small fraction of the products would actually be in a child's mouth, this procedure is likely to overestimate the amount of DEHP released. In their risk assessment, CPSC (5) made some adjustment for this overestimation by assuming that release from the portion that would not be in a child's mouth occurs at the rate seen in the absence of squeezing. However, a problem still remains: it is unlikely that the effects of the squeezing stimulus applied during the ITRI experiments are confined strictly to the area being squeezed, the mouthed area, as this assumption implies. Some of the effects of squeezing are almost certain to be transferred through the PVC and are likely to increase the rate of DEHP leaching from an area much greater in size that that mouthed by a child. Thus, CPSC's adjustment to the leaching data almost certainly overestimated the amount of DEHP that would be ingested by a child.

Many other aspects of these experiments add to the uncertainty regarding their appropriateness for estimating the exposure of children to DEHP. When individual pacifiers were tested repeatedly and for different lengths of time, the rate of leaching in μg/h varied up to eightfold for the same pacifier at different times. The choice of 0.16% mucin in saliva as a saliva simulant was made by ITRI "to produce a leaching rate similar to that of human saliva;" but as mentioned above, tests using two samples of human saliva produced leaching rates that differed by more than fivefold. The procedure for squeezing the various children's products was, of course, no more than a crude attempt to imitate some of the mechanical effects that would occur during chewing and sucking and it is not possible to tell how well it simulated the effects of chewing. However, in experiments in which squeezing was performed 30 and 15 times per minute, the rate of leaching differed also by a factor of 2 (114). Because of all these sources of variability, it is impossible to determine how well the laboratory procedures are likely to mimic the actual situation.

The most detailed set of data on leaching is presented in a memorandum written by B. Bhooshan and dated August 24, 1983 (115). This document contains data on nine types of pacifier, four types of teether, and six types of plastic toy that were tested, each with triplicate samples, under the squeezing conditions already mentioned. Leaching from each sample was tested for 22 h on each of three consecutive days. These data illustrate the extreme variability of the results. For example, the amount of DEHP leaching from one individual pacifier of a type containing about 35% DEHP was 104 μg on the first day of testing, 1450 μg on the second day, and 138 μg on the third day. With a different type of pacifier, one sample of which contained 42.4% DEHP, one of the triplicate samples tested released 229–556 μg on the 3 days of testing, while another presumably identical pacifier released 759–4270 μg. Overall, the amount of DEHP released from different pacifiers in 1 day under identical testing conditions varied from a low of 72 μg (sample number F-820-1541-13 on day 3) to 4760 μg (sample number E-815-1338-2 on day 2), a range of 66-fold.

The range in amount of DEHP released from teethers and plastic toys was somewhat less extreme. It was 32-fold for teethers (85.9–2770 μg, both from different samples of the same type of teether) and 12-fold for toys (94–1123 μg for different toys and 170–1123 μg for the same toy on different days).

These differences in leaching cannot simply be explained on the basis of differences in DEHP content and surface area. The toy with the highest degree of leaching had a lower content of DEHP (29.3%) and a smaller surface area (155.5 cm^2) than that with the lowest degree of leaching (38% DEHP, 198.9 cm^2). Also, the two types of pacifier with the most extreme difference in leaching (66-fold) were very similar in DEHP content (36.9 and 35.4%) and surface area (66.12 and 67.3 cm^2, respectively).

In the face of such unexplained variability, it is difficult to determine how best to use these data to estimate exposure. CPSC's approach in its risk assessment (5) was to separate products into low-release and high-release classes, but considering the wide variation seen with identical products and with the same product at different times, this additional complication seems unwarranted. Furthermore, since the ranges of leaching rates for teethers and toys completely overlap that for pacifiers, and since a child is unlikely to have more than one such item in its mouth at one time, estimating separate leaching rates for pacifiers, teethers, and toys seems unnecessary, since it suggests a level of precision not present in the experimental data.

We have simply estimated the average hourly leaching rate from all 27 pacifiers, 12 teethers, and 18 toys, making no adjustments for surface area, and using this value as a likely worst-case exposure indicator. After correction for appropriate blank values, this gives 662.4 μg/22 h or about 30 μg/h. Since the surface areas of the products tested were 6–7-fold greater for pacifiers and teethers and 10–18-fold greater for toys than the area estimated by CPSC as being subject to mouthing, this estimate is likely to be an overestimate of exposure and hence represents a worst-case estimate. This leaching rate may than be combined with an estimate of the number of hours per day a child might have such a product in its mouth and the number of years during which exposure to these products occurs. In CPSC's risk assessment, the range presented for the total length of exposure per day for all such products was from 6 to 14 h. This seems excessive unless the child sleeps much of the time with a pacifier in its mouth. Unfortunately, as pointed out by CPSC (5), no survey data are available to give a well-supported estimate of exposure.

To provide an estimate of the possible range of exposures and corresponding risks, we consider three possible exposure situations: low, moderate, and high exposures. In the low-exposure situation, we assume oral contact with a pacifier, teether, or plastic toy for an average or 3 h/day for 2 years. For the moderate-exposure scenario, we assume exposure may be for 6 h/day for 2 years. For the high-exposure situation, we assume that exposure may be for 10 h/day for 2 years and 3 h/day for an additional 1 year.

4.2 Exposure Scenario

Using the information on oral exposure discussed above, we now estimate the range of possible children's exposure to DEHP based on the description of low, moderate, and high oral exposure outlined above. Table 9 lists possible exposure scenarios, estimates of total DEHP exposures, and corresponding equivalent daily lifetime doses. The range of equivalent daily lifetime doses is 0.24–0.93 μg/kg·day. We make use of these exposure estimates for risk estimation in the next section.

The following sample calculation illustrates how the human dose estimates in Table 9 were derived. The low-exposure scenario assumes exposure 3 h/day for 2 years. As described in Section 4.1, the average rate of leaching of DEHP in the ITRI studies was 30 μg/h. Hence, total DEHP exposure's

$$30 \, \mu\text{g/h} \times 3 \, \text{h/day} \times 365 \, \text{days/yr} \times 2 \, \text{years}$$

$$= 65{,}700 \, \mu\text{g}$$

TABLE 9. Exposure Scenarios

Scenario	Total DEHP Exposure (mg)	Equivalent Average Daily Lifetime Dose $(\mu g/kg \cdot day)^a$
Low[b]	65.7	0.24
Moderate[c]	131.4	0.49
High[d]	251.8	0.93

[a]Assumes 74-year lifespan and 10-kg body weight. To provide the most conservative estimate of average daily lifetime dose we have made no adjustment for increase in body weight with age.
[b]Oral contact with a pacifier, teether, or toy for 3 h/day for 2 years.
[c]Oral contact with a pacifier, teether, or toy for 6 h/day for 2 years.
[d]Oral contact with a pacifier, teether, or toy for 10 h/day for 2 years, plus 3 h/day for an additional 1 year.

The equivalent average daily lifetime dose is derived as

$$\frac{65,700\,\mu g}{10\,kg} \times \frac{1\,year}{365\,days} \times \frac{1}{74\,years} = 0.24\,\mu g/kg \cdot day,$$

where 10 kg is the approximate body weight, and 74 years is the approximate lifespan. The other values in Table 9 are calculated similarly.

5   RISK CHARACTERIZATION

In this section we combine the estimates of unit cancer risk (UCR) derived in Section 3 with the estimates of human exposure via children's pacifiers, teethers, and toys derived in Section 4. Rather than list all the possible combinations of exposure estimates and UCRs, we present a selection of the possible combinations that gives an indication of the range of possible risks. For each of the three exposure scenarios depicted in Table 9, Tables 10 and 11 list the corresponding estimates of lifetime cancer risk for humans, based on the bioassay data from the sex of each rodent species that was most sensitive to DEHP (gave higher risk). The human risk estimates derived on the basis of the unadjusted DEHP dosage levels are shown in Table 10. The estimates derived using the surrogate target-site dose estimates derived as indicated in Section 3.3.3., and based on the relation between DEHP dose and excretion of DEHP metabolite I by male rats, are also presented (Table 11).

Even the highest estimate of exposure combined with the most conservative UCR value yields a lifetime risk estimate of less than 1×10^{-6} (1 in 1 million). When an attempt is made to make use of the available biological data to define the low-dose risk better, estimates of risk more than 200-fold lower are derived (Table 11). Even these estimates probably overestimate human risk because they do not consider the fact that primates, including humans, are less susceptible to the peroxisome proliferation effects of DEHP and other chemicals that cause the same effect. To the extent that, as we hypothesize, peroxisome proliferation is involved in the mechanism of carcinogenicity of DEHP in

TABLE 10. Estimates of Lifetime Risk to Children Exposed to DEHP through Pacifiers, Teethers, and Toys Based on Unadjusted DEHP Dose Levels[a]

Exposure Estimate[b]	Lifetime Risk Estimate Based on:	
	Male Mouse Data	Female Rat Data
Low	$1.1 \times 10^{-7} (1.6 \times 10^{-7})^c$	$5.1 \times 10^{-8} (1.2 \times 10^{-7})$
Moderate	$2.2 \times 10^{-7} (3.3 \times 10^{-7})$	$1.0 \times 10^{-7} (2.4 \times 10^{-7})$
High	$4.3 \times 10^{-7} (6.2 \times 10^{-7})$	$2.0 \times 10^{-7} (4.6 \times 10^{-7})$

[a]These risk estimates assume that humans and rodents are at equal risk at the same dose level in mg/kg·day.
[b]Low, moderate, and high exposures correspond to 0.24, 0.49, and 0.93 μg DEHP/kg·day, respectively (see Table 9).
[c]Figures in parentheses are upper 95th percentile confidence limits on lifetime risk.

TABLE 11. Estimates of Lifetime Risk to Children Exposed to DEHP through Pacifiers, Teethers, and Toys, Based on Estimated Surrogate Target-Site Dose Levels[a]

Exposure Estimate[b]	Estimated Surrogate Dose (mg/kg·day)[c]	Lifetime Risk Estimate Based on Female Rat Data[d]
Low	1.25×10^{-7}	$1.4 \times 10^{-10} (2.1 \times 10^{-10})^e$
Moderate	3.46×10^{-7}	$4.0 \times 10^{-10} (5.9 \times 10^{-10})$
High	8.65×10^{-7}	$1.0 \times 10^{-9} \ (1.5 \times 10^{-9})$

[a]Surrogate target-site dose calculated as described in Section 3.3.3. These risk estimates assume that humans and rats are at equal risk at the same target-site dose in mg/kg·day and that rats and humans show the same relation between dose of DEHP and target-site dose.
[b]Low, moderate, and high exposures correspond to 0.24, 0.49, and 0.93 μg DEHP/kg·day, respectively (see Table 9).
[c]Derived using the equation: surrogate dose (I mg/kg·day) = $0.0187d^{1.43}$, where d is the estimated dose of DEHP in mg/kg·day.
[d]Risk based on rat data only, because surrogate dose levels are derived from rat data.
[e]Figures in parentheses are upper 95th percentile confidence limits on lifetime risk.

rodents, humans would be expected to be at much lower risk than rodents at the same dose of DEHP.

Table 12 lists the range of estimated childhood exposures to DEHP in comparison to estimates of virtually safe dose (risk $= 10^{-6}$ or 10^{-8}) derived using the Mantel–Bryan procedure from male mouse and female rat data using unadjusted DEHP dose levels and from female rat data using surrogate target-site dose levels as explained in Section 3.3.3. These reveal that the levels of children's exposure to DEHP from pacifiers, teethers, and toys are well below the virtually safe doses.

TABLE 12. Comparison of Estimated Children's Exposure to DEHP with Mantel–Bryan Virtually Safe Dose (VSD) Estimates

	Mantel–Bryan VSD (μg DEHP/kg·day)		
Range of Estimates	Unadjusted Dose[b]		Adjusted Dose[c]
of Children's Exposure			
to DEHP (μg/kg·day)[a]	Male Mouse Data	Female Rat Data	Female Rat Data
0.24–0.93	11.9[d]	46.8[d]	791[d]
	1.6[e]	6.5[e]	198[e]

[a]Exposure estimates from Table 9.
[b]Extrapolation based on applied dose level of DEHP.
[c]Extrapolation based on surrogate target-site dose calculated as described in Section 3.3.3.
[d]Dose corresponding to a risk of 1 in 1 million (10^{-6}).
[e]Dose corresponding to a risk of 1 in 100 million (10^{-8}).

5.1   NOEL/Safety Factor Approach to Risk Assessment

If the mechanism of carcinogenicity of DEHP that has been proposed in Section 3.1 is correct, no increased risk of cancer would occur at exposure levels that do not cause peroxisome proliferation, and subsequent excess peroxide production. Such pathologic effects are of the type normally protected against by the classical toxicological procedure whereby a no observed effect level (NOEL) is identified in animal tests and a safety factor is applied to determine an acceptable daily intake (ADI) for humans (95).

To use this procedure, it is of course necessary to identify a NOEL. Unfortunately, it is not clear if a NOEL has been identified for DEHP. In the phase I validation study conducted as part of the CMA Voluntary TSCA Testing Program (116), groups of 12 male and 12 female F-344 rats were fed diets containing DEHP at 0, 1000, 6000, and 12,000 ppm for 3 weeks. The activity of the enzyme carnitine acetyltransferase, which occurs in the peroxisomes and the mitochondria, showed a dose-related increase in activity at all dose levels after as little as 1 week of treatment. Dose-related effects were also noted on liver weight (increased 20, 66, and 98% in male rats at 3 weeks), serum triglycerides (decreased to 56, 31, and 18% of control in males at 3 weeks), and a cytochemical test (dose-related increase in peroxisome proliferation). Males were affected more than females. These effects were not evident, however, in the animals allowed 2 weeks of recovery after DEHP treatment, indicating that the effects are reversible.

The trade association of the European chemical industry (CEFIC) sponsored a similar study in which groups of male and female Alderly Park SPF-derived albino rats (number unspecified) were fed DEHP at 0, 50, 200, and 1000 mg/kg·day (about 1000, 4000, and 20,000 ppm) for 28 days (117). Liver weight was increased in all treated groups in a dose-related manner. There was a dose-related proliferation of peroxisomes starting at the lowest dose level and a similar proliferation of smooth endoplasmic reticulum.

Morton (58) fed DEHP at various dose levels to groups of 5–12 male Sprague–Dawley rats for 7 days and measured such parameters as liver weight, serum triglyceride level, liver catalase, carnitine acetyltransferase (CAT), carnitine palmitoyltransferase (CPT), and β-oxidation activity. Liver weight was significantly increased in a dose-related manner at DEHP dietary levels of 1000, 2500, and 5000 ppm but not at 50, 100, or 500 ppm. Serum triglyceride levels were significantly reduced in a dose-related manner at all levels tested (50, 500, and 2500 ppm). Catalase activity was increased significantly at 5000 ppm but not at 100 or 1000 ppm. CAT and CPT activities were significantly increased in a dose-related manner at 100, 500, 1000, and 2500 ppm, but not at 50 ppm.

Of perhaps most importance to the present discussion is the liver β-oxidation activity. When total liver β-oxidation activity was measured, significant dose-related increases were seen at 500, 1000, and 5000 ppm and slight but not significant increases were seen at 50 and 100 ppm. Morton (58) also examined β-oxidation activity in isolated mitochondria and peroxisomes after feeding DEHP, at 0, 100, 1000 and 5000 ppm. In peroxisomes, β-oxidation activity was increased significantly only at 5000 ppm, but slight, nonsignificant increases were seen at 100 and 1000 ppm. In isolated mitochondria, β-oxidation activity was increased significantly at 5000 and 1000 ppm and slightly but not significantly at 100 ppm.

In a study recently conducted by the British Industrial Biological Research Association (118), DEHP was fed to groups of five Fischer 344 rats of each sex at dietary levels of 0, 100, 1000, 6000, 12,000, and 25,000 ppm for 21 days. Males and females fed 6000 ppm or more showed significantly increased liver weights and significantly increased peroxisomal β-oxidation activity. Serum triglyceride levels were significantly reduced at the same levels in males. Microsomal lauric acid 11- and 12-hydroxylase activity was significantly increased in males at 1000 ppm and above, as was the number of peroxisomes in the liver. These latter effects were seen in females only at 6000 ppm or more.

In attempting to identify a NOEL from these data, several choices are possible. Based on the dose level causing a significant increase in peroxisomal β-oxidation activity in the studies by Morton (58) and BIBRA (118), a NOEL of 1000 ppm could be identified (about 70 mg/kg·day based on Morton's food consumption and body weight data, or 106 mg/kg·day based on BIBRA data). Based on total liver β-oxidation activity, the NOEL would be set lower, at 100 ppm (about 7 mg/kg·day). A NOEL for all effects of 100 ppm (about 11 mg/kg·day) was identified in the BIBRA study (118). However, a NOEL for all effects cannot be identified from the Morton study (58) since a significant reduction in serum triglyceride level was seen even at the lowest dose of 50 ppm (about 3.5 mg/kg·day), although such an effect was not seen in the BIBRA study at levels below 6000 ppm.

Since these possible NOELs are derived from studies of short-term exposure (7–21 days), estimation of a chronic ADI for humans would typically involve, following EPA (95) or NAS (97) procedures, application of a safety factor of 1000. This would lead to a chronic ADI of between 70 and less than 3.5 μg/kg·day, with the most likely value being 11 μg/kg·day, which is derived from the NOEL for peroxisomal proliferation in the BIBRA study (118). These values are well above the estimated range of children's exposure to DEHP from pacifiers, teethers, and toys of 0.24–0.93 μg/kg·day. The margin of safety is probably larger than is implied above because the 1000-fold safety factor is very conservative since it is clear, as discussed in Section 3.4, that rodents are more sensitive to the effects of DEHP on peroxisome than are humans. Hence, a smaller safety factor than 1000 may be adequate.

6   DISCUSSION

Although it is clear that lifetime exposure of rats and mice to maximum tolerated doses of DEHP causes an increased incidence of liver tumors, there is a substantial body of data, as discussed above, that indicates that the mechanism by which these tumors are apparently induced, involving peroxisome proliferation and excess hydrogen peroxide production, is a secondary one, not related to interaction of DEHP or its metabolites with DNA. Because of this, the use of simple low-dose linear extrapolation models, such as the linearized multistage model favored by the EPA and CPSC, is likely to overestimate risk at low-dose levels. Furthermore, since the peroxisome proliferation response that appears to be involved in the carcinogenic process in rodents does not occur in humans or other primates, any low-dose extrapolation that does not take this finding into account will likely greatly overstate the risk to humans exposed to low levels of DEHP.

In this chapter, we have attempted to make some use of the available biological data to give a more realistic estimate of low-dose risk from DEHP exposure than that obtained by direct linear extrapolation, as performed by CPSC (5), for example.

We have also used different mathematical models, including a threshold model (i.e., NOEL/safety factor), to assess low-dose risk. These procedures produce a range of risk estimates that illustate the uncertainty inherent in this extrapolation. For example, the lifetime daily dose corresponding to a risk of 10^{-6} ranges from 1.5 μg/kg·day, based on the linearized multistage model applied directly to the mouse data, to 791 μg/kg·day, based on the application of the Mantel–Bryan probit model to the rat data, incorporating the surrogate dose adjustment described in Section 3.3.2. These adjustments apply strictly to rats. To the extent that the hypothesized peroxisome proliferation mechanism is involved in the carcinogenicity of DEHP in rodents, the risk to humans would be even less than these values suggest, because humans and other primates are much less responsive to peroxisome proliferation than are rodents (50, 113), and because rodents appear to be inherently hypersusceptible to liver cancer (see Section 3.4.1).

Recognizing the limitations and uncertainties in these low-dose extrapolation procedures, we have attempted to apply them to available estimates of childhood exposure to DEHP resulting from its use in plastic pacifiers, teethers, and toys. By all methods of extrapolation examined, the excess lifetime risk to children is less than 1 in 1 million and is probably less than 1 in 100 million. Alternatively, there is a margin of safety of more than 1000-fold between the lowest daily dose of DEHP causing any effect in experimental animals and the daily dose that children might receive from plastic pacifiers, teethers, and toys. It seems reasonable to conclude that no significant risk exists to children exposed in this way to DEHP.

ACKNOWLEDGMENTS

We thank the members of the Chemical Manufacturers Association Phthalate Esters Panel, particularly Dr. Elizabeth J. Moran, for advice and support in the conduct of this study. We also thank Mary Ann Liebert, Inc. and the *Journal of the American College of Toxicology* for permission to reproduce some of the information discussed in this chapter from our paper "Assessment of possible carcinogenic risk to humans resulting from exposure to di(2-ethylhexyl)phthalate (DEHP)," by D. Turnbull and J. V. Rodricks, *J. Am. Coll. Toxicol.* **4**, 111–145 (1985).

REFERENCES

1. A. D. Little. *Phthalates in Consumer Products*, Contract No. CPSC-C-80-1001. Consumer Product Safety Commission, Washington, DC, 1982.
2. W. L. Guess, J. Jacobs, and J. Autian, A study of polyvinyl chloride blood bag assemblies. I. Alteration or contamination of ACD solutions. *Drug Intell.* **1**, 120 (1967).

3. R. J. Jaeger and R. J. Rubin, 1970. Plasticizers from plastic devices. Extraction, metabolism, and accumulation by biological systems. *Science* **170**, 460–462 (1970).

4. National Toxicology Program, *NTP Technical Report on the Carcinogenesis Bioassay of Di(2-ethylhexyl)phthalate (CAS No. 117-81-7) in F344 Rats and B6C3F Mice (Feed Study)*, NIH Publ. No. 82-1773. NTP, Washington, DC, 1982.

5. Consumer Products Safety Commission, *Children's Chemical Hazards. Risk Assessment on di(2-ethylhexyl)phthalate in Children's Products*. Chemical Hazards Program, Directorate for Health Sciences, CPSC, Washington, DC, 1983.

6. National Academy of Sciences, *Risk Assessment in the Federal Government: Managing the Process*. National Academy Press, Washington, DC, 1983.

7. J. A. Thomas, K. A. Curto, and M. J. Thomas, MEHP/DEHP: Gonadal toxicity and effects on rodent accessory sex organs. *Environ. Health Perspect.* **45**, 85–88 (1982).

8. T. J. B. Gray and S. D. Gangolli, Aspects of the testicular toxicity of phthalate esters. *Environ. Health Perspect.* **65**, 229–235 (1986).

9. L. E. Milkov, M. V. Aldyreva, T. B. Popova, K. A. Lopukhova, Y. L. Makarenko, L. M. Malyar, and T. K. Shakhova, Health status of workers exposed to phthalate plasticizers in the manufacture of artificial leather and films based on PVC resins. *Environ. Health Perspect.* **3**, 175–178 (1973).

10. R. Gilioli, C. Gulgheroni, T. Terrance, G. Fillipini, N. Masseto, and R. Boeri, A neurological electromyographic and electroneurographic study in subjects working at the production of phthalate plasticizers: Preliminary results. *Med. Lav.* **69**, 631 (1978).

11. A. M. Thiess, A. Korte, and I. Fleig, Study of morbidity in BASF workers exposed to di-(2-ethylhexyl)phthalate (DOP). *18th Annu. Meet. Hum. Soc. Ind. Med.* (1978), pp. 137–151.

12. C. P. Carpenter, C. S. Weil, and H. F. Smyth, Chronic oral toxicity of di(2-ethylhexyl) phthalate for rats, guinea pigs and dogs. *Arch. Ind. Hyg. Occup. Med.* **8**, 219–226 (1953).

13. R. S. Harris, H. C. Hodge, E. A. Maynard, and H. J. Blanchet, Jr., Chronic oral toxicity of 2-ethylhexyl phthalate in rats and dogs. *Arch. Ind. Health* **13**, 259–264 (1956).

14. R. Lefaux, *Practical Toxicology of Plastics*. CRC Press, Cleveland, OH, 1968.

15. W. R. Grace and Co., Dioctyl phthalate, Tech. Brochure (1948). As cited in L. G. Krauskopf, Studies on the toxicity of phthalates via ingestion. *Environ. Health Perspect.* **3**, 61–72 (1973).

16. S. Northup, L. Martis, R. Ulbricht, J. Garber, J. Miripol, and T. Schmitz, Comment on the carcinogenic potential of di(2-ethylhexyl) phthalate. *J. Toxicol. Environ. Health* **10**, 493–518 (1982).

17. V. F. Simmon, K. Kauhanen, and R. G. Tardiff, Mutagenic activity of chemicals identified in drinking water. In D. Scott, B. A. Bridges, and F. H. Sobels, Eds., *Progress in Genetic Toxicology*. North-Holland Biomedical Press, Amsterdam, 1977, pp. 249–258.

18. Y. Yagi, K. Tutikawa, and W. Shimoi, Teratogenicity and mutagenicity of a phthalate ester. *Teratology* **14**, 259–260 (1976).

19. R. J. Rubin, W. Kozumbo, and R. Kroll, Ames mutagenic assay of a series of phthalic acid esters: positive response of the dimethyl and diethyl esters in TA100. *Abstr. Pap., 18th Annu. Meet., Soc. Toxicol., New Orleans, LA*, No. 266 (1979).

20. P. E. Kirby, R. F. Pizarello, T. E. Lawlor, S. R. Haworth, and J. R. Hodgson, Evaluation of di-(2-ethylhexyl)phthalate and its major metabolites in the Ames test and L5178Y mouse lymphoma mutagenicity assay. *Environ. Mutagen.* **5**, 657–663 (1982).

21. E. Zeiger, S. Haworth, W. Speck, and K. Mortelmans, Phthalate ester testing in the National Toxicology Program's Environmental Mutagenesis Test Development Program. *Environ. Health Perspect.* **45**, 99–101 (1982).

22. J. Warren, N. D. Lalwani, and J. K. Reddy, Phthalate esters as peroxisome proliferator carcinogens. *Environ. Health Perspect.* **45**, 35–40 (1982).

23. Chemical Manufacturers Association, Phthalate Esters Program Panel Voluntary Test Program Health Effects Testing, Phase I: Validation Results, Volume I, CMA, Washington, DC, 1982.

24. I. Tomita, Y. Nakamura, N. Aoki, and N. Inui, Mutagenic/carcinogenic potential of DEHP and MEHP. *Environ. Health Perspect.* **45**, 119–125 (1982).

25. K. Yoshikawa, A. Tanaka, T. Yamaha, and H. Kurata, Mutagenicity study of nine monoalkyl phthalates and a dialkyl phthalate using Salmonella typhimurium and Escherichia coli. *Food Chem. Toxicol.* **21**, 221–223 (1983).

26. G. D. Divincenzo, W. H. Donish, K. R. Mueller, M. L. Hamilton, and E. D. Barber, Mutagenicity testing of urine from rats dosed with 2-ethylhexanol derived plasticizers. *Environ. Mutagen.* **5**, 471 (1983).

27. A. R. Malcolm, *Mutagenicity and Tumor-promoting Potential of Di(2-ethylhexyl)Phthalate in Chinese Hamster Cells* (draft). Environmental Research Laboratory, U.S. Environmental Protection Agency, Narragansett, RI, 1982.

28. J. E. Hodgson, B. C. Myhr, M. McKeon, and D. J. Brusick, Evaluation of di-(2-ethylhexyl) phthalate and its major metabolites in the primary rat hepatocyte unscheduled DNA synthesis assay. *Environ. Mutagen.* **4**, 388 (1982).

29. B. Butterworth, The genetic toxicology of di(2-ethylhexyl)phthalate (DEHP). *CIIT Act.* **4**, 1–8 (1984).

30. J. H. Turner, J. C. Petricciani, M. L. Crouch, and S. Wenger, An evaluation of the effects of diethylhexyl phthalate (DEHP) on mitotically capable cells in blood packs. *Transfusion (Philadelphia)* **14**, 560–566 (1974).

31. M. A. Stenchever, M. A. Allen, L. Jerominski, and R. V. Petersen, Effects of bis(2-ethylhexyl) phthalate on chromosomes of human leukocytes and human fetal lung cells. *J. Pharm. Sci.* **65**, 1648–1651 (1976).

32. K. Tsuchiya and K. Hattori, A chromosomal study of cultured human leukocytes treated with phthalic acid esters. *Rep. Hokkaido Inst. Public Health* **26**, 114 (1976).

33. S. Abe and M. Sasaki, Chromosome aberrations and sister chromatid exchanges in Chinese hamster cells exposed to various chemicals. *J. Natl. Cancer Inst.* **58**, 1635–1641 (1977).

34. B. J. Phillips, T. E. B. James, and S. D. Gangolli, Genotoxicity studies of di(2-ethylhexyl)phthalate and its metabolites in CHO cells. *Mutat. Res.* **102**, 297–304 (1982).

35. M. Ishidate, Jr. and S. Odashima, Chromosome tests with 134 compounds on Chinese hamster cells in vitro—a screening for chemical carcinogens. *Mutat. Res.* **48**, 337–354 (1977).

36. A. M. Thiess and I. Fleig, Chromosomal studies of employees after exposure to di-2-ethylhexyl phthalate (DOP). *Zentralbl. Arbietsmed., Arbietsschutz Prophyl.* **28**, 351–355 (1978).

37. D. L. Putman, W. A. Moore, L. M. Schechtman, and J. R. Hodgson, Cytogenetic evaluation of di-(2-ethylhexyl) phthalate and its major metabolites in Fischer 344 rats. *Environ. Mutagen.* **5**, 227–231 (1983).

38. A. R. Singh, W. H. Lawrence, and J. Autian, Mutagenic and antifertility sensitivities of mice to di-2-ethylhexyl phthalate (DEHP) and dimethoxy-ethyl phthalate (DMEP). *Toxicol. Appl. Pharmacol.* **29**, 35–46 (1974).

39. J. Autian, Antifertility effects and dominant lethal assays for mutagenic effects of DEHP. *Environ. Health Perspect.* **45**, 115–118 (1982).

40. C. J. Rushbrook, T. A. Jorgenson, and J. R. Hodgson, Dominant lethal study of di(2-ethylhexyl)phthalate and its major metabolites in ICR/SIM mice. *Environ. Mutagen.* **5**, 387 (1982).

41. P. W. Albro, J. T. Corbett, J. L. Schroeder, S. Jordan, and H. B. Matthews, Pharmacokinetics, interactions with macromolecules and species differences in metabolism of DEHP. *Environ. Health Perspect.* **45**, 19–25 (1982).

42. A. von Daniken, W. K. Lutz, R. Jackh, and C. Schlatter, Investigation of the potential for binding of di(2-ethylhexyl)phthalate (DEHP) and di(2-ethylhexyl)adipate (DEHA) to liver DNA in vivo. *Toxicol. Appl. Pharmacol.* **73**, 373–387 (1984).

43. P. W. Albro, J. T. Corbett, J. L. Schroeder, and S. T. Jordan, Incorporation of radioactivity from labelled di-(2-ethylhexyl)phthalate into DNA of rat liver in vivo. *Chem. Biol. Interact.* **44**, 1–16 (1983).

44. J. L. Seed, Mutagenic activity of phthalate esters in bacterial liquid suspension assays. *Environ. Health Perspect.* **45**, 111–114 (1982).

45. G. M. Williams and J. H. Weisburger, Chemical carcinogens. In C. D. Klaassen, M. O. Amdur, and J. Doull, Eds., *Casarett and Doull's Toxicology*, 3rd ed. Macmillan, New York, 1986, pp. 99–173.

46. E. C. Miller, Some current perspectives on chemical carcinogenesis in humans and experimental animals. *Cancer Res.* **38**, 1479–1496 (1978).

47. E. C. Miller and J. A. Miller, Mechanisms of chemical carcinogenesis: Nature of proximate carcinogens and interactions with macromolecules. *Pharmacol. Rev.* **18**, 805–838 (1966).

48. H. P. Shu, D. J. Paustenbach, and F. J. Murray, A critical evaluation of the use of mutagenesis, carcinogenesis, and tumor promotion data in a cancer risk assessment of 2,3,7,8-tetrachlorodibenzo-p-dioxin. *Regul. Toxicol. Pharmacol.* **7**, 57–88 (1987).

49. J. K. Reddy, D. L. Azarnoff, and C. E. Hignite, Hypolipidaemic hepatic peroxisome proliferators form a novel class of chemical carcinogens. *Nature (London)*, **283**, 397–398 (1980).

50. J. K. Reddy and N. D. Lalwani, Carcinogenesis by hepatic peroxisome proliferators: Evaluation of the risk of hypolipidemic drugs and industrial plasticizers to humans. *CRC Crit. Rev. Toxicol.* **12**, 1–58 (1983).

51. C. Masters and R. Holmes, Peroxisomes: New aspects of cell physiology and biochemistry. *Physiol. Rev.* **57**, 816–882 (1977).

52. J. M. Lord, Biogenesis of peroxisomes and glyoxysomes. *Subcell. Biochem.* **7**, 171–211 (1980).

53. N. E. Tolbert, Metabolic pathways in peroxisomes and glyoxisomes. *Annu. Rev. Biochem.* **50**, 133–157 (1981).

54. P. B. Lazarow and C. DeDuve, A fatty acyl-CoA oxidizing system in rat liver peroxisomes; enhancement by clofibrate, a hypolipidemic drug. *Proc. Natl. Acad. Sci. U.S.A.* **73**, 2043–2046 (1976).

55. J. K. Reddy, J. R. Warren, M. K. Reddy, and N. D. Lalwani, Hepatic and renal effects of peroxisome proliferators. *Ann. N.Y. Acad. Sci.* **386**, 81–110 (1982).

56. P. B. Lazarow, Three hypolipidemic drugs increase hepatic palmitoylcoenzyme A oxidation in the rat. *Science* **197**, 580–581 (1977).

57. T. Osumi and T. Hashimoto, Enhancement of fatty acyl-CoA oxidizing activity in rat liver peroxisomes by di-(2-ethylhexyl)phthalate. *J. Biochem.* (*Tokyo*) **83**, 1361–1365 (1978).

58. S. J. Morton, The hepatic effects of dietary di-2-ethylhexyl phthalate, Ph.D. Thesis, Johns Hopkins University, Baltimore, MD (1979).

59. A. E. Ganning and G. Dallner, Induction of peroxisomes and mitochondria by di(2-ethylhexyl)phthalate. *FEBS Lett.* **130**, 77–79 (1981).

60. A. E. Ganning, E. Klasson, A. Bergman, U. Brunk, and G. Dallner, Effect of phthalate ester metabolites on rat liver. *Acta Chem. Scand., Ser. B* **B36**, 563–565 (1982).

61. N. D. Lalwani, M. K. Reddy, S. A. Qureshi, and J. K. Reddy, Development of hepatocellular carcinomas and increased peroxisomal fatty acid β-oxidation in rats fed [4-chloro-6-(2,3-xylidino)-2-pyrimidinylthio] acetic acid (Wy-14643) in the semipurified diet. *Carcinogenesis* (*London*) **2**, 645–650 (1981).

62. E. C. Foerster, T. Fahrenkemper, V. Rabe, P. Graf, and H. Sies, Peroxisomal fatty acid

oxidation as detected by H_2O_2 production in intact perfused rat liver. *Biochem. J.* **196**, 705–712 (1981).

63. K. E. Tomaszewski, D. K. Agarwal, R. L. Melnick, E. J. Rauckman, and W. M. Kluwe, Production and degradation of hydrogen peroxide in liver homogenates prepared from rats or mice treated with di-(2-ethylhexyl)phthalate (DEHP). *Toxicologist* **5**, 213 (1985).

64. W. E. Fahl, N. D. Lalwani, T. Watanabe, S. K. Goel, and J. K. Reddy, DNA damage related to increased hydrogen peroxide generation by hypolipidemic drug-induced liver peroxisomes. *Proc. Natl. Acad. Sci. U.S.A.* **81**, 7827–7830 (1984).

65. J. K. Reddy, N. D. Lalwani, M. K. Reddy, and S. A. Qureshi, Excessive accumulation of autofluorescent lipofuscin in the liver during hepatocarcinogenesis by methyl clofenapate and other hypolipidemic peroxisome proliferators. *Cancer Res.* **42**, 259–266 (1982).

66. B. Chance, H. Sies, and A. Boveris, Hydroperoxide metabolism in mammalian organs. *Physiol. Rev.* **59**, 527–605 (1979).

67. E. Freese, Molecular mechanisms of mutation. *Chem. Mutagens* **1**, 1–56 (1971).

68. R. J. Wang, H. N. Ananthaswamy, B. T. Nixon, P. S. Hartman, and A. Eisenstark, Induction of single-strand DNA breaks in human cells by H_2O_2 formed in near uv (black light)-irradiated medium. *Radiat. Res.* **82**, 269–276 (1980).

69. J. Schoneich, The induction of chromosomal aberrations by hydrogen peroxide in strains of ascites tumors in mice. *Mutat. Res.* **4**, 384–388 (1967).

70. H. F. Stich, L. Wei, and P. Lam, The need for a mammalian test system for mutagens: Action of some reducing agents. *Cancer Lett.* **5**, 199–204 (1978).

71. M. O. Bradley, I. C. Hsu, and C. C. Harris, Relationship between sister chromatid exchange and mutagenicity, toxicity and DNA damage. *Nature (London)* **282**, 318–320 (1979).

72. W. D. MacRae and H. F. Stich, Induction of sister chromatid exchanges in Chinese hamster ovary cells by thiol and hydrazine compounds. *Mutat. Res.* **68**, 351–365 (1979).

73. R. Parshad, W. G. Taylor, K. K. Sanford, R. F. Camalier, R. Gantt, and R. E. Tarone, Fluorescent light-induced chromosome damage in human IMR-90 fibroblasts. Role of hydrogen peroxide and related free radicals. *Mutat. Res.* **73**, 115–124 (1980).

74. G. Speit and W. Vogel, The effect of sulfhydryl compounds on sister chromatid exchanges. II. The question of cell specificity and the role of H_2O_2. *Mutat. Res.* **93**, 175–183 (1982).

75. G. Speit, W. Vogel, and M. Wolf, Characterization of sister chromatid exchange induced by hydrogen peroxide. *Environ. Mutagen* **4**, 135–142 (1982).

76. D. E. Levin, M. Hollstein, M. F. Christman, E. A. Schwiers, and B. N. Ames, A new Salmonella tester strain (TA 102) with A″T base pairs at the site of mutation detects oxidative mutagens. *Proc. Natl. Acad. Sci. U.S.A.* **79**, 7445–7449 (1982).

77. N. Hirota and T. Yokoyama, Enhancing effect of hydrogen peroxide upon duodenal and upper jejunal carcinogenesis in rats. *Gann* **72**, 811–812 (1981).

78. A. Ito, M. Naito, Y. Naito, and H. Watanabe, Induction and characterization of gastro-duodenal lesions in mice given continuous oral administration of hydrogen peroxide. *Gann* **73**, 315–322 (1982).

79. T. J. Slaga, Overview of tumor promotion in animals. *Environ. Health Perspect.* **50**, 3–14 (1983).

80. B. N. Ames, Dietary carcinogens and anticarcinogens. *Science* **221**, 1256–1264 (1983).

81. G. F. Blane and F. Pinaroli, [Fenofibrate: Animal toxicology in relation to side-effects in man.] *Nouv. Presse Med.* **9**, 3737–3746 (1980).

82. P. W. Albro, J. R. Haas, C. C. Peck, D. G. Odam, J. T. Corbett, F. J. Bailey, H. E. Blatt, and B. B. Barrett, Identification of the metabolites of di-(2-ethylhexyl) phthalate in urine from the African green monkey. *Drug Metab. Dispos.* **9**, 223–225 (1981).

83. P. W. Albro, R. Thomas, and L. Fishbein, Metabolism of diethylhexyl phthalate by rats. Isolation and characterization of the urinary metabolites. *J. Chromatogr.* **76**, 321–330 (1973).

84. E. Moran, A. Lington, G. Divincenzo, E. Robinson, M. Chadwick, A. Branfman, M. McComish, and D. Silveira, Species differences in the metabolism of DEHP in monkeys, rats, and mice. *Toxicologist* **5**, 238 (1985).

85. J. Nixon and S. J. Jackson, *Bis(2-Ethylhexyl) Phthalate: A Comparative Subacute Toxicity Study in the Rat and Marmoset*, Rep. No. CTL/690. Prepared for CEFIC (Council European of the Federation of the Industry Chemical), 1982.

86. E. Robinson, A. Lington, G. Divincenzo, M. Chadwick, A. Branfman, D. Silveira, and M. McComish, Non-linearity of metabolism of DEHP with dose and prior exposure. *Toxicologist* **5**, 238 (1985).

87. C. C. Brown, High- to low-dose extrapolation in animals. *ACS Symp. Ser.* **293**, 57–79 (1984).

88. I. C. Munro and D. R. Krewski, Risk assessment and regulatory decision making. *Food Cosmet. Toxicol.* **19**, 549–560 (1981).

89. K. S. Crump, D. G. Hoel, and C. H. Langley, Fundamental carcinogenic processes and their implications for low-dose risk assessment. *Cancer Res.* **36**, 2973–2979 (1976).

90. N. E. Day and C. C. Brown, Multistage models and primary prevention of cancer. *J. Natl. Cancer Inst.* **84**, 977–989 (1980).

91. U.S. Environmental Protection Agency, Guidelines for carcinogen risk assessment. *Fed. Regist.* **51**, 33992–34003 (1986).

92. K. S. Crump and P. W. Crocket, Improved confidence limits for low-dose carcinogenic risk assessment from animal data. *J. Hazard. Mater.* **10**, 419–431 (1985).

93. N. Mantel and W. Bryan, "Safety" testing of carcinogenic agents. *J. Natl. Cancer Inst.* **27**, 455–470 (1961).

94. N. Mantel, N. R. Bohidar, C. C. Brown, J. L. Ciminera, and J. W. Tukey, An improved Mantel-Bryan procedure for "safety" testing of carcinogens. *Cancer Res.* **35**, 865–872 (1975).

95. M. L. Dourson and J. F. Stara, Regulatory history and experimental support of uncertainty (safety) factors. *Regul. Toxicol. Pharmacol.* **3**, 224–238 (1983).

96. A. J. Lehman and O. G. Fitzhugh, 100-Fold margin of safety. *Q. Bull.—Assoc. Food Drug. Off. U.S.* **18**, 33–35 (1954).

97. National Academy of Sciences, *Drinking Water and Health*. NAS, Washington, DC, 1977.

98. P. J. Gehring, P. G. Watanabe, and C. N. Park, Resolution of dose-response toxicity data for chemicals requiring metabolic activation: Example—vinyl chloride. *Toxicol. Appl. Pharmacol.* **44**, 581–591 (1978).

99. M. W. Anderson, D. G. Hoel, and H. L. Kaplan, A general scheme for the incorporation of pharmacokinetics in low-dose risk estimation for chemical carcinogenesis: Example—vinyl chloride. *Toxicol. Appl. Pharmacol.* **55**, 154–161 (1980).

100. A. S. Whittemore, S. C. Grosser, and A. Silvers, Pharmacokinetics in low dose extrapolation using animal cancer data. *Fundam. Appl. Toxicol.* **7**, 183–190 (1986).

101. M. E. Andersen, H. J. Clewell, III, M. L. Gargas, F. A. Smith, and R. H. Reitz, Physiologically based pharmacokinetics and the risk assessment process for methylene chloride. *Toxicol. Appl. Pharmacol.* **87**, 185–205 (1987).

102. J. C. Lhuguenot, A. M. Mitchell, and C. R. Elcombe, Dose- and time-dependency of mono(2-ethylhexyl)phthalate (MEHP) metabolism in primary rat hepatocyte cultures. *Toxicologist* **4**, 96 (1984).

103. J. C. Lhuguenot, E. A. Lock, and C. R. Elcombe, Dose- and time-dependency of mono- and di-(2-ethylhexyl)phthalate (MEHP and DEHP) metabolism in rats. *Toxicologist* **4**, 96 (1984).

104. J. C. Lhuguenot, A. M. Mitchell, G. Milner, E. A. Lock, and C. R. Elcombe, The metabolism of di(2-ethylhexyl)phthalate (DEHP) and mono(2-ethylhexyl)phthalate (MEHP) in rats. In vivo and in vitro dose and time dependency of metabolism. *Toxicol. Appl. Pharmacol.* **80**, 11–22 (1985).

105. W. H. Butler and P. M. Newberne, Eds., *Mouse Hepatic Neoplasia*. Elsevier, Amsterdam, 1975.

106. D. B. Clayson, International Commission for Protection against Environmental Mutagens and Carcinogens. ICPEMC Working Paper 2/3: Carcinogens and carcinogenesis enhancers. *Mutat. Res.* **86**, 217–229 (1981).

107. K. Ogawa, T. Onoe, and M. Takeuchi, Spontaneous occurrence of γ-glutamyl transpeptidase-positive hepatocytic foci in 105-week-old Wistar and 72-week-old Fischer 344 male rats. *J. Natl. Cancer Inst.* **67**, 407–412 (1981).

108. J. M. Ward, Increased susceptibility of livers of aged F344/NCr rats to the effects of phenobarbital on the incidence, morphology, and histochemistry of hepatocellular foci and neoplasms. *J. Natl. Cancer. Inst.* **71**, 815–823 (1983).

109. R. Schulte-Hermann, I. Timmermann-Trosiener, and J. Schuppler, Promotion of sponta-neous preoplastic cells in rat liver as a possible explanation of tumor production by nonmutagenic compounds. *Cancer Res.* **43**, 839–844 (1983).

110. I. F. H. Purchase, Inter-species comparisons of carcinogenicity. *Br. J. Cancer* **41**, 454–468 (1980).

111. R. A. Griesemer and C. Cueto, Jr., Toward a classification scheme for degrees of experimental evidence for the carcinogenicity of chemicals for animals. *IARC Sci. Publ.* **27**, 259–281 (1980).

112. International Agency for Research on Cancer, *Chemicals and Industrial Processes and Industries Associated with Cancer in Humans*, IARC Monogr., Vol. 1–29, IARC Monogr. Suppl. 4. IARC, Lyon, France, 1982.

113. C. R. Elcombe and A. M. Mitchell, Peroxisome proliferation due to di(2-ethylhexyl) phtha-late (DEHP): Species differences and possible mechanisms. *Environ. Health Perspect.* **70**, 211–219 (1986).

114. Inhalation Toxicology Research Institute, *Phthalate Ester Migration from Polyvinyl Chloride Consumer Products*, Phase I final report. Submitted to U.S. Consumer Product Safety Commission, Washington, DC, August 23, 1983.

115. B. Bhooshan, Consumer Products Safety Commission. Memorandum describing results of Phase II DEHP leaching studies conducted by Inhalation Toxicology Research Institute, August 24, 1983.

116. Midwest Research Institute, *Toxicological Effects of Diethylhexyl Phthalate*, Final Report, MRI Proj. No. 7343-B. Phthalate Esters Program Panel, Voluntary Test Program, Health Effects Testing, Phase I: Validation Results, Vol. II. Chemical Manufacturers Association, Washington, DC, 1982.

117. R. H. Hinton, S. C. Price, D. Hall. P. Grasso, and F. Mitchell, *Report to CEFIC on a 28-Day Dose and Time Response Study on Di-ethylhexyl Phthalate in Rats*, Study 5/81/TX. Robens Institute of Industrial and Environmental Health and Safety, University of Surrey, Guildford, Surrey, England, 1982.

118. British Industrial Biological Research Association, *A 21 Day Dose-response Study of Di(2-ethylhexyl) Phthalate in Rats*, Rep. No. 0512/1/84 (draft.) BIBRA, Carshalton, Surrey, England, July, 1984.

G

ASSESSING THE RISKS TO WILDLIFE

27

An Environmental Risk Assessment of a Pesticide

Gary M. Rand

FMC Corporation, Princeton, New Jersey

1 INTRODUCTION

Carbofuran is a broad-spectrum reversible anticholinesterase carbamate insecticide/nematicide principally used for the control of soil and foliar pests. It is available in granular and flowable formulations. In order for carbofuran, or any pesticide, to be approved for registration in the United States the U.S. Environmental Protection Agency (EPA) requires under the Federal Insecticide Fungicide and Rodenticide Act (FIFRA or P.L. 95396) that certain toxicology, environmental, product/residue chemistry, and ecological effects data be submitted. These data are used by the U.S. EPA for determining the potential hazards to humans and the environment (including nontarget birds, wild mammals, fish, and aquatic invertebrates). Before registration, the manufacturer (or registrant) must show that a pesticide "when used in accordance with widespread and commonly recognized practice will not generally cause unreasonable adverse effects on the environment" [P.L. 95396, Section 3 (c)(5)(D)]. Unreasonable adverse effects means "any unreasonable risk to man or the environment, taking into account the economic, social and environmental costs and benefits of the use of the pesticide" [P.L. 95396, Section 2 (bb)]. An environmental or *ecological* risk assessment must be conducted to assess unreasonable risks to the environment. This type of assessment is directed at the area of *ecotoxicology*, which is the study of the adverse effects of toxic substances on organisms of nonhuman, nontarget species, including endangered or threatened species. This is a relatively young science that is rapidly evolving. State-of-the-art techniques have not been adequately developed and validated for risk assessment in this area as they have in mammalian toxicology. Ecological risk assessments are difficult to conduct because the concern is the protection of a myriad of species in the environment, which may ultimately be affected by not only a chemical but a host of other nonchemically oriented elements as a result of the complexities and interactions of aquatic and terrestrial communities.

Toxicology data to date indicate that although carbofuran is acutely toxic to mammalian species, neither carbofuran nor its metabolites have been demonstrated to be oncogenic, teratogenic, fetotoxic, or mutagenic in various species. In general, the risk associated with human exposure to carbofuran is minimal compared to the risk associated with exposure to organophosphate pesticides, a group of compounds with a similar mode of action (1). Furthermore, there is a significant "margin of safety" for carbofuran in that there is "a large range of doses between the dosage that produces mild illness and the dosage that produces death" (1). This represents a distinct advantage over many organophosphate pesticides whose inhibition of acetylcholinesterase is not reversible (1).

The available ecotoxicology data indicate that carbofuran is acutely toxic to wildlife, especially birds (1). Data from laboratory and field studies with birds and the use history of carbofuran show that application of granular carbofuran results in mortality of certain avian species, including both passerines and raptors (1, 2). Although existing data show that these effects are not excessive, widespread, long-lasting, or likely to diminish wildlife resources, in 1985 the U.S. EPA initiated a Special Review of all granular formulations of pesticide products containing the active ingredient carbofuran. The EPA's rationale for the Special Review was that "carbofuran is highly, acutely toxic to birds when used on field corn, sorghum, rice fields and all other agricultural and non-agricultural sites, and meets or exceeds the existing risk criterion for acute avian toxicity" described in the *Federal Register* [40 CFR 162.11 (a) (3) (i) (B) (2)]. This criterion mandates that a Special Review shall be conducted if a pesticide" occurs as a residue immediately following application in, or on the feed of an avian species, representative of the species likely to be exposed to such feed in amounts equivalent to the average daily intake of such representative species, at levels equal to or greater than the subacute dietary LC_{50} measured in avian test animals as specified in the Registration Guidelines."

Although the regulation can be applied only to foliar application (flowable formulation), which produces residues on bird food, it is understood that the granular formulation does not produce appreciable residues on bird foods. However, there is good evidence that birds consume lethal quantities of carbofuran granules. The U.S. EPA believed that ingestion of the carbofuran granules produced "widespread avian mortality" in treated fields and that the regulatory intent of the dietary trigger was exceeded for the major agricultural uses of granular carbofuran (e.g., corn). The EPA reviewed the existing data base on the granular formulation of carbofuran and concluded that it is "highly toxic to birds and its use results in significant fatalities of many small species of birds and also secondary poisoning of birds of prey."

This chapter presents on environmental risk assessment of carbofuran—a pesticide registered for use on a variety of agricultural crops in the United States. This assessment is unique to other chapters in this text since it addresses the area of ecotoxicology. The assessment evaluates the potential impact of carbofuran on nontarget organisms that inhabit aquatic and terrestrial ecosystems. The methods used in this chapter should be applicable to other assessments where pesticides are intentionally applied over land and water.

1.1   Special Review Process

The term Special Review is the name now used by the EPA for the process previously called the Rebuttable Presumption Against Registration (RPAR) process. Modifications to the process are proposed in the new Special Review regulations (50 FR 12183). Among the modifications to the process are new risk assessment criteria.

Before a product can be registered, the registrant of the pesticide must prove that the material can be used without "unreasonable adverse effects on the environment." If at any time the EPA determines that a pesticide no longer meets the standard for registration, the Administrator of the EPA may cancel the registration under Section 6 of FIFRA.

The EPA has provided the administrative process for evaluating whether a pesticide satisfies or continues to satisfy the statutory standard for registration. The Special Review process provides a formal procedure through which the EPA may gather and evaluate information about the risks and benefits of a pesticide's use. It also provides a means by which the public may comment on and participate in the EPA's decisionmaking process. The regulations governing this process are set forth in 40 CFR 162.11.

A Special Review is begun when the EPA determines that a pesticide meets or exceeds one or more of the risk criteria set out in the regulations [40 CFR 162.11 (a)(3)]. The EPA generally announces the beginning of the Special Review in the *Federal Register*. Registrants and other interested parties are invited to review the basis for the EPA's decision to initiate the Special Review and to submit data and information that rebut or support the EPA's determination of risk. Commentors may also suggest methods to reduce risk of the pesticide.

If risk issues are not satisfactorily resolved, the EPA will proceed to evaluate the risks and benefits of the pesticide in order to determine whether to propose regulatory actions to reduce the risks. If the EPA determines that the risk of use exceeds the benefits, it will issue a Notice of Intent to Cancel the registration of products intended for such use. The Notice may state the intention to cancel registrations outright or may require certain changes in the composition, packaging, application methods, and/or labeling of the product. The changes would be intended to reduce the risks to levels that, when considered against the benefits, will not pose "unreasonable adverse effects to man or the environment."

1.2   General Ecotoxicology and Environmental Testing Requirements in FIFRA

There are a number of differences between classical mammalian toxicology and ecotoxicology (Table 1). Ecotoxicology is a complex, multidisciplinary science. The ecotoxicology of any chemical may be considered as a sequence of interactions and effects controlled by the toxicity and physicochemical properties of the chemical (Fig. 1). Any assessment of an agricultural chemical must take into account, in a quantitative way, each of the distinct abiotic (i.e., physicochemical) and biotic (i.e., organismal) processes involved. Toxicological events in the environment are thus controlled by the chemical and physical properties of the chemical agent.

A pesticide may be intentionally released into the environment and subject to physical dispersal into the atomsphere, water, soil, and/or sediment. Other chemicals accidentally released are subject to similar processes.

The amount or quantity of the chemical including the forms and site of such releases must be clearly known if the subsequent behavior of the chemical is to be understood. The chemical may then be transported geographically and into the biota and perhaps chemically modified or transformed and degraded by abiotic processes (e.g., hydrolysis, photolysis) or more often by microorganisms present in the environment. The resulting degradation products may have different environmental behavior patterns and toxic properties. The degradation products may be innocuous or they may have a greater detrimental impact than the parent chemical. The final parameter that determines the likelihood of an adverse effect is that of exposure. The nature of the target organisms (e.g., birds, fish, terrestrial invertebrates) must be identified along with the type of exposure (i.e., acute, chronic, intermittent) in order to assess risk.

Wildlife and aquatic species may elicit a variety of responses due to the presence of a xenobiotic including an immediate overt response (convulsions or death) to covert,

TABLE 1. Differences between Mammalian and Aquatic/Avian Toxicology (or Ecotoxicology)

Mammalian Toxicology	Ecotoxicology (Aquatic/Avian Toxicology)
Objective: to protect humans	Objective: to protect populations of many diverse species
Must almost always rely on animal models since experimentation with humans is not feasible	Can experiment directly on species of concern
Species of interest (humans) is known; thus, degree of extrapolation is certain	Not able to identify and test all species of concern; thus, degree of extrapolation is uncertain
Test organisms are warm-blooded (body temperature is relatively uniform and nearly independent of environmental temperature); thus, toxicity is predictable	Test organisms (aquatic) live in a variable environment and are cold-blooded (body temperature); thus, toxicity may not be sufficiently predictable
The dose of a test chemical usually can be measured directly and accurately and administered by a number of routes	The "dose" is known only in terms of the chemical's concentration in water (for aquatic organisms) and the length of exposure to it; the actual "absorbed dose" is sometimes determined experimentally using bioconcentration and metabolism studies
Extensive basic research has been conducted; emphasis has been on understanding mechanisms of toxic action	Little basic research has been conducted; emphasis has been on measuring toxic effects and generating numbers, with an eye toward regulatory needs
Test methods are well developed, their usefulness and limits well understood	Test methods are either relatively new or generally not formalized (standardized); their usefulness in many cases is uncertain

sublethal effects such as reduced growth, impaired reproduction, and altered behavior. The actual ecosystem itself of which the wildlife and aquatic species are an integral part can react in a variety of structural or functional ways to the effects on the component organisms. Changes may occur in species diversity or in their interactions or in energy flows. The responses of an individual organism, population, or community to the chemical over time and the significance of these responses relative to other background responses is a critical aspect of the assessment.

A rational ecotoxicological assessment must consider many factors in a quantitative and integrated way. All toxicology data must be evaluated in light of data on the transport, distribution, transformation, and ultimate fate of the chemical in the aquatic and terrestrial environments.

The EPA has established guidelines on the kinds of data that must be submitted on each chemical to support the registration requirements of pesticides under FIFRA. The data submitted enable the EPA to make regulatory judgments with respect to the safety of each pesticide. The guidelines include sections detailing what data are required and when they are required. The standard for conducting acceptable tests, guidance on the evaluation and reporting of data, and examples of acceptable protocols can also be obtained from the EPA.

The data requirements for registration are presented in 40 CFR Part 158 (Pesticide

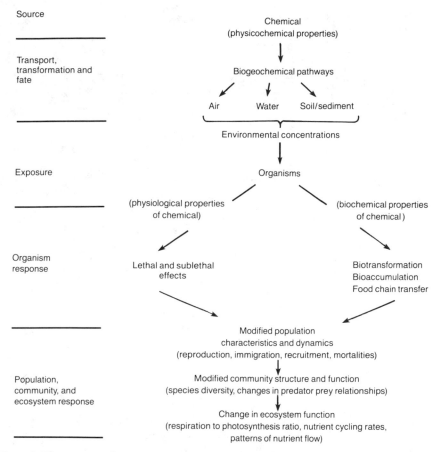

Figure 1. The sequence of events leading to the effects of a chemical at different levels of organization.

Registration; Proposed Data Requirements) and are intended to generate information necessary to address concerns pertaining to the identity, composition, potential adverse effects, and environmental fate of each pesticide. Subdivisions E (Hazard and Evaluation; Wildlife and Aquatic Organisms) and N (Environmental Fate) of the guidelines are briefly discussed below because of their relevance to the environmental risk assessment process.

Subdivision E provides guidelines for testing the effects of pesticides on wildlife and aquatic organisms. The data requirements presented in 158.145 pertain to Subdivision E (see Table 2). These data will be used by the U.S. EPA for determining potential hazards to nontarget birds, wild mammals, fish, and aquatic invertebrates. A tier testing scheme is followed. The initial data are used for the following:

- To define acute toxicity (i.e., LC_{50}, EC_{50}, LD_{50}) of the active ingredient of each chemical to different aquatic and terrestrial organisms.
- To compare toxicity data with actual or estimated environmental concentrations (EECs) to assess potential impacts.

TABLE 2. 158.145 Wildlife and Aquatic Organism Data Requirements[a]

Kind of Data Required	Terrestrial Food Crop	Terrestrial Nonfood	Aquatic Food Crop	Aquatic Nonfood	Greenhouse Food Crop	Greenhouse Nonfood	Forestry	Domestic Outdoor	Indoor	Data to Support MP	Data to Support EP	Guidelines Reference Number
Avian and Mammalian Testing												
Avian oral LD_{50}[b]	(R)	(R)	(R)	(R)	(CR)	(CR)	(R)	(R)	(CR)	TGAI	TGAI	71-1
Avian dietary LC_{50}[b]	(R)	(R)	(R)	(R)	(CR)	(CR)	(R)	(R)	(CR)	TGAI	TGAI	71-2
Wild mammal toxicity[c]	(CR)	(CR)	(CR)	(CR)			(CR)	(CR)		TGAI	TGAI	71-3
Avian reproduction[d]	(CR)	(CR)	(CR)	(CR)			(CR)	(CR)		TGAI	TGAI	71-4
Simulated and actual field testing[b]—mammals and birds	(CR)	(CR)	(CR)	(CR)			(CR)	(CR)		TEP	TEP	71-5
Aquatic Organism Testing												
Freshwater fish LC_{50}[b,e]	(R)	(R)	(R)	(R)	(CR)	(CR)	(R)	(R)	(CR)	TGAI	TGAI	72-1
Acute LC_{50} freshwater invertebrates[b,e]	(R)	(R)	(R)	(R)	(CR)	(CR)	(R)	(R)	(CR)	TGAI	TGAI	72-2
Acute LC_{50} estuarine and marine organisms[e,f]	(CR)	(CR)	(CR)	(CR)			(CR)	(CR)		TGAI	TGAI	72-3
Fish early life stage and aquatic invertebrate life cycle[g]	(CR)	(CR)	(CR)	(CR)			(CR)	(CR)		TGAI	TGAI	72-4
Fish, life cycle[h]	(CR)	(CR)	(CR)	(CR)			(CR)	(CR)		TGAI	TGAI	72-5
Aquatic organism accumulation[c]	(CR)	(CR)	(CR)	(CR)			(CR)	(CR)		TGAI, PAI, or degradation product	TGAI, PAI, or degradation product	72-6
Simulated or actual field testing aquatic organisms[i]	(CR)	(CR)	(CR)	(CR)			(CR)	(CR)		TEP	TEP	72-7

a Sections 158.50 and 158.100 describe how to use this table to determine the environmental fate data requirements and the substances to be tested. *Key:* R = required; CR = conditionally required; parentheses (i.e., (R), (CR)) indicate requirements that apply when an experimental use permit is being sought; TGAI = technical grade of the active ingredient; PAIRA = "pure" active ingredient—radiolabeled; TEP = typical end-use product; EP = end-use product.

b Tests for pesticides intended solely for indoor application will be required on a case-by-case basis, depending on use pattern, production volume, and other pertinent factors.

c Tests required on a case-by-case basis depending on the results of lower tier studies such as acute and subacute testing, intended use pattern, and pertinent environmental fate characteristics.

d Data required if one or more of the following criteria are met: (i) The pesticide or any of its major metabolites or degradation products, especially preceding or during the breeding season. (ii) The pesticide or any of its major metabolites of degradation products are stable in the environment to the extent that potentially toxic amounts may persist in avian feed. (iii) The pesticide or any of its major metabolites or degradation products is stored or accumulated in plant or animal tissues, as indicated by its octanol–water partition coefficient, accumulation studies, metabolic release and retention studies, or as indicated by structural similarity to known bioaccumulative chemicals. (iv) Any other information, such as that derived from mammalian reproduction studies, that indicates that reproduction in terrestrial vertebrates may be adversely affected by the anticipated use of the pesticide product. *Note:* Prior to conducting this test to support the registration of an avicide, the applicant should consult the U.S. EPA.

e Data from testing with the applicant's end-use product or a typical end-use product is required to support the registration of each end-use product which meets any one of the following conditions: (i) the end-use pesticide will be introduced directly into an aquatic environment when used as directed; (ii) the LC_{50} or EC_{50} of the technical grade of active ingredient is equal to or less than the maximum expected environmental concentration (MEEC) or the estimated environmental concentration (EEC) in the aquatic environment when the end-use pesticide is used as directed; or (iii) an ingredient in the end-use formulation other than the active ingredient is expected to enhance the toxicity of the active ingredient or to cause toxicity to aquatic organisms.

f Data required if the product is intended for direct application to the estuarine or marine environment, or the product is expected to enter this environment in significant concentrations because of its expected use or mobility pattern.

g Data from fish early life-stage tests or life-cycle tests with aquatic invertebrates (on whichever species is most sensitive to the pesticide as determined from the results of the acute toxicity tests) are required if the product is applied directly to water or expected to be transported to water from the intended use site, and when any one or more of the following conditions apply: (i) if the pesticide is intended for use such that it presence in water is likely to be continuous or recurrent regardless of toxicity; or (ii) if any LC_{50} or EC_{50} value determined in acute toxicity testing is less than 1 mg/L; or (iii) if the estimated environmental concentration in water is equal to or greater than 0.01 of any EC_{50} or LC_{50} determined in acute toxicity testing; or (iv) if the actual or estimated environmental concentration in water resulting from use is less than 0.01 of any EC_{50} or LC_{50} determined in acute toxicity testing and if the following conditions exist: (a) studies of other organisms indicate the reproductive physiology of fish and/or invertebrates may be affected; or (b) physiochemical properties indicate cumulative effects; or (c) the pesticide is persistent in water (e.g. half-life in water greater than 4 days).

h Data are required if end-use product is intended to be applied directly to water or expected to transport to water from the intended use site, and when any of the following conditions apply: (i) if the estimated environmental concentration is equal to or greater than one-tenth of the no-effect level in the fish early life-stage or invertebrate life-cycle test; or (ii) if studies of other organisms indicate the reproductive physiology of fish may be affected.

i Required if significant concentrations of the active ingredient and/or its principal degradation products are likely to occur in aquatic environments and may accumulate in aquatic organisms.

- To provide data that determine the need for precautionary label statements to minimize the potential adverse effects to wildlife and aquatic organisms.
- To indicate the need for further laboratory and/or field studies.

Additional tests (i.e., avian, fish, and invertebrate reproduction and life cycle studies) are required when the basic ecotoxicology effects data along with the fate data suggest possible long-term problems. These additional data are used for the following:

- To estimate potential chronic effects in light of estimated or actual environmental concentrations.
- To determine if additional field or laboratory data are needed to assess hazard. Simulated or actual field studies are required on some chemicals to develop data on aquatic and wildlife species in natural or simulated systems.

Field studies are used to confirm experimentally the safety of a material under anticipated conditions of use (i.e., at the label use rate, frequency, and typical method of application). The necessity for conducting field studies is greatest if the margin between chronic toxicological effects and environmental exposure concentrations is narrow (i.e., margin of safety is low). In addition, if a material is applied directly to water, field data may be necessary to confirm that the material has no significant adverse effect on the structure or functioning of the ecosystem.

Figures 2, 3, and 4 illustrate the tier testing scheme for avian wildlife, wild mammals, and aquatic organisms, respectively. These figures do not constitute the requirements or when each test is required; this information is contained in 40 CFR 158.145 (see Table 2).

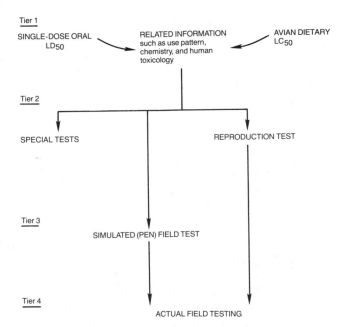

Figure 2. Tier testing scheme in FIFRA for avian wildlife.

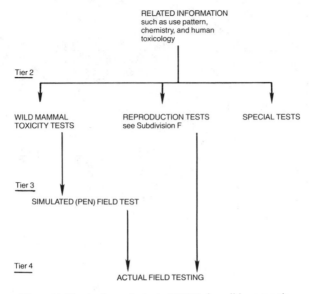

Tier 1

RELATED INFORMATION
such as use pattern,
chemistry, and human
toxicology

Tier 2

WILD MAMMAL
TOXICITY TESTS

REPRODUCTION TESTS
see Subdivision F

SPECIAL TESTS

Tier 3

SIMULATED (PEN) FIELD TEST

Tier 4

ACTUAL FIELD TESTING

Figure 3. Tier testing scheme in FIFRA for wild mammals.

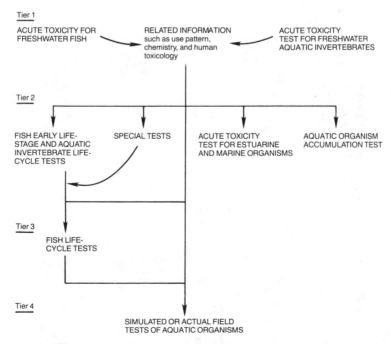

Tier 1

ACUTE TOXICITY FOR
FRESHWATER FISH

RELATED INFORMATION
such as use pattern,
chemistry, and human
toxicology

ACUTE TOXICITY
TEST FOR FRESHWATER
AQUATIC INVERTEBRATES

Tier 2

FISH EARLY LIFE-
STAGE AND AQUATIC
INVERTEBRATE LIFE-
CYCLE TESTS

SPECIAL TESTS

ACUTE TOXICITY
TEST FOR ESTUARINE
AND MARINE ORGANISMS

AQUATIC ORGANISM
ACCUMULATION TEST

Tier 3

FISH LIFE-
CYCLE TESTS

Tier 4

SIMULATED OR ACTUAL FIELD
TESTS OF AQUATIC ORGANISMS

Figure 4. Tier testing scheme in FIFRA for aquatic organisms.

TABLE 3. 158.130 Environmental Fate Data Requirements[a]

Kind of Data Required	Environmental Fate Data Requirements: General Use Patterns									Test Substance		Guidelines Reference Number
	Terrestrial		Aquatic		Greenhouse		Forestry	Domestic Outdoor	Indoor	Data to Support MP	Data to Support EP	
	Food Crop	Nonfood	Food Crop	Nonfood	Food Crop	Nonfood						
Degradation Studies—Laboratory												
Hydrolysis	(R)	(R)	(R)	(R)	(R)	(R)	(R)	(R)		TGAI or PAIRA	TGAI or PAIRA	161-1
Photodegradtion												
In water	R	R	R	R			R			TGAI or PAIRA	TGAI or PAIRA	161-2
On soil[b]	CR						CR			TGAI or PAIRA	TGAI or PAIRA	161-3
In air[c]	CR									TGAI or PAIRA	TGAI or PAIRA	161-4
Metabolism Studies—Laboratory												
Aerobic soil	(R)	(R)			R	R	(R)	R		TGAI or PAIRA	TGAI or PAIRA	162-1
Anaerobic soil[d]	R									TGAI or PAIRA	TGAI or PAIRA	162-2
Anaerobic aquatic			R	R						TGAI or PAIRA	TGAI or PAIRA	162-3
Aerobic aquatic			(R)	(R)						TGAI or PAIRA	TGAI or PAIRA	162-4
Mobility Studies												
Leaching (adsorption/desorption)	(R)	(R)	(R)		(R)	(R)	(R)	(R)		TGAI or PAIRA	TGAI or PAIRA	163-1
Volatility												
(Lab)[c]	(CR)				(CR)	(CR)				TEP	TEP	163-2
(Field)[c]	(CR)				(CR)	(CR)				TEP	TEP	163-3

Dissipation Studies—Field

Study								Guideline Ref. No.
Soil	(R)	(R)		TEP	(R)	TEP	(R)	163-1
Aquatic (sediment)	(R)	(R)		TEP		TEP		164-2
Forestry			R	TEP		TEP		164-3
Combination and tank mixes[c]	CR	(CR)						164-4
Soil, long-term[e]	CR			TEP		TEP		164-5

Accumulation Studies

Study								Guideline Ref. No.
Rotational crops								
(Confined)[f]	(CR)	(CR)		PAIRA		PAIRA		165-1
(Field)[g]	(CR)	(CR)		TEP		TEP		165-2
Irregated crops[h]	(CR)	(CR)	(CR)	TEP		TEP		165-3
In fish[i,j]	(CR)	(CR)	(CR)	TGAI or PAIRA		TGAI or PAIRA		165-5
In aquatic nontarget organisms[i,j]	(CR)	(CR)		TEP		TEP		165-5

[a] Sections 158.50 and 158.100 describe how to use this table to determine the environmental fate data requirements and the substances to be tested. *Key*: R = required; CR = conditionally required; parentheses (i.e., (R), (CR)) indicate requirements that apply when an experimental use permit is being sought; TGAI = technical grade of the active ingredient; PAIRA = "pure" active ingredient—radiolabeled; TEP = typical end-use product; EP = end-use product.

[b] Not required if use involves application to soils solely by injection of the product into the soil or by incorporation of the product into the soil upon application.

[c] Required on case-by-case basis depending on product use pattern and other pertinent factors.

[d] Not required if anaerobic aquatic metabolism study has been conducted.

[e] Required if pesticide residues do not readily dissipate in soil.

[f] Confined accumulation study is required when it is reasonably foreseeable that any food or feed crop may be subsequently planted on the site of pesticide application.

[g] Field accumulated study is required if significant pesticide residue is likely to be present in soil at time of plant crop, as evidence by residue data obtained from confined accumulation study.

[h] Required if it is reasonably foreseeable that water at treated site may be used for irrigation purposes.

[i] Required if significant concentrations of the active ingredient and/or its principal degradation products are likely to occur in aquatic environments and may accumulate in aquatic organisms.

[j] Required unless tolerance or action level for fish has been granted.

The environmental fate data are used as part of the criteria along with the effects data to trigger or move from one tier to the next higher tier.

Acceptable protocols and the evaluation/interpretation of data are well documented for most of the laboratory ecotoxicology studies. However, the methodology for the conduct and interpretation of field studies is in its early stages of development. This is not surprising since the science of ecotoxicology has not had a long history and quite often the fundamental basics in aquatic and terrestrial ecology are not widely understood. Nonetheless, the manufacturers must conduct field studies for certain chemicals if they are to be registered. However, these studies are often conducted with much frustration by the registrants because field testing is a rapidly evolving area.

The data requirements for environmental fate (Subdivision N) are presented in 158.130 (see Table 3). This subdivision provides guidance to develop data on the fate of pesticides in the environment through degradation, metabolism, mobility, dissipation, and accumulation. These data provide information on:

- The most important degradation routes.
- The potential half-life and persistence in different environmental compartments (soil, sediment, water, air).
- The dissipation and mobility of the material, which environmental compartments and organisms will most likely be exposed, and potential environmental concentrations.

When conducting an environmental hazard assessment it is assumed that the toxicological effects data are to be interpreted in relation to the fate data and the actual or estimated exposure concentrations of the chemical in the environment.

2   CHEMICAL IDENTIFICATION

2.1   Identity, Physicochemical Properties and Uses of Carbofuran

Carbofuran (2, 3-dimethyl-7-benzofuranyl methylcarbamate) is a broad-spectrum carbamate insecticide/nematicide used for the control of soil-borne and foliar pests. Technical carbofuran is a white crystalline solid. The formula and physicochemical properties are illustrated in Table 4.

Carbofuran was developed in the United States in the 1960s by FMC Corporation and introduced for use in 1967. The material has demonstrated effective control against approximately 300 economic pests on more than 40 crops throughout the world. It provides plant protection through both contact and systemic action. When applied to the soil, carbofuran is absorbed by the plant roots and it moves systemically through the plant via the vascular system, controlling both foliar and root-feeding pests. Foliar applications control insects by both contact action and as a stomach poison by ingestion of treated plant parts.

Manufacturing use products (MUPs) include a 75, 85, and 90% dust base (DB). Commercial formulations of carbofuran include various granular (G) formulations (% w/w carbofuran: 2G, 3G, 5G, 10G, and 15G), a 75% (w/w carbofuran) wettable powder (WP), and a 4-lb/gal flowable (4F) concentrate for use in sprays.

2.2   Mode of Action

Carbofuran elicits its toxic effects by inhibition of acetylcholinesterase (AChE) activity in plasma, brain, or erythrocytes (1). Although experimental evidence suggests that

TABLE 4. Chemical and Physical Properties of Carbofuran

Registered trademark names:	Furadan®, Cristofuran®, Curaterr®, Pillar furan®, Yaltox®	
Common name:	Carbofuran	
Chemical name:	2, 3-Dihydro-2, 2-dimethyl-7-benzofuranyl methylcarbamate	
Empirical formula:	$C_{12}H_{15}NO_3$	
Molecular weight:	221.26	
Appearance:	Tan crystalline solid	
Odor:	Slightly phenolic	
Density:	1.180 at 20°C	
Melting point:	Pure 153–154°C	
	Technical 150–152°C	
Solubility at 25°C:	Water 700 ppm	
	Organic solvents	%w/w
	n-Methyl-2-pyrrolidone	30
	Dimethylformamide	27
	Dimethyl sulfoxide	25
	Acetone	15
	Acetonitrile	14
	Methylene chloride	12
	Cyclohexanone	9
	Benzene	4
	Ethanol	4
	Xylene	<1
	Petroleum ether	<1
	Kerosene	<1
	HAN solvents	<1
Vapor pressure:	2×10^{-5} mm Hg at 33°C	
Stability:	Unstable in alkaline media	
	Degrades at temperatures > 130°C	

carbamate insecticides are toxic because of their ability to inhibit AChE activity in birds, fish, and mammals, the precise biochemical mechanism for the inhibition is not fully known. Compounds that possess an electrophilic carbon, such as the acyl carbon of carbofuran, interact with the basic group of the esteratic site of the enzyme (i.e., AChE) and thus cause competitive inhibition (3). One favored explanation for the interaction of carbamate insecticides with AChE has been discussed by Kuhr and Dorough (4). The overall reaction does not destroy AChE but it does result in the hydrolysis of the insecticide molecule. In the case of carbamates, the half-life of decarbamylation has been estimated to be 30–40 min (5, 6). Thus, provided the exposure is terminated, carbamylated enzyme would begin to recover in a few minutes and would be virtually restored to normal activity, within several hours.

For comparative purposes, organophosphorus compounds inhibit AChE based on phosphorylation of the esteratic site, namely, the serine hydroxyl group. The phosphorylated enzyme is considerably less susceptible to hydrolysis. Consequently, recovery from organophosphorus poisoning is much slower than recovery from carbamate intoxication. Because of these reaction differences, carbamates and organophosphates have been termed *reversible* and *irreversible* inhibitors of AChE, respectively (1). These terms are not entirely correct since the destruction of reversible inhibitors does not occur during the course of a reaction but carbamates undergo hydrolysis, and, because phosphorylated AChE eventually hydrolyzes, the enzyme recovers or "reverses" as well (4).

3 METABOLISM AND MAMMALIAN TOXICOLOGY

3.1 Metabolism of Carbofuran

Carbamates in general undergo metabolic reactions in vivo involving oxidation, reduction, hydrolysis, and conjugation. In mammals, the liver is the primary organ involved in these reactions where the responsible enzymes are associated with the smooth endoplasmic reticulum of liver cells (7).

Metabolism of carbofuran is similar in the rat, mouse, cow, and hen (8–12). The metabolism in plants, animals, and insects is illustrated in Fig. 5. For example, in the hen after carbofuran was administered compounds II, III, and IV were observed in the liver in free and conjugated forms. In the feces, in addition to the foregoing, compounds VI, VII, VIII, and IX and five unknowns were found (12). Mouse liver enzyme preparations degraded carbofuran to at least seven organosoluble metabolites. Three were identified as 3-hydroxycarbofuran, 3-ketocarbofuran, and N-hydroxymethyl carbofuran (13). Alfalfa containing carbofuran residues in the form of glycosides of 3-hydroxycarbofuran (V), 2, 3-dihydro-3, 7-dihydroxy-2, 2-dimethyl benzofuran (XIII), and 2, 3-dihydro-7-hydroxy-2, 2-dimethyl-3-oxobenzofuran (XIV) was fed to rats. Urine contained the glucuronides and sulfate compounds XIII, XIV, XXI, and XXII and the glucuronide of 3-hydroxycarbofuran (V). Carbofuran was metabolized and excreted as the glucuronides and sulfates: compounds V, XII, XIII, XX, and XXI (14).

Carbofuran is almost completely metabolized via oxidation at ring carbon number 3 (3-hydroxycarbofuran, 3-ketocarbofuran) and hydrolytic cleavage of the ester linkage to yield the 7-hydroxy metabolites (3-hydroxy-7-phenol, 3-keto-7-phenol, and 7-phenol); in addition, minor amounts of other related metabolites are excreted as glucuronide or sulfate conjugates.

3.2 Absorption, Transport, and Distribution

Carbofuran is rapidly absorbed and distributed following oral administration to mice and rats. For example, 67% of the administered labeled dose in fasted mice was absorbed within 60 min; peak levels were present in the blood within 35–40 min and tissue levels indicated rapid distribution (15). Absorption and distribution were also rapid following oral administration of radiolabeled carbofuran (50 mg/kg) in the rat; peak plasma levels were reported within 7 min and were followed by even tissue distribution (16). Peak levels of radiolabeled material were detected in the blood of the rat (1 mg/kg) and cow (0.52 and 1.0 mg/kg) within 2 h after treatment (8, 11). In dermal absorption studies in mice with ^{14}C-ring-labeled carbofuran in acetone, 72% penetrated through the skin within 15 min (17). Within 8 h, 73% was found in excretory products and 12% was found in the carcass; the stomach and intestines contained about 3% each, and the liver and blood contained 1.0 and 0.8%, respectively. In acute inhalation studies with rats (nose only) exposed to an aerosol of radiolabeled carbofuran in ethanol (1.2 μg/L, 50 min) absorption was more rapid and cholinesterase inhibition was greater per μg/kg than for the oral route (18).

3.3 Excretion

Carbofuran is rapidly eliminated in the urine of mice (10), rats (8, 16), cows (11), and hens (12) following oral administration. Within 24 h, about 70% of the administered dose of ^{14}C-ring-labeled carbofuran was excreted in the urine with about 2% in the feces (8). For a

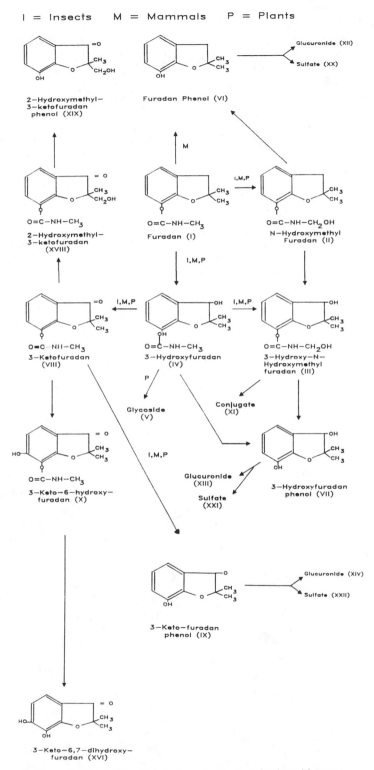

I = Insects   M = Mammals   P = Plants

Figure 5. Metabolism of carbofuran in plants, animals and insects.

lacatating cow receiving a single oral dose, 94% of the dose appeared in the urine within 72 h while only 0.2 and 0.7% were removed via milk and feces, respectively (11). Fasted mice excreted 24 and 6% of the administered oral dose in the urine and expired CO_2, respectively, within 60 min after administration (15). Elimination of the parent compound is less rapid in laying hens. After 24 h, 66% of the administered oral dose was eliminated of which 72% was hydrolyzed (12). A total of 80% of the dose was eliminated after 10 days. Residues in eggs were present at a peak of 0.13 ppm carbofuran equivalents by day 4, and except for liver (0.19 ppm) and kidneys (0.19 ppm), tissues contained less than 0.1 ppm by 24 h.

In studies conducted with ^{14}C-carbonyl-labeled carbofuran, degradation of the carbonyl group results in loss of radiolabel in expired CO_2 and consequent incorporation of $^{14}CO_2$ into body constituents. Following oral administration of 0.4 mg/kg [^{14}C]carbonyl carbofuran to rats, Dorough (8) found 40% radiolabel excreted in expired CO_2 within 12 h and 30% radiolabel in the urine (compared to 72% in urine with ^{14}C-ring-labeled carbofuran). In laying hens, an estimated 54% of the administered dose had been hydrolyzed to phenolic products within 6 h (12). After 24 h, 66% of the dose was eliminated of which 72% was hydrolyzed. A total of 80% of the dose was eliminated after 10 days. Major excreta metabolites were 3-keto-7-phenol, 3-hydroxy-7-phenol, 7-phenol, and 3-hydroxycarbofuran.

Studies in the lactating cow indicate that, following administration of a single oral dose of carbofuran, approximately 0.2% of the administered dose is eliminated in the milk within 24 h. The major hydrolytic products of carbofuran found were conjugated 3-keto-7-phenol and 3-hydroxycarbofuran; only 0.001% of the parent compound, carbofuran, was found (11). For a cow given single doses of carbofuran, 3-hydroxycarbofuran, and carbofuran residues contained in alfalfa, levels of up to 2.5% radiolabeled carbofuran and 0.7% carbofuran residues were excreted in milk after 4 days and most of the administered dose was in the urine (14). Metabolism of carbofuran, 3-hydroxycarbofuran, and carbofuran alfalfa residues were similar.

3.4   Acute Toxicity (Response to Single Doses)—Mammals

Acute toxicity of carbofuran is directly related to inhibition of acetylcholinesterase activity, which is similar in all animals (1). Clinical signs of toxicity are dose related and usually include salivation, lacrimation and tremors and may progress to miosis, diarrhea, emesis, dyspnea, convulsions, and ultimately death. The effects of single acute doses are

TABLE 5. Single-Dose LD_{50} for Carbofuran

Species	Route	LD_{50} (mg/kg)	Formulation	Reference
Rat (M, F)	Oral	7.8–34.5	Technical[a]	1
Mouse	Oral	2.0[b]	Technical	19
Dog	Oral	19	Technical	20
Rabbit (M, F)	Dermal	> 2000	Technical 3G, 5G, 10G, 15G, 4F	21
Guinea pig (M, F)	Inhalation	0.043[c]	75 WP	20

[a]Solution in corn oil.
[b]Three-day observation period.
[c]Inhalation, LC_{50} (mg/L).

similar to repeated doses. Table 5 (19–21) illustrates that carbofuran is highly toxic (LD_{50} is less than 35 mg/kg) via oral administration but relatively nontoxic when administered by the dermal route. The granular and flowable formulations are typically less toxic than the technical grade compound, which may be due to the binding of the active ingredient to the inert matrices of the formula, resulting in decreased availability of the compound for absorption. Inhalation exposure is unlikely because of the physicochemical nature of carbofuran (low vapor pressure and moderate water solubility); however, carbofuran is highly toxic as a dust or aerosol if the particles are in the respirable range.

3.5 Irritation/Sensitization—Mammals

In dermal sensitization studies carbofuran was nonsensitizing (1). Carbofuran and Furadan ® formulations are neither skin nor eye irritants (21).

3.6 Carcinogenicity, Mutagenicity, and Teratogenicity in Mammals

No evidence of oncogenicity was observed in mice and rats during chronic 2-year feeding studies with carbofuran (22). Results of a battery of mutagenicity assays (gene mutation, chromosome aberration, and primary DNA damage/repair studies) indicate that carbofuran is not genotoxic (22). The negative results from the mutagenicity studies concur with the absence of carcinogenicity established in the 2-year feeding studies. Carbofuran was not teratogenic in studies with rats and rabbits (22). In addition, carbofuran did not cause reproductive toxicity in a three-generation study with rats (22).

3.7 Oral Exposure—Human

In a laboratory experiment, adult male volunteers were administered a single oral dose of 0.05, 0.10, or 0.25 mg/kg carbofuran (23). Reversible inhibition of erythrocyte cholinesterase activity was observed at the two high-dose levels. Clinical symptomology at 0.10 mg/kg included headache whereas at 0.25 mg/kg salivation, abdominal pain, drowsiness, dizziness, and vomiting were evident. All symptoms subsided and volunteers recovered. No clinical symptomology was observed at 0.05 mg/kg.

3.8 Accidential and Intentional Poisoning—Human

The morning following an accidental misapplication of a flowable formulation of carbofuran to a cornfield, approximately 150 workers entered the treated field to detassel the corn. Symptoms of nausea and dizziness began to appear, and 74 workers reported to the hospital, 45 of which received medical attention. Twenty-nine were admitted to the hospital and one remained overnight. Treatment included atropine sulfate (24).

There were 83 cases of carbofuran intoxication in 1974 in the province of Saskatchewan during a grasshopper control spraying program (1). All individuals exhibiting symptoms of carbofuran poisoning were reported to have not been following the recommended safety procedures for handling carbofuran (i.e., the use of respirator and gloves). Safety information was distributed and all individuals stated that although they were aware of the information, they were complacent. Doctors estimated that 30 of the cases were "anxiety" or "psychosomatic." Most cases were treated with atropine. Some people required hospitalization but all were released within 48 h; the majority of cases were treated as outpatients. No long-term effects were reported. In one case of carbofuran poisoning, a man was completely "saturated" with the pesticide when a hose on his equipment burst. After 48 h of atropine and oxygen administration, he was released from the hospital. Signs of intoxication including respiratory distress had disappeared (1).

Case reports of occupational exposure illustrate the fairly rapid onset of symptoms and corresponding rapid recovery (with and without atropine treatment) resulting from moderate carbofuran intoxication (20).

3.9   Use Experience—Human

Early symptoms of carbofuran poisoning include headache, lightheadedness, weakness, and nausea. Later signs and symptoms are constriction of the pupils (i.e., miosis; may be preceded by a transient dilation), blurred vision, abdominal cramps, excessive salivation and perspiration, diarrhea, and vomiting. Symptomology has not progressed beyond this point in experiences during manufacturing, formulation, and application (20, 21). There are no known chronic effects to humans from carbofuran exposure.

4   ENVIRONMENTAL FATE AND ECOTOXICOLOGY

4.1   Hydrolysis

Carbofuran is stable in water at acid and neutral pH in the absence of light but it hydrolyzes rapidly with increasing pH (1). For example, at a pH of 6 (at 25°C) the hydrolytic half-life is approximately 350 days, whereas at pH levels of 7, 8, and 9 the half-lives (at 25°C) are about 35, 6, and 0.60 days, respectively. Hydrolytic rate constants and half-lives were determined for carbofuran and its related metabolites (10). Studies were conducted in phosphate buffer at pH 9.5. The results indicate that carbofuran is more stable than the metabolites (i.e., 3-hydroxy-, 3-keto-N-hydromethyl-, 3-keto-N-hydro-xymethyl-, carbofuran). The rate of hydrolysis also increases with increasing temperature such that each 1°C increase is reportedly estimated to produce a 35% increase in the hydrolysis rate at ambient temperatures. In all hydrolysis studies conducted, the major product is 7-phenol, which is the least toxic carbofuran metabolite.

If hydrolysis is the major environmental degradation route for carbofuran, its persistence in the aquatic environment would likely be increased with low temperatures and acidic pH levels. The primary phenolic product, a 7-phenol, is much less persistent than carbofuran, disappearing by volatilization and by further photodegradation to polar products.

4.2   Photolysis

Carbofuran degradation in water and soil is enhanced in the presence of sunlight. Carbofuran undergoes photodecomposition in aqueous solutions during exposure to light in the 300–400-nm range (1). The decomposition of carbofuran in distilled irradiated water under aerobic conditions at pH 7 (initial concentration 5 mg/L) followed first-order kinetics with a half-life of 5.6 days. When irradiated with benzophenone (photosensitizer) the half-life was 1.8 days, suggesting that a triplet or singlet oxygen was involved in the reaction. Based on these findings, it was concluded that the rate at which carbofuran undergoes photodecomposition in water is such that "accumulation in water exposed to sunlight is not likely to be a problem" (1).

Silica gel and soil experiments irradiating ^{14}C-labeled carbofuran on thin plates illustrated that the half-life was less than 1 week.

The primary photoproduct of carbofuran in the above studies was 7-phenol.

4.3 Volatility

Vapor pressure data indicate that carbofuran and its carbamate metabolites are nonvolatile (1, 21). Carbofuran has a vapor pressure of 3.4×10^{-6} mm Hg while 3-hydroxycarbofuran and 3-ketocarbofuran are approximately 2.0×10^{-7} mm Hg at 25°C. Based on the solubility (700 mg/L) and vapor pressure of carbofuran at 25°C (3.4×10^{-6}), it is not likely that volatilization contributes significantly to the losses of carbofuran from aquatic environments after mixing or from soil surfaces.

4.4 Soil Adsorption

In adsorption studies with five different soil types (e.g., sand, sandy loam, silt loam, clay loam, muck) and a wide range of textural characteristics, soil adsorption isotherms indicated that carbofuran did not bind significantly to any of the soils examined (1).

In leaching studies with seven soil types, data show that the parent compound exhibits a fair degree of mobility in sand and sandy loam soil. This mobility was retarded in muck and clay loam. Field studies, however, have shown that little carbofuran moved outside the top soil layer (i.e., 0–7.6 cm) over 120 days (1).

Sorption is unlikely to contribute significantly to the disappearance of carbofuran from the water phase in an aquatic ecosystem. Thus at soil–water equilibration, concentrations of carbofuran in sediment are expected to be similar to those in the water.

4.5 Microbial Degradation

The role of soil bacteria in carbofuran degradation is still unclear. Under acidic and neutral pH conditions, the degradation of carbofuran in soil and water is strongly affected by microbial decomposition. Strains of actinomycetes and fungi have been shown to metabolize carbofuran actively to at least eight different metabolites (25). More recently, metabolism of carbofuran has been demonstrated with a *Pseudomonas* sp. isolate and sterilized soils did not show evidence of carbofuran degradation (26). On the other hand, several investigators believe that microbial processes play a negligible role in carbofuran metabolism (1).

The evidence suggests that hydrolysis and photolysis are the major factors that contribute to the dissipation of carbofuran in the environment.

4.6 Field Studies

Several field studies support the rapid rate of disappearance of carbofuran in the aquatic environment. In an Illinois study (1), water runoff from a watershed treated with granular carbofuran at 4.48 kg active/ha yielded residues of 1.1 mg/L (ppm) in a pond (pH unspecified). The concentration of carbofuran in the pond water was reported to have declined to less than 0.07 mg/L within 16 days post-treatment. In another study conducted in Alberta, Canada, an alkaline pond (pH 8.2) was sprayed by aircraft with the flowable formulation of carbofuran at 0.14 kg active/ha (1). Initial maximum residues of 4.3 μg/L (ppb) declined to approximately 0.3 μg/L within 8 days. Furthermore, rice paddy water from post-flood application of carbofuran to rice paddy fields in California (1.0 lb active/acre) and Louisiana (0.6 lb active/acre) were monitored for dissipation of carbofuran (27). Postflood residue analysis indicated that the half-life in water from a California rice paddy and a Louisiana rice paddy were approximately less than 2 days and less than 4 days, respectively.

4.7   Plant Metabolism

Metabolism of carbofuran in plants is similar to that in animals (see Fig. 5). Metabolites differ only in the types of conjugate formed (i.e., glycosides in plants versus glucuronides and sulfates in animals). The major degradative pathways of carbofuran, which account for the observed plant residues, have been reasonably well characterized (8, 10, 17, 28). The primary transformation product in most plants is 3-hydroxycarbofuran—a considerable portion of which has been reported to be in the form of glycosidic conjugates (17, 28, 29). Glycosides of carbofuran phenol have also been reported. Alfalfa plants grown in soil treated with 18 mg of ring-[^{14}C] or 9 mg of carbonyl-[^{14}C]carbofuran were found to contain metabolites identified as glycosides of 3-hydroxycarbofuran (37.3%) and 2, 3-dihydro-3, 7-dihydroxy-2, 2-dimethyl-3-oxobenzofuran. Identical products were found in bean plants treated in a similar manner (14).

The unconjugated 3-hydroxycarbofuran is first oxidized to 3-ketocarbofuran and this product is rapidly hydrolyzed to the much less toxic 3-hydroxycarbofuran phenol (10, 29). Therefore, 3-ketocarbofuran will not likely be detected as a terminal residue in plants above trace levels.

Several other degradation products of carbofuran have generally been found in trace amounts in plant tissues but appear to be of less toxicological significance. In some instances, it is not clear whether the carbamate and phenolic terminal residues are formed in the soil and are subsequently taken up by the plants or whether they are generated within the plants. It is, however, clearly evident that the conversion of parent compound to 3-hydroxycarbofuran is not one generated in soil since it is rarely detected in soils above trace levels (30).

4.8   Aquatic Organisms—Acute and Chronic Toxicities

In acute laboratory tests with aquatic organisms, LC$_{50}$ values for carbofuran ranged from 130 to 14,000 ppb in tests of 72–96 h of continuous exposure (Table 6) (31–41). The Dungeness crab and waterflea (*Daphnia*) were the most sensitive, followed by fish and worms, which were the most tolerant.

A 14-day flow-through toxicity study was conducted to determine the LC$_{50}$ (and lethal threshold concentration or incipient LC$_{50}$) and/or EC$_{50}$ (and incipient EC$_{50}$ for sublethal responses) for rainbow trout (*Salmo gairdneri*) when continuously exposed to technical grade carbofuran (27). The LC$_{50}$ could not be estimated because at the highest exposure of 391 μg/L the mortality was only 35%. However, an EC$_{50}$ (effective concentration to produce a sublethal response to 50% of the test population) based on loss of equilibrium was determined since over 65% of the fish at the highest concentration exhibited loss of equilibrium. The 24-h EC$_{50}$ values for days 1–8 ranged from 268 to 128 μg/L, respectively. An incipient EC$_{50}$ value of approximately 150 μg/L was attained by day 5. Behavioral observations throughout the study indicated that mortality was preceded by loss of equilibrium in the three highest exposure test groups (98–39/μg/L). Significant body weight effects were also noted in these three groups. No abnormalities were found in the

TABLE 6. Acute Toxicities (LC$_{50}$'s) of Carbofuran to Aquatic Organisms

Type of Water and Species Tested	Time (h)	LC$_{50}$[a] (ppb)	Reference
Fresh Water			
Yellow perch,			
Perca flavescens	96	147	31
Green sunfish,			
Lepomis cyanellus	72	160	32
Lake trout,			
Salvelinus namaycush	96	164	31
Bluegill,			
Lepomis macrochirus	96	240	31
Channel catfish,			
Ictalurus punctatus	96	248	31
Static test, tapwater	96	1,420	33
Partial media replacement	96	510	33
Rice paddy water with history[b]	96	130	33
Rice paddy water with no prior history[b]	96	370	33
African catfish,			
Mystus vittatus	96	310	34
Rainbow trout,			
Salmo gairdneri	96	380	31
Crayfish,			
Procambarus acutus acutus	96	500	35
Mosquitofish,			
Gambusia affinis	72	520	36
Coho salmon,			
Oncorhychus kisutch	96	530	31
Indian carp,			
Saccobranchus fossilis	96	547	37
Brown trout,			
Salmo trutta	96	560	31
Fathead minnow,			
Pimephales promelas	96	872	31
Water flea,			
Daphnia magna	48	38	27
Annelid worm,			
Limnodrilus hoffmeisterei	96	11,000	38
Annelid worm,			
Tubifex tubifex	96	14,000	38
Marine			
Dungeness crab, *Cancer magister*			
Larva	96	2.5	39
Adult	96	190	39
Sheepshead minnow,			
Cyprinodon variegatus	96	386	40
C. variegatus	3,144	49	40
Bivalve molusks			
Cockle, *Clinocardium nuttali*	96	3,750	41
Clam, *Macoma nasuta*	96	17,000	41
Mussel, *Mytilus edulis*	96	22,000	41
Clam, *Rangia cuneata*	96	125,000	41

[a]Concentrations shown are in micrograms of carbofuran per liter of medium (ppb).
[b]Rice paddy water from rice paddies with and without a history of pesticide application, as shown.

56- and 34 μg/L test groups. The no-effect concentration in this study for carbofuran to rainbow trout for 14 days of continuous exposure was 56 μg/L (criterion is loss of equilibrium).

A 90-day posthatch early life stage toxicity study was conducted to estimate the maximum acceptable toxicant concentration (MATC or safe concentration) for rainbow trout continuously exposed to technical grade carbofuran (27). Eggs and subsequently the trout fry were exposed continuously in a flow-through system for a total of 101 days to measured concentrations (with acetone carrier) ranging from 7.16 to 88.7 μg/L. Hatchability of treated eggs after 14 days was not different from the controls and fry survival between hatch and 30 days of exposure was not affected. Fry growth (i.e., standard length) was significantly reduced after 30 days of exposure to 88.7 μg/L and at 56.7 and 88.7 μg/L after 60, 75, and 90 days of exposure when compared to controls. Fry growth (i.e., wet weight) was significantly reduced at 56.7 and 88.7 μg/L after 75 days. After 90 days, only trout fry at 88.7 μg/L had significantly reduced wet weights. Based on the results of this study, the MATC limits for carbofuran and rainbow trout were estimated to be between 24.8 (NOEC or no observed effect concentration) and 56.7 μg/L (LOEC or lowest observed effect concentration).

Parrish et al. (40) conducted an early life stage toxicity study with sheepshead minnows (*Cyprinodon variegatus*). At concentrations up to 99 μg/L, carbofuran did not significantly affect the growth of parent fish or the number of eggs produced but mortality of fry from fish exposed to 23 and 49 μg/L was greater than that of the controls. The MATC limits for carbofuran and sheepshead minnow were between 15 and 23 μg/L. This is similar to the previous study with rainbow trout and that of Caldwell (39), who demonstrated that adult Dungeness crabs (*Cancer magister*) showed no deleterious effects on growth, survival, or reproduction during exposure to 25 μg/L of carbofuran for 69 days.

A chronic 21-day (life cycle) toxicity study was conducted to estimate the MATC limits for *Daphnia magna* continuously exposed to carbofuran technical at measured concentrations (with acetone carrier) ranging from 1.7 to 27 μg/L (26). Adult survival, adult length, and total young produced per adult per day after 21 days exposure to carbofuran at 27 μg/L were significantly reduced. Mortality was 82% at this concentration but no other treatment groups exhibited greater than 7% mortality. Neither the length of the surviving adults, nor adult survival, nor young produced per adult per reproductive day were significantly affected at any other exposure concentration. Based on the results of this *Daphnia* life cycle study, the MATC limits for carbofuran were estimated to be between 9.8 and 27 μg/L.

Carbofuran is not expected to accumulate in aquatic organisms. The potential bioaccumulation in fish can be examined on the basis of the correlation between bioconcentration factor (BCF) and the octanol–water partition coefficient (P_{ow}) of the material (i.e., $\log BCF = 0.542 \log P_{ow} + 0.124$; Neely et al. (42)). The P_{ow} of carbofuran is reported to be 17 (1). The BCF (concentration in tissue/concentration in water) for carbofuran is approximately 6. This estimate of the BCF is similar to the value reported in a study using bluegills (1, 27). The data indicate that bluegill continuously exposed to a mean concentration of 0.066 mg/L [^{14}C]carbofuran reached equilibrium in 1–3 days of exposure and maintained this throughout the remainder of the 28-day exposure. Tissue concentrations of carbofuran averaged about five times that in the water. Upon cessation of exposure in uncontaminated water, clearance of carbofuran from the tissues was consistent with the expected pattern of first-order kinetics. The clearance half-life was less than 1 week. The results obtained using a lower exposure concentration of carbofuran in water did not follow the accumulation model for fish; that is, the BCF and clearance pattern obtained were not consistent with first-order kinetics.

In a bioaccumulation study using a model ecosystem, ^{14}C-ring-labeled carbofuran was applied to sandy loam soil and aged for 30 days (1). After 30 days of aging, the tanks holding the soil were filled with water and were allowed to equilibrate for 3 days. Channel catfish (*Ictalurus punctatus*) were then introduced into the system. Concentrations in the water (0.14 mg/L) were constant throughout a 37-day exposure period. The bioconcentration factors in whole fish, muscle, viscera, and carcass were 2.6, 1.0, 15, and 1.5, respectively. These findings indicate that after equilibrium was established (10 days), most of the carbofuran was concentrated in the nonedible portions of the fish (i.e., carcass and viscera). After the 37-day period, some fish were transferred to other uncontaminated tanks for a 14-day depuration period. By the third day, the fish had eliminated greater than 89, 97, 81, and 93% of the C-residues measured in the muscle, viscera, carcass, and on a whole fish basis.

Negligible accumulations of carbofuran were observed in egg masses of the caddisfly (*Triaenoidus tardus*) during immersion for 120 h in water containing 8 µg/L carbofuran (43). Rapid equilibrium and low accumulation were also reported for the sheepshead minnow; in a 28-day flow-through study, maximum tissue concentrations were measured between days 3 and 10 when upper concentration factors of 5–20 × were recorded (40).

4.9   Birds—Acute and Chronic Toxicities

Birds can be exposed to carbofuran by several different routes, including exposure to direct spray, ingestion of contaminated food, and direct ingestion of granules. However, the literature indicates that the major route of exposure for birds is through ingestion of exposed granules that are not properly incorporated during application.

Acute oral toxicities of carbofuran to birds range from 238 ppb (µg/kg BW) for whistling-ducks to 38,900 ppb for domestic chickens (Table 7) (44–47). Waterfowl are the most sensitive group to carbofuran technical while gallinaceous birds are the least sensitive; passerines are intermediate in their sensitivity. Carbofuran administered to birds in the diet for 5 days, plus 3 days postexposure on untreated diet, produced LC_{50} values of 21–1459 ppm dietary carbofuran; younger birds were more sensitive than older ones (Table 8) (48, 49). The dietary inclusion studies support the oral toxicity studies in that mallard are among the most sensitive birds to carbofuran. It is evident from acute toxicity studies with the technical grade material that carbofuran is acutely toxic to birds.

The acute toxicity of carbofuran granules (i.e., Furadan ®10G, 10% carbofuran by weight) to house sparrows (*Passer domesticus*) and red-winged blackbirds (*Agelaius phoeniceus*) was also studied in the laboratory (50). The studies demonstrated that ingestion of a single carbofuran granule is fatal to either species.

Acute symptoms of carbofuran poisoning in birds, which may persist for up to 7 days, include a loss in muscular coordination, head nodding, vocal sounds, salivation, tears, diarrhea, immobility with wings spread, labored breathing, eye pupil constriction, arching of back, and arching of neck over back; death may occur within 5 min after ingestion (44).

Laboratory studies show that chronic dietary exposure to carbofuran does not affect reproductive performance in bobwhite quail and mallard duck at concentrations several orders of magnitude higher than typical field residue levels (27). Bobwhite quail and mallard duck were exposed to dietary inclusion of carbofuran technical up to 180 and 10 ppm, respectively, daily over a 24 (mallard) to 26 (bobwhite) week period, which

TABLE 7. Acute Oral Toxicities of Carbofuran to Birds

Species Tested	LD$_{50}$[a]	Reference
Fulvous whistling-duck,		
Dendrocygna bicolor	238	44
Mallard, *Anas platyrhynchos*		
Age 36 h	280–480	45
Age 7 days	530–740	45
Age 30 days	410–640	45
Age 3–4 months	320–500	44
Age 6 months	330–520	45
Red-winged blackbird,		
Agelaius phoeniceus	422	46
Quelea, *Quelea quelea*	422–562	46
House finch,		
Carpodacus mexicanus	750	46
Japanese quail,		
Coturnix japonica	1,300–2,100	47
House sparrow,		
Passer domesticus	1,330	46
Common grackle,		
Quiscalus quiscula	1,330–3,160	46
Rock dove,		
Columba livia	1,330	46
Brown-headed cowbird,		
Molothrus ater	1,330	46
Ring-necked pheasant,		
Phasianus colchicus	2,380–7,220	44
Northern bobwhite,		
Colinus virginianus	3,640–6,990	44
European starling,		
Sturnus vulgaris	5,620	46
Domestic chicken,		
Gallus gallus	25,000–38,900	1

[a] Concentrations shown are in micrograms of carbofuran administered per kilogram of body weight (ppb) in a single dose fatal to 50% within 14 days.

included both pre- and post-egg production. There were no marked differences between treatments in the overall development and hatching of eggs laid or in the survivability of the offspring.

4.9.1   *Field Studies.*

The granular formulation of carbofuran is used on corn and other crops in the United States. Although product uses and labels require soil incorporation or covering of the granules, exposed granules may still occur with currently used equipment (51). Granules well incorporated into the soil are less likely to be picked up by birds than granules that remain on the surface. Carbofuran granules are most often applied in-furrow or in bands. Band application produces more exposed granules than in-furrow application. However, an accidental spillage (e.g., at turning rows) by farmers may produce significantly more exposure to birds than evenly distributed granules regardless of application technique. Granules from either the carbofuran 10G or 15G formulation can

TABLE 8. Toxicity^a (LC$_{50}$) of Dietary Carbofuran to Birds

Organism	Concentration^b	Reference
Mallard	190	48
Ring-necked pheasant	573	48
Japanese quail		
Age 1 day	140–471	49
Age 7 days	436–1103	49
Age 10–14 days	438	48
Age 14 days	586–1004	49
Age 21 days	779–1459	49

^{a}Five-day dietary exposure followed by 3-day untreated diet.
^{b}Concentration of carbofuran in diet, in mg/kg (ppm) fresh weight.

be ingested along with grit or food material by birds. The particle size of the granules is similar in size (0.2–1.5 mm) to grit consumed by small birds such as house sparrows (52). There is thus a potential that birds feeding in treated fields will consume granules. The flowable formulation of carbofuran (Furadan® 4F) presents a secondary potential source of exposure to birds either through direct contact with spray during application (i.e., by ground or aerial) or via ingestion of food contaminated with residues from the spray.

Waterfowl kills in the United States and Canada have been reported with both the granular and flowable formulations (1, 53). The exact nature and type of application or misapplication (i.e., overexposure, either accidental or intentional) is not known in all cases. However, since restrictions have been placed on the label concerning the use of carbofuran near waterfowl, reports of waterfowl kills have subsided when the material is applied according to the use label.

A review of the avian field studies with the granular formulations follows. The flowable formulation is not discussed but it should be noted that the one field study conducted with this formulation on alfalfa at a maximum field rate demonstrates minimal risk to bird species. The review below is composed of either field monitoring studies, which monitor mainly for dead birds (carcasses), or field experiments, which are designed to answer a host of questions. Unfortunately, the data generated by field studies are difficult to interpret and many of the methods used to monitor biological endpoints have not been adequately addressed or validated for the purpose of assessing chemically induced stress on birds. This is not surprising since the science of avian toxicology like ecotoxicology has not had a long history and many of the general basics in avian ecology and behavior are not clearly understood.

The reviews discussed below are on studies used by the U.S. EPA to initiate the Special Review in which they concluded that "carbofuran in its granular formulation is highly toxic to birds" and its use results in "significant fatalities of many small species of birds, widespread avian mortality, significant local, regional or national population reductions in non-target organisms or fatality to members of endangered species." It should be noted, however, that only one field study actually demonstrated significant adverse effects on birds but this study for reasons discussed below was conducted under a worst-case scenario and therefore is not representative of a typical application.

The first study was conducted in Utah where Furadan® 10G and 15G formulations were applied as a band (7 in. wide) at planting at a maximum use rate (greater than 3 lb active/acre) to corn (2). Each treatment contained three replicate test plots and three replicate control plots were also included in the experimental design. This study represented a worst-case scenario. A total of 911 dead birds were found on corn plots (254 acres) during organized carcass searches with approximately 91% (831) of those being a single species (i.e., horned larks). A total of 504 birds were killed on 10G test plots, but the difference was not statistically significant (the remaining 34 birds were found on control plots that were adjacent to treated plots). Other bird species that were found dead included 21 yellow-headed blackbirds, 19 Brown-headed cowbirds, and 19 mourning doves. Four predatory birds were found dead (i.e., two ravens, one marsh hawk, and one short eared owl) and analysis of stomach contents indicated that these fatalities may have resulted from secondary exposure (i.e., consumption of smaller birds that had ingested carbofuran granules). Several birds exhibited atypical behavior, which involved the inability to fly or uncoordinated motion while sitting, standing, or walking. These signs are typical symptoms associated with acetylcholinesterase (AChE) inhibition. Although significant total bird mortality occurred in treated areas compared to controls in this study, analysis of bird density estimates on the test plots themselves showed no significant differences between Furadan-treated areas and the controls.

In considering this study to assess the potential hazard of Furadan granules to birds, the following factors must be considered: (i) rate of application, (ii) cultural practices (and deviations from normal cultural practices at the study site), (iii) crop stand and its relation to the affected species, (iv) key species population levels in the test area, and (v) behavioral habits of the key species. Each of these areas is discussed below.

Rate of Application.   The rate used was equivalent to a maximum labeled use rate of 3 lb active/acre. This clearly represents a worst-case application scenario since the rate most often used by corn farmers is 1.0 lb active/acre. The worst-case situation is typically recommended for most field study requirements in FIFRA. It is evident that the higher rate would result in a much higher probability of a bird picking up granules, leading to the potential for significantly greater mortality than would be expected under more common use rate conditions. In other avian field monitoring studies where Furadan granules were applied to corn at more conventional rates of 1.0 lb active/acre, significantly lower levels of bird mortality have occurred adding substantiation to this contention. These studies are discussed later.

Cultural Practices.   In those instances where concentrations of granules did occur on the soil surface as a result of normal (i.e., at loading, at end rows during turning) agricultural practices, no attempt was made to cover or incorporate them. This was part of the recommended worst-case scenario. Although spillage of granules may occur, a normal practice would be for the farmer, at a minimum, to cover the spills by moving soil with his foot. In addition, since end rows become compacted due to planter turning, a normal practice for growers is to retill this area before making final passes on the end-row areas. The retilling thus results in incorporation of exposed granules. It is evident once again that practices utilized in the Utah study resulted in atypical conditions, thus contributing to the unusually high avian mortality.

Crop Stand.   The rainfall indicated that no significant rain occurred until 54 days after planting. Corn growth was less than optimal as demonstrated by stand counts. Horned larks, the primary species affected in this study, are ground birds; they are almost never seen where the vegetation is high. The low corn stand resulted in an environment that was particularly conducive to unexpectedly high foraging by horned larks on test plots and the resulting horned lark mortalities.

Population Levels of Horned Larks. Test plots were selected for insecticide treatments because they bordered nonagricultural areas, which maximized habitat available for cover and residence habitat for passerine species. Many border areas were overgrazed, encouraging the production of annual weeds that are food resources for birds. Horned lark populations were particularly prevalent in these areas.

Behavioral Habits of Horned Larks. The literature indicates that horned larks pick up food and nest on the ground. These habits coupled with the study factors previously discussed enhance the probability of unusually high levels of horned lark mortalities.

The mortalities observed in this study were not a normal occurrence since they have never been documented. Furadan granules have been used extensively for over 17 years and no such incident has ever been noted. In addition, background survey (Breeding Bird Survey) information currently available demonstrates that populations of species commonly observed in or near cornfields (e.g., blackbirds, robins, lark spp.) have not declined (54). For example, horned larks were the seventh most common bird recorded in the Breeding Bird Survey (55). The other bird species (e.g., cowbirds, morning doves) found dead in low numbers in this study are common species and have generally demonstrated stable populations. Extrapolation of these data to other areas is not appropriate because the study area was uniquely selected and the results are also unique to the circumstances and location of the study. The Utah site is not typical of Midwest cornfield habitats.

In a second study, 15 cornfields (total 195 ha) in Maryland were treated with Furadan 10G at planting in seed furrow (1.12 kg active/ha) (56). Carcass searches were conducted within 1 day of treatment and 3–4 days posttreatment. Some songbirds were found dead but only five (two American robins, one blackbird, one Savannah sparrow, one grasshopper sparrow) contained carbofuran. The partial remains of four American robins and one common grackle were also found dead, but the cause of death was unknown. Two other birds were found exhibiting abnormal behavior indicative of carbofuran poisoning. The authors indicate that granules were exposed in furrows because of spillage, during loading, and at row ends when the planter was lifted out of the furrow. Surface granules in furrows were hard to find after it rained, but in turn areas the granules were visible for 21 days. The authors also stated that bird mortalities may occur regularly with a potential mortality approaching 1 million.

There were no pretreatment observations in this study to establish baseline on the types and diversity of avian species common to this area and the incidence of "naturally occurring" mortalities. Furthermore, there were no "control" fields monitored concurrently with treated fields. These are crucial parts of a sound experimental design. The study therefore does not compare mortality of birds before and after treatment nor does it indicate the numerical significance of these mortalities compared to typical background populations of these species.

The number (5) of confirmed carbofuran-related mortalities and the number (17) of speculated sublethal carbofuran poisonings in birds killed in this study are insignificant compared to naturally occurring bird mortalities (i.e., from predation, disease, parasites) and to population trends of these species. According to the Breeding Bird Survey (BBS) (54), most of these bird species displayed population increases in states where Furadan granules are used. Some of these species showed population declines in the BBS but declines were related to weather and artificial changes (i.e., habitat destruction) and not chemicals. Furthermore, some of these birds species are involved in large management programs to control their populations to prevent their depredations on crops (57). It should also be noted that no raptor mortalities were found and none of the above avian species found dead were part of the National List of species exhibiting evidence of unstable or decreasing population trends in significant portions of their ranges (58).

The information presented in this study along with the discussion on natural population trends clearly shows that the low numbers of mortality reported here are not biologically significant, should not affect populations of birds, and do not demonstrate that Furadan granules produce unreasonable adverse effects in the environment.

In a study in the Southeast in 1977 at four sites, a modified Powr-Till seeder was evaluated for applying carbofuran (Furadan 10G) to pine seed orchards to improve incorporation of granules to limit bird mortality (59). Study plots were divided into two plots—a plot treated with the Powr-Till seeder and a second plot where check and hand treatments were located. Rows were disked after seeder application to cover spillage. After hand application, exposed granules were covered with pine straw or wood chips. To evaluate how much the Powr-Till seeder minimized bird mortalities versus the hand application, bird mortality observations were conducted before (baseline) and after treatment.

A total of 96 birds were found dead at the four sites (total 117 acres). Possible secondary poisoning of two loggerhead shrikes (one dead, one sick) were also noted. No other raptors were found dead or moribund. Crop dissections of dead birds revealed carbofuran particles in only a few of the birds. Bird mortality was minimal with the Powr-Till seeder as noted by the authors. Mortalities noted as a result of hand application are not surprising since incorporation was not according to the current use directions on Furadan labels.

Flickinger et al. (60) conducted a study in 1970 and 1973–1975 on the effects of Furadan 3G to wildlife in and near rice fields on the Texas Gulf Coast. Five study areas were selected, which varied in size and soil type and which previously had bird mortalities from aldrin/dieldrin poisoning. Aerial applications (0.5 lb/acre) began in May after the peak of northward migration of birds. Treatments were made while water drained from rice fields into ditches and canals. Searches were conducted before and after treatment. Pen tests in the field were also conducted with fulvous whistling ducks and mallards in treated and untreated fields.

Results indicate that carbofuran was absorbed in clay soil within 1.5 h, whereas in sandy soil the granules remained on the surface for over 24 h. Four sandpipers and one red-winged blackbird were found dead; one blackbird was sick, but flew away. All sandpipers contained granules in their stomachs. In one site, 1500 birds were found feeding in the field before and after treatment but no treatment effects were observed. In the pen studies, there were no signs of intoxication in either ducks or mallards and fulvous duck populations increased by 80% during the time period covering the study. In addition, no bird mortality was reported by local people after Furadan® 3G replaced aldrin although many reports were received when aldrin was in use.

Several problems in the design make it difficult to assess the potential hazard of Furadan 3G application to rice field agroecosystems. The authors have not presented comparative population data between Furadan-treated and -untreated (control) areas before and after treatment. Baseline data are critical to understand the effects of the chemical. Since the authors have stated the study areas had a history of aldrin use, residue analysis should have included aldrin. The authors have insufficient residue information regarding the dead sandpipers and moribund and dead blackbirds.

While there were deficiencies with the study design, the total number of mortalities and/or moribund birds was low over a multiyear period at typical use rates on rice. In addition, no raptor mortalities were recorded. This study supports other studies with low avian mortalities on corn at typical use rates.

The four field studies (2, 56, 59, 60) previously discussed were cited by the U.S. EPA in their initiation of the Special Review. A 2-year avian field study conducted in Wisconsin was not mentioned in the Special Review (61). This study was a multiyear field monitoring study on corn at typical use rates. Cornfields were observed up to 5 days after application of Furadan granules (1.0 lb active/acre) as a 7-in. band and in-furrow. Corn seeds were treated and other rootworm insecticides/herbicides were also used. Over one-third of each of the treated fields had granules visible, usually at row ends.

In 1972, field inspections were made in 74 cornfields covering 1118 acres. Birds commonly observed in and near the cornfields included blackbirds, robins, sparrows, larks, wrens, meadow larks, bobolinks, pigeons, swallows, killdeers, and crows. Eleven dead birds and three dead field mice were found in eight fields treated with rootworm insecticides; seven of the fields had been treated with Furadan and one with Dasanit (fensulfothion, an organophosphate). Among the dead birds were three red-winged blackbirds, two robins, one bluebird, one catbird, one sparrow, and two unidentified birds. In 1973, field inspections were made in 51 cornfields covering 865.2 acres. Six birds (one sparrow, one cowbird, two blackbirds, and two robins) and one mole were found dead in three fields treated with rootworm insecticides; two of the fields had been treated with Furadan and one with Dasanit. Tissue analysis for carbofuran was not conducted in dead animals because there was an insufficient amount of tissue sample. From one to five birds and small mammals were found dead, within 2 weeks of application, in only 9 of 115 cornfields treated with corn rootworm insecticides. The observers found 1 dead bird per 100 acreas surveyed and 1 dead mammal per 45 acres surveyed. No dead birds or mammals were found on 10 fields without rootworm insecticide applications. Evidence was insufficient to prove or disprove that insecticides killed the small number of birds and mammals collected.

Although the experimental design/technique deficiencies noted in the discussion of other field studies are also present in this study, it is relevant, nevertheless, that this 2-year study supports all other incidental findings of avian mortality in the field (56, 59, 60) with typical use rates for carbofuran granules. If significant mortalities were a direct result of carbofuran exposure in birds after application, it should have been observed in this study. Furthermore, if secondary poisoning of raptors was a problem, it also should have been evident in this study—yet no raptor mortalities were observed.

Several incidents of secondary poisoning in bald eagles have been reported in the state of Virginia in the past few years but in only a few cases has laboratory analysis confirmed the presence of carbofuran. This information is not documented in the open literature. The only other documentation on secondary poisoning of raptors is on two red-shouldered hawks found sick on a cornfield in Maryland treated once with Furadan 10G, at plant, in seed furrow (1.12 kg a.i./ha) (79). One female hawk was suffering from carbamate intoxication and was subsequently sacrificed for analysis. A second less affected hawk was nursed in the laboratory and then released the following day. The female hawk contained 47 μg of Furadan in the gastrointestinal tract and 49.6 μg in the tissue. Based on residues in the digestive tract of the female hawk and the nature of the toxic symptoms, the author concluded that the two hawks were poisoned by Furadan acquired from ingesting small vertebrate prey. The author concluded that, based on his field searches of approximately 345 ha during 1980–1982, several thousand raptors may be affected over the 3 million ha of corn treated with granular carbofuran. This has not been substantiated either in the open literature or through communications with farmers.

In this study, it is difficult to ascertain how the author can proposed any credible or reasonably accurate extrapolation to red-shouldered hawk populations for 3 million acres of corn when only 1 hawk died in this study. There were no available published reports found in the literature concerning the population impact of any chemical on raptors other than the organochlorines, mercury, thallium sulfate (62), and the organophosphates (63). In general, carbamates have not been implicated in producing significant mortalities or population effects in raptors. Other factors have led to population declines of red-shouldered hawks such as habitat alteration (64, 65). Newton (62) states that for raptors, three factors cause declines (or limiting numbers), namely: restriction and degradation of habitat, persecution by humans, and contamination by toxic chemicals (viz., organochlorines, mercury, thallium).

5   USE OF ALTERNATIVE CHEMICALS AND BENEFITS

The U.S. EPA in the Special Review document for carbufuran suggested likely alternatives for the control of corn rootworm in field corn at times of planting. These chemicals were terbufos (Counter®), fonofos (Dyfonate®), chlorpyrifos (Lorsban®), fensulfothion (Dasanit®), phorate (Thimet®), trimethacarb (Broot®), isofenfos (Amaze®), ethoprop (Mocap®), and carbofuran flowable (Furadan® 4F).

The alternative insecticides are all acutely toxic to birds. The acute toxicity (LD_{50}) for these insecticides, for various bird species, is illustrated in Tables 9 (66) and 10 (67). In general, the technical grade was more toxic than the granular formulation. Ingestion of 10 granules or less of any one of the alternatives (except isofenfos and trimethacarb) could be lethal to small passerines such as house sparrows and red-winged blackbirds (50). The available literature indicates that granular formulations of trimethacarb were not tested with birds.

Out of the nine insecticides suggested as alternatives, two are carbamates (carbofuran and trimethacarb) and the remaining seven are organophosphates. Organophosphates may present a greater secondary hazard to raptors than the carbamates since they irreversibly inhibit acetylcholinesterase, are more slowly metabolized, have greater half-lives, and generally have more toxic metabolites than carbamates (5). Secondary poisonings from organophosphate insecticides have been reported in the literature (63, 68–70). The severity of organophosphate poisoning in birds is potentially more biologically significant than the impact of any carbamate on birds. For example, other effects of organophosphate pesticides on birds have been noted experimentally (71–73) and include impairment of feeding, thermoregulation, salt gland and endocrine gland function, nesting behavior, and reproduction.

The documentation above substantiates the potential risk to birds associated with exposure to the alternative insecticides—a risk that appears to be significantly greater with organophosphates than carbamates.

Information concerning human effects, and the potential for dermal exposure during loading, shows that this is also important in assessing risk. Furadan granular formulations are at least 4- to 100-fold less toxic by the dermal route of exposure than are other available competitive granular formulations (terbufos, phorate, ethoprop). No clinical signs of toxicity were observed following exposure of animals to granular formulations of

TABLE 9. Acute Oral LD$_{50}$ of Technical Grade and Granular Formulations of Insecticides to Adult Bobwhite

	Formulation	LD$_{50}$ (mg/kg)	95% CI
Dithiophosphate			
Terbufos	Technical	15	12–19
(Counter)	15G	26[a]	20–34
Fonofos	Technical	12	10–14
(Dyfonate)	20G	14	12–17
Phorate	Technical	7	4–11
(Thimet)	15G	21[a]	14–31
Thiophosphate			
Chlorpyrifos	Technical	32	24–43
(Lorsban)	15G	108[a]	80–145
Fensulfothion	Technical	1.2	1.0–1.6
(Dasanit)	15G	2.4[a]	2.0–2.9
Isofenfos	Technical	13	10–16
(Amaze)	15G	19	15–23
Ethoprop[b]	Technical	4.2[c]	
(Mocap)	10G	4.8[c]	
Carbamate			
Carbofuran	Technical	12	7–19
(Furdan)	10G	12	9–16

[a]Significantly different from technical grade.
[b]From Balcomb et al. (50).
[c]LD$_{50}$ values for house sparrows.
Source: Hill and Camardese (66).

carbofuran even at the highest dose tested of 2000 mg/kg. The lower dermal toxicity of carbofuran indicates a reduced risk to the user.

The EPA has also named Furadan 4F as a likely alternative to granular formulations of carbofuran. Furadan 4F is an effective soil-applied insecticide; however, it is a Hazard Category I Product (Danger—Poison), whereas Furadan granules are a Hazard Category II Product (Warning). Use of Furadan 4F will thus result in more exposure (liquid spray versus granules) and although it can safely be handled extra safety cautions are needed.

Granular formulations of carbofuran, marketed under the trademark Furadan® (3G, 5G, 10G, and 15G), have benefits to both the grower and to the environment. The material provides effective control of a broad spectrum of plant-damaging nematodes and insects. To growers the net result is increased profits as a result of higher yields from production of a high-quality marketable commodity. Other benefits include the following: the use of granular formulations of Furadan eliminates exposure of mixers/applicators to more toxic liquid pesticides, the need for less foliar pesticides because of the systemic activity of Furadan, reduced exposure to people, plants, and animals offsite because drift is eliminated with soil application of Furadan granules, reduced impact to valuable

TABLE 10. Acute Oral LD$_{50}$ (in mg/kg) for the Technical grades of Several Insecticides to Five Avian Species[a]

	Coturnix Quail	Common Pigeon	Starling	Common Grackle	Red-Winged Blackbird
Organophosphate					
Chlorpyrifos	13.3	10	75	5.62	13.3M
(Lorsban)	(7.5–23.7)[b]	(5.62–17.8)	(NC)[c]	(3.16–10.0)	
Fensulfothion	1.78F	0.56	0.56	0.42	0.24M
(Dasanit)	(1.00–3.16)	(0.32–1.00)	(0.32–1.00)	(NC)	(NC)
Ethoprop	7.50F	13.3	7.50	10.0	4.21M
(Mocap)	(NC)	(NC)	(NC)	(5.6–17.8)	(NC)
Carbamate					
Carbofuran	3.16F	1.33	5.62	1.33	0.42M
	(1.78–5.62)	(NC)	(3.16–10.0)	(NC)	(NC)

[a]The birds are mixed sexes unless specified as F or M.
[b]Numbers in parentheses are confidence intervals with $p = 0.05$.
[c]NC—not calculated.
Source: Schafer and Brunton (67).

beneficial insect populations, which are often severely impacted by foliar pesticides, less use of a multitude of pesticides since Furadan has a broad spectrum of activity, and fewer applications of Furadan granules are needed since it does the same job as several alternative foliar pesticides that are applied repeatedly.

6 ECOTOXICOLOGY HAZARD ASSESSMENT

6.1 Aquatic Organisms

Laboratory studies indicate that carbofuran is both acutely and chronically toxic to fish and aquatic invertebrates. However, laboratory studies expose organisms to constant, continuous concentrations of the material, thus exemplifying worst-case conditions. Aquatic organisms in the natural environment are rarely if ever exposed to constant concentrations of any foreign chemical, especially carbofuran. As a result of natural dilution and degradation, the half-life of carbofuran in typical ambient surface waters (at pH 8) is approximately 1 week or less. This is supported by laboratory and field environmental chemistry data. Although carbofuran is acutely toxic to aquatic organisms, based on environmental fate studies, the hazard associated with its long-term exposure should be minimal since it would not remain in the environment long enough to produce the effects noted in the laboratory studies.

6.2 Birds

Laboratory studies indicate that carbofuran is acutely toxic to birds. However, chronic laboratory studies indicate that carbofuran is not cumulatively toxic and it does not affect reproductive performance in birds. These laboratory studies are only a means of estimating relative toxicity; they should not be used alone to assess hazard to birds since field studies at typical use rates are the "real indicators" of potential adverse impacts and population effects. Field studies show a low number of bird mortalities in a limited number of bird species when common application practices are followed. The low number of bird mortalities reported in all field studies (i.e., when carbofuran is used at typical use rates) is not biologically significant if consideration is given to the following: the percentage of naturally occurring mortalities (due to weather, predation, disease, and food supply) in wild bird populations, the incredible reproductive potential of wild birds, and background population trends of birds. Mortality resulting from exposure of birds to carbofuran is a very small number in comparison to the mortality for wild birds as a result of natural causes.

The field studies and population survey studies show that the low number of birds demonstrating acute effects does not result in population reductions of avian species. This is supported by the U.S. EPA's Pesticide Incident Monitoring System reports through September 1979, which do not document any significant incidents to wild birds resulting from the use of Furadan granules on agronomic crops. Furthermore, Furadan granules have been registered for use since 1969 without the citing of a major avian incident on agronomic crops such as corn, sorghum, or rice.

Based on the available biological/toxicological information it may be concluded that (i) carbofuran exposure will not produce significant changes in populations of wild birds, and (ii) the low number of raptor mortalities related to carbofuran shows that the potential for secondary poisoning is minimal.

Therefore, carbofuran exposure does not pose an unreasonable hazard to nontarget birds on agricultural crops.

REFERENCES

1. National Research Council of Canada, *Carbofuran: Criteria for Interpreting the Effects of its use on Environmental Quality.* NRC Associate Committee on Scientific Criteria for Environmental Quality, 1979.

2. G. M. Booth, M. W. Carter, C. D. Jorgensen, C. M. White, and R. C. Whitmore, *Effects of Furadan Formulations 10G and 15G on Avian Populations Associated with Cornfields.* A study conducted by Brigham Young University for FMC Corporation. Discussed in the "Special Review Position Document I" and in the FMC response to this document.

3. F. Bergmann, I. B. Wilson, and D. Nachmansohn, Acetylcholinesterase. IX. Structural features determining the inhibition by amino acids and related compounds. *J. Biol. Chem.* **186**, 693–703 (1950).

4. R. J. Kuhr and H. W. Dorough, *Carbamate Insecticides: Chemistry, Biochemistry and Toxicology.* CRC Press, Cleveland, OH, 1976.

5. R. D. Obrien, *Insecticides: Action and Metabolism.* Academic Press, New York, 1967.

6. E. Reiner and W. N. Aldridge, Effects of pH on inhibition and spontaneous reactivation of acetylcholinesterace treated with esters of phosphoric acids and of carbamic acids. *Biochem. J.* **105**, 171–179 (1967).

7. A. J. Ryan, The metabolism of pesticidal carbamates. *CRC Crit. Rev. Toxicol.* **1**, 33–54 (1971).

8. H. W. Dorough, Metabolism of Furadan (NIA-10242) in rats and houseflies. *J. Agric. Food Chem.* **16**, 319–325 (1968).

9. T. C. Marshall and H. W. Dorough, Biliary excretion of carbamate insecticides in the rat. *Pestic. Biochem. Physiol.* **11**, 56–63 (1979).

10. R. L. Metcalf, C. Fukuto, C. Collins, K. Borek, S. Abd-El-Aziz, R. Munoz, and C. C. Cassil, Metabolism of 2,2-dimethyl-2,3-dihydrobenzofuranyl-7-N-methylcarbamate (Furadan) in plants, insects and mammals. *J. Agric. Food Chem.* **16**, 300–309 (1968).

11. G. W. Ivie and H. W. Dorough, Furadan-^{14}C metabolism in a lactating cow. *J. Agric. Food Chem.* **16**, 849–855 (1968).

12. B. W. Hicks, H. W. Dorough, and R. B. Davis, Fate of carbofuran in laying hens. *J. Econ. Entomol.* **63**, 1108–1111 (1970).

13. S. P. Shrivastava, G. P. Georghion, R. L. Metcalf, and T. R. Fukuto, Carbamate resistance in mosquitos. The metabolism of propoxur by susceptible and resistant larvae of *Culex pipiens fatigans. Bull. W.H.O.* **42**, 931–942 (1970).

14. J. B. Knaak, D. M. Munger, and J. F. McCarthy, The metabolism of Carbofuran alfalfa residue in the rat. *Abstr. Pap., 158th Meet. Am. Chem. Soc.* (1970), Pestic. 16.

15. S. M. Ahdaya, R. J. Monroe, and F. E. Guthrie, Absorption and distribution of intubated insecticides in fasted mice. *Pestic. Biochem. Physiol.* **16**, 38–46 (1981).

16. P. W. Ferguson, M. S. Dey, S. A. Jewell, and R. I. Krieger, Carbofuran metabolism and toxicity in the rat. *Fundam. Appl. Toxicol.* **4**, 14–21 (1984).

17. P. V. Shah, R. J. Monroe, and F. E. Guthrie, Comparative rates of dermal penetration of insecticides in mice. *Toxicol. Appl. Pharmacol.* **59**, 414–423 (1981).

18. P. W. Ferguson, S. A. Jewell, R. I. Krieger, and O. G. Raabe, Carbofuran disposition in the rat after aerosol inhalation. *Environ. Toxicol. Chem.* **1**, 248–258 (1982).

19. M. A. H. Fahmy, T. R. Fukuto, R. O. Meyers, and R. B. March, The selective toxicity of new N-phosphorothioyl carbamate esters. *J. Agric. Food Chem.* **18**, 793–796 (1970).

20. J. S. Tobin, Carbofuran: A new carbamate insecticide. *J. Occup. Med.* **12**, 16–19 (1970).

21. FMC Corporation, *Furadan Product Manual.* FMC Corporation, Philadelphia, PA, 1986.

22. Personal communication. To Dr Gary Rand.

23. Federal Register, *Fed. Regist.* **50**(219), 46986–46987 (1985).

24. U.S. Environmental Protection Agency, *Summary for Reported Incidents Involving Carbofuran, Pesticide Incident Monitoring*, Rep. No. 109. USEPA, Washington, DC, 1978.

25. I. H. Williams, H. S. Pepin, and M. J. Brown, Degradation of carbofuran by soil microorganisms. *Bull. Environ. Contam. Toxicol.* **15**, 242 (1976).

26. A. Felsot, J. V. Maddox, and W. Bruce, Enhanced microbial degradation of carbofuran in soils with histories of Furadan use. *Bull. Environ. Contam. Toxicol.* **26**, 781–788 (1981).

27. G. M. Rand and J. R. DeProspo, *Environmental Toxicology of Carbofuran.* Presented at the Fourth Annual Meeting of the Society of Environmental Toxicology and Chemistry, 1983.

28. R. J. Ashworth and T. J. Sheets, Metabolism of carbofuran in tobacco. *J. Agric. Food Chem.* **20**, 407–412 (1972).

29. S. K. Kapoor and R. L. Kalra, Uptake and metabolism of carbofuran in maize plants. *J. Food Sci. Technol.* **12**, 227–230 (1975).

30. J. H. Caro, H. P. Freeman, D. E. Gloteflety, N. C. Turner, and W. M. Edwards, Dissipation of soil incorporated carbofuran in the field. *J. Agric. Food Chem.* **21**, 1010–1015 (1973).

31. W. W. Johnson and M. T. Finley, Handbook of acute toxicity of chemicals to fish and aquatic invertebrates. Summaries of toxicity tests conducted at Columbia National Fisheries Research Laboratory, 1965-78. *U.S. Fish Wildl. Serv., Resour. Publ.* **137** (1980).

32. W. A. Brungs, R. A. Carlson, W. B. Horning, II, H. H. McCormick, R. L. Spehar, and J. D. Yount, Effects of pollution on freshwater fish. *J. Water Pollut. Control Fed.* **50**, 1582–1637 (1978).

33. K. W. Brown, D. C. Anderson, S. G. Jones, L. E. Deuel, and J. D. Price, The relative toxicity of four pesticides in tap water and water from flooded rice paddies. *Int. J. Environ. Stud.* **14**, 49–54 (1979).

34. S. R. Verma, S. Rani, S. K. Bansal, and R. C. Dalela, Effects of the pesticides thiotox, dichlorvos and carbofuran on the test fish *Mystus vittatus. Water Air Soil Pollut.* **13**, 229–234 (1980).

35. M. L. Cheah, J. W. Avault, Jr., and J. B. Graves, Acute toxicity of selected rice pesticides to crayfish *Procambarus clarkii. Prog. Fish-Cult.* **42**, 169–172 (1980).

36. R. B. Davey, M. V. Meisch, and F. L. Carter, Toxicity of five ricefield pesticides to the mosquito fish, *Gambusia affinis*, and green sunfish, *Lepomis cyanellus*, under laboratory and field conditions. *Environ. Entomol.* **5**, 1053–1056 (1976).

37. S. R. Verma, S. K. Bansal, A. K. Gupta, N. Pal, A. K. Tyagi, M. C. Bhatnagar, V. Kumar, and R. C. Dalela, Bioassay trials with twenty-three pesticides to a fresh water teleost, *Saccobranchus fossilis. Water Res.* **16**, 525–529 (1982).

38. N. K. Dad, S. A. Qureshi, and V. K. Pandya, Acute toxicity of two insecticides to tubificid worms, *Tubifex tubifex and Limnodrilus hoffmeisteri. Environ. Int.* **7**, 361–363 (1982).

39. R. S. Caldwell, Biological effects of pesticides on the dungeness crab. *U.S. Environ. Prot. Agency Rep.* **600/3-77-131** (1977).

40. P. R. Parrish, E. E. Dyar, M. A. Lindberg, C. M. Shanika, and J. M. Enos, Chronic toxicity of methoxychlor, malathian and carbofuran to sheepshead minnows *(Cyprinodon variegatus)*, *U.S. Environ. Prot. Agency Rep.* **600/3-77-059** (1977).

41. H. R. Zakour, Toxicity, uptake and metabolism of the N-methylcarbamate pesticide carbofuran by the freshwater mollusc *Glebula rotundata* (Lamarck). Ph.D. Thesis, Rice University, Houston, TX (1980).

42. W. B. Neeley, D. R. Branson, and G. E. Blau, Partition co-efficient to measure bioconcentration potential of organic chemicals in fish. *Environ. Sci. Technol.* **8**, 1113–1115 (1974).

43. D. Belluck and A. Felsot, Bioconcentration of pesticides by egg masses of the caddis fly, *Triaenodes tardus Milue. Bull. Environ. Contamin. Toxicol.* **26**, 299–306 (1981).

44. R. K. Tucker and D. G. Crabtree, Handbook of toxicity of pesticides to Wildlife. *U.S. Fish Wildl. Serv., Resour. Publ.* **84** (1970).

45. R. H. Hudson, R. K. Tucker, and M. A. Haegele, Effect of age on sensitivity: Acute oral toxicity of 14 pesticides to mallard ducks of several ages. *Toxicol. Appl. Pharmacol.* **22**, 556–561 (1972).

46. E. W. Schafer, Jr., W. A. Bowles, Jr., and J. Hurlbert, The acute oral toxicity, repellency, and hazard potential of 998 chemicals to one or more species of wild and domestic birds. *Arch. Environ. Contam. Toxicol.* **12**, 355–382 (1983).

47. M. Sherman and E. Ross, Acute and subacute toxicity of Japanese quail to the Carbamate insecticides, carbofuran and SD 8530. *Poult. Sci.* **48**, 2013–2018 (1968).

48. E. F. Hill, R. G. Heath, J. W. Spann, and J. S. Williams, Lethal dietary toxicities of environmental pollutants to birds. *U.S. Fish Wildl. Serv., Spec. Sci. Rep.: Wildl.* **191** (1975).

49. E. F. Hill and M. B. Camardese, Subacute toxicity testing with young birds: Response in relation to ages and interest variability of LC_{50} estimates. *ASTM Spec. Tech. Publ.* **STP 757**, 41–65 (1982).

50. R. Balcomb, R. Stevens, and C. Bowen, II, Toxicity of 16 granular insecticides to wild-caught songbirds. *Bull. Environ. Contam. Toxicol.* **33**, 302–307 (1984).

51. D. C. Erbach and J. J. Tollefson, Granular insecticide application for corn rootworm control. *Trans. ASAE* **26**, 696–699 (1983).

52. W. Keil, Investigations on food of house and tree-sparrows in a cereal growing area during winter. In S. C. Kendeigh and J. Panowski, Eds., *Productivity, Population Dynamics and Systematics of Granivorous Birds.* PWN-Polish Scientific Publications, Warsaw, 1973, p. 253.

53. R. Eisler, Carbofuran hazards to fish, wildlife, and invertebrates: A synoptic review. *U.S. Fish Wildl. Serv., Rep.* **PB 86-12688**, 5 (1985).

54. C. S. Robbins, D. Bystrak, and P. J. Geissler, *The Breeding Bird Survey: Its First Fifteen Years, 1965–1979.* U.S. Fish and Wildlife Service, Laurel, MD, 1986.

55. R. A. Dolbeer and R. A. Stehn, Population status of blackbirds and starlings in North America, 1966–1981. In D. J. Decker, Ed., *Proceedings of the First Eastern Wildlife Damage Control Conference.* Itaca, NY, 1983, p. 51.

56. R. Balcomb, C. A. Bowen, II, D. Wright, and M. Law, Effects on Wildlife of at-planting corn applications of granular carbofuran. *J. Wildl. Manage.* **48**, 1353–1359 (1984).

57. E. W. Schafer, Potential primary and secondary hazards of avicides. In D. O. Clark, Ed., *Proceedings of the Eleventh Vertebrate Pest Conference.* University of California, Davis, 1984, p. 217.

58. U.S. Fish and Wildlife Service, *Nongame Migratory Bird Species with Unstable or Decreasing Population Trends in the United States.* Report prepared by the Office of Migratory Bird Management and Patuxent Wildlife Research Center, U.S. Fish and Wildlife Service, Washington, DC, 1982.

59. N. A. Overgard, D. F. Walsh, G. D. Hertel, L. R. Braber, R. E. Major, and J. E. Gates, Evaluation of modified Powr-till seeder soil incorporation to provide insect control and minimize bird mortality. *U.S. Fish Wildl. Serv., Res. Publ.* **R8-TP3** (1983).

60. E. L. Flickinger, K. A. King, W. F. Stout, and M. M. Mohn, Wildlife hazards from Furadan 3G applications to rice in Texas. *J. Wildl. Manage.* **44**, 190–197 (1980).

61. S. J. Kleinert, *A Study on Potential Hazard of Insecticide Granules to Birds.* A paper presented for the 28th Annual Wisconsin Pest Control Conference with Industry, Madison, WI, 1974.

62. I. Newton, *Population Ecology of Raptors.* Buteo Books, SD, 1979.

63. H. Mendelssohn and U. Paz, Mass mortalities of birds of prey caused byazodrin, an organophosphate insecticide. *Biol. Conserv.* **11**, 163–170 (1970).

64. W. E. C. Todd, *Birds of Western Pennsylvania.* Univ. of Pittsburg Press, Pittsburg, PA, 1940.

65. S. F. Cohen, The distribution of the Western redshouldered hawk (*Buteo lineatus elegans* (assin)). M.A. Thesis, California State College, Long Beach (1970).

66. E. F. Hill and M. B. Camardese, Toxicity of anticholinesterase insecticides to birds: Technical grade versus granular formulations. *Ecotoxicol. Environ. Saf.* **8**, 551–563 (1984).

67. E. W. Schafer and R. B. Brunton, Indicator bird species for toxicity determination: Is the technique usable in test method development? *ASTM Spec. Tech. Publ.* **STP 680**, 157–168 (1979).

68. J. A. Mills, Some observations on the effects of field applications of fensulfothion and parathion on bird and mammal populations. *Proc. N.Z. Ecol. Soc.* **20**, 65–71 (1973).

69. E. F. Hill and V. M. Mendenhall, Secondary poisoning of barn owls with famphur, an organophosphate insecticide. *J. Wildl. Manage.* **44**, 676–681 (1980).

70. D. H. White, K. A. King, C. A. Mitchell, E. F. Hill, and T. G. Lamont, Parathion causing secondary poisoning in a Laughing Gull breeding colony. *Bull. Environ. Contam. Toxicol.* **23**, 281–284 (1974).

28

Examination of Potential Risks from Exposure to Dioxin in Sludge Used to Reclaim Abandoned Strip Mines

Russell E. Keenan, Mary M. Sauer, Frank H. Lawrence, Elizabeth R. Rand, and David W. Crawford
Envirologic Data Incorporated, Portland, Maine

1   INTRODUCTION

The production of pulp and paper uses several standard manufacturing processes in which water is used as a medium of transport, a cleaning agent, a solvent or mixer, and an agent in the fiber-to-fiber bonding reaction during paper manufacture. Throughout these processes, wastewaters are generated, recycled, and eventually discharged to the mill's waste treatment plant (1).

The pulp and paper mill described in this case study is typical of many such facilities in that it treats approximately 28 million gallons of waste process water per day (2). The primary wastewater treatment used by this mill involves a sedimentation process. The solids produced from sedimentation are called primary sludge.

Secondary water treatment begins with the addition of nitrogen and phosphorus to the wastewater after much of the fiber and other solids have been removed in the primary clarification process (3). The added nitrogen and phosphorus support microorganisms that use the organic matter in sludge as a carbon source. This activity increases the microbial mass that is settled out and, in most processes, is known as activated sludge. After dewatering, the material is called secondary sludge. In this case, the primary and secondary sludges are combined and dewatered to approximately 27–30% solids content. Each day, this process results in the generation of approximately 800 wet tons of dewatered paper mill sludge.

Agricultural land application of sludge as a low-cost fertilizer and soil conditioner has been a valuable, accepted practice for a number of years (4). Sludge contains nutrients that are required for plant growth—namely, nitrogen, phosphorus, potassium, calcium, and minor trace elements. Sludge is high in organic matter, which when added to the soil improves both its structure and water-holding capacity. In addition, the fibrous nature of a paper mill sludge retards runoff and erosion.

The sludge produced from this Midwestern pulp and paper mill is composed primarily of cellulose fiber, clay, lime, and other materials used in pulp and paper manufacturing and possesses properties making it an excellent soil substitute for reclaiming abandoned mine lands (2, 3). Sludge may be applied directly to the mine land surface with no incorporation (typically on steep grades) or may be incorporated with mine spoil to a depth of about 6 in. The amended spoil is seeded with grasses and legumes. Application of the paper mill sludge to the acidic spoil supports vegetative growth and acts to neutralize acidic conditions that often exist on mine lands (3).

Recently, trace concentrations of 2, 3, 7, 8-tetrachlorodibenzo-p-dioxin (2, 3, 7, 8-TCDD) were measured in sludge samples from this mill. Levels of 2, 3, 7, 8-TCDD in three sludge samples taken prior to land application ranged from none detected to approximately 10 parts per trillion (ppt) on a dry weight basis (2). The 2, 3, 7, 8-TCDD congener is one of a family of 75 polychlorinated dibenzo-p-dioxins (PCDDs) and 135 related polychlorinated dibenzofurans (PCDFs) (5). To date, only one sludge sample from this mill has been tested for other PCDD and PCDF congeners. Results of the PCDD and PCDF analyses on sludge samples are summarized in Table 1.

The presence of 2, 3, 7, 8-TCDD and other congeners in sludge used for mine reclamation has raised concerns over the potential public health impacts. Concerns have been based principally on 2, 3, 7, 8-TCDD's persistence in the environment, its long biological half-life in mammals (including humans), and its high acute toxicity and carcinogenicity in laboratory animals (5–9). Assessment of the potential risks related to PCDDs and PCDFs in sludge is clearly important to the future of the mine reclamation program and to the paper industry as it seeks environmentally sound disposal options.

Risk assessment, as defined by the National Academy of Sciences, is the characterization of the probability of potentially adverse health effects from human exposures to

TABLE 1. Results of PCDD and PCDF Analysis of Sludge Samples Taken Prior to Land Application: Dry Weight Basis (ppt)

	Sample		
Congener	1	2[a]	3
2, 3, 7, 8-TCDD	5.0	ND[b] (28.5)	10.7
Total PeCDDs		ND (26.7)	
Total HxCDDs		ND (24.5)	
Total HpCDDs		ND (111)	
Total OCDDs		273	
2, 3, 7, 8-TCDF[c]		101	
Total PeCDFs		ND (36.3)	
Total HxCDFs		ND (36.3)	
Total HpCDFs		ND (72.9)	
Total OCDFs		ND (246)	

[a]Dry weight figures for all groups except 2, 3, 7, 8-TCDD were calculated from wet weight figures provided by laboratory using a factor based on relations between 2, 3, 7, 8-TCDD dry weight and wet weight laboratory results.
[b]ND = none detected. Numerals in parentheses are the limits of detection.
[c]May include contributions from other TCDF isomers.

environmental hazards (10). The risk assessment process is usually divided into four major steps: hazard identification, dose–response assessment, exposure assessment, and risk characterization (10, 11).

Hazard identification is the process of determining whether exposure to an agent can cause an increase in the incidence of a health condition or effect (10). A qualitative assessment, it contains a weight-of-evidence review of the relevant biological and chemical information to determine whether or not an agent may pose a hazard (11).

Dose–response assessment is the process of characterizing the relation between the dose of an agent and the incidence of an adverse health effect in exposed populations (10). Oftentimes, an extrapolation must be made from high to low doses and from animal to human exposures. In accordance with the U.S. Environmental Protection Agency's (EPA's) Guidelines for Carcinogenic Risk Assessment (11), the dose–response assessment should describe and justify the methods of extrapolation and provide a description of the uncertainty inherent in these methods.

Exposure assessment is the process of measuring or estimating the intensity, frequency, and duration of human exposures to an agent in the environment. The exposure assessment may estimate either actual or hypothetical exposures. In general, the exposure assessment describes the magnitude, duration, timing, and route of exposure; the size, nature, and subpopulations of humans exposed; and the uncertainties in all estimates.

Risk characterization is the process of obtaining a quantitative estimate of risk (11). The risk characterization step is performed by combining the exposure and dose–response assessments, including the uncertainties identified in the preceding steps. The discussion of the underlying assumptions and associated uncertainties provides insight into the degree to which the numerical estimates are likely to reflect the true magnitude of human risk.

In this investigation the EPA's Guidelines for Carcinogen Risk Assessment (11) were followed as a general framework and guide for conducting the study. The assessment of carcinogenic risk from exposure to 2, 3, 7, 8-TCDD in the sludge is the principal focus of this analysis. Nearly all risk assessments to date have indicated that when the concerns about cancer are resolved, the potential risk posed by 2, 3, 7, 8-TCDD's other toxicities are also de minimis (insignificant). The acute hazard is not an issue because exposure to the low levels of 2, 3, 7, 8-TCDD in the sludge are well below acutely toxic levels.

This study assesses the potential risk for the extreme and highly improbable case of a family "homesteading" on a mine site area reclaimed with sludge. This analysis is based on the highly improbable scenario of people possibly building homes on a reclaimed mine site area at some point in the future. If this were to take place, individuals might reside year-round on the reclaimed mine site and could potentially use this land to raise dairy and beef cattle, hunt game, and raise a garden crop—for a lifetime of 70 years. At the present time, the exposures depicted in this report exist solely as hypothetical ones that might be possible. In short, individuals are not known to be currently exposed through these routes or at the levels described in this report.

Lifetime incremental cancer risks were calculated based on the assumption that 2, 3, 7, 8-TCDD and its equivalents in the sludge are at an upper-limit concentration of 35 ppt. The basis for this figure is the only complete congener analysis of sludge from this mill and a calculation of toxic equivalency using the interim toxicity equivalence procedures of the U.S. EPA (12). The toxicity equivalence approach is a hazard weighting scheme whereby PCDD and PCDF congeners are each assigned a toxicity equivalence factor (TEF) relating the toxicity of a particular congener to the toxicity of 2, 3, 7, 8-TCDD (termed TCDD for the remainder of this chapter) (12).

In order to calculate the TCDD toxic equivalents level discussed above, a value of one-half of the detection limit was assumed for nondetectable congeners, rather than assuming a value of zero. The EPA (12) procedures do not discuss a methodology for calculating TEFs when the substance is not detected. The method used in this analysis conservatively assumes that some level of the substance is present and arbitrarily sets that level at one-half of the detection limit when it is not detectable. In addition, it was assumed that all congeners in each homologue group contained chlorine substitutions at the 2, 3, 7, and 8 positions. This assumption provides an upper-bound, most conservative estimate of toxicity (12).

In addition to developing lifetime incremental cancer risk estimates for exposures to a TCDD equivalent concentration of 35 ppt in the sludge, numerical results of the risk assessment were expressed as concentrations of TCDD equivalents in the sludge and soil corresponding to a preselected maximum incremental lifetime cancer risk of 1 in 1 million (1×10^{-6}). For each route of exposure, these calculated concentrations of TCDD equivalents in sludge or soil are called *virtually safe concentrations*. Each virtually safe concentration was estimated to result in a human exposure no greater than the virtually safe dose for TCDD and its equivalents. The 1×10^{-6} risk level was selected to represent a level of acceptable or de minimis risk to the general population.

Several composite scenarios were also developed to show the risk for an individual who may incur more than one route of exposure. The probability of lifetime exposures through the routes examined are discussed along with the uncertainties and conservatism of the risk assessment approach.

Currently, federal regulatory standards do not exist for dioxin in soils or sludges. A number of reports, however, have sought to address the issue of acceptable levels of dioxin in soil based on a risk assessment approach. Kimbrough et al. (13) of the Centers for Disease Control (CDC) determined that a concentration of 1 ppb TCDD in residential soil is a reasonable level at which to begin consideration of action to limit human exposure. Soil concentrations of TCDD ranging from 6.2 to 79 ppt were projected to produce maximum allowable residues in beef, pork, and milk (13). Paustenbach et al. (14) evaluated the use of the CDC approach to set limits for TCDD in residential soil and soil within industrial areas, and they found that soil concentrations of TCDD considerably in excess of 1 ppb should be acceptable. Fries (15) reexamined the potential health risks from dioxin in sludges applied to agricultural lands. Eschenroeder et al. (16) examined the human health risks related to soil amended with sewage sludge contaminated with PCDDs and PCDFs, which originated as impurities of pentachlorophenol. The U.S. EPA (17) also has developed a methodology for estimating human exposure and cancer risk related to TCDD-contaminated soil.

Several states have recently promulgated or are developing standards or guidelines for dioxin in sludges and soils (18–20). The state of Maine (18) adopted a maximum allowable concentration limit in land-applied sludge of 250 ppt TCDD equivalents. The maximum allowable soil concentration limit for sites where sludges are landspread was set at 27 ppt TCDD equivalents. The Ohio EPA (19) has set a maximum concentration limit of 100 ppt TCDD equivalents in soil in its guidelines for the land application of paper mill sludge.

We have assessed the human health risks and impacts on terrestrial wildlife associated with exposure to dioxin from the land application of wastewater treatment plant sludges in the state of Maine (21–23). The Maine Department of Environmental Protection evaluated these analyses for the purpose of setting dioxin standards (18). In support of state regulatory proceedings in the Midwest, Envirologic Data (24) assessed the potential risks to human health associated with exposure to dioxin in sludge used to reclaim abandoned strip mines. This chapter describes a revision of that assessment. Results of the analysis presented in this chapter are examined in light of recent regulatory action and the findings of some of the studies described above.

2 HAZARD IDENTIFICATION

2.1 Physical and Chemical Properties

An understanding of TCDD's physical and chemical properties is important in evaluating the environmental behavior of dioxin in soil and sludge. TCDD has a molecular weight of 322. It is practically insoluble in water (25) but is slightly soluble in most organic solvents (26). TCDD is therefore considered a lipophilic compound, exhibiting a higher degree of solubility in fats and oils than in water, evident in TCDD's high octanol–water partition coefficient (K_{ow}) (25). Because TCDD is lipophilic, it will tend to accumulate in fatty tissues of exposed organisms (27). TCDD also displays a high soil–water partition coefficient (K_{oc}) (25), suggesting that TCDD in soil is strongly sorbed to soil particles, rather than being washed out with percolating water. TCDD is fairly stable to the action of acids, bases, oxidation, reduction, and heat (5). It is susceptible to photodegradation in the presence of ultraviolet light (28, 29). Although TCDD exhibits a very low vapor pressure (2.02×10^{-7} Pa at 25°C), this compound demonstrates volatility at ambient soil temperatures (30).

2.2 Animal Health Effects

The toxicity of TCDD in animals has been extensively examined in a number of acute, subchronic, and chronic studies (13). TCDD is absorbed through the gastrointestinal (GI) tract with absorption fractions reported to range from 50 to 86% in feeding and gavage experiments, depending on the vehicle matrix (31–34). Soil-borne TCDD typically is absorbed by the GI tract to a lesser extent (35–39).

Once absorbed, TCDD is rapidly distributed to tissues with a high lipid content and is typically found localized in the liver or adipose (fat) tissue, depending on the species (40). Excretion of TCDD is slow, with the elimination half-life in animals reported to range from about 10 days for the hamster (34) to about 1 year for the monkey (41).

The acute toxicity of TCDD exhibits more than a 1000-fold range of response among different species. The acute LD_{50} in guinea pigs is reported to be 0.6 μg/kg body weight compared to a range of 1157–5051 μg/kg in the hamster (6). Symptoms of acute lethal poisoning have included severe weight loss and thymic atrophy with death occurring up to 47 days after exposure (42, 43). TCDD has been shown to cause an acnegenic skin response in certain species (42). Hepatic toxicity is a prominent component of TCDD toxicity in rats, mice, and rabbits (42). TCDD also has the potential to alter significantly the immune response in animals (44).

TCDD is a potent inducer of microsomal enzymes including aryl hydrocarbon hydroxylase (AHH) (13, 42, 45). Enzyme induction is a very sensitive, yet nonspecific, indicator of dioxin exposure. TCDD binds to the Ah receptor, a soluble cytosolic protein within the cell, with the Ah receptor–TCDD complex then entering the nucleus and initiating enzyme induction (13, 45–47). The Ah-receptor-mediated model has been postulated to have a role in the toxicity of TCDD (45–48). In addition, interactions between the TCDD–Ah receptor complex and an epidermal growth factor (EGF) receptor may play a role in the toxicity of TCDD (49, 50).

TCDD has induced teratogenic, fetotoxic, and other reproductive-related effects in mice, rats, and monkeys (13, 51,52). TCDD has demonstrated a lack of mutagenic activity in virtually all tests (53).

TCDD is carcinogenic in rats and mice and induces a number of different tumor types, although the liver is the primary target tissue (7, 8). TCDD has been shown to be a potent promoter of liver tumors in the rat (54). TCDD also has been shown to be a tumor promoter in the skin of hairless mice (55). There is little evidence to suggest that TCDD acts as a tumor initiator (13, 47, 53–55).

2.3   Human Health Effects

The health effects of TCDD in animals are well documented; however, their applicability to predicting human health effects is unclear. The available data on human exposure is more abundant than for most chemicals, and it comes primarily from occupational exposures and industrial accidents (56). The levels of TCDD to which people were exposed are much greater than those that could typically be encountered in the environment. The interpretation of many of these studies is difficult because of the uncertainty regarding the level of exposure and by concomitant exposures to other chemicals (56).

The half-life of TCDD in humans is not known precisely, but Poiger and Schlatter (57) have calculated a half-life of about 5 years based on a study involving a single human volunteer. Nearly complete absorption of TCDD from the gastrointestinal tract was demonstrated in this study. Jones et al. (58) cited the data by Poiger and Schlatter (57) as evidence that the effective retention period for TCDD is much longer than 1 year; although it is unlikely to be much longer than 5 years.

Chloracne is the most consistent adverse effect in humans and is the hallmark of exposure to TCDD (59). This effect has been observed in cases of both acute and chronic exposure to TCDD in significant concentrations and can be induced following systemic uptake or dermal exposure (42, 59). Chloracne can be caused by exposure to numerous other chlorinated aromatic hydrocarbons (13), although TCDD appears to be the most potent chloracnegen (59). The American Medical Association (56) noted that workplace exposures involving substances like 2, 4, 5-T and its contaminant TCDD have led to definable and measurable effects on specific organ systems. Health effects that have been observed in individuals exposed to substances contaminated with TCDD include porphyria cutanea tarda, hyperpigmentation, hirsutism, altered liver function, and neurological problems (60–63). Generally, these reports are derived from case histories or clinical surveys in which the incidence in control groups was not assessed and exposure to other chemicals occurred. In addition, most workplace exposures have involved high concentrations of TCDD as a result of production processes, leaks, or explosions.

A number of epidemiological studies have been conducted on persons exposed to TCDD from industrial accidents, occupational contact, or herbicide use. Reviews of the epidemiologic data base can be found in EPA (52), AMA (56), and NCASI (64). Case–control studies of workers in Sweden exposed to phenoxy herbicides or chloro-phenols reported a statistically significant increased risk of soft-tissue sarcomas and malignant lymphomas (65–67). These results have not been confirmed in other epidemio-logic studies of herbicide exposure and were recently considered too inconclusive to affect regulatory policy dramatically (68). A cohort study of Swedish agricultural and forestry workers did not show a significantly increased relative risk of soft-tissue sarcoma when compared to Swedish men employed in other industries, even though the agricultural and forestry workers' exposures to phenoxy acids are assumed to be greater than those of other occupational groups (69).

New Zealand case–control studies of soft-tissue sarcoma found no evidence for a relation with occupational exposure to phenoxy herbicides (70–72). The authors concluded that the New Zealand findings suggest that it is unlikely that 2, 4, 5-T, or its contaminant TCDD, causes soft-tissue sarcoma in humans at the exposure levels encountered in ground spraying (72). Pearce et al. (73) reported that agricultural workers were at increased risk of developing non-Hodgkin's lymphoma in a New Zealand case–control study. In the second interview phase of this study, no significant difference between cases and controls were observed regarding potential exposure to phenoxy herbicides or chlorophenols (74). Hoar et al. (75), in an NCI case–control study of agricultural use of herbicides in Kansas, demonstrated an association between the use of phenoxyacetic acid herbicides, specifically 2, 4,-D, and non-Hodgkin's lymphoma; an association was not found with soft-tissue sarcoma or Hodgkin's disease. However, 2, 4-D does not contain TCDD (75).

Potential reproductive and teratogenic effects also have been examined in studies of individuals exposed to herbicides. In a study of professional herbicide sprayers in New Zealand, Smith et al. (76) found no statistically significant increase in the risk of miscarriages or birth defects.

While epidemiologic studies of Vietnam veterans exposed to Agent Orange and other herbicides are still underway, results of some studies have been reported. Wolfe et al. (77) has reported that the Air Force Ranch Hand study, to date, has provided insufficient evidence to support a cause and effect relation between herbicide exposure and health effects. Kang et al. (78) found no significant association between soft-tissue sarcoma and previous military service in Vietnam, in a case comparison group study. A New York State study was reported to find no statistically significant association between soft-tissue sarcoma and either Vietnam service or general military service (79).

Erickson et al. (80) reported the results of a CDC case–control study as evidence that Vietnam veterans, in general, are at no greater risk than other men at fathering babies with serious structural birth defects, when all types of birth defects are considered in the aggregate. An Australian case–control study of veterans reported no association between exposure and adverse pregnancy outcome and suggested that the risk of siring a malformed child was no higher for Australian Vietnam veterans compared to other Australian males (81–83). The AMA (56) has concluded that, while studies are still underway, results to date on Vietnam veterans exposed to Agent Orange have not demonstrated a clear relation between exposure and serious illness.

Workers in the chemical manufacturing industry have also been the subject of epidemiologic studies. Suskind (59) reported results of a study of workers exposed to TCDD during an accident involving 2, 4, 5-T manufacturing at a chemical plant in Nitro, West Virginia. An increased risk was not found on a long-term basis for overall mortality, cardiovascular disease, hepatic disease, renal disease, central or peripheral nerve problems, reproductive problems, or birth defects among either exposed workers or among workers who developed chloracne. Based on a review of dioxin exposure studies, Suskind (59) indicated that sufficient exposure to TCDD can induce chloracne, but systemic effects such as peripheral neuritis and transient hepatic dysfunction have occurred only in association with, and subsequent to, chloracne. A Dow Chemical Company cohort mortality study of 2192 chemical workers with potential occupational exposure to TCDD, and/or other higher chlorinated dioxins, found no statistically significant increased overall mortality or cancer mortality relative to mortality among U.S. white males (84). In a survey of reproductive events of wives of chemical workers exposed to chlorinated dioxins, overall, no statistically significant associations were found between adverse pregnancy outcomes and paternal dioxin exposure (85).

In conclusion, the only consistently demonstrated long-term health effect related to TCDD exposure has been chloracne. The epidemiologic evidence relating exposure to substances contaminated with TCDD and cancer in humans has been termed contradictory (86). The types of cancer for which the strongest positive associations have been reported include soft-tissue sarcoma (66, 67) and malignant lymphoma (65). Other epidemiologic studies, however, have not confirmed the positive association reported between phenoxy herbicide or chlorophenol exposure and soft-tissue sarcoma or lymphoma shown in Swedish studies (69–72, 74). It is not appropriate to conclude that herbicides or chlorophenols containing TCDD cause cancer in humans on the basis of results of several Swedish studies due to the lack of confirming evidence from other epidemiologic studies and the limitations associated with these studies.

2.4   TCDD Levels in Adipose Tissue

Numerous studies have reported background levels of TCDD in the adipose tissue of individuals with no known exposure to TCDD (87–92). These observations suggest that exposure to TCDD is widespread in the populations tested; however, the data are variable with some nondetectable levels. Mean background levels have been reported to range from about 3 to 10 ppt (87–89, 92). Sielken (93) found that evidence from North America suggests that TCDD levels in human adipose tissue have a log–normal distribution and are positively correlated with age. Sielken (93) also notes that among the observed U.S. background TCDD levels in adipose tissue, more than 10% were greater than 12 ppt.

TCDD levels in adipose tissue of Vietnam veterans were reported to range from a few ppt to as high as 99 ppt in fat, with a mean of 8.3 ppt (94). Samples of fat tissues from citizens of southern Vietnam, believed to have been exposed to Agent Orange, contained levels of TCDD ranging from 4 to 79 ppt, with a mean of 22 ppt (95). TCDD levels measured in blood fat of 10 veterans who handled Agent Orange in the late 1960s averaged 48 ppt (96). Preliminary results of blood fat measurements in 444 Vietnam veterans, who served in areas where Agent Orange was sprayed, showed a median level of TCDD of 3.8 ppt. This figure was virtually identical to the non-Vietnam veteran median of 3.9 ppt (97). The biological or medical significance of dioxin in fat tissues in both unexposed and exposed individuals is not known at this time.

3   DOSE–RESPONSE ASSESSMENT

3.1   Cancer Potency Determination

The relation between the dose of TCDD and the probability of inducing a carcinogenic effect is characterized in this chapter. Carcinogenic incidence data resulting from high doses of TCDD administered to animals in laboratory experiments were extrapolated to low-level human exposures. Dose–response extrapolation is only one component of the quantitative risk assessment process (11). Yet it is clear that choices, assumptions, and judgments made in the dose–response assessment have a significant impact on the results of the risk assessment, and hence on risk management decisions (14, 98). Therefore, consideration of the validity of the dose–response extrapolation is addressed in this analysis.

The EPA (52), the Centers for Disease Control (13), and the Food and Drug Administration (99) have performed risk assessments of TCDD. The EPA and CDC used the multistage model (100) to estimate the dose–response relation for low-level human exposures based on data obtained in rodents at high doses. In contrast, the FDA (99) employed a linear interpolation model. Each of these models assumes that there is no threshold for carcinogenesis; that is, any dose, no matter how small, will result in some level of risk (53). The basic purpose of these models is to estimate the maximum possible linear slope (the 95% upper confidence limit) of the dose–response curve in the low-dose range. This estimated slope constitutes the cancer potency, also termed q_1^* in the multistage model. The larger the value of the cancer potency, the greater the potential to induce cancer at a given dose.

Potency estimates for TCDD have been based on studies of Sprague–Dawley rats fed TCDD in the diet at 0.001–0.1 μg/kg·day (7), Osborne–Mendel rats administered 0.01–0.5 μg/kg·wk, and B6C3F$_1$ mice administered 0.01–0.5 (male) or 0.04–2.0 μg/kg·wk (female) TCDD by gavage (8). Animals administered TCDD exhibited increased incidence of a wide range of tumor types including those of the liver, subcutaneous tissue, tongue, nasal turbinate/hard palate, or lung, depending on the particular study.

The cancer potency figure used by the EPA, 1.56×10^5 (mg/kg·day)$^{-1}$, produced by the multistage model, was based on the geometric mean of two pathologists' (Dr. Kociba and Dr. Squire) interpretations of the tissue slides from the Kociba et al. (7) data for female rats using pooled tumor types. This is the most conservative estimate of TCDD's potency of those calculated by the three agencies (13, 52, 99). It is derived from data on the most sensitive combination of species, strain, and sex of laboratory animals tested. The EPA (52) also has estimated cancer potencies based on the National Toxicology Program/National Cancer Institute studies; but none was as conservative as that mentioned above.

The CDC (13) examined bioassay data from NTP (8) and Kociba et al. (7). The CDC did not report actual potency figures in their analysis; rather, they reported virtually safe doses (VSDs) for a range of sensitivities (i.e., from the most sensitive species/strain/sex/tumor type combination to the least sensitive species/strain/sex/tumor type combination) (13). We calculated the cancer potencies corresponding to the VSDs reported by the CDC and obtained a range from 7.0×10^2 to 3.6×10^4 (mg/kg·day)$^{-1}$.

In addition to the full range of potency figures calculated from the CDC's VSD data, we also calculated the CDC cancer potency figure corresponding to the combination of the most sensitive tumor type in the least sensitive species, strain, and sex of laboratory animal tested. Specifically, this cancer potency figure was derived by examining the CDC data on VSDs for each of the six subpopulations of laboratory animals tested, Sprague–Dawley female and male rats, Osborne–Mendel female and male rats, and B6C3F$_1$ female and male mice. The lowest of the 95% lower confidence bounds for the VSD for each of the six subpopulations were compared (i.e., the most conservative VSD in each group, therefore the most sensitive tumor type). Of these, the highest VSD was associated with the B6C3F$_1$ female mouse data for lymphoma and leukemia (making this species and sex the least sensitive). We calculated the cancer potency figure associated with this VSD from the CDC analysis, resulting in a potency of 1.8×10^3 (mg/kg·day)$^{-1}$.

The FDA used a cancer potency estimate of 1.75×10^4 (mg/kg·day)$^{-1}$ based on the Kociba et al. (7) rat data to support advisory levels for TCDD in Great Lakes fish. The FDA concluded that fish with levels of 50 ppt TCDD should not be consumed and

TABLE 2. Cancer Potency Figures and Corresponding Virtually Safe Doses (VSDs) for 2, 3, 7, 8-TCDD

	Acceptable Incremental Cancer Risk	Cancer Potency[a] $(mg/kg \cdot day)^{-1}$	VSD[a] $(fg/kg \cdot day)$
EPA	1×10^{-6}	1.56×10^5	6.4
	1×10^{-5}	Same	64
CDC	1×10^{-6}	$3.6 \times 10^4 - 7 \times 10^2$	28–1,400
	1×10^{-5}	Same	280–14,000
FDA	1×10^{-6}	1.75×10^4	57
	1×10^{-5}	Same	570
Estimate used in this analysis:			
	1×10^{-6}	1.7×10^4	60
	1×10^{-5}	Same	600

[a]All figures (cancer potencies or VSDs) calculated from agency data were rounded to two significant figures. For the EPA and FDA, VSDs at acceptable cancer risks of 1×10^{-6} and 1×10^{-5} were calculated from cancer potencies used by the two agencies. For the CDC, cancer potencies were calculated from VSDs. Equation for calculation: acceptable incremental cancer risk = VSD × cancer potency.

25–50 ppt should not be consumed more than twice a month (99, 101). Previous to this analysis, the FDA had used a no observed effect level (NOEL) approach to support development of the advisory levels (102).

A comparison of the cancer potency figures developed by the three agencies reveals considerable differences among the estimates (Table 2). The EPA potency figure exceeds the most conservative CDC figure by a factor of 4 and exceeds the FDA figure by a factor of 9. Yet these particular potency figures were all derived from the same data set, the female rat data of the Kociba et al. (7) study. Even greater differences between estimated potencies can be seen if one compares the EPA potency, $1.56 \times 10^5 (mg/kg \cdot day)^{-1}$, with the lower end of the CDC potency range, $7.0 \times 10^2 (mg/kg \cdot day)^{-1}$. The EPA potency is approximately 223 times larger than this CDC figure.

The differences among the three agencies' cancer modeling analyses are largely due to differences in data interpretation and calculation. The FDA used only the Kociba histopathological diagnosis; the EPA used both the Kociba and Squire results in their analyses, while the more conservative of the CDC figures is based on the Squire results (103). The EPA pooled tumor types, while CDC analyzed each tumor types separately with the liver tumor analysis for female rats comprising the most conservative analysis. Because almost all animals with tumors of any type also had liver tumors, this difference in approach between EPA and CDC has little impact on these agencies' most conservative potency and VSD determinations. While the EPA and FDA used the administered dose in the model, the CDC used the liver TCDD concentration for female rats with liver tumors. The EPA adjusted for high early mortality in female rats while the CDC and FDA did not make this adjustment.

An additional factor that has a large effect on the magnitude of the human cancer potency estimate is the choice of animal to human correction factor. Whereas the EPA extrapolated from rat to human using the assumption that dose per unit body surface area is an equivalent dose between species, the CDC and FDA assumed dose per unit body weight (103). If the EPA had used the same methodology as the CDC and FDA, the EPA cancer potency figure of $1.56 \times 10^5 \,(\text{mg/kg·day})^{-1}$ would have been reduced by a factor of 5.4, resulting in $2.9 \times 10^4 \,(\text{mg/kg·day})^{-1}$, a figure similar to the more conservative CDC estimate.

Based on our consideration of the various analyses, we have identified a best estimate of a reasonably conservative potency for the purpose of this risk assessment. We estimated a cancer potency figure for TCDD by computing the geometric mean of a range of potencies: the EPA potency of $1.56 \times 10^5 \,(\text{mg/kg·day})^{-1}$ and the potency from CDC of $1.8 \times 10^3 \,(\text{mg/kg·day})^{-1}$, which corresponds to the analysis of female mouse data for lymphoma and leukemia. The high end of the range represents the most conservative (EPA) analysis of the female Sprague–Dawley rat tumor data, principally liver tumors, therefore essentially the most sensitive tumor type. The low end of the range represents a slightly less conservative (CDC) analysis of the most sensitive tumor type (lymphoma and leukemia) in the least sensitive species and sex tested, B6C3F$_1$ female mice. The geometric mean cancer potency computed from this range is $1.7 \times 10^4 \,(\text{mg/kg·day})^{-1}$. Our approach is summarized in Fig. 1. For comparison, cancer potency figures developed by the EPA, CDC, and FDA are shown in Fig. 2 and Table 2, along with our geometric mean cancer potency estimate.

Support for our approach is based partly on the premise that TCDD may be less toxic (i.e., less carcinogenic) in humans than in the most sensitive animal species tested. Although limited data are available regarding the differential susceptibility between laboratory animal species and humans, studies by Kligman and Rowe indicate that humans are less sensitive to TCDD's chloracnegenic effects than the rabbit ear (104, 105). Also relevant are the findings of human epidemiologic studies. Although TCDD clearly has been demonstrated to be carcinogenic in laboratory animals, there is little epidemiologic evidence for an association between human exposure to TCDD and cancer.

Additional support for our averaging approach, rather than use of the most conservative EPA potency alone, is based on the appropriateness of adjustments for dose between rodents and humans used in the agency analyses. As explained previously, only the EPA extrapolated from rodent to human cancer potency by applying a surface area scaling factor. The CDC and FDA assumed that dose per unit body weight is the appropriate scaling factor. As a surrogate for relative rates of metabolism between species, the surface area scaling factor is inappropriate for poorly metabolized chemicals such as TCDD. In an interspecies comparison of carcinogenic potency for approximately 70 chemicals, the use of a body weight correction factor gave good interspecies correlations between potencies (106). In our geometric mean approach, we have used one potency based on a surface area scaling factor (EPA) and one potency based on a body weight scaling factor (CDC).

The best estimate cancer potency of $1.7 \times 10^4 \,(\text{mg/kg·day})^{-1}$, computed for this risk assessment, is almost identical to the FDA cancer potency of $1.75 \times 10^4 \,(\text{mg/kg·day})^{-1}$. The FDA potency is based on the Kociba et al. (7) rat study, which employed the most sensitive sex, strain, and tumor type. The FDA extrapolation model assumed a linear dose–response relation between the upper 95% confidence limit on the lowest dose that elicited a significant response and the origin. This method has the advantage that it does not attempt to force a fit to the data. We believe that the FDA cancer potency estimate is fully protective of public health. The similarity of the FDA potency to our best estimate, geometric mean potency, therefore lends additional support to the use of our potency for this risk assessment.

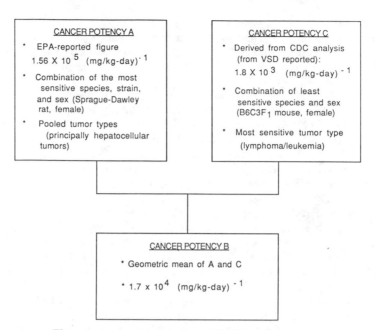

Figure 1. Approach to selection of TCDD cancer potency.

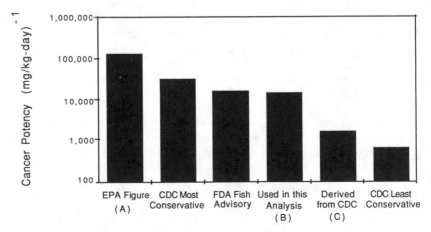

Figure 2. Cancer potency estimates for 2, 3, 7, 8-TCDD.

946

3.2 Appropriateness of Dose–Response Model

The appropriateness of the dose–response analyses used for TCDD is explored in this section. First, Sielken's (98) analysis of the problems associated with the modeling of the Kociba et al. (7) rat data by federal agencies is reviewed. Second, the use of a nonthreshold mathematical model for TCDD by U.S. regulatory agencies is considered, and alternative approaches are briefly discussed.

Sielken's (98) reanalysis of TCDD's virtually safe dose provides support for our selection of a lower cancer potency than that estimated by the EPA. Sielken (98) showed that when the multistage model is fitted to the Kociba et al. (7) data on rat liver tumors, trade-offs inherent in curve fitting may lead to questionable fits in the low-dose area. Estimated tumor response rates, compared to observed response rates, were too large at the lowest nonzero experimental dose level and too small at the intermediate dose level. Sielken showed that the presence or absence of experimental data at the lowest experimental dose produces very little effect on the shape of the fitted model curve and produces only a very small change to the estimated value of the VSD. Sielken identified a saturation-like phenomenon within the dose–response relation at the highest dose level and noted that it is impossible for the multistage model to portray both this phenomenon at the higher doses and the observed nonlinearity at the lowest dose levels. In the fitting process, the behavior of the curve at the lower doses is essentially ignored while the relative flatness of the curve at higher doses is depicted. Sielken (98) excluded the highest dose level from the analysis and developed the fitted model estimate of the VSD (at a 1×10^{-6} risk level) for the probability of hepatocellular neoplastic nodule or carcinoma in a female rat to be 140 pg/kg·day (140,000 fg/kg·day) in the diet. Using the usual confidence limit procedure for the multistage model, Sielken (98) calculated the 95% statistical lower confidence limit for this VSD to be 22 fg/kg·day, which is 6400 times smaller than the fitted model value for the VSD. Sielken noted that the procedure used to construct 95% confidence limits on the VSD is very nonresponsive to the experimental data and that the confidence limits may be very far away from the fitted model values. Sielken's analysis clearly demonstrates that results of mathematical modeling of the TCDD cancer bioassay data are very sensitive to modeling assumptions and that the agency analyses may considerably overestimate TCDD's cancer potency. Sielken's approach has been critically evaluated and discussed in detail (107, 108).

Evidence showing that TCDD may act as a cancer promoter rather than as an initiator suggests that the nonthreshold dose–response assessment used by regulatory agencies in the United States likely overestimates potential carcinogenic risks (53). Carcinogens may roughly be divided into two categories—initiators and promoters. An initiator, if not already electrophilic, undergoes metabolic transformation to an electrophile and reacts covalently with DNA (109). Once a cell is initiated, it incorporates a critical amount of DNA damage into its replicating genome, which may be locked into the cell for as long as the cell line continues to reproduce. A promoter acts to increase the tumorigenic response to an initiator when applied after the initiator (109). Promoters require prolonged and repeated exposure or persistence in the body before tumor formation in animals, whereas for tumor initiators, short-term exposure may cause tumors (53). While tumor initiation is regarded as an irreversible event, tumor promotion may be reversible upon removal of the promoter, when the tumor has not progressed to an advanced state (53).

Explicit in the difference between promoters and initiators is the ability to interact with DNA. TCDD has been shown to be nonmutagenic based on the preponderance of data from bacterial mutagenesis tests and has been shown not to bind to DNA to any appreciable extent (53). These data indicate that TCDD is not genotoxic; that is, it does not interact directly with DNA.

Pitot et al. (54) and Poland et al. (55) have demonstrated TCDD's tumor-promoting activity. Many promoters, including TCDD, affect cellular growth and differentiation and alter a number of cell membrane properties (110). Tumor promoters, in contrast to initiator and genotoxic carcinogens, may display a threshold in their dose response (109). If this is true for TCDD, the multistage model, which assumes a linear nonthreshold response, will overestimate the incremental cancer risk associated with TCDD exposure.

Authorities on TCDD risk assessment have raised the issue of the appropriateness of the use of the multistage model, given that TCDD acts as a promoter. In the CDC's risk assessment of TCDD in residential soil (13), the authors note that the dose–response curve for promoters may not be linear, thus resulting in an overestimate of the risk. They also state, however, that a scientific data base that would allow the use of less conservative models did not exist.

In a recent paper, Shu et al. (53) examined the scientific literature on TCDD's lack of mutagenicity and its impact on risk assessment. The authors show that the mechanism data on TCDD strongly support the hypothesis that tumor development is based on a promotional mechanism and not on initiation. Thus, they believe that risk estimates at low doses using currently formulated linear low-dose extrapolation models are not supported by the scientific evidence on initiation. The authors conclude that alternate means of evaluating TCDD risk should be investigated.

Kolbye (111) noted that linear extrapolation may be appropriate for electrophilic, highly genotoxic compounds, but that it has little meaning for secondary carcinogens, including TCDD. Weisburger and Williams (112) have pointed out the importance of distinguishing between whether a substance acts through a genotoxic or nongenotoxic (epigenetic) mechanism. The action of epigenetic agents usually requires their presence at high levels for a long time and is reversible up to a certain point. The different fundamental mechanisms of operation between genotoxic and epigenetic agents require that distinct types of risk analysis be performed (112).

Recently, the EPA convened a special advisory committee to study dioxin (113). They described TCDD's mechanisms of toxicity as follows:

> There is no evidence that TCDD or its metabolites alter the structure of DNA, but TCDD is carcinogenic in at least two rodent species. It acts as a potent promoting agent in at least two different tissues in two different species, but there is no evidence for initiation activity in any species.

Also pertinent is a statement from the committee's conclusions regarding human health risk assessment:

> Mechanistic models should be used for quantitative risk estimation for TCDD and related compounds. Such methods should consider epidemiological data, sex–species susceptibility, the promoting action of TCDD, and its pharmacokinetic properties in predicting risks for exposed populations.

Based on increasing evidence and support for the threshold model and the lack of evidence for the appropriateness of a nonthreshold model for TCDD, several agencies outside the United States have used the safety factor (threshold) approach and developed allowable daily intakes (ADIs) for TCDD. Shu et al. (53) point out that risk assessments incorporating a threshold approach more accurately reflect the scientific understanding of the mechanism of action of TCDD than those that assume a nonthreshold (initiation) mechanism. Allowable daily intakes are derived from no observed effect levels (NOELs) with application of a safety (uncertainty) factor. The Ontario Ministry of the Environment (5) calculated a maximum allowable daily intake for humans of 10 pg/kg·day based on a NOEL of 1 ng/kg·day (1000 pg/kg·day) and a safety factor of 100. The State Institute of National Health (SINH) in The Netherlands obtained a maximum ADI of 4 pg/kg·day based on a NOEL of 1 ng/kg·day and a safety factor of 250 (114).

The EPA (103), while not using the ADI approach in their risk assessment, calculated an ADI at 1 pg/kg·day based on a LOAEL of 1 ng/kg·day and a safety factor of 1000. The FDA, prior to their linear model approach discussed earlier in this section (99), had originally used a safety factor approach to support advisory levels for TCDD in fish. The FDA (99) calculated a TCDD exposure level of 13 pg/kg·day from consuming fish containing 25 ppt TCDD at the 99th percentile of U.S. fish consumption. The FDA noted that this exposure level was less than $\frac{1}{70}$th of the animal NOEL of 1 ng/kg·day. This approach was used to support 25 ppt TCDD as a "safe" level in Great Lakes fish. The selection of appropriate safety factors has been reviewed by Calabrese (115) and others.

Allowable daily intakes estimated for TCDD generally range from 1 to 10 pg/kg·day (1000 to 10,000 fg/kg·day). These figures can be compared to the full range of agency virtually safe doses, at 1×10^{-6} and 1×10^{-5} cancer risks, of 6.4–14,000 fg/kg·day and to our best estimate VSD of 60–600 fg/kg·day (Table 2).

Based on a comprehensive examination of the data on TCDD, we conclude that the scientific basis for using a linear, nonthreshold model for low-dose risk extrapolation is that the mechanism of TCDD-induced carcinogenicity is not completely understood; therefore, a conservative approach has been adopted by U.S. federal agencies. At the same time, it seems appropriate the U.S. regulatory agencies should press on with the development of alternative threshold models for promoters like TCDD, in the interest of fostering informed risk management decisions.

We have selected a nonthreshold model for use in this risk analysis. Yet, at the same time, we have attempted to develop a reasonable approach to cancer potency determination. Our approach, as outlined in Section 3.1, seems justified based on the following considerations:

- The potential for humans to be less susceptible to TCDD toxicity compared to the most sensitive laboratory animal species tested.
- The questionable fit of the multistage model to the Kociba et al. (7) data set in the low-dose region, possibly resulting in considerable overestimates of TCDD's cancer potency.
- The questionable appropriateness of using the linear nonthreshold model for TCDD, given the evidence that TCDD acts as a cancer promoter.

4 EXPOSURE ASSESSMENT

4.1 Exposure Scenarios

Exposure assessment is the process of measuring or estimating the intensity, frequency, and duration of human exposures to an agent in the environment. Important parameters for estimating exposure include the concentration of the chemical, the degree to which the chemical is free to migrate from the substrate, and the magnitude, duration, and frequency of contact. In addition, it is critical that an estimate be made of the agent's bioavailability through each potential exposure pathway. Potential human absorption and bioavailability of the chemical are functions of many complex variables and are oftentimes poorly defined.

The purpose of this risk analysis, as originally performed to support the development of environmental standards, was to estimate the maximum hypothetical exposure for individuals residing in mine site areas reclaimed with sludge containing dioxin. Exposures were estimated for an individual who resides on a sludge-reclaimed mine site; uses the land for raising dairy and beef cattle; hunts game from contaminated land; raises vegetables; and eats meat, milk, and vegetables from this farm only, for a lifetime of 70 years. At this time, no such individual exists, and it is highly unlikely that this combination of scenarios would ever be realized, even if the land were to be used in this manner.

Exposure scenarios were divided into the following four general categories:

1. *Residential contact*
   Dermal uptake
   Oral uptake of soil
   Dust inhalation
2. *Hunting of game species*
   Wild turkey consumption
   Venison consumption
3. *Milk and beef consumption*
   Cattle grazed on reclaimed mine site
   Cattle fed hay grown on reclaimed mine site
4. *Vegetable consumption* (family garden)
   Corn consumption

The routes of exposure to TCDD for residents are skin contact, soil ingestion, and dust inhalation. These exposure scenarios apply to an individual who resides year-round on a reclaimed mine site and not to an individual who may only occasionally enter the reclaimed mine site area. Less frequent visitation would produce a correspondingly lesser exposure.

Hunting of game species whose territories have overlapped with sludge-reclaimed mine sites may be the most likely scenario of exposure since these areas will, in all probability, return to a natural state. In fact, this may constitute the only source of exposure, particularly if residential or agricultural development does not occur on reclaimed mine areas. White-tailed deer and wild turkey were selected for this analysis based on their importance as game species in the geographical area studied here.

Consumption of milk and beef may be an important route of exposure if cattle are grazed or fed hay grown on reclaimed mine sites. As noted earlier, TCDD is a lipophilic compound (27), which may accumulate in milk or beef fat (13). In addition, crops raised for human consumption on reclaimed mine sites constitute potential sources of exposure. Corn, an above ground crop, was examined in this analysis.

We selected these exposure scenarios to represent a reasonable range of possible exposure pathways of concern. Of course, other game species and crop types also could have been assessed, if there were no limitations on the size and scope of this project.

This analysis did not examine the potential impact on fish because the use of paper mill sludge on the abandoned mine lands serves to minimize surface runoff into bodies of water. This paper mill sludge behaves as a cake sludge, containing at least 20–30% total solids as opposed to a slurry sludge, which contains only 2–8% total solids (116). Cake sludge, fibrous in nature and containing a high percentage of clay and claylike materials, exhibits excellent cohesive properties.

In addition, sludge is high in organic matter, which when added to the soil improves both its structure and water-holding capacity. The beneficial effects of these properties at reducing erosion and sediment losses in soil are well documented (117). Sediment loss has been shown to be inversely related to organic matter content and degree of aggregation. Paper mill sludge may also stabilize soils against erosion forces by protecting the soil surface from raindrop impact.

Nutrient concentrations in runoff water and sediment from sludge-treated soils are generally higher than from untreated soils; yet the total amount of nutrients delivered to a waterway from a sludge application site is likely to be less than that originating from an untreated area (117). This is due to a decrease in the total quantity of sediment transport and erosion from a sludge-amended soil as compared to an untreated area. The ability of paper mill sludge to control erosion and stabilize slopes has been shown at abandoned strip mine reclamation projects where it has been used very successfully for this purpose (118). One study has indicated that a sludge layer can be 99% effective at reducing erosion on roadside plots compared to unprotected control plots based on its ability to reduce runoff velocity and to absorb moisture (119).

4.2 Sludge Application Model

Paper mill sludge is either topdressed or incorporated with native soil when it is applied to agricultural or forest lands. For the reclamation of abandoned strip mines, incorporation of sludge with coal mine spoil to a depth of about 6 in. represents a more typical application practice than direct application to the surface. Direct application (topdressing) is usually limited to steep slopes and in areas where native material is not available for mixing. The soil incorporation method is the one examined in this analysis.

Sludge used for mine reclamation is generally applied at about 100 dry tons/acre (120). At a soil weight of 1000 dry tons/acre·6 in., and assuming a mixing depth of 6 in., application of 100 dry tons sludge/acre results in a mixing rate of 1:9 in the top 6 in. This ratio was factored into the calculation, as was the maximum average TCDD toxic equivalent concentration of 35 ppt in the sludge, to yield an initial TCDD equivalent concentration of 3.5 ppt in the soil.

Exposure estimates presented in the following sections were based on 70 years of exposure, with the exception of a 5-year exposure in the case of soil ingestion by children. An environmental half-life for TCDD of 10 years was used in estimating exposures. Young (121) has suggested that the half-life for TCDD in soil might be about 10–12 years, but recent research suggests that at the soil surface, the half-life is much shorter due to volatilization and photodegradation (30, 122). Half-life considerations are important because human exposure through ingestion, inhalation, and dermal contact is virtually always to the TCDD contained at the soil surface and not to that contained at lower depths (14).

Consideration must be given to the timing of potential exposures relative to sludge application. In the case of hunting, exposure of deer or wild turkey to the sludge-reclaimed

TABLE 3. Description of Sludge and Soil Concentrations of TCDD and Its Equivalents Used in Exposure Assessment

Exposure Category	Sludge TCDD Equivalents Level (ppt)	Initial Soil-TCDD Equivalents Level after Application (ppt)	Initial Soil-TCDD Level at Start of Exposure (ppt)	70-year Average Soil-TCDD Equivalents Level (ppt)	5-year Average Soil-TCDD Equivalents Level (ppt)
Residential contact	35	3.5	3.0	0.65	2.7
Hunting of game species	35	3.5	3.5	0.74	
Milk and beef consumption (grazed)	35	3.5	3.0	0.65	
Milk and beef consumption (hay-fed)	35	3.5	3.0	0.65	
Vegetable consumption	35	3.5	3.0	0.65	

mine site area could occur shortly after application. Therefore, for wildlife, a latency period is not assumed between sludge application and initial exposure. In all other exposure categories, however, some minimum latency period would be expected. For exposure through residential contact, direct grazing of cattle, raising hay for cattle feed, and crops for human consumption, a minimum period of 2 years was assumed before any activity leading to exposure could possibly occur. This represents the period of state control over the reclamation sites (2). In reality, the length of time between sludge application and initial exposure will almost certainly be much greater than 2 years for these exposure categories.

By assuming a half-life of 10 years, 70-year and 5-year average soil concentrations of TCDD and its equivalents were calculated and are shown in Table 3. These average contaminant levels were used in the exposure and risk calculations presented in the following sections.

4.3 Exposure Models

Potential exposures were calculated for an adult weighing 70 kg (154 lb) (123), except for soil ingestion, which was based on a child weighing 17 kg (37 lb) (17). A 70-year exposure period was assumed for all scenarios except soil ingestion, which was assumed to occur only for a child aged 2–6. Soil ingestion by adults was considered to be insignificant, based on a review of the relevant literature by Paustenbach et al. (14). Exposures were calculated as lifetime average daily doses (LADDs). Exposure models and equations are described in the following sections.

4.3.1 Residential Contact. Dermal contact, inhalation, and soil ingestion may contribute to residential contact both indoors and outdoors. Exposure parameters are summarized for these routes in Tables 4–8.

4.3.1.1 Dermal Uptake. In addition to dermal contact with outdoor soil, dermal contact with household dust may contribute to TCDD exposure due to the tracking-in of outdoor soil contaminated with TCDD. It was estimated that household dust con-

TABLE 4. Dermal Uptake

Parameter	Value
Indoor dust–TCDD factor	75% Soil–TCDD level
Outdoor soil contact rate	1 mg/cm^2·day
Indoor dust contact rate	0.03 mg/cm^2·day
Exposed surface area	
Outdoor, age 2–12	Both hands, legs, feet
age 13–70	Both hands, most of forearms
Indoor	Both hands
Exposure duration	
Outdoor	5 days/week, 6 months/year, 70 years
Indoor	365 days/year, 70 years
Bioavailability	1%

TABLE 5. Calculation of Outdoor Lifetime Soil Accumulation

Age	Surface Area Child/Adult[a]	Surface Area Child (2½-yr-old)[b]	(Exposed[c] (cm²)	Soil Contact Rate (g/cm²·day)	Exposure Duration (days)	Soil Load on Skin[d] (g)
1	—	—	—	—	0	0
2	0.30	0.91	1,911	0.001	130	248
3	0.36	1.09	2,289	0.001	130	298
4	0.40	1.21	2,541	0.001	130	330
5	0.43	1.30	2,730	0.001	130	355
6	0.45	1.36	2,856	0.001	130	371
7	0.47	1.42	2,982	0.001	130	388
8	0.50	1.52	3,192	0.001	130	415
9	0.52	1.58	3,318	0.001	130	431
10	0.55	1.67	3,507	0.001	130	456
11	0.58	1.76	3,696	0.001	130	480
12	0.61	1.85	3,885	0.001	130	505
13	0.65	—	1,105	0.001	130	144
14	0.70	—	1,190	0.001	130	155
15	0.76	—	1,292	0.001	130	168
16	0.82	—	1,394	0.001	130	181
17	0.87	—	1,479	0.001	130	192
18	0.90	—	1,530	0.001	130	199
19	0.94	—	1,598	0.001	130	208
20	0.96	—	1,632	0.001	130	212
21–70	1.00	—	1,700	0.001	6500	11,050
					Total	16,786

[a]Derived from ICRP (123).
[b]Calculated from ratios given in previous column.
[c]For ages 2–12, calculated using a figure of 2100 cm² representing both hands, legs, and feet exposed for a 2½-yr-old from Hawley (125) using appropriate surface area ratio from previous column. For ages 21–70, 1700 cm² represents both hands and most of forearms (Hawley, 125). Ages 13–20 figures calculated from 1700 cm² using appropriate surface area ratio.
[d]Exposed surface area × contact rate × exposure duration.

centrations of TCDD are approximately 75% of outdoor soil-TCDD concentrations. This estimate was based on a study of lead contamination in the vicinity of smelters in Toronto (124, 125), in which lead concentrations were measured in house dust and compared with that in garden soil. This figure of 75% assumes that a portion of the indoor dust is generated inside the house from activities such as smoking, cooking, wearing of fabrics, or from use of powders and sprays (125), and that the transport into the house of soil from outside would be reduced during winter months. The 75% factor is similar to a factor of 80% used by Hawley (125) for the soil composition of household dust.

The amount of soil or dust that will accumulate on the skin depends on the exposed skin surface area and the soil/dust contact rate, which in turn depends on a number of factors such as soil type, soil moisture, daily activities, and age. For outdoor activities, a skin contact rate of 1 mg soil/cm² surface area per day was selected based on studies of soil accumulation on children's hands (17). It was estimated that this value also pertains to other exposed skin of the body (17).

A dermal contact rate of 0.03 mg dust/cm² surface area per day was estimated for

TABLE 6. Calculation of Indoor Lifetime Soil Accumulation

Age	Surface Area Child/Adult[a]	Exposed[b] (cm²)	Dust Contact Rate (g/cm²·day)	Exposure Duration (days)	Dust Load on Skin[c] (g)
1	0.22	200	0.00003	365	2.2
2	0.30	273	0.00003	365	3.0
3	0.36	328	0.00003	365	3.6
4	0.40	364	0.00003	365	4.0
5	0.43	391	0.00003	365	4.3
6	0.45	410	0.00003	365	4.5
7	0.47	428	0.00003	365	4.7
8	0.50	455	0.00003	365	5.0
9	0.52	473	0.00003	365	5.2
10	0.55	501	0.00003	365	5.5
11	0.58	528	0.00003	365	5.8
12	0.61	555	0.00003	365	6.1
13	0.65	592	0.00003	365	6.5
14	0.70	637	0.00003	365	7.0
15	0.76	692	0.00003	365	7.6
16	0.82	746	0.00003	365	8.2
17	0.87	792	0.00003	365	8.7
18	0.90	819	0.00003	365	9.0
19	0.94	855	0.00003	365	9.4
20	0.96	874	0.00003	365	9.6
21–70	1.00	910	0.00003	18,250	498.2
				Total	618

[a]Derived from ICRP (123).
[b]Based on surface area of both hands of 910 cm² for adult (Hawley, 125). Figures at other ages calculated using appropriate surface area ratio.
[c]Exposed surface area × contact rate × exposure duration.

indoor activities based on data from Solomon and Hartford (126) as discussed by Hawley (125). Hawley (125) calculated average dust values on bare floors from data on lead and cadmium in household dust to be 320 and 290 mg/m², respectively, or about 0.03 mg/cm². It was assumed that this level of dust would be contacted by the exposed skin surface in 1 day. For exposure outdoors, exposed surfaces for 2–12-year-old children were assumed to consist of both hands, legs, and feet based on significant play activity in close contact with the soil. For people 13–70 years old, it was assumed that exposed skin surfaces consisted of both hands and most of the forearms, based on yard and garden work and assuming that gloves were not worn (adapted from Hawley, 125). For indoor exposure, exposed surfaces were assumed to consist of an area equivalent to that of both hands for all age groups. These assumptions surely overestimate the actual dermal exposure. Calculations for outdoor soil and indoor dust accumulation are shown in Tables 5 and 6, respectively.

The duration of potential outdoor exposure on reclaimed mine lands was estimated at 5 days/week, 6 months/year, for 70 years—essentially during warm-weather months. Indoor exposure was calculated based on 365 days of exposure per year for 70 years.

TABLE 7. Inhalation

Parameter	Value
TSPs in outdoor air	$40\,\mu g/m^3$
Percentage of TSPs comprised of resuspended local soil	50%
Percentage of TSPs in indoor air compared to outdoor air	75%
Respiratory rate	
8-h working light activity	$9.6\,m^3$
8-h nonoccupational activity	$9.6\,m^3$
8-h resting	$3.6\,m^3$
	$\overline{22.8\,m^3}$
Exposure duration	
Outdoor	8 h/day, 5 days/week, mid-April to mid-October, for 70 years
Indoor	16 h/day, mid-April to mid-October when also outdoors, or 24 h/day on all days when not outdoors, for 70 years
Bioavailability	38%

TABLE 8. Oral Uptake of Soil

Parameter	Value
Indoor dust-TCDD factor	75% Soil-TCDD level
Soil ingestion rate	100 mg/day
Dust ingestion rate	25 mg/day
Exposure duration	
Outdoor	5 days/week, mid-April to mid-October, for 5 years
Indoor	365 days/year for 5 years
Bioavailability	40%

Obviously, these exposure durations overestimate realistic exposures; an individual might be expected to spend a considerable amount of time away from the residence, for example, at the workplace, and few persons garden each day.

About 1% of the TCDD in soil or dust was estimated to be absorbed through the skin, based on data from Poiger and Schlatter (35) and Shu et al. (127). In the study by Poiger and Schlatter (35), at the lowest dose tested (26 ng), about 0.05% of TCDD applied dermally in a soil paste to rats reached the liver. At the two higher doses, the percentages of administered dose found in the liver were 1.7 and 2.2%. Actually, the total absorbed dose would have been greater than the percentages reported by Poiger and Schlatter for the liver alone. Our review of the literature indicates that total absorbed dose may be approximately two times as great as that measured in the liver. A figure of 1% for dermal absorption of TCDD was selected by Kimbrough et al. (13) based on Poiger and Schlatter's data; and this appears reasonable, especially for low soil-TCDD concentrations.

The bioavailability of TCDD, according to the Poiger and Schlatter study, appeared to decrease with decreasing concentrations (14).

Shu et al. (127) found 0.79% of the administered dose in the liver following a 24-h contact duration with environmentally contaminated soil at 123 ppb TCDD (dose equal to 125 ng/kg). In order to examine the effect of length of contact of TCDD with soil, Shu et al. (127) also used a recently prepared laboratory contaminated soil at 100 ppb TCDD and found 0.73% of the administered dose in the liver after a 24-h contact duration. Thus, the degree of uptake did not appear to be affected by the length of time that TCDD had been in contact with the soil (i.e., the aging of environmentally contaminated Times Beach, Missouri, soil appeared to be of no consequence compared to the recently contaminated laboratory soil). Shu et al. (127) calculated a mean of 0.76% of the administered dose in the liver from the two experiments. This figure was used to calculate a dermal bioavailability figure of 1.5% relative to the liver level of TCDD administered orally in corn oil, adjusted for unabsorbed dose.

In addition to aging, several other parameters that may potentially affect dermal absorption were studied, including duration of dermal exposure, dose of TCDD, and presence of crankcase oil as a co-contaminant. The rate of dermal penetration of [^{3}H]TCDD following a 4-h contact period with the skin was found to be approximately 60% of that following a 24-h contact (administered dose found in liver was 0.62% and 1.00% for 4- and 24-h contacts, respectively). Dermal uptake did not appear to be significantly influenced by the concentration of TCDD in the soil. Doses tested were 12.5 and 125 ng TCDD/kg, corresponding to concentrations of TCDD in the soil of 10 and 100 ppb, respectively. Variations in oil concentration also did not have a significant impact on absorption.

The use of a 1% bioavailability figure in this analysis probably overestimates exposure because the actual human soil-to-skin contact durations are considerably less than 24 h—the duration of contact used in the rat experiments on which the bioavailability estimate is based. Also, the bioavailability of TCDD to humans may be overstated by the rat data because rodent skin is generally more permeable than human skin for a number of compounds (128, 129).

The formulas for calculating dermal exposure as lifetime average daily dose (LADD) are

$$E_{\text{dermal, outdoor}} = CAB\left(\frac{1}{L}\right)\left(\frac{1}{W}\right) \tag{1}$$

and

$$E_{\text{dermal, indoor}} = CIAB\left(\frac{1}{L}\right)\left(\frac{1}{W}\right), \tag{2}$$

where E = exposure, LADD (pg/kg·day)
C = concentration of TCDD in soil averaged over exposure period (pg/g)
I = indoor dust-TCDD factor
A = accumulated dust or soil over lifetime (g)
B = bioavailability of TCDD
L = lifetime (days)
W = body weight (kg).

Use of these equations is illustrated in the following example.

Illustrative Example 1. Calculating a Lifetime Average Daily Dose (LADD) for Dermal Contact

Given. A hypothetical individual was assumed to reside year-round for a lifetime in a house built on an abandoned mine site reclaimed with sludge. Exposure was calculated as the daily dose averaged over a lifetime (70 years) of exposure, using Eqs. (1) and (2). Because it is the lifetime average daily dose that we calculated, the concentration of TCDD used in Eqs. (1) and (2) was the concentration of soil-TCDD and its equivalents averaged over 70 years of exposure. As explained earlier, it was assumed, for the purpose of this analysis, that the sludge used to reclaim the abandoned mine site contained an initial concentration of 35 ppt TCDD and its equivalents. Assuming a 1:9 dilution of sludge with mine spoil and a minimum 2-year latency period before the site is developed for residential use, the resulting 70-year average soil concentration of TCDD and equivalents was calculated at 0.65 ppt, as shown in Table 3. Thus a figure of 0.65 ppt (pg/g) was used in these calculations to represent the dioxin content of outdoor soil. Indoor dust was assumed to contain TCDD at 75% of the outdoor soil-TCDD level.

Soil and dust accumulations on the skin over the 70 years of exposure were calculated to be 16,786 and 618 g, respectively. The amounts were calculated as the product of exposed skin surface area, soil or dust contact rate, and exposure duration, as shown in Tables 5 and 6. Of the dioxin present in the soil or dust that accumulated on the skin, only 1% was assumed to be absorbed into the body. The absorbed lifetime dose of TCDD was then divided by the lifetime of exposure (70 years $\times$ 365 days/year = 25,550 days) and body weight of 70 kg to result in a daily dose of TCDD averaged over a lifetime, on a per kg body weight basis.

Solution. Using the assumptions outlined above, solution of Eq. (1) and (2) provided estimates of lifetime average daily dose.

$$E_{\text{dermal, outdoor}} = \left(0.65\frac{\text{pg}}{\text{g}}\right)(16,786\,\text{g})(0.01)\left(\frac{1}{25,550\,\text{days}}\right)\left(\frac{1}{70\,\text{kg}}\right)$$

$$= 6.1 \times 10^{-5}\,\text{pg/kg·day},$$

$$E_{\text{dermal, indoor}} = \left(0.65\frac{\text{pg}}{\text{g}}\right)(0.75)(618\,\text{g})(0.01)\left(\frac{1}{25,550\,\text{days}}\right)\left(\frac{1}{70\,\text{kg}}\right)$$

$$= 1.7 \times 10^{-6}\,\text{pg/kg·day},$$

$$E_{\text{dermal, total}} = 6.1 \times 10^{-5} + 1.7 \times 10^{-6}\,\text{pg/kg·day}$$

$$= 6.3 \times 10^{-5}\,\text{pg/kg·day}.$$

4.3.1.2   Inhalation. In addition to skin contact, an individual residing on a reclaimed mine site may incur TCDD exposure through inhalation of airborne dust containing TCDD resuspended from the soil. Modeling parameters are summarized in Table 7. Because of dilution with ambient air in the outdoor environment, exposure via the inhalation of resuspended soil particles is expected to be small. Exposure to TCDD volatilized from the soil is believed to be an insignificant pathway as compared to resuspended dust, and it was not modeled in this analysis. Any volatilization of TCDD from the surface layer would probably occur mainly during the first summer following sludge application, based on a model developed by Freeman and Schroy (30).

A total suspended particulate (TSP) concentration in outdoor air of $40 \, \mu g/m^3$ was assumed for the mine site areas. This was based on 1985 annual average TSP data for a city located near the mine reclamation area (120). The level of airborne TSPs derived from resuspended local soil was estimated to be no more than 50% based on the analysis of particulate data by Trijonis et al. (130), showing that nearly half of all inhalable particulate mass in St. Louis, Missouri, consisted of mostly dust-related crustal material. This estimate may considerably overstate true levels because vegetation on the reclaimed mine sites tightly covers the soil and allows little opportunity for resuspension of soil particles. Typically, no more than 50% of TSPs are respirable (less than $10 \, \mu m$ in diameter) (14, 131). However, all TSPs derived from resuspended local soil were assumed to be respirable for the purpose of this analysis. In order to estimate the concentration of TCDD in the air, it was assumed that the concentration of TCDD associated with suspended particulates is the same as that in the soil. The indoor TSP level that is comprised of local soil was set at 75% of the outdoor TSP comprised of resuspended local soil (16, 125).

Respiratory rates for light and resting activity are given in Table 7 (123). A resident was estimated to spend about 8 h/day, 5 days/week, for 6 months/year (mid-April to mid-October) in outdoor activities on reclaimed mine land. All remaining time was assumed to be spent indoors.

Not all the TCDD associated with respired particles is absorbed by the body. A bioavailability fraction of 38% was used for the inhalation of TCDD-contaminated particles. This fraction was derived based on the following assumptions. It was assumed that 25% of all inhaled particles are exhaled, 25% are deposited in lower respiratory passages (of which half are retained and half eliminated from the lungs and swallowed), and 50% are deposited in upper respiratory passages and swallowed (14, 17). Of the particles swallowed, it was assumed that about 40% might be absorbed in the GI tract (based on the bioavailability of TCDD adsorbed onto soil particles, discussed in Section 4.3.1.3).

The equations for calculating exposure through inhalation are

$$E_{\text{inhalation, outdoor}} = CT_sF_cTR_rDB\left(\frac{1}{L}\right)\left(\frac{1}{W}\right) \tag{3}$$

and

$$E_{\text{inhalation, indoor}} = CI_tT_sF_cTR_rDB\left(\frac{1}{L}\right)\left(\frac{1}{W}\right), \tag{4}$$

where E = exposure, LADD (pg/kg·day)
$\quad\quad C$ = concentration of TCDD in soil averaged over exposure period (pg/g)
$\quad\quad T_s$ = TSPs comprised of resuspended local soil
$\quad\quad F_c$ = conversion factor, $1 \times 10^{-6} \, g/\mu g$
$\quad\quad I_t$ = indoor TSP factor
$\quad\quad T$ = TSP in outdoor air ($\mu g/m^3$)
$\quad\quad R_r$ = respiratory rate (m^3/day)
$\quad\quad D$ = exposure duration (days)
$\quad\quad B$ = bioavailability
$\quad\quad L$ = lifetime (days)
$\quad\quad W$ = body weight (kg).

The following example illustrates the use of these equations.

Illustrative Example 2. Calculating a Lifetime Average Daily Dose (LADD) for Inhalation

Given. A hypothetical individual was assumed to reside year-round for a lifetime in a house built on an abandoned mine site reclaimed with sludge. As in the dermal uptake calculation, the daily dose averaged over a lifetime of exposure was calculated. The initial concentration of 35 ppt TCDD and its equivalents in the sludge was calculated to give a concentration of 0.65 ppt in the soil averaged over the 70-year exposure period, as explained previously. It was assumed that this individual is exposed to an average outdoor TSP level of $40\,\mu g/m^3$, of which 50% is composed of resuspended local soil. When indoors, it was assumed that the resident was exposed to an airborne dust level 75% of that in the outdoor air. The person was estimated to spend 8 h/day for 130 days (5 days/week for 6 months) outdoors on the site. All remaining time was spent inside the house. Of the TCDD inhaled by the individual on soil or dust particles, 38% was assumed to be absorbed into the body.

Solution. Outdoor and indoor exposures were calculated using Eqs. (3) and (4) as shown below. The indoor and outdoor exposures were then added to estimate total lifetime average daily dose through inhalation:

$$E_{\text{inhalation, outdoor}} = \left(0.65\frac{\text{pg}}{\text{g}}\right)(0.5)\left(1\times10^{-6}\frac{\text{g}}{\mu\text{g}}\right)\left(40\frac{\mu\text{g}}{\text{m}^3}\right)\left(9.6\frac{\text{m}^3}{\text{day}}\right)$$

$$\times\left(130\frac{\text{days}}{\text{year}}\times70\,\text{years}\right)(0.38)\left(\frac{1}{25{,}550\,\text{days}}\right)\left(\frac{1}{70\,\text{kg}}\right)$$

$$= 2.4\times10^{-7}\,\text{pg/kg·day},$$

$$E_{\text{inhalation, indoor}} = \left(0.65\frac{\text{pg}}{\text{g}}\right)(0.75)(0.5)\left(1\times10^{-6}\frac{\text{g}}{\mu\text{g}}\right)\left(40\frac{\mu\text{g}}{\text{m}^3}\right)$$

$$\times\left[\left(13.2\frac{\text{m}^3}{\text{day}}\times130\frac{\text{days}}{\text{year}}\right)+\left(22.8\frac{\text{m}^3}{\text{day}}\times235\frac{\text{days}}{\text{year}}\right)\right]$$

$$\times(70\,\text{years})(0.38)\left(\frac{1}{25{,}550\,\text{days}}\right)\left(\frac{1}{70\,\text{kg}}\right)$$

$$= 1.5\times10^{-6}\,\text{pg/kg·day},$$

$$E_{\text{inhalation, total}} = 2.4\times10^{-7}+1.0\times10^{-6}\,\text{pg/kg·day}$$

$$= 1.2\times10^{-6}\,\text{pg/kg·day}.$$

4.3.1.3 Oral Uptake of Soil. Soil ingestion by children was the third residential contact scenario examined. Modeling parameters are summarized in Table 8. As in the skin contact scenario, the indoor dust-TCDD concentration was projected to be 75% of the outdoor soil-TCDD concentration. The rate of soil ingestion for a child aged 2–6 years was estimated based on a review of relevant literature (14, 17, 125, 132–136). Although estimates of soil ingestion have ranged from about 50 to 250 mg/day, 100 mg/day appears to be a reasonable estimate for outdoor soil ingestion by children. Ingestion of indoor dust was estimated at about 25% of the outdoor rate, or 25 mg/day. Ingestion of between 3 and 100 mg/day of household dust was estimated by Hawley (125), depending on the age of the child and the season of the year. Outdoor soil ingestion was projected to occur 5 days/week for 6 months/year from mid-April to mid-October for a child aged 2–6. Household dust ingestion was assumed to occur year-round.

Binding of TCDD to sludge particles reduces the bioavailability of TCDD in the GI tract compared to TCDD in a solvent or food medium. A bioavailability figure of 40% was used in this analysis based on a review of the experimental data regarding bioavailability of soil-borne TCDD. Poiger and Schlatter (35) dosed rats by gavage with laboratory contaminated soil that had been in contact with [^{3}H]TCDD for either 10–15 h or for 8 days (doses ranging from 12.7 to 22.9 ng TCDD) and determined the percentage of administered dose remaining in the liver after 24 h. For soil that had been in contact with TCDD for 10–15 h, 24% of the administered dose was found in the liver. For soil that had been in contact with TCDD for 8 days, 16% of the TCDD was found in the liver. These figures can be compared to absorption after oral administration of 14.7 ng TCDD using 50% ethanol as the vehicle; 36.7% of the total dose was found in the liver after 24 h. Thus, administration of the TCDD in a soil matrix reduced accumulation in the liver to about half of that observed from administration of TCDD in 50% ethanol. Efficiency of absorption appeared to decrease with increasing time of soil-to-TCDD contact (35).

McConnell et al. (137) measured liver concentrations in guinea pigs and rats and AHH induction in rats following ingestion of in situ TCDD-contaminated Missouri soil. At the highest dose tested in rats (about 5 µg TCDD/kg), liver concentrations were twice as high in rats fed TCDD in corn oil (40.8 ppb) compared to rats given TCDD in contaminated soil (20.3 ppb); yet AHH induction was similar between the two groups. The guinea pig data were unreliable for the purpose of estimating bioavailability (39, 137). McConnell et al. (137) concluded that absorption of TCDD in soil appears highly efficient in the guinea pig and rat, but they did not calculate bioavailability percentages.

Lucier et al. (36), after reexamining the McConnell et al. (137) rat data, concluded that the oral bioavailability of TCDD in soil was approximately 50%, based on liver-TCDD concentrations measured at the high dose (about 5 µg TCDD/kg). Examination of the liver concentrations at the next lower dose (about 1 µg TCDD/kg) indicates a 25% bioavailability. These data suggest that bioavailability of soil-TCDD was dose dependent in this study (14).

Umbreit et al. (138) observed TCDD toxicity in guinea pigs and AHH induction in rats following oral doses of in situ TCDD-contaminated Times Beach, Missouri, soil and Newark, New Jersey, manufacturing site soil. The results showed that both soils induced similar levels of AHH activity in rats (at total doses of 10 or 40 µg/kg), yet in guinea pigs (at 1–10 µg/kg) the Newark soil produced much lower toxicity than did the Times Beach soil. The authors suggested that the differences in bioavailability between the two soils (as indicated by toxicity differences) may be related to different soil compositions and the presence of aqueous versus waste oil components (138).

In another study, Umbreit et al. (37) measured liver-TCDD concentrations in guinea pigs fed the same New Jersey manufacturing site soil and a New Jersey metal salvage yard soil at doses ranging from 0.32 to 12 µg/kg. Comparing the resulting liver-TCDD concentrations to those in the positive controls (decontaminated soil spiked with TCDD for 1 h), Umbreit et al. calculated a bioavailability of less than 0.5% for the manufacturing site soil and 21.3% for the salvage yard soil.

These estimates of oral bioavailability, however, have been found to contain serious methodological shortcomings (39). Hepatic concentrations of TCDD in the positive control and experimental animals were obtained at different times and the positive control animals suffered severe toxicity. Therefore, in large part, differences in toxicity and pharmacokinetics, rather than in bioavailability, are reflected by the Umbreit et al. (37) bioavailability estimates.

Bonaccorsi et al. (38) studied the bioavailability of in situ TCDD-contaminated Seveso soil and laboratory contaminated soil in rabbits. They compared liver concentrations after oral doses of Seveso soil with a comparable dose of TCDD in alcohol and found the absorption of Seveso soil-borne TCDD to be, on average, 68% lower than that of solvent-borne TCDD at the 80 ng/day dose level (with a 99% confidence interval ranging from 40 to 95%). At the same dose, absorption of laboratory contaminated soil was found to be, on average, 44% lower than that of solvent-borne TCDD (with a 99% confidence interval ranging from 19 to 68%). Differences in uptake of TCDD from laboratory contaminated soil relative to solvent appeared to be more evident at higher doses of TCDD.

Assuming that liver concentrations represent 70% of the body burden in rats (31), the EPA Exposure Assessment Group (17) used 8-day data from Poiger and Schlatter to calculate a total GI tract absorption of 20–26%. Kimbrough et al. (13) used a 30% bioavailability figure in the CDC risk assessment based on data from McConnell et al. (137) and Poiger and Schlatter (35). Lucier et al. (36) attributed a 25–50% bioavailability to the McConnell et al. (137) rat data, while Umbreit et al. (37, 138) attributed an 85% bioavailability to the McConnell et al. (137) data. Umbreit et al. (37, 138) did not discuss how this percentage was derived. Umbreit has since indicated that the percentage is too high and is currently reanalyzing the bioavailability calculations (139). As pointed out by Shu et al. (39), the Umbreit et al. (37, 138) recalculations of bioavailability based on the guinea pig data of McConnell et al. (137) were inaccurate and were based on data that are inappropriate to estimating oral bioavailability.

Paustenbach et al. (14) concluded that 30% bioavailability of TCDD in soil in the GI tract is likely to be an upper estimate and that 10% bioavailability may be a more reasonable estimate given the low concentrations of TCDD in the environment and the subsequent small daily oral dose anticipated for many contaminated sites (e.g., small bolus dose as compared to that used in the animal studies).

In a recent paper, Shu et al. (39) investigated the oral bioavailability of TCDD from environmentally contaminated soil from Times Beach, Missouri. The percentage of the administered dose found in the liver 24 h after dosing increased with increasing dose for both the soil and corn oil vehicles. Doses ranged from 2.0 to 1450 ng TCDD/kg. Oral bioavailability of soil-bound TCDD was calculated at 37–49% with a mean of 43%. Calculations were performed by comparing the percentage of administered dose which appears in the liver of rats administered soil-bound TCDD to that of rats given TCDD in corn oil. The percentage of administered dose in the liver of rats given TCDD in corn oil was adjusted to reflect unabsorbed TCDD, which has been estimated to be about 30% (140). In the absence of this adjustment, the calculated mean oral bioavailability would be somewhat greater than 43%. The oral bioavailability of soil-bound TCDD did not appear to be affected by the approximately 500-fold difference in administered dose in this study.

The variation in oral bioavailability figures reported in the literature may be due to several factors. Investigators have examined bioavailability using either AHH induction or actual liver concentrations of TCDD. The amount of soil or TCDD administered to the test animals varies among studies. The organic content of the soils and the length of TCDD contact with soil have also differed markedly from study to study. In addition, the presence of co-contaminants may affect bioavailability.

Examination of the experimental data clearly shows that bioavailability of soil-borne TCDD is not as great as that obtained through dosing via organic solvents. Given the absence of data on the bioavailability of TCDD in the particular sludge–soil mixture that is the subject of this analysis, data on other soils can be used to develop a reasonable figure. Disregarding the oral bioavailability figures calculated by Umbreit et al. (37, 138) because of methodological shortcomings, reported oral bioavailability figures for environmentally contaminated soils obtained from Seveso and Missouri ranged from about 25 to over 50%. Based on these data, a bioavailability figure of 40% appears to be a reasonable estimate for TCDD in the sludge examined in this analysis, given the high organic content, relatively small quantities of soil ingested, and low levels of TCDD in the sludge.

Soil ingestion is believed to be significant for only 5 years. Therefore, the daily exposure over the 5-year period should be averaged over a lifetime of 70 years in order to calculate lifetime incremental cancer risks.

The formulas for calculating exposure through outdoor soil and indoor dust uptake are

$$E_{\text{soil uptake}} = CR_i F_c DB \left(\frac{1}{L}\right)\left(\frac{1}{W}\right) \tag{5}$$

and

$$E_{\text{dust uptake}} = CIR_i F_c DB \left(\frac{1}{L}\right)\left(\frac{1}{W}\right), \tag{6}$$

where E = exposure, LADD (pg/kg·day)
   C = concentration of TCDD in soil averaged over exposure period (pg/g)
   I = indoor dust-TCDD factor
   R_i = rate for soil or dust ingestion (mg/day)
   F_c = conversion factor, 1×10^{-3} g/mg
   D = exposure duration (days)
   B = bioavailability
   L = lifetime (days)
   W = body weight (kg).

An example calculation follows.

Illustrative Example 3. Calculating a Lifetime Average Daily Dose (LADD) for Soil Uptake

Given. A hypothetical individual was assumed to reside year-round in a house built on an abandoned mine site reclaimed with sludge. This individual was assumed to reside on the site as a child aged 2–6 years, starting 2 years following mine reclamation with sludge. The 5-year average soil-TCDD concentration corresponding to this scenario was calculated to be 2.7 ppt (Table 3). The indoor dust-TCDD concentration was calculated at 75% of this level. The child was assumed to ingest soil at the rate of 100 mg/day for 5 days/week, 6 months/year, for 5 years and 25 mg/day of dust for 365 days/year for 5 years. Forty percent of the TCDD ingested was assumed to be absorbed into the body. An average body weight of 17 kg was assumed.

Solution. Based on the assumptions described above, soil and dust uptake were calculated using Eqs. (5) and (6). Outdoor and indoor exposures were then added to calculate the child's total lifetime average daily dose of TCDD through this route:

$$E_{\text{soil uptake}} = \left(2.7\frac{\text{pg}}{\text{g}}\right)\left(100\frac{\text{mg}}{\text{day}}\right)\left(1\times10^{-3}\frac{\text{g}}{\text{mg}}\right)$$

$$\times\left(130\frac{\text{days}}{\text{year}}\times5\text{ years}\right)(0.4)\left(\frac{1}{25{,}000\text{ days}}\right)\left(\frac{1}{17\text{ kg}}\right)$$

$$= 1.6\times10^{-4}\text{ pg/kg·day},$$

$$E_{\text{dust uptake}} = \left(2.7\frac{\text{pg}}{\text{g}}\right)(0.75)\left(25\frac{\text{mg}}{\text{day}}\right)\left(1\times10^{-3}\frac{\text{g}}{\text{mg}}\right)$$

$$\times\left(365\frac{\text{days}}{\text{year}}\times5\text{ years}\right)(0.4)\left(\frac{1}{25{,}550\text{ days}}\right)\left(\frac{1}{17\text{ kg}}\right)$$

$$= 8.5\times10^{-5}\text{ pg/kg·day},$$

$$E_{\text{soil \& dust uptake}} = 1.6\times10^{-4}+8.5\times10^{-5}\text{ pg/kg·day}$$

$$= 2.5\times10^{-4}\text{ pg/kg·day}.$$

4.3.2 Hunting of Game Species.

Sportsmen hunting in the area of reclaimed mine sites may kill and consume game species that inhabit these areas. A number of game species can be found in this part of the state, including white-tailed deer, eastern wild turkey, cottontail rabbit, squirrel, ruffed grouse, and bobwhite quail. The white-tailed deer and eastern wild turkey were selected for this analysis because of their importance to area hunters.

4.3.2.1 Human Uptake from Wild Turkey.

The woodlands around the mine reclamation area in southeast Ohio provide good habitat for the eastern wild turkey. Turkeys inhabiting a sludge-reclaimed mine site have some potential for exposure to TCDD in the sludge, and therefore hunters of wild turkey have potential for exposure. Exposure modeling parameters are summarized in Table 9.

Birds, in general, may potentially be exposed to TCDD in soil through consumption of worms, insects, vegetation, or possibly through soil ingestion by dusting of feathers and

TABLE 9. Human Uptake from Wild Turkey

Parameter	Value
Daily total food consumption for turkey	200 g/day
Grass component of total turkey diet	15%
Grass consumption from reclaimed mine site compared to total	8%
Soil-TCDD uptake coefficient for grasses	0.1%
Insect component (with significant soil contact) of total turkey diet	0.6%
Insect consumption from reclaimed mine site compared to total	8%
Insect bioaccumulation factor for TCDD in soil	100%
Bioavailability of TCDD in grass/insects to turkey	86%
Body weight for turkey	6.4 kg
Estimated half-life for whole-body elimination of TCDD in turkey	60 days
Turkey consumption rate/exposure duration	0.4 kg/day for 5 days/year, 70 years
Bioavailability of TCDD in turkey to humans	100%

subsequent preening or by adherence of soil particles to seeds, insects, and so on. Young and Cockerham (141) reported finding TCDD in livers and stomachs of southern meadowlarks, mourning doves, and Savannah sparrows from a test area within Eglin Air Force Base, Florida, that had been sprayed with herbicides containing TCDD. Southern meadowlarks showed the highest accumulated levels with average liver concentrations greater than the mean soil-TCDD concentrations in the surrounding area. This was attributed to preening of feathers and consumption of soil-borne insects with adhered soil particles (141). It is not possible to relate these data directly to wild turkey on reclaimed mine sites because of the differences in feeding habits, habitats, soil type, vegetation cover, and so on.

A 6.4-kg (14-lb) turkey was estimated to consume about 200 g/day of food, of which about 85% or greater is plant matter, depending on the season and location (142–144). The type of plant matter consumed depends largely on habitat and may vary considerably with season of year (144). Types of plant food include mast (oak, beech, pine), fruits (dogwood, grape, cherry, gum, persimmon, juniper), seeds (native grasses and sedges, corn, oats, weeds), and greens consisting of grass and grasslike plants as well as some annual and perennial forbs (144). In a literature review of the feeding habits of the eastern wild turkey, Korshgen (144) reported that weighted average data from turkey crops and stomach analyses showed that acorns comprised almost 32% of wild turkey fall and winter diets (% volume basis) while all-season droppings analyses indicated an average acorn consumption of nearly 17% of total food (% volume basis).

Grasses constitute an important food for the eastern turkey, especially during winter and spring (144). Grass leaves made up 14.8% of the turkey diet in a Pennsylvania study and 12.3% in a West Virginia study on a volume basis from droppings analyses (144). Combined data throughout the eastern turkey's range, based on crop and stomach analyses, showed that grass leaves were 3.6% of all food while droppings contained grass leaves as 16.5% of all food. During winter and spring seasons, grass leaves constituted 3.1 and 17.6%, respectively, of total diet by volume in the Pennsylvania study. Based on these data and on similarities between the forest cover types of southeast Ohio and the Pennsylvania and West Virginia habitats, it was estimated that 15% of the total diet consists of grasses, and it was assumed that grasses were grown in the sludge-reclaimed mine area.

Wild turkeys are hunted in late April to early May in Ohio. Breeding activities generally occur mid-March to mid-April with eggs laid by mid-April (143). The annual range of the eastern wild turkey may vary from 1000 to 4000 acres depending on the season of the year and food availability (142, 144). An average range, with an area of about 2500 acres, could theoretically encompass one large reclaimed mine site of about 200 acres in size. It was assumed that consumption of grass from the reclaimed mine site compared to the total range can be estimated by the ratio of the area of a 200-acre mine site to the 2500-acre range, or about 8%. Of course, it is very unlikely that the range for all turkeys bagged by an individual over a 70-year lifetime would encompass a sludge-reclaimed mine site.

Grasses growing on the reclaimed site were estimated to take up about 0.1% TCDD from the soil; that is, the TCDD concentration in the grass would be 0.1% of the soil-TCDD concentration. Data specific to uptake of TCDD by grasses were inadequate to predict an uptake coefficient for this analysis. Therefore, data on uptake in aboveground parts of several plant species were used to develop the 0.1% estimate. Wipf et al. (145) found a level of 8 ppt TCDD in corn sheaths, compared to 10,000 ppt in soil, 1 year following the Seveso, Italy, accident in the fall of 1977. TCDD was not detected in the cob and kernels. A percent uptake of about 0.08% can be inferred from their data. However, the authors noted that TCDD in the corn sheaths may in fact have been due to contamination from local dust rather than true uptake. In less contaminated areas where soil-TCDD concentrations ranged from 2 to 200 ppt, no TCDD was detected in vegetation grown close to the ground 1 year following the Seveso accident. Plant types analyzed included grass, silverbeet, millet, sage, cauliflower, chicory, cabbage, and cucumber. One year later, in the fall of 1978, following plowing in one of these zones, oats, peas, and vetch grown in this soil showed no measurable levels of TCDD. Soil-TCDD concentrations were probably less than 10 ppt throughout, based on soil samples taken the following summer of 1979. Wheat and rye samples analyzed in the same zone in the summer of 1980 all showed no detectable TCDD.

In a controlled greenhouse study, Facchetti et al. (146) examined absorption of TCDD by maize and bean plants from soil containing 1–752 ppt TCDD. Soil consisted of Seveso-contaminated soil mixed with Seveso-noncontaminated soil. While high adsorption of TCDD by the roots was observed, no significant increase of TCDD in the parts aboveground was shown, either as a function of time or with the increase in TCDD concentration. In maize plants cultivated in outdoor greenhouses, percent uptakes ranging from 0.13 to 0.16% can be inferred, while in bean plants grown under similar conditions, percent uptakes ranging from 0.11 to 0.29% can be inferred from the data. Facchetti et al. (146) observed that plants grown in soil containing 1 ppt TCDD displayed tissue-TCDD concentrations that varied with their location. Concentrations were greater for those plants grown near the pots containing contaminated soil, or grown in the indoor greenhouse with no air aspiration. Facchetti et al. (146) concluded that the aboveground parts of these plants were contaminated by evaporation of TCDD from the polluted soil rather than true uptake. For the plants grown in TCDD-contaminated soil, plant uptake was on the order of a few ppt and did not appear to increase with increasing soil-TCDD concentration. Based on these and other data, Fries (15) noted that the uptake and translocation of TCDD in plants used for animal feed are not significant routes of exposure for grazing or confined animals. Studies of other halogenated hydrocarbons have generally shown that contamination of aerial parts of plants is principally from surface contamination due to dust or redeposition of volatilized material from the soil (15). Fries reported that work on PBBs shows that surface contamination from dust gathered during harvest of forage crops provides a negligible contribution to residues in harvested feed, with concentrations in feed of less than 1% of that in soil.

At first inspection, a recent greenhouse study of maize and bean plants (147) seems to indicate that a larger plant uptake coefficient may be more appropriate than the figure of 0.1% employed in this analysis. Several shortcomings, however, are associated with the Sacchi et al. (147) study (148, 149). First, the authors failed to report uptake values for nontreated control plants (150). Sacchi et al. (147) indicated that some cross-contamination had occurred when plants grown in soil containing 3300 ppt TCDD were raised in close proximity to plants grown in uncontaminated soil. There is no indication in the description of the other experiments conducted by these authors whether the treatments consisting of relatively high soil-TCDD concentrations were physically located away from the treatments of relatively low TCDD levels. Depending on how close the pots were to one another, there may have been cross-contamination, which would have exaggerated the uptake values for the plants grown in soils of low TCDD concentration (148, 150).

Second, the authors (147) reported that varying amounts of tritium-labeled TCDD were sprayed onto the soil. Presumably, an organic solvent was used since TCDD is only very slightly soluble in water. It is very likely that the solvent would not rapidly evaporate, particularly if it were mixed with peat and soil under the conditions of the study (151).

Trace levels of solvent that remain in the soil would make the TCDD much more bioavailable for plant uptake and translocation than under normal field conditions. This circumstance also provides a greater opportunity for evaporation and subsequent adherence to the aerial portion of the plants, thereby resulting in higher measured concentrations of TCDD in plant material.

It was observed that the TCDD measured in the aerial plant parts in the Sacchi et al. (147) study did not increase in proportion with increasing soil concentrations of the contaminant. This is further evidence in favor of the volatilization theory, as stated by Facchetti et al. (146), rather than true plant uptake and translocation. In exposure modeling and risk assessment, it is important to use data collected under conditions that are most comparable to actual field situations. This is particularly true with respect to estimating plant uptake coefficients, as there may be more volatilization and redeposition on plants in a confined atmosphere than in the field where there is greater air movement (150).

It appears that Sacchi et al. (147) were aware of the possibility of volatilization and redeposition of TCDD into plant tissue as a phenomenon that might confound their results. However, they discounted this mechanism as being responsible for the increased levels of TCDD observed in the aerial portions of bean plants. Their opinion was based on data reported for one experimental trial in which plants were grown in hydroponic culture containing tritium-labeled water. As mentioned earlier, TCDD is only very slightly soluble in water. Presumably, the dioxin was dissolved in an organic solvent, followed by the use of a solubilizing surfactant to disperse the hydrophobic substance in the water-based nutrient solution. Under these experimental conditions, the potential TCDD uptake and translocation by plants would be greatly increased over field conditions in which the dioxin is tightly bound to soils of high organic content.

Finally, results based on studies using tritium-labeled TCDD can be misleading because the tritium can be exchanged from one molecule to another (148, 149). The phenomenon of chemiluminescence may produce spurious counts; thus, measurements of radioactivity for detecting dioxin may be greatly inaccurate. According to Fries (148), the authors offered no indication that they used procedures to minimize this potential problem. Without background values from nontreated control samples, it is impossible to determine if chemiluminescence occurred. If it did, the amount of TCDD taken up by the plant would be overestimated and the error would be reflected to the greatest extent in the samples of relatively low concentration.

Young (121) examined plant concentrations of TCDD on a test grid at Eglin Air Force Base and reported "typical" data for grasses, small broadleaf plants, and soil sampled from 0.5-m^2 plots. Young reported that the concentrations observed in the aboveground vegetation may reflect soil particle contamination as these plants were perennial species. However, the full range of results and methodologies employed in this study were not reported. Therefore, we judged the data inadequate for the purpose of predicting plant uptake of TCDD.

Cocucci et al. (152) measured TCDD contamination in underground and aerial parts of carrots, potatoes, onions, and narcissus grown in Seveso soil containing TCDD. New aerial parts showed lower TCDD concentrations than underground organs. While TCDD levels in aerial parts (0.84–2.2 ppt) were significant compared to soil-TCDD levels (2.7–8.3 ppt), these data must be interpreted carefully. All four plant types examined have underground organs that may make absorption and translocation kinetics very different from that of grasses. In addition, plants were sampled in the spring following the explosion of the trichlorophenol reactor. New vegetative activity sampled in the spring was sustained by underground organs formed in the preceding year, at which time the plants were exposed to the toxic rain. We therefore feel that the data reported in this study are inadequate for predicting uptake of TCDD in plants.

In conclusion, based on the laboratory and field experiments conducted to date, a soil-TCDD uptake coefficient of 0.1% for aboveground parts of plants, including grasses, in the field appears reasonable for use in this analysis. It seems probable that contaminations via soil particles, dust, and volatilization potentially are more significant than true uptake and translocation of TCDD from the soil, which appear to be quite minor. The significance of these pathways of contamination would be a worthwhile subject for further work in field studies of wild and cultivated plants at low soil-TCDD concentrations.

Insects are of primary importance to the diet of young turkeys, but their diet changes as they grow older (143). For adult turkeys, combined data from regions throughout the eastern United States indicate that animal foods, mostly insects, comprise between 1 and 2% by volume of winter and spring diets, 9% of summer, and 14% of fall diets based on crops, stomachs, or droppings analyses (144). In a Pennsylvania study, up to 0.7% of the winter and spring diets and between 6.2 and 6.9% of the summer and fall diets of wild turkeys were found to consist of animal foods, mostly insects, measured as percent volume based on crops, stomachs, or droppings analyses. An annual average of about 3% can be calculated based on the Pennsylvania data. Insects comprise a larger percentage of total diet in the southern U.S. area of the wild turkey's range (144). On an annual basis, animal foods in the turkey's diet reportedly consist mainly of grasshoppers, walking-sticks, and other straight-winged insects (144). These data indicate that insects comprise only a small proportion of the adult turkey's diet, especially in the winter and spring seasons. In this analysis, we estimated that 8% of the insects consumed derive from the reclaimed mine site, based on the same reasoning as described for grass consumption by turkeys.

Not all insects on a reclaimed site will come into close contact with the soil, thereby reducing the potential for accumulating TCDD through uptake or soil adherence, especially given the dense vegetation cover. Data on the proportion of soil-borne insects relative to other insects in the wild turkey diet were unavailable. Results of a Virginia study, based on crop and stomach analyses, indicated that 267 species of animal foods comprised 5.3% of all food in the wild turkey diet (144). Almost all the animal food was composed of insects (4.7% of all food), of which about one-half consisted of grasshoppers (2.2%) and one-third consisted of Diptera fly larvae. Korshgen (144) reported that the principal animal foods in the wild turkey diet, based on eastern U.S. combined data, are mainly grasshoppers, stink bugs, June beetles, ground beetles, and snout beetles in the summer, and principally grasshoppers in the fall. Walking-sticks may occasionally become even more important than grasshoppers during autumn (144). Adult grasshoppers and walking-sticks, which probably comprise the largest percentage of total insect mass on an annual basis, are unlikely to incur significant contact with the soil on reclaimed mine sites because of their life habits and the dense grass cover. We estimated for this analysis that about 20% of the insect component of the wild turkey diet may come into close enough contact with the soil on a reclaimed mine site to incur significant exposure to TCDD in the soil. The 20% factor was applied to the 3% average insect component in the diet shown in the Pennsylvania study to give a 0.6% insect component (with significant soil contact) in the turkey diet.

Data on TCDD levels in insects are limited. Young and Cockerham (141) reported TCDD concentrations in crickets (18–26 ppt), a composite of soil- and plant-borne insects (40 ppt), burrows spiders (115 ppt), and insect grubs (238 ppt) taken from a test area at Eglin Air Force Base, Florida. TCDD was not detected in grasshoppers. The grasshopper and composite insect samples appear to have been taken from a large grid with soil-TCDD concentrations ranging from less than 10 to 470 ppt with a median of 30 ppt and a mean of about 115 ppt (153). Only 3 of 26 samples showed concentrations greater than 100 ppt. The sampling location for other insects was not reported.

Based on the median soil concentration of 30 ppt TCDD and the median insect concentration of 40 ppt TCDD, it can be assumed that insects reach body levels similar to the soil levels. While acknowledging the uncertainty in this extrapolation, these data suggest a bioaccumulation factor (BCF) of about 1. Based on the experiment at Eglin, it can be inferred that insects in the area of reclamation will contain TCDD at about the same concentration as in the soil amended with sludge. Therefore, the 0.6% insect matter of the total diet was assumed to contain the same concentration of TCDD as that found in the soil. This considers the sum of true uptake by the insect as well as soil adherence to the insects.

Bioavailability of TCDD in grasses or insects to the wild turkey was estimated at 86%. This figure represents the upper end of the range of about 50–86% reported for absorption of TCDD from feeding or gavage studies of laboratory animals (31–34). Data were unavailable regarding bioavailability of TCDD specific to birds.

The wild turkey's daily dioxin exposure and resulting body burden must be estimated before the hunter's oral exposure can be estimated. The estimated body burden of the turkey does not represent a single turkey's uptake, but rather an average for turkeys caught throughout the 70-year hunting period. The turkey's average daily uptake of TCDD (and its equivalents) is

$$E = [(CFG_d G_c G_u) + (CFI_d I_c I_b)]B\left(\frac{1}{W}\right), \tag{7}$$

where E = exposure, average daily dose (pg/kg·day)
  C = concentration of TCDD in soil averaged over 70-year exposure period
  F = food consumption (g/day)
  G_d = grass component of diet
  G_c = grass consumption factor
  G_u = soil-TCDD uptake coefficient for grasses
  I_d = insect component of diet
  I_c = insect consumption factor
  I_b = insect bioaccumulation factor
  B = bioavailability
  W = body weight (kg).

Illustrative Example 4. Estimating Daily Ingestion of TCDD by Wild Turkey

Given. Turkeys were assumed to inhabit the mine site area at anytime during a 70-year period following application of sludge containing 35 ppt TCDD and its equivalents. Due to mixing with soil and degradation over time, a 70-year average concentration of TCDD and its equivalents was calculated to be 0.74 ppt (Table 3). The hypothetical turkey weighing 6.4 kg that is the subject of this example was thus exposed to soil containing 0.74 ppt. In the first part of the equation, uptake of TCDD through consumption of grasses was calculated based on a total food consumption rate of 200 g/day, of which 15% consists of grasses. Only 8% of grass consumed was assumed to be growing on the sludge-reclaimed mine site. The dioxin concentration in the grass that the turkey consumes was assumed to be 0.1% of the soil level, or 0.00074 ppt. The turkey's exposure through insect consumption also was calculated. While the turkey consumes 3% of its total diet as insects, only 20% of that, or 0.6% of the total diet, is believed to come into close contact with the soil. Of the insects consumed by this turkey, only 8% were assumed to come from the sludge-reclaimed mine site. The insects consumed were assumed to contain the same level of dioxin as the soil, or 0.74 ppt. Of the TCDD ingested by the turkey, 86% was assumed to be absorbed into the body.

Solution. Exposure was calculated using Eq. (7).

$$E = \{[(0.74 \text{ pg/g})(200 \text{ g/day})(0.15)(0.08)(0.001)]$$

$$+ [(0.74 \text{ pg/g})(200 \text{ g/day})(0.006)(0.08)(1)]\}(0.86)\left(\frac{1}{6.4 \text{ kg}}\right)$$

$$= 9.8 \times 10^{-3} \text{ pg/kg·day}.$$

The turkey of this analysis, exposed to a soil-TCDD level representing an average over the 70-year period following sludge application, was estimated to incur a daily dose of 9.8×10^{-3} pg/kg of body weight. The estimated average daily uptake of TCDD by the turkey was used to calculate an average (or steady-state) body burden level of TCDD in the wild turkey, that is, a steady-state level at which intake equals excretion. Studies with rats have indicated that the retention and elimination of TCDD follow a first-order process (31, 32). The steady-state body burden levels of TCDD resulting from continuous uptake can be estimated (5) using

$$S = \frac{1.443 E t_{1/2}}{t}, \tag{8}$$

where S = steady-state body burden level (pg/kg)
E = exposure, average daily dose (pg/kg·day)
$t_{1/2}$ = half-life (days)
t = time interval between exposures (1 day for daily continuous exposure).

Information regarding the half-life of TCDD in birds was unavailable. Half-lives for whole-body elimination of TCDD from other animal species have been reported: 30 days in the guinea pig, 31 days in the rat, 17–37 days in the mouse, 11–15 days in the hamster, and 365 days in the monkey (5). For the purpose of this analysis, a half-life of 60 days was assumed for the wild turkey; this figure is about twice that of the half-lives reported for rodents. The procedure to estimate the steady-state body burden of TCDD in turkeys is illustrated in the following example.

Illustrative Example 5. Estimating Steady-State Body Burden of TCDD for the Wild Turkey

Given. For the hypothetical turkey, a daily dose of 9.8×10^{-3} pg/kg·day was calculated in Example 4. A half-life of 60 days for TCDD in the turkey and continuous (i.e., everyday) ingestion of TCDD were assumed.

Solution. The steady-state body burden of TCDD was calculated using Eq. (8).

$$S = \frac{(1.443)(9.8 \times 10^{-3} \text{ pg/kg·day})(60 \text{ days})}{1}$$

$$= 8.5 \times 10^{-1} \text{ pg/kg}.$$

The TCDD was assumed to be evenly distributed throughout the turkey for the purpose of this analysis. In actuality, TCDD would most likely accumulate in the liver and fat tissues; and thus the turkey meat would have a lower concentration than that presented here. Based on this analysis, turkey meat from this bird would contain 8.5×10^{-1} pg TCDD/kg and its equivalents.

Based on the Ohio hunting limit of one wild turkey per year, turkey consumption for an individual living in this area can be estimated. A 6.4-kg (14-lb) turkey is expected to yield about 4.1–4.5 kg (9–10 lb) of turkey meat (154). For a family of three persons, one turkey might provide up to four meals, giving an average consumption figure of about 0.4 kg/day (0.9 lb/day) for 5 days/year. A 100% bioavailability figure was used for the TCDD in turkey because the laboratory studies on which the TCDD cancer potency is based were conducted with similar oral routes of administration (feeding and gavage). The formula for calculating the potential uptake of TCDD by humans is

$$E_{\text{turkey consumption}} = SR_c DB \left(\frac{1}{W}\right)\left(\frac{1}{L}\right), \tag{9}$$

where E = exposure, LADD (pg/kg·day)
$\quad S$ = steady-state TCDD level in turkey (pg/g)
$\quad R_c$ = consumption rate (kg/day)
$\quad D$ = exposure duration (days)
$\quad B$ = bioavailability
$\quad W$ = body weight (kg)
$\quad L$ = lifetime (days).

Illustrative Example 6. Calculating Human Exposure through Wild Turkey Consumption

Given. Uptake was calculated in this example for a 70-kg individual who bags 1 turkey/year for 70 years. Rather than estimate the TCDD concentration in each turkey over the 70-year period, an "average" turkey exposed to the 70-year average TCDD concentration in the soil was assumed to have been eaten each year. The TCDD concentration in the turkey meat was 8.5×10^{-1} pg/kg, as estimated in Example 5. The individual hunter, or member of the family, was assumed to consume 0.4 kg/day of turkey meat for 5 days/year, for 70 years. All the TCDD ingested was estimated to be bioavailable.

Solution. The lifetime average daily dose was calculated using Eq. (9).

$$E = \left(8.5 \times 10^{-1}\frac{\text{pg}}{\text{kg}}\right)\left(0.4\frac{\text{kg}}{\text{day}}\right)\left(5\frac{\text{days}}{\text{year}} \times 70 \text{ years}\right)(1)\left(\frac{1}{70 \text{ kg}}\right)\left(\frac{1}{25,550 \text{ days}}\right)$$

$$= 6.6 \times 10^{-5} \text{ pg/kg·day}.$$

Due to species differences, the wild turkey exposure assessment cannot be extrapolated directly to other game bird species. Ohio hunting restrictions for ruffed grouse and bobwhite quail are six birds per hunting season compared to one wild turkey. Because of their lower body weights, grouse and quail consume a larger percentage of body weight in food per day compared to wild turkey. Like the wild turkey, the ruffed grouse and bobwhite quail primarily consume plant matter (142, 143), although the insect component may comprise a more significant part of their total diet than that of the wild turkey. In spite of these differences, human exposure through consumption of these other bird species is almost certainly insignificant.

4.3.2.2   Human Uptake from Venison Meat.   The potential for human exposure to TCDD through the consumption of venison is addressed in the following paragraphs. Modeling parameters are summarized in Table 10.

Deer inhabiting areas around reclaimed mine sites could be exposed to TCDD in sludge through ingestion of grass or soil. Deer investigated in the southeast Ohio hill counties were found to consume principally, in decreasing order of importance by weight, wild crab apple, corn, honeysuckle leaves and stems, sumac seeds and stems, grapes, acorns, persimmon fruit, pokeweed, fungi, and cinquefoil leaves (155). Ohio deer are not heavily dependent on hardwood browse during any season of the year (155). Only trace quantities of grasses were found in deer rumens, but collectively, grasses and herbaceous perennials were important food items, accounting for about 7–10% by dry weight of their annual diet. Based on the above data, the grass component of the total deer diet was assumed to be 10%. The percentage of grass potentially consumed from a reclaimed mine site compared to the total grass consumed was estimated at 15%. This figure was based on a ratio of 200 acres, representing the potential area of one large reclaimed mine site, to 1280 acres (2 mi^2), representing the approximate home range or territory of white-tailed deer. As before, it was assumed that grasses contain 0.1% of the soil concentration of TCDD.

Data on soil ingestion by deer were unavailable. It was assumed that some soil might be pulled up when browsing on grasses and other perennials. The soil component of the deer diet was estimated at 1.5% of the grass consumption, or 0.15% of the total diet. Based on the Healy (156) study, New Zealand cows grazed on pasture year-round were estimated to consume about 3% of their total dry matter intake as soil during warm-weather months. Based on the differences in feeding habits between deer and cattle, deer were conservatively estimated to consume about 50% of the soil ingested percentage that had been estimated

TABLE 10. Human Uptake from Venison

Parameter	Value
Grass component of total deer diet	10%
Grass consumption from reclaimed mine site compared to total	15%
Soil-TCDD uptake coefficient for grasses	0.1%
Ratio of TCDD concentration in venison fat to TCDD concentration in diet	5
Soil component of total deer diet	0.15%
Soil intake from reclaimed mine site compared to total	15%
Venison fat consumption rate	1 g/day
Exposure duration	365 days/year, 70 years
Bioavailability of TCDD in venison to humans	100%

for cattle—about 1.5% of total grass consumption. Only 15% of the total soil ingested was assumed to derive from a reclaimed mine site, based on the same reasoning as applied to grass consumption.

Data on the relation between the concentration of TCDD in the diet and the resulting steady-state body burden of TCDD in deer were unavailable. Therefore, data available for cattle have been used to estimate the steady-state body burden of TCDD in deer. TCDD levels in beef fat of cattle given feed containing 24 ppt TCDD for 28 days were shown to be about 4 times the dietary levels of TCDD (157). It is likely that this factor would have reached 5 in a longer study (15).

Based on these data, the ratio of the TCDD concentration in the venison fat to the TCDD concentration in the grass component of the deer diet was assumed to be 5. This ratio of 5 was applied similarly to the soil-TCDD concentration to estimate the steady-state body burden in venison fat resulting from ingestion of soil.

Based on a hunting restriction of one deer per year in Ohio, and an estimated weight of 45 kg venison per deer (142), a two-person family was assumed to consume the venison from one deer in a year at a rate of about 60 g/day per person. Assuming that venison contains 1.4% fat (142), the rate of venison fat consumption over the course of 1 year was estimated at 1 g/day.

The equation for calculating TCDD uptake through venison consumption is

$$E_{\text{venison consumption}} = [(CG_uG_dG_cR_t) + (CS_dS_iR_t)]$$
$$\times VDB\left(\frac{1}{W}\right)\left(\frac{1}{L}\right), \qquad (10)$$

where E = exposure, LADD (pg/kg·day)
  C = concentration of TCDD in soil averaged over 70-year exposure period (pg/g)
  G_u = soil-TCDD uptake coefficient for grasses
  G_d = grass component of diet
  G_c = grass consumption factor
  R_t = ratio of TCDD concentration in venison fat to that in diet
  S_d = soil component of diet
  S_i = soil intake factor
  V = venison fat consumption rate (g/day)
  D = exposure duration (days)
  B = bioavailability
  W = body weight (kg)
  L = lifetime (days).

Illustrative Example 7. Calculating Human Uptake of TCDD through Venison Consumption

Given. An individual was assumed to consume venison each year for 70 years from deer that inhabit an area encompassing a mine site reclaimed with sludge. First, the steady-state body burden of TCDD resulting from consumption of grasses and soil by the deer was estimated. As in the wild turkey example, each deer was assumed to be exposed to the 70-year average soil-TCDD equivalent concentration of 0.74 ppt, based on an initial concentration of 35 ppt TCDD and its equivalents in the sludge (Table 3). To calculate the body burden related to the consumption of grasses, the grass was assumed to contain 0.1%

of the concentration of TCDD in the soil. Ten percent of the total diet was assumed to be grass, and only 15% of the total grass consumed grew on the reclaimed mine site. The steady-state body burden of TCDD in the venison fat, through the grass consumption pathway, was assumed to be a factor of 5 times the concentration of TCDD in the grass.

Similarly, the body burden of TCDD related to ingestion of soil was estimated at a factor 5 times the concentration of TCDD in the soil. Soil was assumed to comprise only 0.15% of the total deer diet, and 15% of the total soil consumed was assumed to derive from a reclaimed mine site. Finally, uptake by an individual consuming venison was calculated based on a consumption rate of 1 g of venison fat per day, each day for 70 years. All the TCDD in the venison fat was assumed to be absorbed through the GI tract of this individual.

Solution. The lifetime average daily dose to an individual who consumes venison meat from deer that inhabit areas of mine sites reclaimed with sludge containing 35 ppt TCDD and its equivalents was calculated using Eq. (10):

$$
\begin{aligned}
E_{\text{venison consumption}} = &\left\{ \left[\left(0.74 \frac{\text{pg}}{\text{g}} \right)(0.001)(0.1)(0.15)(5) \right] \right. \\
&+ \left. \left[\left(0.74 \frac{\text{pg}}{\text{g}} \right)(0.0015)(0.15)(5) \right] \right\} \\
&\times \left(1 \frac{\text{g}}{\text{day}} \right) \left(365 \frac{\text{days}}{\text{year}} \times 70 \text{ years} \right)(1)\left(\frac{1}{70 \text{ kg}} \right)\left(\frac{1}{25{,}550 \text{ days}} \right) \\
&= (5.6 \times 10^{-5} + 8.3 \times 10^{-4} \text{ pg/g})(1.4 \times 10^{-2} \text{ g/kg·day}) \\
&= 1.3 \times 10^{-5} \text{ pg/kg·day.}
\end{aligned}
$$

4.3.3   Milk Consumption. The amount of TCDD taken up by humans through milk consumption was estimated for two separate exposure pathways by which dairy cows might be exposed to TCDD in sludge. Specifically, we examined the feeding of hay grown on the reclaimed mine site to cattle that are not grazed and the grazing of cattle on the reclaimed mine site. Exposure parameters for the two pathways are summarized in Table 11.

TABLE 11. Milk Consumption

Parameter	Value
Ratio of TCDD concentration in milk fat to TCDD concentration in diet	4
Supplemental feeding factor	67%
Soil-TCDD uptake coefficient for grasses	0.1%
Soil intake factor	3%
Consumption factor	
Hay-fed cattle	100%
Grazed cattle	25%
Milk fat consumption rate	11 g/day
Bioavailability, TCDD in milk	100%
Exposure duration	365 days/year, 70 years

TCDD present in cattle feed is selectively distributed to fat tissue, including milk fat in lactating dairy cows. Jensen and Hummel (158) fed commercial feed spiked with TCDD to lactating dairy cows. Three cows were each given feed containing TCDD at 5, 15, 50, or 150 ppt for 14 days consecutively at each concentration, and at 500 ppt for 21 days, for a total exposure period of 11 weeks. TCDD residues in milk ranged from nondetectable at the 5-ppt diet concentration to 89 ppt at the 500-ppt diet concentration. TCDD residues in milk increased in proportion to the TCDD in the diet. We calculated an average ratio of TCDD in the milk to TCDD in the feed of 0.145 based on the Jensen and Hummel (158) residue data where cows had been on a specific feeding regimen for at least 12 days. Jensen and Hummel (158) did not report the fat content of the milk examined in this study. Therefore, we assumed an average fat content of 3.7% for whole milk, the average percentage of fat in milk produced in Ohio in 1985 (159). At this fat content, and assuming that all TCDD in the milk had concentrated in the milk fat, we calculated a ratio of TCDD in the milk fat to TCDD in the feed of 4.

In the case of the hay-feeding exposure pathway, we assumed that hay grown on reclaimed mine site areas was fed to dairy cattle on a year-round basis. No direct grazing on reclaimed mine site pastures was included in this pathway. Supplemental feeding generally comprises about one-third of the total feed intake for hay-fed cattle [based on information obtained from the Ohio Agricultural Extension Service (160)]. In our analysis, the supplemental feeding factor reduces the amount of hay potentially containing TCDD to 67% of the total feed consumed. A farmer was assumed to consume milk for 365 days/year for 70 years. All milk consumed by the farmer under this exposure pathway was derived from the cattle fed hay grown on the mine site, thus the 100% consumption factor as shown in Table 11.

For the grazing exposure pathway, dairy cattle were estimated to graze for about 3 months. This analysis is conservative for lactating dairy cows that, in general, are rarely pastured (15). As in the hay-feeding exposure pathway, the amounts of grasses and soil consumed from the mine site area during the grazing period were reduced to 67% of total intake based on supplemental feeding. A farmer was assumed to consume milk for 365 days/year for 70 days, but only 25% of all milk consumed year-round was derived from cattle grazed on sludge-reclaimed mine sites where the sludge contains TCDD. The rationale behind this percentage is given in the following paragraphs.

At the beginning of the summer grazing period, the TCDD level in milk fat was assumed to be essentially zero. Several weeks of exposure are then necessary before a steady-state TCDD level is approached. Fries (161) noted that the milk fat concentrations of similar compounds, polychlorinated biphenyls (PCBs), approached steady state in about 3 weeks. When grazing on sludge-amended pastures ceases at the end of the 3-month period, the milk fat TCDD level will decrease at a rate corresponding to the elimination half-life of TCDD, reported to be about 41 days by Jensen and Hummel (158). In the following 9 months (about 274 days) with no additional TCDD exposure, the milk fat TCDD level is expected to decrease by one-half every 41 days, resulting in about 1% of the steady-state level reached during the grazing period.

In the exposure calculations, application of the 25% consumption factor can be related to the milk consumed by the farmer during the 3-month grazing period compared to the full year. If cows are actually grazed for a full 3 months, then the actual duration of a farmer's exposure might be somewhat longer than the 3 months, due to lingering milk fat TCDD levels following cessation of grazing. However, 3 months is used as an approximation, assuming about 2 months of exposure at steady-state TCDD levels and the equivalent of 1 month of steady-state exposure composed of lower TCDD levels both pre-steady-state and postexposure. Additional justification for this rationale is based on the likelihood that some milk consumed during this period is almost certainly purchased from outside sources, and that even where all milk is derived from grazed cattle, it is virtually inconceivable that all cattle would be grazed on sludge-reclaimed mine sites.

For the grasses and hay consumed by dairy cattle, a soil-TCDD uptake coefficient of 0.1% was used as explained in a previous section. For the grazing scenario, dairy cattle grazed on sludge-reclaimed mine site pastures are expected to ingest a certain amount of soil. Based on data on New Zealand dairy cattle, soil intake during warm-weather months was estimated to constitute about 3% of the total dry matter intake (156). The average soil ingestion for cows from six farms was 0.4 kg/day compared to a total dry matter intake estimated at about 12 kg/day. Cows in this study received no supplemental feed and were grazed the entire year. While the proportion of soil in cattle diet increases as forage quality and quantity decreases (15), it was assumed that cattle would be grazed on mine site areas only during the warm-weather months of the year.

Milk fat consumption was estimated at 11 g/day based on a milk consumption figure of 305 g/day (about 1.3 cups/day), the U.S. average per capita consumption in 1981 (162), and a 3.7% fat level [percentage of fat in all milk produced in Ohio in 1985 (159)].

The formulas for calculating TCDD uptake through milk consumption are

Hay-feeding

$$E_{\text{milk}} = CG_u R_t S_f C_f R_c BD\left(\frac{1}{L}\right)\left(\frac{1}{W}\right) \tag{11}$$

Grazing

$$E_{\text{milk}} = [(CG_u R_t S_f) + (CS_i R_t S_f)]$$
$$\times C_f R_c BD\left(\frac{1}{L}\right)\left(\frac{1}{W}\right), \tag{12}$$

where E = exposure, LADD (pg/kg·day)
$\quad C$ = concentration of TCDD in soil averaged over exposure period (pg/g)
$\quad G_u$ = grass uptake coefficient for TCDD in soil
$\quad S_i$ = soil intake factor
$\quad R_t$ = ratio of TCDD concentration in milk fat to TCDD concentration in diet
$\quad S_f$ = supplemental feeding factor
$\quad C_f$ = consumption factor
$\quad R_c$ = consumption rate (g/day)
$\quad B$ = bioavailability
$\quad D$ = exposure duration (days)
$\quad L$ = lifetime (days)
$\quad W$ = body weight (kg).

Illustrative Example 8. Calculating Human Uptake of TCDD from Consumption of Milk from Cows Fed Hay Grown on a Sludge-Reclaimed Mine Site

Given. Dairy cows were assumed to be fed hay year-round, all hay grown on former mine sites reclaimed with sludge. However, the hay was estimated to constitute only 67% of the total feed, with the remainder provided by feeding supplements. Because the individual was assumed to consume milk for 70 years through this exposure pathway, the 70-year average soil-TCDD equivalent concentration of 0.65 ppt, corresponding to an initial concentration of 35 ppt TCDD and its equivalents in the sludge (Table 3), was used to calculate exposure. Grasses were assumed to contain 0.1% of the concentration of TCDD in the soil. The steady-state concentration of TCDD in the milk fat was estimated to be 4 times greater than the concentration of TCDD in the grasses. Consumption of milk fat was assumed to occur at a rate of 11 g/day. All the TCDD contained in the milk fat was assumed to be bioavailable.

Solution. The lifetime average daily dose was calculated using Eq. (11) and the assumptions outlined above:

$$E_{milk} = \left(0.65 \frac{pg}{g}\right)(0.001)(4)(0.67)(1)\left(11 \frac{g}{day}\right)(1)$$

$$\times (25{,}550 \text{ days})\left(\frac{1}{25{,}550 \text{ days}}\right)\left(\frac{1}{70 \text{ kg}}\right)$$

$$= 2.7 \times 10^{-4} \text{ pg/kg·day}.$$

Illustrative Example 9. Calculating Human Uptake of TCDD from Consumption of Milk from Cows Grazed on Sludge-Reclaimed Mine Site Pasture

Given. In this exposure pathway, it was assumed that TCDD may be taken up by the cow through consumption of pasture grasses or through direct ingestion of soil. For the first case, the steady-state concentration of TCDD in the milk fat was calculated in a similar fashion to that of the calculations in Example 8, assuming a 70-year average soil concentration of 0.65 ppt TCDD equivalents, a 0.1% soil-TCDD uptake coefficient for grasses, a factor of 4 relating TCDD in the milk fat to TCDD in the diet, and a supplemental feeding factor of 67%. In the second case of direct soil ingestion, soil was assumed to constitute 3% of the diet. This factor was therefore applied to the ratio of TCDD in milk fat to TCDD in diet of 4, the supplemental feeding factor of 67%, along with a soil-TCDD concentration of 0.65 ppt, to calculate the resulting steady-state concentration of TCDD in the milk fat. The two components of steady-state concentration were added. To this figure was applied a consumption factor of 25%; that is, only 25% of all milk consumed by the individual over 70 years was assumed to derive directly from dairy cows grazed on sludge-reclaimed mine sites. Milk fat consumption was estimated at 11 g/day for 70 years.

Solution. The lifetime average daily dose was calculated using Eq. (12) and the assumptions outlined above:

$$E_{milk} = \left\{\left[\left(0.65 \frac{pg}{g}\right)(0.001)(4)(0.67)\right] + \left[\left(0.65 \frac{pg}{g}\right)(0.03)(4)(0.67)\right]\right\}$$

$$\times (0.25)\left(11 \frac{g}{day}\right)(1)(25{,}550 \text{ days})\left(\frac{1}{25{,}550 \text{ days}}\right)\left(\frac{1}{70 \text{ kg}}\right)$$

$$= 2.1 \times 10^{-3} \text{ pg/kg·day}.$$

4.3.4   Beef Consumption. The amount of TCDD taken up by humans through beef consumption was estimated for two separate exposure pathways. Similar to the analysis of milk consumption, we examined the uptake of TCDD and its equivalents by cattle fed hay that had been grown on the reclaimed mine site. These animals were not grazed, however. In the second pathway, we estimated TCDD uptake by grazing cattle on the reclaimed mine site. Exposure parameters for the two pathways are summarized in Table 12.

The distribution of TCDD to the fat of cattle fed TCDD in commercial feed was examined by Jensen et al. (157). Seven beef cattle were given feed containing 24 ppt TCDD for 28 days. TCDD residue found in fat tissue ranged from not detected to 95 ppt. The TCDD concentration in the fat was approximately 4 times higher than the TCDD concentration in the diet. It is likely that this factor may have reached 5 in a longer study in which steady-state conditions would have been achieved (15). Bovard et al. (163) found a residue/diet factor of 3.8 in cattle fed heptachlor for 712 days where steady-state conditions had been reached. In a 160-day feeding experiment in which nonlactating heifers were fed 1, 2, 3, 6, 8, 9-HxCDD, 1, 2, 3, 4, 6, 7, 8-HpCDD, OCDD, 1, 2, 3, 4, 6, 7, 8-HpCDF, or OCDF, body fat/diet factors of 0.05–2.1 were demonstrated (164).

As in the analysis of milk consumption in the hay-feeding exposure pathway, beef cattle were assumed to be fed hay that had been grown on reclaimed mine site areas on a year-round basis. Again, a supplemental feeding factor of 67% was applied. A farmer was assumed to consume beef for 365 days/year for 70 years, and all beef consumed by the farmer was derived from cattle fed hay grown on the mine site.

For the grazing exposure pathway, beef cattle were estimated to graze for about 5 months/year. Similar to the hay-feeding exposure pathway, the amounts of grasses and soil ingested from the mine site area during the grazing period were reduced to 67% of the total intake based on supplemental feeding. Again, a farmer was assumed to consume beef for 365 days/year for 70 years. However, only 50% of all beef consumed year-round was estimated to derive from cattle grazed on sludge-reclaimed mine sites where the sludge contains TCDD. Supporting rationale for this value is given in the following paragraph.

Beef fat residues tend to reflect average dietary concentrations over long periods of intake (161). Whereas milk fat residues of PCBs may approach steady state in a matter of weeks, Fries (161) noted that beef fat concentrations of an organic pesticide, heptachlor, took 280 days (40 weeks) to reach steady state. Heptachlor is a high molecular weight,

TABLE 12. Beef Consumption

Parameter	Value
Ratio of TCDD concentration in beef fat to TCDD concentration in diet	5
Supplemental feeding factor	67%
Soil-TCDD uptake coefficient for grasses	0.1%
Soil intake factor	3%
Consumption factor	
Hay-fed cattle	100%
Grazed cattle	50%
Beef fat consumption rate	12.6 g/day
Bioavailability, TCDD in beef	100%
Exposure duration	365 days/year, 70 years

chlorinated compound that is insoluble in water but soluble in organic solvents. If we assume TCDD exhibits behavior similar to that of heptachlor, the tissue residue of TCDD at the end of a 5-month grazing period may not have reached a steady-state level. At the end of the grazing period, exposure ceases and beef fat levels will decrease at a rate corresponding to the elimination half-life of TCDD in beef fat, calculated to be 115 days by Jensen et al. (157). In the following 7 months (about 213 days) with no additional TCDD exposure, the TCDD residue in the fat is expected to decrease by one-half every 115 days, resulting in about 25% of the maximum level that was reached at the end of the grazing period. As mentioned, the concentration of TCDD in beef fat was approximately 4 times greater than that in the diet at the end of a 28-day exposure (157). For the purpose of this analysis, a reasonable hypothesis projects that a concentration in the fat about 5 times greater than the TCDD concentration in the diet approximates the tissue residue of TCDD at steady state. Accumulation from year to year is unlikely to be a significant factor, due to the shorter period of summer grazing (5 months maximum), compared to nongrazing (7 months) in Ohio, significantly reducing residues during the nongrazing period.

The 50% beef consumption factor essentially represents the percentage of total beef consumed in a year, derived from cattle slaughtered near the end of the grazing period on TCDD-contaminated sludge-reclaimed mine sites. That is, cattle are assumed to be slaughtered at a time in which their fat tissues would contain maximum TCDD levels. If slaughtering occurred during the nongrazing period, TCDD levels would be lower. The remaining 50% of beef consumed was assumed to derive from either nongrazed cattle or cattle grazed on pasture on which TCDD-contaminated sludge had not been applied. This estimate appears reasonable, although it is clear that a particular farmer's actual exposure would depend on when the animal was slaughtered in relation to the grazing period and the proportion of beef consumed from animals that were not grazed on reclaimed mine sites. We believe that, in reality, only a small fraction of a farmer's uptake is from the farmer's own meat supply. Thus, our analysis considerably overstates the potential for uptake.

For grasses or hay consumed by beef cattle in both exposure pathways, a soil-TCDD uptake coefficient of 0.1% was used, similar to the analysis of milk consumption. In the case of grazed cattle, soil intake again was assumed to constitute 3% of the total dry matter intake (156). Beef fat consumption was estimated at 12.6 g/day based on a typical beef consumption rate of 105 g/day (about $\frac{1}{4}$ lb) at a 12% fat content (13).

The formulas for calculating TCDD uptake through beef consumption are

Hay-feeding

$$E_{\text{beef}} = C G_u R_t S_f C_f R_c BD \left(\frac{1}{L}\right)\left(\frac{1}{W}\right) \tag{13}$$

Grazing

$$E_{\text{beef}} = [(C G_u R_t S_f) + (C S_i R_t S_f)]$$
$$\times C_f R_c BD \left(\frac{1}{L}\right)\left(\frac{1}{W}\right), \tag{14}$$

where E = exposure, LADD (pg/kg·day)

C = concentration of TCDD in soil averaged over exposure period (pg/g)

G_u = grass uptake coefficient for TCDD in soil

S_i = soil intake factor
R_t = ratio of TCDD concentration in beef fat to TCDD concentration in diet
S_f = supplemental feeding factor
C_f = consumption factor
R_c = consumption rate (g/day)
B = bioavailability
D = exposure duration (days)
L = lifetime (days)
W = body weight (kg).

Illustrative Example 10. Calculating Human Uptake of TCDD from Consumption of Beef from Cattle Fed Hay Grown on a Sludge-Reclaimed Mine Site

Given. As in Example 8, beef cattle were assumed to be fed hay year-round, all hay grown on former mine sites reclaimed with sludge, and hay constituting 67% of the total feed. A 70-year average soil-TCDD equivalent concentration of 0.65 ppt was used to calculate exposure. Grasses were assumed to contain 0.1% of the soil-TCDD concentration. The steady-state concentration of TCDD in the fat was estimated at a factor of 5 times the concentration of TCDD in the grasses. A farmer was assumed to consume beef fat at a rate of 12.6 g/day for 70 years, only from cattle that had been fed hay grown on a sludge-reclaimed mine site.

Solution. The lifetime average daily dose was calculated using Eq. (13):

$$E_{\text{beef}} = \left(0.65\,\frac{\text{pg}}{\text{g}}\right)(0.001)(5)(0.67)(1)\left(12.6\,\frac{\text{g}}{\text{day}}\right)(1)$$
$$\times (25{,}550\,\text{days})\left(\frac{1}{25{,}550\,\text{days}}\right)\left(\frac{1}{70\,\text{kg}}\right)$$
$$= 3.9 \times 10^{-4}\,\text{pg/kg·day}.$$

Illustrative Example 11. Calculating Human Uptake of TCDD from Consumption of Milk from Cattle Grazed on Sludge-Reclaimed Mine Site Pasture

Given. As in Example 9, cattle may be exposed to TCDD through consumption of pasture grasses or ingestion of soil directly. In the first case, a 70-year average soil-TCDD equivalent concentration of 0.65 ppt was used and grasses were assumed to contain 0.1% of the soil-TCDD concentration. The steady-state concentration of TCDD in the fat was estimated at a factor of 5 times the TCDD concentration in the grasses or soil. Again, a supplemental feeding factor of 67% was used. In the case of direct soil ingestion, soil was assumed to constitute 3% of the diet. This factor was used with the ratio of TCDD in fat to TCDD in diet of 5, the supplemental feeding factor of 67%, and the soil-TCDD concentration of 0.65 ppt to calculate the resulting steady-state concentration of TCDD in the fat. To the sum of the two components of steady-state concentration was applied a consumption factor of 50%; that is, 50% of all beef consumed by this individual over 70 years was assumed to derive directly from beef cattle grazed on sludge-reclaimed mine sites. The farmer was assumed to ingest 12.6 g/day of beef fat for 70 years.

Solution. The lifetime average daily dose was calculated using Eq. (14):

$$E_{\text{beef}} = \left\{ \left[\left(0.65\frac{\text{pg}}{\text{g}}\right)(0.001)(5)(0.67) \right] + \left[\left(0.65\frac{\text{pg}}{\text{g}}\right)(0.03)(5)(0.67) \right] \right\}$$

$$\times (0.5)\left(12.6\frac{\text{g}}{\text{day}}\right)(1)(25{,}550\,\text{days})\left(\frac{1}{25{,}550\,\text{days}}\right)\left(\frac{1}{70\,\text{kg}}\right)$$

$$= 6.1 \times 10^{-3}\,\text{pg/kg·day}.$$

4.3.5 Vegetable Consumption.
Crops raised for human consumption on reclaimed mine sites may conceivably represent a potential source of exposure. Using corn as a model for an aboveground family garden crop, uptake through consumption of corn was assessed. Modeling parameters are summarized in Table 13. Limited data are available to characterize uptake of TCDD from the soil into corn kernels. Wipf et al. (145) found no detectable traces of TCDD in corn kernels from corn grown on TCDD-contaminated Seveso soil 1 year following the explosion in Seveso, Italy. From these data, we calculated the maximum possible hypothetical uptake based on the detection limit of 0.8 ppt TCDD in corn kernels relative to the measured TCDD level in the soil of 10,000 ppt. This resulted in an estimated uptake of 0.008% for use in this analysis.

The garden soil was assumed to consist of the paper mill sludge thoroughly mixed with mine spoil as described in Section 4.2. All corn consumed by an individual was estimated to have been grown in the mine site garden. Corn consumption was estimated at 250 g/day fresh corn for 30 days in the summer and 100 g/day frozen corn once per week for the remainder of the year (48 days). The weighted average of the two consumption figures was calculated to equal approximately 160 g/day for those days on which corn is consumed, 78 days each year for 70 years.

The formula for calculating exposure is

$$E_{\text{corn}} = CUC_f R_c BD\left(\frac{1}{L}\right)\left(\frac{1}{W}\right), \tag{15}$$

where E = exposure, LADD (pg/kg·day)
C = concentration of TCDD in soil averaged over exposure period (pg/g)
U = corn uptake coefficient for TCDD in soil
C_f = consumption factor
R_c = consumption rate (g/day)
B = bioavailability
D = exposure duration (days)

TABLE 13. Corn Consumption

Parameter	Value
Soil-TCDD uptake coefficient for corn	0.008%
Corn consumption from home garden factor	100%
Consumption rate	160 g/day
Bioavailability	100%
Exposure duration	78 days/year, 70 years

$L =$ lifetime (days)
$W =$ body weight (kg).

Illustrative Example 12. Calculating Human Uptake of TCDD from Consumption of Corn

Given. A home gardener was assumed to consume corn exclusively from the home garden for 70 years. Therefore, the 70-year average concentration of TCDD and its equivalents in the soil was used to calculate uptake. Corn kernels were estimated to contain 0.008% of the soil-TCDD concentration. The farmer was assumed to ingest 160 g/day of corn for 78 days/year each year.

Solution. The lifetime average daily dose of TCDD from corn consumption was calculated using Eq. (15):

$$
E_{corn} = \left(0.65 \frac{pg}{g} \right)(0.00008)(1)\left(160 \frac{g}{day} \right)(1)
$$
$$
\times \left(78 \frac{days}{year} \times 70 \, years \right)\left(\frac{1}{25{,}550 \, days} \right)\left(\frac{1}{70 \, kg} \right)
$$
$$
= 2.5 \times 10^{-5} \, pg/kg \cdot day.
$$

4.4   Estimation of Dose

Human uptake of TCDD and its equivalents, expressed as lifetime average daily doses for the described exposure pathways, are given in Table 14. The LADDs shown correspond to an initial level of 35 ppt TCDD equivalents in the sludge used to reclaim the abandoned strip mine sites. This sludge-TCDD equivalent level is reduced in the process of incorporation with mine spoil and degradation over the period of exposure.

TABLE 14. Lifetime Average Daily Doses Associated with Initial Sludge-TCDD Equivalent Level of 35 ppt

Exposure Pathway	LADD (pg/kg·day)
Residential contact	
Dermal uptake	6.3×10^{-5}
Inhalation	1.2×10^{-6}
Oral uptake of soil[a]	2.5×10^{-4}
Hunting of game species	
Wild turkey	6.6×10^{-5}
Venison	1.3×10^{-5}
Milk and beef consumption	
Hay-feeding: Milk	2.7×10^{-4}
Beef	3.9×10^{-4}
Grazing: Milk	2.1×10^{-3}
Beef	6.1×10^{-3}
Vegetable consumption	
Corn	2.5×10^{-5}

[a]Average daily dose during the 5-year period of exposure would be 3.5×10^{-3} pg/kg·day.

5 RISK ASSESSMENT

The results of the quantitative risk assessment are expressed as the additional risk, over the course of a 70-year lifetime, of contracting cancer over and above the background risk level (about 1 in 4) that already exists from all causes. Lifetime incremental cancer risks associated with the lifetime average daily doses shown in Table 14 were calculated as the product of the LADD and cancer potency:

$$R = EC_pF_c, \tag{16}$$

where R = risk
  E = exposure, lifetime average daily dose (pg/kg·day)
  C_p = cancer potency (mg/kg·day)$^{-1}$
  F_c = conversion factor, 10^{-9} mg/pg.

This method of calculation is a valid approximation of extra risk at low doses (52). The risk calculation is illustrated by the following example in which the lifetime incremental cancer risk related to skin contact was calculated.

Illustrative Example 13. Calculating Lifetime Incremental Cancer Risk Related to Skin Contact

Given. In Example 1, we estimated the lifetime average daily dose to an individual who incurs significant skin contact with soil on reclaimed mine sites to be 6.3×10^{-5} pg/kg·day. We developed a best estimate of cancer potency for TCDD of 1.7×10^4 (mg/kg·day)$^{-1}$ as described in Section 3.1.

Solution. The lifetime incremental cancer risk associated with skin contact was estimated using Eq. (16):

$$\text{Risk} = (6.3 \times 10^{-5}\,\text{pg/kg·day})[1.7 \times 10^4\,(\text{mg/kg·day})^{-1}](10^{-9}\,\text{mg/pg})$$
$$= 1.1 \times 10^{-9}.$$

The cancer potency figure used to calculate risk represents the geometric mean of two potency figures, each representing an upper bound on potency; that is, the potency is not likely to be greater but may very well be lower. Uptake was calculated essentially for the most highly exposed individual in the population hypothetically using the reclaimed mine sites for residential purposes and farming. Application of an upper bound cancer potency figure to the lifetime dose estimates thus results in estimates of an upper limit on individual risk, rather than a point estimate, or most likely value of risk.

Upper bounds of lifetime incremental cancer risks for individual scenarios are shown in Table 15. All individual risk levels are less than 1×10^{-6}. Upper bounds of lifetime incremental cancer risks range from the lowest risk of 2.0×10^{-11} for the inhalation pathway to the highest risk of 1.0×10^{-7} for the grazing beef pathway. Calculated cancer risks were based on 70-year exposure durations for all scenarios except soil ingestion by children. If actual exposures were of shorter duration, they would be associated with proportionately lower risks.

In addition to estimating risks corresponding to an initial sludge-TCDD concentration

TABLE 15. Risk Assessment Results

Exposure Pathway	Lifetime Incremental Cancer Risk Corresponding to Sludge at 35 ppt TCDD Equivalents	Virtually Safe Concentration of TCDD Equivalents in Soil[a] (ppt)	Virtually Safe Concentration of TCDD Equivalents in Sludge[b] (ppt)
Residential contact			
Dermal uptake	1.1×10^{-9}	3,200	32,000
Inhalation	2.0×10^{-11}	170,000	1,700,000
Oral uptake of soil	4.3×10^{-9}	810	8,100
Hunting of game species			
Wild turkey	1.1×10^{-9}	3,200	32,000
Venison	2.2×10^{-10}	16,000	160,000
Milk and beef consumption			
Hay-feeding: Milk	4.6×10^{-9}	760	7,600
Beef	6.6×10^{-9}	530	5,300
Grazing: Milk	3.6×10^{-8}	97	970
Beef	1.0×10^{-7}	35	350
Vegetable consumption			
Corn	4.3×10^{-10}	8,100	81,000

[a]Corresponds to virtually safe concentration of TCDD equivalents in soil immediately after application at a 1×10^{-6} risk level.
[b]Corresponds to a 1×10^{-6} risk level.

of 35 ppt TCDD equivalents, "reverse" calculations also were performed to estimate initial soil-TCDD and initial sludge-TCDD concentrations at a specified incremental cancer risk level of 1×10^{-6}. For each route of exposure, these calculated concentrations of TCDD equivalents in sludge or soil are called *virtually safe concentrations*. The formulas are

$$C_v = C_i R_a \left(\frac{1}{R} \right), \tag{17}$$

where C_v = virtually safe concentration of TCDD equivalents in soil at 1×10^{-6} risk level
       C_i = initial soil-TCDD equivalent concentration (pg/g)
      R_a = acceptable risk level, 1×10^{-6}
      R = risk

and

$$S_v = C_v F, \tag{18}$$

where S_v = virtually safe concentration of TCDD equivalents in sludge at 1×10^{-6} risk level
      C_v = virtually safe concentration of TCDD equivalents in soil at 1×10^{-6} risk level
      F = factor relating initial soil-TCDD equivalent concentration to sludge-TCDD equivalent concentration.

    Essentially, Eq. (17) represents the solution of the equating of the two ratios: (i) the ratio of the risk we estimated for a given exposure pathway to the corresponding initial soil-

TCDD concentration, and (ii) the ratio of the acceptable risk level to the virtually safe concentration of TCDD in soil. Equation (18) relates the virtually safe concentration of TCDD in the soil to that in sludge. These calculations are illustrated in the following example.

Illustrative Example 14. Calculating Virtually Safe Concentrations of Initial Soil-TCDD Equivalents and Sludge-TCDD Equivalents at a 1×10^{-6} Risk Level for Skin Contact

Given. A 1.1×10^{-9} incremental cancer risk level was calculated in Example 13 for skin contact using an initial soil-TCDD equivalent concentration of 3.5 ppt (before the 2-year latency period) based on the corresponding initial sludge-TCDD equivalent concentration of 35 ppt. An acceptable risk level of 1×10^{-6} was selected in order to estimate the virtually safe concentration of TCDD and its equivalents in the soil and sludge.

Solution. Using Eqs. (17) and (18), we calculated the virtually safe concentrations of TCDD and its equivalents in the soil and sludge, respectively:

$$C_v = (3.5\,\text{pg/g})(1 \times 10^{-6})\left(\frac{1}{1.1 \times 10^{-9}}\right)$$

$$= 3200\,\text{pg/g}$$

and

$$S_v = (3200\,\text{pg/g})(10)$$

$$= 32{,}000\,\text{pg/g}.$$

Virtually safe concentrations of TCDD and its equivalents in the soil (immediately after application) and sludge corresponding to a preselected, maximum incremental lifetime cancer risk of 1×10^{-6} are shown in Table 15. The lowest virtually safe concentrations correspond to the exposure pathway that displayed the highest risk level, the grazing-beef exposure pathway. We estimated virtually safe concentrations of TCDD equivalents in the sludge ranging from 350 to 1,700,000 ppt, depending on the exposure pathway examined. The corresponding virtually safe concentrations estimated for the soil ranged from 35 to 170,000 ppt.

It is also possible to develop composite exposures where more than one route of exposure is conceivable. It is of course unrealistic to total all exposure routes together because the probability of all routes occurring to one individual for the lifetime of exposure used in this analysis would be negligible, or virtually impossible. Even the probability of any one of the exposure pathways occurring for a 70-year period is extremely small. Furthermore, there is no regulatory precedent which would suggest that such a conservative analysis be used to demonstrate that one person's exposure would not result in more than a 1×10^{-6} risk level. In fact, as discussed by Travis et al. (165), recent regulatory action by the EPA and others suggests that for small-population risks, the de minimis risk is considered to be a 1×10^{-4} lifetime risk.

Nevertheless, we have developed several composite scenarios representing various combinations of routes: (i) residential contact including dermal uptake, inhalation, and oral uptake of soil, (ii) hunting of game species including wild turkey and deer, (iii) a total composite including all routes, with the exception of the hay-fed-beef and grazing-cow milk exposure pathways. Both types of beef and milk exposure pathways could not be included in the composite because exposure would then be double-counted. The hay-fed-cow milk and grazing-beef pathways were selected for the composite scenario to represent a reasonably worst-case situation. Risk assessment results for the composite scenarios are given in Table 16. It is important to recognize the limitations of the composite exposure approach, particularly when these types of result are used in risk management settings. The summing of all conceivable exposure pathways will compound the conservatism inherent in each individual analysis, thus producing an unrealistic portrayal of the actual risk.

A lifetime incremental cancer risk level of 1×10^{-6} (1 in 1 million) was used in this analysis to represent a level of incremental risk that is clearly considered acceptable (de minimis) by state and federal regulatory agencies. A recent analysis of risk decisions in federal regulatory agencies indicates that individual lifetime risks to the general population greater than 1×10^{-6}, and sometimes up to more than 1×10^{-4}, have been determined to be acceptable because of the small size of the exposed population or because of cost or feasibility constraints (166).

In a review of cancer risk management, Travis et al. (165) found that regulatory action was never taken for individual risk levels below 1×10^{-4} when small-population effects were involved. The level of acceptable risk dropped to 1×10^{-6} only for effects involving exposure to the total U.S. population. These analyses demonstrate that our selection of a 1×10^{-6} risk level for use in this analysis is extremely conservative given the very small population that will ever potentially be exposed to TCDD in the reclaimed mine sites.

In order to place these risk levels into perspective, consider the average annual per capita risks of mortality for activities such as smoking (3×10^{-3}), motor vehicle accidents (2×10^{-4}), swimming (3×10^{-5}), and being struck by lightning (5×10^{-7}) (167). When multiplied by a lifetime period at risk, the risks of all these activities are much greater than a lifetime incremental cancer risk level of 1×10^{-6}.

TABLE 16. Risk Assessment Results: Composite Exposure Pathways

Exposure Pathway	Lifetime Incremental Cancer Risk Corresponding to Sludge at 35 ppt TCDD Equivalents	Virtually Safe Concentration of TCDD Equivalents in Soil (ppt)	Virtually Safe Concentration of TCDD Equivalents in Sludge (ppt)
Residential contact	5.4×10^{-9}	650	6,500
Dermal uptake			
Inhalation			
Oral uptake of soil			
Hunting of game species	1.3×10^{-9}	2,700	27,000
Wild turkey			
Venison			
Milk and beef consumption			
Hay-feeding: Milk			
Grazing: Beef			
Vegetable consumption			
Corn			
Total composite	1.1×10^{-7}	31	310

6   CONCLUSIONS

Upper bounds for lifetime incremental cancer risks for the individual scenarios of exposure examined in this chapter ranged from 2.0×10^{-11} for inhalation to 1.0×10^{-7} for the consumption of beef from cattle grazed on reclaimed mine site pastures. These risk levels correspond to a concentration of 35 ppt TCDD equivalents in the sludge applied to the mine site. Based on the limited data available to characterize PCDD and PCDF content of this sludge, the concentration of 35 ppt TCDD equivalents appears to represent a reasonable estimate for use in this analysis. The risk calculations indicate that exposure to sludge on reclaimed mine sites presents an insignificant risk to human health at the dioxin levels tested and under the scenarios examined in this report. Examination of the virtually safe concentrations that we calculated for TCDD equivalents in the sludge (Tables 15 and 16) indicates that levels 10 times higher than 35 ppt TCDD equivalents would still present no more than a 1×10^{-6} risk for any exposure pathway examined.

Results of our risk assessment can be examined in relation to recent regulatory action and the findings of similar studies. The most conservative virtually safe concentration in sludge of 310 ppt for the total composite of the various exposure pathways (Table 16) is not dissimilar to the state of Maine's maximum allowable concentration limit in landspread sludge of 250 ppt TCDD equivalents. Of course, while the two figures are similar in magnitude, the bases of the analyses are not identical. Our analysis also supports Ohio's maximum permissible concentration of 100 ppt TCDD equivalents for soil to which sludges are applied on a one-time basis.

We estimated a virtually safe concentration of TCDD equivalents in the soil of about 650 ppt for residential exposure pathways (dermal uptake, inhalation, and oral uptake of soil). This figure can be compared to the Kimbrough et al. (13) estimate of 1 ppb TCDD in residential soil as a reasonable level at which to begin consideration of action to limit human exposure. Compared to soil-TCDD concentrations of 6.2–79 ppt projected to produce maximum allowable residues in beef, pork, and milk (13), use of a different approach resulted in our estimates of virtually safe concentrations in the soil of 35–760 ppt TCDD equivalents for consumption of milk and beef.

Our analyses of risks associated with exposure to dioxin in sludges used for agricultural land application in the state of Maine (21–23) also demonstrated no significant risk from sludges containing low levels of TCDD. A number of significant differences exist between these analyses and the analysis presented in this chapter, especially regarding the sludge-to-soil application modeling. Even given these differences, allowable average TCDD levels in the soil and sludge calculated at a 1×10^{-6} risk level in the analyses of Maine sludges are not dissimilar to the virtually safe concentrations calculated for similar exposure pathways in this chapter. Eschenroeder et al. (16) also examined the health risks of human exposure to soil amended with sludges containing low concentrations of PCDDs and PCDFs and found no unreasonable risk to human health.

The risk estimates presented in this chapter represent hypothetical risk levels based on the assumption that people are actually living on the reclaimed mine sites or using the land to hunt or graze livestock. Exposures were assumed to start either immediately or 2 years following application and extend for 70 years, except for soil ingestion by children, which was assumed to occur for 5 years. It is obvious that the probability of such exposures actually occurring is extremely small. Thus, these risks represent an extreme upper bound of possible risk, not the most likely risk. It also is important to recognize the distinction in risk assessment between hypothetical risks as calculated in this analysis and actual risks, such as those calculated from accident statistics. The latter risks are based on actual measured events and outcomes rather than possible outcomes based on mathematical interpretation of bioassay results.

The purpose of this analysis was to identify upper bounds of hypothetical risks that could be related to the use of sludge for mine site reclamation, not actual risks. The calculated upper bounds of risk can then be used in a risk management setting to aid in determining appropriate levels of regulatory concern. Risk managers must integrate the results of the risk assessment with socioeconomic, technical, political, and other considerations in order to develop, analyze, and compare regulatory options and make a decision on the appropriate regulatory response (10, 11, 168).

It is also important to recognize the uncertainties and conservatism inherent in these risk calculations. The risk assessment process used in this analysis assumes that animal data on TCDD carcinogenicity can be used to make an adequate prediction of human response at much lower dose levels; specifically, doses about 10,000,000 times less than those actually tested. This extrapolation, accomplished via a nonthreshold mathematical model, introduces a good deal of uncertainty that can only produce risk estimates that are greater than, rather than less than, estimates of the true risk. For example, we derived a potency factor for TCDD from data on the most sensitive tumor types in bioassays of several species and strains of laboratory animals. This derivation, although a slight departure from the ultraconservatism of the U.S. EPA figure, still represents a conservative approach to TCDD risk estimation, given the problems with fit of the female rat liver data to the model (98) and evidence supporting a threshold effect for TCDD based on its action as a cancer promoter rather than as an initiator.

Uncertainty, only in the direction of overstating the true risks, was also introduced through the use of toxic equivalency factors developed by the U.S. EPA, since it is not clearly established experimentally that toxic equivalency correlates with carcinogenic equivalency. In addition, a number of factors in the exposure analysis were based solely on TCDD data, and it is not clear whether these factors can be extrapolated to other congeners using the toxic equivalency procedure; although it is quite likely that they are fairly accurate.

The sludge application model used in this analysis also contributed some uncertainty to the final risk estimates. It was assumed that all sludge is incorporated with mine spoil at a 1:9 dilution. In some cases, however, incorporation is not possible and sludge must be applied directly to the surface. Because these cases comprise only a small percentage of total application area, we believe that use of the incorporation model better portrays typical mine site reclamation practice.

Numerous exposure factors had to be estimated in this analysis in order to calculate risks. In some cases, limited data bases contributed to uncertainty in the estimate used. As an example, the age-specific soil contact rate for exposed skin was estimated from several studies of soil accumulation on children's hands. The contact rate estimate contains the uncertainty of the original data on which it was based, as well as the uncertainty of the extrapolation from child to adult and from hands to other body areas.

We believe that the response to uncertainty should not consist solely of selecting the "most conservative" set of factors possible, but rather should ideally consist of a balanced weighting of the evidence. However, in this analysis, we have almost certainly overstated, and perhaps unrealistically portrayed, possible risks. An alternate risk analysis could be based on the "most likely" set of assumptions and thereby demonstrate the impact of our selection of numerous worst-case parameters.

Although it is virtually certain that the combination of exposure pathways examined in this assessment will never be realized, the results of this study illustrate the de minimis nature of the potential risks that have been identified and elevated to the level of public debate. Results of this risk analysis clearly show that a paper mill sludge used to reclaim abandoned mine sites presents an insignificant risk to the health of individuals that might reside on the reclaimed mine site areas or use the land to hunt or to graze livestock, for a full lifetime of exposure. Concentrations of TCDD equivalents in sludge below about 400 ppt present no significant threat to human health under any of the exposure pathways examined in this analysis. We believe that even higher levels would not present a significant risk, given the conservative exposure modeling performed in this analysis and the selection of a very conservative level of acceptable risk.

While this chapter presents an analysis of the health risks related to the application of one specific pulp and paper mill sludge, under identical exposure pathways, the risk assessment may be generalized and appropriately used to assess the risks associated with low concentrations of dioxin in sludges produced at other similar pulp and paper mill facilities. In light of the regulatory precedent for assessing the significance of small-population effects (165, 166), clearly the issue of low concentrations of dioxin in sludges used to reclaim abandoned strip mines is de minimis. For risk management purposes, this low level of hypothetical risk associated with the use of a paper mill sludge containing low concentrations of dioxin for mine site reclamation should be balanced against the risks that may be associated with unreclaimed mine sites, the cost–benefit and risk–benefit of placing the sludges elsewhere, and the cost–benefit of continuing to produce paper to meet the needs of consumers throughout the world.

REFERENCES

1. National Council of Paper Industry for Air and Stream Improvement, Inc., *Pulp and Papermill Sludges in Maine: A Characterization Study*, NCASI Tech. Bull. 447. NCASI, New York, NY, 1984.

2. Client, *Sludge Management Plan*, 1986.

3. M. E. Watson and H. A. J. Hoitink, Long term effects of papermill sludge in stripmine reclamation. *Ohio Rep.*, March-April (1985).

4. U.S. Environmental Protection Agency, *Use and Disposal of Municipal Wastewater Sludge*, EPA-625/10-84-003. Environmental Regulations and Technology, USEPA, Washington, DC, 1984.

5. Ontario Ministry of the Environment, *Scientific Criteria Document for Standard Development No. 4–84 Polychlorinated Dibenzo-p-dioxins (PCDDs) and Polychlorinated Dibenzofurans (PCDFs)*. OME, Ontario, Canada, 1985.

6. R. J. Kociba and O. Cabey, Comparative toxicity and biologic activity of chlorinated dibenzo-p-dioxins and furans relative to 2, 3, 7, 8-tetrachlorodibenzo-p-dioxin (TCDD). *Chemosphere* **14**, 649–660 (1985).

7. R. J. Kociba, D. G. Keyes, J. E. Beyer et al., Results of a two-year chronic toxicity and oncogenicity study of 2, 3, 7, 8-tetrachlorodibenzo-p-dioxin in rats. *Toxicol. Appl. Pharmacol.* **46**, 279–303 (1978).

8. National Toxicology Program, *Carcinogenesis Bioassay of 2, 3, 7, 8-Tetrachlorodibenzo-p-dioxin (CAS No. 1746-01-6) in Osborne-Mendel Rats and B6C3F1 Mice (Gavage Study)*, Tech. Rep. Ser. No. 209. NTP, Research Triangle Park, NC, 1982.

9. H. Poiger and C. Schlatter, Pharmacokinetics of 2, 3, 7, 8-TCDD in man. *Chemosphere* **15**, 1489–1494 (1986).

10. National Research Council, *Risk Assessment in the Federal Government: Managing the Process*. National Academy Press, Washington, DC, 1983.

11. U.S. Environmental Protection Agency, Guidelines for carcinogen risk assessment. *Fed. Regist.* **51**, 33992–34003 (1986).

12. U.S. Environmental Protection Agency, *Interim Procedures for Estimating Risks Associated with Exposures to Mixtures of Chlorinated Dibenzo-p-Dioxins and Dibenzofurans (CDDs and CDFs)*, EPA/625/3-87/012. Risk Assessment Forum, USEPA, Washington, DC, 1987.

13. R. D. Kimbrough, M. Falk, P. Stehr, and G. Fries, Health implications of 2,3,7,8-tetrachlorodibenzodioxin (TCDD) contamination of residential soil. *J. Toxicol. Environ. Health* **14**, 47–93 (1984).

14. D. J. Paustenbach, H. P. Shu, and F. J. Murray, A critical examination of assumptions used in risk assessments of dioxin contaminated soil. *Regul. Toxicol. Pharmacol.* **6**, 284–307 (1986).

15. G. F. Fries, Assessment of potential residues in foods derived from animals exposed to TCDD-contaminated soil. *Chemosphere* (to be published).

16. A. E. Eschenroeder, R. J. Jaeger, J. J. Ospital, and C. P. Doyle, Health risk analysis of human exposures to soil amended with sewage sludge contaminated with polychlorinated dibenzodioxins and dibenzofurans. *Vet. Hum. Toxicol.* **28**, 435–442 (1986).

17. U.S. Environmental Protection Agency. *Risk Analysis of TCDD Contaminated Soil*, EPA-600/8-84-031. Exposure Assessment Group, USEPA, Washington, DC, 1984.

18. Maine Department of Environmental Protection. *Interim Standards for Sludge and Residuals Containing Polychlorinated Dibenzo-p-dioxins and Polychlorinated Dibenzofurans (PCDDs and PCDFs)*, Part D, Amendment to Chapter 567, *Rules for Land Application of Sludge and Residuals*. MDEP, Augusta 1986.

19. Ohio Environmental Protection Agency, *Guidelines for Land Application of Paper Mill Sludge*. EPA, OH, April 30, 1987.

20. Wisconsin Department of Health and Social Services, *Human Exposure Assessment for Dioxin Contaminated Papermill Sludge Amended to Soils*. WDHSC, Madison January 23, 1987.

21. F. Lawrence, *Health Risk Assessment Related to Exposure to Dioxin from Land Application of Wastewater Sludges*, Testimony presented at public hearing before Maine Board of Environmental Protection regarding proposed amendment to Chapter 567 dioxin standards *Rules for Land Application of Sludge and Residuals*. Envirologic Data, Portland, ME, March 19, 1986.

22. R. E. Keenan, *Potential Impacts of Wildlife from Dioxin Containing Sludges*, Testimony presented to the Board of Environmental Protection, State of Maine, in public hearing, April 16. Envirologic Data, Portland, ME, 1986.

23. National Council of Paper Industry for Air and Stream Improvement, Inc., *Assessment of Human Health Risks Related to Exposure to Dioxin from Land Application of Wastewater Sludge in Maine*, NCASI Tech. Bull. 525. New York, NY prepared by Envirologic Data, Portland, ME, 1987.

24. Envirologic Data, *Assessment of Human Health Risks and Potential Impacts on Terrestrial Wildlife Related to Exposure to Dioxin from Strip Mine Reclamation with Bypro® Papermill Sludges in Southeast Ohio*. Envirologic Data, Portland, ME, 1986.

25. L. Marple, R. Brunck, B. Berridge, and L. Throop, Comparison of experimental and calculated physical constants for 2,3,7,8-tetrachlorodibenzo-p-dioxin. *Ext. Abstr. Am. Chem. Soc. Meet., New York*, pp. 124–127 (1986).

26. J. M. Schroy, F. D. Hileman, and S. C. Ching, Physical/chemical properties of 2,3,7,8-TCDD. *Chemosphere* **14**, 877–880 (1985).

27. H. B. Matthews and L. S. Birnbaum, Factors affecting the disposition and persistence of halogenated furans and dioxins. In R. E. Tucker, A. C. Young, and A. P. Gray, Eds., *Human and Environmental Risks of Chlorinated Dioxins and Related Compounds*. Plenum Press, New York, 1983.

28. D. G. Crosby, K. W. Moilanen, and A. S. Wong, Environmental generation and degradation of dibenzodioxins and dibenzofurans. *Environ. Health Perspect.* **5**, 259–266 (1973).

29. J. M. Schroy, F. D. Hileman, and S. Ching, Physical/chemical properties of 2, 3, 7, 8-tetrachloro-dibenzo-p-dioxin. *ASTM Spec. Tech. Publ.* **891**, 409–421 (1985).

30. R. A. Freeman and J. M. Schroy, Environmental mobility of dioxins. *ASTM Spec. Tech. Publ.* **891**, 422–439 (1985).

31. G. Fries and G. Marrow, Retention and excretion of 2, 3, 7, 8-tetrachlorodibenzo-p-dioxin by rats. *J. Agric. Food Chem.* **23**, 265–269 (1975).

32. J. Q. Rose, J. C. Ramsey, T. H. Wentzler, R. A. Hummel, and P. J. Gehring, The fate of 2, 3, 7, 8-tetrachlorodibenzo-p-dioxin following single and repeated oral doses to the rat. *Toxicol. Appl. Pharmacol.* **36**, 209–226 (1976).

33. W. N. Piper, R. Q. Rose, and P. J. Gehring, Excretion and tissue distribution of 2, 3, 7, 8-tetrachlorodibenzo-p-dioxin in the rat. *Environ. Health Perspect.* **5**, 241–244 (1973).

34. J. R. Olson, T. A. Gasiewicz, and R. A. Neal, Tissue distribution, excretion and metabolism of 2, 3, 7, 8-tetrachlorodibenzo-p-dioxin (TCDD) in the Golden Syrian hamster. *Toxicol. Appl. Pharmacol.* **56**, 78–95 (1980).

35. H. Poiger and C. Schlatter, Influence of solvents and adsorbents on dermal and intestinal adsorption of TCDD. *Food Cosmet. Toxicol.* **18**, 477–481 (1980).

36. G. Lucier, R. Rumbaugh, Z. McCoy, R. Hass, D. Harvan, and P. Albro, Ingestion of soil contaminated with 2, 3, 7, 8-tetrachlorodibenzo-p-dioxin (TCDD) alters hepatic enzyme activities in rats. *Fundam. Appl. Toxicol.* **6**, 364–371 (1986).

37. T. H. Umbreit, E. J. Hesse, and M. A. Gallo, Bioavailability of dioxin in soil from a 2, 4, 5-T manufacturing site. *Science* **232**, 497–499 (1986).

38. A. Bonaccorsi, A. di Domenico, R. Fanelli, F. Merli, R. Motta, R. Vanzati, and G. Zapponi, The influence of soil particle adsorption on 2, 3, 7, 8-tetrachlorodibenzo-p-dioxin biological uptake in the rabbit. *Arch. Toxicol., Suppl.* **7**, 431–434 (1984).

39. H. Shu, D. Paustenbach, J. Murray, L. Marple, B. Brunck, D. Dei Rossi, and P. Teitelbaum, Bioavailability of soil-bound TCDD: Oral bioavailability in the rat. *Fundam. Appl. Toxicol.* **10**, 648–654 (1988).

40. T. A. Gasiewicz, J. R. Olson, L. H. Geiger, and R. A. Neal, Absorption, distribution and metabolism of 2, 3, 7, 8-tetrachlorodibenzodioxin (TCDD) in experimental animals. In R. E. Tucker, A. L. Young, and A. P. Gray, Eds., *Human and Environmental Risks of Chlorinated Dioxins and Related Compounds.* Plenum Press, New York, 1983.

41. W. P. McNulty, K. A. Nielsen-Smith, J. O. Lay, Jr., D. L. Lippstreu, N. L. Kangas, P. A. Lyon, and M. L. Gross, Persistence of TCDD in monkey adipose tissue. *Food Chem. Toxicol.* **20**, 985–987 (1982).

42. R. J. Kociba and B. A. Schwetz, Toxicity of 2, 3, 7, 8-tetrachlorodibenzo-p-dioxin (TCDD). *Drug Metab. Rev.* **13**, 387–406 (1982).

43. J. R. Olson, M. A. Holscher, and R. A. Neal, Toxicity of 2, 3, 7, 8-tetrachlorodibenzo-p-dioxin in the Golden Syrian hamster. *Toxicol. Appl. Pharmacol.* **55**, 67–78 (1980).

44. J. Dean and R. Kimbrough, Immunotoxicity of the chlorinated dibenzodioxins and dibenzofurans. In J. A. Moore Ed., *Report of the Dioxin Update Committee.* Convened by EPA Office of Pesticide and Toxic Substances, Dioxin Update Conference, July 1–2, 1986.

45. A. Poland, J. Knutson, and E. Glover, A consideration of the mechanism of action of 2, 3, 7, 8-tetrachlorodibenzo-p-dioxin and related halogenated aromatic hydrocarbons. In R. E. Tucker, A. L. Young, and A. P. Gray, Eds., *Human and Environmental Risks of Chlorinated Dioxins and Related Compounds.* Plenum Press, New York, 1983.

46. E. Roberts, N. Shear, and A. Okey, The Ah receptor and dioxin toxicity: From rodent to human tissues. *Chemosphere* **14**, 661–674 (1985).

47. A. Poland, Mechanism of action. In J. A. Moore, Ed., *Report of the Dioxin Update Committee.*

Convened by EPA Office of Pesticides and Toxic Substances, Dioxin Update Conference, July 1–2, 1986.

48. A. Poland and J. Knutson, 2, 3, 7, 8-tetrachlorodibenzo-p-dioxin and related halogenated aromatic hydrocarbons: Examination of the mechanisms of toxicity. *Annu. Rev. Pharmacol. Toxicol.* **22**, 517–554 (1982).

49. W. Greenlee, R. Osbourne, K. Dold, L. Hudson, and W. Toscano, Toxicity of chlorinated aromatic compounds in animals and humans: *In vitro* approaches to toxic mechanisms and risk assessments. *Environ Health Perspect.* **60**, 69–76 (1985).

50. B. Madhukar, D. Brewster, and F. Matsumura, Effects of *in vivo* administered 2, 3, 7, 8-tetrachlorodibenzo-p-dioxin on receptor binding of epidermal growth factor in hepatic plasmal membrane of rat, guinea pig, mouse, and hamster. *Proc. Natl. Acad. Sci. U.S.A.* **81**, 7407–7411 (1984).

51. F. J. Murray, F. A. Smith, K. D. Nitschke, C. G. Humiston, R. J. Kociba, and B. A. Schwetz, Three-generation reproduction study of rats given 2, 3, 7, 8-tetrachlorodibenzo-p-dioxin (TCDD) in the diet. *Toxicol. Appl. Pharmacol.* **50**, 241–252 (1979).

52. U.S. Environmental Protection Agency, *Health Assessment Document for Polychlorinated Dibenzo-p-dioxins*, EPA/600/8-84/014F. Office of Health and Environmental Assessment, USEPA, Washington, DC, 1985.

53. H. P. Shu, D. J. Paustenbach, and F. J. Murray, A critical evaluation of the use of mutagenesis, carcinogenesis, and tumor promotion data in a cancer risk assessment of 2, 3, 7, 8-tetrachlorodibenzo-p-dioxin. *Regul. Toxicol. Pharmacol.* **7**, 57–88 (1987).

54. H. C. Pitot, T. Goldsworthy, H. A. Campbell, and A. Poland, Quantitative evaluation of the promotion by 2, 3, 7, 8-tetrachlorodibenzo-p-dioxin of hepatocarcinogenesis from diethylnitrosamine. *Cancer Res.* **40**, 3616–3620 (1980).

55. A. Poland, D. Palen, and E. Glover, Tumor promotion by TCDD in skin of HRS/J hairless mice. *Nature (London)* **300**, 271–273 (1982).

56. American Medical Association, *The Health Effects of "Agent Orange" and Polychlorinated Dioxin Contaminants: An Update, 1984*, Tech. Rep. Council on Scientific Affairs, Advisory Panel on Toxic Substances, AMA, Chicago, IL, 1984 (updated 1985).

57. H. Poiger and C. Schlatter, Pharmakokinetics of 2, 3, 7, 8-TCDD in man. *Chemosphere* **15**, 1489–1494 (1986).

58. K. Jones, I. Nisbet, C. Knoheim, F. Hasselriis, D. Sussman, D. Lipsky, C. Kemp, and J. Hahn, A peer review of the paper *Environmental Levels and Health Effects of PCDD'S and PCDF'S* (as amended by Commoner, Webster, and Shapiro, submitted to Dioxin '85, Bayreuth, FRG, September, 1985). Prepared for Government Refuse Collections and Disposal Association, 1986.

59. R. R. Suskind, Chloracne, 'The hallmark of dioxin intoxication.' *Scand. J. Work Environ. Health* **11**, 165–171 (1985).

60. J. Bleiberg, M. Wallen, R. Brodkin, and I. L. Applebaum, Industrially acquired porphyria. *Arch. Dermatol.* **89**, 793–797 (1964).

61. J. Pazderova-Vejlupkova, M. Nemcorva, J. Pickova, L. Jirasek, and E. Lukas, The development and prognosis of chronic introxication by tetrachlorodibenzo-p-dioxin in men. *Arch. Environ. Health* **36**, 5–11 (1981).

62. R. Singer, M. Moses, J. Valiciukas, R. Lilis, and I. J. Selikoff, Nerve condition velocity of studies of workers employed in the manufacture of phenoxy herbicides. *Environ. Res.* **29**, 297–311 (1982).

63. M. Moses, R. Lilis, K. D. Crow, J. Thornton, A. Fischbein, H. A. Anderson, and I. J. Selikoff, Health status of workers with past exposure to 2, 3, 7, 8-tetrachlorodibenzo-p-dioxin in the manufacture of 2, 4, 5-trichlorophenoxyacetic acid: Comparison of findings with and without chloracne. *Am. J. Ind. Med.* **5**, 161–182 (1984).

64. National Council of Paper Industry for Air and Stream Improvement, Inc., *Dioxin: A Critical Review of Its Distribution, Mechanism of Action, Impacts on Human Health, and the Setting of Acceptable Exposure Limits*, NCASI Tech. Bull. 524, New York, NY, 1987.

65. L. Hardell, M. Eriksson, P. Lenner, and E. Lundgren, Malignant lymphoma and exposure to chemicals, especially organic solvents, chlorophenols and phenoxyacetic acids; a case control study. *Br. J. Cancer* **43**, 169–176 (1981).

66. M. Ericksson, L. Hardell, N. Berg, T. Moller, and O. Axelson, Soft-tissue sarcomas and exposure to chemical substances: A case-referrent study. *Br. J. Ind. Med.* **38**, 27–33 (1981).

67. L. Hardell and A. Sandstrom, Case-control study: Soft-tissue sarcomas and exposure to phenoxyacetic acids or chlorophenols. *Br. J. Cancer* **39**, 711–717 (1979).

68. *Evatt P. Royal Commission on the Use and Effects of Chemical Agents on Australian Personnel in Vietnam*: Final Report, Vols. 1–9. AGPS, Canberra, 1985; through W. Hall, The Agent Orange controversy after the Evatt Royal Commission. *Med. J. Aust.* **145**, 219–225 (1986).

69. K. Wiklund and L. Holm, Soft tissue sarcoma risk in Swedish agricultural and forestry workers. *JNCI, J. Natl. Cancer Inst.* **76**, 229–234 (1986).

70. A. H. Smith, D. O. Fisher, N. Pearce, and C. A. Teague, Do agricultural chemicals cause soft tissue sarcoma? Initial findings of a case-control study in New Zealand. *Commun. Health Stud.* **6**, 114–119 (1982).

71. A. H. Smith, D. O. Fisher, H. J. Giles, and N. Pearce, The New Zealand soft tissue sarcoma case-control study. Interview findings concerning phenoxyacetic acid exposure. *Chemosphere* **12**, 565–571 (1983).

72. A. H. Smith and N. E. Pearce, Update on soft tissue sarcoma and phenoxyherbicides in New Zealand. *Chemosphere* **15**, 1795–1798 (1986).

73. N. E. Pearce, A. H. Smith, and D. O. Fisher, Malignant lymphoma and multiple myeloma linked with agricultural occupations in a New Zealand cancer registry-based study. *Am. J. Epidemiol.* **121**, 225–237 (1985).

74. N. E. Pearce, A. H. Smith, J. K. Howard, R. A. Sheppard, H. J. Giles, and C. A. Teague, Non-Hodgkin's lymphoma and exposure to phenoxyherbicides, chlorophenols, fencing work, and meat works employment. *Br. J. Ind. Med.* **43**, 75–83 (1986).

75. S. Hoar, A. Blair, F. Holmes, C. Boysen, R. Robel, R. Hoover, and J. Fraumeni, Agricultural herbicide use and risk of lymphoma and soft-tissue sarcoma. *J. Am. Med. Assoc.* **256**, 1141–1147 (1986).

76. A. H. Smith, D. O. Fisher, N. Pearce, and C. J. Chapman, Congenital defects and miscarriages among New Zealand 2, 4, 5-T sprayers. *Arch. Environ. Health* **37**, 197–200 (1982).

77. W. Wolfe, G. Lathrop, R. Albanese, and P. Moynahan, An epidemiological investigation of health effects in Air Force personnel following exposure to herbicides and associated dioxins. *Chemosphere* **14**, 707–716 (1985).

78. H. K. Kang, L. Weatherbee, P. Breslin, Y. Lee, and B. M. Shepard, Soft tissue sarcomas and military service in Vietnam: A case comparison group analysis of hospital patients. *J. Occup. Med.* **28**, 1215–1218 (1986).

79. P. Greenwald, B. Kovasznag, D. N. Collins, and G. Therriault, Sarcomas of soft tissue after Vietnam service. *J. Natl. Cancer Inst.* **73**, 1107–1109 (1984).

80. J. Erickson, J. Mulinare, P. McClain, T. Fitch, L. James, A. McClearn, and M. Adams, Vietnam veterans' risks for fathering babies with birth defects. *J. Am. Med. Assoc.* **252**, 903–912 (1984).

81. B. Armstrong, "Australians report no link between service in Vietnam and birth defects among offspring. *Epidemiol. Monit.* **3**, 1 (1983).

82. A. Lipson, W. Gaffey, and F. LaVecchio, Agent Orange and birth defects. Letter to the Editor. *N. Engl. J. Med.* **309**, 491–492 (1983).

83. Minister of Veterans' Affairs, *Case-Control Study of Congenital Anomalies and Vietnam Service (Birth Defects Study)*, Australian Government Publishing Service, 1983; through AMA, *The Health Effects of "Agent Orange" and Polychlorinated Dioxin Contaminants: An Update, 1984*, 1984 (updated 1985).

84. M. G. Ott, R. A. Olson, R. R. Cook, and G. G. Bond, Cohort mortality study of chemical workers with potential exposure to the higher chlorinated dioxins. *J. Occup. Med.* **29**, 422–429 (1987).

85. J. C. Townsend, K. M. Bodner, P. F. D. Van Peenen, R. D. Olson, and R. R. Cook, Survey of reproductive events of wives of employees exposed to chlorinated dioxins. *Am. J. Epidemiol.* **115**, 695–713 (1982).

86. A. Blair, Review of the epidemiologic data regarding dioxin and cancer. In J. A. Moore, Ed., *Report of the Dioxin Update Committee*. Convened by EPA Office of Pesticide and Toxic Substances, Dioxin Update Conference, July 1–2, 1986. Updated in May 1988. U.S. EPA, Waterside Mall, M Street, Washington, D.C.

87. M. Graham, F. Hileman, D. Kirk, J. Wendling, and J. Wilson, Background human exposure TO 2, 3, 7, 8-TCDD. *Chemosphere* **14**, 925–928 (1985).

88. D. Patterson, R. Hoffman, L. Needham, D. Roberts, J. Bagby, J. Pirkle, H. Falk, E. Sampson, and V. Honk, 2, 3, 7, 8-tetrachlorodibenzo-p-dioxin levels in adipose tissue of exposed and control persons in Missouri: An interim report. *J. Am. Med. Assoc.* **256**, 2683–2686 (1986).

89. J. Ryan, R. Lizotte, and B. Lau, Chlorinated dibenzo-p-dioxins and chlorinated dibenzo-furans in Canadian human adipose tissue. *Chemosphere* **14**, 697–706 (1985).

90. J. Ryan, A. Schecter, R. Lizotte, W. Sun, and L. Miller, Tissue distribution of dioxins and furans in humans from the general population. *Chemosphere* **14**, 929–932 (1985).

91. A. Schecter, J. Ryan, R. Lizotte, W. Sun, L. Miller, G. Gitlitz, and M. Bogdasarian, Chlorinated dibenzodioxins and dibenzofurans in human adipose tissue from exposed and control New York State patients. *Chemosphere* **14**, 933–937 (1985).

92. M. Nygren, C. Rappe, G. Lindstrom, M. Hansson, P. Bergqvist, S. Marklund, L. Domellof, L. Hardell, and M. Olsson, Identification of 2, 3, 7, 8-substituted polychlorinated dioxins and dibenzofurans in environmental and human samples. In C. Rappe, G. Choudhary, and L. H. Keith, Eds., *Chlorinated Dioxins and Dibenzofurans in Perspective*. Lewis Publishers, Chelsea, MI, 1986, pp. 17–34.

93. R. L. Sielken, Statistical evaluations reflecting the skewness in the distribution of TCDD levels in human adipose tissue. *Chemosphere* **16(8–9)**, 2135–2140 (1987).

94. L. Hobson, L. Lee, M. Gross, and A. Young, Dioxin in body fat and health status: A feasibility study. *Ext. Abstr., Div. Environ. Chem., Am. Chem. Soc.* **23**, 91–93 (1983); through A. Young and L. Cockerham, Fate of TCDD in field ecosystems—Assessment and significance for human exposures. In M. Kamrin and P. Rogers, Eds., *Dioxins in the Environment*. Hemisphere New York, 1985, pp. 153–171.

95. A. J. Schecter, J. J. Ryan, M. Gross, N. C. A. Weerasinghe, and J. D. Constable, Chlorinated dioxins and dibenzofurans in human adipose tissues from Vietnam, 1983–84. In C. Rappe, G. Choudhary, and L. H. Keith, Eds., *Chlorinated Dioxins and Dibenzofurans in Perspective*, Lewis Publishers, Chelsea, MI, 1986, pp. 35–50.

96. P. C, Kahn, Unpublished data cited in New York Times, *Researchers Report Finding Telltale Signs of Agent Orange*, Thursday, September 18, 1986.

97. Centers for Disease Control, Serum dioxin in Vietnam-era Veterans—Preliminary report. *MMWR* **36**, 470–475 (1987).

98. R. L. Sielken, Quantitative cancer risk assessments for 2, 3, 7, 8-tetrachlorodibenzo-p-dioxin (TCDD). *Food Chem. Toxicol.* **25**, 257–267 (1987).

99. Food and Drug Administration, Statement by Sanford A. Miller, Ph.D., Director, Bureau of Foods, before the subcommittee on Natural Resources, Agriculture, Research and

Environment, Committee on Science and Technology, U.S. House of Representatives, June 30, 1983.

100. R. B. Howe and K. S. Crump, *Global 82, A Computer Program to Extrapolate Quantal Animal Toxicity Data to Low Doses*. Prepared for Office of Carcinogen Standards, Occupational Safety and Health Administration, 1982.

101. R. Scheuplein, Proposed Food and Drug Administration approach to tolerance-setting for dioxins in food. In W. Lowrance, Ed., *Public Health Risks of the Dioxins*. W. Kaufman, Inc., Los Altos, CA, 1984, pp. 367–372.

102. F. Cordle, Use of epidemiology in the regulation of dioxins in the food supply. In F. Coulston and F. Pocchiari, Eds., *Accidental Exposure to Dioxins, Human Health Aspects*, Academic Press, New York, 1983, pp. 245–256.

103. U.S. Environmental Protection Agency, *Ambient Water Quality Criteria for 2,3,7,8-Tetrachlorodibenzo-p-dioxin*, EPA 440/5-84-007. Office of Water Regulations and Standards, USEPA, Washington, DC, 1984.

104. V. K. Rowe, Direct Testimony of Dr. V. K. Rowe before the U.S. Environmental Protection Agency, Exhibit 865, FIFRA Docket Nos. 415 et al., November 13, 1980.

105. F. Tschirley, Dioxin. *Sci. Am.* **254**(2), 29–35 (1986).

106. E. Crouch and R. Wilson, Interspecies comparison of carcinogenic potency. *J. Toxicol. Environ. Health* **5**, 1095–1118 (1979).

107. K. S. Crump, A critical evaluation of Sielken's dose response assessment for TCDD. *Food Chem. Toxicol.* **26**, 77–79 (1988).

108. R. L. Sielken, Jr., A response to Crump's evaluation of Sielken's dose-response assessment for TCDD. *Food Chem. Toxicol.* **26**, 79–83 (1988).

109. G. Williams and J. Weisburger, Chemical carcinogens. In C. Klaassen, M. Amdur, and J. Doull, Eds., *Casarett and Doull's Toxicology: The Basic Science of Poisons*. New York, 1986, pp. 99–173.

110. I. Weinstein, Dioxins as carcinogenic promoters. In W. Lowrance, Ed., *Public Health Risks of the Dioxins*. W. Kaufman, Inc., Los Altos, CA, 1984, pp. 155–160.

111. A. Kolbye, Jr., Mechanisms of carcinogenesis related to TCDD. In F. Coulston and F. Pocchiari, Eds., *Accidental Exposure to Dioxins, Human Health Aspects*. Academic Press, New York, 1983, pp. 191–199.

112. J. H. Weisburger and G. M. Williams, The decision-point approach for systematic carcinogen testing. *Food Cosmet. Toxicol.* **19**, 561–566 (1981).

113. Dioxin Update Committee, *Report of the Dioxin Update Committee*. Convened by EPA Office of Pesticides and Toxic Substances, Dioxin Update Conference, July 1–2, 1986.

114. C. van der Heijden, A. Knaap, P. Kramers, and M. van Logten, *Evaluation of the Carcinogenicity and Mutagenicity of 2,3,7,8-Tetrachlorodibenzo-1,4-Dioxin (TCDD); Classification and No-Effect Level*, Rep. DOC/LCM 300/292. State Institute of National Health, Bilthoven, The Netherlands, 1982.

115. E. J. Calabrese, *Principles of Animal Extrapolation*. Wiley, New York, 1983.

116. R. K. White, Select the right land application system for your needs. *Biocycle*, March/April, pp. 24–27 (1982).

117. E. J. Kladivko and D. W. Nelson, Surface runoff from sludge-amended soils. *J.—Water Pollut. Control Fed.* **15**, 100–110 (1979).

118. Client, *Utilization of Pulp and Paper Mill Sludge as Sanitary Landfill Cover Material*, 1983.

119. State of Alaska, *Highway Right-of-Way Sludge Disposal*. State of Alaska Department of Transportation and Public Facilities, Research Station, Fairbanks, Alaska, 1986.

120. Client, Personal communication to Envirologic Data (1987).

121. A. Young, Long-term studies on the persistence and movement of TCDD in a natural ecosystem. *Environ. Sci. Res.* **26**, 173–190 (1983).

122. A. F. Yanders, *Environmental Fate of Dioxin*. Presented at the Maine Department of Environmental Protection Dioxin Workshop, Augusta, February 4, 1987.

123. International Commission on Radiological Protection, *Report of the Task Group on Reference Man*, ICRP Publ. 23. Pergamon, Oxford, 1975.

124. T. M. Roberts, W. Gizyn, and T. C. Hutchinson, Lead contamination of air, soil, vegetation and people in the vicinity of secondary lead smelters. *Trace Substances Environ. Health* **8**, 155–166 (1974).

125. J. Hawley, Assessment of health risk from exposure to contaminated soil. *Risk Anal.* **5**, 289–302 (1985).

126. R. L. Solomon and J. W. Hartford, Lead and cadmium in dusts and soils in a small urban community. *Environ. Sci. Technol.* **10**, 773–777 (1976).

127. H. Shu, P. Teitelbaum, A. S. Webb, L. Marple, B. Brunck, D. Dei Rossi, J. Murray, and D. Paustenbach, Bioavailability of soil-bound TCDD: Dermal bioavailability in the rat. *Fundam. Appl. Toxicol.* **10**, 335–343.

128. R. C. Wester and P. K. Noonan, Relevance of animal models for percutaneous absorption. *Int. J. Pharm.* **7**, 99–110 (1980).

129. R. Wester and H. Maibach, Cutaneous pharmakokinetics: 10 steps to percutaneous absorption. *Drug Metab. Rev.* **14**, 169–205 (1983).

130. J. Trijonis, J. Eldon, J. Gins, and G. Berglund, *Analysis of the St. Louis RAMS Ambient Particulate Data*, Vol. 1, *Final Report*, EPA-450/4-80-006a. Prepared for U.S. Environmental Protection Agency, Research Triangle Park, NC, 1980.

131. U.S. Environmental Protection Agency, *Review of the National Ambient Air Quality Standards for Particulate Matter: Updated Assessment of Scientific and Technical Information, Draft Addendum to the 1982 OAQPS Staff Paper*. Office of Air Quality Planning and Standards, USEPA, Research Triangle Park, NC, 1986.

132. M. Lepow et al., Role of airborne lead in increased body burden of lead in Hartford children. *Environ. Health Perspect.* **6**, 99–102 (1974).

133. M. Lepow et al., Investigations into sources of lead in the environment of urban children. *Environ. Res.* **10**, 415–426 (1975).

134. M. Duggan and S. Williams, Lead-in-dust in city streets. *Sci. Total Environ.* **7**, 91–97 (1977).

135. J. van Wijnen, P. Clausing, and B. Brunekreef, *A Method for Estimating Soil Ingestion of Young Children*. Abstract presented at Dioxin '86, Japan, 1986.

136. P. Clausing, B. Brunekreef, and J. van Wijnen, A method for estimating soil ingestion by children. *Inter. Arch. Occup. Environ. Health* **59**, 73–82 (1987).

137. E. McConnell, G. Lucier, R. Rambaugh, P. Albro, D. Harvan, J. Hass, and M. Harris, Dioxin in soil: Bioavailability after ingestion by rats and guinea pigs. *Science* **223**, 1077–1079 (1984).

138. T. H. Umbreit, E. J. Hesse, and M. A. Gallo, *Differential Bioavailability of TCDD from Contaminated Soils from Times Beach, Missouri and Nework, New Jersey*, Prepr. ext. abstr. Presented before American Chemical Society, New York, April 1986.

139. T. H. Umbreit, Personal communication to Envirologic Data (1987).

140. W. N. Piper, J. Q. Rose, and P. J. Gehring, Excretion and tissue distribution of 2,3,7,8-tetrachlorodibenzo-p-dioxin in the rat. In E. H. Blair, Ed., *Chlorodioxins—Origin and Fate*. American Chemical Society, Washington, DC, 1973, pp. 85–91.

141. A. L. Young and L. G. Cockerham, Fate of TCDD in field ecosystems—Assessment and significance for human exposures. In M. A. Kamrin and P. W. Rodgers, Eds., *Dioxins in the Environment*. Hemisphere, New York, 1985, pp. 153–171.

142. Environmental Research and Technology, *Summary of Information on Wildlife Species on Mine Lands*. Unpublished tables and data transmitted to Envirologic Data by ERT, Fort Collins, CO, 1986.

143. L. L. Rue, Wild turkey. In *Game Birds of North America*. Harper, New York, 1973.

144. L. Korshgen, Feeding habits and foods. In A. Schorger, Ed., *The Wild Turkey*. Univ. of Oklahoma Press, Tulsa, 1966, pp. 137–198.

145. H. Wipf, E. Homberger, N. Neuner, U. Ranalder, W. Vetter, and J. Vuilleumier, TCDD levels in soil and plant samples from the Seveso area. In O. Hutzinger et al., Eds., *Chlorinated Dioxins and Related Compounds*. Pergamon, New York, 1982, pp. 115–126.

146. S. Facchetti, A. Balasso, C. Fichtner, G. Frare, A. Leoni, C. Mauri, and M. Vasconi, Studies on the absorption of TCDD by plant species. In C. Rappe, G. Choudhary, and L. H. Keith, Eds., *Chlorinated Dioxins and Dibenzofurans in Perspective*. Lewis Publishers, Chelsea, MI, 1986, pp. 225–235.

147. G. A. Sacchi, P. Vigano, G. Fortunati and S. M. Cocucci, Accumulation of 2, 3, 7, 8-tetrachlorodibenzo-p-dioxin from soil and nutrient solution by bean and maize plants. *Experientia* **42**, 586–588 (1986).

148. G. F. Fries, *Memorandum to Bryce J. Sproul, Maine Department of Environmental Protection, Regarding Uptake and Translocation of TCDD by Plants*. U.S.D.A. Agric. Res. Serv., Beltsville, MD, 1986.

149. A. F. Yanders, *Memorandum to Bryce J. Sproul, Maine Department of Environmental Protection, Regarding Uptake and Translocation of TCDD by Plants*. University of Missouri, Environmental Trace Substances Research Center, Columbia, 1986.

150. G. F. Fries, *Letter to R. Keenan, Envirologic Data, Regarding Uptake of TCDD by Plants*. U.S.D.A., Agric. Res. Serv., Beltsville, MD, 1986.

151. R. D. Kimbrough, *Memorandum to Bryce J. Sproul, Maine Department of Environmental Protection, Regarding Review of Article on Plant Uptake, Sampling Methodology, and Interim Dioxin Standards for Sludges*. Centers for Disease Control, Atlanta, GA, 1986.

152. S. Cocucci, F. DiGerolamo, A. Verderio, A. Cavallero, G. Colli, A. Gorni, G. Invernizzi and L. Luciani, Absorption and translocation of tetrachlorodibenzo-p-dioxin by plants from polluted soil. *Experientia* **35**, 482–484 (1979).

153. F. D. Bartleson, D. D. Harrison, and J. D. Morgan, *Field Studies of Wildlife Exposed to TCDD Contaminated Soils*, AFATL-TR-75-49. Eglin Air Force Base, FL, 1975.

154. K. Morrow, Ohio Department of Natural Resources, Division of Wildlife, personal communication to Envirologic Data (1986).

155. C. M. Nizon, M. W. McClain, and K. R. Russell, Deer food habits and range characteristics in Ohio. *J. Wild. Manage.* **34**, 870–886 (1970).

156. W. Healy, Ingestion of soil by dairy cows. *N.Z. J. Agric. Res.* **11**, 487–499 (1968).

157. D. Jensen, R. Hummel, N. Mahle, C. Kocher, and H. Higgins, Residue study on beef cattle consuming 2, 3, 7, 8-tetrachlorodibenzo-p-dioxin. *J. Agric. Food Chem.* **29**, 265–268 (1981).

158. D. Jensen and R. Hummel, Secretion of TCDD in milk and cream following the feeding of TCDD to lactating dairy cows. *Bull. Environ. Contam. Toxicol.* **29**, 440–446 (1982).

159. Ohio Department of Agriculture. *Ohio Agricultural Statistics*. ODA, Columbus OH, 1985.

160. P. Spike, Ohio Agricultural Extension Service, personal communication to Envirologic Data (1986).

161. G. Fries, Potential polychlorinated biphenyl residues in animal products from application of contaminated sewage sludge to land. *J. Environ. Qual.* **11**, 14–20 (1982).

162. Maine Department of Agriculture, *Maine Agricultural Statistics 1983–1984*. Food and Rural Resources, MDA Augusta, ME, 1984.

163. K. P. Bovard, J. P. Fontenot, and B. M. Priode, Accumulation and dissipation of heptachlor residues in fattening steers. *J. Anim. Sci.* **33**, 127–132 (1971).

164. C. E. Parker, W. A. Jones, II. B. Matthews, E. E. McConnell, and J. R. Hass, The chronic toxicity of technical and analytic pentachlorophenol in cattle: Chemical analysis of tissues. *Toxicol. Appl. Pharmacol.* **55**, 359–369 (1980).

165. C. C. Travis, S. Richter, E. A. C. Crouch, P. Wilson, and E. D. Klema, Cancer risk management; a review of 132 federal regulatory decisions. *Environ. Sci. Technol.* **21**, 415–420 (1987).

166. J. V. Rodricks, S. M. Brett, and G. C. Wrenn, *Significant Risk Decisions in Federal Regulatory Agencies.* Environ Corporation, Washington, DC, 1987.

167. E. Crouch and R. Wilson, *Risk/Benefit Analysis.* Ballinger, Cambridge, MA, 1982.

168. Office of Science and Technology Policy, Chemical carcinogens: a review of the science and its associated principles. *Fed. Regist.* **50**, 10372–10442 (1985).

169. G. F. Fries and D. J. Paustenbach. A critical evaluation of factors used in assessing incinerator emissions as a potential source of TCDD in foods of animal origin. 7th Inter Dioxin Symposion, *Las, Vegas, NV. abstract RC-05.*

29

Endangerment Assessment for the Bald Eagle Population near the Sand Springs Petrochemical Complex Superfund Site

Lisa C. Gandy
National Hazardous Materials Training Center, Division of Interdisciplinary Toxicology, University of Arkansas for Medical Sciences, Little Rock, Arkansas

1 INTRODUCTION

In 1987 an endangerment assessment was conducted as part of the Remedial Investigation/Feasibility Study (RI/FS) phase of remediation for a U.S. Environmental Protection Agency (U.S. EPA) Superfund site in Oklahoma. This endangerment assessment was unique because it included an endangerment assessment for the bald eagle (*Haliaeetus leucocephalus*), a federally protected endangered species (1). Although the Comprehensive Environmental Response, Compensation and Liability Act of 1980 (2) and the Federal Water Pollution Control Act (3) dictate that the damages or potential damages to natural resources, including land, fish, wildlife, biota, air, water, groundwater, and drinking water supplies (4), must be assessed, damages to wildlife and other biota are not typically included as part of the site endangerment assessment conducted during the RI/FS. The natural resource damage assessment, which is conducted by the appropriate trustees designated under the National Oil and Hazardous Substance Pollution Contingency Plan (5), or Section 311(f) (5) of the Federal Water Pollution Control Act, typically takes place during site closure (6, 7). As a result, risk assessments or endangerment assessments on endangered avian species, such as the bald eagle, are rare.

Although the complete endangerment assessment for this Superfund site characterized the risks to both human populations and the bald eagle population, this chapter focuses specifically on the bald eagle endangerment assessment. The objective of the bald eagle assessment was to determine if the chemicals present at the site currently impact, or have the potential to affect adversely, the bald eagle population near the site.

Unlike endangerment assessments for human populations, endangerment assessments for endangered species often lack a significant amount of critical data necessary to conduct a quantitative risk assessment. This assessment for the bald eagle population near the

999

Oklahoma Superfund site was not exempt from this problem, thus necessitating a qualitative characterization of risk.

It is anticipated that this chapter may serve as a model for future endangerment assessments of endangered species. It identifies the critical areas where analytical data are needed to provide a better assessment of the hazards to avian populations from chemical contaminants. It also points out the necessity, under the Federal Endangered Species Act of 1973 (8), of considering the effects of chemical contaminants not only on the endangered populations but also on the habitats that are critical to their survival.

2 SITE OVERVIEW

2.1 Location

The Sand Springs Petrochemical Complex is a U.S. EPA Superfund site located in Sand Springs, Oklahoma. Located in northeast Oklahoma, the Sand Springs Petrochemical Complex lies on the outskirts of the city of Sand Springs. The site is bounded on the east by Sand Springs Wastewater Treatment Plant, on the west by the Sand Springs Railway Company tracks, and on the south by the Arkansas River (Figs. 1 and 2). The Arkansas River levee traverses the site and provides access to the southern portion of the site. Several small businesses and light industries currently operate on the site.

2.2 Site History

The Sand Springs Petrochemical Complex Superfund site was the home of a large petroleum refining operation from approximately 1930 to 1949. The Sinclair Oil

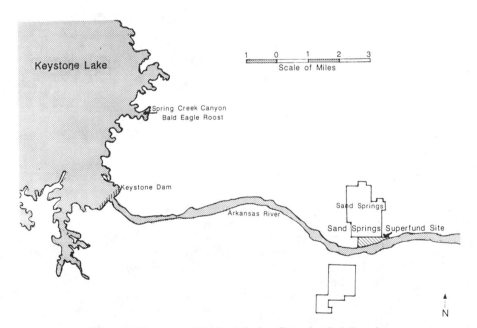

Figure 1. Plan view of the Sand Springs Petrochemical Complex.

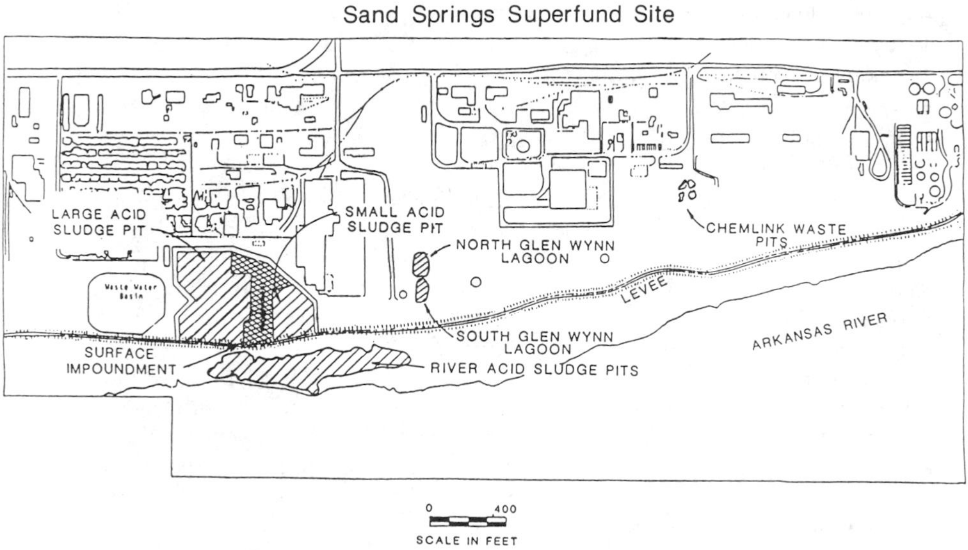

Sand Springs Superfund Site

Figure 2. Geological elevation view of the Sand Springs Petrochemical Complex.

Corporation operated the refinery until refinery operations ceased in 1949. By October 1953 all but 38 of the 2000 acres of refinery property had been sold to the Sand Springs Home, a charitable organization. From 1949 through 1986, several businesses and industries leased and/or purchased tracts of land on the original refinery property from the Sand Springs Home. Many of these businesses are currently operating on the Sand Springs site.

In 1969 the Sinclair Oil Corporation merged with the Atlantic Richfield Company and the 38-acre tract of land still retained by the Sinclair Oil Corporation was absorbed in the merger. In 1986 this 38-acre tract of land was sold to a company that currently operates on the site.

Operations at the site over this 50-year period include oil refining, solvent recycling, waste oil recycling, and other light industrial operations. The operations at the Sand Springs Petrochemical Complex site over this 50-year period have resulted in the generation of large volumes of hazardous wastes, waste oil, and other hazardous substances. Included in these hazardous substances and wastes are various volatile and nonvolatile organics, chlorinated solvents, and sludges containing heavy metals. These chemicals were stored or disposed of in drums, tanks, unlined pits, or lagoons or were buried onsite. Poor operation resulted in the contamination of groundwater and the high potential for runoff contamination offsite.

2.3   Sources of Chemical Contamination

The ranking of the Sand Springs Petrochemical Complex site as a Superfund site is due to the presence of the following defined sources of contamination:

1. A large acid sludge pit and a small acid sludge pit that have been in existence since the original refinery operation.

2. A 400-ft-long, 100-ft-wide surface impoundment located between these two sludge pits.
3. River acid sludge pits located to the south of the main pits and on the river side of the Arkansas River levee.
4. The north Glen Wynn lagoon and the south Glen Wynn lagoon.
5. Four acid pits located in the eastern third of the site.

The large, the small, and the river acid sludge pits are the result of refining operations. These unlined pits contain sulfuric acid sludge with concentrations of heavy metals such as chromium and lead and with a pH of 2.5. Over the years, this sulfuric acid sludge has seeped into the Arkansas River. Groundwater contamination is also likely from these pits. Surface water runoff occurs from these acid sludge pits, drains into a storm sewer on the site, and subsequently is emptied into the Arkansas River.

In 1980 the liquid from the surface impoundment located between the large and small acid pits was analyzed by the U.S. EPA Field Investigation Team (FIT). Analyses revealed a pH between 1.5 and 2.1 for the surface impoundment liquid and the presence of chrysene, anthracene, phenanthrene, pyrene, benzene, 1, 1-difluorotetrachloroethane, toluene, phenol, nitrobenzene, and fluoronapthalene. The surface impoundment represents a potential source for groundwater contamination.

The Glen Wynn lagoons are located in the center of the Sand Springs Petrochemical site on a portion of the original refinery site. The Glen Wynn lagoons are part of the Glen Wynn operation, a solvent recycling facility. The liquids in the south Glen Wynn lagoon are estimated to be 2 ft deep and liquids in the north lagoon are estimated to be approximately 1.7 ft deep. South lagoon samples collected by U.S. EPA FIT personnel in 1982 showed significant contamination by chlorinated volatiles, benzene, toluene, and numerous long-chain aliphatic hydrocarbons indicative of oils. Lead and zinc levels were also high. The north lagoon samples showed similar types of contaminants as the south lagoon. Sediments from the north lagoon, however, showed higher levels of volatile organics and metals, and a PCB concentration of 20 ppm was found. Both Glen Wynn lagoons are likely sources for groundwater contamination. Surface water runoff from the lagoons drains into a storm sewer on the site and empties into the Arkansas River.

2.4   Overview of Chemical Contamination

Chemical contamination at the Sand Springs Petrochemical Complex is extensive. More than 76 chemicals were measured above analytical detection limits in sludge samples alone. The large number of chemicals present at the site makes the assessment of the potential health risks to both human and animal populations in the surrounding areas a difficult, if not impossible, task. Therefore, in accordance with U.S. EPA guidelines (9), the compounds or group of compounds posing the greatest potential risk to human health and to the environment were used to assess the potential public health and wildlife hazards of this site. These compounds are referred to throughout this chapter as the *indicator chemicals.*

3   INDICATOR CHEMICALS

3.1   Selection

The selection of the indicator chemicals for the Sand Springs Petrochemical Complex endangerment assessment was based on the analytical data for samples collected in five environmental media during the remedial investigation: sludge, liquid waste, surface water, air, and sediment (10). The criteria, assumptions, and methods used for the selection of the indicator chemicals followed those outlined in the U.S. EPA guidelines (9). A brief synopsis of the methods and assumptions used to select the indicator chemicals is provided; however, a more detailed explanation of selection process of indicator chemicals for this site can be found in Mathes (11).

Lists of chemicals in each of the five environmental media listed above were enumerated. The toxicological class of each chemical, such as potential carcinogen or noncarcinogen, was determined when possible. Rating values indicating severity of toxicological effects of noncarcinogens, and water, soil, and air toxicity constants, as defined in the U.S. EPA *Superfund Public Health Evaluation Manual* (9), were obtained when possible from the U.S. EPA (9). Mean concentration values of each chemical in each of the five media listed above were determined and used as representations of the concentrations of chemicals within each environmental medium.

Chemicals were separated into two groups based on toxicological class: potential carcinogen or noncarcinogen. Mean and maximum concentrations of each chemical in each of the five environmental media were multiplied by the corresponding toxicity constant (9) to obtain an indicator score. For each chemical, the separate indicator scores for each medium were summed for both mean and maximum concentrations. Chemicals were then ranked according to total indicator score in both the potential carcinogen and noncarcinogen categories. The 13 chemicals with the highest indicator scores in both the potential carcinogen and noncarcinogen groups were enumerated.

Chemicals for which no water, soil, or air toxicity constants were available or chemicals for which toxicological class was unidentifiable remained within the list of chemicals for final evaluation. The evaluation of these chemicals was based on structure–toxicity relationships, environmental persistence, and prevalence of the chemical at the site (11).

Final selection of the indicator chemicals was determined by the magnitude of the indicator scores, an evaluation of the chemical's environmental fate and transport characteristics, prevalence of a particular chemical in each environmental medium at the site, and data on ambient levels of each chemical in media throughout the United States. As a result of the criteria used for the selection of the indicator compounds, several of the higher ranking potentially carcinogenic and noncarcinogenic chemicals found at this site were eliminated as possible indicator chemicals.

3.2 Indicator Chemicals Selected for the Endangerment Assessment

Seven chemicals were chosen as the indicator chemicals for the Sand Springs Petrochemical Complex endangerment assessment. This group of seven compounds consists of the following five chemical contaminants: lead, cadmium, trichloroethylene, tetrachloro ethylene, and benzene; and the following two chemical classes: the polycyclic aromatic hydrocarbons (PAHs) and the alkyl benzenes.

4 BALD EAGLE HAZARD ASSESSMENT

4.1 Status of Bald Eagles in Oklahoma

Oklahoma is an important wintering area for the bald eagle, *Haliaeetus leucocephalus*. It consistently ranks among the top 10 wintering sites for bald eagles in the lower 48 states (12). According to a 1962 National Audubon Society study, which assessed the relative size of bald eagle populations throughout the country, the state of Oklahoma ranked fourth or fifth in the study (13).

The large number of bald eagles present in the state of Oklahoma during the winter is principally due to the large number of open, unfrozen lakes, rivers, and reservoirs; plentiful supplies of food; and relatively mild winter temperatures (12). Bald eagles have been reported at almost all bodies of water in the state during the winter months (13, 14). Bald eagle populations of 25 or more eagles exist at approximately 20 locations throughout the state, including Keystone Reservoir located approximately 7–7.5 mi upstream from the Sand Springs Petrochemical Complex (15, 16).

4.2   Characteristics and Biology of the Bald Eagle

4.2.1   *Physical Characteristics and Endangered Status.*   The bald eagle is physically one of the largest migratory and predatory bird species in the world. It has a 6.5–7 ft wingspan, is 3–3.5 ft tall, and can weigh 8–15 pounds. The bald eagle, endemic to North America, was first listed as an endangered species in 1967. In 1978 the bald eagle was listed by the U.S. Fish and Wildlife Service as an endangered species in 43 states including Oklahoma (1, 12). Today the bald eagle is listed as endangered or threatened throughout most of its range. It is unlisted in Alaska were approximately 10,000 still breed (12).

4.2.2   *Taxonomy and Migratory Behavior.*   Two subspecies of bald eagles have been identified in North America. The northern subspecies, *Haliaeetus leucocephalus* ssp. *alascanus*, breeds in the northern United States and southern Canada and migrates south in the winter. The southern subspecies, *Haliaeetus leucocephalus* ssp. *leucocephalus*, breeds primarily in the lower Mississippi states to Baja California, the Gulf Coast, and Florida (17).

The state of Oklahoma lies within both the wintering range of the northern subspecies and the breeding and wintering range of the southern subspecies. The bald eagles of the southern race, however, have not been reported as having successfully bred in Oklahoma in over 10 years (12, 13). Although it is the northern subspecies that is believed to overwinter in Oklahoma, the birds in Oklahoma display taxonomic characteristics intermediate between the two subspecies.

Bald eagles have been tagged and recaptured by the Office of Migratory Bird Management (OMBM) in Laurel, Maryland, in order to identify the subspecies, migratory patterns, and nesting range of the wintering bald eagles in Oklahoma (13). The OMBM's studies indicated that Oklahoma's bald eagle populations nest primarily in the western Great Lakes states (Wisconsin, Minnesota, Michigan, and the Dakotas) and in southern central Canada (Ontario, Saskatchewan, and Manitoba) (18). OMBM's studies confirm the belief that it is primarily the northern subspecies that overwinters in the state of Oklahoma.

Bald eagles begin arriving in Oklahoma from late October to mid-late November (12, 13). They typically leave Oklahoma in March and return to the same nesting sites year after year. Reports indicate, however, that bald eagles have arrived in Oklahoma as early as September and have left the state as late as May (13).

4.2.3   *Wintering and Feeding Behavior.*   During the breeding or nesting season, bald eagles exhibit extreme territorial behavior. In contrast to the territorial behavior exhibited during the nesting season, bald eagles become quite sociable during the wintering season

TABLE 1. **Prey Items Collected beneath Feeding Trees along Salt Fork River, December 1973 to February 1974**

Prey Item	Number Found	Percentage
Whole or parts of gizzard shad	39	82.2
Canada goose	7	14.6
Mallard duck	1	2.1
Green-winged teal	1	2.1
Total	48	100.0

Source: Modified from Lish and Lewis (14).

and roost in large numbers (12). Communal roosts are typically established in large trees with open crowns and stout lateral limbs. Trees having these characteristics provide maneuverability and easy entry and exit for this 6–7 ft wingspan bird.

In Oklahoma, cottonwoods (*Populus deltoides*), sycamores (*Platanus occidentalis*), and oaks (*Quercus spp.*) are the preferred roost tree species (13, 14, 19). In most cases, roost trees are located within approximately 1 km of feeding areas; however, eagles have been known to feed as far as 24–32 km from roost sites (13, 20). Generally, bald eagles will only feed great distances from their night roost sites when no suitable roost trees are available near feeding areas and/or when human disturbance at roosting sites is high, forcing eagles to relocate to more remote roosting sites.

The effects of human presence and activities on bald eagles are not fully known; however, it is generally agreed that bald eagles are sensitive to human activities and human disturbances (1, 12, 13, 18, 21). Bald eagles exhibit considerable variation in responses to human activity depending on the type, frequency, duration of activity, extent of modification of the physical environment, time in the bird's reproductive cycle, and an individual bird's accommodation to disturbance. Some bald eagles will tolerate human presence until it reaches a critical point or threshold level (21). Out of necessity, bald eagles seem to be more tolerant of human disturbance at their feeding areas than at their roosting or nesting sites (13, 19).

Bald eagles generally feed in the early morning hours. Although bald eagles feed primarily on fish, they are also opportunists that eat whatever is available (22). As winter progresses and food becomes scarce, their diet often changes from fish to include dead or injured waterfowl or small mammals (13, 14) (Table 1).

4.3 Sand Springs/Keystone Reservoir Bald Eagle Populations

The bald eagle population at Keystone Reservoir, 7–7.5 mi upstream from the Sand Springs Superfund site, has significantly increased in size from 1979 to 1983. During this 4-year period, the number of bald eagles wintering at Keystone Reservoir rose from 13 to 45. Eagle counts at Keystone from 1983 to 1986, however, indicate a decline in the number of eagles at this site (13, 14–16). The establishment of a second roost site when the Keystone Reservoir froze in the early 1980s is a possible explanation for this decline in numbers (23, 24). Reports suggest that this second roost site can be found at Leonard, approximately 30 mi downstream from the Sand Springs site. Evidence confirming the location of this second roost site, however, is not available (23, 25).

Bald eagle populations in the area of the Sand Springs Petrochemical Complex roost primarily at the Tulsa Audubon Society Wildlife Preserve in Spring Creek Canyon on the northeastern side of Keystone Reservoir. This population feeds primarily in two locations close to the roost site: below Keystone Dam, to approximately 1 km (0.6 mi) below the dam, and at the confluence of the Salt Fork branch of the Arkansas River and Keystone Lake, 8 mi upstream from the Sand Springs Petrochemical Complex.

These two sites near the Keystone Reservoir are the preferred local feeding sites because of their abundant supplies of food. Since the confluence of a river and a lake is the most productive area of a body of water, the confluence of the Arkansas River and Keystone Lake has been a natural source of food for the Keystone bald eagle populations. Conversely, the 1968 construction of the Keystone Dam increased the availability of food for the bald eagles and for waterfowl (13, 14, 18). This enhancement of food supplies below the dam is largely due to fish being pulled through the turbines, injured or killed, and released below the dam. Both of these local feeding areas are also relatively shallow and subject to occasional flooding. This flooding has led to little urbanization and has resulted in a moderate to low amount of disturbance to the eagle populations during feeding.

Disturbance in the area below the dam, however, is increasing. Nevertheless, the abundance of dead or injured fish released below the dam seems to compensate for increasing human population densities and disturbance (14).

Very little feeding occurs elsewhere along the Arkansas River. A 1975 report on bald eagle feeding activity in this area (13) indicated that approximately 91% of the feeding activity for the populations at Keystone occurred below the dam while approximately 9% occurred further downstream.

4.4   Diet of the Keystone Bald Eagle Population

The principal component of the diet of the bald eagle populations near the Sand Springs site is the fish species, *Dorosoma cepedianum*, commonly known as gizzard shad. However, as winter progresses and food becomes scarce, their diet often changes to include dead or injured waterfowl, such as Canada geese (*Branta canadensis*) and mallard ducks (*Anas platyrhynchos*) (14). While rodents and other small mammals comprise a large part of the bald eagle diet in many locations in Oklahoma (13, 14), no evidence exists that the eagles in the Keystone area feed on small mammals such as the eastern cottontail (*Sylvilagus floridanus*) and the Plains pocket gopher (*Geomys bursarius*) (26).

Although bald eagles have not been observed feeding from the Arkansas River directly adjacent to the Sand Springs Petrochemical Complex (26), they have been observed in trees on the Sand Spring Petrochemical site and sitting on sand bars adjacent to the site. Also, Shalaway (19) reported that bald eagles were seen both perching and flying just north of the proposed Shenandoah Housing Development, which lies to the southeast of the Sand Springs Petrochemical Complex and directly south of the Arkansas River. Additionally, potential bald eagle habitat exists along the banks of the Arkansas River approximately $\frac{1}{4}$ mi from the Sand Springs Petrochemical Complex (27).

The habitat use and feeding behavior of bald eagles described above are important to determine whether bald eagle populations at Sand Springs will be a target for chemical contamination by the Sand Springs Petrochemical Complex. In addition to the chemical, physical, and toxicological properties of the contaminant(s), and information on the levels of the contamination in the environment, the information on the biology of the bald eagle is used to determine the possible route (such as inhalation, ingestion, and dermal contact) and extent of exposure. Subsequently, the potential risk to the bald eagle populations near the Sand Springs Petrochemical Complex can be assessed.

4.5 Toxicological Studies in Avian Species

4.5.1 General Overview. A significant number of toxicological studies have been conducted on avian species, such as the bobwhite, ring-neck pheasant, Japanese quail, Coturnix quail, mallard, common pigeon, red-winged blackbird, starling, cowbird, grackle, and the scaleless hen (28–33). These studies predominantly examined the toxicological and reproductive effects of pesticides, pesticide metabolites, or chemosterilants on bird species. Several of these studies have examined the effects of DDT, its most persistent metabolite dichlorodiphenyldichloroethylene (DDE), and other persistent pesticides on egg-shell thinning and reproduction in reptors including the bald eagle (34, 35).

4.5.2 Toxicities of Indicator Chemicals in Bald Eagle. An investigation of the literature, however, reveals little data on the toxicological effects of the individual seven indicator chemicals at the Sand Springs Petrochemical Complex [lead, cadmium, polycyclic aromatic hydrocarbons (PAHs), trichloroethylene, tetrachloroethylene, benzene, and the alkyl benzenes] on bald eagles, other raptors, or avian species in general. A few studies have examined the toxicological effects of lead on bald eagles, other raptors, and waterfowl (22, 36, 37); however, little of these data are derived from studies on lead toxicity to bald eagles as a result of lead in the environment. Available information on lead toxicity to bald eagles comes principally from investigations of lead poisoning due to lead shot or to the ingestion of lead shot from injured or dead game or waterfowl. Furthermore, these studies are descriptive in nature, focusing primarily on lead concentrations found in various organs and on acute toxicosis symptoms in both acute and fatal lead poisoning cases. No experimental data on dose–response relations, mechanism of lead toxicity, or chronic and subchronic toxicities in eagles or in birds were generated from these studies. Nevertheless, a summary of these studies on lead toxicosis in bald eagles and other birds follows.

4.5.3 Lead Toxicity Studies in Bald Eagles and Other Birds. Bald eagles having acute lead poisoning exhibited symptoms such as an inability to maintain an upright position, paralysis of the wings and legs resulting in the reluctance or inability to fly and the sagging of wings by the side, marked emaciation, foul breath odor, green watery feces, bile staining of the gastrointestinal tract, and blindness (22, 36–38). In all studies except one, when any or all of these symptoms were present, mortality resulted in 6 days to 3 weeks. Thus, acute exposure to lead at sufficient doses may be fatal to bald eagles in several days to several weeks. The rate of mortality due to lead poisoning, however, is dependent on the condition of the bird, the diet of the bird, and other environmental conditions (37).

An investigation of the effects of lead shot on five bald eagles fed 10 No. 4 lead pellets per dosage over a period of 10 months in 1978 and 1979 (only two birds were dosed at one time) resulted in four fatalities and severe blindness in a fifth bald eagle (38). The concentration of lead in the livers of the four deceased eagles ranged from 11 to 27 ppm compared to the control bald eagle, which had 0.4 ppm. All birds are exposed to low amounts of lead in their food resulting in measurable amounts of lead in hard and soft tissues—thus recordable levels in the control bird (37). In the fifth and blinded bald eagle, the level of lead in the liver was 3.6 ppm.

Chemical analysis of liver and kidney tissues of a deceased immature bald eagle by Jacobson et al. (37) revealed 22.9 and 11.3 ppm lead, respectively. Lead concentrations as low as 14.9 and 10.8 ppm in the liver and kidney, respectively, were reported as fatal to a juvenile bald eagle (36). Redig et al. (36) also investigated lead toxicosis in other raptors and reported concentrations of lead in the liver and kidney as high as 57 and 78 ppm, respectively, in a female prairie falcon which died within 6 days. In mallard ducks, lead content exceeding a range of 6–20 ppm in the liver and kidney and 3 ppm in the brain indicated acute exposure to lead (37, 39).

Studies of lead content in the clotted blood from the heart of mallard ducks by Longcore et al. (39) reveal 10 ppm as acutely toxic to mallards. Blood levels in bald eagles captured over a 3-year period by the Minnesota Department of Natural Resources (as cited in 22) ranged from 0.4 to 17 ppm. These concentrations are within the range and above the threshold blood level that produce specific effects in humans (11). The mean blood level was five times higher than those found in unexposed birds. However, no information describing the health of the birds was reported.

4.6   Potential Exposure Sources

Many of the potential human exposure routes for chemicals from the Sand Springs Petrochemical Complex also exist as possibilities for the bald eagle. These include inhalation of volatilized chemicals in the air, inhalation of dust from contaminated soils, dermal exposure to contaminated surface waters and soils, and ingestion of contaminated surface waters and soils. In addition, since the eagles near the Sand Springs Petrochemical Complex derive a major portion of their food supply from fish in the Arkansas River, migration of chemicals into the river and their bioconcentration in fish may provide a significant indirect route of exposure.

When the location and behavior of the bald eagle, as well as the nature of the site and surroundings, are taken into consideration, some of these potential exposure sources appear much more realistic than others.

4.7   Potential Exposure Pathways

As indicated in Section 4.3, the wintering bald eagle population closest to the Sand Springs Superfund site is located at the Tulsa Audubon Society Wildlife Preserve in Spring Creek Canyon. This roost site is located approximately 7–8 mi from the Sand Springs Petrochemical Complex. Approximately 91% of this population feeds below Keystone Dam, which lies upstream from the Sand Springs Superfund site. The remaining 9% of the eagles feed lower downstream, which is closer to the Sand Springs site. Bald eagle activity around the Sand Springs Petrochemical Complex is observed only occasionally. This is not surprising since the Sand Springs site is near an area of significant human population and has no particular attributes with respect to feeding or roosting sites. Because bald eagles are only occasionally observed near the Sand Springs Petrochemical Complex, the threat of exposure through onsite ingestion of contaminated soil or water must be considered an infrequent or low possibility.

Dermal absorption through contact with contaminated soil must also be regarded as unlikely since bald eagles typically perch and roost in trees rather than on the ground. The most likely potential and complete pathways for exposure are represented by inhalation of volatilized chemicals and contaminated dusts, ingestion or dermal absorption of offsite contaminated surface water, and ingestion of fish and water from the Arkansas River.

4.8   Evaluation of Potential Exposure

4.8.1   Inhalation Exposure. The most important factor that diminishes the bald eagle population's potential risk from inhalation exposure is the distance of the bald eagle roost and feeding areas from the Sand Springs site. While it is true that air concentrations of some of the volatile chemicals measured at the site exceed exposure guidelines calculated for humans (11), these concentrations rapidly diminish by dilution with distance from the site. Similarly, the migration of dust is rather limited, and concentrations of contaminated dust arriving at the principal roosting and feeding grounds is expected to be infinitesimal. Although bald eagles may fly above the site, during which they might receive measurable exposures, these exposures will most likely be negligible. This conclusion is based on the fact that the number of bald eagle sightings in the immediate vicinity is small and that the probability that the duration of exposure is in all likelihood brief as a result of high human activity in this area. While some inhalation exposure to volatilized chemicals or contaminated dusts from the site is possible, the exact magnitude of this exposure is not known. It is certain, however, that the magnitude of such exposure is not great enough to raise serious concerns for this endangered species.

4.8.2   Dermal Exposure. Because the prospect of dermal exposure of bald eagles at the Sand Springs Petrochemical Complex is highly unlikely, the assessment of potential dermal exposure is primarily based on a scenario in which migration of chemicals through groundwater or surface water results in contamination of the Arkansas River. Dermal exposure of bald eagles to river water may occur during feeding. Typical bald eagle feeding behavior takes place as follows. Bald eagles perch in large trees to watch for prey; when prey are spotted, eagles dive from their perches and swoop down to their prey with legs and talons exposed; fish or waterfowl are pulled directly out of the water or directly from flight as is sometimes the case with injured waterfowl. Dermal absorption of chemical contaminants by bald eagles during feeding will occur primarily through exposed legs and talons. The rate of absorption through these surfaces, however, is most likely quite low since these parts of the bird repel water and are covered in thick leathery skin.

Even if the rate of dermal absorption were high, it does not appear that the eagles would be exposed to significant concentrations of chemical contaminants. Virtually all feeding activity of the eagles occurs upstream from the facility where the concentration of environmental contaminants is at background levels. Observed feeding behavior along the Arkansas River to date indicates that no feeding activity has been recorded adjacent to or downstream from the Sand Springs site. The possibility certainly exists that there is some unobserved feeding activity downstream, or that feeding patterns may change in the future to incorporate some downstream sites.

The analytical data at present are inadequate to evaluate whether the concentrations of chemicals of concern at the Sand Springs Superfund site are elevated downstream. However, the flow of the Arkansas River is such that there will undoubtedly be substantial dilution of any chemicals reaching the river. The potential for dermal absorption is therefore regarded as small.

4.8.3   Exposure via Ingestion. Exposure from ingestion may occur from contaminated water or food, although the probability of this occurring at the Sand Springs site is considered remote. The same factors that limit dermal absorption, such as the current location of bald eagle feeding areas with respect to the Sand Springs site and the downstream dilution of any migrating chemicals, also limit exposure potential by ingestion of river water. Like dermal absorption, exposure by this route is not considered to pose a hazard to the eagle population.

Low concentrations of chemicals downstream from the Sand Springs site may pose a problem if there is bioconcentration or bioaccumulation in eagle food source such as fish. Ingestion of contaminated food and bioaccumulation of contaminants have been the primary exposure routes in raptors for environmental contaminants (36) and should be considered carefully in this situation. The important factors to consider are the identity, concentration, bioconcentration, and bioaccumulation tendencies of the chemicals involved.

The concentrations of the indicator chemicals in the Arkansas River, if present at all, are expected to be very small (see Section 4.8.2). Furthermore, the indicator compounds at the site do not possess the characteristic of significant bioaccumulation. For example, lead, cadmium, trichloroethylene, tetrachloroethylene, and the alkyl benzenes all have relatively low bioaccumulation factors. The PAHs, while highly lipophilic, also do not tend to accumulate in aquatic species. This absence of accumulation by PAHs is usually attributed to a rapid rate of metabolism and elimination.

The absence of demonstrated chemical migration from the site to the Arkansas River, in conjunction with the high probability that any such migration would be followed by extensive dilution, the apparent absence of significant amounts of chemicals having high bioaccumulation characteristics, and the absence of feeding in areas adjacent to or immediately downstream from this Superfund site, strongly indicates that the ingestion of fish does not pose a hazard for the bald eagles.

4.9 Potential Hazards to Bald Eagle Habitat

Under the Federal Endangered Species Act of 1973, both the endangered species and the habitat critical to the survival of the species are protected (8). When assessing the potential hazards or risks of chemical contamination on endangered species, it is important to recognize that survival and reproduction are only one dimension of endangered species population dynamics (34). The availability of habitat is also an important element of population stability for endangered species; therefore, the effects of habitat loss on endangered species must be addressed.

For the Sand Springs site, if heavy metals or other chemical contaminants are persistent in the soil along the banks of the river adjacent to the site, the potential loss of bald eagle habitat from heavy metal or chemical contamination must be assessed. Heavy metal toxicity in plants is well documented (40–42); however, less information is available on the effects of other toxic chemicals such as benzenes, trichloroethylene, tetrachloroethylene, and the alkyl benzenes on plant species. Contamination of soils by zinc, lead, and cadmium results in the reduction of root growth and leaf expansion, causing vegetation to become chlorotic and depauperate in size (40). Additionally, heavy metal deposition in soils has prevented the revegetation of many areas where vegetation was destroyed by sulfur dioxide emissions from nearby smelting operations (43). Thus, if heavy metal contamination of the banks along the river adjacent to the Sand Springs Petrochemical site is a problem, it may inhibit seedling establishment, increase sapling mortality, preclude roost tree replacement, and result in the ultimate decline and loss of critical bald eagle habitat.

No data are currently available, however, on the concentrations or levels of contaminants along the banks adjacent to this site. Any determination of the potential risks from this site to the bald eagle habitat cannot be made without this information. Therefore, for future assessments of hazards to endangered species and their habitats to be complete, the remedial investigation must include sampling regimes that will provide the necessary data to evaluate the potential effects of contamination on the endangered species habitat.

4.10 Summary of the Hazard Assessment for Bald Eagle Populations

The level of chemical contamination present at the Sand Springs Petrochemical Complex seems to pose little threat to the bald eagle populations that inhabit the area. The likelihood that any hazard exists from direct contact with the sediment, sludge, soil, or surface water; from inhalation of the air near the site; or from direct contact with the water of the Arkansas River directly adjacent to the site is quite low. The only potential hazard to the bald eagle population near the site exists from the possible accumulation of site contaminants in the food source of the bald eagles. This potential risk, however, is expected to be minimal based on the low bioaccumulation of the indicator chemicals. Coupled with information on the overall low frequency of bald eagle feeding in this area and on the probable low levels of chemical contamination in the water, the available data indicate that this potential hazard is quite low.

An inherent weakness in this bald eagle hazard assessment is that it has been based on qualitative data because of the lack of quantitative information from river water sampling, fish tissue sampling, sediment sampling data, and duration and frequency of potential exposures. Thus, the exact level of exposure to each of the indicator chemicals is unknown. The use of qualitative data to assess risk, although sufficient in this study, results in a high degree of uncertainty in the assessment.

To be better able to identify the potential hazard to the bald eagle populations near Sand Springs Petrochemical Complex through the food chain, more quantitative data are necessary. Sediment sampling data to determine the extent of chemical contamination in the river sediments, levels of bioaccumulation in fish and other aquatic organisms in the Arkansas River near the site, and detailed data on bald eagle feeding locations, frequency of feeding, and quantities of fish ingested are necessary for an accurate risk evaluation. Even with these data, however, an accurate determination of a safe level of exposure to these indicator chemicals is difficult. This determination is difficult because of the deficiency of basic toxicological research and accumulated data addressing the chronic hazards of these chemicals to this species.

It is equally important to consider habitat preservation when assessing the hazard to the bald eagle populations near the Sand Springs site. Under the Federal Endangered Species Act of 1973 (8), both the endangered species and the habitat critical to the survival of the species are protected. If the persistence of heavy metals in the soil is a problem at the site or along the banks adjacent to the site, the hazard to eagle habitat along the banks must be considered. Heavy metal contamination of the soils in the vicinity of the roost trees may result in roost tree mortality and in the toxicity to and mortality of seedlings necessary for roost tree replacement.

REFERENCES

1. U.S. Department of the Interior, U.S. Fish and Wildlife Service, Determination of certain bald eagle populations as endangered or threatened. *Fed. Regist.* **43**(31), 6230–6233 (1978).

2. Public law 95–510, *Comprehensive Environmental Response, Compensation, and Liability Act of 1980*, Title I, Sect. 111 (h) (2), 1980.

3. The Federal Water Pollution Control Act, *33 U.S.C.* 1321, Sect. 311, 1972.

4. Public law 95–510, *Comprehensive Environmental Response, Compensation, and Liability Act of 1980*, Title I, Sect. 101(16), 1980.

5. *National Oil and Hazardous Substances Pollution Contingency Plan*, 40 Code of Federal Regulations, Sect. 300.72. U.S. Government Printing Offices, Washington, DC, 1986.

6. P. Douglas, U.S. Fish and Wildlife Service, personal communication to Lisa Gandy (1987).

7. W. W. Johnson, U.S. Fish and Wildlife Service, personal communication to Lisa Gandy (1987).

8. Public Law 93–205, *Endangered Species Act of 1973*, Sect. 7, 1973.

9. U.S. Environmental Protection Agency, *Superfund Public Health Evaluation Manual*. Office of Emergency and Remedial Response, USEPA, Washington, DC, 1986.

10. J. Mathes & Associates, Inc., *Remedial Investigation Report for the Sand Springs Petrochemical Complex.* 1986.

11. J. Mathes & Associates, Inc., *Endangerment Assessment for the Operable Unit of the Sand Springs Petrochemical Complex Superfund Site Tulsa County, Oklahoma,* Contract No. 60636. Prepared under contract for the Oklahoma Department of Health, Tulsa, 1987.

12. Oklahoma Department of Wildlife Conservation, *The Bald Eagle in Oklahoma*, pamphlet. ODWC, 1986.

13. J. W. Lish, Status and ecology of Bald Eagles and nesting of Golden Eagles in Oklahoma. M. S. Thesis, Oklahoma State University, Stillwater (1975).

14. J. W. Lish and J. C. Lewis, Status and ecology of Bald Eagles wintering in Oklahoma. *Proc. 29th Annu. Conf. Southeast. Assoc. Game and Fish Comm.* (1975), pp. 415–423.

15. Oklahoma Cooperative Wildlife Research Unit, *Summary Midwinter Bald Eagle Surveys.* OCWRU, 1979–1986.

16. Tulsa Audubon Society, *Oklahoma Blad Eagle Counts Raw Data.* TAS, Tulsa, OK, 1979–1987.

17. American Ornithologist Union, *Check-list of North American Birds.* Lord Baltimore Press, Baltimore, MD, 1957.

18. J. Crowley and N. Garrison, *Bald Ealges of Keystone Resevoir (Northeastern Oklahoma): A Plea for Habitat Conservation,* A Tulsa Audubon Society Publication, Tulsa, OK, 1978.

19. S. Shalaway, Biological assessment of impact of Shenandoah development on wintering Bald Eagles. In *Final Environmental Impact Statement for Shenandoah Development, Sand Springs, Tulsa County, Oklahoma,* Appendix B. Department of Housing and Urban Development, Fort Worth Regional Office, Fort Worth, TX, 1983, pp. 1–7.

20. J. F. Swisher, Jr., Roosting area of the Bald Eagle in northern Utah. *Wilson Bull.* **76**, 186–187 (1964).

21. U.S. Fish and Wildlife Service, Region 4, *Management Guidlines for the Bald Eagle in the Southeast Region.* USTWS, Washington, DC, 1987, p. 1.

22. J. P. Cohn, Lead shot poisons Bald Eagles. *BioScience* **35**(8), 474–476 (1985).

23. Personal communication from Mr. Bruce Ewing, Bald Eagle Committee Chairman, Tulsa Audubon Society (1987).

24. Personal communication from Mr. Kent Wire, Past Chairman Bald Eagle Committee, Tulsa Audubon Socitey (1987).

25. Personal communication from Mr. James Lish, Oklahoma Cooperative Wildlife Research Unit, Oklahoma State University, Stillwater (1987).

26. Personal communication from Mr. Jim Andreason, Biologist, Oklahoma Department of Wildlife Conservation, Oklahoma City (1987).

27. Letter to the U.S. Environmental Protection Agency from the Oklahoma Department of Wildlife Conservation, Oklahoma City, June, 1983.

28. R. G. Heath and J. W. Spann, Reproduction and related residues in birds fed mirex. In W. B. Deichmann, Ed., *Pesticides and the Environment: A Continuing Controversy.* Intercontinental Medical Book Corporation, New York, 1973.

29. R. K. Tucker and M. A. Haegele, Comparative and acute oral toxicity of pesticides to six species of birds. *Toxicol. Appl. Pharmacol.* **20**, 57–65 (1971).

30. W. H. Stickel, J. A. Galyen, R. A. Dyrland, and D. L. Hughes, Toxicity and persistence of mirex in birds. In W. B. Deichmann, Ed., *Pesticides and the Environment: A Continuing Controversy.* Intercontinental Medical Book Corporation, New York, 1973.

31. E. W. Schafer, The acute oral toxicity of 369 pesticidal, pharmaceutical, and other chemicals to wild birds. *Toxicol. Appl. Pharmacol.* **21**, 315–330 (1972).

32. E. W. Schafer, Jr., R. B. Brunton, E. C. Schafer, and G. Chavez, Effects of 77 chemicals on reproduction in male and female coturnix quail. *Ecotoxicol. Environ.* **6**, 149–156 (1982).

33. B. W. Wilson, C. M. Cisson, W. R. Randall, J. E. Woodrow, J. N. Seiber, and J. B. Knaak, Organophosphate risk assessment: Field testing of DEF with the scaleless chicken. *Bull. Environ. Contam. Toxicol.* **24**, 921–928 (1980).

34. J. W. Grier, Ban of DDT and subsequent recovery of reproduction in Bald Eagles. *Science* **218**, 1232–1234 (1982).

35. S. N. Wiemeyer, T. G. Lamont, C. M. Bunck, C. R. Sindelar, F. G. Gramlich, J. D. Fraser, and M. A. Byrd, Organochlorine pesticide, polychlorobiphenyl, and mercury residues in Bald Eagle eggs-1969-70-and their relationships to shell thinning and reproduction. *Arch. Environ. Contam. Toxicol.* **13**, 529–549 (1984).

36. P. T. Redig, C. M. Stowe, D. M. Barnes, and T. D. Àrent, Lead toxicosis in raptors. *J. Am. Vet. Med. Assoc.* **177**(9), 941–943 (1980).

37. E. Jacobson, J. W. Carpenter, and M. Novilla, Suspected lead toxicosis in a Bald Eagle. *J. Am. Vet. Med. Assoc.* **171**(9), 952–954 (1977).

38. O. H. Pattee, S. N. Wiemeyer, B. M. Mulhorn, L. Sileo, and J. W. Carpenter, Experimental lead shot poisoning in Bald Eagles, *Haliaeetus leucocephalus. J. Wildl. Manage* **45**(3), 806–810 (1981).

39. J. R. Longcore, R. Andrews, L. N. Locke, G. E. Bagley, and L. T. Young, Significance of lead residues in mallard tissues. *U.S. Fish Wildl. Serv., Spec. Sci. Rep.: Wildl.* **182**, 1–24 (1974).

40. K. Mengel and E. A. Kirkby, *Principles of Plant Nutrition*, International Potash Institute, Bern, Switzerland, 1978, pp. 509–520.

41. R. K. Brewer, Lead. In H. D. Chapman, Ed., *Diagnostic Criteria for Plants and Soils.* Division of Agricultural Sciences, University of California, 1966, pp. 213–217.

42. A. L. Page, T. J. Ganji, and M. S. Joshi, Lead quantities in plants, soils, and air near some major highways in southern California. *Hilgardia* **41**, 1–3 (1971).

43. L. Friberg, M. Piscator, G. F. Norberg, and T. Kjellstrom, Eds., *Cadmium in the Environment*, 2nd ed. CRC Press, Cleveland, OH, 1974.

H

RISK MANAGEMENT

30

Legal and Philosophical Aspects of Risk Analysis

Louis Anthony Cox, Jr.
US West Advanced Technologies, Englewood, Colorado

Paolo F. Ricci
Lawrence Berkeley Laboratory, University of California, Berkeley, California

A risky economic or technological activity, such as the production, transportation, distribution, or use of an industrial chemical or a consumer product, typically represents an intersection of many economic transactions and processes within a social and political framework. *Social risk management cannot be understood apart from the context of these social processes*: risk management decisions and policies are interwoven with social decision processes and with issues of responsibility, accountability, and political representation. As stated in Chapter 2, judgments of acceptability for risky activities are not just a matter of numbers but draw on the judicial, regulatory, and political mechanisms through which social choices are made and enforced.

In this chapter, some of the fundamental factors that must be considered when evaluating risk acceptability are discussed. The concepts of *voluntariness, equity*, procedural *legitimacy*, treatment of *uncertainty*, and psychological *perceptions* are reviewed. The discussion emphasizes concepts and guiding principles for risk managers. Concepts that should be considered by decisionmakers are presented even when (as for risk equity) the formal theory is insufficiently developed to give quantitative calculations for taking all relevant factors into account. Some of the real-world practices that reflect these underlying principles are also presented. The intent is to provide the reader with an introduction to the nonquantitative issues that must be considered in translating the results of a quantitative risk assessment into implications for policy or action.

1 VOLUNTARINESS

Social decisions based on the informed preferences of those affected, constrained only by respect for individual rights and liberties, is an ideal that is central to normative political theories in Western societies (1, 2). Sensitivity to this cultural preference has been the basis for accepting *voluntary and informed consent* as a key determinant in assessing risk acceptability. In a society that values individual liberties, a risk that an individual is willing to take may be acceptable at a higher level than a quantitatively similar risk imposed on an individual by another party over which the individual has little or no control (3, 4).

Many of our individual activities, as well as society's expectations regarding safety and responsibility, are influenced by the degree of voluntariness or imposition, as determined through (i) the affected party's initial freedom to choose or reject an activity and (ii) the individual's ability to control its progress or aftermath. For example, an individual may be entitled to smoke cigarettes in private, creating enormous health risks for himself, and yet be forbidden to smoke in public, where he would impose much smaller risks (via secondary smoke inhalation) on others.

The full concept of voluntariness in determining the acceptability of a risk, and especially for acceptance of uncertain risks, is far more subtle and complex than such examples initially suggest. For example, the distinction between ex ante and ex post risk assessments, and the fact that uncertain risks evolve over time (since the passage of time is itself informative, as shown in Chapter 2, raise important questions about the meaning of voluntariness over time. Varying degrees of voluntariness can be distinguished, depending on how much is known and how much is controllable about the risks of an activity as time passes.

1.1   Voluntary Individual Choices

A truly voluntary activity (resulting in risk) is one that an individual is free and able to reject without penalty, that an individual can control while undertaking, and whose risks are fully known or easily discoverable (4). Sport parachuting is a good example. If any of these conditions are violated, the concept of voluntariness becomes strained. For example, workers may be "free" to reject participation in a hazardous occupational activity, but if doing so poses a threat to their jobs, then accepting the activity is not entirely voluntary for them, and should not be interpreted as a sign that its risk is "acceptable". Similarly, longtime cigarette smokers may in principle be "free" to give up smoking, but if they were incompletely informed about its risks when they began and are not able to give it up without physiological and psychological trauma, then the extent to which it remains a truly "voluntary" activity, especially if they would like to and have tried to quit, is debatable (5). Voluntariness is not a one-dimensional concept when an individual's own preferences may be divided.

A second type of voluntariness applies to an activity that individuals are initially free to reject without penalty, but over which they lose control once it has begun. Drinking, smoking, and other addictive activities are examples, as is elective cosmetic surgery. From a social risk management point of view, such activities may be viewed as "voluntary" insofar as the affected parties initially choose to expose themselves to the risks: no one else imposes the risks of these activities on them. But where advertisements and deliberate inducements by others play a major role in the initial decision to participate, the idea of pure voluntariness is again compromised.

Third, there are activities, such as driving a car to work, that individuals may have little choice but to participate in, but whose risks they can to a large extent control through prudence and skill. The perception of *controllability* of risks, even when it is illusory, plays a large role in individual judgments of risk acceptability (6). Risks that are not within the control of an individual may be tolerated relatively cheerfully if they are of natural origin (like lightning, earthquakes, volcanic eruptions, or cosmic radiation) and yet be bitterly contested if they are imposed by human activities [like industrial explosions, hazardous waste leakage, or radiation from the nuclear fuel cycle (3)]. Human tolerances for quantitatively similar risks can vary widely depending on whether the activities or sources producing them are seen as violating the rights of those affected.

Finally, there is the belief, made explicit in the statutory language of regulatory agencies such as the Consumer Product Safety Commission [see (4)], that a truly free choice requires the participants to have full *information* about what is being chosen. Consumers who buy a risky product because they have been lied to about its risks would not ordinarily be considered to have "voluntarily accepted" the risks of the product: they did not know what they were accepting. Right-to-know and duty-to-warn legislation make explicit the notion that a lack of equality in information about the potential risks of an economic transaction (such as employment in a hazardous occupation or purchase of a product) should not be allowed as a basis for reaching mutual "acceptance" of the transaction. It is the symmetry, rather than the absolute quality, of information that is important in this context. If neither the buyer nor the seller of a product knows its risks, then the buyer may still be said to have "voluntarily" assumed the (uncertain) risks of the product, as long as the seller disclosed all the relevant information available. Thus there can be a social dimension in defining voluntariness.

Example 1. Duty to Warn in Tort Law. The common law in this country, as well as various legislative actions by the Consumer Product Safety Commission (CPSC) and the Occupational Safety and Health Administration (OSHA), clearly recognize that an employer or manufacturer has a duty to warn employees or consumers, respectively, of potential occupational or consumption risks that the manufacturer may know about and that are not patent or that cannot be understood on the basis of common knowledge. Whether a firm must warn its employees or consumers about *unknown* risks, however, is less clear. In *Besheda* v. *Johns-Mansville Products Corp.* (Supreme Court of New Jersey, 1982, 90 N.J. 191, 47 A.2d 539), for example, the question was raised of whether a manufacturer (in this case, of asbestos products) has a duty to warn customers of a risk that is unknown at the time of sale. The New Jersey Supreme Court held that even though this duty does not reasonably arise under negligence law, strict product liability can still be imposed in retrospect because it would be unfair to avoid compensating innocent plaintiffs when manufacturers and distributors are better able to bear the unforeseen costs. However, such reasoning, which mixes economic welfare arguments (who is best able to bear the costs of an unanticipated loss?) with deontological arguments (what are each party's duties and legal obligations?) has come under sharp criticism and has provoked calls for tort law reform in recent years (7). After all, it is also unfair to force manufacturers to compensate plaintiffs for risks that they could not reasonably have foreseen and that were voluntarily accepted.

So far, we have discussed voluntariness as it applies to individual choices. Risk management decisions usually involve social choice, however. These choices involve multiple parties and partially conflicting interests participating in, or being represented in, the decision process. The concept of voluntary acceptance of risky activities must be expanded when multiple decisionmakers participate in the acceptance decision. The following subsections further develop the concept of voluntary choice for group decisions.

1.2 Voluntary Bilateral Agreement

The simplest case of joint decisionmaking involves voluntary agreement on a transaction between two economic agents, with either party free and able to withhold agreement if he so chooses. The transaction will not be consummated unless both parties expect to gain from it and voluntarily agree to it. Even in this simplest case, however, asymmetries in the private information about risks available to the different parties can create ambiguities about the degree of voluntary acceptability.

Example 2. Unequal Knowledge Regarding Product Hazard. A manufacturer wishes to sell a product to a consumer. The manufacturer is concerned that the product may be defective and that it may cause damage to the consumer. The manufacturer is aware, but the consumer is not, that the probability of a product defect is $p = 0.01$. The consumer knows only that half of all manufacturers provide "low-quality" products with $p = 0.09$, while half provide high-quality products with $p = 0.01$. The customer's maximum acceptable probability of defect in exchange for the product benefits is 0.03. What inefficiencies might arise in these circumstances, and how can regulatory or legal measures be used to improve economic efficiency?

Solution. To the consumer, given his information about product qualities, the probability that this manufacturer's product will prove defective is $(0.5)(0.01) + (0.5)(0.09) = 0.05$, which is unacceptable. There is thus an economic inefficiency: the consumer will refuse to buy the manufacturer's product even though he would consider its risks acceptable if he knew what the manufacturer knows. Both parties might expect to gain from the sale if they could credibly share their private information.

If manufacturers are allowed to assume and are able to afford high liability for product defects, then economic efficiency (i.e., consummation of mutually beneficial transactions) may be restored. Manufacturers of low-risk products can afford to bear greater product liability than can manufacturers of high-risk products, thus sending a market "signal" to the customer that reveals that they are low-risk producers. This is one way in which legal liability can be used to promote economic efficiency—by driving high-risk producers out of the market. Alternatively, a regulatory standard that is enforceable by the government and that prevents low-quality products from being sold can give customers the assurance they need to be willing to buy the product. In practice, limitations on corporate liability, wealth constraints, and other institutional factors (e.g., the fact that liability may be determined retrospectively by the courts rather than prospectively through agreements between buyers and sellers) can prevent manufacturers from using liability to signal their private information about product quality to consumers (8–10).

Example 2 illustrates the intermixture of purely objective aspects of risk (viz., the fact that the manufacturer's product has a 0.01 probability of defect) with socioeconomic and institutional constraints on who knows, or can find out, the critical data in determining the final "acceptability" of a risk to those who must make the acceptability decision. As another example, if it becomes technically feasible for manufacturers to screen their products more accurately for defects, then uncertain risks that were formerly considered "acceptable" may now become considered "unacceptable" unless they are screened. The ability of one party to take additional care at reasonable cost, rather than simply the probable magnitude and severity of adverse consequences, helps to determine the "acceptability" of a risky transaction.

1.3 Indirect Agreement

In the case of bilateral agreements, with either party free to reject any proposed risky transaction unless the sharing of risks and benefits is acceptable, the idea of "voluntary" acceptance of risk is relatively straightforward. When more than two people are involved, and the preferences of individuals may conflict with the preferences of the majority involved in a risk acceptance decision, the idea of voluntariness becomes more complex. Does a voluntary precommitment to abide by the results of a group decision process make one a voluntary acceptor of all its decisions? This is a matter of definition. It makes plain the connection between issues of voluntariness and of legitimacy of process in reaching collective decisions about acceptability.

Individuals may be said to accept a risk *indirectly voluntarily* if they voluntarily accept a social decision process that in turn leads to social acceptance of it. Conversely, if they deny the legitimacy of the process and find the risk individually unacceptable, then they may react to it as they would to any other nonvoluntary, imposed risk. It is only necessary to consider the recent history of nuclear power or hazardous facility siting in this country to appreciate the close connection between (i) the perceived legitimacy of processes for determining acceptability and (ii) the perception of voluntary participation in judging acceptability (11, 15).

The idea of voluntary commitment to a social decision process is essential to understanding voluntariness over time. Individuals may agree to abide by the results of a social decision process (e.g., majority rule) because they expect to gain from the process on average, even though they may dislike particular decisions. From this standpoint, acceptability of each particular risky prospect is not a very well-defined or relevant issue. Rather, acceptability and equity of the portfolio of risks accepted by the process as it is applied over time become the key items to evaluate (12, 13). For example, a hazardous facility siting decision that would be "unacceptable" to neighbors of the site in isolation may become acceptable to them when it is seen as part of a portfolio of social risk management decisions that includes siting some other facility far away.

1.4   Implicit Acceptance

Still further from the ordinary notion of voluntary acceptance of risk is the idea that a decisionmaker or decisionmaking body (e.g., a regulatory agency) has an obligation to take those actions that the members of society *would* choose (via an appropriate legitimate collective choice process) if they had the same information as the decisionmakers. In this view, it is individual preferences for *consequences* rather than for *acts* or social decisions that should be the ultimate basis for social choice. Actual social choices are made by combining these individual preferences for consequences with the best available scientific information about the probable consequences of different choices. Individuals are represented in the decisionmaking process by their preferences for outcomes, rather than by their beliefs about the best ways to achieve them.

Individuals may be said to *accept implicitly* a risky prospect if they accept explicitly the decision process used to combine individual preferences for consequences with scientific information about probable consequences to reach a social decision of acceptability, even if they do not accept explicitly (and may not even know about) the scientific information fed into this process. The decisionmakers participating in the process believe that those they represent would agree with their risk acceptance decisions if they had (and understood) the same information as the decisionmakers (2).

Of course, whether implicit acceptance "feels" like at least indirectly voluntary acceptance (i.e., acceptance via legitimate representation) to those being represented depends not only on the perceived legitimacy of the decisionmaking process but also on the extent to which those being represented *trust* those representing them to identify and apply appropriate scientific information.

As the interaction between individuals and social decision processes becomes more important in defining acceptability of a risk, the concept of voluntariness becomes increasingly intermixed with other issues used to evaluate social decision processes— issues of equity and fairness, legitimacy, trust under ignorance and uncertainty, and perception. These issues are explored separately.

2   RISK EQUITY AND FAIRNESS

A second key set of factors affecting the acceptability of a risky activity concerns the *fairness and equity* of the distribution of its risks and benefits. For risks (unlike, say, income distribution) the concept of equity is complicated by the fact that risk–benefit distributions that are fair and equitable ex ante may turn out to be inequitable (though not perhaps unfair) ex post (14).

Intuitively, a distribution of risks and benefits flowing from some activity appears to be unfairly distributed if those who bear the risks do not receive the benefits. More generally, a situation in which individual benefits are not distributed in proportion to individual risks (assuming that both are measured on ratio scales) appears on the face of it to be potentially unfair. For example, a situation in which one community bears all the risks from a facility that N communities use and receive benefits from might appear patently unfair. However, modern theories of distributional justice, fairness, and equity suggest that, where risks are concerned, it is not possible to judge whether a distribution of benefits is fair just by looking at it: it is also important to understand how it came about (15, 16).

This is the essential distinction between state-based and process-based notions of justice (15). A state of affairs (e.g., a risk–benefit distribution) that appears unfair may be considered defensible if it arose through a sequence of justice-preserving changes in an initially fair state. On the other hand, when just processes do produce unjust states (e.g., highly asymmetric risk–benefit distributions), corrective actions by the state may be required to restore the balance. Corrective, as opposed to distributive, justice provides the active link between process-based and state-based conceptions of fair distribution (15).

Example 3. Efficiency and Fairness in Facility Siting. Suppose that N communities in a state must jointly agree on where to site a hazardous waste disposal facility that all expect to use, but that none wants to host. What social decision procedures might the communities use to decide where to site the facility? What trade-offs between efficiency and fairness do alternative decision procedures imply?

Solution. Over a dozen proposals and variations have been advanced in the economics and game theory literatures to address this type of multiple-decisionmaker problem (12, 13, 17–26). The three alternative approaches discussed below illustrate some of the main elements in this broad range of possibilities.

A. A Lottery. One possible decision procedure would be to decide by lottery which community is assigned the facility, with each community being equally likely to be selected. This procedure is not likely to be economically efficient: it will probably not assign the facility to the community that would mind it least, for example. But it might very well be considered a fair procedure.

Ex ante, the expected social utility to each community from agreeing to participate in the lottery might be $B - R/N$, where B denotes the economic value of being able to use the facility to dispose of hazardous wastes locally (in state) and R is the social disutility from having the facility sited in the community. Even though the risk–benefit combination (R, B) may be unacceptable to every community, so that the benefits of local disposal are outweighed by its perceived risks for each community by itself, the combination $(R/N, B)$, representing the ex ante expected risk–benefit combination from participation in the lottery, may be acceptable to everyone. That is, everyone may be willing to participate in the lottery and to commit to abiding by its outcome, expecting ex ante to gain thereby, even though the loser may regret the outcome ex post. Even though the ex post distribution of risks and benefits will be asymmetric, if it arose from voluntary participation in a fair lottery then it may still be regarded as fair. Had the same distribution arisen by other means, however—for example, if community X were assigned the facility because it was less successful than the other $N - 1$ communities in exerting political influence on state decisionmakers—then it might be regarded as unfair.

B. *Negotiated Compensation.* The pure lottery procedure is simplistic. Actual risk management decisions seldom use explicit randomization to assure fairness, although there may be a trend in that direction as nontraditional approaches to dispute resolution are sought (19, 24). Moreover, assignment by lottery may fail to exploit opportunities for mutual expected gain through a system of ex ante *compensation payments* (24). For example, it may be possible for $N - 1$ communities to pay the Nth community to accept willingly the facility in exchange for a combination of ex ante payments, perhaps in the form of new schools and parks and insurance against ill health effects. How such socially compensated risk-bearing agreements should be negotiated or arbitrated depends on social objectives for trade-offs between fairness, efficiency, and community rights and duties. For example, should a very poor community be allowed to accept very risky facilities based on its willingness to accept compensation? What floors on payments and what ceilings on risks are required to prevent unethical exploitation of poorer communities by richer ones? Economic efficiency, defined solely in terms of willingness to pay and willingness to accept payment, may conflict with ethical principles of justice.

C. *Bidding Procedures* (21–23). A final approach that has been tried (with incomplete success) in Massachusetts (19) involves a *bidding process* wherein communities express the strength of their preferences through announced compensation amounts that they would be willing to pay to avoid the facility (or that they would accept to take the facility). These announced amounts are then used to select a site, to collect payments from the other $N - 1$ communities, and to compensate the community to which the facility is assigned. Under some strong economic assumptions, for example, that expressed bids are not distorted by unequal wealth or by asymmetric information about the true risks of the facility, such procedures can lead to outcomes that balance "fairness" (in an appropriately defined sense emphasizing symmetry among players) and economic efficiency. However, when each community has private information about its own true preferences, strategic behavior (in which communities distort their announced willingness to pay or to accept payment) may make it impossible to achieve an efficient outcome (21–23, 25). Bidding mechanisms for reaching social agreement on the acceptability of risky activities and the distribution of their risks and benefits continue to be the focus of both theoretical and empirical research (26, 27).

As the facility siting example suggests, the perceived equity of risk distributions is often closely tied up with issues of procedural legitimacy and ex ante voluntary commitment to a decision process over time. There are other ways to evaluate risk equity issues, however. Legal and regulatory constraints help protect individuals from inequities in individual risk arising from inequities in the distribution of bargaining power in economic transactions.

For example, a manufacturer may not expose employees to high levels of hazardous substances just because they will (or can be made to) agree to accept the risks in exchange for money. Nor can a consumer sell the right to sue for personal injury arising from product defects. Uniformly applicable EPA, OSHA, and product liability standards help decouple inequities in health risk exposure from possible asymmetries in economic bargaining position or market power.

Risk equity also depends on the *identifiability* of victims. Suppose that it is known that an activity will cause cancer in approximately 1 out of every 1 million people exposed—namely, only in people having a particular enzyme deficiency that manifests itself only in terms of vastly heightened susceptibility to certain carcinogens. If every member of the population is judged to be a priori equally likely to have the deficiency, then the risk may be considered equitably distributed. On the other hand, if it turns out that only members of a certain race, or of certain ethnic communities, or only those having certain other physical ailments (e.g., an allergy to sunshine, carried on the same gene as the hypothesized enzyme deficiency) are susceptible, then the same risk may be considered to be very inequitably distributed—perhaps "unacceptably" so. It is not the expected number of occurrences per million person-years of exposure in the whole population that counts in determining equity, but the way that this risk density is distributed among identifiable subsets of the population. This depends on what individuals know about their own response "types," as discussed in Chapter 2. The same objective frequency distribution of individual risks may be acceptable if no individual knows where he falls in the frequency distribution, but it may be unacceptable if those who fall at the high end know it and must live with the knowledge.

Equity issues are important because they can affect the way that risk management decisions are made. For example, in assessing the chronic health risks from energy-producing facilities, it is common practice to assess the expected number of illnesses and fatalities in the surrounding population due to pollution emitted by the facility (28). Both expected effects per hundred thousand people exposed and expected total effects may be estimated. However, such risks are usually not equitably distributed: neighbors of the power plant may be exposed to substantially greater risks than most of the population included in the risk calculations. To take this inequity in risk into account, a risk manager deciding whether to purchase additional pollution reduction equipment may wish to assign greater weight to the preferences (e.g., the willingness to pay) of people living closer to the power plant. Use of such "equity weights" can help compensate in the social decisionmaking process (e.g., cost–risk–benefit analysis) for inequities in the distribution of risks and benefits (29).

While there is no well-developed formal or mathematical theory that describes risk equity, as yet, there is a recent and growing literature that seeks to apply decision analysis methods to these issues (30–32). Much of this literature has been flawed by the assumption that probability distributions over numbers of fatalities adequately capture the idea of social risk, without taking into account the knowledge that individuals have of their own risks over time. Despite recent theoretical progress in identifying trade-offs and differences in concepts of equity (32), the field of risk analysis has not yet identified criteria that are apt to be of much practical use to real decisionmakers in formalizing trade-offs between risk magnitude and risk equity in real situations.

2.1 Maximally Threatened Individuals

In practice, the individual risk to the *maximally threatened* individual (i.e., to the maximally exposed individual, if no individual knows his own response "type") is often given special status in regulatory language and in risk analyses conducted by regulatory agencies. One reason is that if the individual risk to the maximally threatened individual can be shown to be "acceptably" small, then it might seem plausible that the risk to the entire population is also acceptable, since no other individual in it bears a higher risk. We have reviewed various points of view in this chapter and Chapter 2 that suggest that such reasoning alone is inadequate: population risk and individual risk must be assessed separately, taking procedural and distributional aspects of the population risk into account.

The identity of the maximally threatened individual will in general depend on the information set that is used to calculate risks (see Chapter 2). At one extreme, perfect information would show (at least in a competing risks model) a whole set of maximally threatened individuals, namely, precisely those individuals who will in fact be damaged. Risks calculated with respect to imperfect information—as all real risks are—will confound objective individual risk with information about individuals.

The idea of a maximally exposed, or maximally threatened, individual is also not well suited for taking into account background risks. Who is more "threatened" by a risk: an individual whose hazard rate is increased from 0.01 to 0.02, or an individual whose hazard rate is increased from 0.02 to 0.03? The former represents 50 years of lost life expectancy (with it being considerably more likely than not that the loss will be greater than its expected value), while the second represents only a 17-year reduction in life expectancy. On the other hand, with less expected life left, the second individual might be thought to suffer more for each additional expected year lost.

Deciding who is the most damaged by a risk involves questions of risk equity and risk attitude toward probability distributions over remaining life, as well as questions about whose risk attitude is to be used when different individuals have different risk attitudes. It may be that individual A would prefer an increase in hazard rate from 0.02 to 0.03 to an increase from 0.01 to 0.02, while individual B might have the opposite preferences. Which (if either) set of preferences is to be used to identify the "most harmed" individual and to evaluate the harm (diminished expected utility) done to different individuals by a new population risk is a policy question with no easy answer.

There is another possible reason for focusing on the risk to the maximally threatened individual. A very simple model of *individual rights* based on a social contract argument might hold that an individual should be protected by the state against all man-made risks of more than a certain size, where the threshold at which her rights become violated (and hence legal intervention is justified) may depend on the total risk to which she is exposed and on factors such as whether the risk is imposed without consent or is "voluntary" in one or more of the senses discussed above. According to this view, the allowable level of risk that one agent may impose on another can be determined in principle by considering the greatest level that individuals would mutually agree to allow each other, starting from a symmetric (i.e., equitable) initial state in which either no one was allowed to create risks for anyone else, or in which everyone could create risks without restriction (15).

2.2 Rights-Based Criteria

More realistically, a *rights-based criterion* of acceptability for risky activities requires balancing the rights of individuals to engage in activities (even though other individuals may be exposed to some risk thereby) against the rights of individuals not to have risks imposed on them (even though enforcing this restriction may interfere with the behavior of others). How the balance should be struck in particular cases—say, in a dispute between a homeowner and an industrial plant operator, where the plant creates only very small risks to the homeowner—depends on what theory of *initial entitlements* is accepted. Is the homeowner initially (i.e., before settlement) entitled to zero risk, or is the plant operator initially entitled to engage in "reasonably" safe production activities? If the conflict is settled through a negotiated or adjudicated compensation agreement, then the "fair" terms of agreement will depend on the hypothesized initial (presumably "fair") system of entitlements.

Presumptions about entitlement affect both the definition of deontologically "acceptable" risk levels and the evaluation of the fairness of compensation arrangements for those on whom risk is imposed. It should be noted that any system of entitlements is apt to be inconsistent with pure economic efficiency, since those who own rights to resources (e.g., clean air) by entitlement are not necessarily those who value them most, and since reallocation of entitlements through compensation negotiations imposes dead-weight costs (17).

The evolution of legal doctrine vis-à-vis responsibility for and social acceptability of risky activities has shown a gradual, though by no means complete, clarification and partial resolution of the practical ambiguities left by abstract theories of rights, duties, and entitlements. No single unified theory has emerged or seems likely to do so [despite some recent ambitious efforts in law and economics (7, 17, 33, 34)], and it seems inevitable that important decisions regarding ex post responsibility and compensation for risks that were ex ante uncertain or unforeseen will continue to require subjective value judgments to fill in the gaps left by prescriptive theory.

3   PROCEDURAL LEGITIMACY: LEGAL AND REGULATORY PERSPECTIVES

Society has a range of instruments for managing chronic health and safety risks through loss reduction, loss prevention, and loss spreading or sharing. These instruments include private and social insurance, tort liability, worker's compensation, health, safety, and environmental regulation, negotiated compensation agreements (settled by the participants out of court, e.g., using alternative dispute resolution programs established by states), environmental law and legislation, and voluntary self-regulation of standards and practices by industry groups and associations. These mechanisms often overlap. For example, the settlement of the well-publicized Agent Orange cases involves aspects of tort litigation, negotiated settlement, and social insurance (7).

Previous subsections have already stressed the importance of procedural legitimacy and its interactions with issues of voluntariness and equity in determining the social acceptability of public decision procedures that permit or accept risky activities. In the remainder of this subsection, we examine current legal and regulatory approaches to the control of risky activities.

3.1   The Problem of Proof

Legal acceptability of an activity is based on answers to fundamental questions posed by affected members of the public, by regulators, and by industry. One such question that has been the object of heated debate in recent years is the following: *How can disputes be adjudicated and defensible policy decisions be made in the absence of adequate scientific information and knowledge about causal mechanisms?* A central issue is that of "proof" in cases where it is not clear whether a risk is being imposed, or where the magnitude of the putative risks created by an activity are highly uncertain. (Recall from Chapter 2 that uncertainties of six orders of magnitude are not unusual.) Not only must the legal definition of proof be refined when neither plaintiff nor defendant can do more than speculate about the probable causal mechanisms that may have contributed to the plaintiff's injury, but traditional standards for assigning the burden of proof must also be rethought. It is no longer sufficient to ask for a "but-for" or "more likely than not" standard of proof when causal mechanisms are unknown, or when the defendant's estimated share in causation of the plaintiff's injury varies randomly with the amount of research done (and perhaps with which side is doing it!) (35).

In traditional administrative law, for example, the burden of proof is placed on the proponent of action—the agency calling for a change in the status quo. This amounts to an assumption that those who might be subjected to regulation are "innocent" until proved "guilty;" that is, an economic agent should not be regulated until the regulating agency can prove that the agent is creating a risk of harm to someone. However, this allocation can be changed by statute: if an *uncertain* risk, that might or might not exist, is itself considered unacceptable, then economic agents who may be creating such risks can be treated as guilty (i.e., can be regulated) until they can prove themselves innocent. The Federal Insecticide, Fungicide, and Rodenticide Act (FIFRA), for example, places the burden of proof on registrants. Similarly, the Food and Drug Administration (FDA) requires pharmaceutical manufacturers to demonstrate that a new drug is safe and effective before allowing it to be sold.

3.2   Cost–Risk–Benefit Analysis

A strictly economically "rational" approach, based on cost–risk–benefit analysis, for setting standards of proof and for allocating the burden of proof would require balancing three factors: (i) the costs and informativeness of additional safety research (e.g., resource requirements per unit reduction in uncertainty), (ii) the losses (e.g., number of preventable fatalities per year) from falsely withholding a product (e.g., a vaccine or other drug) from the market if in fact it is safe and effective, and (iii) the losses (e.g., number of additional fatalities) from falsely permitting a product to be marketed if in fact it is not safe and effective. These factors would determine the *probability* of safety that would have to be demonstrated in order to justify releasing a new product.

If the costs of acquiring relevant information were to fall, then the required acceptance threshold for probability of safety would rise, other things being equal. In other words, stronger evidence of safety must be presented to justify a decision to release a new product when evidence about the product's risks is relatively easy to obtain. Similarly, as the ratio of the expected damages from incorrectly withholding versus incorrectly releasing the product increases, the acceptance threshold for probability of safety would decrease, other things being equal. The worse the relative consequences of a certain kind of error, the more care one should take to avoid it, even if this means raising the probability of the reverse, less grievous, error.

Finally, the allocation of burden of proof would be based on who (e.g., manufacturers or federal agencies) is the cheapest information producer, and on consideration of the incentives to manufacturers to produce socially beneficial products, given the burden of proof (7, 33).

These sorts of trade-offs, and the consequential balancing of different objectives in determining the acceptability of an uncertain risk, are implied by the principles of

TABLE 1. Synopsis of Selected Criteria for Regulating Public, Occupational, and Environmental Exposure

Criteria	Implication	Remarks
Zero risk	Absolute control, through ban (substances demonstrated to be carcinogenic are banned). Substances must be generally shown to be safe [*Certified Color Mftrs.* v. *Mathews*, 543 F2d 284 (CA DC 1976)].	Delaney Clause to the Federal Food, Drug, and Cosmetic Act (approval of food related additives) (FDA), 21 USC Sec. 348(c)(3)(A); also see 21 USC Sec. 376(b)(5)(B) and 21 USC Sec. 3606(d)(1)(H).
To the extent feasible	"Capable of being done." Cost–benefit analysis is inappropriate; emphasis on human life and workers' health protection against toxic or harmful agents. Economic feasibility is the standard.	(OSHA) Section 6(b)(5), 21 USC Sec. 655(b)(5) and *American Textile Manufacturers Association* v. *Donovan*, 101 SCt 2478 (1981).
De minimis	Level of risk that can be ignored. From the Common Law maxim, *de minimis non curat lex*: the law does not concern itself with trifles.	In *EDF* v. *EP. 4*, 636 F2d 1267 (CA DC 1980), a case involving the Clean Air Act and TSCA, the court held that the agency can "overlook circumstances that in context may... be *de minimis*," but "it must find the concentration at which there are only trivial benefits to be derived from regulation." [Also see *Monsanto* v. *Kennedy*, 613 F2d 947 (CA DC 1979).]
Natural standard	Risks from naturally occurring events serve as a benchmark for created events.	Pervades the law and human behavior.
Unreasonable risks	Considers costs and benefits of proposed action to reduce risk. Balancing of costs and benefits may include cost of burden imposed by regulation, probability of harm, and severity of harm.	(TSCA)5(f), 15 USC Sec. 2604(f).
Significant risk	No explicit consideration of costs or benefits but technology forcing. Significance is determined case-by-case; the agency must find such significance before proceeding further, *Ind.*—*Union Dept. AFL-CIO* v. *Am. Petroleum Institute*, 449 US 609, 642 (1980).	Highest degree of safety is called for (OSHA) Sec. (6)(b)(5), 29 USC 655(b)(5).

1028

TABLE 1 (*Continued*)

Criteria	Implication	Remarks
Adequate margin of safety	Air pollutants (e.g., SO_2, CO, TSP, HC). Protects health of the less resistant segments of population. No consideration of costs or benefits are required to justify environmental standard, but some (e.g., 0.005% of population at risk from airborne lead) can be at risk after imposing standard.	Clean Air Act for Primary and Secondary National Ambient Air Quality Standards. (CAA Sections 108, 109, 42 USC §§7408, 7409). Also see *Lead Industrial Association Inc.* v. *EPA.* 647 F2d 1130 (CA DC), *cert. denied* 449 US 1042 (1980).
Reasonably necessary or appropriate	Cost and benefit balancing with substantive evidence requirement (relevant to safety issues rather than carcinogens) against "risk of material health impairment." Particularly applicable to standards that do not involve toxic agents.	See (TSCA) Sec. 4(f), 15 USC 2603(f) and §(5)(f), 15 USC 2604(f).
Ample margin of safety	Air pollutants not covered under CAA Sections 108, 109 (e.g., Be, Hg, asbestos). Emphasis on serious or incapacitating illness or mortality. No explicit consideration of costs or benefits to justify ambient air quality standards. Practical application include best available technology (BAT) and some form of risk–benefit or cost–benefit trade-off.	Includes consideration of risk remaining after BAT control of pollutant. Clean Air Act, Sec. 112 for hazardous pollutants.
As low as reasonably achievable (ALARA)	Individual and societal risks: the former on a low annual probability; the latter at the expected value. The consequences may be raised to either 1.0 or other exponent > 1.0, depending on nature of consequence (e.g., cancers of delayed deaths).	Societal risk set at a limit; ALARA cost-effectiveness to further reduce societal risk.

economically rational decision analysis. But such balancing is at odds with the spirit of rights-based or legal duty-based acceptability criteria (16). For example, if the FDA's duty is seen as being protection of consumers against preventable man-made risks, regardless of the cost–risk–benefit consequences, then it makes sense for the agency to insist on demonstrations of safety and effectiveness, even when doing so means that some useful products will never be brought to market (4). Other regulatory bodies face similar issues in deciding what shall be the basis of their regulatory policies, as reflected in their evidentiary requirements for acceptance or permission of uncertain risks. Table 1 gives several examples of different legislative intents, agency criteria, and court interpretations for the bases of risk regulation (36).

3.3 Alternatives to Proof

When the relation between a suspected cause and an adverse effect is only scientific hypothesis, as is typically the case for diseases characterized by long latency periods, low exposures, and multiple competing or contributing causal factors, meeting the burden of proof can be difficult or impossible. An agency often attempts to adopt "conservative" approaches to solve the resulting complex issues. A well-known example among risk assessors is the use of a linear dose–response extrapolation in evaluating bioassay data. Such approaches deliberately seek to yield conservative, or unrealistically high, projected incidence rates of adverse effects. If an agency's mandate is to ensure that no unacceptably high risk slips by, then such as approach is merely prudent. If the agency is intended to balance risks, information costs, and benefits in deciding whether to permit an uncertain risk, however, then deliberately distorting the risk component is undesirable: it cannot contribute to a more rational balancing of conflicting goals. Conservative approaches can be challenged and overturned by the reviewing courts, who may clarify the intended basis for regulation in the process (see Table 1).

The fact that legal theory (and underlying theories of justice) provides only guidance, rather than determining unique solutions, to problems of risk acceptability is reflected in the ambiguity of statutory language dealing with the management of uncertain risks. For example, one legislative mandate to the Administrator of the United States Environmental Protection Agency (EPA) is to issue standards to protect the public against severe health effects when an agent is found to "significantly contribute to an increase in mortality" [Clean Air Act, as amended, 112(a) (1)]. Yet, although the same agency is involved, the Toxic Substances Control Act (TSCA) [15 U.S. Code, Sec. 2605(a)] calls for more of a balancing approach, guarding "adequately" against "unreasonable risk of injury" with the "least burdensome requirements." Similar language can be found in FIFRA [7 U.S. Code, Sec. 136(bb).] But the practical meanings and operational definitions of these vague terms are often left for the courts to decide.

3.4 What is Significant Risk

The issue most frequently relegated to the courts is: What is "significant" risk of harm or "adequate" protection against it? This is just the question of acceptability for uncertain risks in thin disguise. If an agency promulgates a standard, and if the standard leads to litigation, then the reviewing courts must determine or define the intent of Congress as expressed in the enabling legislation behind the regulation. For example, the U.S. Supreme Court, in a decision involving the Occupational Safety and Health Administration's (OSHA's) rule-making for exposure to benzene in the workplace, held that "OSHA must develop better evidence of carcinogenesis for benzene" before applying regulatory restrictions based on suspected but unproven risks [*Industrial Union Department, AFL-CIO* v. *American Petroleum Institute*, 100 S. Ct. 2844, 66L. Ed. 2nd 268 (1980)]. This is an example of the "innocent until proved guilty" approach to regulation of uncertain risks. The Court further held that assumptions about carcinogens should be supported by "reputable scientific thought" rather than ad hoc conservative guesses. In the same finding, however, the Court noted that the concept of significant risk is not a "mathematical straightjacket," and that "OSHA ... is not required to support findings of significant risk with anything approaching scientific certainty." Such careful hedging of language and interpretation allows room for different approaches, based on alternative consequential, deontological, or pragmatic theories, to the social management of uncertain risks. It can be interpreted as a sign that the underlying risk acceptability problems cannot be resolved clearly and decisively by legal reasoning alone.

Even when a standard of proof or evidence has been established at the level of guiding verbal criteria, as in Table 1, the practical problem of deciding whether a particular data set meets the standard must be solved. How legally convincing is a given scientific data set, and what quantitative data indicate "significant" risks? The courts have come to recognize that there are two complementary issues to be decided in establishing significance. First is the *statistical significance* of the evidence suggesting that a health risk exists. For example, a given study may support the hypothesis that exposure to substance X causes carcinomas in laboratory mice at the 15% statistical significance level (85% confidence level), but not at the 5% significance level (95% confidence level) due to sample size limitations. More generally, the *strength of the evidence* supporting a hypothesis that a health risk is posed by a substance or activity must be assessed, whether by statistical methods or more general evaluation of causal reasoning.

Second, if an effect exists, there is the question of whether it is "significant" in the sense of being *large enough to require remedial control action*. As an example, the Food and Drug Administration (FDA) has adopted a threshold of 10^{-6} individual lifetime cancer risk as an administrative standard of "insignificant risk" for application to products such as color additives in hair dyes. Any risk smaller than this is considered "insignificant" in the pragmatic sense of not requiring action by the agency. However, the burden of showing that an additive poses "insignificant" risks (by this definition) is placed on the manufacturer.

In general, numerical thresholds for triggering agency action have been phrased in terms of absolute risk levels and have not allowed for uncertainty about risks as part of the statement of the threshold (36). For example, the FDA could have adopted a definition of insignificance for uncertain risks that might have had the form "probability of at least 90% that the individual lifetime cancer risk is no greater than 10^{-6}." More generally, a criterion of the form "no more than x% chance of risk greater than y," where there is a range of allowable trade-offs between x and y, could be used to define a concept of "significance" that addresses both the statistical issue of uncertainty in data (statistical significance) and the management issue of desirable thresholds for intervention.

In the court system, these two aspects of significance have been addressed somewhat separately through discussions of what constitutes "substantial evidence" and what constitutes "significant risk." For example, the 5th Circuit Court of Appeals in 1983 addressed the problem of what constitutes "substantial evidence" of adverse health effects in its review of the evidence presented by the Consumer Product Safety Commission (CPSC) on the cancer risks from formaldehyde gas produced by urea-formaldehyde foam insulation [*Gulf South Insulation* v. *Consumer Product Safety Commission*, F01 F.2d 1137

(5th Cir., 1983)]. The CPSC had proposed to ban the product, based on evidence from an animal study that suggested that the human risk of nasal carcinomas from exposure could be "up to" 51 carcinomas per million persons exposed, depending on the extrapolation method used. (The presumed duration of exposure is not made explicit here.) This estimate was based on a single animal study of approximately 240 laboratory rats.

The court concluded that, given the many uncertainties in this type of risk assessment (see Chapter 2), "the Commission's cancer prediction of up to 51 in a million provides... no basis for review under the substantial evidence standard." The statistical evidence could not rule out with sufficiently high confidence the *possibility* that there was in fact no adverse effect from exposure, even through it made plausible the alternative hypothesis that an effect was there. The situation was somewhat similar to tossing a coin ten times and getting eight heads: the observed evidence does not then conclusively *prove* that the coin is biased in favor of heads, although it certainly makes that conjecture plausible. Biological evidence in risk assessment is similarly apt to be suggestive rather than conclusive, and the courts must then decide what constitutes sufficiently good evidence to justify action.

The idea of significant evidence of significant effects as the criterion for significant risk, as in the "$x\%$ probability of a risk greater than y" formula, has been presented by the courts on some occasions. For example, in the 1980 *Industrial Union* case cited above, the Supreme Court held that "the burden was on the agency to show that on the basis of substantial evidence, it is at least more likely than not that long-term exposure to 10 ppm of benzene presents a significant risk of material health impairment." This explicit linking of the substantial evidence and significant risk concepts in determining whether regulatory intervention is justified reflects an awareness that regulatory risk management deals with highly uncertain risks, and that guiding language must be formulated to address uncertainty as well as risk magnitude.

A final example illustrating the role of the legal system in establishing the legitimacy of regulatory decisions concerns a 10th Circuit Court of Appeals decision on the meaning of "significant risk" (which the U.S. Supreme Court, in the benzene cancer risk decision, had held is to be established on a case-by-case basis). In the case of *Kerr-McGee Nuclear Corp.* v. *NRC* [673 F. 2d 1124 (10th Cir. 1982)], the court's opinion noted that the Nuclear Regulatory Commission (NRC), in its Final Generic Environmental Impact Statement, had estimated that, among other adverse effects, the release of radon from uncontrolled uranium mill tailings "would cause 5.4 additional cancer deaths in the United States between 1979 and 2000." (Note that the uncertainty about this number, although essential to any full and correct presentation of risk estimates, is not included in this statement.) This estimated risk was deemed minimal: it corresponded to only 1 cancer death in 50 million, as compared to a rate from natural background radiation of perhaps 50 in 1 million, for the population of the United States. However, for the residents and workers nearby uncontrolled tailings, the risk of premature death from cancer was estimated to be approximately 1 per 2600 person-lifetimes of exposure. This measure, though crude (e.g., leaving unestimated the person-years of life that would be lost), was considered by the court to be a "satisfactory basis" for establishing that uncontrolled uranium mill tailings pose an unacceptable public health risk.

The court asserted that bounding the population risk "somewhere between 1 in 2000 and 1 in 50 million" constituted a reasonable and appropriate exercise of the NRC's powers, and that "erring on the side of caution" is appropriate when there is scientific uncertainty. Over the past few years, such statements have been subjected to increasingly critical scrutiny by legal scholars as the enormous social costs of using conservative risk estimates to ban products or to assess liability have become more apparent (7, 37).

4 UNCERTAINTY

Chapter 2 surveyed some of the principal sources of uncertainty in health risk assessment. Factors such as unknown causal mechanisms, uncertain exposures, omitted or unobservable explanatory variables, sampling variability, population heterogeneity, model uncertainty (e.g., for statistical dose–response models), and conceptual ambiguities (e.g., over the concept of causation in the presence of interacting factors) were identified as major contributors to the very wide variability in scientific results aimed at estimating the health effects of suspected hazards.

Highly uncertain risk estimates abound in nearly all fields of applied risk analysis, from assessments of carcinogenic risks for chemicals to accident rates in transportation and other industries to public health effects of power plant emissions (38). Risk assessment and risk management cannot be cleanly separated for such uncertain risks. For example, the decision of when to stop collecting information and act is a risk *management* problem, while expressing the residual uncertainty about risk at the time that the transition from research to action is made is part of the risk *assessment* process. Balancing the estimated but uncertain health costs of delayed action against the costs of inappropriate action based on inadequate information involves both risk assessment and risk management. Management decisions limit the accuracy of risk assessments by deciding when "enough" evidence is available to move forward.

In very simple situations, the trade-offs involved can be formulated explicitly and analyzed mathematically using techniques such as the sequential probability ratio test of statistical decision theory (39). In most practical applications, however, the balance between possible costs of waiting, costs of research, and costs of erroneous decisions can not be made on any formal basis, but must rely on the heuristic wisdom and willingness to gamble of the decisionmaker(s).

The existence of high variability in actual consequences even when risks, or underlying probabilities, are fixed and known has sometimes prompted the use of acceptability criteria for the plausible upper bounds of consequences. (These plausible upper bounds are sometimes given names such as the upper 99% confidence limit, although they actually refer to a quantile of an assumed probability distribution for consequences, rather that to statistical confidence limits of estimates in the conventional statistical sense.) For example, instead of defining an acceptable risk for some activity, such as operation of a power plant for a year, as fewer than 1 expected early fatality per 1 million people exposed, one could require that the *probability* of more than 1 early fatality must be smaller than 1 in 1 million. More generally, boundaries of acceptability for known risks can be defined in terms of *limit lines* specifying the maximum acceptable consequence at each probability level.

From a decision-analytic point of view, however, it does not make sense to define a maximum acceptable probability for a given level of consequence—or, equivalently, a maximum acceptable consequence for a given level of probability—in isolation. It is the whole probability distribution over all consequence levels simultaneously that counts in determining the acceptability of a risky prospect. Trading off higher probabilities of bad consequences against lower probabilities of worse ones, or against higher probabilities of better ones, will produce an infinite variety of equally valid (mutually indifferent) limit lines. Thus, unique limit lines that in any sense represent a "maximum acceptable distribution" cannot be defined. Moreover, which trade-offs are acceptable, in the sense of leading to equally preferred overall probability distributions for consequences, depends on the assessor's subjective attitudes regarding aversion to factors such as risk, anxiety, disappointment, and regret.

Example 4. Impact of Regret-Aversion on Risk Management Decisions. Suppose that a public decisionmaker must decide whether to approve release of a vaccine that has demonstrable benefits but that also, according to some scientific speculation, might create some risk of a certain kind of disease among those exposed to it. Assume that the risk is currently unquantifiable; its very existence is uncertain. How might the decisionmaker's current choice be affected by her beliefs about what information will become available in the future? What factors might she take into account in reaching a present decision?

Solution. The decisionmaker might be willing to risk releasing the vaccine, in the absence of substantial evidence that it creates a health risk, if she feels certain that, whether or not the postulated risk exists, its health effects will forever be undetectable. Given the inevitable noise in epidemiological data, inability to detect even substantial increases in the risk of a common health effect is not unlikely. On the other hand, the same decisionmaker, given the same current scientific information about the likelihood of risks from the vaccine, might be unwilling to risk releasing it if the postulated health effect were a "signature disease" that could easily and unambiguously be traced to the vaccine. One explanation for this change in choice, given differences in anticipated information about effects, is avoidance of *decision regret* and self-recrimination (41). Similarly, an individual may be more willing to accept the risk of cigarette smoking if he knows that any future cancers cannot be proved to have resulted from smoking, as opposed to, say, medical radiation.

Although the terms regret, anxiety, and disappointment name emotions, the phenomena they describe refer not to purely psychological or perceptual aspects of risk but to objective properties of the risks themselves. The potential for regret depends on the extent to which different decisions can lead to differently valued consequences (42). The potential for disappointment depends on how far actual observable consequences can stray from their expected values (43). And the potential for anxiety is created by delayed resolution of uncertainty about possible adverse consequences, with the magnitude of the delay and the possible severity of the consequences both contributing to anxiety. All three are objective properties of the random process generating consequences and information about consequences.

How individuals respond to such factors in evaluating risks, however, is a matter of individual psychology. Different rational individuals can disagree about the relative desirabilities of risky prospects, even though they share identical preferences for deterministic consequences and identical beliefs about the probable consequences of each prospect. The problem therefore arises of deciding what attitudes to take in making social judgments of risk acceptability on behalf of groups of individuals whose personal attitudes toward them differ. For example, should society ever be more (or less) risk averse than any of its members? Such questions require theories of *preference aggregation*, explaining how social preferences should depend on the preferences of the members of society.

Preference aggregation theories in the literature on applied welfare economics (25), political economy and public finance, and collective choice developed over the past 30 years have led to the following important conclusions:

1. In general, there is no satisfactory way of aggregating *ordinal* individual preferences for *acts* to achieve an aggregate social preference ordering for acts (25, 44).

2. Individual preferences for *consequences* can, under fairly mild conditions, be aggregated by (possibly weighted) summation of individual utility functions to give a utilitarian social utility function (45–47).

3. Individual preferences for *acts* cannot, in general, be combined into a coherent social utility function for acts. Instead, the "acceptability" of a risk to a group will depend on the opportunities for ex ante *risk sharing*, for example, through insurance (20).

4. If individual risks can be traded ex ante, as in the case of financial risks trading on a stock market, then differences in individual risk attitudes (or beliefs) can lead to risk spreading and trading through transactions from which all participants expect to gain. In other words, the *process* of risk management through market mechanisms can make risks "acceptable" that would not be if their initial distribution could not be changed through market transactions (20, 48).

Of course, individual health and safety risks cannot be traded like shares on a stock market. Also, insurance markets for irreversible, nontransferrable harms behave differently from insurance markets for purely financial risks. While individuals will, according to traditional economic analysis, fully insure themselves in financial markets, so that they are indifferent between occurrence and nonoccurrence of the insured damage, they may not fully insure in situations involving irreversible losses, even if full monetary compensation is possible (48). Health and life insurance markets often offer only certain amounts of insurance at certain prices, so that individuals cannot fully express their preferences by selecting from an infinitely rich menu of alternatives. Nonetheless, the economic analysis of market risks suggests that mechanisms such as private and social insurance and compensation schemes that allow individuals to redistribute their risks to take advantage of differences in their preferences and attitudes can make risk–benefit combinations collectively "acceptable" that would not be in the absence of such transfers.

In summary, subjective attitudes toward uncertainty and toward the experience of living under uncertainty can importantly affect individual evaluations of risky prospects, and hence individual judgments of the "acceptability" of a risk–benefit combination. Known risks produce uncertain consequences and may be ranked differently by individuals with different degrees of risk aversion for consequences. Uncertain risks may become more accurately revealed as time passes and may be ranked differently ex ante by individuals with different degrees of aversion for disappointment, regret, and anxiety. When different individuals have different risk attitudes, processes that allow them to exploit these differences through ex ante mutually desired exchange agreements can make a risk mutually acceptable that would be unacceptable in the absence of such agreements. It is not necessary for society to pass judgment on the validity of different subjective risk attitudes or to select a single attitude for use in social decisions, when risk management through voluntary insurance and compensation transactions can solve the acceptability problem.

5 RISK PERCEPTIONS

How risks are perceived by the public depends on a variety of psychological and perceptual factors that are not usually included in risk analysis reports, and that may easily be overlooked by public decisionmakers charged with the responsibility of making centralized decisions about risk acceptability. Whether such perceptual issues *should* be overlooked in favor of a strictly "rational" appraisal of risks, costs, and benefits is discussed further below. However, it is important for public decisionmakers to understandard the factors affecting public perceptions of risk, if only to make them more effective in communicating their understanding of risk problems and the rationales for their decisions.

5.1 Empirical Evidence on Risk Perception

Behavioral psychology has in this decade made a number of startling contributions to our understanding of how people think about risky prospects—what concerns and affects them in making choices. Three especially relevant sets of findings are as follows:

1. Given a choice between two monetary lotteries with different probability distributions over gains and losses, people do not necessarily *choose* the one that they describe as being the more *valuable* (59).

2. Individuals often appraise risky prospects not in terms of probability distributions over *final consequences* (e.g., asset position at the end of the experiment), as required by traditional normative models of rational choice behavior, but in terms of probable *gains and losses* relative to some psychologically determined reference point or aspiration level (49). Moreover, how this reference point is set may depend on how the risky prospect is described (50). For example, describing consequences in terms of number of lives saved instead of in terms of number of fatalities can reverse majority preferences for alternative risk control options. The choice between a small, certain loss and a potentially larger, uncertain loss will shift in favor of the former if it is called an "insurance premium" instead of a "small certain loss."

3. Perceptions of technological risks are affected at least as much by two groups of perceptual factors, sometimes referred to in the aggregate as the "dread" and "unknown risk" factors, as they are by objective frequencies and magnitudes. Subjective rankings of hazards in terms of likelihood of being killed by them show that people tend to underestimate the contributions of common diseases and to overestimate the contributions of striking or unusual hazards, such as accidents and homicides, to overall mortality rates. In general, the perceived "riskiness' of a technological hazard is in increasing function of the "dread" and "unknown risk" factors (51).

The important contributors to these risk perception factors include aspects of voluntariness, magnitude, and equity (for the dread factor) and uncertainty (for the unknown risk factor). The more a hazard is seen as being uncontrollable, unavoidable, involuntary, or inequitable, the higher is its dread score. Similarly, the more it is perceived as creating risks that are new, unknown to science or to those exposed, unobservable, and with long-delayed (i.e., hidden) consequences, the more risky it is likely to appear, through the contribution of the unknown risk factor. Of course, different people weigh these factors differently in coming up with their overall perceptions of the riskiness of a hazard. But the set of factors that are important in determining relative perceptions of risk go well beyond the statistical frequency, magnitude, and uncertainty of effects.

5.2 Treatment of Perceptions and Preferences in Policymaking

Individual perceptions and preferences regarding risks can be changeable, overly sensitive to erroneous impressions, and unreliable. This raises crucial questions for public policymakers: when public perceptions and statistical realities conflict, is it the public decisionmaker's duty to *represent* the views and preferences of members of society, or to *protect* what he considers to be their true best interests? How can she draw the line between responsibility and paternalism when she perceives public preferences as being based on inaccurate perceptions? And how can decisionmakers overcome flaws and inconsistencies in their own perceptions and decision processes?

Institutional practices have evolved in part to answer these questions. Court hearings and regulatory proceedings often provide members of the public with the opportunities to state their views or to challenge current policies and presuppositions. At the same time, the courts have the authority to permit (i.e., accept on behalf of society) risky activities if, after hearing the arguments and perceptions of opposing groups or individuals, they still feel that the risks created are acceptable. Legislative and regulatory decisions result from involved processes in which conflicting preferences and perceptions can be debated, refined in light of new scientific evidence or arguments, and eventually resolved, pending review by the courts.

The question of what preferences (e.g., preferences based on what information, expertise, or perceptions) should be granted status in formal decision procedures is continually being answered. While it seems clear that individual preferences based on beliefs commonly regarded as false should not guide public decisions, it is less clear how preferences based on extreme, possibly morbid, individual risk aversion or sensitivity to "dread" factors should be treated. Ultimately, the social acceptance of a risky activity over the objections of its opponents is defined by the acceptability of the social decision process on which acceptance of the activity is based. The acceptability, or legitimacy, of this process to individuals may in turn depend on how fully and fairly it considers and responds to their perceptions before reaching a decision.

This concludes our review of the major factors contributing to judgments of risk acceptability. Although we have emphasized the five issues of voluntariness, equity, procedural legitimacy, uncertainty, and risk perceptions, it should be clear that these are not five distinct areas but rather are overlapping perspectives for viewing the components of risk acceptability.

6   TOWARD ACCEPTABILITY CRITERIA FOR CHRONIC HEALTH RISKS

There is great demand among regulatory agencies and those who care about public policy for clear, numerical standards for judging the acceptability of risks. Numerical thresholds are greatly to be desired. They could reduce ambiguity and debate at the regulatory level, clarify the responsibilities of economic agents, and provide useful points of departure for court deliberations if necessary. However, defensible numerical criteria are hard to come by. Protection of individual rights, legitimacy of process, equity of risk–benefit distribution, appropriate prudence in the absence of knowledge, and other key elements of social risk acceptability judgments do not lend themselves well to numerical representations.

Inevitably, numerical criteria have been and will continue to be proposed. It is far easier to compare numbers than to evaluate social decision processes. In the remainder of this chapter, we therefore review recent proposals for numerical standards of acceptable risk and comment on possible foundations and magnitudes for acceptable risk thresholds. In addition, we summarize some constructive suggestions and criteria for making acceptable risk judgments even in the absence of numerical decision rules.

6.1   Cost–Risk–Benefit Analysis for Known Risks

The simplest case for acceptability decisions occurs when the chronic health risks of an activity are known. When the set of risks produced by a technological or economic activity is known, their "acceptability," from the standpoint of purely economic rationality, depends only on what it would cost to reduce or control them. Any chronic health risk that can be eliminated without cost is unacceptable.

A very common practice is to evaluate risk control measures in terms of *dollars spent per statistical life saved*. This leads naturally to the following economic logic for evaluating acceptable risks:

Step 1. Evaluate the dollar value per statistical life saved that those at risk (e.g., workers in a hazardous occupation) place on their own lives. This can be attempted through either *expressed preference* (survey) or *revealed preference* (personal expenditures on insurance and risk-reducing measures) approaches. A plausible value for the 1980s might be $500,000 per statistical life saved.

Step 2. Evaluate the dollar costs of alternative control options, including the option of banning the activity if that is a possibility. Include the dollar value of benefits foregone (i.e., opportunity costs) along with the direct costs of control in calculating the total economic cost to society of each option.

Step 3. Implement those control options whose benefits (expected lives saved times imputed dollar value per statistical life saved, from step 1) exceed their costs.

Step 4. A risk is said to be *acceptable*, within this paradigm, if the costs of further controlling it exceed the benefits from further control, for each remaining (unimplemented) control option. The numerical criterion for risk acceptability will take the form "accept risk X if and only if the cost-per-statistical life saved of controlling it by the most cost-effective method exceeds $500,000 (or some other appropriate cutoff level.)" Debate then centers on choice of the appropriate cutoff level.

This economic cost–risk–benefit analysis approach has a superficial appearance of objectivity and rationality that many policy analysts find attractive. Many excellent economists consider some version of it useful and valid as a guide for determining acceptability of risks, and considerable econometric experience and debate have been brought to bear on the problems of estimating life values in step 1 and net economic costs of control in step 2 (52). Current legal, economic, public policy, and risk analysis journals contain many examples of applications of this approach.

However, there are also powerful arguments against the assumptions and conceptual framework of cost–risk–benefit analysis and against the validity of its conclusions as guides to policy. One line of attack holds that the approach ignores protection of rights, adjustments for equity, legitimacy of process, and other important factors beyond its narrow scope. Other criticisms rest on the same economic grounds as cost–risk–benefit analysis itself. Perhaps the most important of these is that *dollars are not spent to save statistical lives but to purchase reductions in risk*.

Consider the difference between (i) a risk control measure that reduces annual fatality probabilities in population A from 0.9 to 0.8 and (ii) a measure that reduces annual fatality probabilities in population B from 0.2 to 0.1. If populations A and B are the same size (and recruit new members to fill gaps left by fatalities, so that they remain the same size), then both measures save the same expected numbers of lives per year. But risk-averse individuals may be expected to be willing to pay more for a 0.1 reduction in risk starting from a high base level of risk than starting from a lower base level (53). This may help explain the often cited "anomaly" whereby society seems willing to spend vastly more to save identifiable victims (trapped miners, children needing transplants) who will surely die without help than to save, with equal certainty on a statistical basis, the anonymous victims of transportation accidents or hazardous products or practices. Ex post savings in lives do not adequately reflect ex ante reductions in risks unless adjustments for background risk levels are made.

Even if all risks are small enough so that adjustments for differences in background levels can be ignored, the difference between purchasing reductions in risk and purchasing statistical lives remains important. As mentioned previously, analysis of individual insurance purchasing decisions shows that risk-averse individuals may *not* fully insure themselves where irreversible losses are involved. Imputing individuals' economic valuations of their own lives from their revealed safety-purchasing or insurance-purchasing behavior can therefore produce misleading conclusions. It is quite conceivable that individuals may place *infinite* dollar value on their own lives (in the sense that their fatality risk versus dollar compensation indifference curve goes to infinity on the dollar axis as it approaches some finite asymptotic value, corresponding to "maximum compensable risk," on the risk axis) and yet still be willing to spend only moderate amounts to reduce, or to insure themselves against, small fatality risks (54).

A third class of objections to the cost risk–benefit analysis paradigm for defining acceptable risks is that *the willingness of individuals to pay for reductions in risk depends on their income levels, their expectations, and the hypothesized method of financing.* It is not clear that society should use the same life values for individuals in a group as they appear to use for themselves. For example, low-income workers in a hazardous occupation (e.g., coal miners) who are accustomed to (and who may even have come to accept as unavoidable) early disease-related deaths may express lower willingness-to-pay values for improvements in safety than workers of better health and higher economic status in other occupations. But this does not mean that they do, or that society should, value their lives any less highly.

The amount that a group is collectively willing to pay for a reduction in health and safety risks may reflect the proposed financing scheme (or the members' implicit assumptions about financing if no explicit financing scheme is proposed). Consider inviting N individuals to submit "bids" for the maximum amounts they would be willing to pay for a risk control measure, with the understanding that it will be undertaken if and only if the sum of all bids exceeds its cost. This procedure may elicit one result (combined willingness to pay) if each individual is required to pay the amount of his bid if the project is undertaken, and a very different result if each individual is required to pay only $1/N$th of the total cost (18, 25).

Despite these criticisms, the cost–risk–benefit analysis approach contains valuable elements. Balancing the costs against the benefits of risk control measures is clearly necessary for any efficient allocation of resources. Ignoring such balancing, for example, in favor of strict rights-based or other categorical criteria, implies accepting more or higher risks than are theoretically necessary, because scarce resources will not be allocated where they are expected to do the most good. In addition, the approach correctly points out that *unavoidable risks* (e.g., those from cosmic rays, which cannot be controlled at any reasonable cost) or *necessary benefits* from an activity (e.g., those from eating) can make risks pragmatically acceptable regardless of their magnitudes. However, to implement fully the cost–risk–benefit analysis approach, it is necessary to develop better measures of the benefits from risk reduction than the conventional one of expected number of statistical lives saved.

6.2 Acceptability of Uncertain Risks: The de Minimis Approach

The cost–risk–benefit analysis approach to risk acceptability is intended to guide trade-offs between known control costs, including foregone benefits, and corresponding known risk reductions. When risks are uncertain, a different set of issues must be confronted, centering on the three-way trade-off among costs of risk research, costs of risk control (including foregone economic benefits), and the uncertain benefits of possible risk reductions resulting from control. These issues are usually too difficult to treat rigorously. It is not always clear which cost–risk–uncertainty combinations are most desirable or what qualitative changes would improve the situation.

It may initially seem that lower control costs or better information (i.e., reduced uncertainty) about risks are always desirable. However, if risk management is decentralized, better information or reduced control costs may degrade the performance of the risk management process by making choices that were easy more difficult, or by making risk-sharing transactions impossible. For example, in a group of risk-averse individuals mutually insuring each other against a hazard (e.g., house fires or cancers), each individual would be willing to pay to *prevent* the discovery and disclosure of public information about who the victims will be (e.g., whose houses will burn or who is most likely to get cancer). Such information would undermine the basis for insurance, diminishing everyone's *ex ante* expected utility. This is one case in which everyone would prefer that better information about risks not be made available (48).

Similarly, when no individual knows his own risk, but only the population distribution of risks, it may be relatively easy to achieve agreement on social risk management policies. But revealing to individuals where they fall in the overall distribution can create unconquerable conflicts of interest.

Given the complexities involved in managing (i.e., researching and controlling) uncertain risks, no simple numerical criteria for acceptability appear likely to be able to express a fully "rational" risk management policy. Recognizing this, risk analysts have sought the next best thing: simple numerical screening criteria capable of identifying at least *some* uncertain risks as acceptable, while allowing less clear cases to be passed on for more elaborate consideration and decisionmaking. An important example of this screening approach that has received considerable attention in recent years is the development of proposed de minimis standards for risk regulation, as discussed in Chapter 33.

De minimis standards are an example of an *action threshold* approach to risk management: below the de minimis risk threshold, regulatory action is not triggered (either because the threat is considered trivial or for some other reason). Regulatory action thresholds are usually proposed not directly for risks, which may be unobservable, but for the more easily measurable dose, exposure, or concentration variables that give rise to risks. For example, if the effect of power plant emissions is to shift the cumulative survival probability distributions of exposed individuals leftward, it might be very hard to conceive of or to articulate what possible sets of shifts might be "acceptable" in exchange for the production of power. It is much easier to state and enforce limits on ambient concentrations or directly on emission rates.

Several possible bases for exposure thresholds below which no action will be taken have been suggested in the literature. Well-known ones, and some criticisms of them, include the following (4):

1. *Biological thresholds.* A number of diseases, *not* including most cancers, can be assumed to have minimal dose or exposure thresholds that are required to trigger them. Doses or exposures below these levels have no harmful effects and may therefore be excluded from regulatory intervention.

2. *Comparison to existing background levels.* An ad hoc basis for setting de minimis thresholds that has been proposed with surprising frequency is to limit newly created exposures to a few percent of the natural or background level. This reflects a presumption that what is is acceptable and has no explicit justification in terms of costs and benefits of possible controls.

3. *No observable empirical effect.* Another proposal that seems difficult to justify is that exposures should be limited to levels at which no noticeable effects are observed. This might be characterized uncharitably as a "what you don't see can't hurt you" approach: given the enormous uncertainties in risk assessment and the typical impossibility of making precise and confident risk estimates by epidemiological, experimental, or model-based means, especially for effects with long latency periods or affecting sensitive subpopulations, it is possible that even catastrophic public health effects could be hidden by the "noise" in empirical data.

An alternative, economic approach to setting regulatory action thresholds is based on the view that the primary purpose of a de minimis threshold is to act as a screen for the cases that a regulatory agency must review, helping to focus agency resources where they are likely to be most useful. If it is assumed that (i) very small exposures tend to allow only very small benefits to be achieved from control; but that (ii) control costs tend to decline less rapidly than benefits for sufficiently small risks (e.g., because of fixed administrative cost components); and if it is further assumed that (iii) these statistical tendencies hold with enough regularity in the population of cases presented to an agency for resolution so that the costs of discovering exceptions outweigh the resulting benefits of more accurate control, then the use of a threshold screening policy can be reconciled with an economic cost–risk–benefit rationale for efficient allocation of agency resources. Chapter 33 considers regulatory action thresholds further in the specific context of proposed de minimis levels.

7   CONCLUSION: THE PORTFOLIO MANAGEMENT APPROACH TO RISK ACCEPTABILITY

Risks that are acceptable today may not be acceptable in the near future. New scientific information, improved ability to control risks, or changes in risk attitudes may make a formerly acceptable risk no longer acceptable. The idea that decisions of risk acceptability are dynamic and provisional and must be monitored and adapted over time suggests a similar approach to the definition of acceptable risk by regulatory agencies. In short, for a resource-limited regulatory agency, *the acceptability of a risky activity at any time depends on the current context of risky activities and control opportunities in which it is embedded.* This view provides a useful perspective for integrating the risk acceptability issues discussed in this chapter into a broader framework for organizing social risk management decisions.

An agency's approach to risk management can be thought of metaphorically in terms of its management of several lists of risky activities or prospects (55). On one list are *known problems* waiting for consideration and regulatory action. A second list consists of *suspected problems* in need of investigation, and possibly action. Finally, there are two (perhaps dismally short) lists: one of *solved problems* that have been investigated and for which regulatory solutions have been established and must now be monitored and enforced; and one for *nonproblems*, meaning suspected problems that have been investigated and found not to be problems after all (e.g., because the chemicals involved have been shown to produce zero health effects at ambient levels). Each list is sorted (perhaps heuristically) in rough order of the decreasing priority of the problems on it. As suspected problems are investigated, and uncertainties about their risks are resolved, they may move down in the priority list for suspected problems until further current investigation is unwarranted; or they may be moved down off the suspected problem list altogether and onto the nonproblem list; or they may move up until they are pushed off the suspected problem list and inserted into the known problem list, awaiting remedial action. Typically, one group of interested parties will follow a problem through the investigation, disposition, and resolution stages, and perhaps even participate in postresolution monitoring and enforcement. But the overall flow of risk management can usefully be viewed as one of allocating resources to processing the problems on different lists.

Each year, the agency must choose how to allocate its limited resources to process the pending problems on the first three lists. This creates certain trade-offs. Is it better to spend resources addressing another known problem or investigating another suspected one? At what point do the unknown risks from failing to explore items on the suspected problems list outweigh the losses from deferring action on known problems? And how should the pending problems within each list be ordered in terms of priority?

The concept of acceptable risk can help with these agenda-setting issues. The only permanently acceptable risks are those that get moved to the nonproblem list, assuming that there are no classification errors. However, within any given time horizon, there are known and suspected problems that are so far down on their corresponding priority lists that they will not be addressed until long after the many higher-priority problems that dominate them and that occupy current attention have been resolved. Such problems pose *provisionally acceptable* risks: risks that are acceptable until more important ones have been resolved. In practice, new problems for investigation and resolution are continually being created by industrial society as new products and technologies emerge. Each new problem or potential problem must be inserted into an appropriate priority position on the known problem or suspected problem list as it is identified. If the rate at which problems that supersede suspected problem X in priority are generated is greater than the rate at which they can be investigated, then problem X will remain provisionally acceptable. Whether risky activities that are currently classified as provisionally acceptable are permitted, pending processing, depends on whether risks are viewed as "guilty until proved innocent" or as "innocent until proved guilty."

This list-processing analogy for social risk management has applications beyond the choices and policies of regulatory agencies. For example, parts of the legislative and court systems can be described in similar terms. However, the ways in which problems are generated and inserted into the lists of outstanding cases to be considered are quite different and typically reflect the decentralized efforts of multiple (possibly opposed) agents rather than the largely centralized efforts of a few public decisionmakers. Rather than agency pull, in which problems are actively sought in order to protect the public, public push may bring risk management problems onto the court or legislative agenda.

The criteria by which priorities are set within outstanding problem lists may also be quite different, emphasizing protection of individual rights and definition and enforcement of risk management duties, rather than careful shepherding of agency resources. Since many of the costs of legal disputes are borne by the affected parties, a distributed set of risk–benefit comparisons is built into the selection of disputes for resolution by litigation (56).

Of course, the individual risks, costs, and potential benefits of a case may differ from the social ones, with concern over the financial risks of litigation being intermixed with concern over possible health risks. Moreover, the individual benefits of winning a case may be smaller than or different from the social benefits. Litigation that might be socially worthwhile as a tool of risk management may not be undertaken if individuals do not expect to gain from pursuing it, and conversely (37, 57). Thus, reactive social risk management by the legal system is very much a complement to, rather than a substitute for, proactive risk management by regulatory agencies.

Nonetheless, the same concepts of acceptable and provisionally acceptable risks levels—as reflecting the agenda-setting criteria for social risk management decision processes, rather than any intrinsic or absolute features of the risk situations—apply. The implication of this view is that acceptable risk thresholds are generally temporary, changing criteria that can only be understood and defended in terms of underlying social decision processes.

The list-processing, or problem portfolio, model is least applicable to highly decentralized risk management processes, such as individual insurance and consumption purchases. When individuals are able to customize their own risk portfolios to reflect personal risk attitudes and preferences, the idea of a generically applicable "acceptable" risk level is no longer useful. Different individuals may accept different risks.

The concept is more useful on the manufacturer's side, where the decentralized allocation by companies of corporate resources to risk research and control for products and work environments can be held to a common set of standards by law and regulation. Each company is held responsible for researching and controlling its own portfolio of risks in accord with socially acceptable standards. It is in this context that the idea of publicly stated levels of acceptable risk, for use by producers in their own risk management decisions, is most important. Without such clear ex ante guidance, manufacturers may be unwilling to produce socially beneficial but risky products (e.g., certain vaccines), for fear of legal liability should the courts decide in retrospect, after the risks have been revealed, that the initial production activity was "unacceptably" risky (37).

Standards or acceptability thresholds can be adopted for guiding decentralized private-sector resource allocation decisions as well as centralized regulatory ones. It is tempting to cite specific numerical bounds for different types of risk—for example, a maximum individual excess lifetime fatality or cancer probability of 10^{-4} for occupational risks from all occupational exposures (assuming full disclosure and informed consent by the worker); 10^{-6} for less controllable risks, such as treatment of public drinking water or discharge of air pollutants; and 10^{-3} for sale of products such as cigarettes to fully informed, willing consumers. However, such numbers are not truly adequate. Useful standards would have to specify allowable uncertainty as well as allowable risk and must recognize that most risks are not satisfactorily describable by single numbers but rather by survival time distributions, hazard functions, and the other tools introduced in Chapter 2.

In summary, the idea of acceptable risk thresholds seems easiest to justify as a device for constraining and guiding regulatory risk management efforts. It is less clearly applicable to the private decisions of economic agents (consumers or producers), where the availability of detailed case-specific information about costs, uncertainties, and benefits makes it reasonable to expect and require more careful and detailed approaches to risk management. Although the need for simple, concrete, easily operationalized standards of acceptable risks for guiding private sector health and safety risk management decisions cannot be denied, it seems unlikely that this need can be met without ignoring some important aspects of risk and uncertainty.

The acceptability of risks is not an easy question and in general may not have answers that are both easy to apply and fully defensible on rational or moral grounds. Exceptions may occur for some industries or classes of risk, however, where useful de minimis bounds, for example, can perhaps be established. The most realistic view of risk acceptability for the practitioner may be that it is a property of risk management decision processes, rather than of risky activities or situations. Proposed risk acceptability criteria must therefore be evaluated within the framework of the underlying risk management decision processes that they support. Acceptability of a technological risk is not only a matter of risk statistics and objective numbers, but of social processes and of trade-offs that society is willing to make to achieve the overall goal of decisions that are *on average* reasonably fair, efficient, workable, and acceptable.

REFERENCES

1. J. S. Mill, *On Liberty*, Watts Pub., London, UK (1903).

2. D. VanDeVeer, *Paternalistic Intervention: The Moral Bounds of Benevolence*. Princeton Univ. Press, Princeton, NJ, 1986, esp. Chaps. 2, 4, and 6.

3. C. Starr and C. Whipple, A perspective on health and safety risk analysis. *Manage. Sci.* **30**(4), 452–463 (1984).

4. W. W. Lowrance, *Of Acceptable Risk: Science and the Determination of Safety*. Morgan Kaufman, Los Altos, CA, 1976.

5. T. C. Schelling, *Choice and Consequences*. Harvard Univ. Press, Cambridge, MA, 1984.

6. P. Slovic, B. Fishhoff, and S. Lichtenstein, Facts and fears: Understanding perceived risk. In R. Schwing and W. A. Albers, Jr., Eds., *Societal Risk Assessment: How Safe is Safe Enough?* Plenum Press, New York, 1980.

7. R. A. Epstein, The legal and insurance dynamics of mass tort litigation. *J. Leg. Stud.* **13**, 3 (1984).

8. S. Matthews and A. Postlewaithe, Quality testing and disclosure. *Rand J. Econ.* **16**(3), 328–340 (1985).

9. C. Shapiro, Consumer information, product quality, and seller reputation. *Bell J. Econ.* **13**, 20–35 (1982).

10. S. Shavell, Risk sharing and incentives in the principal and agent relationship. *Bell J. Econ.* **10**, 55–73 (1979).

11. M. C. Olson, *Unacceptable Risk: The Nuclear Power Controversey*. Bantam Books, New York, 1976.

12. K. Chatterjee, Disagreement in bargaining: Models with incomplete information. In A. E. Roth, Ed., *Game-Theoretic Models of Bargaining*. Cambridge Univ. Press, London and New York, 1985.

13. R. E. Kasperson and J. X. Kasperson, *Determining the Acceptability of Risk: Ethical and Policy Issues*, Repr. No. 41. Center for Technology, Environment, and Development (CENTED), Clark University, Worcester, MA, 1984.

14. R. L. Keeney, Utility functions for equity and public risk. *Manage. Sci.* **26**(4), 345–353 (1980).

15. R. Nozick, *Anarchy, State, and Utopia.* Basic Books, New York, 1974.

16. C. Fried, *Right and Wrong.* Harvard Univ. Press, Cambridge, MA, 1978.

17. W. Samuelson, A comment on the Coase theorem. In A. E. Roth, Ed., *Game-Theoretic Models of Bargaining.* Cambridge Univ. Press, Cambridge, MA, 1985.

18. H. Raiffa, *The Art and Science of Negotiation.* Harvard Univ. Press, Cambridge, MA, 1982.

19. H. Raiffa, Environmental conflict resolution. In H. Raiffa, Ed., *The Art and Science of Negotiation,* Harvard Univ. Press, Cambridge, MA, 1982. Chap. 21 pp. 310–317.

20. H. Raiffa, *Decision Analysis.* Addison–Wesley, Reading, MA, 1968.

21. R. B. Myerson and M. A. Satterthwaite, Efficient mechanisms for bilateral trading. *J. Econ. Theory* **29**, 265–281 (1983).

22. B. Holmstrom and R. B. Myerson, Efficient and durable decision rules with incomplete information. *Econometrica* **51**(6), 1799–1819 (1983).

23. P. Milgrom and J. Roberts, Relying on the information of interested parties. *Rand J. Econ.* **17**(1), 18–32 (1986).

24. H. Kunreuther et al., A decision-process perspective on risk and policy analysis. *Manage. Sci.* **30**(4), 475–485 (1984).

25. J. R. Green and J. J. Laffont, *Incentives in Public Decision Making.* North-Holland, New York, 1979.

26. C. R. Plott, Rational choice in experimental markets. *J. Business* **59**(4, pt. 2), S301–S327 (1986).

27. E. Hoffman and M. L. Spitzer, Entitlements, rights, and fairness: Some experimental results. *J. Leg. Stud.* **14**, 259–298 (1985).

28. Arthur D. Little, Inc., *Analysis of Routine Occupational Risks Associated with Selected Electrical Energy Systems,* Rep. RP 1772-1. Electric Power Research Institute (EPRI), Palo Alto, CA, 1985.

29. H. W. Brock, The problem of utility weights in group preference aggregation. *Oper. Res.* **28**(1), 176–187 (1980).

30. R. L. Keeney, Equity and public risk. *Oper. Res.* **28**, 527–534 (1980).

31. R. L. Keeney and R. L. Winkler, Evaluating decision strategies for equity of public risks. *Oper. Res.* **33**(5), 955–970 (1985).

32. P. C. Fishburn, Equity axioms for public risks. *Oper. Res.* **32**(4), 901–908 (1984).

33. W. M. Landes and R. A. Posner, Causation in tort law: An economic approach. *J. Leg. Stud.* **12**(1), 109–134 (1983).

34. W. Y. Oi, Tort law as a regulatory regime: A comment on Landes and Posner. *J. Leg. Stud.* **13**(3), 435–440 (1984).

35. L. A. Bebchuck, Litigation and settlement under imperfect information. *Rand J. Econ.* **15**(3), 404–415 (1984).

36. P. F. Ricci and L. A. Cox, Jr., Acceptability of chronic health risks. *Toxics Law Rep.* **1**(35), 986–1001 (1987).

37. K. S. Abraham and R. A. Merrill, Scientific uncertainty in the courts. *Issues Sci. Technol.,* Winter, pp. 93–107 (1986).

38. L. A. Cox, Jr., Sources of artifactual uncertainty in risk analysis. *Risk Anal.* **2**(3), 121–135 (1982).

39. D. Bertsekas, *Dynamic Programming and Stochastic Control.* Academic Press, New York, 1976.

40. R. F. Griffiths (Ed.), *Dealing with Risk.* Manchester Univ. Press, Great Britain, 1981, esp. Chap. 4.

41. R. Sugden, Regret, recrimination, and rationality. In L. Daboni et al., Eds., *Recent Developments in the Foundations of Utility and Risk Theory.* Reidel, Boston, MA, 1984.

42. D. E. Bell, Risk premiums for decision regret. *Manag. Sci.* **29**(10), 1156–1166 (1983).

43. D. E. Bell, Disappointment in decision making under uncertainty. *Oper. Res.* **30**(5), 1–27 (1982).

44. K. J. Arrow, *Social Choice and Individual Values*, 2nd ed. Yale Univ. Press, New Haven, CT, 1963.

45. C. Kirkwood, Pareto optimal and equity in social decision analysis. *IEEE Trans. Syst., Man, Cybernet.* **SMC-9**(2), 89–91 (1979).

46. R. L. Keeney and C. Kirkwood, Group decision making using cardinal social welfare functions. *Manage. Sci.* **22**(4), 430–437 (1975).

47. J. C. Harsanyi, Cardinal welfare, individualistic ethics, and interpersonal comparisons of utility. *J. Political Econ.* (1952). Reprinted in E. S. Phelps (Ed.), *Economic Justice*. Penguin Books, Baltimore, MD, 1973.

48. J. Hirschleifer and J. G. Riley, The analytics of uncertainty and information—An expository survey. *J. Econ. Literature* **17**, 1375–1421 (1979).

49. D. Kahneman and A. Tversky, Prospect theory: An analysis of decision under risk. *Econometrica* **47**, 263–291 (1979).

50. A. Tversky and D. Kahneman, Rational choice and the framing of decisions. *J. Business* **59**(4, pt 2), S251–S278 (1986).

51. P. Slovic, Perception of risk. *Science* **236**, 236–285 (1987).

52. W. K. Viscusi, *Risk by Choice: Regulating Health and Safety in the Workplace*. Harvard Univ. Press, Cambridge, MA, 1983.

53. M. C. Weinstein et al., The economic value of changing mortality probabilities: A decision-theoretic approach. *Q. J. Econ.* pp. 373–396 (1980).

54. R. A. Howard, On fates comparable to death. *Manage. Sci.* **30**(4), 407–422 (1984).

55. J. Mumpower, An analysis of the *de minimis* strategy for risk management. *Risk Anal.* **6**(4), 437–446 (1986).

56. J. F. Reinganum and L. L. Wilde, Settlement, litigation, and the allocation of litigation costs. *Rand J. Econ.* **17**(4), 557–566 (1986).

57. S. Shavell, The social vs. the private incentive to bring suit in a costly legal system. *J. Leg. Stud.* **11**, 333–339 (1982).

58. M. E. Ames, *Outcome Uncertain: Science and the Political Process*. Communications Press, Washington, DC, 1978, esp. Chap. 3.

59. P. Slovic and S. Lichtenstein, Preference reversals: A broader perspective. *Am. Econ. Rev.* **73**, 596–605 (1983).

31

A Decision-Oriented Framework for Evaluating Environmental Risk Management Strategies: A Case Study of Lead in Gasoline

D. Krewski
Health Protection Branch, Health & Welfare Canada, Ottawa, Ontario, Canada

A. Oxman and G. W. Torrance
Department of Clinical Epidemiology and Biostatistics, McMaster University, Hamilton, Ontario, Canada

1 INTRODUCTION

The process of risk assessment and risk management has been the subject of intensive study in recent years (Royal Society Study Group, 1983; National Research Council, 1983; World Health Organization, 1985). These discussions have highlighted scientific approaches to the identification of environmental hazards, the means available for their control, and the optimal allocation of societal resources for the management of risk (Krewski, 1987). A systematic review of the main elements of risk assessment and risk management has recently been conducted by Krewski and Birkwood (1987).

The scientific enterprise of hazard identification relies largely on toxicological studies conducted in the laboratory and epidemiological studies of human populations (Krewski et al., 1982; Somers and Krewski, 1982). Statistical analysis of these data, coupled with information on levels of exposure, can then provide estimates of the associated level of risk (Munro and Krewski, 1981; Krewski et al., 1984, 1987).

Once a hazard has been identified, a variety of regulatory, economic, advisory, or technological risk management strategies may be invoked to protect human health and preserve environmental quality (Krewski and Birkwood, 1988). The selection of the most appropriate means of responding to a specific problem can be difficult, requiring evaluation of a wide range of factors (Somers, 1983, 1984). In addition to the scientific data on risk, extrascientific factors involving socioeconomic and political considerations can also be important. Because of the complexity of many decisions, a well-defined framework within which different risk management options may be evaluated can thus be of great value (Torrance and Krewski, 1987).

In this chapter, we present a decision-oriented framework that may be applied to provide a comprehensive assessment of environmental hazard control programs. The proposed model takes into account the health, environmental, social, and financial consequences of the option under consideration. This framework is not intended to provide a systematic approach leading to clear-cut decisions on environmental hazards, but rather as a mechanism for approaching environmental problems in a logical and comprehensive manner. Such an approach is of use in objectively evaluating all the available data and summarizing the results in a form that will assist decisionmakers in reaching the best possible solution to the problem at hand. Even when a decision cannot be reached, the analyses proposed here can be of value in identifying information gaps or important uncertainties that need to be addressed.

To illustrate how our framework may be applied, we review the analyses conducted in the United Kingdom, Canada, and the United States concerning the levels of lead to be permitted in gasoline (Southwood, 1983; McMullen et al., 1984; Schwartz et al., 1985). This is done not for the purpose of determining the most appropriate course of action to be followed on this issue, but rather to illustrate the use of our model in the evaluation of different risk management strategies. The health effects of lead are well documented [Environmental Protection Agency (EPA), 1986], with lead in gasoline representing a major source of exposure to lead. This case is of particular interest because the three analyses considered adopt different viewpoints and reach different conclusions. The reasons for this are identified by examining these evaluations within the context of our decision model.

2   A FRAMEWORK FOR EVALUATING RISK MANAGEMENT STRATEGIES

2.1   Risk Management Options

Risk management options may be broadly classified as regulatory, economic, advisory, or technological (Krewski and Birkwood, 1988). Unlike regulation, which invokes strict criteria to be enforced by regulatory authorities, economic approaches to risk management rely largely on economic incentives and disincentives to reduce the levels of anthropogenic pollutants introduced into the environment. Advisory options for risk management rely on the provision of advice to promote risk avoidance. New technological developments may also be used for pollution abatement without being required by direct regulation. These options are not mutually exclusive, as illustrated by the use of all four approaches in controlling industrial emission of sulfur dioxide into the atmosphere in Canada (Burnett et al., 1988).

A decision-oriented assessment of risk requires that there be at least two alternative courses of action under consideration. If there is only one possible course of action, there is no need for a decision, and no need for an analysis. In the simplest case, one of the alternatives is the status quo, while the other alternative is the new risk management strategy under consideration. The assessment is then based on the incremental impacts of the new approach as compared to the existing situation.

Frequently, there are more than two alternatives under consideration. In addition, each alternative can also be considered at several different levels of intensity. For example, three possible approaches to responding to a particular environmental hazard could be to do nothing, to launch a public information program, or to impose formal regulations. Public information programs may be implemented at different levels of vigor and expense, while regulations can be invoked at different levels of stringency. Multiple alternatives with multiple levels of scale within each alternative add to the complexity of the analysis but do not change the fundamental approach.

2.2 A Decision Framework

A comprehensive assessment of a risk management strategy requires that all relevant impacts be given proper consideration (Drummond et al., 1987). As illustrated in Fig. 1, a hazard control program may have an incremental impact on human health, the environment, or social structure (Oxman et al., 1987). There may also be important economic consequences that flow from them. In addition, there will generally be direct financial consequences due to the cost of the program itself.

Health effects are the impacts that a decision will have on human health, expressed in terms of criteria such as injury, disease, and mortality. Environmental consequences are the effects on the ecosystem in which we live, including both transient and persistent adverse effects on our natural environment. Social consequences are reflected in changes in social relationships such as employment rates. As discussed below, the health, environmental, and social impacts of a decision can have subsequent economic consequences. In addition, consideration needs to be given to the direct financial consequences of a decision

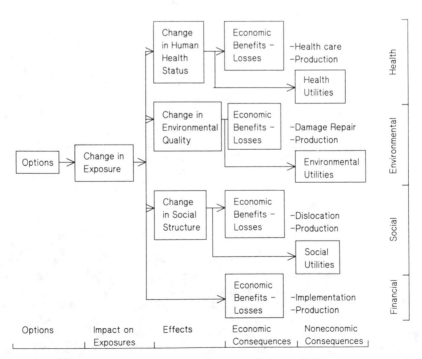

Figure 1. A decision oriented framework for evaluating environmental risk management strategies.

such as the economic costs or benefits of developing, designing, and implementing a given risk management program.

To carry out a particular analysis, all the elements in Fig. 1 should be addressed. In order to provide some general guidance in this regard, we briefly discuss each of these elements in turn.

2.3 Exposure Assessment

The intent of the environmental hazard control program is to reduce the risk of damage to human health, to the environment, and to social structure by reducing exposure to the hazard. Levels of exposure to environmental hazards and changes in those levels can be measured in a variety of ways (Neely and Blau, 1985). For example, toxic chemicals may exist in the biosphere either as naturally occurring substances or as a result of human activities. Surveys of environmental quality can be used to evaluate the presence of chemicals in the general environment, including those present in air and water (Munn, 1981; Gilbert, 1987). These compounds may result in subsequent human exposure via inhalation or the consumption of drinking water. Ingestion of food additives and contaminants can be evaluated directly using data on food consumption patterns (Nutrition Canada, 1974) coupled with information on the levels of these chemicals in food (Food Safety Council, 1978).

Occupational exposures can be assessed using a variety of monitoring instruments, including personal monitors carried by individual workers. Biological monitoring can also be used to confirm chemical exposure via the detection of the parent compound or certain metabolites in urine or other tissue samples, although the specificity of this approach remains to be established (Tannenbaum and Skipper, 1984).

2.4 Effects

A reduction in exposure to an environmental hazard should lead to beneficial effects. This can occur in three domains: human health, the environment, and social structure. In our framework, the elements shown in the effects column represent outcome changes measured in natural physical units. Beneficial health effects would be measured in terms of the number of lives saved, life years gained, reduction in disease occurrence rates, reduction in disability days or hospitalization days, or reduction in restricted activity days (Drummond et al., 1987). Examples of environmental outcomes include increases in air clarity, reduction of air odors, increases in water clarity, reductions in ambient noise levels, and increases in park acreage. Social outcomes include reductions in unemployment and reductions in worker dislocation.

2.5 Economic Consequences

Effects within all three domains will generally have economic implications (Thompson, 1985). For example, improvements in health status will lead to reductions in future health care expenditures and increases in workplace productivity. Both are positive economic benefits. Similarly, improvements in environmental quality can lead to economic gains. For example, a reduction in acidic deposition can produce economic benefits by reducing the amount of repair that may be required to restore damaged buildings while increasing the productivity of forests and lakes. In the social domain, reductions in worker dislocation can lead to economic gains by averting the corresponding dislocation costs and the associated reductions in workplace productivity.

In addition to these economic consequences, there are generally direct economic costs or benefits associated with many risk management options. For example, a regulatory program to reduce stack emissions by using scrubbers would incur certain implementation costs (to develop, promulgate, and monitor the regulation) and increased production costs due to reduced efficiency and yield.

The net economic consequence may be assessed by aggregating across the various components. Because some components will be gains and others losses, it is often difficult to establish in advance whether the net economic consequences of regulation will be positive or negative.

2.6 Noneconomic Consequences

Regardless of their economic consequences, improvements in human health, environmental quality, and social structure are beneficial in their own right (Thompson, 1986). These improvements may be measured using different utility functions. The concept of utility is used to represent the strength of preference for particular outcomes. Thus, improved outcomes are reflected by increased utilities. The utility approach is particularly useful when there are multiple effects within each domain. For example, in the health domain it is common that an improvement will result both in fewer deaths and less morbidity. Utilities offer a method to aggregate these two disparate effects into one measure (Sackett and Torrance, 1978; Kaplan et al., 1979; Weinstein, 1981; Kaplan and Bush, 1982; Churchill et al., 1984).

In the case of health, utilities are cardinal values that are assigned to each health state on a scale that is established by assigning a value of 1.0 to being healthy and 0.0 to being dead. Utility values reflect the quality of the health state and allow morbidity and mortality to be combined into a single weighted measure called quality adjusted life years (QALYs) gained (Weinstein and Stason, 1977; Wilkins and Adams, 1978; Dillard, 1983).

Similar measures of utility can be applied to environmental and social effects. Although there has been little empirical work in these domains, the principles remain the same as for health effects. The best and worst possible outcomes are respectively assigned utilities of 1.0 and 0.0., and the intermediate outcomes are assessed relative to these two anchors.

2.7 Decision Analysis

Strategies for controlling environmental hazards can be evaluated using cost–effectiveness analysis (CEA), cost–utility analysis (CUA), or cost–benefit analysis (CBA) (Drummond et al., 1987; Torrance and Krewski, 1987). These techniques are simply different methods of aggregating the data from Fig. 1 to assist in decisionmaking.

Cost–effectiveness analysis (CEA) may be based on the cost required either to reduce exposure or to cause positive effects. If little is known about the linkage between exposure reduction and improvements in health, environmental quality, or social structure, it may be wise to restrict the analysis to exposure reduction only. In this way, alternative programs can be compared using CEA to determine the alternative with the lowest cost per unit reduction in exposure.

The exposure reduction approach was used by Logan et al. (1981) to compare the cost effectiveness of alternative programs to reduce blood pressure and hypertension. Thus, rather than attempting to estimate the possible ultimate health impact in terms of cardiovascular disease, Logan restricted his measures to a reduction of blood pressure.

With CEA, the financial cost of the program in dollars is compared to the consequences of the program in nondollar units by means of a cost–effectiveness ratio. If there are several alternatives directed at the same type of effect, this approach can identify which of those is the most cost effective.

Cost–utility analysis (CUA) is simply a special form of cost–effectiveness analysis in which the measure of effect is quality adjusted life years gained. The advantage of CUA over CEA is that it uses a common unit of measurement for all programs and thus allows a greater degree of generalization.

In cost–benefit analysis (CBA), all costs and consequences are converted to dollars and summarized in the net benefit figure. A program is considered to be cost beneficial if the net benefit is positive. If there are multiple alternatives, the one with the largest net benefit is the best.

Other analyses are also possible (Torrance and Krewski, 1987). Risk–benefit analysis (RBA), for example, is similar to CBA except that no attempt is made to quantify human health effects. In addition to the economic factors discussed above, socioeconomic impact analysis (SEIA) considers nonallocative economic effects such as those involving market structure, international trade, or inflation.

3 A CASE STUDY: REDUCING LEAD IN GASOLINE

3.1 Health Effects of Lead

The health effects of lead have been studied extensively and are well documented (EPA, 1986; Hare, 1986). In particular, toxic effects of lead are directed against heme synthesis, the kidney, and the nervous system (Niebor and Sanford, 1985). Children appear to be more sensitive than adults to lead poisoning. It is the health effects of lead in children that have been the primary concern in considerations of lead additives in gasoline, particularly neurobehavioral and cognitive effects (EPA, 1986). Other clinical effects that are of concern include anemia in children (Schwartz et al., 1985) and teratogenic effects (Needleman et al., 1984).

Recently, concern has been raised over the neuropsychiatric effects of lead in adults with occupational exposure to lead at serum levels as low as $40\,\mu g/dL$ (Cullen et al., 1983; Rosen et al., 1983; Campara et al., 1984; Mantere et al., 1984; Schottenfeld and Cullen, 1984), although these effects have generally not played a major role in considerations of lead in gasoline. However, recent studies have demonstrated an association between blood lead levels and blood pressure, which is a major cause of cardiovascular morbidity and premature mortality (Pocock et al., 1984; Harlan et al., 1985; Kirkby and Gyntelberg, 1985; Kromhout et al., 1985). The hypothesis that lead causes increased blood pressure is biologically plausible and it is supported by experimental studies in animals. However, both the magnitude of the effect and the strength of the evidence are still disputed (Hare, 1986, p. 341).

The fact that lead in gasoline is a major source of exposure to lead comes from a number of epidemiologic studies (EPA, 1986), as well as from the Isotopic Lead Experiment in northern Italy, which has attempted to estimate the portion of human lead from gasoline by analyzing the ratios of two isotopes of lead. Lead emissions from automobiles are probably responsible for 20% of the lead burden of most adults and 35% or more in

TABLE 1. Risk Management Options for Reducing Lead in Gasoline Considered in United Kingdom, Canada, and the United States

Country	Goal	Options	Major Consequences Considered in Quantitative Analysis	Method of Analysis	Recommendation	Comments
United Kingdom	Human health improvement	$0.4 \, g/L^a$ $0.4 \, g/L$ + filters $0.15 \, g/L$ $0 g/L$ (unleaded)	Emission rates Financial costs of lead reduction	Scorecard	Reduce or eliminate lead in gasoline	Economic valuation of effects viewed as highly uncertain
Canada	Human health improvement	$0.77 \, g/L^a$ $0.29 \, g/L$ $0.15 \, g/L$ $0 g/L$ (unleaded) $0 g/L$ (except heavy trucks) Filter (nonvehicles only) Filter (new and retrofit)	Emission rates Social effects Financial costs of lead reduction	CEA	No specific recommendation	Nonallocative economic effects considered Industry and government cost estimates differed markedly
United States	Human health improvement	$0.29 \, g/L^a$ $0.026 \, g/L$	Health effects Environmental effects Financial costs of lead reduction	CBA	Reduce lead levels in gasoline to $0.026 \, g/L$	Health care and premature mortality monetarized Environmental effects monetarized

^{a}Status quo (baseline).

1053

children. As such, reducing the levels of lead in gasoline can have an appreciable impact on total exposure.

3.2   Reducing Lead in Gasoline

As summarized in Table 1, the United Kingdom, Canada, and the United States have all recently evaluated the economic consequences of reducing or eliminating lead in gasoline (Southwood, 1983; McMullen et al., 1984; Schwartz et al., 1985). It should be noted that these three evaluations have been selected to illustrate the different approaches taken within the context of our decision framework. Thus, it should be emphasized that we are not attempting an exhaustive review of these evaluations or of the costs and benefits of reducing lead in gasoline in general. Rather, it is our intention to use these data to study the decision criteria underlying each case.

3.2.1   *United Kingdom.*   In the United Kingdom, the Department of Transport set up a Working Party on Lead in Petrol (WORLIP) in December 1978 comprised of government officials and specialists from the oil and automotive industries. Its goal was to assess the feasibility, effectiveness, and costs of various options for reducing lead emissions from vehicles. The Working Party submitted a detailed analysis of five options for reducing lead in gasoline in July 1979. Their analysis of three of these options is included in the Ninth Report of the Royal Commission on Environmental Pollution on Lead in the Environment (Southwood, 1983). The report addresses the following issues: the sources of lead pollution and pathways to humans, lead pollution and wildlife, methods of reducing lead in the environment and human uptake, and technical and economic implications of different options for reducing or eliminating lead from gasoline.

The economic analysis presented in the Royal Commission's report uses a scorecard approach. The consequences considered include additional crude oil requirements, additional gasoline production costs, car manufacturers' costs, total additional costs, extra cost to motorists, and forecast percent reduction in lead emissions. The unleaded option is recommended, based on a lack of compelling arguments for the retention of leaded gasoline.

3.2.2   *Canada.*   Under the Canadian Clean Air Act, which was promulgated on November 1, 1971, regulations were issued for lead-free gasoline effective July 1, 1974 and for leaded gasoline effective January 1, 1976. The latter prescribes a maximum permissible concentration of lead in leaded gasoline of $0.77 \, g/L$. Concern for environmental quality was the basis for further assessment of automotive lead emissions and of possible means to reduce these emissions.

Six options to reduce automotive lead emissions were investigated by the Environmental Protection Service of the Department of the Environment. The Department published their Socio-economic Impact Analysis of Lead Phase-down Control Options in February 1984 (McMullen et al., 1984). The Canadian evaluation is based on a cost–effectiveness analysis, in which the cost per tonne reduction of lead emissions is calculated. Nonallocative costs are considered separately. The ranking of the six options evaluated in the Canadian analysis is sensitive to the cost estimates used. Specifically, the differences in cost effectiveness of the options not only change in magnitude but in direction, depending on whether the government or the industry estimates of costs are used. The fact that no final recommendation was made is due in part to this discrepancy.

3.2.3   United States. The Clean Air Act of 1963 gives the Administrator of the Environmental Protection Agency (EPA) broad authority to control or prohibit the manufacture or sale of any fuel additive if (i) its emission products cause or contribute to air pollution which may be reasonably anticipated to endanger the public health or welfare, or if (ii) they will impair to a significant degree the performance of any emission control device or system in general use. In August 1984 the EPA recommended a reduction of lead in gasoline based on both of these concerns. The recommendations made by the EPA were part of a series of actions taken by the Agency over the previous 11 years to address the health and environmental hazards posed by lead in gasoline. The Final Regulatory Impact Analysis for this reduction was published by the EPA in February 1985 (Schwartz et al., 1985).

The U.S. evaluation is based on a cost–benefit analysis. The net benefits of reducing lead in gasoline are calculated with and without the estimated benefits from a reduction in blood pressure due to reduced lead levels. Different assumptions are made regarding "misfueling," or the misuse of leaded gasoline in cars equipped with catalytic converters. The U.S. report strongly advocates a reduction to 0.026 g/L.

Although all three evaluations conclude that further reductions (or elimination) of lead in gasoline are desirable, the U.S. evaluation concludes that further reducing lead in gasoline would have economic benefits, the U.K. evaluation concludes that there would be economic losses, and the Canadian evaluation concludes that there might be either benefits or losses. The three evaluations use different methodologies, and without some guidelines for assessing them, it is difficult to interpret the differences in their findings. Thus, we review these three evaluations in terms of the general framework introduced in Section 2.

3.3   Options Considered

The primary options considered for reducing lead in each of these evaluations are listed in Table 1. Note that there are different baselines to which the alternatives are compared, and the alternatives being considered are different. While this accounts in part for the differences in the findings of the three evaluations, there are other differences between the evaluations that may be even more important.

Two additional options are discussed in the U.K. report but not analyzed in detail: a reduction to 0.15 g/L coupled with the use of lead filters and the encouragement of greater use of diesel and other alternatives to gasoline. Detailed analyses of reductions to lead levels below 0.15 g/L but above zero were not performed on the grounds that at levels below 0.15 g/L, the value of lead as an octane booster would be only marginal, that many existing car engines would begin to develop valve recession problems, and that it would become prohibitively expensive to maintain present octane values. This is in contrast to the U.S. EPA report, which makes no such claims and presents a detailed evaluation of reducing lead levels to 0.026 g/L.

Two additional options are discussed briefly in the Canadian report: a special excise tax and a "pool" approach. The excise tax would be used to reduce or eliminate the price differential between leaded and lead-free gasoline, thereby decreasing the ratio of leaded to lead-free gasoline sold. The pool approach involves the establishment of limits on the lead content on the total volume (leaded and lead-free) of gasoline produced.

In addition to the 0.026 g/L option evaluated in the U.S. report, an alternative level of

0.052 g/L was also considered by the U.S. EPA, and the benefits and costs of these two alternatives were compared. The U.S EPA is also currently considering a ban on lead in gasoline equivalent to the "unleaded" alternative for the United Kingdom and Canada listed in Table 1. A complete ban was not promulgated in 1985 because of concern that certain engines may rely on lead for protection against valve-seat recession. This issue is considered in the separate Regulatory Impact Analysis noted above. Other options considered by the EPA but not formally analyzed include public education, stepped-up enforcement of existing regulations, and marketable permits and pollution charges (see Krewski and Birkwood, 1988, for a more detailed discussion of these risk management strategies).

3.4 Exposures

Although exposure to lead is of primary interest in evaluating strategies for reducing lead in gasoline, the options being evaluated also have impacts on other exposures. Decreasing the amount of lead in gasoline reduces emissions of other pollutants, including hydrocarbons, nitrogen oxides, and carbon monoxide. Most of these reductions results from decreased "misfueling," or the misuse of leaded fuel in vehicles equipped with pollution-control catalysts.

The U.K. evaluation considers the potential for new exposures that could occur with alternatives that might be used to replace lead in gasoline. In particular, consideration is given to the manganese compound MMT, an antiknock additive. The potential for increased emissions of aromatic hydrocarbons resulting from the use of higher octane components such as benzene is also discussed.

Differences in the degree of consideration given to hazards other than lead is in part due to the different circumstances in the three countries. Catalytic converters to reduce emissions of carbon monoxide, hydrocarbons, and nitrogen oxides are used in the exhaust systems of most cars in the United States to meet emission limits and are used on new light-duty vehicles in Canada as of September 1, 1987. These devices are deactivated by lead, this being the principal reason why unleaded gasoline is required by law to be available in the United States and is available commercially in Canada. Catalytic converters are not used in the United Kingdom where emission limits are less stringent and more easily met with smaller fuel-efficient cars. Thus, unleaded gasoline is not available there.

3.5 Effects

The evaluations carried out in the United Kingdom, Canada, and the United States differed substantially with respect to the health, environmental, social, and financial consequences considered quantitatively. The main differences in each of these four categories are outlined below.

3.5.1 Health Effects. The U.S. study is the only one of the three evaluations that quantified the health effects of reducing lead in gasoline and the only one that considered the effects of lead on blood pressure. Although both the U.K. and U.S. studies considered effects from substitute additives and changes in refining processes, there are important differences in their assessments. The U.S. study postulates a net decrease in benzene emissions due to less misfueling (and consequently more efficient removal of benzene from exhaust by catalytic converters), whereas the U.K. study (given that catalytic converters are not used in the United Kingdom) postulates an increase in benzene emissions due to increased benzene in gasoline from the postulated changes in refining processes. The U.S. study includes possible financial consequences of MMT, which is banned in unleaded gasoline in the United States due to its adverse effects on tailpipe hydrocarbon emissions.

3.5.2   Environmental Effects. The U.S. evaluation is the only one that quantitatively considers the environmental consequences of reducing lead in gasoline. The consequences that are evaluated are the impacts of increased emissions of nitrous oxides and other pollutants due to misfueling. These include reductions in ozone levels, increases in acidic deposition, and the fading of textile dyes. Although the U.K. evaluation does discuss the impacts of lead on plants and animals, these consequences are not included in the formal evaluation of options for reducing lead in gasoline.

3.5.3   Social Effects. The Canadian study is the only one of the three that considers the social impacts of reducing lead in gasoline. These include impacts on employment, possible plant closures, and changes in the distribution of income due to potential effects on the automotive parts aftermarket (as a result of reduced maintenance and purchases of replacement parts), lead additive manufacturers, and the lead and petroleum industries.

Both the U.K. and Canadian studies address impacts on oil imports and balance of payments in the discussion. This is essentially a question of economic distribution on an international level. Strategies to control environmental hazards can have important impacts on international trade, which can be important in many public policy decisions. While such considerations should not be ignored, a discussion of international economics is beyond the scope of this chapter. In the case of reducing lead in gasoline, both the United States and Canada considered these impacts to be extremely difficult or impossible to estimate.

3.5.4   Financial Effects. All three evaluations consider the financial benefits from reduced automobile maintenance, although they use different assumptions. Maintenance benefits are realized as a result of reductions in the combustion products of lead alkyls which cause fouling of spark plugs, reduced corrosion of exhaust systems and engines from the by-products of lead and the lead scavengers, and a reduction in the required frequency of oil changes. Eliminating lead in gasoline also increases fuel economy by reducing the fouling of spark plugs and by allowing the engine to be tuned for optimum efficiency, with the catalytic converter controlling emissions. Fuel savings are analyzed quantitatively in both the U.S. and Canadian studies, although not on the same basis. Fuel savings are discussed but not quantified in the U.K. Study.

All three evaluations consider the impact of reducing or eliminating lead on the costs of oil refining. Only the Canadian study assesses the financial impact on the lead industry. Although both the U.K. and Canadian studies consider costs to the automotive industry, the costs analyzed are notably different due to the disparate uses of catalytic converters, the availability of lead-free gasoline, and the compression ratios (and octane requirements) of cars in the two countries.

3.6   Consequences

The U.S. study is the only one of the three evaluations that attempts to quantify health and environmental effects in economic terms. For health effects in children, only the economic consequences (the costs of medical care and compensatory education) are valued. The value of neurological and behavioral changes per se (i.e., the utility value of the reduced quality of life for injured children and their families) is not estimated or included in the analysis. For this and other reasons, it is suggested that childrens' health benefits may be underestimated.

The economic consequences of a potential reduction in the incidence of hypertension (and subsequently the incidence of stroke and myocardial infarction due to hypertension) are also calculated, taking into account both medical care expenses and lost production. Changes in the quality of life such as pain and suffering from strokes are not valued, although mortality is. Several studies of the value of preventing a premature death based on willingness to pay are cited. The values noted range from $0.4 to $7 million per statistical life saved. A value of $1 million, taken from the lower end of that range, is used in the analysis.

The health and environmental effects of reductions of other pollutants (from a reduction in misfueling) are also valued and a detailed description of the methods used is provided. The values of the environmental and health effects of reductions in pollutants other than lead are aggregated and shown as benefits from a reduction in "conventional pollutants" in the summary.

3.7 Decision Analysis

The three reports use different decision analytic methods. The U.K. analysis uses a scorecard approach, the Canadian analysis is based on cost effectiveness, and the U.S. analysis uses a cost–benefit approach.

The U.K. analysis calculates the expected percentage reduction in lead levels and reports this together with the expected costs. The estimated annual cost is 7–8 (1978) British pounds per motorist for the 0.15 g/L option (approximately $30–40 U.S. 1987), and 17–18 pounds for the zero-lead option (approximately $70–90 U.S. 1987). These two options involve reductions of 62 and 100% of (1971) lead emissions, respectively. The net total costs are 844 million pounds for the 0.15 g/L option and 826 million pounds for the unleaded option (approximately $240 million and $230 million U.S. 1987) annually over 20 years. The unleaded option is recommended based on a lack of compelling arguments for the retention of leaded gasoline. The economic analysis is largely discounted because of "so many imponderables" in the estimates.

The Canadian analysis calculates the cost per tonne reduction of lead emissions. The estimates for the lead-free option range from a benefit of $910 (1983) Canadian per tonne to a cost of $14,605 per tonne. The total net benefit or cost ranges from a benefit of $105 million to a cost of $1681 million in 1987 U.S. dollars. This corresponds to a benefit of approximately $200 million or a cost of $3 billion over 20 years. The estimates for the 0.15 g/L option range from a cost of $2010 (1983) Canadian per tonne to a cost of $15,450 per tonne. The range in the total net cost in 1987 U.S. dollars is approximately $350 million to $2700 million. No final recommendation is made in the Canadian report.

The U.S. analysis calculates the net benefits of reducing lead in gasoline with and without the blood pressure benefits. The estimated net benefits, not including blood-pressure-related benefits, range from $4.1 billion (U.S. 1983) if the proposed change has no impact on misfueling to $6.7 billion if the rule eliminates all misfueling (approximately $5.7 and $9.4 billion U.S. 1987). The net benefits are estimated to be $5.9 billion assuming partial misfueling (approximately $8.3 billion U.S. 1987). If the blood pressure benefits are included, the net benefits are much higher—$33.4 billion under the partial misfueling assumption (approximately $47 billion U.S. 1987). The estimate of the net benefits from the financial consequences alone (maintenance + fuel economy − refining costs) under the

partial misfueling assumption is $2246 million (over $3 billion U.S. 1987 over 7.5 years).
The U.S. report strongly advocates a reduction to 0.026 g/L.

3.8   Other Considerations

All three studies note conflicts and uncertainties in the source data and frequently use data
from two or more sources to indicate a range of values, to calculate an average, or to
conduct a sensitivity analysis. The estimated maintenance savings per g/L reduction of
lead in gasoline range from essentially zero in the United Kingdom to approximately $50
million per year in Canada to nearly $3 billion in the United States.

When critical data elements are uncertain, it is generally useful to explore the impact on
the conclusion of using different plausible values. No formal sensitivity analyses are
presented in the U.K. report, although the impacts of many of the assumptions on the
analysis were considered. In the Canadian study, there is a large disparity between
government and industry estimates of refining costs, and results are presented using both
sets of estimates. This large difference arises from industry's inclusion of the capital costs of
plant modifications required to meet the production of gasoline with a reduced lead
content. The government estimates exclude such costs on the grounds that capital
investment would be required for plant modernization regardless of the decision taken on
lead in gasoline.

The U.S. study presents a range of sensitivity analyses on the estimates of the financial
consequences. Sensitivity analyses are also presented for the health and environmental
benefits, although the scope of the sensitivity analyses is more limited. For example, only
one value is used for estimating the value of preventing a premature death, and no
estimates are included in the analysis for the value of reduced morbidity. None of the three
analyses varies the discount rate or the analytic horizon.

The practicality of the alternatives considered was addressed in all three reports,
although the major considerations are quite different in the three studies. A primary
concern in the U.K. study was complying with European Economic Community (EEC)
standards and negotiating with other EEC member states over new standards. In addition,
major changes in the automotive industry needed to be considered given the lack of lead-
free gasoline in the United Kingdom and differences in automobile standards. Major
concerns in the Canadian study were effects on employment and possible plant closures. In
addition, all three studies noted additional options but did not analyze them in detail
because they were not considered feasible or implementable. For example, the U.S. EPA
considered public education regarding misfueling, stepped-up enforcement, and market-
oriented alternatives including marketable permits and pollution charges as potential
options but found them to be impractical.

4   SUMMARY AND CONCLUSIONS

In this chapter, we have presented a decision-oriented framework for the evaluation of
environmental risk management strategies. This framework takes into account effects on
human health, the environment, and social structure, as well as the financial costs of
establishing the risk management program itself. Traditional methods of program
evaluation such as CEA and CBA were shown to arise as special cases.

To explore the utility of this general framework, existing evaluations of alternative
ways of reducing the level of lead in gasoline conducted in the United Kingdom, Canada,

and the United States were examined. The objective of this review was not to select the most appropriate approach to reducing lead in gasoline, but to test the utility of our framework in practice as a means of facilitating improved decisionmaking.

All three reports review the toxicity of lead and concur that it is highly toxic even at low levels of exposure. There are, however, differences between the evaluations. The Canadian report concludes that the primary health benefit of reducing lead in gasoline will be a reduction of risk for neurological and behavioral changes in young children. Neither the U.K. nor Canadian report considers the effects of lead on blood pressure, and neither evaluation attempts to value the health effects, the environmental effects, or the economic consequences of the health and environmental effects associated with reducing lead in gasoline.

The three evaluations use fundamentally different methods in their detailed analysis of the main options considered for reducing lead in gasoline. The U.K. study uses a scorecard approach, whereas cost–effectiveness and cost–benefit analyses are employed by Canada and the United States, respectively. The U.S. analysis is the most quantitative of the three, placing a monetary value on both health and environmental impacts. The U.K. analysis is the least quantitative, viewing such economic valuations as being highly uncertain. This uncertainty is apparent in the Canadian analysis, in which the cost–effectiveness ratios differ widely depending on whether industry or government cost estimates are used.

That the three evaluations reach different conclusions is perhaps not surprising. To begin with, the baseline conditions and options considered are different. This, coupled with the different methods of analysis and degree of quantitation of the major health, environmental, social, and financial impacts, leads to distinctly different recommendations. By reviewing these analyses within our framework, the reasons for those differences become clear.

This case study demonstrates that the detailed evaluations carried out in these three countries all fall within the framework provided by our model. Furthermore, this case study has served to highlight several points with respect to the systematic evaluation of environmental risk management strategies.

First, many assumptions and judgments are incorporated into an economic analysis, and there is generally a great deal of uncertainty with respect to many of the estimates that are used. Thus, important assumptions should be clearly identified in an analysis, and sensitivity analyses of key assumptions should be conducted to assess the robustness of the conclusions reached for these assumptions.

Second, analyses of environmental risk management programs are complex. The framework presented in this chapter can be used as an aid to sort out this complexity. In particular, this framework can be used systematically to identify, measure, and value *all* important costs and consequences of a decision. If each important consequence or decision criterion is itemized and concisely displayed, decisionmakers can quickly determine which consequences have been estimated and whether important consequences have been left out of the analysis. If consequences are aggregated, the relative contribution of each component can be assessed. This last point is illustrated in the U.S. evaluation, where adult blood pressure has a major impact on the final result and fuel economy has a relatively minor impact.

Finally, it is important to appreciate that even in cases where a formal quantitative analysis is not done to aid in decisionmaking, the same factors discussed here must be taken into account, implicitly if not explicitly. Some decisions may be easy to make, as in cases where the costs are small and the risks are high. In these cases, a detailed analysis of the type proposed here would be of little value to the decisionmaking process, and would in fact be a waste of time and resources. On the other hand, there is a large number of decisions regarding environmental hazards where the costs, the potential consequences, and the associated uncertainties are substantial. The greater the complexity of the decision, the greater the value of explicating and clarifying the assumptions and judgments made by following a systematic framework such as that described here.

REFERENCES

Burnett, R., Krewski, D., Birkwood, P. L., and Franklin, C. A. (1988). Health risks from transported air pollution. In C. D. Fowle, L. Grima, and R. Munn, Eds., *Information Needs for Risk Management*. Institute for Environmental Studies, University of Toronto, Toronto, Canada (in press).

Campara, P., D'Andrea, F., Micciolo, R., Savonitto, C., Tansella, M., and Zimmermann–Tansella, Ch. (1984). Psychological performance of workers with blood-lead concentration below the current threshold limit value. *Int. Arch. Occup. Environ. Health* **53**, 233–246.

Churchill, D. N., Morgan, J., and Torrance, G. W. (1984). Quality of life in end-stage renal disease. *Peritoneal Dial. Bull.* **4**, 20–23.

Cullen, M. R., Robins, J. M., and Eskenazi, B. (1983). Adult inorganic lead intoxication: Presentation of 31 new cases and a review of recent advances in the literature. *Medicine (Baltimore)* **62**, 221–247.

Dillard, S. (1983). *Durée ou qualité de la vie?* Ministère du Communication, Quebec.

Drummond, M. F., Stoddard, G. L., and Torrance, G. W. (1987). *Methods for the Economic Evaluation of Health Care Programmes.* Oxford Univ. Press, London and New York.

Environmental Protection Agency (EPA) (1986). *Review of the National Ambient Air Quality Standards for Lead: Assessment of Scientific and Technical Information.* USEPA, Research Triangle Park, NC.

Food Safety Council (1978). Proposed system for food safety assessment. Chapter 4. Human exposure assessment. *Food Cosmet. Toxicol.* **16**, Suppl. 2, 25–28.

Gilbert, R. O. (1987). *Statistical Methods in Environmental Pollution Monitoring.* Van Nostrand-Reinhold, New York.

Hare, F. K. (Chairman) (1986). *Lead in the Canadian Environment: Science and Regulation.* Final Report of the Commission on Lead in the Environment, Royal Society of Canada, Ottawa.

Harlan, W. R., Landis, J. R., Schmouder, R. L., Goldstein, N. G., and Harlan, L. C. (1985). Blood lead and blood pressure. *JAMA, J. Am. Med. Assoc.* **253**, 530–534.

Kaplan, R. M., and Bush, J. W. (1982). Health related quality of life measurement for evaluation research and policy analysis. *Health Psychol.* **1**, 61–80.

Kaplan, R. M., Bush, J. W., and Berry, C. C. (1979). Health status index: Category rating versus magnitude estimation for measuring levels of well-being. *Med. Care* **17**, 501–525.

Kirkby, H., and Gyntelberg, F. (1985). Blood pressure and other cardiovascular risk factors of long-term exposure to lead. *Scand. J. Work Environ. Health* **11**, 15–19.

Krewski, D. (1987). Risk and risk management: Issues and approaches. In R. S. McColl, Ed., *Environmental Health Risks: Assessment and Management.* Univ. of Waterloo Press, Waterloo, pp. 29–51.

Krewski, D., and Birkwood, P. (1987). Risk assessment and risk management. *Risk. Abstr.* **4**, 53–61.

Krewski, D., and Birkwood, P. (1988). Regulatory and nonregulatory options for risk management. In *Risk Management: Estimation, Evaluation and Assessment.* Univ. Of Waterloo Press, Waterloo (in press).

Krewski, D., Clayson, D., and McCullough, R. S. (1982). Identification and measurement of risk. In I. Burton, C. D. Fowle, and R. S. McCullough Eds., *Living with Risk: Environmental Risk Management in Canada*. Institute for Environmental Studies, University of Toronto, pp. 7–23.

Krewski, D., Brown, C., and Murdoch, D. (1984). Determining "safe" levels of exposure: Safety factors or mathematical models? *Fundam. Appl. Toxicol.* **4**, S383–S394.

Krewski, D., Murdoch, D., and Withey, J. R. (1987). The application of pharmacokinetic data in carcinogenic risk assessment. In *Pharmacokinetics in Risk Assessment, Drinking Water and Health*, Vol. 8. National Academy Press, Washington, DC., pp. 441–468.

Kromhout, D., Wibowo, A. A. E., Herber, R. F. M., Dalderup, L. M., Heerdink, H., de Lezenne Coulander, C., and Zielhuis, R. L. (1985). Trace metals and coronary heart disease risk indicators in 152 elderly men (the Zutphen Study). *Am. J. Epidemiol.* **122**, 378–385.

Logan, A. G., Milne, B. J., Achber, C., Campbell, W. P., and Haynes, R. B. (1981). Cost-effectiveness of a worksite hypertension program. *Hypertension* **3**, 211–218.

Mantere, P., Hanninen, H., Henberg, S., and Luukkonen, R. (1984). A prospective follow-up study on psychological effects in workers exposed to low levels of lead. *Scand. J. Work Environ. Health* **10**, 43–50.

McMullen, J., Ahuja, Wong, W., and Struthers, L. (1984). *Socio-economic Impact Analysis of Lead Phase-down Control Options*. Environmental Protection Service, Environment Canada, Ottawa.

Munn, R. E. (1981). *The Design of Air Quality Monitoring Networks*. Macmillan, London.

Munro, I. C., and Krewski, D. R. (1981). Risk assessment and regulatory decision making. *Food Cosmet. Toxicol.* **19**, 549–560.

National Research Council, Committee on the Institutional Means for Assessment of Risks to Public Health (1983). *Risk Assessment in the Federal Government, Managing the Process*. National Academy Press, Washington, DC.

Needleman, H. L., Rabinowitz, M., Leviton, A., Linn, S., and Schoenbaum, S. (1984). The relationship between prenatal exposure to lead and congenital anomalies. *JAMA, J. Am. Med. Assoc.* **251**, 2956–2959.

Neely, W. B., and Blau, G. E. (Eds.) (1985). *Environmental Exposure from Chemicals*, Vols. 1 and 2. CRC Press, Boca Raton, FL.

Niebor, E., and Sanford, W. E. (1985). Essential, toxic and therapeutic functions of metals (including determinants of reactivity). In E. Hodgson, Jr., Ed., *Reviews in Biochemical Toxicology*. New York, p. 205.

Nutrition Canada (1974). *Food Consumption Patterns Report*. Health & Welfare Canada, Ottawa.

Oxman, A. D., Torrance, G. W., Garland, W. J., and Shannon, H. S. (1987). *Nuclear Safety in Ontario: A Comprehensive Framework for Decision-Making and Critical Review of Quantitative Analyses*. Submission to Ontario Nuclear Safety Review, McMaster University, Hamilton, Ontario, Canada.

Pocock, S. J., Shaper, A. G., Ashby, D., Delves, T., and Whitehead, T. P. (1984). Blood lead concentration, blood pressure, and renal function. *Br. Med. J.* **289**, 872–874.

Rosen, I., Wildt, K., Gullberg, B., and Berlin, M. (1983). Neuro-physiological effects of lead exposure. *Scand. J. Work Environ. Health* **9**, 431–441.

Royal Society Study Group (1983). *Risk Assessment: A Study Group Report*. Royal Society, London.

Sackett, D. L., and Torrance, G. W. (1978). The utility of different health states as perceived by the general public. *J. Chronic Dis.* **31**, 697–704.

Schottenfeld, R. S., and Cullen, M. R. (1984). Organic affective illness associated with lead intoxication. *Am. J. Psychiatry* **141**, 1423–1426.

Schwartz, J., Pitcher, H., Levin, R., Ostro, B., and Nichols, A. L. (1985). *Costs and Benefits of*

Reducing Lead in Gasoline, Final Regulatory Impact Analysis, Publ. No. EPA 230-05-85-006. Environmental Protection Agency, Washington, DC.

Somers, E. (1983). Environmental health risk management in Canada. *Regul. Toxicol. Pharmacol.* **3**, 75–81.

Somers, E. (1984). Risk estimation for environmental chemicals as a basis for decision making. *Regul. Toxicol. Pharmacol.* **4**, 99–106.

Somers, E., and Krewski, D. (1982). Risks from environmental chemicals. In J. T. Rogers, and D. V. Bates, Eds., *Risk: A Symposium on the Assessment and Perception of Risk to Human Health in Canada*. Royal Society of Canada, Ottawa, pp. 43–51.

Southwood, T. R. E. (Chairman) (1983). *Lead in the Environment*, 9th Rep. Royal Commission on Environmental Pollution, H.M. Stationers Office, London.

Tannenbaum, S. R., and Skipper, P. L. (1984). Biological aspects to the evaluation of risk: Dosimetry of carcinogens in man. *Fundam. Appl. Toxicol.* **4**, 5367–5373.

Thompson, M. S. (1985). Measuring health benefits. In D. B. Clayson, D. Krewski, and I. C. Munro, Eds., *Toxicological Risk Asressment, Vol. II, General Criteria and Case Studies*, CRC Press, Boca Raton, FL, pp. 97–108.

Thompson, M. S. (1986). Willingness to pay and accept risks to cure chronic disease. *Am. J. Public Health* **76**, 392–396.

Torrance, G. W., and Krewski, D. (1985/86). Economic evaluation of toxic chemical control programs. *Toxic Subst. J.* **7**, 53–71.

Weinstein, M. C. (1981). Economic assessments of medical practices and technologies. *Med. Decis. Making* **1**, 309–330.

Weinstein, M. C., and Stason, W. B. (1977). Foundations of cost-effectiveness analysis for health and medical practices. *N. Engl. J. Med.* **296**, 716–721.

Wilkins, R., and Adams, O. B. (1978). *Healthfulness of Life*. Institute for Research on Public Policy. Montreal, Canada.

World Health Organization (1985). *Risk Management in Chemical Safety*, ICP/CEH 506/m01 56881. European Regional Program on Chemical Safety, WHO, Geneva.

32

Regulating Coke Oven Emissions

Lester B. Lave

*Graduate School of Industrial Administration, Carnegier–Mellon University,
Pittsburgh, Pennsylvania*

Beth A. Leonard

McKinsey & Company, Pittsburgh, PA

INTRODUCTION

Assessing the cancer hazard to workers and the public has come to occupy a central role in regulatory decisionmaking. Risk analysis techniques have been used to quantify the probability of cancer from exposure to chemicals in air, water, food, soil, and the workplace. Recently, the Environmental Protection Agency (EPA) proposed a new regulation concerning coke oven emissions, in order to protect surrounding residents. The EPA's risk analysis of this hazard is controversial and needs to be understood in some detail to arrive at a judgment as to whether current levels of emissions pose a nontrivial risk to those residing around coke ovens (EPA 1987a).

The history of governmental regulations involving coke oven emissions has been marred by a failure to coordinate the efforts of the EPA (which attempts to protect the public) with efforts by the Occupational Safety and Health Administration (OSHA) (which attempts to protect workers). The risk assessments of the two agencies have been inconsistent; the regulations of the two agencies display even less consistency, even down to the level of what is regulated and what constitutes a violation. These inconsistencies affect the cost and efficacy of the EPA's proposed standard.

This chapter addresses the technology for coking coal and abating the emissions of this process. We then examine the history of regulation of the industry. The risk assessments of both OSHA and EPA are reviewed as well as the EPA's regulatory impact analysis. We find there are substantial problems with the EPA's analysis of risk and regulatory impacts; their recommended option—the proposed regulation—makes little sense.

THE TECHNOLOGY OF MAKING COKE

Making coal into coke requires heating coal to high temperatures in a chamber without oxygen (to prevent combustion) (EPA, 1987a). Impurities are volatilized, leaving almost

1064

pure carbon. This coke is used principally as a reducing agent in steelmaking. Coke oven gases are extremely toxic since they contain more than 10,000 different chemicals as gases, condensable vapors, and particles, including coal tars, sulfur oxides, hydroaromatic compounds, paraffins, olefins, phenol, nitrogen-containing compounds, and carbon monoxide. Some of these chemicals are potent carcinogens. The gases are released as coal is dumped into the ovens during the process called *charging*. In addition, gases leak through imperfect seals around doors and piping, when the coke is removed from the oven, and as the coke is cooled by *quenching*.

Prior to the early 20th century, *beehive* technology dominated coke production. The name refers to the circular, doomed structure of these firebrick ovens. Coal entered the beehive through an opening in the middle of the dome, which then served as the discharge point for the *foul gases* developed during the coking process (EPA, 1987b). Unlike later ovens, emissions were completely uncontrolled and discharged directly to the atmosphere. Furthermore, air was admitted to the chamber in controlled amounts for the purpose of actually burning the volatiles to produce heat for continued distillation. The coking process itself took from 48 to 72 h. Once the coking process was complete, the coke was pushed out of the oven through a door at the base of the structure into a quenching car where it was cooled with water.

There were several problems with beehive ovens. First, only very specific types and grades of coal could be used to form coke since the process was largely uncontrolled. Second, these ovens produced excessive air pollution.

The Europeans developed and constructed alternative coking processes as the higher-quality coking coals were depleted, and as the techniques used in gas-producing retorts were applied to coking facilities. Because of the relative abundance of high-quality coking coal, the United States lagged in the development and implementation of new techniques. The evolution consisted of three major components: (i) the separation of coking and heating into distinct compartments, (ii) the containment of waste gases and exclusion of air from the system, and (iii) the use of the waste gases as the primary heat source for continued distillation. From the mid-19th century through the beginning of the 20th century, coking technology changed and *by-product* ovens were built.

By-product batteries, as they now exist, consist of rows of very narrow (12–22 in.) coking chambers flanked on either side by heating flues. Coal is introduced through lids in the top of the battery and is then leveled using a leveling bar to ensure uniformity of distillation. The unit is then closed, and heated gases are passed through the heating flues on either side of the coking chamber. To permit the escape of volatiles during the coking process, an opening is located at one or both ends of the coking chamber. These openings are fitted with offtake valves, which are connected to the gas-collecting main for the battery. The entire system is under positive pressure, forcing the gases to circulate and preventing oxygen from entering. The coking process takes from 16 to 20 h. Once completed, both side doors of the coking chamber are opened and a mechanical pusher shoves the coke into a quench car. From there it is taken to the quench tower where the coke is cooled with water.

The movement from beehives to by-product ovens marked a movement from free discharge of gases into the atmosphere to a relatively contained system. Emissions from these contained systems still occur, however. When the coal is introduced into the coking chamber, large volumes of gas are physically displaced, some of which exits through the open lid where the coal is entering. During the coking process itself, the positive pressure in the system creates leaks from any connections that are not completely sealed—through lids, side doors, or offtake valves. After coking is completed, emissions occur when the side doors are opened to allow the pusher to remove the coke.

REGULATING COKE OVEN EMISSIONS

The health hazards posed by coke oven emissions have led to their regulation by two federal agencies and numerous state and local authorities. Emissions from coke ovens have been regulated for years, first from the viewpoint of damage to the health of workers, then as a source of suspended particles and sulfur oxides to ambient air. More recently, the EPA has proposed to regulate the emissions as a "hazardous air pollutant" to those living near coke ovens (under Sec. 112 of the Clean Air Act) (EPA, 1987a). OSHA and EPA have investigated coke oven emissions several times since creation of the agencies (Briggs and Lave, 1982; EPA, 1987b). They have sought to find an acceptable balance between the inherent problems of making coke, the cost of abating emissions, the economic condition of the steel industry, and the perceived damage to workers' health and the environment. Over time, the perceived threat to public health has increased with the collection of better data documenting the high incidence of cancer among coke over workers. At the same time, the economic condition of the steel industry has declined, making it more likely that stringent emissions regulations would lead to the closing of many coke ovens and would increase the economic pressure on the steel industry (EPA, 1987b).

OSHA Regulation

In 1969, under powers granted him by the Contract Work Hours Standard Act of 1962, the Secretary of Labor adopted a coal tar pitch volatiles (CTPV) threshold limit value (TLV) of $0.2 \, mg/m^3$ of air for worker exposure in federally funded employment (this section is based on Briggs and Lave, 1982). When OSHA was created in 1970, it adopted this standard for all workers, along with many other standards that had been applied only to workers in federally funded employment.

In June 1971, the American Iron and Steel Institute (AISI) petitioned the secretary of labor to develop a less stringent standard specifically applicable to coke oven emissions. A month later the United Steelworkers of America filed a petition requesting a more stringent standard. Both petitions were denied by the Department of Labor in September of 1971, pending further research by the National Institute of Occupational Safety and Health (NIOSH), a research agency within the Department of Health, Education, and Welfare that was created to suggest guidelines and offer advice to OSHA, an agency within the Department of Labor.

NIOSH and the steel industry jointly funded epidemiologic studies of steel workers (Lloyd, et al., 1971). These studies uncovered a large increase in cancer incidence among coke oven workers, particularly of lung cancer. Subsequent studies focused on coke oven workers and managed to estimate the exposure to CTPV and the excessive risk associated with high exposure (Redmond et al., 1972, 1976; Mazumdar et al., 1975). Extensive data analyses were conducted; these were presented at rule-making hearings. Estimates of the number of workers affected and the expected number of excess deaths, as well as data on the cost and feasibility of engineering controls to meet the standards, were presented (Briggs and Lave, 1982). A NIOSH report was published in February 1973, and a Standards Advisory Committee was subsequently established in August 1974. The committee's report was submitted to the Secretary of Labor in May 1975. Two months later a proposed standard was published in the *Federal Register*. OSHA conducted hearings on the proposed standard between November 1975 and May 1976. The final standard of 0.15 mg/m³ was published on October 22, 1976 and became effective January 20, 1977. The industry was given until January 20, 1980 to come into full compliance with the standard.

The regulation established a permissible exposure limit of 0.15 mg of the benzene-soluble fraction (benzene-soluble organics or BSO) of CTPV per cubic meter of air, when collected over any 8-h period. In addition, the rule required the adoption of both engineering controls and work practice rules at each coke oven battery, even if the exposure level were below 0.15 mg/m³. If these specified controls and work practices did not reduce emissions below that level, employers were required to install other (nonspecified) controls as necessary. Employees were to be afforded respiratory protection by personal air filtration devices whenever the exposure limit was exceeded. As promulgated, the standard also required employers to engage in research to develop new technologies to reduce emissions.

Two points should be kept in mind when evaluating the OSHA standard. First, in direct contrast to the EPA standard described below, OSHA specified the goals and the process of achieving them. In particular, OSHA's regulations consist of exact descriptions of the technologies to be employed, the recordkeeping and written procedures to support those technologies, and mandated reporting to OSHA. This regulation can be characterized as a "design standard;" that is, employers were told precisely what steps to take. In contrast, the EPA has proposed a "performance standard" in which they specify the desired outcome and let company management figure out how to meet the standard.

OSHA specified that even if these design criteria did not result in satisfactory reductions, there was performance standard to met; OSHA determined the maximum permissible exposure and required companies to find some way to meet it. Thus, OSHA mandated that employers find new technologies to reach the acceptable exposure limit, a regulatory principle known as technology forcing (Briggs and Lave, 1982). If compliance with OSHA'a design standard did not ensure sufficient emissions reductions, the burden then fell upon the industry to find new technologies to reach the performance standard.

In December 1976, the AISI and the American Coke and Chemical Institute applied to the Secretary of Labor for a stay of the effective date of certain of the standard's provisions. The petition was denied in January 1977. Next, the two institutes and a number of steel companies sought judicial review of the standard in the Third Circuit Court of Appeals. The three principal claims were: (i) the exposure limit of 0.15 mg/m³ was invalid because there was no substantial evidence of either health effects requiring this standard or the technical feasibility of attaining this limit, (ii) the Secretary of Labor had exceeded his statutory powers, and (iii) there was no substantial evidence to support the need for specified mandated controls and procedures (Briggs and Lave, 1982).

The case was argued before the Third Circuit Court of Appeals on January 5, 1978. The court upheld the Secretary's determination that coke oven emissions are carcinogenic and thus necessitate development of a standard. It also upheld the standard requiring engineering controls and the exposure limit of 0.15 mg/m³. However, the Court held that the Secretary had exceeded his authority by requiring employers to conduct research on engineering and work practice controls, by imposing quantitative fit tests for respirators, and by applying the standard to employees who did not work at coke ovens.

Petitions for a writ of certiorari to the U.S. Supreme Court were filed by the AISI and Republic Steel Corporation in December 1978. The Court agreed to hear the appeal, but later the plaintiffs withdrew their petitions, apparently believing they had little chance of winning and fearing a related ruling on benzene would be changed to their disadvantage.

Once the petition was withdrawn, industry implicitly accepted the regulation and committed itself to comply. In point of fact, OSHA's actual measurements of BSO taken at a number of coke plants suggest that the industry is still woefully out of compliance. For example, from April 1979 to July 1981, OSHA inspections revealed that 48% of samples (205/422) were above the standard of 0.15 mg/m^3. Since the standard became effective in January 1977, these inspections occurred at least 18 months after it was in effect. With 48% of samples above the standard, the industry was clearly not in general compliance. Since OSHA did not act to impose large fines or attempt to close coke ovens violating the standard, OSHA tacitly accepted the situation and condoned these worker exposures.

OSHA's consultant estimated that the annual cost of complying with the coke oven standard would be in excess of $200 million. The Business Roundtable conducted a study to document the cost of regulation to member companies. The study found that steel companies reported spending $5–7 million in 1977 to comply with the coke oven standard. While the companies may have been slow in ordering control equipment and initiating their abatement program, it is revealing that so little was spent. In short, the industry has not yet complied with the standard and OSHA has tacitly acceded.

Perhaps the primary reason why neither OSHA nor EPA has demanded stringent controls is the poor economic condition of the steel industry. Between 90 and 95% of the coke produced in the United States is used to produce steel (EPA, 1987). As steel production has declined, coke production has also been cut drastically. Over the last 15 years, coke production in this country has dropped by over 60%. Over the same period, the number of operating coke plants has declined from 62 to 36. This is an industry that is experiencing massive economic hardship.

When OSHA first started regulating this industry in the early 1970s, the steel industry and consequently the coke industry were experiencing an era of massive prosperity. In 1976, when OSHA developed its regulation, the steel industry was described as "large, stable, and profitable" 1976, p. 46748). In fact, despite the $200 million to $1.28 billion annual price tag on this standard, "none of the steel industry spokesmen testified that the proposed standard... would imperil the existence of the coke industry in the United States" (OSHA, 1976, p. 46748). By 1987, the steel industry had experienced years of decline and it was evident that stringent emissions standards would result in plant closures and hardship to the industry.

The EPA explored three options for regulation. The standard proposed by the EPA would cost less than $20 million per year and "would add one more battery to the group of 14 batteries (out of a total of 43 in the country) that are currently operating at marginal costs greater than the price of coke" (EPA, 1987a, p. 13593). Enforcement of this standard would weaken the industry.

EPA Regulation

The EPA has been working on its standard for general population exposures to coke oven gases for about 10 years. As early as 1979, a draft risk analysis was published. In April 1982, the EPA announced the availability of draft health assessment documents for coke oven emissions. Four public meetings to review drafts of this document were held between August 1982 and September 1983. However, the EPA did not add coke oven emissions to the list of hazardous air pollutants (under Sec. 112 of the Clean Air Act) until September 1984. At that time, the EPA indicated that emission standards for wet-coal charged by-product coke oven batteries would be proposed in the spring of 1985. Such standards were issued in April 1987.

Identifying which individual chemicals in coke oven gases cause the observed increase in cancer incidence is extremely difficult. The gases change with the composition of the coal; the chemical composition changes as the gases cool and age, since they react rapidly with other gases. The full-scale process cannot be duplicated in a laboratory. Thus, some *indicator substance* must be selected to characterize the level of emissions from an oven. For years, the indicator substance chosen by toxicologists has been benzopyrene or an aggregate of chemicals, either coal tar pitch volatiles (CTPV) or benzene-soluble organics (BSO). The EPA breaks this tradition by establishing "visible emissions" as the indicator.

One serious problem that this creates is that the EPA's proposed standards depend heavily on risk assessment which is based on levels of BSO, while the regulation is based on visible emissions of yellow-brown smoke. The EPA (1987, p. 327) writes: "Opacity is a crude indicator of the concentration of pollutants." The EPA's specific standard would regulate emissions based on two criteria—allowable length of visible emissions periods during charging of the battery and permissible percentages of doors, lids, and offtakes with visible emissions due to leaks. Actual measurements under existing standards range from 11 to 32 s of visible emissions per charge, 4 to 12% leaking doors (PLD), 1 to 5% leaking lids (PLL), and 4 to 10% leaking offtakes (PLO). The EPA's proposed standard would limit visible emissions during charging to 16 s and would require no more than 10 PLD, 3 PLL, and 6 PLO.

While there are many technical difficulties in measuring coke oven emissions and controlling leaks, the EPA's proposed standard represents a step backward from the earlier OSHA standard. It does not define the concentration limit designed to protect the surrounding population from the carcinogenic gases. Instead, it sets a standard for visible emissions at the coke oven (EPA, 1987a) which is not clearly correlated to increased levels of risk for the community.

A second shortcoming of the EPA proposal is that it focuses on "fugitive" emissions, those from leaks around doors and offtakes, rather than the emissions from stacks or during the charging, pushing of the coke, or quenching. As mentioned above, emissions may occur during several stages of the process, from any of a multitude of openings in the battery, and may not be consistent from one charge to the next. The fugitive nature of the emissions makes control technologies difficult and expensive.

Finally, the cost to reduce exposure under the EPA standard is very high. This was a problem faced by OSHA as well. The lung cancer risk faced by workers is significant (perhaps 10% of the most exposed workers might develop lung cancer) by the standards of the regulatory agencies and requires regulatory attention (Byrd and Lave, 1987). At the same time, controlling emissions was estimated to be extremely costly (more than $200 million per year). As a result, the expense per lung cancer averted was estimated to be greatly in excess of $1 million. The debate over the OSHA standard had to do with whether the workers should be protected; although the risk was large enough ordinarily to require action, the cost per lung cancer averted was greater than that usually faced by the agency, creating questions of efficiency. Spending $200 million per year in an industry such as cotton textiles could prevent many more cancers. The same theme arises in the proposed EPA standard, although at a lower risk level. According to the EPA's assessment, the upper bound estimate is large enough that the risk is significant and the situation demands action. However, the cost per cancer averted is estimated to be more than $1 million; more than the amount that federal regulatory agencies usually require (Travis et al., 1987).

The history of regulation in this industry reflects, in part, the difficulties associated with setting a meaningful standard for fugitive emissions. Standards often appear arbitrary; specific reductions in emissions due to different types of control technology are almost impossible to generalize. The bands of uncertainty concerning estimated health consequences are inordinately large, again due to the specificity of any measurements to that particular oven for that particular charge. All these factors have forced an increasing reliance on risk assessment in an attempt to clarify the trade-offs inherent in regulating this industry.

Contradictions Between OSHA and EPA

The approach that EPA and OSHA have taken to regulate this industry is marked by inconsistencies and contradictions. OSHA stated that

> if a well defined and controlled procedure is used, the results of BSFTPM [benzene soluble fraction of total particulate matter, equivalent to BSO–benzene soluble organics] exposure measurements are reasonably accurate and reproducible. The test is relatively simple and can be carried out by all employers large or small. Most employers already have considerable experience with this test, and some have been using it since 1967, including use in connection with the present standard for CTPV. (OSHA, 1976, pp. 46752–46753)

OSHA considered the use of a visible emissions standard and rejected it:

> In this regard it should be noted that a permissible exposure limit is an objective requirement, whereas questions as to what constitutes a visible emission are subjective. Moreover, there are risk data available regarding various levels of exposure to BFSTPM [BSO] whereas no such data exists for visible emissions. (OSHA, 1976, p. 46754)

In stark contrast, the EPA concluded:

> Because of the technological difficulty of collecting and measuring emissions from coke-oven batteries...a mass emission limitation for coke ovens was technologically and economically impracticable. Instead, the Agency found limits based on visible emissions to be the only feasible means of measuring coke oven emissions. (EPA, 1987a, p. 13590).

The EPA does not seem to have evaluated the reasonableness of a standard based on anticipated concentrations in the vicinity around the plant, although such measurements were made and compared to predictions from their human exposure model (a model developed to predict concentrations in areas near batteries based on emissions levels at the plant).

These contradictions result from many factors, beginning with different statutory goals and organization, different approaches to carrying out their statutory mandate, and different economic and regulatory environments when the agencies were designing the regulations. The contradictions also reflect an unfortunate lack of communication between the agencies. Whatever the causes, these contradictions represent a misallocation of resources that could have been better used elsewhere. There is nothing in the EPA regulation not already required by the OSHA regulation. If OSHA had enforced its own regulation, the EPA would not have found sufficient hazard to justify additional regulation.

Effective regulation requires the EPA and OSHA to coordinate their efforts. For example, a control strategy that relies on personal protective devices would reduce the exposure of the worker population without affecting general population exposure; a control strategy that limited the time any individual worker could spend at a coke oven would reduce the individual worker risk without reducing the risks to the general public. At some coke ovens, the ovens and quenching process have been enclosed within a shed, thus reducing general public exposure while increasing worker exposure. The total benefit of a particular control strategy cannot be properly evaluated unless both *at-risk* populations are considered. Unless coke oven regulation is designed with both the public and workers in mind, agencies will continue to reduce the risks to their target population with little or no consideration of the effects on the other population. Instead of reducing total emissions and curing both problems, each agency will be pushing the industry to suboptimize and perhaps even to spend money on changes that will have to be dismantled because they are benefitting one party at the expense of the other.

HEALTH EFFECTS OF COKE OVEN GASES

Scientific evidence including epidemiologic surveys, animal studies, and chemical analyses all support the finding that coke oven emissions are carcinogenic in humans at exposure levels encountered by coke oven workers in the 1950s. Among the diseases associated with CTPV are lung and urinary tract cancers, skin tumors, and nonmalignant respiratory diseases such as bronchitis and emphysema (Lloyd, et al., 1971; Redmond et al., 1972). The increased incidence of these diseases is well established and relatively well documented for coke oven workers.

While there is no doubt that coke oven workers are at increased risk of lung cancer, there is substantial doubt that people residing near coke ovens are at significantly greater risk. Measurements of CTPV in surrounding areas show that concentrations are more than a factor of 100 lower than those experienced by the most exposed workers. The epidemiologic studies do not show (and would not be expected to show) a statistically significant increase in cancer risk for even the coke oven workers exposed at low levels. Since these exposure levels are still much greater than those for the surrounding population, there is some direct indication that nearby residents may not be at significant risk. After doing a careful study for AISI, Lamm (1982) testified that a "significantly increased risk of lung cancer in the community from coke oven emissions in the ambient air is questionable." Thus, there is a fundamental issue about whether there is any risk to the surrounding population and thus a reason for any new EPA regulation.

A second reason that the public may not be at elevated risk from coke ovens is that the emissions are at an extremely high temperature and cool before they reach the surrounding community. The gases change rapidly and radically as they cool; gases condense forming small particles, large particles settle out, and the compounds oxidize. Thus, what coke oven workers breathe is likely to be substantially different from what nearby residents breathe. For example, the hot gases are extremely irritating to workers' respiratory tracts. After the gases have cooled, oxidized, and been diluted, they are much less irritating.

Epidemiologic studies of nearby residents could not reveal a statistically significant increase in lung or total cancer incidence unless the actual risk was much greater than that estimated by the EPA. Even if the population were subjected to exposures that produced an increase in cancers equal to the upper bound risk calculated by the EPA, an increase of 1 cancer per 1000 residents over their lives, this represents only a 2% increase in the cancer rate. This rate is much too small to detect using epidemiology. Is a 2% or smaller increase in the lung cancer rate for the most exposed population worth all the effort of an EPA regulation? We discuss risk goals below.

Assessing the Public Health Risk

NIOSH and the steel industry conducted an elaborate, ongoing epidemiologic study that discovered and quantified the excess cancer risks for coke oven workers (Lloyd, 1971; Redmond et al., 1972, 1976; Mazumdar et al., 1975). These epidemiologic studies are the basis of the OSHA and EPA risk analyses. Several difficulties need to be discussed explicitly, since each affects the risk analysis. We emphasize that this risk analysis is almost unique in having human data on both dose (although dose is inferred from 1960 data) and outcome (excess cancers) in the work setting of interest. Although there are uncertainties, they are small relative to the more usual case where no human data are available. In all but a few cases, it is only by assumption in extrapolating from rodent studies that a chemical is classified as a human carcinogen; the International Agency for Research on Cancer lists only 23 chemicals (or groups of chemicals) as having adequate human data to conclude that the chemical is a carcinogen.

Unfortunately, the coke oven studies share the shortcoming of many epidemiology studies in that they collected no data on cigarette smoking habits or on exposure levels for each workers. To remedy the lack of smoking data, Redmond et al. (1972) assumed that coke oven workers had smoking habits identical to those of other steel workers. Some assumption is needed since cigarette smoking vastly increases the relative risk of lung cancer, both by itself and in conjunction with other carcinogens. Even minor differences in the smoking histories of coke oven workers and steel workers more generally could imply that the risk estimates are biased. In particular, coke oven workers had dirtier, less desirable jobs than other steel workers, received generally lower pay, and a higher proportion of these workers were blacks. Such factors suggest the smoking rate would be higher for coke oven workers, which would suggest that too much risk is ascribed to coke oven gases and too little to their smoking habits.

The EPA (1984) has stated that any variation in smoking rates between coke oven workers and steel workers more generally is unlikely to overturn the fundamental result that coke oven emissions have increased lung cancer rates in workers. We agree with this conclusion. However, even a relatively small increase in smoking rates for coke oven workers compared to steel workers more generally would exert a major bias in the EPA's risk analysis. In particular, if coke oven workers smoke somewhat more cigarettes per day or for more years of their lives, the true risks to the surrounding population would be much smaller than the EPA estimates.

The lack of exposure data has been accounted for by assuming that CTPV levels observed in several coke ovens in 1960 characterize the exposures that these workers have received, by job category (Fannick et al., 1972; Mazumdar et al., 1975). In particular, the assumption has been made that coke ovens were no dirtier in the 1940s and 1950s and no cleaner more recently. The assumption seems doubtful since, after World War II, there was growing concern for worker health and safety and so it seems likely that conditions in coke ovens gradually improved. Furthermore, from the end of the depression to the end of the 1950s, the demand for steel was high. It seems evident that workers generally put in much more than 40 h each week and often there was no time or material to perform preventive maintenance or nonessential repairs. Thus, it seems likely that the additional number of hours worked and greater emissions from the ovens meant that workers received much greater exposures than the 1960 measurements suggest. If so, the actual dose is greater than the estimated dose and the risk estimates are biased upward. Thus, the cancer rates estimated from these data probably overstate the risks to people residing around coke ovens in the 1980s.

OSHA and EPA Approaches to Estimating the Low-Dose Response

The data on work history, along with the assumption that exposure levels have not changed over time, allow characterization of each worker's exposure. Cause of death data for each worker can be used to find the excess number of cancers in the population. With data on date of first exposure, length of exposure, total exposure, and whether the worker eventually died of cancer, it is possible to estimate a dose–response relation. Land (1976) estimated a dose–response relation for OSHA, and the EPA's (1984) Carcinogen Assessment Group and Lamm (1982b) reestimated the relation, although only the Land data were used in the reestimation.

The four major questions in estimating a relation are (i) the functional form to be used, (ii) the assumed lag between exposure and manifestation of the disease, (iii) whether to use the upper part of the 95% confidence interval rather than the maximum likelihood estimates from the dose–response relation, and (iv) whether to incorporate additional conservative assumptions regarding exposure. Lamm (1982, 1983) presents a good overview of the issues as well as detailed criticism of the EPA's method.

Coke ovens' workers are subjected to much greater exposures than surrounding residents. Thus, the dose–response relationship is estimated for these high exposure levels. Since the people residing near coke ovens are exposed to coke oven gases at exposures $\frac{1}{100}$ or less than workers, estimating the incidence of lung cancer for this population requires extrapolating the estimated dose–response relation far outside the range of observed exposure levels. Even a minor error in specifying the functional form of the dose–response relation could lead to a major error when extrapolating far outside the range of observed data.

The EPA is aware of this potential for error and has developed a procedure that is highly unlikely to underestimate the risk.

> This means that, unless there is specific, explicit information of the contrary, we will use the model that gives the highest risk at environmental levels of exposure, subject to the constraints that the model have an acceptable scientific basis and be consistent with the observed data. Therefore, our estimates should be viewed as plausible upper bounds of risk. (EPA, 1987, p. 156).

In other words, when there is inherent uncertainty, as in extrapolating estimates far outside the range of observed data, the EPA has tried to develop methods that will not underestimate the risk, and thus should be overestimating the risk by large amounts in most cases.

For example, the EPA refuses to choose the functional form (for the dose–response relation) that fits the data best:

> The maximum likelihood model cannot be regarded as a very prudent method of estimating risk at low exposure levels, especially when the experimental evidence indicates it is almost as likely that the risks are five orders of magnitude higher. We cannot simply use the best-fitting model to obtain our risk estimates without having the potential for seriously underestimating the true risk. (EPA, 1987, p. 154).

Instead, the EPA chooses the functional form that gives the greatest risk level. Even for this function, they do not choose the maximum likelihood estimates. Rather, the EPA calculates a 95% confidence interval around the parameters and chooses the upper bound of this interval to calculate population risk.

The EPA has built in a number of other conservative assumptions that should ensure that risk is not being underestimated when there is uncertainty. The EPA assumed that the coke ovens will continue operating into the indefinite future at full capacity 90% of the time, an assumption that is not consistent with the decline in the steel industry. They also assume that the population residing near the coke oven will experience the estimated outdoor ambient concentration of BSO 24 h/day for all of their lives. For this to be possible, people would have to eat, sleep, and work on their porches for 70 years of life. A building provides a barrier that keeps 20–40% of the outdoor pollutants outside. Since people only spend a couple hours a day outdoors, the EPA assumption is a large exaggeration of exposure. Furthermore, people usually leave the neighborhood to attend school, to seek medical care, shop, work, and vacation. Thus, it is evident that the EPA estimate of exposure is intended to be an upper bound of the range of possible exposures that residents may experience; whether it is a *plausible* upper bound is the question. If the assumed exposures are many times greater than people actually experience, the estimated cancer risks would be many times higher than they should be and the basis for the proposed new regulation would disappear.

A range of possible dose–response relationships for the epidemiologic data have been proposed. There is no compelling theoretical reason to select one of these forms as being more appropriate in this case. Thus, Land (1976), the EPA (1984), and Lamm (1982) estimate and present a range of different low-dose extrapolation models. Several of the models presented fit the data about equally well. Within the observed range of exposures, the models have similar implications concerning the implied increase in lung cancer incidence. However, for exposures 100 times smaller than those observed for workers, the models have quite different implications. Thus, estimating the response in the general population is sensitive to the choice of low-dose extrapolation model.

Land (1976) deals with the lag between exposure and manifestation of cancer in two ways. First, he assumes decreasing weighting factors for the 5 years of exposure just before

TABLE 1. Goodness of Fit of Cumulative Dose, Additive Risk Model, with Potency Being Age Dependent

	Linear	1.5	Quadratic	2.5	Cubic
			X^2 *Values (df = 12)*		
Zero lag	10.52	6.43	4.98	5.0	5.89
5-Year lag	12.62	9.96	10.08	11.71	14.21
10-Year lag	11.44	7.81	7.66	9.40	12.25
15-Year lag	9.47	9.22	11.23	14.13	17.32
			p Values		
Zero lag	0.56	0.89	0.96	0.96	0.92
5-Year lag	0.39	0.62	0.62	0.46	0.28
10-Year lag	0.48	0.80	0.81	0.67	0.42
15-Year lag	0.66	0.68	0.51	0.29	0.14

Source: Lamm (1982), Table 6.

death. Thus, exposure in the year before death is given almost no weight, that 2 years before death is given a bit more weight, and so on. Second, he assumes there is a further lag or latency period of up to 15 years in length. For example, for a lag of 15 years, the most recent 15 years of exposure would be disregarded in calculating total exposure, and the 5 years of exposure before that would be subject to declining weights. The basis for the assumption is that this additional lag is totally irrelevant in causing the cancer. This assumption seems questionable; for cigarette smoking, a 15-year lag would imply that the most recent 15 years of smoking exposure were irrelevant in causing lung cancer. Thus, after someone quit smoking, the risk of lung cancer should continue to rise for 15 years before leveling off or dropping (since relevant cumulative exposure would continue to increase). Cigarette smokers who quit immediately experience a leveling off of lung cancer risk and then a decrease in risk after 5–10 years, implying there is little or no lag. Supporting this notion are the findings of Land (1976) and Lamm (1982, 1983) that the model that fits the coke oven data best in one with zero lag.

Land (1976) estimated both the linear and quadratic forms and found that the quadratic, zero-lag relation fit the data best. Lamm (1982) fits a number of different functional forms and lag periods as shown in Table 1. A linear relation never fits the data as well as relation with exponents in the range of 2–3. For a linear relation, the best fit is obtained with a 15-year lag. However, for an exponent of 2–3, either the best fit occurs at a zero lag or a zero lag is about as good as the fit for a longer lag.

In nearly all cases, and for this study of coke ovens, the EPA (1984) rejected the nonlinear dose–response relation. The rejection is not based on scientific data or biological theory. Rather, they are attempting to ensure that they do not underestimate the risks. Thus, the EPA cites an example where a few changes in the data can produce large changes in the estimated coefficients and the implied risks at low exposure levels. Unfortunately, when the data base is small, changes in critical data points can produce precisely this result. However, the question is whether there is a reason to believe that errors of observation or missing data would be such as to bias the risk estimates downward. After all, a few changes in critical points could indicate that nearby residents are at essentially no risk. In short, the EPA has attempted to design risk estimation procedures that will not underestimate the true risks and will probably overstate them by a large margin.

The EPA approach is an arbitrary one in the name of prudent public health protection. Certainly, protecting public health calls for prudence. Unfortunately, the arbitrary approach of the EPA focuses on one part of the process, the low-dose response, and makes some arbitrary assumptions, such as the linear specification and the 95% confidence interval. A more systematic examination would look at possible errors in all aspects of the estimation and control and seek a conservative policy rather than being extremely conservative on one aspect (the functional form of the dose–response relation) and ignoring other espects. In this case, for example, the EPA biased the risk estimates downward by tending to underestimate the levels of CPTV in the surrounding communities.

Lamm has calculated the risks for a lifetime exposure to $1 \mu g/m^3$ of CTPV as shown in Table 2. Reading down the table, introducing a 10-year lag increases the risk by about 30%. Given the other problems, this is a trivial change. Reading across the top row, each increase of 0.5 in the exponent decreases the risk level by roughly a factor of 10. Thus, the linear form implies a risk of 1 cancer per 1000 lifetimes, the quadratic form implies 5.8 cancers per million lifetimes, and the cubic form 2.9 cancers per hundred-million lifetimes.

For the nonlinear relation, the higher the background level of CTPV, the greater will be

TABLE 2. Expected Cancer Deaths for 100 Million People Exposed for Their Lifetimes to 1 μg/m³ CTPV

	Linear	1.5	Quadratic	2.5	Cubic
		Excess Risk			
Zero lag					
Zero background	102,000	7,900	581	41	3
4 μg/m³ background[a]	101,000	21,500	5,230	990	176
10-Year lag					
Zero background	134,000	11,400	924	72	6
4 μg/m³ background[a]	133,000	36,300	8,320	1,730	341
		Relative Risk			
Zero lag					
Zero background	1.0226	1.0018	1.0001	1.0000	1.0000
4 μg/m³ background[a]	1.0206	1.0055	1.0012	1.0002	1.0000
10-Year lag					
Zero background	1.0296	1.0025	1.0002	1.0000	1.0000
4 μg/m³ background	1.0263	1.0079	1.0018	1.0004	1.0001

[a]Measured as BSO.
Source: Lamm (1982), Table 7.

the effects of 1 μg of CTPV. Thus, having a background level of 4 μg/m³ implies that the quadratic form gives an estimated cancer rate of 0.5 per million rather than 5 per million.

The bottom half of the table gives the relative risks of the increased exposure. The linear form implies a 2% increase in cancer risk; even this risk level is far too small to be detected in an epidemiologic study. The quadratic form implies a 0.01–0.1% increase, depending on the background level of CTPV. The relative risks of the cubic form are two orders of magnitude smaller.

The EPA's risk estimation procedure can be improved. Lamm's analysis is extremely helpful in putting the EPA estimates and the risks more generally into perspective. Which estimates are more valid or scientifically defensible depends on how one treats the coke oven worker data and how conservative a set of assumptions are deemed to be appropriate. We believe that the epidemiologists ought to do the best job they can in establishing the basic data on incidence of cancer and exposure, rather than being constrained by arbitrary policies designed to overestimate risks. Furthermore, they ought to estimate the standard deviation or range of expected errors about their data. Then the biometricians should estimate a range of dose–response relation exploring the effect of the range of possible errors. The data should be taken seriously in the sense that relation which do not fit it well or which fit it less well than others should be discarded. The aim of the analysis should be a best estimate of incidence of cancer in the affected population, along with a frequency distribution of the range of effects that might occur if the possible errors in the data are accounted for. This approach, while requiring somewhat more time and resources, would give a much more systematic view of risks to the exposed population. In light of the public health risks and enormous expenditure on control required by proposed regulations, devoting the time and resources to getting good risk estimates seems warranted.

COST EFFECTIVENESS OF THE STANDARDS

Under the EPA's assumptions that coke ovens operate at full capacity 90% of the time, they estimate that 720 Mg/yr of BSO would be released under current conditions. They appear to be assuming that OSHA standards will continue to be enforced to their current levels (i.e., not enforced) and that no new enforcement or new standards will be introduced.

The EPA has considered three control options. The first would require maintenance efforts to seal doors and offtakes better. The second would also require moderate capital expenditures to control emissions. The third would require rebuilding coke ovens.

The first option would reduce total emissions to 450 Mg/yr and cost $7 million per year. The EPA estimates that it would reduce the number of respiratory cancer deaths from 6.9 to 4.3/yr, a reduction of 2.6/yr. In addition, the lifetime risk for those most at risk would fall from 3.4 per 100 people to 1.6 per 100 people. The second control option would reduce total emissions to 420 Mg/yr at a cost of $19.3 million per year, or a reduction of 30 Mg/yr at a cost increase of $12.3 million per year, compared to option 1. Cancer deaths would fall to 4.0/yr, a reduction of 0.3 deaths compared to option 1. Those at highest risk would find their lifetime risks fell from 1.6 per 100 (option 1) to 1.4 per 100. Option 3 would reduce emissions to 100 Mg/yr at a cost of perhaps $500 million in capital costs or an implied annual cost of about $100 million. Thus, option 3 reduces emissions by 320 Mg/yr and increases costs $81 million per year over option 2. The number of cancer deaths due to coke oven emissions would be estimated to fall to 0.9/yr, a reduction of 3.1/yr compared to option 2. Those at highest risk would have their incidence of cancer fall from 14 per 1000 to 3 per 1000 lifetimes.

The EPA recommends the middle option with more maintenance work to seal doors or moderate capital expenditures to replace the worst equipment. It is interesting to calculate the cost effectiveness of each of the options compared to the previous option, bearing in mind all the caveats above about the upper bound nature of the estimates. Option 1 is estimated to save 2.6 lives per year at a cost of $7 million per year, or about $2.7 million per life saved. If the maximum likelihood estimate of the number of cancers averted were used instead of the 95% upper bound, the risks would be reduced by more than a factor of 10. If so, the cost would be more than $27 million per cancer averted. Option 2 saves an additional 0.3 deaths at an additional cost of $12.3 million or $41 million per life saved. Similarly, if the maximum likelihood estimate were used instead of the 95% upper bound, risks would be reduced by at least a factor of 10 and the cost would be more than $410 million per cancer averted. Option 3 is estimated to prevent 3.1 premature deaths at an additional cost of $81 million, or a cost of $26 million per life saved. If the maximum likelihood estimate were used, the cost per premature cancer averted would be more than $260 million.

The plausible upper bound approach to estimating risk may mislead the public and EPA decisionmakers. Presumably, in setting policy one wants to look at the expected number of lives saved, not the plausible upper bound estimate. The number of conservative assumptions made at each stage by the EPA leads us to believe that the risks to people residing near coke ovens may be zero and probably are two orders of magnitude lower than those of the EPA's upper bound. If so, the cost per cancer averted would be two orders of magnitude greater than those calculated above: $270 million for option 1, $4100 million for the incremental benefit of option 2, and $2600 million for the incremental benefit of option 3.

After considering the various options, the EPA chose option 2. The rationale for this choice is unclear and it certainly cannot be supported. Option 1 is a modest program that does not cost much and reduces the risk little. Presumably, it is rejected because it accomplishes too little risk reduction. If the EPA is taking action because it believes the risks to the public are too high, option 2 is an inadequate remedy because it still leaves them very high. Rather, the rationale seems to have more to do with what the industry is able to afford than the risk reduction benefits. Option 3 seems to be rejected because it requires very large investments to rebuild coke ovens, something that is unlikely to occur in a deteriorating steel industry, especially when future technology may obviate the need for coke.

CONCLUSION

The EPA's proposed regulation seems unjustified. As summarized in Table 3, the risk assessment procedure is extremely conservative, for example, in underestimating the dose received by coke oven workers, overestimating the exposure of the public, and making extreme assumptions in the low-dose extrapolation. If the EPA were overstating risks by merely a factor of 2, the basis for the regulation would disappear. There are many places in the analysis that would each suggest risks are being overstated by more than a factor of 2.

The control option recommended appears to be seeking lower risks and higher expenditures per cancer averted than are usually required by the EPA (Milvy, 1986; Travis

TABLE 3. Summary of Risk Analysis

Assumptions in Epidemiology

Worker exposure characterized by 1960 measurements: worker exposure is probably higher, which means risks are overestimated.

Coke oven workers assumed to smoke no more than other steel workers: they probably did smoke more and so risks are overestimated.

Assumptions in Risk Analysis

No threshold dose–response relation: cool, transformed, diluted emissions may pose no significant health risks to public.

Linear dose–response relation: quadratic model fits data better and so risks are overstated by a large amount.

Coke ovens assumed to operate at 90% of capacity: in a declining industry, this leads to overestimating exposures and thus risks.

People assumed to be exposed to outside air for every minute of their lives: in fact, they rarely are exposed to this air and thus risks are overstated.

Exposure characterized by diffusion models rather than actual measurements: exposures are probably understated and thus risks are understated.

Assumptions in Standards

Visible emissions standard since EPA assumptions of emissions cannot be measured: OSHA standard requires measuring emissions.

No coordination of EPA standard with existing OSHA standard.

EPA selected option 2, which has a much greater cost per cancer prevented than other EPA standards.

---

et al., 1987; Byrd and Lave, 1987). Similarly, the cost-effectiveness of the standard in terms of the cost of preventing a premature death is greater than most EPA decisions. Yet one cannot help but get the impression in reading the *Federal Register* notice that if the industry were booming and highly profitable, the EPA would have recommended option 3. For example, the EPA proposed a highly protective benzene standard for an industry that could afford it (Bartman, 1982).

OSHA has published regulations to protect the health of coke oven employees. The EPA has developed a proposed regulation to protect the general population living near these facilities. The process of standard setting for this industry reflects a general lack of communication and coordination between these two agencies, resulting in inconsistencies and contradictions and a general overstatement of the benefits to be derived from regulation. Since the agencies have turned their attention to coke ovens at different times, demanding different standards, the industry has a feeling of being embattled and wondering who is in charge. The real issue is not the need for a new EPA regulation; rather, it is enforcing existing regulations and handling explicitly the joint protection of workers and the public in a coordinated manner.

The only intellectually satisfactory solution is to regulate by industry, rather than by environmental medium or whether the risk is to workers or the general public. However, trying to bring each part of the EPA together with OSHA within a single agency is unlikely to produce an outcome that is either effective or likely to please the public. Short of bringing the agencies together, attention from the White House or Office of Management and Budget (OMB) might have forced OSHA and EPA to work on regulating coke ovens at the same time and to emphasize approaches that would simultaneously lower exposure to workers and the public. Alternatively, the OMB might have required the EPA to demonstrate that new regulations were required even if OSHA enforced existing regulations. The White House or Congress must exercise oversight responsibility when more than a single agency, or even when more than one group within a single agency, are acting to regulate the same aspects of an industry.

GLOSSARY

API	American Petroleum Institute
AISI	American Iron and Steel Institute
EPA	Environmental Protection Agency
OSHA	Occupational Safety and Health Administration
BSO	benzene-soluble organics
CTPV	coal tar pitch volatiles
BSFTPM	benzene-soluble fraction of total particulate matter; equivalent to BSO
PLL	percentage of leaking lids
PLD	percentage of leaking doors
PLO	percentage of leaking offtakes
mg	milligrams
$\mu g/m^3$	micrograms per cubic meter
Mg	megagrams

ACKNOWLEDGMENTS

This work was supported in part by National Science Foundation grant SES-8715564. We thank Steven Lamm for providing us with extensive unpublished material and for answering our questions. For helpful discussions we thank John Mendeloff, Harold Paxton, Morton Corn, Michael Wright, and Philip Masciantonio.

REFERENCES

Bartman, T. R. (1982). Regulating benzene. In L. B. Lave, Ed., *Quantitative Risk Assessment in Regulation*. Brookings Institution, Washington, DC.

Briggs, D. D., and Lave, L. B. (1982). Regulating coke oven emissions. In L. B. Lave, Ed., *Quantitative Risk Assessment in Regulation*. Brookings Institution, Washington, DC, 1982.

Byrd, D., and Lave, L. B. (1987a). Significant risk is not the antonym of de minimis risk. In C. Whipple, Ed., *De Minimis Risk*. Plenum Press, New York.

Byrd, D., and Lave, L. B. (1987b). Narrowing the range: A framework for risk regulators. *Issues Sci. Technol.* **3**, 92–100.

Environmental Protection Agency (1984). *Carcinogen Assessment of Coke Oven Emissions*. EPA, Washington, DC.

Environmental Protection Agency (1987a). National emission standards for hazardous air pollutants: Coke oven emissions from wet-coal charged by-product coke oven batteries; proposed rule and notice of public hearing. *Fed. Regist.* **52**(78), 13586—13606 (1987).

Environmental Protection Agency (1987b). *Coke Oven Emissions from Wet-Coal Charged By-Product Coke Oven Batteries—Background Information for Proposed Standards*, Draft EIS. EPA, Research Triangle Park, NC, April 1987.

Fannick, N., Gonshor, L. T., and Shockley, J., Jr. (1972). Exposure to coal tar pitch volatiles at coke ovens. *Am. Ind. Hyg. Assoc. J.* **33**, 461–468.

Lamm, S. H. (1982a). *Statement of Dr. Steven H. Lamm on the Draft Carcinogen Assessment of Coke Oven Emissions Before the Environmental Health Committee*. Environment Protection Agency, Washington, DC, August 3, 1982.

Lamm, S. H. (1982b). *Evaluation of the Carcinogen Assessment Group's Revised Carcinogen Assessment of Coke Oven Emissions*. CEOH, Washington, DC, December 9, 1982.

Lamm, S. H. (1983a). *Supplemental Report of Dose-Response Analysis for Community Exposure to Coke Oven Emissions in the Ambient Air*. CEOH, Washington, DC, March 15, 1983.

Lamm, S. H. (1983b). *Comments on Carcinogen Assessment Group's Quantitative Section of the Carcinogen Assessment of Coke Oven Emissions, EPA-CAG*. CEOH, Washington, DC, September 23, 1983.

Land C. E. (1976). Presentation to OSHA Hearings on Coke Oven Standards, May 4, 1976.

Lloyd, J. W. (1971). Long-term mortality study of steelworkers. V. Respiratory cancer in coke plant workers. *J. Occup. Med.* **13**, 53–68.

Mazumdar, S., Redmond, C., Sollecito, W., and Sussman, N. (1975). An epidemiological study of exposure to coal tar pitch volatiles among coke oven workers. *J. Air Pollut. Control Assoc.* **25**, 382–389.

Milvy, P. (1986). A general guideline for management of risk from carcinogens. *Risk Anal.* **6**, 60–80.

Occupational Safety and Health Administration (OSHA) (1976). Exposure to coke oven emissions. *Fed. Regist.* **41**(206) (1976).

Redmond, C. K., Ciocco, A., Lloyd, J. W., and Rush, H. W. (1972). Long-term mortality study of steelworkers. VI. Mortality from malignant neoplasms among coke oven workers. *J. Occup. Med.* **14**, 621–629.

Redmond, C. R., Strobino, B. R., and Cypess, R. H. (1976). Cancer experience among coke by-product workers. *Ann. N.Y. Acad. Sci.* **271**, 102–115.

Travis, C. C., Richter, S. A., Crouch, E. A. C., Wilson, R., and Klema, E. D. (1987). Cancer risk management: A review of 132 federal regulatory decisions. *Environ. Sci. Technol.* **21**, 415–420.

33

Ranking Possible Carcinogens: One Approach to Risk Management*

Bruce N. Ames

Department of Biochemistry, University of California, Berkeley, California

Renae Magaw and Lois Swirsky Gold

Biology and Medicine Division, Lawrence Berkeley Laboratory, Berkeley, California

INTRODUCTION

Epidemiologists estimate that at least 70% of human cancer would, in principle, be preventable if the main risk and antirisk factors could be identified (1). This is because the incidence of specific types of cancer differs markedly in different parts of the world where people have different life-styles. For example, colon and breast cancer, which are among the major types of cancer in the United States, are quite rare among Japanese in Japan, but not among Japanese-Americans. Epidemiologists are providing important clues about the specific causes of human cancer, despite inherent methodological difficulties. They have identified tobacco as an avoidable cause of about 30% of all U.S. cancer deaths and of an even larger number of deaths from other causes (1, 2). Less specifically, dietary factors, or their absence, have been suggested in many studies to contribute to a substantial proportion of cancer deaths, though the intertwined risk and antirisk factors are being identified only slowly (1, 3, 4). High fat intake may be a major contributor to colon cancer, though the evidence is not as definitive as that for the role of saturated fat in heart disease or of tobacco in lung cancer. Alcoholic beverage consumption, particularly by smokers, has been estimated to contribute to about 3% of U.S. cancer deaths (1) and to an even larger number of deaths from other causes. Progress in prevention has been made for some occupational factors, such as asbestos, to which workers used to be heavily exposed, with delayed effects that still contribute to about 2% of U.S. cancer deaths (1, 5). Prevention may also become possible for hormone-related cancers such as breast cancer (1, 6) or virus-

*Reprinted from Bruce N. Ames, Renae Magaw, and Lois Swirsky Gold, Ranking Possible Carcinogenic Hazards, *Science* **236**, 271–280 (1987). Copyright © 1987 AAAs.

related cancers such as liver cancer (hepatitis B) and cancer of the cervix (papilloma virus HPV16) (1, 7).

Animal bioassays and in vitro studies are also providing clues as to which carcinogens and mutagens might be contributing to human cancer. However, the evaluation of carcinogenicity in rodents is expensive and the extrapolation to humans is difficult (8– 11). We will use the term "possible hazard" for estimates based on rodent cancer tests and "risk" for those based on human cancer data (10).

Extrapolation from the results of rodent cancer tests done at high doses to effects on humans exposed to low doses is routinely attempted by regulatory agencies when formulating policies attempting to prevent future cancer. There is little sound scientific basis for this type of extrapolation, in part due to our lack of knowledge about mechanisms of cancer induction, and it is viewed with great unease by many epidemiologists and toxicologists (5, 9–11). Nevertheless, to be prudent in regulatory policy, and in the absence of good human data (almost always the case), some reliance on animal cancer tests is unavoidable. The best use of them should be made even though few, if any, of the main avoidable causes of human cancer have typically been the types of synthetic chemicals that are being tested in animals (10). Human cancer may, in part, involve agents such as hepatitis B virus, which causes chronic inflammation; changes in hormonal status; deficiencies in normal protective factors (such as selenium or β-carotene) against endogenous carcinogens (12); lack of other anticarcinogens (such as dietary fiber or calcium) (4); or dietary imbalances such as excess consumption of fat (3, 4, 12) or salt (13).

There is a need for more balance in animal cancer testing to emphasize the foregoing factors and natural chemicals as well as synthetic chemicals (12). There is increasing evidence that our normal diet contains many rodent carcinogens, all perfectly natural or traditional (e.g., from the cooking of food) (12), and that no human diet can be entirely free of mutagens or agents that can be carcinogenic in rodent systems. We need to identify the important causes of human cancer among the vast number of minimal risks. This requires knowledge of both the amounts of a substance to which humans are exposed and its carcinogenic potency.

Animal cancer tests can be analyzed quantitatively to give an estimate of the relative carcinogenic potencies of the chemicals tested. We have previously published our Carcinogenic Potency Database, which showed that rodent carcinogens vary in potency by more than 10 millionfold (14).

This chapter attempts to achieve some perspective on the plethora of possible hazards to humans from exposure to known rodent carcinogens by establishing a scale of the possible hazards for the amounts of various common carcinogens to which humans might be chronically exposed. We view the value of our calculations not as providing a basis for absolute human risk assessment, but as a guide to priority setting. One problem with this type of analysis is that few of the many natural chemicals we are exposed to in very large amounts (relative to synthetic chemicals) have been tested in animals for carcinogenicity. Thus, our knowledge of the background levels of human exposure to animal carcinogens is fragmentary, biased in favor of synthetic chemicals, and limited by our lack of knowledge of human exposures.

RANKING OF POSSIBLE CARCINOGENIC HAZARDS

Since carcinogens differ enormously in potency, a comparison of possible hazards from various carcinogens ingested by humans must take this into account. The measure of

Table 1. Ranking Possible Carcinogenic Hazards

Possible Hazard: HERP (%)[a]	Daily Human Exposure[b]	Carcinogen Dose per 70-kg Person	Potency of Carcinogen: TD$_{50}$ (mg/kg)[c]		References
			Rats	Mice	
Environmental Pollution					
0.001*	Tap water, 1 L	Chloroform, 83 µg (U.S. average)	(119)	90	96
0.004*	Well water, 1 L contaminated (worst well in Silicon Valley)	Trichloroethylene, 2800 µg	(−)	941	97
0.0004*	Well water, 1 L contaminated, Woburn	Trichloroethylene, 267 µg	(−)	941	98
0.0002*		Chloroform, 12 µg	(119)	90	
0.0003*		Tetrachloroethylene, 21 µg	101	(126)	
0.008*	Swimming pool, 1 h (for child)	Chloroform, 250 µg (average pool)	(119)	90	99
0.6	Conventional home air (14 h/day)	Formaldehyde, 598 µg	1.5	(44)	100
0.004		Benzene, 155 µg	(157)	53	
2.1	Mobile home air (14 h/day)	Formaldehyde, 2.2 mg	1.5	(44)	28
Pesticide and Other Residues					
0.0002*	PCBs: daily dietary intake	PCBs, 0.2 µg (U.S. average)	1.7	(9.6)	101
0.0003*	DDE/DDT: daily dietary intake	DDE, 2.2 µg (U.S. average)	(−)	13	16
0.0004	EDB: daily dietary intake (from grains and grain products)	Ethylene dibromide, 0.42 µg (U.S. average)	1.5	(5.1)	102
Natural Pesticides and Dietary Toxins					
0.003	Bacon, cooked (100 g)	Dimethylnitrosamine, 0.3 µg	(0.2)	0.2	40
0.006	Sake (250 mL)	Diethylnitrosamine, 0.1 µg	0.02	(+)	
0.003		Urethane, 43 µg	(41)	22	24
0.03	Comfrey herb tea, 1 cup	Symphytine, 38 µg (750 µg of pyrrolizidine alkaloids)	1.9	(?)	103
0.03	Peanut butter (32 g; one sandwich)	Aflatoxin, 64 ng (U.S. average, 2 ppb)	0.003	(+)	18
0.06	Dried squid, broiled in gas oven (54 g)	Dimethylnitrosamine, 7.9 µg	(0.2)	0.2	37
0.07	Brown mustard (5 g)	Allyl isothiocyanate, 4.6 mg	96	(−)	47
0.1	Basil (1 g of dried leaf)	Estragole, 3.8 mg	(?)	52	48

HERP (%)	Daily human exposure	Carcinogen and dose per 70 kg	Potency (TD₅₀)		Reference
0.1	Mushroom, one raw (15 g) (*Agaricus bisporus*)	Mixture of hydrazines, and so forth	(?)	20,300	104
0.2	Natural root beer (12 oz; 354 mL) (now banned)	Safrole, 6.6 mg	(436)	56	105
0.008	Beer, before 1979 (12 oz; 354 mL)	Dimethylnitrosamine, 1 µg	(0.2)	0.2	38
2.8*	Beer (12 oz; 354 mL)	Ethyl alcohol, 18 ml	9110	(?)	23
4.7*	Wine (250 mL)	Ethyl alcohol, 30 ml	9110	(?)	23
6.2	Comfrey-pepsin tablets (nine daily)	Comfrey root, 2700 mg	626	(?)	103
1.3	Comfrey-pepsin tablets (nine daily)	Symphytine, 1.8 mg	1.9		
	Food Additives				
0.0002	AF-2: daily dietary intake before banning	AF-2 (furylfuramide), 4.8 µg	29	(131)	44
0.06*	Diet cola (12 ounces; 354 mL)	Saccharin, 95 mg	2143	(−)	106
	Drugs				
[0.3]	Phenacetin pill (average dose)	Phenacetin, 300 mg	1246	(2137)	51
[5.6]	Metronidazole (therapeutic dose)	Metronidazole, 2000 mg	(542)	506	107
[14]	Isoniazid (prophylactic dose)	Isoniazid, 300 mg	(150)	30	108
16*	Phenobarbital, one sleeping pill	Phenobarbital, 60 mg	(+)	5.5	50
17*	Clofibrate (average daily dose)	Clofibrate, 2000 mg	169	(?)	52
	Occupational Exposure				
5.8	Formaldehyde: workers' average daily intake	Formaldehyde, 6.1 mg	1.5	(44)	109
140	EDB: workers' daily intake (high exposure)	Ethylene dibromide, 150 mg	1.5	(5.1)	55

[a]Asterisks indicate HERP from carcinogens thought to be nongenotoxic. The amount of rodent carcinogen indicated under carcinogen dose is divided by 70 kg to give a milligram per kilogram of human exposure, and this human dose is given as the percentage of the TD_{50} dose in the rodent (in milligrams per kilogram) to calculate the human exposure/rodent potency index (HERP).

[b]We have tried to use average or reasonable daily intakes to facilitate comparisons. In several cases, such as contaminated well water or factory exposure to EDB, this is difficult to determine, and we give the value for the worst found and indicate pertinent information in the References and Notes. The calculations assume a daily dose for a lifetime; where drugs are normally taken for only a short period, we have bracketed the HERP value. For inhalation exposures we assume an inhalation of 9 600 L/8 h for the workplace and 10,800 L/14 h for indoor air at home.

[c]A number in parentheses indicates a TD_{50} value not used in HERP calculation because it is the less sensitive species; (−) = negative in cancer test. (+) = positive for carcinogenicity in test(s) not suitable for calculating a TD_{50}; (?) = is not adequately tested for carcinogenicity. TD_{50} values shown are averages calculated by taking the harmonic mean of the TD_{50}'s of the positive tests in that species from the Carcinogenic Potency Database. Results are similar if the lowest TD_{50} value (most potent) is used instead. For each test the target site with the lowest TD_{50} value has been used. The average TD_{50} has been calculated separately for rats and mice, and the more sensitive species is used for calculating the possible hazard. The database, with references to the source of the cancer tests, is complete for tests published through 1984 and for the National Toxicology Program bioassays through June 1986 (14). We have not indicated the route of exposure or target sites or other particulars of each test, although these are reported in the database.

potency that we have developed, the TD_{50}, is the daily dose rate (in milligrams per kilogram) to halve the percentage of tumor-free animals by the end of a standard lifetime (14). Since the TD_{50} (analogous to the LD_{50}) is a dose rate, the lower the TD_{50} value the more potent the carcinogen. To calculate our index of possible hazard we express each human exposure (daily lifetime dose in milligrams per kilogram) as a percentage of the rodent TD_{50} dose (in milligrams per kilogram) for each carcinogen. We call this percentage HERP [human exposure dose/rodent potency dose]. The TD_{50} values are taken from our ongoing Carcinogenic Potency Database (currently 3500 experiments on 975 chemicals), which reports the TD_{50} values estimated from experiments in animals (14). Human exposures have been estimated from the literature as indicated. As rodent data are all calculated on the basis of lifetime exposure at the indicated daily dose rate (14), the human exposure data are similarly expressed as lifelong daily dose rates even though the human exposure is likely to be less than daily for a lifetime.

It would be a mistake to use our HERP index as a direct estimate of human hazard. First, at low dose rates human susceptibility may differ systematically from rodent susceptibility. Second, the general shape of the dose–response relation is not known. A linear dose response has been the dominant assumption in regulating carcinogens for many years, but this may not be correct. If the dose responses are not linear but are actually quadratic or hockey-stick shaped or show a threshold, then the actual hazard at low dose rates might be much less than the HERP values would suggest. An additional difficulty is that it may be necessary to deal with carcinogens that differ in their mechanisms of action and thus in their dose–response relation. We have therefore put an asterisk next to HERP values for carcinogens that do not appear to be active through a genotoxic (DNA damaging or mutagenic) mechanism (15) so that comparisons can be made within the genotoxic or nongenotoxic classes.

Table 1 presents our HERP calculations of possible cancer hazards in order to compare them within several categories so that, for example, pollutants of possible concern can be compared to natural carcinogens in the diet. A convenient reference point is the possible hazard from the carcinogen chloroform in a liter of average (U.S.) chlorinated tap water, which is close to a HERP of 0.001%. Chloroform is a by-product of water chlorination, which protects us from pathogenic viruses and bacteria.

Contaminated Water

The possible hazards from carcinogens in contaminated well water [e.g., Santa Clara ("Silicon") Valley, California, or Woburn, Massachusetts] should be compared to the possible hazard of ordinary tap water (Table 1). Of 35 wells shut down in Santa Clara Valley because of their supposed carcinogenic hazard, only two have HERP values greater than ordinary tap water. Well water is not usually chlorinated and typically lacks the chloroform present in chlorinated tap water. Water from the most polluted well (HERP = 0.004% per liter for trichloroethylene), as indicated in Table 1, has a HERP value orders of magnitude less than for the carcinogens in an equal volume of cola, beer, or wine. Its HERP value is also much lower than that of many of the common natural foods that are listed in Table 1, such as the average peanut butter sandwich. Caveats for any comparisons are given below. Since the consumption of tap water is only about 1 or 2 L/day, the animal evidence provides no good reason to expect that chlorination of water or current levels of synthetic pollution of water pose a significant carcinogenic hazard.

Pesticide Residues

Intake of synthetic pesticide residues from food in the United States, including residues of industrial chemicals such as polychlorinated biphenyls (PCBs), averages about 150 μg/day. Most (105 μg) of this intake is composed of three chemicals (ethylhexyl diphenyl phosphate, malathion, and chlorpropham) shown to be noncarcinogenic in tests in rodents (16). A carcinogenic pesticide residue in food of possible concern is DDE, the principal metabolite (> 90%) of DDT (16). The average U.S. daily intake of DDE from DDT (HERP = 0.0003%) is equivalent to the HERP of the chloroform in one glass of tap water and thus appears to be insignificant compared to the background of natural carcinogens in our diet (Table 1). Even daily consumption of 100 times the average intake of DDE/DDT or PCBs would produce a possible hazard that is small compared to other common exposures shown in Table 1.

Nature's Pesticides

We are ingesting in our diet at least 10,000 times more by weight of natural pesticides than of synthetic pesticide residues (12). These are natural "toxic chemicals" that have an enormous variety of chemical structures, appear to be present in all plants, and serve to protect plants against fungi, insects, and animal predators (12). Though only a few are present in each plant species, they commonly make up 5–10% of the plant's dry weight (12). There has been relatively little interest in the toxicology or carcinogenicity of these compounds until quite recently, although they are by far the main source of "toxic chemicals" ingested by humans. Only a few dozen of the thousands present in the human diet have been tested in animal bioassays, and only some of these tests are adequate for estimating potency in rodents (14). A sizable proportion of those that have been tested are carcinogens, and many others have been shown to be mutagens (12), so it is probable that many more will be found to be carcinogens if tested. Those shown in Table 1 are estragole (HERP = 0.1% for a daily 1 g of dried basil), safrole (HERP = 0.2% for a daily natural root beer), symphytine (a pyrrolizidine alkaloid, 0.03% for a daily cup of comfrey tea), comfrey tablets sold in health food stores (6.2% for a daily dose), hydrazines in mushrooms (0.1% for one daily raw mushroom), and allyl isothiocyanate (0.07% for a daily 5 g of brown mustrad).

Plants commonly produce very much larger amounts of their natural toxins when damaged by insects or fungi (12). For example, psoralens, light-activated carcinogens in celery, increase 100-fold when the plants are damaged by mold and, in fact, can cause an occupational disease in celery-pickers and in produce-checkers at supermarkets (12, 17).

Mold synthesize a wide variety of toxins, apparently as antibiotics in the microbiological struggle for survival: over 300 mycotoxins have been described (18). They are common pollutants of human food, particularly in the tropics. A considerable percentage of those tested have been shown to be mutagens and carcinogens: some, such as aflatoxin and sterigmatocystin, are among the most potent known rodent carcinogens. The potency of aflatoxin in different species varies widely; thus, a bias may exist as the HERP uses the most sensitive species. The aflatoxin content of U.S. peanut butter averages 2 ppb, which corresponds to a HERP of 0.03% for the peanut butter in an average sandwich (Table 1). The Food and Drug Administration (FDA) allows 10 times this level (HERP = 0.3%), and certain foods can often exceed the allowable limit (18). Aflatoxin contaminates wheat, corn (perhaps the main source of dietary aflatoxin in the United States), and nuts, as well as a wide variety of stored carbohydrate foodstuffs. A carcinogenic, though less potent, metabolite of alfatoxin is found in milk from cows that eat moldy grain.

There is epidemiologic evidence that aflatoxin is a human carcinogen. High intake in the tropics is associated with a high rate of liver cancer, at least among those chronically infected with the Hepatitis B virus (19, 20). Considering the potency of those mold toxins that have been tested and the widespread contamination of food with molds, they may represent the most significant carcinogenic pollution of the food supply in developing countries. Such pollution is much less severe in industrialized countries, due to refrigeration and modern techniques of agriculture and storage, including use of synthetic pesticides and fumigants.

Food Preparation

Preparation of foods and beverages can also produce carinogens. Alcohol has been shown to be a human carcinogen in numerous epidemiologic studies (1, 21). Both alcohol and acetaldehyde, its major metabolite, are carcinogens in rats (22, 23). The carcinogenic potency of ethyl alcohol in rats is remarkably low (23), and it is among the weakest carcinogens in our database. However, human intake of alcohol is very high (about 18 g per beer), so that the possible hazards shown in Table 1 for beer and wine are large (HERP = 2.8% for a daily beer). The possible hazard of alcohol is enormous relative to that from the intake of synthetic chemical residues. If alcohol (20), trichloroethylene, DDT, and other presumptive nongenotoxic carcinogens are active at high doses because they are tumor promoters, the risk from low doses may be minimal.

Other carcinogens are present in beverages and prepared foods. Urethane (ethyl carbamate), a particularly well-studied rodent carcinogen, is formed from ethyl alcohol and carbamyl phosphate during a variety of fermentations and is present in Japanese sake (HERP = 0.003%), many types of wine and beer, and in smaller amounts in yogurt and bread (24). Another fermentation product, the dicarbonyl aldehyde methylglyoxal, is a potent mutagen and was isolated as the main mutagen in coffee (about 250 μg in one cup). It was recently shown to be a carcinogen, though not in a test suitable for calculating a TD_{50} (25). Methylglyoxal is also present in a variety of other foods, such as tomato puree (25, 26). Diacetyl (2, 3-butanedione), a closely related dicarbonyl compound, is a fermentation product in wine and a number of other foods and is responsible for the aroma of butter. Diacetyl is a mutagen (27) but has not been tested for carcinogenicity.

Formaldehyde, another natural carcinogenic and mutagenic aldehyde, is also present in many common foods (22, 26–28). Formaldehyde gas caused cancer only in the nasal turbinates of the nose-breathing rodents and even though formaldehyde is genotoxic, the dose response was nonlinear (28, 29). Hexamethylenetetramine, which decomposes to formaldehyde in the stomach, was negative in feeding studies (30). The effects of oral versus inhalation exposure for formaldehyde remain to be evaluated more thoroughly.

As formaldehyde is almost ubiquitous in foods, one can visualize various formaldehyde-rich scenarios. Daily consumption of shrimp (HERP = 0.09% per 100 g) (31), a sandwich (HERP of two slices of bread = 0.4%) (22), a cola (HERP = 2.7%) (32), and a beer (HERP = 0.2%) (32) in various combinations could provide as much formaldehyde as living in some mobile homes (HERP = 2.1%; Table 1). Formaldehyde is also generated in animals metabolically, for example, from methoxy compounds that humans ingest in considerable amounts from plants. The level of formaldehyde reported in normal human blood is strikingly high (about 100 μM or 3000 ppb) (33) suggesting that detoxification mechanisms are important.

The cooking of food generates a variety of mutagens and carcinogens. Nine heterocyclic amines, isolated on the basis of their mutagenicity from proteins or amino acids that were heated in ways that occur in cooking, have now been tested; all have been shown to be potent carcinogens in rodents (34). Many others are still being isolated and characterized (34). An approximate HERP of 0.02% has been calculated by Sugimura et al. for the daily intake of these nine carcinogens (34). Three mutagenic nitropyrenes present in diesel exhaust have now been shown to be carcinogens (35), but the intake of these carcinogenic nitropyrenes has been estimated to be much higher from grilled chicken than from air pollution (34, 36). The total amount of browned and burnt material eaten in a typical day is at least several hundred times more than that inhaled from severe air pollution (12).

Gas flames generate NO_2, which can form both the carcinogenic nitropyrenes (35, 36) and the potently carcinogenic nitrosamines in food cooked in gas ovens, such as fish or squid (HERP = 0.06%; Table 1) (37). We suspect that food cooked in gas ovens may be a major source of dietary nitrosamines and nitropyrenes, though it is not clear how significant a risk these post. Nitrosamines were ubiquitous in beer and ale (HERP = 0.008%) and were formed from NO_2 in the gas-flame-heated air used to dry the malt. However, the industry has switched to indirect heating, which resulted in markedly lower levels (<1 ppb) of dimethylnitrosamine (38). The dimethylnitrosamine found in human urine is thought to be formed in part from NO_2 inhaled from kitchen air (39). Cooked bacon contains several nitrosamines (HERP = 0.009%). (40).

Oxidation Reactions

Oxidation of fats and vegetable oils occurs during cooking and also spontaneously if antioxidant levels are low. The result is the formation of peroxides, epoxides, and aldehydes, all of which appear to be rodent carcinogens (8, 12, 27). Fatty acid hydroperoxides (present in oxidized oils) and cholesterol epoxide have been shown to be rodent carcinogens (though not in tests suitable for calculating a TD_{50}). Dried eggs contain about 25 ppm of cholesterol epoxide (a sizable amount), a result of the oxidation of cholesterol by the NO_2 in the drying air that is warmed by gas flames (12).

Normal oxidation reactions in fruit (such as browning in a cut apple) also involve production of peroxides. Hydrogen peroxide is a mutagenic rodent carcinogen that is generated by oxidation of natural phenolic compounds that are quite widespread in edible plants. A cup of coffee contains about 750 μg of hydrogen peroxide (25); however, since hydrogen peroxide is a very weak carcinogen (similar in potency to alcohol), the HERP for drinking a daily cup of coffee would be very low [comparable to DDE/DDT, PCBs, or ethylene dibromide (EDB) dietary intakes]. Hydrogen peroxide is also generated in our normal metabolism; human blood contains about 5 μM hydrogen peroxide and 0.3 μM of the cholesterol ester of fatty acid hydroperoxide (41). Endogenous oxidants such as hydrogen peroxide may make a major contribution to cancer and aging (42).

Caloric Intake

Caloric intake, which could be considered the most striking rodent carcinogen ever discovered, is discussed remarkably little in relation to human cancer. It has been known for about 40 years that increasing the food intake in rats and mice by about 20% above optimal causes a remarkable decrease in longevity and a striking increase in endocrine and mammary tumors (43). In humans, obesity (associated with high caloric intake) leads to increased levels of circulating estrogens, a significant cause of endometrial and gallbladder cancer. The effects of moderate obesity on other types of human cancer are less clear (1).

Food Additives

Food additives are currently screened for carcinogenicity before use if they are synthetic compounds. AF-2 (HERP = 0.0002%), a food perservative, was banned in Japan (44). Saccharin (HERP = 0.06%) is currently used in the United States (the dose response in rats, however, is clearly sublinear) (45). The possible hazard of diethylstilbestrol residues in meat from treated farm animals seems miniscule relative to endogenous estrogenic hormones and plant estrogens (46). Some natural carcinogens are also widely used as additives, such as allyl isothiocyanate (47), estragole (48), and alcohol (23).

Air Pollution

A person inhales about 20,000 L of air in a day; thus, even modest contamination of the atmosphere can result in inhalation of appreciable doses of a pollutant. This can be seen in the possible hazard in mobile homes from formaldehyde (HERP = 2.1%) or in conventional homes from formaldehyde (HERP = 0.6%) or benzene (HERP = 0.004%; Table 1). Indoor air pollution is, in general, worse than outdoor air pollution, partly because of cigarette smoke. The most important indoor air pollutant may be radon gas. Radon is a natural radioactive gas that is present in the soil, gets trapped in houses, and gives rise to radioactive decay products that are known to be carcinogenic for humans (49). It has been estimated that in 1 million homes in the United States the level of exposure of products of radon decay may be higher than that received by today's uranium miners. Two particularly contaminated houses were found that had a risk estimated to be equivalent to receiving about 1200 chest x-rays a day (49). Approximately 10% of the lung cancer in the United States has been tentatively attributed to radon pollution in houses (49). Many of these cancers might be preventable since the most hazardous houses can be identified and modified to minimize radon contamination.

General outdoor air pollution appears to be a small risk relative to the pollution inhaled by a smoker: one must breathe Los Angeles smog for a year to inhale the same amount of burnt material that a smoker (two packs) inhales in a day (12), though air pollution is inhaled starting from birth. It is difficult to determine cancer risk from outdoor air pollution since epidemiologists must accurately control for smoking and radon.

Drugs

Some common drugs shown in Table 1 give fairly high HERP percentages, primarily because the dose ingested is high. However, since most medicinal drugs are used for only short periods while the HERP index is a daily dose rate for a lifetime, the possible hazard would usually be markedly less. We emphasize this in Table 1 by bracketing the numbers for these shorter exposures. Phenobarbital (HERP = 16%) was investigated thoroughly in humans who had taken it for decades, and there was no convincing evidence that it caused cancer (50). There is evidence of increased renal cancer in long-term human ingestion of phenacetin, an analgesic (51). Acetaminophen, a metabolite of phenacetin, is one of the most widely used over-the-counter pain killers. Clofibrate (HERP = 17%) is used as a hypolipidemic agent and is thought to be carcinogenic in rodents because it induces hydrogen peroxide production through peroxisome proliferation (52).

Occupational Exposures

Occupational exposures can be remarkably high, particularly for volatile carcinogens, because about 10,000 L of air are inhaled in a working day. For formaldehyde, the exposure to an average worker (HERP = 5.8%) is higher than most dietary intakes. For a number of volatile industrial carcinogens, the ratio of the permitted exposure limit [U.S. Occupational Safety and Health Administration (OSHA)] in milligrams per kilogram to the TD_{50} has been calculated; several are close to the TD_{50} in rodents and about two-thirds have permitted HERP values > 1% (53). The possible hazard estimated for the actual exposure levels of the most heavily exposed EDB workers is remarkably high, HERP = 140% (Table 1). Though the dose may have been somewhat overestimated (54), it was still comparable to the dose causing cancer in half the rodents. An epidemologic study of these heavily exposed EDB workers who inhaled EDB for over a decade did not show any increase in cancer, though because of the limited duration of exposure and the relatively small numbers of people monitored the study would not have detected a small effect (54, 55). OSHA still permits exposures above the TD_{50} level. California, however, lowered the permitted level over 100-fold in 1981. In contrast with these heavy workplace exposures, the Environmental Protection Agency (EPA) has banned the use of EDB for fumigation because of the residue levels found in grain (HERP = 0.0004%).

UNCERTAINTIES IN RELYING ON ANIMAL CANCER TESTS FOR HUMAN PREDICTION

Species Variation

Though we list a possible hazard if a chemical is a carcinogen in a rat but not in a mouse (or vice versa), this lack of agreement raises the possibility that the risk to humans is nonexistent. Of 392 chemicals in our database tested in both rats and mice, 226 were carcinogens in at least one test, but 96 of these were positive in the mouse and negative in the rat or vice versa (56). This discordance occurs despite the fact that rats and mice are very closely related and have short life spans. Qualitative extrapolation of cancer risks from rats or mice to humans, a very dissimilar long-lived species, is unlikely to be as reliable. Conversely, important human carcinogens may not be detected in standard tests in rodents; this was true for a long time for both tobacco smoke and alcohol, the two largest identified causes of neoplastic death in the United States.

For many of the chemicals considered rodent carcinogens, there may be negative as well as positive tests. It is difficult to deal with negative results satisfactorily for several reasons, including the fact that some chemicals are tested only once or twice, while others are tested many times. The HERP index ignores negative tests. Where there is species variation in potency, use of the more sensitive species, as is generally done and as is done here, could introduce a tendency to overestimate possible hazards; however, for most chemicals that are positive in both species, the potency is similar in rats and mice (57). The HERP may provide a rough correlate of human hazard from chemical exposure; however, for a given chemical, to the extent that the potency in humans differs from the potency in rodents, the relative hazard would be different.

Quantitative Uncertainties

Quantitative extrapolation from rodents to humans, particularly at low doses, is guesswork that we have no way of validating (1, 5, 10, 11, 58). It is guesswork because of lack of knowledge in at least six major areas: (i) the basic mechanisms of carcinogenicity; (ii) the relation of cancer, aging, and life span (1, 10, 42, 59); (iii) the timing and order of the steps in the carcinogenic process that are being accelerated; (iv) species differences in metabolism and pharmacokinetics; (v) species differences in anticarcinogens and other defenses (1, 60); and (vi) human heterogeneity—for example, pigmentation affects susceptibility to skin cancer from ultraviolet light. These sources of uncertainty are so numerous, and so substantial, that only empirical data will resolve them, and little of this is available.

Uncertainties Due to Mechanism in Multistage Carcinogenesis

Several steps (stages) are involved in chemical carcinogenesis, and the dose–response curve for a carcinogen might depend on the particular stage(s) it accelerates (58), with multiplicative effects if several stages are affected. This multiplicative effect is consistent with the observation in human cancer that synergistic effects are common. The three steps of carcinogenesis that have been analyzed in most detail are initiation (mutation), promotion, and progression, and we discuss these as an aid to understanding aspects of the dose–response relation.

Mutation (or DNA damage) as one stage of the carcinogenic process is supported by various lines of evidence: association of active forms of carcinogens with mutagens (61), the changes in DNA sequence of oncogenes (62), genetic predisposition to cancer in human diseases such as retinoblastoma (63) or DNA-repair deficiency diseases such as xeroderma pigmentosum (64). The idea that genotoxic carcinogens might show a linear dose–response relation might be plausible if only the mutation step of carcinogenesis was accelerated and if the induction of repair and defense enzymes was not a significant factor (65).

Promotion, another step in carcinogenesis, appears to involve cell proliferation, or perhaps particular types of cell proliferation (66), and dose–response relations with apparent thresholds, as indicated by various lines of evidence. (i) The work of Trosko et al. (67) shows promotion of carcinogenesis due to interference with cell–cell communication causing cell proliferation. (ii) Rajewsky's studies and other work indicate that initiation by some carcinogenic agents appears to require proliferating target cells (68). (iii) The work of Farber et al. (69) on liver carcinogenesis supports the idea that cell proliferation (caused by partial hepatectomy or cell killing) can be an important aspect of hepatocarcinogenesis. They have also shown for several chemicals that hepatic cell killing shows a toxic threshold with dose. (iv) Work on carcinogenesis in the pancreas, bladder, stomach (70), and other tissues (58) is also consistent with results on the liver (71, 72) though the effect of cell proliferation might be different in tissues that normally proliferate. (v) The work of Mirsalis et al. (71) suggests that a variety of nongenotoxic agents are hepatocarcinogens in the $B6C3F_1$ mouse (commonly used in cancer tests) because of their toxicity. Other studies on chloroform and trichloroethylene also support this interpretation (72, 73). Cell proliferation resulting from the cell killing in the mouse liver shows a threshold with dose (71). Also relevant is the extraordinarily high spontaneous rates of liver tumors (21% carcinomas, 10% adenomas) in the male $B6C3F_1$ mouse (74). These spontaneous tumors have a mutant *ras* oncogene, and thus the livers in these mice appear to be highly initiated (mutated) to start with (75). (vi) As Weinberg (62) has pointed out, "oncogene-bearing cells surrounded by normal neighbors do not grow into a large mass if they carry only a single oncogene. But if the normal neighbors are removed ... by killing them with a cytotoxic drug... then a single oncogene often suffices." (vii) Cell killing, as well as mutation, appears to be an important aspect of radiation carcinogenesis (76).

Promotion has also been linked to the production of oxygen radicals, such as from phagocytic cells (77). Since chronic cell killing would usually involve inflammatory reactions caused by neutrophils, one would commonly expect chemicals tested at the maximally tolerated dose (MTD) to be promoters because of the chronic inflammation.

Progression, another step in carcinogenesis, leading to selection for invasiveness and metastases, is not well understood but can be accelerated by oxygen radicals (78).

Chronic cell toxicity caused by dosing at the MTD in rodent cancer bioassay thus not only could cause inflammation and cell proliferation, but also should be somewhat mutagenic and clastogenic to neighboring cells because of the release of oxygen radicals from phagocytosis (12, 79, 80). The respiratory burst from phagocytic neutrophils releases the same oxidative mutagens produced by radiation (77, 79). Thus, animal cancer tests done at the MTD of a chemical might commonly stimulate all three steps in carcinogenesis and be positive because the chemical caused chronic cell killing and inflammation with some mutagenesis. Some of the considerable human evidence for chronic inflammation contributing to carcinogenesis and also some evidence for and against a general effect of inflammation and cytotoxicity in rodent carcinogenesis have been discussed (81).

Another set of observations may also bear on the question of toxicity and extrapolation. Wilson, et al. (82) have pointed out that among carcinogens one can predict the potency in high-dose animal cancer experiments from the toxicity (the LD_{50}) of the chemical, though one cannot predict whether the substance is a carcinogen. We have shown that carcinogenic potency values are bounded by the MTD (57). The evidence from our database suggests that the relation between TD_{50} and MTD has a biological as well as a statistical basis (57). We postulate that a just sublethal level of a carcinogen causes cell death, which allows neighboring cells to proliferate, and also causes oxygen radical production from phagocytosis and thus chronic inflammation, both important aspects of the carcinogenic process (57). The generality of this relation and its basis needs further study.

If most animal cancer tests done at the MTD are partially measuring cell killing and consequent cell proliferation and phagocytic oxygen radical damage as steps in the carcinogenic process, one might predict that the dose–response curves would generally be nonlinear. For those experiments in our database for which life table data (14) were available, a detailed analysis (83) shows that the dose–response relation are more often consistent with a quadratic (or cubic) model than with a linear model.

Experimentally, it is very difficult to discriminate between the various extrapolation models at low doses (11, 58). However, evidence to support the idea that a nonlinear dose–response relation is the norm is accumulating for many nongenotoxic and some genotoxic carcinogens. Dose–response curves for saccharin (45), butylated hydroxyanisole [BHA (84)], and a variety of other nongenotoxic carcinogens appear to be nonlinear (85). Formaldehyde, a genotoxic carcinogen, also has a nonlinear dose response (28, 29). The data for both bladder and liver tumors in the large-scale study on acetylaminofluorene a genotoxic chemical, could fit a hockey-stick-shaped curve, though a linear model, with a decreased effect at lower dose rates when the total dose is kept constant (86), has not been ruled out.

Carcinogens effective at both mutating and killing cells (which includes most mutagens) could be "complete" carcinogens and therefore possibly more worrisome at doses far below the MTD than carcinogens acting mainly by causing cell killing or proliferation (15). Thus, all carcinogens are not likely to be directly comparable, and a dose of 1/100 the TD_{50} (HERP = 1%) might be much more of a carcinogenic hazard for the genotoxic carcinogens dimethylnitrosamine or aflatoxin than for the apparently nongenotoxic carcinogens trichloroethylene, PCBs, or alcohol (HERP values marked with asterisks in Table 1). Short-term tests for mutagenicity (61, 87) can have a role to play, not only in understanding mechanisms but also in getting a more realistic view of the background levels of potential genotoxic carcinogens in the world. Knowledge of mechanism of action and comparative metabolism in rodents and humans might help when estimating the relative importance of various low-dose exposures.

Human cancer, except in some occupational or medicinal drug exposures, is not from high (just subtoxic) exposures to a single chemical but is rather from several risk factors often combined with a lack of antirisk factors (60), for example, aflatoxin (a potent mutagen) combined with an agent causing cell proliferation, such as hepatitis B virus (19). High salt [a possible risk factor in stomach cancer (13)] and high fat [a possible risk factor in colon cancer (4)] both appear to be effective in causing cell killing and cell proliferation.

Risk from carcinogenesis is not linear with time. For example, among regular cigarette smokers the excess annual lung cancer incidence is approximately proportional to the fourth power of the duration of smoking (88). Thus, if human exposures in Table 1 are much shorter than the lifetime exposure, the possible hazard may be markedly less than linearly proportional.

A key question about animal cancer tests and regulatory policy is the percentage of tested chemicals that will prove to be carcinogens (89). Among the 392 chemicals in our database that were tested in both rats and mice, 58% are positive in at least one species (14). For the 64 "natural" substances in the group, the proportion of positive results is similar (45%) to the proportion of positive results in the synthetic group (60%). One explanation offered for the high proportion of positive results is that more suspicious chemicals are being tested (e.g., relatives of known carcinogens), but we do not know if the percentage of positives would be low among less suspicious chemicals. If toxicity is important in carcinogenicity, as we have argued, then at the MTD a high percentage of all chemicals might be classified as "carcinogens."

THE BACKGROUND OF NATURAL CARCINOGENS

The object of the chapter is not to do risk assessment on naturally occurring carcinogens or to worry people unduly about an occasional raw mushroom or beer, but to put the possible hazard of synthetic carcinogens in proper perspective and to point out that we lack the knowledge to do low-dose "risk assessment." We also are almost completely ignorant of the carcinogenic potential of the enormous background of natural chemicals in the world. For example, chloinesterase inhibitors are a common class of pesticides, both synthetic and natural. Solanine and chaconine (the main alkaloids in potatoes) are cholinesterase inhibitors and were introduced generally into the human diet about 400 years ago with dissemination of the potato from the Andes. They can be detected in the blood of almost all people (12, 90). Total alkaloids are present at a level of 15,000 μg per 200-g potato with not a large safety factor about sixfold from the toxic level for humans (91). Neither alkaloid has been tested for carcinogenicity. By contrast, malathion, the main synthetic organophosphate cholinesterase inhibitor in our diet (17 μg/day) (16), is not a carcinogen in rodents.

The idea that nature is benign and that evolution has allowed us to cope perfectly with the toxic chemicals in the natural world is not compelling for several reasons. (i) There is no reason to think that natural selection should eliminate the hazard of carcinogenicity of a plant toxin that causes cancer in old age past the reproductive age, though there could be selection for resistance to the acute effects of particular carcinogens. For example, aflatoxin, a mold toxin that presumably arose early in evolution, causes cancer in trout, rats, mice, and monkeys, and probably people, though the species are not equally sensitive. Many of the common metal salts are carcinogens (such as lead, cadmium, beryllium nickel, chromium, selenium, and arsenic) despite their presence during all of evolution. (ii) Given the enormous variety of plant toxins, most of our defenses may be general defenses against acute effects, such as shedding the surface lining of cells of our digestive and respiratory systems every day; protecting these surfaces with a mucin layer; having detoxifying enzymes that are often inducible, such as cytochrome P-450, conjugating enzymes, and glutathione transferses; and having DNA repair enzymes, which would be useful against a wide variety of ingested toxic chemicals, both natural and synthetic. Some human cancer may be caused by interfering with these normal protective systems. (iii) The human diet has changed drastically in the last few thousand years, and most of us are eating plants (such as coffee, potatoes, tomatoes, and kiwi fruit) that our ancestors did not. (iv) Normal metabolism produces radiomimetic mutagens and carcinogens, such as hydrogen peroxide and other reactive forms of oxygen. Though we have defenses against these agents, they still may be major contributors to aging and cancer. A wide variety of external agents may disturb this balance between damage and defense (12, 42).

IMPLICATIONS FOR DECISIONMAKING

For all of these considerations, our scale is not a scale of risks to humans but is only a way of setting priorities for concern, which should also take into account the numbers of people exposed. It should be emphasized that it is a linear scale and thus may overestimate low potential hazards if, as we argue above, linearity is not the normal case, or if nongenotoxic carcinogens are not of very much concern at doses much below the toxic dose.

Thus, it is not scientifically credible to use the results from rodent tests done at the MTD to estimate directly human risks at low doses. For example, an EPA risk assessment (92) based on a succession of worst-case assumptions (several of which are unique to EDB) concluded that EDB residues in grain (HERP = 0.0004%) could cause 3 cases of cancer in 1000 people (about 1% of all U.S. cancer). A consequence was the banning of the main fumigant in the country. It would be more reasonable to compare the possible hazard of EDB residues to that of other common possible hazards. For example, the aflatoxin in the average peanut butter sandwich, or a raw mushroom, are 75 and 200 times, respectively, the possible hazard of EDB. Before banning EDB, a useful substance with rather low residue levels, it might be reasonable to consider whether the hazards of the alternatives, such as food irradiation, or the consequences of banning, such as increased mold contamination of grain, pose less risk to society. Also, there is a disparity between OSHA not regulating worker exposures at a HERP of 140%, while the EPA bans the substance at a HERP of 0.0004%. In addition, the FDA allows a possible hazard up to a HERP of 0.3% for peanut butter (20 ppb), and there is no warning about buying comfrey pills.

Because of the large background of low-level carcinogenic and other (93) hazards, and the high costs of regulation, priority setting is a critical first step. It is important not to divert society's attention away from the few really serious hazards, such as tobacco or saturated fat for heart disease, by the pursuit of hundreds of minor or nonexistent hazards. Our knowledge is also more certain about the enormous toll of tobacco—about 350,000 deaths per year (1, 2).

There are many trade-offs to be made in all technologies. Trichloroethylene and tetra-chloroethylene (perchloroethylene) replaced hazardous flamming solvents. Modern synthetic pesticides displaced lead arsenate, which was a major pesticide before the modern chemical era. Lead and arsenic are both natural carcinogens. There is also a choice to be made between using synthetic pesticides and raising the level of plants' natural toxins by breeding. It is not clear that the latter approach, even where feasible, is preferable. For example, plant breeders produced an insect-resistant potato, which has to be withdrawn from the market because of its acute toxicity to humans due to a high level of the natural plant toxins solanine and chaconine (12).

This analysis on the levels of synthetic pollutants in drinking water and of synthetic pesticide residues in foods suggests that this pollution is likely to be a minimal carcinogenic hazard relative to the background of natural carcinogens. This result is consistent with the epidemiologic evidence (1). Obviously, prudence is desirable with regard to pollution, but we do need to work out some balance between chemophobia with its high costs to the national wealth and sensible management of industrial chemicals (94).

Human life expectancy continues to lengthen in industrial countries and the longest life expectancy in the world is in Japan, an extremely crowded and industrialized country. U.S. cancer death rates, except for lung cancer due to tobacco and melanoma due to ultraviolet light, are not on the whole increasing and have mostly been steady for 50 years. New progress in cancer research, molecular biology, epidemiology, and bio-chemical epidemiology (95) will probably continue to increase the understanding necessary for lengthening life span and decreasing cancer death rates.

REFERENCES

1. R. Doll and R. Peto, *The Causes of Cancer* (Oxford Univ. Press, Oxford, England, 1981).
2. *Smoking and Health: A Report of the Surgeon General*, Department of Health, Education and Welfare Publication No. (PHS) 79-50066 (Office of the Assistant Secretary for Health, Washington, DC, 1979).
3. G. J. Hopkins and K. K. Carroll, *J. Environ. Pathol. Toxicol. Oncol.* **5**, 279 (1985); J. V. Joossens, M. J. Hill, J. Geboers, Eds., *Diet and Human Carcinogenesis* (Elsevier, Amsterdam, 1985); I. Knudsen, Ed., *Genetic Toxicology of the Diet* (Liss, New York, 1986); Committee on Diet, Nutrition and Cancer, Assembly of Life Sciences, National Research Council, *Diet, Nutrition and Cancer* (National Academy Press, Washington, DC, 1982).
4. R. P. Bird, R. Schneider, D. Stamp, W. R. Bruce, *Carcinogenesis* **7**, 1657 (1986); H. L. Newmark et al., in *Large Bowel Cancer*, vol. 3 in *Cancer Research Monographs*, A. J. Mastromarino and M. G. Brattain, Eds. (Praeger, New York, 1985), pp. 102–130; E. A. Jacobson, H. L. Newmark, E. Bright-See, G. McKeown-Eyssen, W. R. Bruce, *Nutr. Rep. Int.* **30**, 1049 (1984); M. Buset, M. Lipkin, S. Winawer, S. Swaroop, E. Friedman, *Cancer Res.* **46**, 5426 (1986).
5. D. G. Hoel, R. A. Merrill, F. P. Perera, Eds., *Banbury Report 19. Risk Quantitation and Regulatory Policy* (Cold Spring Laboratory, Cold Spring Harbor, NY, 1985).
6. B. E. Henderson et al., *Cancer Res.* **42**, 3232 (1982).
7. R. Peto and H. zur Hausen, Eds., *Banbury Report 21. Viral Etiology of Cervical Cancer* (Cold Spring Harbor Laboratory, Cold Spring Habor, NY, 1986); F.-S. Yeh et al., *Cancer Res.* **45**, 872 (1985).

8. International Agency for Research on Cancer, *IARC Monographs on the Evaluation of the Carcinogenic Risk of Chemicals to Humans* (International Agency for Research on Cancer, Lyon, France, 1985), vol. 39.

9. D. A. Freedman and H. Zeisel, *From Mouse to Man: The Quantitative Assessment of Cancer Risks* (Tech. Rep. No. 79, Department of Statistics, University of California, Berkeley, 1987).

10. R. Peto, in *Assessment of Risk from Low-Level Exposure to Radiation and Chemicals*, A. D. Woodhead, C. J. Shellabarger, V. Pond, A. Hollaender, Eds. (Plenum, New York and London, 1985), pp. 3–16.

11. S. W. Samuels and R. H. Adamson, *J. Natl. Cancer Inst.* **74**, 945 (1985); E. J. Calabrese, *Drug Metab. Rev.* **15**, 505 (1984).

12. B. N. Ames, *Science* **221**, 1256 (1983); *ibid.* **224**, 668, 757 (1984).

13. H. Ohgaki et al., *Gann* **75**, 1053 (1984); S. S. Mirvish, *J. Natl. Cancer Inst.* **71**, 630 (1983); J. V. Joossens and J. Geboers, in *Frontiers in Gastrointestinal Cancer*, B. Levin and R. H. Riddell, Eds. (Elsevier, Amsterdam, 1984), pp. 167–183; T. Hirayama, *Jpn. J. Clin. Oncol.* **14**, 159 (1984); C. Furihata et al., *Biochem. Biophys. Res. Commun.* **121**, 1027 (1984).

14. R. Peto, M. C. Pike, L. Bernstein, L. S. Gold, B. N. Ames, *Environ. Health Perspect.* **58**, 1 (1984); L. S. Gold et al., *ibid.*, p. 9; L. S. Gold et al., *ibid.* **67**, 161 (1986); L. S. Gold et al., *ibid.*, in press.

15. G. M. Williams and J. H. Weisburger, in *Casavett and Doull's Taxicology. The Basic Science of Poisons*, C. D. Klaassen, M. O. Amdur, J. Doull, Eds. (Macmillan, New York, ed. 3, 1986), chap. 5, pp. 99–172; B. E. Butterworth and T. J. Slaga, Eds., *Banbury Report 25. Non-Genotoxic Mechanisms in Carcinogenesis* (Cold Spring Harbor Laboratory, Cold Spring Harbor, NY, 1987).

16. The FDA has estimated the average U.S. dietary intake of 70 pesticides, herbicides, and industrial chemicals for 1981/1982 [M. J. Gartrell, J. C. Craun, D. S. Podrebarac, E. L. Gunderson, *J. Assoc. Off. Anal. Chem.* **69**, 146 (1986)]. The negative test on 2-ethylhexyl diphenyl phosphate is in J. Treon, F. Dutra, F. Cleveland, *Arch. Ind. Hyg. Occup. Med.* **8**, 170 (1953).

17. R. C. Beier et al., *Food Chem. Toxicol.* **21**, 163 (1983).

18. L. Stoloff, M. Castegnaro, P. Scott, I. K. O'Neill, H. Bartsch, Eds., *Some Mycotoxins*, vol. 5 in *Environmental Carcinogens. Selected Methods of Analysis* (IARC Scientific Publ. No. 44, International Agency for Research on Cancer, Lyon, France, 1982); H. Mori et al., *Cancer Res.* **44**, 2918 (1984); R. Röschenthaler, E. E. Creppy, G. Dirheimer, *J. Toxicol.-Toxin Rev.* **3**, 53 (1984); W. F. O. Marasas, N. P. J. Kriek, J. E. Fincham, S. J. van Rensburg, *Int. J. Cancer* **34**, 383 (1984); *Environmental Health Criteria 11: Mycotoxins* (World Health Organization, Geneva, Switzerland, 1979), pp. 21–85; W. F. Busby et al., in *Chemical Carcinogens*, C. E. Searle, Ed. (ACS Monograph 182, American Chemical Society, Washington, DC, ed. 2, 1984), vol. 2, pp. 944–1136.

19. S. J. Van Rensburg et al., *Br. J. Cancer* **51**, 713 (1985); S. N. Zaman et al., *Lancet* **1985-I**, 1357 (1985); H. Austin et al., *Cancer Res.* **46**, 962 (1986).

20. A. Takada, J. Nei, S. Takase, Y. Matsuda, *Hepatology* **6**, 65 (1986).

21. J. M. Elwood et al., *Int. J. Cancer* **34**, 603 (1984).

22. Aldehydes and ketones are largely responsible for the aroma and flavor of bread [Y. Y. Linko, J. A. Johnson, B. S. Miller, *Cereal Chemistry* **39**, 468 (1962)]. In freshly baked bread, formaldehyde (370 μg per two slices of bread) accounts for 2.5% of the total carbonyl compounds [K. Lorenz and J. Maga, *J. Agric. Food Chem.* **20**, 211 (1972)]. Acetaldehyde, which is present in bread at about twice the level of formaldehyde, is a carcinogen in rats [R. A. Woutersen, L. M. Appelman, V. J. Feron, C. A. Vanderheijden, *Toxicology* **31**, 123 (1984)] and a DNA cross-linking agent in human cells [B. Lambert, Y. Chen, S.-M. He, M. Sten, *Mutat. Res.* **146**, 301 (1985)].

23. Ethyl alcohol contents of wine and beer were assumed to be 12% and 5%, respectively. The TD_{50} calculation is based on M. J. Radike, K. L. Stemmer, E. Bingham, *Environ. Health Perspect.* **41**, 59 (1981). Rats exposed to 5% ethyl alcohol in drinking water for 30 months had increased incidences of endocrine and liver tumors.

24. C. S. Ough, *J. Agric. Food Chem.* **24**, 323 (1976). Urethane is also carcinogenic in hamsters and rhesus monkeys.

25. Y. Fujita. K. Wakabayashi, M. Nagao. T. Sugimura, *Mutat. Res.* **144**, 227 (1985); M. Nagao, Y. Fujita, T. Sugimura, in *IARC Workshop*, in press.

26. M. Petro-Turza and I. Szarfoldi-Szalma, *Acta Alimentaria* **11**, 75 (1982).

27. L. J. Marnett et al., *Mutat. Res.* **148**, 25 (1985).

28. Formaldehyde in air samples taken from all the mobile homes examined ranged from 50 to 660 ppb mean, 167 ppb) [T. H. Connor, J. C. Theiss, H. A. Hanna, D. K. Monteith, T. S. Matney, *Toxicol. Lett.* **25**, 33 (1985)]. The important role of cell toxicity and cell proliferation in formaldehyde carcinogenesis is discussed in T. B. Starr and J. E. Gibson [*Annu. Rev. Pharmacol. Taxicol.* **25**, 745 (1985)].

29. J. A. Swenberg et al., *Carcinogenesis* **4**, 945 (1983).

30. G. Della Porta, M. I. Colnaghi, G. Parmiani, *Food Cosmet. Taxicol.* **6**, 707 (1968).

31. Formaldehyde develops postmortem in marine fish and crustaceans, probably through the metabolism of trimethylamine oxide. The average level found in shrimp from four U.S. markets was 94 mg/kg [T. Radford and D. E. Dalsis, *J. Agric. Food Chem.* **30**, 600 (1982)]. Formaldehyde is found in remarkably high concentrations (300 ppm, HERP = 29% per 100 g) in Japanese shrimp that have been bleached with a sulfite solution [A. Yoshida and M. Imaida, *J. Food Hygienic Soc. Japan* **21**, 288 (1980)].

32. J. F. Lawrence and J. R. Iyengar, *Int. J. Environ. Anal. Chem.* **15**, 47 (1983).

33. H. d'A. Heek et al., *Am. Ind. Hyg. Assoc. J.* **46**, 1 (1985).

34. T. Sugimura et al., in *Genetic Taxicology of the Diet*, I. Knudsen, Ed. (Liss, New York, 1986), pp. 85–107; T. Sugimura, *Science* **233**, 312 (1986).

35. H. Ohgaki et al., *Cancer Lett.* **25**, 239 (1985).

36. T. Kinouchi, H. Tsutsui, Y. Ohnishi, *Mutat. Res.* **171**, 105 (1986).

37. T. Kawabata et al., in *N-Nitroso Compounds: Analysis, Formation and Occurrence*, E. A. Walker, L. Griciute, M. Castegnaro, M. Borzsonyl, Eds. (IARC Scientific Publ. No. 31, International Agency for Research on Cancer, Lyon, France, 1980), pp. 481–490; T. Maki, Y. Tamura, Y. Shimamura, and Y. Naoi [*Bull. Environ. Contam. Toxicol.* **25**, 257 (1980)] have surveyed Japanese food for nitrosamines.

38. T. Fazio, D. C. Havery, J. W. Howard, in *N-Nitroso Compounds: Analysis Formation and Occurrence*, E. A. Walker, L. Griciute, M. Castegnaro, M. Borzsonyi, Eds. (IARC Scientific Publ. No. 31, International Agency for Research on Cancer, Lyon, France, 1980), pp. 419–435; R. Preussmann and G. Eisenbrand, in *Chemical Carcinogenesis*, C. E. Searle, Ed. (ACS Monograph 182, American Chemical Society, Washington, DC, ed. 2, 1984), vol. 2, pp. 829–868; D. C. Havery, J. H. Hotchkiss, T. Fazio, *J. Food Sci.* **46**, 501 (1981).

39. W. A. Garland et al., *Cancer Res.* **46**, 5392 (1986).

40. E. A. Walker, L. Griciute, M. Castegnaro, M. Borzsonyi, Eds., *N-Nitroso Compounds: Analysis, Formation and Occurrence* (IARC Scientific Publ. No. 31, International Agency for Research on Cancer, Lyon, France, 1980), pp. 457–463; B. Spiegelhalder, G. Eisenbrand, R. Preussmann, *Oncology* **37**, 211 (1980); R. A. Scanlan and S. R. Tannenbaum, Eds., *N-Nitroso Compounds* (ACS Symposium Series No. 174, American Chemical Society, Washington, DC, 1981), pp. 165–180. Nitrosamines are formed in cured meats through reactions of secondary amines with nitrites added during the manufacturing process. One survey of bacon commercially available in Canada identified N-nitrosodimethylamine (DMN), N-nitrosodiethylamine (DEN), and N-nitrosopyrrolidine (NPYR) in most samples tested, with average levels of 3.4, 1.0, and 9.3 ppb, respectively. The cooked-out fat from the bacon

samples contained DMN and NPYR at average levels of 6.4 and 21.9 ppb, respectively [N. P. Sen, S. Seaman, W. F. Miles, *J. Agric. Food Chem.* **27**, 1354 (1979); R. A. Scanlan, *Cancer Res.* **43**, 2435s (1983)]. The Average levels of NPYR in cooked bacon have decreased since 1971 because of reduced levels of nitrite and increased levels of ascorbate used in bacon curing mixtures [D. C. Havery, T. Fazio, J. W. Howard, *J. Assoc. Off. Anal. Chem.* **61**, 1379 (1978)].

41. Y. Yamamoto et al., *Anal. Biochem.* **160**, 7 (1987).

42. B. N. Ames and R. L. Saul, in *Theories of Carcinogenesis*, O. H. Iversen, Ed. (Hemisphere, New York, in press); R. Cathcart, E. Schwiers, R. L. Saul, B. N. Ames, *Proc. Natl. Acad. Sci. U.S.A.* **81**, 5633 (1984).

43. B. P. Yu, E. J. Masoro, I. Murata, H. A. Bertrand, F. T. Lynd, *J. Gerontol.* **37**, 130 (1982); F. J. C. Roe, *Proc. Nutr. Soc.* **40**, 57 (1981); *Nature (London)* **303**, 657 (1983); M. J. Tucker, *Int. J. Cancer* **23**, 803 (1979).

44. Y. Tazima, *Environ. Health Perspect.* **29**, 183 (1979); M. Kinebuchi, T. Kawachi, N. Matsukura, T. Sugimura, *Food Cosmet. Toxicol.* **17**, 339 (1979).

45. F. W. Carlborg, *Food Chem. Toxicol.* **23**, 499 (1985).

46. T. H. Jukes, *Am. Stat.* **36**, 273 (1982); *J. Am. Med. Assoc.* **229**, 1920 (1974).

47. Allyl isothiocyanate (AITC) is the major flavor ingredient, and natural pesticide, of brown mustard and also occurs naturally in varying concentrations in cabbage, kale, broccoli, cauliflower, and horseradish [Y. M. Ioannou, L. T. Burka, H. B. Matthews, *Toxicol. Appl. Pharmacol.* **75**, 173 (1984)]. It is present in the plant's volatile oil as the glucoside sinigrin. (The primary flavor ingredient of yellow mustard is p-hydroxybenzyl isothiocyanate.) The AITC yield from brown mustard is approximately 0.9% by weight, assuming all of the sinigrin is converted to AITC [A. Y. Leung, *Encyclopedia of Common Natural Ingredients Used in Food, Drugs and Cosmetics* (Wiley, New York, 1980), pp. 238–241]. Synthetic AITC is used in nonalcoholic beverages, candy, baked goods, meats, condiments, and syrups at average levels ranging from 0.02 to 88 ppm [T. E. Furia and B. Nicolo, Eds., *Fenaroli's Handbook of Flavor Ingredients*, (CRC Press, Cleveland, OH, 2 ed., 1975), vol. 1, p. 19].

48. Estragole, one of numerous safrole-like compounds in plants, is present in the volatile oils of many edible plants, including basil, tarragon, bay, anise, and fennel, as well as in pine oil and turpentine [A. Y. Leung, *Encyclopedia of Common Natural Ingredients Used in Food, Drugs, and Cosmetics* (Wiley, New York, 1980)]. Dried basil has a volatile oil content of about 1.5 to 3.0$, which contains (on average) 25$ estragole [H. B. Heath, *Source Book of Flavors* (AVI, Westport, CT, 1981), pp. 222–223]. Estragole is used commercially in spice, anise, licorice, and fruit flavors. It is added to beverages, candy, baked goods, chewing gums, ice creams, and condiments at average levels ranging from 2 to 150 ppm [NAS/NRC Food Protection Committee, Food and Nutrition Board, *Chemicals Used in Food Processing* (NAS/NRC Publ. No. 1274, National Academy of Sciences, Washington, DC, 1965), p. 114].

49. The estimation of risk is from human data on uranium miners and estimates of intake. E. P. Radford, *Environ. Health Perspect.* **62**, 281 (1985); A. V. Nero et al., *Science* **234**, 992 (1986); A. V. Nero, *Technol. Rev.* **89**, 28 (1986); R. Hanley, *The New York Times*, 10 March 1986, p. 17.

50. The average daily adult dose of phenobarbital for sleep induction is 100 to 320 mg (HERP = 26 to 83%), though its use is declining [AMA Division of Drugs, *AMA Drug Evaluations* (American Medical Association, Chicago, IL, ed. 5, 1983), pp. 201–202]. The TD_{50} data in the table is for phenobarbital, which, so far, has been shown to be carcinogenic only in mice; the sodium salt of phenobarbital is carcinogenic in both rats and mice. Human studies on phenobar bital and cancer are reviewed in A. E. M. McLean, H. E. Driver, D. Lowe, I. Sutherland, *Toxicol. Lett.* **31** (suppl.), 200 (1986).

51. Phenacetin use has gradually decreased following reports of urinary bladder and kidney tumors in heavy users [J. M. Piper, J. Tonascia, G. M. Matanoski, *N. Engl. J. Med.* **313**, 292 (1985)]. Phenacetin also induces urinary bladder and kidney tumors in rats and mice.

52. The human dose of clofibrate is 2 g per day for many years [R. J. Havel and J. P. Kane, *Annu. Rev. Med.* **33** 417 (1982)]. The role of clofibrate as a peroxisome proliferator is reviewed in J. K. Reddy and N. D. Lalwani [*CRC Crit. Rev. Taxicol.* **12**, 1 (1983)]. An epidemiologic study is in World Health Organization Report, *Lancet* **1984-II**, 600 (1984).

53. L. S. Gold, G. Backman, N. K. Hooper, R. Peto, *Lawrence Berkely Laboratory Report 23161* (1987); N. K. Hooper and L. S. Gold, in *Monitoring of Occupational Genotaxicants*, M. Sorsa and H. Norppa, Eds. (Liss, New York, 1986), pp. 217–228; K. Hooper and L. S. Gold, in *Cancer Prevention: Strategies in the Workplace*, C. Becker, Ed. (Hemisphere, Washington, DC, 1985), pp. 1–11.

54. California Department of Health Services, *EDB Criteria Document* (1985).

55. M. G. Ott, H. C. Scharnweber, R. R. Langner, *Br. J. Ind. Med.* **37**, 163 (1980); J. C. Ramsey, C. N. Park, M. G. Ott, P. J. Gehring, *Taxicol. Appl. Pharmacol.* **47**, 411 (1978). This has been disputed (54). The carcinogen dose reported in the table assumes a time-weighted average air concentration of 3 ppm and an 8 hour workday 5 days per week for 50 weeks per year for life.

56. R. Magaw, L. S. Gold, L. Bernstein, T. H. Slone, B. N. Ames, in preparation.

57. L. Bernstein, L. S. Gold, B. N. Ames, M. C. Pike, D. G. Hoel, *Fundam. Appl. Toxicol.* **5**, 79 (1985); L. Bernstein, L. S. Gold, B. N. Ames, M. C. Pike, D. G. Hoel, *Risk Anal.* **5**, 263 (1985).

58. D. B. Clayson, *Toxicol. Pathol.* **13**, 119 (1985); D. B. Clayson, *Mutat. Res.*, in press.

59. R. Peto, S. E. Parish, R. G. Gray, in *Age-Related Factors in Carcinogenesis*, A. Likhachev, V. Anisimov, R. Montesano, Eds. (IARC Scientific Publ. No. 58, International Agency for Research on Cancer, Lyon, France, 1985), pp. 43–53.

60. D. M. Shankel, P. Hartman, T. Kada, A. Hollaender, Eds., *Antimutagenesis and Anticarcinogenesis: Mechanisms* (Plenum, New York, 1986.

61. B. N. Ames and J. McCann, *Cancer Res.* **41**, 4192 (1981).

62. R. A. Weinberg, *Science* **230**, 770 (1985).

63. A. G. Knudson, Jr., *Cancer Res.* **45**, 1437 (1985).

64. J. E. Cleaver, in *Genes and Cancer*, J. M. Bishop, J. D. Rowley, M. Greaves, Eds. (Liss, New York, 1984), pp. 117–135.

65. A. D. Woodhead, C. J. Shellabarger, V. Pond, A Hollaender, Eds., *Assessment of Risk from Low-Level Exposure to Radiation and Chemicals: A Critical Overview* (Plenum, New York, 1985).

66. J. Cairns, *Nature (London)* **255**, 197 (1975); C. C. Harris and T. Sun, *Carcinogenesis* **5**, 697 (1984); A. M. Edwards and C. M. Lucas, *Biochem. Biophys. Res. Commun.* **131**, 103 (1985); H. Tsuda et al., *Cancer Res.* **39**, 4491 (1979); W. H. Haese and E. Bueding, *J. Pharmacol. Exp. Ther.* **197**, 703 (1976).

67. J. E. Trosko and C. C. Chang, in *Methods for Estimating Risk of Chemical Injury: Human and Non-Human Biota and Ecosystems*, V. B. Vouk, G. C. Butler, D. G. Hoel, D. B. Peakall, Eds. (Wiley, New York, 1985), pp. 181–200; J. E. Trosko and C. C. Chang, in *Assessment of Risk from Low-Level Exposure to Radiation and Chemicals: A Critical Overview*, A. D. Woodhead, C. J. Shellabarger, V. Pond, A. Hollaender, Eds. (Plenum, New York, 1985), pp. 261–284; H. Yamasaki, *Toxicol. Pathol.* **14**, 363 (1986).

68. M. F. Rajewsky, in *Age-Related Factors in Carcinogenesis*, A. Likhachev, V. Anisimov, R. Montesano, Eds. (IARC Scientific Publ. No. 58, International Agency for Research on Cancer, Lyon, France, 1985), pp. 215–224; V. Kinsel, G. Furstenberger, H. Loehrke, F. Marks, *Carcinogenesis* **7**, 779 (1986).

69. E. Farber, *Cancer Res.* **44**, 5463 (1984); E. Farber, S. Parker, M. Gruenstein, *ibid.* **36**, 3879 (1976).

70. A. Denda, S. Inui, M. Sunagawa, S. Takahashi, Y. Konishi, *Gann* **69**, 633 (1978); R. Hasegawa and S. M. Cohen, *Cancer Lett.* **30**, 261 (1986); R. Hasegawa, S. M. Cohen, M. St. John, M. Cano,

L. B. Ellwein, *Carcinogenesis* **7**, 633 (1986); B. I. Ghanayem, R. R. Maronpot, H. B. Matthews, *Toxicology* **6**, 189 (1986).

71. J. C. Mirsalis et al., *Carcinogenesis* **6**, 1521 (1985); J. C. Mirsalis et al., *Environ. Mutag.* **8** (suppl. 6), 55 (1986); J. Mirsalis et al., Abstract for Fourth International Conference on Environmental Mutagens, held 24–28 June in Stockholm, Sweden (1985).

72. W. T. Stott, R. H. Reitz, A. M. Schumann, P. G. Watanabe, *Food Cosmet. Toxicol.* **19**, 567 (1981).

73. D. H. Moore, L. F. Chasseaud, S. K. Majeed, D. E. Prentice, F. J. C. Roe, *ibid.* **20**, 951 (1982).

74. J. K. Haseman, J. Huff, G. A. Boorman, *Toxicol. Pathol* **12**, 126 (1984); R. E. Tarone, K. C. Chu, J. M. Ward, *J. Natl. Cancer Inst.* **66**, 1175 (1981).

75. S. H. Reynolds, S. J. Stowers, R. R. Maronpot, M. W. Anderson, S. A. Aaronson, *Proc. Natl. Acad. Sci. U.S.A.* **83**, 33 (1986); T. R. Fox and P. G. Watanabe, *Science* **228**, 596 (1985).

76. T. D. Jones, *Health Phys.* **4**, 533 (1984); J. B. Little, A. R. Kennedy, R. B. McGandy, *Radiat. Res.* **103**, 293 (1985).

77. T. W. Kensler and B. G. Taffe, *Adv. Free Radical Biol. Med.* **2**, 347 (1986); P. A. Cerutti, in *UCLA Symposium on Molecular and Biology Growth Factors, Tumor Promoters and Cancer Genes*, in press; P. A. Cerutti, in *Biochemical and Molecular Epidemiology of Cancer*, vol. 40 of UCLA Symposium on Molecular and Cellular Biology, C. Harris, Ed. (Liss, New York, 1986), p. 167; in *Theories of Carcinogenesis*, O. H. Iversen, Ed. (Hemisphere, New York, in press); H. C. Birnboim, *Carcinogenesis* **7**, 1511 (1986); K. Frenkel and K. Chrzan, *ibid.* **8**, 455 (1987).

78. J. Rotstein, J. O. O'Connell, T. Slaga, *Proc. Assoc. Cancer Res.* **27**, 143 (1986); J. S. O'Connell, A. J. P. Klein-Szanto, J. DiGiovanni, J. W. Fries, T. J. Slaga, *Cancer Res.* **46**, 2863 (1986); J. S. O'Connell, J. B. Rotstein, T. J. Slaga, in *Banbury Report 25. Non-Genotoxic Mechanisms in Carcinogenesis*, B. E. Butterworth and T. J. Slaga, Eds. (Cold Spring Harbor Laboratory, Cold Spring Harbor, NY, 1987).

79. M. A. Trush, J. L. Seed, T. W. Kensler, *Proc. Natl. Acad. Sci. U.S.A.* **82**, 5194 (1985); A. I. Tauber and B. M. Babior, *Adv. Free-Radical Biol. Med.* **1**, 265 (1985); G. J. Chellman, J. S. Bus, P. K. Working, *Proc. Natl. Acad. Sci. U.S.A.* **83**, 8087 (1986).

80. I. U. Schraufstatter et al., *Proc. Natl. Acad. Sci. U.S.A.* **83**, 4908 (1986); M. O. Bradley, in *Basic and Applied Mutagenesis*, A. Muhammed and R. C. von Borstel, Eds. (Plenum, New York, 1985), pp. 99–109.

81. L. Diamond, T. G. O'Brien, W. M. Baird, *Adv. Cancer Res.* **32**, 1 (1980); D. Schmahl, *J. Cancer Res. Clin. Oncol.* **109**, 260 (1985); O. H. Iversen and E. G. Astrup, *Cancer Invest.* **2**, 51 (1984); A. Hagiwara and J. M. Ward, *Fundam. Appl. Toxicol.* **7**, 376 (1986); J. M. Ward, in *Carcinogenesis and Mutagenesis Testing*, J. F. Douglas, Ed. (Humana, Clifton, NJ, 1984), pp. 97–100.

82. L. Zeise, R. Wilson, E. Crouch, *Risk Analysis* **4**, 187 (1984); L. Zeise, E. A. C. Crouch, R. Wilson, *ibid.* **5**, 265 (1985); L. Zeise, E. A. C. Crouch, R. Wilson, *J. Am. College Toxicol.* **5**, 137 (1986).

83. D. Hoel, personal communication.

84. N. Ito, S. Fukushima, A. Hagiwara, M. Shibata, T. Ogiso, *J. Natl. Cancer Inst.* **70**, 343 (1983).

85. F. W. Carlborg, *Food Chem. Toxic.* **20**, 219 (1982); *Food Cosmet. Toxicol.* **19**, 255 (1981).

86. K. G. Brown and D. G. Hoel, *Fundam. Appl. Toxicol.* **3**, 470 (1983); N. A. Littlefield and D. W. Gaylor, *J. Toxicol. Environ. Health* **15**, 545 (1985).

87. J. Ashby, *Mutagenesis* **1**, 3 (1986).

88. R. Doll, *Cancer Res.* **38**, 3573 (1978); ———— and R. Peto, *J. Epidemiol. Community Health* **32**, 303 (1978).

89. J. E. Huff, E. E. McConnell, J. K. Haseman, *Environ. Mutagenesis* **7**, 427 (1985); H. S. Rosenkranz, *ibid.*, p. 428.

90. M. H. Harvey, B. A. Morris, M. McMillan, V. Marks, *Human Toxicol.* **4**, 503 (1985).

91. S. J. Jadhav, R. P. Sharma, D. K. Salunkhe, *CRC Crit. Rev. Toxicol.* **9**, 21 (1981).

92. Environmental Protection Agency, *Poisition Document* **4** (Special Pesticide Review Division, Environmental Protection Agency, Arlington, VA, 1983).

93. R. Wilson and E. Crouch, *Risk/Benefit Analysis* (Ballinger, Cambridge, MA, 1982); W. F. Allman *Science 85* **6**, 30 (1985).

94. P. Huber, *Regulation*, **33** (March/April 1984); C. Whipple, *ibid.* **9**, 37 (1985).

95. B. A. Bridges, B. E. Butterworth, I. B. Weinstein, Eds., *Banbury Report 13. Indicators of Genotoxic Exposure.* (Cold Spring Harbor Laboratory, Cold Spring Harbor, NY, 1982); P. E. Enterline, Ed., Fifth Annual Symposium on Environmental Epidemiology, *Environ. Health Perspect.* **62**, 239 (1985).

96. A national survey of U.S. drinking water supplies identified the concentrations of about 20 organic compounds. The mean total trihalomethane concentration was 117 µg/liter, with the major component, chloroform, present at a mean concentration of 83 µg/liter (83 ppb). Raw water that is relatively free of organic matter results in drinking water relatively free of trihalomethanes after chlorination. These studies are reviewed in S. J. Williamson, *The Science of the Total Environment* **18**, 187 (1981).

97. Public and private drinking water wells in Santa Clara Valley, California, have been found to be contaminated with a variety of halogenated hydrocarbons in small amounts. Among 19 public water system wells, the most commonly found contaminants were 1, 1, 1-trichloroethane (TCA), and 1, 1, 2-trichloro-1, 2, 2-trifluoroethane (Freon-113). TCA was found in 15 wells generally at concentrations of less than 30 ppb, though one well contained up to 8800 ppb, and Freon-113 was found in six wells at concentrations up to 12 ppb. Neither chemical has been adequately tested for carcinogenicity in long-term bioassays. In addition to these compounds, three wells also contained carcinogenic compounds at low concentrations. Water from public supply wells may be mixed with treated surface water before delivery, thus the concentrations of these compounds that people actually receive may be somewhat reduced. Thirty-five private drinking water supply wells were examined; the major contaminant was the carcinogen trichloroethylene (TCE), at levels up to 2800 ppb. TCA and Freon-113 were also found in some wells, at maximum levels of 24 ppb and 40 ppb, respectively. Though fewer people drink from private water wells, the contaminant concentrations may be higher because the water is not mixed with water from other sources [California Department of Health Services, California Regional Water Quality Control Board 2, Santa Clara County Public Health Department, Santa Clara Valley Water District, U.S. Environmental protection Agency, *Ground Water and Drinking Water in the Santa Clara Valley: A White Paper* (1984), table 8]. Trichloroethylene may not be a carcinogen in humans at low doses [R. D. Kimbrough, F. L. Mitchell, V. N. Houk, *J. Toxicol. Environ. Health* **15**, 369 (1985)].

98. Contaminated drinking water in the area of Woburn, Massachusetts, was found to contain 267 ppb trichloroethylene, 21 ppb tetrachloroethylene, 12 ppb chloroform, 22 ppb trichlorotrifluoroethane, and 28 ppb 1, 2-*trans*-dichloroethylene [S. W. Lagakos, B. J. Wessen, M. Zelen, *J. Am. Stat. Assoc.* **81**, 583 (1986)].

99. The amount of chloroform absorbed by a 6-year-old child in a chlorinated freshwater swimming pool has been estimated [J. A. Beech, *Med. Hypotheses* **6**, 303 (1980)]. Table 1 refers to the chloroform in an average pool (134 µg/liter) and for a 37-kg child. Three other trihalomethanes were identified in these freshwater pools: bromoform, bromodichloromethane and chlorodibromomethane. U. Lahl, J. Vondusze, B. Gabel, B. Stachel, W. Thiemann [*Water Res.* **15**, 803 (1981)] have estimated absorption in covered swimming pools.

100. J. McCann, L. Horn, J. Girman, A. V. Nero, in *Short-Term Bioassays in the Analysis of Complex Environmental Mixtures*, V. S. Sandhu, D. M. De Marini, M. J. Mass, M. M. Moore, J. L. Mumford, Eds. (Plenum, New York, in press). This estimate (Table 1) for formaldehyde in conventional homes, excludes foam-insulated houses and mobile homes. The figure is a

mean of the median or mean of the reported samples in each paper. For benzene, the figure is a mean of all reported median or mean samples. The level of benzene in Los Angeles outdoor air is similar (U.S. EPA Office of Air Quality Planning and Standards, EPA 450/4-86-012, 1986).

101. The average adult daily PCB intake from food estimated by the FDA in fiscal years 1981/1982 was 0.2 μg/day (16). Many slightly different PCB mixtures have been studied in long-term animal cancer bioassays; the calculation of TD_{50} was from a test of Aroclor 1260 which was more potent than other PCBs (14).

102. The average consumption of EDB residues in grains has been estimated by the EPA for adults as 0.006 μg kg^{-1} day^{-1} and for children as 0.013 μg kg^{-1} day^{-1} [U.S. EPA Office of Pesticide Programs, *Ethylene Dibromide (EDB) Scientific Support and Decision Document for Grain and Grain Milling Fumigation Uses* (8 February 1984)].

103. The leaves and roots of Russian comfrey are widely sold in health food stores and are consumed as a medicinal herb or salad plant or are brewed as a tea. Comfrey leaf has been shown to contain 0.01 to 0.15%, by weight, total pyrrolizidine alkaloids, with an average level of 0.05% for intermediate size leaves [C. C. J. Culvenor, J. A. Edgar, J. L. Frahn, L. W. Smith, *Aust. J. Chem.* **33**, 1105 (1980)]. The main pyrrolizidine alkaloids present in comfrey leaves are echimidine and 7-acetyllycopsamine, neither of which has been tested for carcinogenicity. Almost all tested 1, 2-unsaturated pyrrolizidine alkaloids have been shown to be genotoxic and carcinogenic [H. Mori et al., *Cancer Res.* **45**, 3125 (1985)]. Symphytine accounts for 5% of the total alkaloid in the leaves and has been shown to be carcinogenic [C. C. J. Culvenor et al., *Experientia* **36**, 377 (1980)]. We assume that 1.5 g of intermediate size leaves are used per cup of comfrey tea (Table 1). The primary alkaloids in comfrey root are symphytine (0.67 g per kilogram of root) and echmidine (0.5 g per kilogram of root) [T. Furuya and M. Hikichi, *Phytochemistry* **10**, 2217 (1971)]. Comfrey-pepsin tablets (300 mg of root per tablet) have a recommended dose of one to three tables three times per day. Comfrey roots and leaves both induce liver tumors in rats [I. Hirono, H. Mori, M. Haga, *J. Natl. Cancer Inst.* **61**, 865 (1978)], and the TD_{50} value is based on these results. Those pyrrolizidine alkaloids tested have been found to be at least as potent as carcinogens such as symphytine. If the other pyrrolizidine alkaloids in comfrey were as potent carcinogens as symphytine, the possible hazard of a daily cup of tea would be HERP = 0.6% and that of a daily nine tablets would be HERP = 7.3%.

104. *Agaricus bisporus* is the most commonly eaten mushroom in the United States with an estimated annual consumption of 340 million kilograms in 1984–85. Mushrooms contain various hydrazine compounds, some of which have been shown to cause tumors in mice. Raw mushrooms fed over a lifetime to male and female mice induced bone, forestomach, liver, and lung tumors [B. Toth and J. Erickson, *Cancer Res.* **46**, 4007 (1986)]. The 15-g raw mushroom is given as wet weight. The TD_{50} value based on the above report is expressed as dry weight of mushrooms so as to be comparable to other values for TD_{50} in Table 1; 90% of a mushroom is assumed to be water. A second mushroom, *Gyromitra esculenta*, has been similarly studied and found to contain a mixture of carcinogenic hydrazines [B. Toth, *J. Environ. Sci. Health* **C2**, 51 (1984)]. These mushrooms are eaten in considerable quantities in several countries, though less frequently in the United States.

105. Safrole is the main component (up to 90%) of oil of sassafras, formerly used as the main flavor ingredient in root beer [J. B. Wilson, *J. Assoc. Off. Anal. Chem.* **42**, 696 (1959); A. Y. Leung, *Encyclopedia of Common Natural Ingredients Used in Food, Drugs and Cosmetics* (Wiley, New York, 1980)]. In 1960, safrole and safrole-containing sassafras oils were banned from use in foods in the United States [*Fed. Regist.* **25**, 12412 (1960)]. Safrole is also naturally present in the oils of sweet basil, cinnamon leaf, nutmeg, and pepper.

106. Diet cola available in a local market contains 7.9 mg of sodium saccharin per fluid ounce.

107. Metronidazole is considered to be the drug of choice for trichomonal and *Gardnerella* infections [AMA Division of Drugs, *AMA Drug Evaluations* (American Medical Association, Chicago, IL, ed. 5, 1983), pp. 1717 and 1802].

108. Isoniazid is used both prophylactically and as a treatment for active tuberculosis. The adult prophylactic dose (300 mg daily) is continued for 1 year [AMA Division of Drugs, *AMA Drug Evaluations* (American Medical Association, Chicago, IL, ed. **5**, 1983), pp. 1766–1777].

109. D. M. Siegal, V. H. Frankos, M. A. Schneiderman, *Reg. Toxicol. Pharmacol.* **3**, 355 (1983).

110. Supported by NCI Outstanding Investigator Grant CA39910 to B.N.A., NIEHS Center Grant ES01896, and NIEHS/DOE Interagency Agreement 222-Y01-ES-10066. We are indebted to numerous colleagues for criticisms, particularly W. Havender, R. Peto, J. Cairns, J. Miller, E. Miller, D. B. Clayson, J. McCann, and F. J. C. Roe.

34

Nonpessimistic Risk Assessment and de Minimis Risk as Risk Management Tools

Chris Whipple
Electric Power Research Institute, Palo Alto, California

HISTORICAL BACKGROUND

The attention given to technological and environmental health risks has been increasing over the past two decades (1). Where once environmental problems were dealt with on a case-by-case basis after environmental damage or health harm became apparent, the approach taken since the National Environmental Policy Act was passed in 1969 has been to prevent technological and environmental risks from being created or overlooked. A major current emphasis in environmental management where health risks are concerned is in avoiding health impacts by predictive analysis and testing. This holds for existing risks as well as new risks. A trial-and-error risk management is no longer acceptable for controlling environmental health risks.

A major aspect of this change in objective has been the expanded use of quantitative risk assessment for regulation and other means of risk management. For environmental health risks, direct epidemiological evidence of health risk is used when available, but often such information is not available except for exposures much higher than those of current interest. In these cases, the need is for risk assessment methods that provide estimates of risks to humans even where no direct evidence of effects in humans exists. The toxicological methods that have been used for this purpose, most notably for carcinogens, are controversial because the uncertainty associated with the risk estimates is large. For technological risks such as those from accidents at chemical plants or nuclear power plants, alternatives to trial-and-error risk management have also been demanded. A variety of systems analysis methods collectively known as probabilistic risk assessment have been used in such analyses.

Before the increase in attention to environmental and technological risk issues, risk management was the domain of the technical specialist. Consequently, approaches to the management of environmental and technological risks developed within various professional communities, with considerable variation in the approaches taken. The major similarity in the philosophy of risk management in disparate areas, for example, between

1105

food safety and nuclear power plant safety, was that in both areas, professional judgment was applied in using various standards and practices historically accepted within the profession involved (2).

In both engineering and toxicology, it is commonplace and traditional to use safety factors. In engineering, safety factors typically are based on structural strength versus anticipated loads; the safety factor is the ratio of estimated strength to the largest load that might be experienced. Analogously, in toxicology it is traditional to limit human exposures to a small fraction of the lowest level at which adverse effects are observed (3).

It is often easier to reduce risk through use of a safety factor to a negligible level than to estimate its level. This is particularly true for low-level exposures to chemicals, where risks are highly uncertain. But safety factors, or engineering standards based on safety factors, are not without their drawbacks (4). Safety factors can lead to extreme variations in investment for risk avoidance. The relation between a safety factor and risk is usually hard to determine, and the trade-offs between risk and design factors such as cost are difficult to evaluate. As an example, consider the design of a bridge. Clearly, a safety factor of 5 produces a bridge less likely to fail than does a safety factor of 3, but at higher cost. The cost implications of alternate safety factors can usually be calculated, but the risk associated with various safety factors is generally not known.

In addition to lack of a simple relation between safety factors and risk, there is a lack of standardization on safety factors. One safety factor might apply to a bridge, another to a dam, and a third to the strength of an airplane's wings. While there are obvious reasons for variation (e.g., an airplane must be light enough to fly, a dam does not), balancing such considerations is highly judgmental.

There are several additional drawbacks to safety factors (4). A risk-based approach, in comparison to a safety factor/engineering standard approach, can improve safety priorities. For example, the major emphasis of nuclear power plant safety work (before probabilistic analysis of nuclear plants became widespread) was on a postulated accident known as a large-break loss of cooling accident (LOCA). Risk analyses have consistently found this accident to be a small contributor to overall plant risk, and safety resources once spent for work to assess and reduce large-break LOCA risk have been reallocated to more important issues. Similarly, primary emphasis in dam safety is avoidance of a flood that flows over the top of a dam; spillways are designed to make this extremely unlikely. But failure from overtopping is relatively rare for large engineered dams; more often dams fail because of seepage and construction defects (5).

A second limitation of safety factors, both in engineering and toxicology, is that their application generally presumes that a threshold between "safe" and "dangerous" exists and that the use of a safety factor makes things "safe." This assumption is reasonably good for many risks—for example, stresses on airplane wings and exposure to chemicals posing the risk of acute poisoning—but is not suitable for carcinogens and other risks where no "safe" threshold can be presumed.

Because of the drawbacks with safety factors noted here and because so many risks of current concern involve carcinogens, risk management is becoming increasingly risk based (6). An aspect of this transition is that the technical isolation between various risk areas is disappearing for several reasons. Under a safety factor approach, standards evolve within a specific technical community. In contrast, for a risk-based approach, risk standards can be developed through the comparative evaluation of risk regulation in different arenas, for example, food safety, environmental protection, and engineering. Case studies of risk management decisions involving passive restraints, cotton dust, waterborne carcinogens, and sulfur dioxide (7) and of saccharin, nuclear power, automobiles, swine flu immunization, and several other issues (8) reveal the value of risk assessment in risk management decisionmaking. They also illustrate many of the practical problems of risk management, for example, in dealing with issues where the scientific capability to assess risk is poor.

It is frequently the case that a risk management practice can be justified in one area by recognition of its historical acceptance in another. For example, the FDA and EPA both defend their targeted levels of protection by comparison to accepted background risks from food or the environment. The issue of historical patterns of risk acceptance has been discussed in some detail by Starr in his influential paper on social risk (9), and by Fischhoff et al. (10). Starr refers to the use of historical levels of risk as a guide to risk management as revealed preferences; Fischhoff et al. describe this approach as "bootstrapping." One aspect of risk management that cuts across most risks is the concept and definition of de minimis risk; this topic is described in detail in this chapter.

CONVERGENCE IN APPROACHES TO CARCINOGEN RISK MANAGEMENT

Regulation of exposure to carcinogenic agents is the responsibility of numerous government agencies. The same chemical may be regulated by OSHA to control workplace exposures, by the FDA to control public exposures through the food supply, and by the EPA as an environmental hazard. While the pathway and magnitude of exposure differ by regulatory context, each agency has a common interest in the evidence regarding the carcinogenicity of the substance.

As the trend from the classification of substances as carcinogens or noncarcinogens toward the quantitative estimation of carcinogenic potential has continued, the federal agencies have tried to coordinate their approaches to assess the risks from potentially carcinogenic agents. The consensus of a major effort conducted by the Office of Science and Technology Policy (11) is described as follows:

> The purpose of this document is to: (1) Articulate a view of carcinogenesis that scientists generally hold in common today (Part II); and (2) draw upon this understanding to compose, as was done here by senior scientists from a number of Federal agencies, a series of general principles that can be used to establish specific guidelines for assessing carcinogenic risk (Part I). Because of present gaps in understanding, the principles contain statements of what is generally accepted as fact as well as judgmental (science policy) decisions on unresolved issues, and there has been however an attempt to clearly distinguish between the different types of information presented....

> Similar documents...have been produced in the past, e.g., in the late 1970s and early 1980s several agencies of the Federal government produced statements directed toward providing a consistent basis for a general Federal cancer policy. This document should be seen, in the broad view, as part of an ongoing process, on behalf of the Federal government, that strives to periodically update and review current understanding of carcinogenesis and the scientific process of how this information is utilized.

Consistency in the assessment of cancer risks does not necessarily require that a common regulatory approach be applied. The regulatory mandate varies widely in the scope of considerations and the approach taken. At one extreme is the apparently simple rule embodied in the Delaney Amendment: it prohibits the addition of any substance found to be carcinogenic to food. At the opposite end of the spectrum, other regulations regarding risks require balancing of control costs and benefits.

Despite these apparent differences in regulatory structure, regulatory responses are becoming less diverse with time. Two institutional factors that help promote increasing consistency in the regulation of carcinogens are (i) the interagency coordination on scientific aspects of risk and (ii) the requirement that agencies analyze regulatory costs and benefits and that they base their decisions on such analysis to the extent permitted by the enabling statutes for each agency. An additional factor is that because carcinogens pose common risk management problems for regulators, agencies need to respond in similar ways.

ISSUES IN A MORE CONSISTENT APPROACH TO USE RISK ASSESSMENT

Consistency in risk management does not mean consistency in risk. Risk management actions depend on specific contextual factors that must be recognized and retained in any effort to increase consistency. Consistency as used here refers to commonality in the risk management process and logic. The point is to try to benefit from experience where the common features of a risk make it possible to do so, without neglecting important differences in risks and risk management opportunities. Despite the contextual factors that influence risk management, common patterns are emerging in approaches to risk regulation. Basic elements in the use of risk assessment in risk management decisions listed here, and discussed in greater detail below, include treatment of alternate risks, consistency of assumptions in risk assessment, pessimistic risk assessment in response to uncertainty, and risk management and social values.

Consideration of Alternate Risks

Health or safety regulation can reduce risk. Or it can simply transfer risk from one technology to another, or from one person to the next (12). We ban some technologies or practices on grounds of risk, only to see less desirable and, in many cases, more hazardous alternatives chosen. William Havender has noted (13), for example, that the alternatives to the pesticide EDB may not be safer than EDB and that these had not been studied to the same degree as EDB at the time of the EDB ban.

The removal of one risk often leads to the substitution of another. However, regulatory responsibility and authority are often distributed such that comparison of alternative risks is difficult. For example, the risks from electricity generation are regulated by several different agencies, depending on the technology of generation. The Nuclear Regulatory Commission oversees and regulates nuclear power plants, the EPA sets standards governing coal plants, and various other agencies control the safety of hydroelectric dams.

Even where the regulatory responsibilities for alternative risks are not spread between multiple institutions, the fact that different risks are considered at different times and that the state of scientific evidence is rarely equal makes it difficult to recognize that risk management often involves choosing one risk over another. Examples of failures to consider alternate risks are not hard to find. The decision by the FDA to ban cyclamates, which led to the increased use of saccharin, is an example where the alternate risks were considered separately (the saccharin/cyclamate example is described in more detail below).

The failure to consider alternate risks in risk management decisions is symptomatic of a more general failure to consider undesirable secondary effects from risk management. Regulators often seem to assume that, as Peter Huber puts it (14), "new products and processes generally add to the risk burden of our environment." In fact, he correctly points out that "most new products do not 'add to,' they substitute for." The process can be seen at work in such major human endeavors as the provision of energy, transportation, and food. In the energy area, for example, new power plants are built to more stringent standards and are usually located at more remote sites than old plants. When a new coal or nuclear plant begins operation, it displaces the power (and risk) produced by older, more polluting plants. Richard Wilson of Harvard analyzed this phenomenon and concluded in 1979 (15) that new electricity sources offer net health benefits. Yet this conclusion is rarely reflected in current regulatory decisions governing coal or nuclear power. New plants are stalled for years over risk issues that are small compared to the existing risks in the supply system that new plants could displace.

Many additional examples where alternative risks were ignored can be found (12). A classic example is TRIS, the fire-retardant chemical. In the early 1970s, the Consumer Product Safety Commission hurriedly adopted a rule requiring manufacturers to treat children's pajamas with the chemical. Only after the rule had been implemented—some 5 years later—did concern shift to the potential cancer risk from absorbing TRIS through the skin. Furthermore, after TRIS was benned it was learned that the substitute flame retardants were less effective and possibly more hazardous.

Also in the 1970s, weatherstripping programs were instituted to save energy. This conservation was motivated in part by a desire to avoid the environmental and health risks associated with expanded domestic production, and in part by concerns regarding the political risks associated with imports. The potential for increased exposure to indoor pollutants, radon in particular, was not considered. It now appears that the increase in radon exposure resulting from a 20% reduction in air infiltration increases lifetime lung cancer risk, perhaps by up to as many as 200 additional cases per million exposed (16).

It is conventional wisdom that reducing public risk is never free. It is less often recognized that reducing public risk often means creating occupational risk. An example from the French nuclear power program provides a perfect illustration (17). In 1981, Jacques Lombard and Francis Fagnani analyzed the trade-offs between public and occupational protection involved in selecting systems to control liquid and gaseous effluents during normal operations of nuclear power plants. Nine systems were analyzed, six of which are used in French reactors. In eight of the nine, the installers or monitors of the control systems suffered a radiation dose that exceeded the reduction in public radiation dose—in two cases by a ratio of 400:1.

Inconsistent Assumptions in Risk Assessment

Uncertainties are large when attempting to estimate many health risks, and these are often irreducible given the current state of science. One consideration both to the response to uncertainty and to the value of a framework that considers alternative risks is that relative risk is often more relevant to risk management than is absolute risk. For example, when the issue is the choice between similar risks (e.g., between the use of two chemicals both found to produce cancer in animals at high doses), the decision may be to prohibit the use of the substance judged to pose the greater risk and to permit use of the safer substance. In such cases, it is important to assess those risks consistently.

Cyclamate and saccharin provide a good example of the importance of consistency in risk assessment. The absolute degree of human risk posed by these substances is not known, but high-dose animal tests seem to show more danger from saccharin than from cyclamate (18). Based on these test results, Canada has banned saccharin but permitted the use of cyclamate. In the United States, cyclamate use is prohibited but saccharin use is permitted. This is the case because the two substances were considered separately, several years apart, without the application of a consistent method for interpreting evidence regarding risk.

The cyclamate/saccharin example illustrates another potential type of problem in risk management. Under the view that overestimation of risks leads to risk reduction, extreme assumptions were applied to the data regarding cyclamate (18). A different, less conservative analysis was applied to saccharin. Had consistent criteria for risk assessment been applied it would have been clear that of the two artificial sweeteners, cyclamate was safer. As noted above, consistency in risk assessment methods is important for comparison of the relative risks from alternatives.

Pessimistic Risk Assessment in Response to Uncertainty

Pessimistic, plausible upper bound, or *worst-case* estimates are sometimes referred to as *conservative* estimates, based on the premise that pessimism in risk assessment—that is, the use of assumptions that lead to high estimates of risk—is protective of public health. But this is not true when risk transfers are likely. Adopting worst-case assumptions about one substance or technology can amount to adopting best-case assumptions about a substance that may in fact be worse. At the very least, such an approach diverts resources from more beneficial ends (12).

Where alternate risks are assessed using dissimilar risk assessment methods, it is not possible to use consistent assumptions in risk assessment because the estimation of alternate risks may have no assumptions in common. If pessimistic assumptions are used in such cases, it is unlikely that a common degree of pessimism is achieved across alternate risks. For example, decisions about the use of mammography for early diagnosis of breast cancer involve a trade-off between the risks from radiation exposures received in mammography and the risks from undiagnosed breast cancer if mammography is not performed. The risk estimates for breast cancer and for the effectiveness of mammography in detecing breast cancer derive from actual population data on the incidence of breast cancer. The estimates for the risks of low doses of radiation received in mammography are based on extrapolations from high doses and dose rates, particularly from the observed cancer risks among Japanese exposed to radiation from atomic bombs (19–21). In this case, pessimistic assumptions are not protective; overestimation of radiation risk leads to too little mammography and too much breast cancer.

The artificial sweetener and mammography examples illustrate how intentionally pessimistic assumptions—that is, assumptions that are expected to overestimate the actual risk—produce undesirable outcomes when the issue is to choose between alternate risks.

But because risk analysts and agency standard setters generally focus on one risk at a time, a single risk focus is a natural frame of reference. From the perspective of a single risk management decision, analytical conservatism appears protective, but the price is hidden. A conservative (i.e., high) risk estimate produces lower risk exposures than would a more realistic estimate. Here, the potential costs of large errors seem to be asymmetrical to the regulator. Risk reduction costs appear to be bounded, while consequences of uncertain risk exposures are potentially much greater than the control measures.

An additional factor encouraging regulatory agencies to make conservatism a matter of policy is how decisions might be judge in hindsight. An overcontrolled risk will probably drop from sight once a decision is implemented and control investments made.

But an undercontrolled risk, possibly discovered through the identification of victims, is far more disturbing for a regulatory agency. Examples include the swine flu vaccine, the Pinto gas tank, and many others (22).

Allocating Scarce Resources

In nearly all cases, risk reductions are limited by available resources. Consequently, the logical objective of risk management decisions is to allocate the scarce resource in a way that maximizes social benefits. Prioritization of the risk management effort, while of little concern for a single risk, becomes important under this viewpoint. Clearly, money or regulatory attention spent on one risk is not available for another, so it is important not to waste resources on trivial risks. It is apparent that conservatism is counterproductive and that risks are increased if resources are shifted from significant risks to small, exaggerated risks. Under this fixed allocation or zero sum scenario, risk reductions are maximized when the cheapest and easiest risk reductions are given highest priority. By shifting resources to uncertain risks, conservative estimates, thought of as "health protective," may very well increase overall the risk to public health and well-being.

Which perspective on regulatory resources is correct? Both have their merits. Regulatory agency actions may be limited by the availability of scientific or administrative resources within their own staffs. But risk management responsibility assigned to the agencies by Congress is fragmented and suggests nothing in the way of an overall ceiling on risk spending. The bulk of control costs come from producers, not regulatory agencies, so agency budgets are not a direct constraint. But while expenditures for risk reduction appear to be variable and flexible, dependent on the perceived appropriate action in each case, there may be a political feedback from the regulated parties that limits the amount of money an agency can require someone to spend. The political emphasis on easing regulatory costs has been illustrated by actions such as Executive Order 12291 (23, 24). A subtler consideration is that, to the extent that the public finds uncertain risks discomforting, greater expenditures for risk control may be politically feasible if funds are directed to deal with uncertain (and unpopular) risks.

Another factor to consider is that regulatory decisionmakers may consider the details of the evidence supporting a risk estimate and compensate for perceived biases in analysis. If regulators discount for perceived conservatism and appropriate adjustments are made, then standards will be the same no matter what risk assessment assumptions are made. Conservative analysis would not lead to more or less stringent standards than would best estimates. It is likely that conservatively estimated risks are discounted in some cases but not in others and it is unlikely that adjustments could be made appropriately and consistently.

For the reasons noted above, it is apparent that conservatism in risk management need not be achieved through conservative risk assessment assumptions. It is possible to use stringent criteria for allowable risk, and less conservative assumptions for estimating risk, and to end up with the current levels of protection on average, but with greater consistency than current practice provides.

If regulators had greater flexibility to vary risk criteria in response to conservatisms in risk assessment, in attractive approach would be to select risk assessment assumptions based on their discriminatory power. Relative risk estimates based on overly conservative assumptions may not distinguish important differences between risk. For example, an increase in benign liver tumors and a decrease in leukemias and mammary gland fibroadenomas have been observed in response to test chemicals in the Fischer 344 rat (25).

Under present assessment methods, a carcinogen that increases benign tumors at one site but reduces malignant tumors at other sites will generally be considered to present the same risk to public health as one that increases the overall burden of malignant tumors. Furthermore, models to extrapolate dose–response curves from bioassays to the low-dose region often incorporate conservative statistical procedures to deal with lack of statistical power. As a result, two chemicals with very different NOELs (no observable effect levels) and slopes may not be estimated to have different risks at environmental exposure levels.

Risk Management and Social Values

In *Unfinished Business: A Comparative Assessment of Environmental Problems*, a general review of environmental problems by the EPA (26), it was concluded that EPA program priorities coincide more closely with public perceptions than with the EPA's estimates of risk. The EPA is careful to point out that this does not mean that current priorities are misaligned; the EPA openly acknowledges that its view of the magnitude of an environmental problem is often not defined by the expected health effects associated with it. The EPA and other agencies understand that agency priorities are frequently politically determined. In short, if the presence of toxic chemicals in groundwater is the major current environmental problem in the public's opinion, it will probably be the EPA's major priority as well.

Current approaches to risk management reflect differences in technological opportunities for risk reductions, professional traditions, and in the level of protection desired by the public, as perceived by risk managers. Many factors beside expected health impacts influence perception and acceptance of risk. For example, research has indicated a social aversion to risks that are involuntary or beyond individual control, risks with catastrophic potential, and risks that are highly uncertain in magnitude (9, 27).

Social aversion to technological or environmental risk is generally expressed as opposition to particular technologies—for example, nuclear power or genetically engineered substances—or concern regarding particular risks such as from chemicals in drinking water. Consequently, social values are likely to emerge through the political process in terms of a desire for rigorous regulation of specific technologies.

Risk management approaches that neglect such social factors and instead focus on minimization of expected losses will conflict with existing social values and perceptions. An explanation for the discrepancy is that an analytical approach in which risk is equated with expected loss fails to correspond with the word "risk" as most people use it. This public definition of riskiness includes many factors beside the probability of loss, for example, uncertainty in effect or outcome and the perceived degree of control (28).

The definition of social objectives for risk management is an inherently political process. The objectives are both complex and potentially in conflict. For example, the objective to minimize mortality and morbidity from some environmental health risk, given available resources, is implicit in much of the economic literature on risk management and the use of cost–benefit analysis is recommended for that purpose. But such an objective conflicts with the objectives of avoiding catastrophes and taking extra measures to deal with highly uncertain risks.

Failure to appreciate the conflicting nature of risk management objectives is commonplace, even among risk analysts and risk managers. As an example, safety goals for nuclear power plants were developed over several years and through workshops sponsored by the NRC. In the early stages of their development, the safety goals reflected an aversion to potentially catastrophic accidents through use of a weighting factor on multiple-fatality accidents. (The weighting factor was of the form that the social cost of an accident was assumed to be proportioned to the number of fatalities raised to power greater than 1; typically 1.2.) Support for this approach disappeared after it was noted that such an approach would lead to increased expected fatalities in comparison to a safety goal without such a risk aversion factor. That is, everyone was in favor of a special emphasis to avoid catastrophic losses, until the conflict between this objective and the goal of minimizing expected losses was raised.

This example illustrates some of the tensions present in risk management. It is not in dispute that risk management should be directed by social values as revealed through the political process. But the degree to which specific public concerns are due to misperceived probabilities of health consequences is difficult to determine. To take the results of the EPA report cited above (26), a central issue is why public opinion is that toxic materials in groundwater pose a greater risk than toxic air pollutants. It may be that this opinion is based on different weighting given to qualitative aspects of these risks; alternatively, this opinion may reflect a perception that more people are harmed by toxic substances in groundwater than in air. Depending on which explanation for public opinion is accepted by risk managers, the priority given to groundwater toxics over air toxics is either a matter of values or the result of a misperception of the health benefits likely to result from attention to these problems.

An aspect of the tensions generated by these alternate explanations is the current emphasis on risk communication. It is no accident that the EPA has been a leader in the work and emphasis in this area. The motivation for this work is the dilemma faced by EPA management: the mission of the EPA is both to limit environmental health damage and to be responsive to Congress and the public. Yet the EPA perceives public priorities to be misplaced and to conflict with its ability to address issues where health benefits would, in the EPA's view, be greater.

A related aspect of this issue is the frequent use of risk comparisons by industry in defense of current practices. At the heart of a risk comparison is the assumption that risk is measured in terms of expected consequences and individual probabilities of harm. By taking this definition for risk and by applying the objective of risk reduction or minimization, priorities are focused on big risks, easily reduced risks, and risks with little associated benefit. Under the public definition of risk, attention is focused on uncertain, catastrophic, new, and dread risks.

Approaches to Deal with Uncertainty

Many risks of current concern have long latency periods or catastrophic potential. Unlike routine accident risks, we should anticipate that risk management decisions will be based on highly uncertain estimates of risks (29). Ideally, risks with delayed or catastrophic effects are best managed prospectively, so that the human costs learning by trial and error can be avoided. If our risk management efforts are successful, we will never have good data for these risks. While the public benefits of regulating risks prospectively are clear, where experience is not a guide, risk management is more difficult. We have been struggling with several such cases for the past decade: nuclear power, chemical carcinogens, and more recently, biotechnologies. The magnitudes of these risks are highly uncertain. One approach to deal with uncertainty about such risks has been to try to reduce it through research. Substantial resources have been expanded to understand these risks, and risk management has been improved by such studies. Despite much effort to estimate risk, where direct human evidence is not available, large uncertainties about risk remain. Research may eventually resolve many questions that now trouble us, and in some cases postponing a decision for research may avoid uncertainty. But many risks are likely to remain uncertain for the foreseeable future.

Estimating the magnitude of risks that cannot be measured directly frequently requires the use of assumptions that cannot be tested empirically. Not only are such risks uncertain, but often the uncertainty cannot be characterized probabilistically. Probability distributions are useful for describing some uncertainties, but this is often not feasible in risk assessment. Often, there is no reasonable method even to assign weights to the plausibility of alternative assumptions. Methods have been developed to elicit subjective descriptions of uncertainty; this raises the question of whose estimates to accept.

Recognition of these uncertainties has at times led to the view that risk assessment is a dubious enterprise, too uncertain to be relied on for risk management decisions. But low-level risks are inherently uncertain regardless of the approach taken to their study. This uncertainty is simply more apparent under some approaches to social risk management than others. For example, the uncertainty associated with applying bioassay results to human risk estimation is frequently cited as a major source of uncertainty in risk assessment for toxic substances. Less often recognized are the uncertainties associated with exposure assessment (30). Given the discomfort that uncertainty causes, it is tempting in some cases to overstate what risk assessment can tell us. The limits to science are imprecise, as are the distinctions between that which is known and that which can reasonably be assumed. For this reason, a technically accurate description of uncertainties is now considered essential in risk assessment.

Risk assessors bridge gaps in knowledge with assumptions. Often, there are many alternative assumptions, each scientifically plausible, with no reasonable basis for choosing among them. For example, an analyst must select a dose–response model for extrapolation to low-dose risk.

The recent National Academy of Sciences report *Risk Assessment in the Federal Government: Managing the Process* (31) endorsed the concept that scientific questions about the degree of risk posed by some exposure or activity should be separated, to the extent feasible, from the policy questions of what risk management steps should be taken. This report clearly describes how science and policy cannot be entirely separated and notes that many seemingly scientific issues such as the assumptions made in a risk assessment have direct relevance to management decision. This is seen by the committee that wrote the report:

> The goal of risk assessment is to describe, as accurately as possible, the possible health consequences of changes in human exposure to a hazardous substance; the need for accuracy implies that the best available scientific knowledge, supplemented as necessary by assumptions that are consistent with science, will be applied.

The difficulty arises when there is no scientific basis to select among alternative assumptions. About the best that risk analysis can provide when this happens is a description of the reasons for uncertainty, an assessment of how critical uncertainties can be lowered, and a collection of estimates based on a range of plausible models. Granger Morgan and his colleagues have taken this approach to describe estimated health effects from sulfur air pollution (32).

DE MINIMIS RISK

A common way to deal with uncertainty is to categorize the smallest risks (often the most uncertain risks) as de minimis risks (33–36). De minimis risks are those judged to be too small to be of social concern or too small to justify the use of risk management resources for control, given other more beneficial opportunities. Properly applied, a de minimis risk concept can help prioritize attention to risk in a socially beneficial way. Granted this approach ignores uncertainty below some low limit; de minimis is in the longstanding tradition of risk management methods, which, when faced with uncertainty, concede that discretion is the better part of valor.

Although the de minimis concept and its application to health risks is not new, the impetus to establish a consistent de minimis approach to risk regulation has increased in recent years for several reasons. First, technologies for identifying risks have improved in several ways. Improvements in analytical chemistry permit the detection of hazardous substances at the part per billion or even part per trillion level; only a decade ago such exposures would have been ignored simply because they would have been undetectable. [Radiation is an exception to this rule, since it has been detectable at low levels for decades. This helps to explain why so many de minimis proposals arose from the radiation protection area.]

Second, our view of the nature of low-level risks has shifted somewhat over the past decade. The view that we face rare but potent carcinogens seems to have given way to the view that carcinogens (at least as determined by high-dose animal tests and by inference from in vitro bioassays) are fairly commonplace and significantly varied in their potencies. Recent work that reveals widespread exposures to natural carcinogens in food (37) has troubling implications for a policy based on elimination of carcinogens as a risk management policy (38) and strengthens the argument to move to a carcinogen management approach that prioritizes regulatory attention based on both carcinogenic potency and exposure.

An impact of the increasing number of candidate substances for regulation and of the apparent need to prioritize regulatory efforts is that case-by-case decisionmaking is seen as too cumbersome. As the regulatory approaches to low-level agents mature, more systematic methods are sought. To regulators, the de minimis approach appears to provide a means of normalizing the process, by providing an alternative to standard setting for substances that pose very low risks. This role is particularly important where an agency has a statutory mandate to deal with a substance or class of substances, but where resources are not available to deal with low-risk and low-priority substances.

In addition to these regulatory incentives for using a de minimis approach, industry is likely to be supportive of a de minimis approach since it defines a threshold for regulatory involvement. The de minimis rule could produce greater predictability in regulation and provide a risk target for avoiding regulation.

To the scientific community, the de minimis approach may provide a policy solution to questions that lie beyond the reach of scientific resolution. This would reduce the pressures for regulatory agencies and their scientific staffs to produce scientific judgments regarding low-level risks where information is unavailable.

A major consideration with the application of a de minimis policy to risk management is the effect that such a policy would have on risks borne by the public or an occupational group, in comparison to the risks produced in the absence of a de minimis policy. Clearly, many small risks that would be formally excluded from regulatory concern under a de minimis approach are unlikely to be regulated under any approach. Exposures to these risks are not the issue, since in such cases the de minimis policy would make no difference. However, a de minimis risk policy could be interpreted as formally legitimating risks that are now permitted on pragmatic ground.

While the risks permitted under a de minimis role would be quantitatively small by definition, the public reaction to such risks may be influenced more strongly by other characteristics of the risk (27). Many of the agents for which the de minimis approach is being considered pose uncertain and carcinogenic risks; these characteristics appear to enhance the degree of public concern to risk. For example, news reports that carcinogenic chemicals have been found in drinking water raise public concern, but because such reports typically do not report concentrations or describe risks quantitatively, the level of concern may have little to do with estimated risk.

De Minimis Risk and Conflicting Social Objectives

In health and safety risk regulation, the conflicting objectives of maximum protection and careful use of scarce resources have produced approaches in which these two objectives are considered in varying degrees. In many cases, economic efficiency is explicitly stated as one of several regulatory goals, and the analytical examination of regulatory costs and benefits is customary or even obligatory. In such cases, the de minimis approach is likely to formalize the practice of ignoring very small risks. For other risks, the regulatory mandate is more strongly focused on protection; in these cases the costs of achieving safety are secondary considerations or not legal considerations at all, at least in principle. In practice, cost considerations do usually influence all decisions to some degree. It seems possible that de minimis is particularly useful, because of its historical legal acceptance (39), to avoid the regulation of trivial risks which a literal reading of the law would require. Under a well-designed de minimis system, the social objective to have a high degree of safety could be met, while at the same time the need to ignore small risks could be recognized. In this role, and under favorable circumstances, de minimis offers the possibility of bringing practical considerations into decisions where very small risks are involved without resorting to the risk–cost trade-offs that many find offensive and that certain laws prohibit. In short, de minimis may, in certain cases, permit us to avoid facing the difficult conflicting objectives contained within our risk value system (40).

On a larger scale, the practical value of a de minimis policy may result from the pressures it creates to reevaluate inconsistencies in the attention applied to various risks. A de minimis risk policy is philosophically consistent with the view expressed by Lord Rothschild (41): "There is no point in getting into a panic about the risks of life until you have compared the risks which worry you with those that don't but perhaps should."

A second basic objective in modern risk regulation is the separation (to the extent that is practical) of questions of science from questions of policy (31). This objective arises from several motivations, notably to permit public participation in the formulation of risk policy without requiring scientific expertise, and to permit scientific debate over the degree of risk to be conducted at a distance from questions of regulatory action. In practice, such separation is difficult to maintain as illustrated by the tendency to use conservative assumptions in risk assessment when uncertainties are large. Such conservatism reflects a societal consensus to err on the side of safety in risk matters. (Whether or not this policy actually promotes safety is addressed below.) This issue of separation is particularly difficult for very low risks, because uncertainties are so great at low levels. For many exposures there is no direct evidence that risk exists; the evidence is simply that risk exists for much higher exposures. Out of prudence we assume that the risks do exist, that thresholds do not exist. The de minimis approach may offer policy thresholds in lieu of scientific thresholds; this addresses difficulties noted by John Gibbons (42):

> A zero-threshold situation leaves the policymaker in a great quandary. As long as there is some threshold level below which there are no ill effects, social equity can be preserved. But if dose and effect have a zero-zero intercept, then the policymaker must talk about determining acceptable risk, which is far more difficult to deal with than no risk.

Individual versus Societal de Minimis Risk Definition

Certainly a society can manage risk to the population as a whole by limiting individual risks. This is, in fact, the approach taken by the Nuclear Regulatory Commission in its proposed safety goals for nuclear power plants (43). Individual risk limits are appropriate in cases where individuals would face relatively high risks. But when individual risks are not inequitably high and the motivation for risk management comes more from having a large number of people facing a low-to-moderate risk, rather than from having a few people at high risk, then individual risk approaches can produce resource misallocations. To take a hypothetical example, a 10^{-6}/yr risk of death to 1000 people produces 10^{-3} expected fatalities per year, equivalent to an expectation of 1 fatality per 1000 years. This same risk of 10^{-6}/yr applied to the entire U.S. population of 230 million produces an expectation of 230 fatalities per year. If a judgment of whether these were de minimis risks hinged on the individual risk, the regulatory response (or nonresponse) is likely to treat these risks comparably. Yet common sense tells us that greater effort and expenditure are justified to save 230 lives than 0.001 lives.

Multiple Sources of Risk

The definition of a de minimis risk should include consideration of the possibility that multiple de minimis exposures could result in a large aggregate risk. For instance, one could conceivably be exposed to the same hazardous material in drinking water, by inhalation, or in a variety of foods. As a practical matter, one or two pathways are likely to dominate exposures, and it seems unlikely that total exposures could be greater than several times the exposure via the most significant pathway. Given the uncertainties in risk estimates at such low levels, this factor seems fairly trivial.

A far more troubling question is posed by the sheer number of risk agents. It would hardly be comforting to learn that although no single chemical in drinking water poses a cancer risk in excess of 10^{-7}/yr, there were 10^6 such chemicals. The problem that this issue poses for the use of de minimis as a regulatory threshold is the degree to which risks are examined and managed singly versus on an aggregated basis.

While the prevalent approach of doing risk analyses on a chemical-specific basis seems to support a de minimis concept on an agent-by-agent basis, other arguments support a de minimis definition for an aggregation of agents. Such an approach provides confidence that the sum of de minimis risks any individual sees is limited by the level of aggregation. Clearly, there are many ways to aggregate: all effluents from a single facility could be considered, or one could consider the risk from substances found in the air, in drinking water, or in food. The Food and Drug Administration, for example, treats this issue through the use of very stringent criteria. Proposed de minimis risk levels for radiation are typically higher than the levels considered by the FDA for food additives, reflecting the fact that there are far fewer sources of radiation than of food additives.

Suggestion for de Minimis Applications

Clearly, many issues must be resolved to develop a workable de minimis policy. Given many contextual issues such as multiple exposures, population at risk, and the degree of confidence in a risk estimate, a basic de minimis risk philosophy will have to be flexible to specific considerations. Proposed de minimis approaches have dealt with some aspects of the problem, notably with the use of risk comparisons to select a de minimis level in a specific context. More effect is needed, however, if the de minimis idea is to be adopted as a generally sound risk management approach. In particular, the aggregation of multiple risks has not received sufficient attention. Two additional issues that deserve attention are the consideration of population risks instead of individual risks, where appropriate, and the idea of de minimis probability.

Finally, it should be recognized that public acceptance of de minimis may be the critical constraint and should be a consideration in any proposed approach. To that end, it may be helpful to think of de minimis risks as those that are of too low a priority to regulate, rather than as acceptably low risks. This distinction, by framing the issue as prioritization rather than acceptability, naturally encourages a comparative risk viewpoint and avoids the difficult question "acceptable to whom?" The proposal to define as de minimis risks those that cannot be measured epidemiologically would avoid creating identifiable victims of a de minimis approach. This approach might be considered a necessary condition for defining a de minimis level; however, it is not sufficient because substantial health risks could meet this requirement.

An additional factor that could promote the acceptability of a de minimis approach is recognition that, in general, de minimis levels apply not to actual known risks but rather to risks of unknown magnitude which are conservatively estimated.

SUMMARY

A significant trend evident in the management of many different public risks is the increased use of risk assessment and risk-based standards in place of professional consensus standards. As this transition progresses, several things occur to provide greater consistency in risk management. First, the scientific aspects of quantitative risk assessment have become the focus of broad research communities, including professional societies and university faculties. For this reason, risk assessment methods and assumptions increasingly reflect a professional consensus rather than the chosen policy of a particular regulatory agency.

The second factor leading to greater consistency in risk management concerns the use of risk-based reasoning to establish safety standards. Agency experiences in setting safety goals, such as at the Nuclear Regulatory Commission, suggest that one aspect of establishing safety goals is comparison with risks and goals used in similar circumstances. This is becoming apparent as the EPA and FDA float proposals to consider risks in the 10^{-6} to 10^{-8} per lifetime range as de minimis risks.

A final factor in leading to increased consistency in risk regulation is the movement from an informal, consensual process to one that follows a legalistic process where the basis for a decision must be documented and defended. The need to provide a decision rationale works in support of analytical approaches and to the detriment of judgmental ones. This analytical emphasis, the result of executive orders, legislative requirements, and court decisions, enhances the standing of those experts in analysis in support of risk management and standard setting. As a professional consensus develops in this analytical community, ideas regarding the preferred approach to risk management problems of various types are emerging; this consensus will undoubtedly exert a pressure for agencies to conform to common practice.

The cumulative effect of these changes is that U.S. regulatory institutions are becoming increasingly similar in their approach. But one should recognize the limits to a standard approach to different risks. There are important contextual details for risk management issues that cannot be reduced to a standard approach. Potential benefits of the emerging changes are better predictability and more efficient prioritization of attention to risk. Public acceptance, built through two-way communication between the public and risk managers, is necessary for these benefits to be realized.

REFERENCES

1. W. W. Lowrance, *Of Acceptable Risk: Science and the Determination of Safety.* Wm. Kaufmann, Inc., Los Altos, CA, 1976.

2. W. Hammer, *Product Safety Management and Engineering*, Prentice-Hall, Englewood Cliffs, NJ, 1980.

3. M. L. Dourson and J. F. Stara, Regulatory history and experimental support of uncertainty (safety) factors. *Regul. Toxicol. Pharmacol.* **3**, 224–238 (1983).

4. M. R. Krouse, Workshop report—Engineering standards versus risk analysis. In Y. Y. Haimes and E. Z. Stakhiv, Eds., *Risk-Based Decision Making in Water Resources.* American Society of Civil Engineers, New York, 1986.

5. R. B. Jansen, *Dams and Public Safety.* U.S. Department of the Interior, Water and Power Resources Service, Washington, DC, 1980.

6. C. C. Travis, S. A. Richter, E. A. C. Crouch, R. Wilson, and E. D. Klema, Cancer risk management: A review of 132 federal regulatory decisions. *Environ. Sci. Technol.* **21**(5) (1987).

7. R. W. Crandall and L. B. Lave (Eds.), *The Scientific Basis of Health and Safety Regulation.* Brookings Institution, Washington, DC, 1981.

8. R. Wilson and E. A. C. Crouch, *Risk/Benefit Analysis.* Ballinger, Cambridge, MA, 1982.

9. C. Starr, Social benefit U.S. technological risk. *Science* **165**, 1232–1238 (1969).

10. B. Fischhoff, S. Lichtenstein, P. Slovic, S. Derby, and R. Keeney, *Acceptable Risk.* Cambridge Univ. Press, London and New York, 1981.

11. Office of Science and Technology Policy, Chemical carcinogens; notice of review of the science and its associated principles. *Fed. Regist.* **49** (100), 21594–21661 (1984).

12. C. Whipple Redistributing risk. *Regulation*, May/June (1985).

13. W. Havender, EDB and the marigold option. *Regulation*, January/February (1984).

14. P. Huber, Exorcists vs. gatekeepers in risk regulation. *Regulation*, November/December (1983).

15. R. Wilson, The Environmental and public health consequences of replacement electricity supply. *Energy* **4**, 81–86 (1979).

16. H. Hurwitz, Jr., The indoor radiological problem in perspective. *Risk Anal.* March, 63–77 (1983).

17. J. Lombard and F. Fagnani, Equity aspects of risk management. *Nucl. Saf.*, September/October (1981).

18. W. Havender, The science and politics of cyclamates. *Public Interest*, Spring, p. 71 (1983).

19. C. E. Land, Estimating cancer risks from low doses of ionizing radiation. *Science* **209**, 1197–1203 (1980).

20. National Research Council, Advisory Committee on the Biological Effects of Ionizing

Radiation, *The Effects on Populations of Exposure to Low Levels of Ionizing Radiation* (BEIR III), NRC, Washington, DC, 1980.

21. J. S. Evans, D. W. Moeller, and D. W. Cooper, *Health Effects Model for Nuclear Power Plant Accident Consequence Analysis*, NUREG/CR-4214, SAND85-7185. Prepared under contract from Sandia National Laboratories for the U.S. Nuclear Regulatory Commission, July 1985.

22. E. W. Lawless, *Technology and Social Shock.* Rutgers Univ. Press, New Brunswick, NJ, 1977.

23. Executive Order 12291, *Fed. Regist.* **46**, 13193–13198 (1981).

24. V. K. Smith (Ed.), *Environmental Policy under Reagan's Executive Order.* Univ. of North Carolina Press, Chapel Hill, 1984.

25. J. K. Haseman, patterns of tumor incidence in two-year cancer bioassay feeding studies in Fischer 344 rats. *Fundam. Appl. Toxicol.* **3**, 1–9 (1983).

26. U.S. Environmental Protection Agency, Office of Policy Analysis and Office of Policy, Planning, and Evaluation, *Unfinished Business: A Comparative Assessment of Environmental problems.* USEPA, Washington, DC, February 1987.

27. B. Fischhoff, P. Slovic, S. Lichtenstein, S. Read, and B. Combs, How safe is safe enough? A psychometric survey of attitudes towards technological risks and benefits. *Policy Sci.* **8**, 127–152 (1978).

28. B. Fischhoff, S. Watson, and C. Hope, Defining risks. *Policy Sci.* **17**, 123–139 (1984).

29. C. G. Whipple, Dealing with uncertainty about risk in risk management. In *Hazards: Technology and Fairness.* National Academy of Engineering, National Academy Press, Washington, DC, 1986.

30. D. J. Paustenbach, H. P. Shu, and F. J. Murray, A critical examination of assumptions used in risk assessments of dioxin contaminated soil. *Regul. Toxicol. Pharmacol.* **6**, 284–307 (1986).

31. National Research Council, Committee on the Institutional Means for Assessment of Risks to Public Health, *Risk Assessment in the Federal Government: Managing the Process.* National Academy Press, Washington, DC, 1983.

32. M. G. Morgan, S. C. Morris, M. Henrion, D. A. L. Amaral, and W. R. Rish, Technical uncertainty in quantitative policy analysis—A sulfur air pollution example. *Risk Anal.* **4**, 201–216 (1984).

33. C. G. Whipple (Ed.), *De Minimis Risk.* Plenum Press, New York, 1987.

34. V. O. Wodicka, Cogitationes de minimis. *Regul. Toxicol. Pharmacol.* **7**, 129–130 (1987).

35. F. E. Young, Risk Assessment: The convergence of science and the law. *Regul. Toxicol. Pharmacol.* **7**, 179–184 (1987).

36. P. W. Huber, Little risks and big fears. *Regul. Toxicol. Pharmacol.* **7**, 200–205 (1987).

37. B. Ames, Dietary carcinogens and anticarcinogens. *Science* **221**, 1256–1264 (1983).

38. S. S. Epstein, J. B. Swartz et al., Letter to *Science* **224** (4650), May 18 (1984), and reply by B. Ames in same issue.

39. J. P. Davis, *The Feasibility of Establishing a "De Minimis" Level of Radiation Dose and A regulatory Cut-off Policy for Nuclear Regulation*, Rep. GP-R-33040. General Physics Corporation, Columbia, MD, 1981; also in Whipple (33).

40. G. Calabresi and P. Bobbitt, *Tragic Choices.* Norton, New York, 1978.

41. N. Lord Rothschild, *Coming to Grips with Risk.* Address presented on BBC Television, November 1978, reprinted in *Wall St. J.*, May 13 (1979).

42. J. Gibbons, Risk assessment at the Office of Technology Assessment, In S. Panem. Ed., *Public Policy, Science and Environmental Risk.* Brookings Institution, Washington, DC, 1983.

43. U.S. Nuclear Regulatory Commission, Office of Policy Evaluation, *Safety Goals for Nuclear Power Plant Operation*, NUREG-0880, Revision 1 for Comment. USNRC, Washington, DC, May 1983.

Index

1121

/

Genotoxicity (*Continued*)
  1,1,1-trichloroethane, 338–339
Geophasia, 300
GLIM, 163–164
GLOBAL82, 876
GLOBAL83, 784
Gloves, time to break-through and permeation rates, 731
Glucose tolerance factor, 580, 584
Glucuronides, 918
Glutathione *S*-transferase, 243–246, 262
Glycol ethers, *see also glycol ethers*
  acute toxicity, 727
  A/D ratio, 752, 756
  cancer risk, 727
  characteristics and use, 727–729
  comparative metabolism, 736–738
  dermal absorption, 754–755
  developmental toxicity, 739
  distribution of industrial hygiene air sam-
    pling data, 747
  evaporation rate, 728
  exposure hazard rating, 729
  mutagenicity, 738–739
  occupational exposure, 729–730, 746–748
    semiconductor industry, 728, 730, 746
  personal protective equipment, 730–731
  sampling and analytical methods, 747
  threshold limit values, 745–746
  time to break-through and permeation
    rates for gloves and solvents, 731
  vapor hazard indices, 729–730
  vapor pressures, 729–730
Glycosides, 918
Goodness of fit, 1075
  chi-square test, 227–228
  quantal response models, 227
Graphical Exposure Modeling Systems, 280
Grazing animals, dioxin, uptake, 314–315
Groundwater:
  cancer risk estimates, 499–500
  concentrations of indicator chemicals, 492
  contaminant discharge into river, 487–490
  environmental concentrations, 288
  exposure to chromium, 591–592
  exposure point concentrations, 281
  exposure routes, 515
  former pesticide production facility,
    473, 476–479
  glaciofluvial:
    areas releasing contaminants to,
      485
    contaminant leaching, 490–493
  lifetime carcinogenic risk, 288

monoalkyl quaternary ammonium compounds, biodegradation, 371–372
probability/year of transfer of high-level
  waste, 564–565
1,1,1-trichloroethane contamination, *see*
  1,1,1-Trichloroethane
wastewater treatment site, 579

Half-life:
  dioxin, 697, 940
    environmental, 309–310
    human, 315–316
  methylmercury, 845, 849, 863
  PCDD, 634–635
Haloalkanes, physiological pharmacokinetic
  model approach, 697
Halogenated aliphatic hydrocarbons:
  vapor pressure, 50
  volatilization, 50
  water solubility, 46
Hanna box model, 282
Hazard, definition, 27
Hazard assessment, 512–513, 735–739
  comparative metabolism, 736–738
  definition, 735
  glycol ethers, 735–739
  mutagenicity, 738–739
Hazard evaluation:
  bendectin, 721–722
  methylmercury, 851–855
  pesticides, 805–812
  teratogenicity, 712–716
Hazard function:
  continuous-time, 129–131
  uncertain individual, 140
Hazard identification, 1–5, 40–43, 1047. See
    also specific properties
  bendectin, 716–721
  candidate tests, 41
  chemical and physical properties, 5
  definition, 30, 937
  di-2-ethylhexyl phthalate, 869–871
  dioxin, 939–942
  environmental fate, 4–5
  methylmercury, 847–851
  sampling and statistical aspects, 3–4
  teratogenicity, 712
Hazard index, 286
Hazardous materials:
  federal legislation, 28
  spill incidents, 434–435
Hazardous Substances List, 435
Hazardous waste sites, *see also* Chromium;
    Superfund health hazards